Nursing Assistant
A Nursing Process Approach

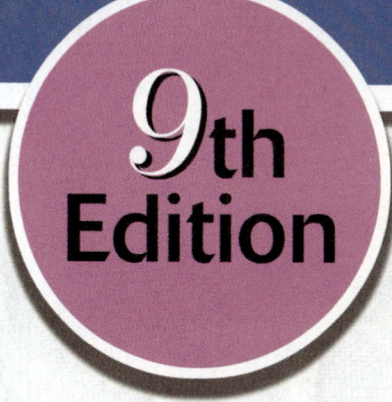

9th Edition

Barbara R. Hegner, MSN, RN
(deceased)

Barbara Acello, MS, RN
Independent nurse consultant and educator

Esther Caldwell, MA, PhD
Consultant in Vocational Education (CA)

THOMSON

DELMAR LEARNING

Australia Canada Mexico Singapore Spain United Kingdom United States

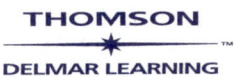

THOMSON
★
DELMAR LEARNING™

Nursing Assistant, A Nursing Process Approach, 9th Edition
by Barbara R. Hegner, Barbara Acello, Esther Caldwell

Vice President, Health Care Business Unit:
William Brottmiller

Editorial Director:
Cathy L. Esperti

Acquisitions Editor:
Marah E. Bellegarde

Developmental Editor:
Marjorie A. Bruce

Marketing Director:
Jennifer McAvey

Marketing Coordinator:
Kip Summerlin

Editorial Assistant:
Erin Adams

Art/Design Coordinator:
Jay Purcell

Project Editor:
Mary Ellen Cox

Production Coordinator:
Bridget Lulay

Library of Congress Cataloging-in-Publication Data
Hegner, Barbara R.
  Nursing assistant: a nursing process approach/Barbara R. Hegner, Barbara Acello, Esther Caldwell.—9th ed.
    p. : cm
  Includes bibliographical references and index.
  ISBN 1-4018-0632-5 (softcover : alk. paper)—ISBN 1-4018-0633-3 (hardcover : alk.paper)
  1. Nurses' aides. 2. Care of the sick. I. Acello, Barbara. II. Caldwell, Esther. III. Title.
  [DNLM: 1. Nurses' Aides. 2. Nursing Care. WY 193 H4644n 2004]
RT84.H45 2004
610.73'06'98—dc21
                                2003051572

International Divisions List

Asia (Including India):
Thomson Learning
60 Albert Street, #15-01
Albert Complex
Singapore 189969
Tel 65 336-6411
Fax 65 336-7411

Australia/New Zealand:
Nelson
102 Dodds Street
South Melbourne
Victoria 3205
Australia
Tel 61 (0)3 9685-4111
Fax 61 (0)3 9685-4199

Latin America:
Thomson Learning
Seneca 53
Colonia Polanco
11560 Mexico, D.F. Mexico
Tel (525) 281-2906
Fax (525) 281-2656

Canada:
Nelson
1120 Birchmount Road
Toronto, Ontario
Canada M1K 5G4
Tel (416) 752-9100
Fax (416) 752-8102

UK/Europe/Middle East/Africa:
Thomson Learning
Berkshire House
1680-173 High Holborn
London WC1V 7AA
United Kingdom
Tel 44 (0)20 497-1422
Fax 44 (0)20 497-1426

Spain (includes Portugal):
Paraninfo
Calle Magallanes 25
28015 Madrid
España
Tel 34 (0)91 446-3350
Fax 34 (0)91 445-6218

brief table of contents

list of tables

contents

SECTION 6

MEASURING AND RECORDING VITAL SIGNS, HEIGHT, AND WEIGHT   281

SECTION 10

OTHER HEALTH CARE SETTINGS   495

SECTION 11

BODY SYSTEMS, COMMON DISORDERS, AND RELATED CARE PROCEDURES   585

SECTION 12

EXPANDED ROLE OF THE NURSING ASSISTANT   781

SECTION 13

RESPONSE TO BASIC EMERGENCIES   851

SECTION 14

MOVING FORWARD   883

BARBARA R. HEGNER

Barbara Robinson Hegner, RN, MSN, was a graduate of a three-year diploma nursing program where direct and total care was the focus. She earned a BSN at Boston College and an MS in nursing from Boston University, with a minor in biologic sciences. She was Professor Emerita of Nursing and Life Sciences at Long Beach City College, Long Beach (CA).

Throughout her professional career, she had a deep interest in both hospital-based and long-term care nursing.

It was Ms. Hegner's belief that to ensure the rights and well-being of all patients and residents requires the care of competent, caring nursing assistants under the supervision of professional nurses. The nursing assistants who provide this care should be thoroughly trained and consistently encouraged, evaluated, and given the opportunity for continued learning. Providing the tools to prepare these health care providers in the most effective and efficient way is the goal of *Nursing Assistant, A Nursing Process Approach,* ninth edition.

BARBARA ACELLO

Barbara Acello, MS, RN, is an independent nurse consultant and educator in Denton, Texas. She is a member of the Texas Nurses' Association, Association of Nurses in AIDS Care, National Association of Directors of Nursing in Long Term Care, and American College of Healthcare Administrators. Mrs. Acello is a proponent and supporter of CNAs. With her husband, she owns and operates a licensed nursing assistant school. She has written many textbooks, journal articles, and other materials related to nursing assistant education. She believes the nursing assistant is the most important caregiver in the health care facility.

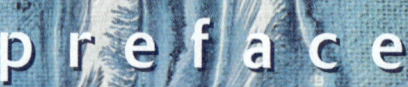

INTRODUCTION

The passage of the Omnibus Budget Reconciliation Act (OBRA) of 1987, which included the Nursing Home Reform Act, was the first federal legislation to address standards for certification of nursing assistants as health care providers in long-term care. This legislation has influenced both the education and practice of all nursing assistants.

Following the enactment of OBRA, the National Council of State Boards of Nursing Inc. developed the Nurse Aide Competency Evaluation Program as the guideline for evaluating nursing assistant education to meet the specific needs of health care consumers. Individual states have developed training programs that meet, and in many cases, exceed the minimum standards of the evaluation program.

Nursing assistants are important members of the nursing team (one part of the interdisciplinary health care team that plans and provides care to clients). Nursing assistants make valuable contributions to the nursing process that the professional nurse follows in assessing the client's needs, planning interventions, implementing care, and evaluating outcomes. Nursing assistants must be helped to see the vital role their accurate observations, reporting skills, and careful attention to instructions plays in the overall success of the nursing care plan. Only then can they recognize their full value as part of the nursing team.

Previous editions of this best-selling text emphasized the importance of treating those entrusted to care as total individuals who possess dignity, have value, and deserve respect. The continuing goal of this text and supplement package is to provide the tools that instructors can use to teach nursing assistants to meet high standards of care. This will enable them to help clients achieve a desirable level of comfort, restoration, and wellness while protecting and respecting clients' rights as health care consumers.

THE FUTURE

The ways in which health care is provided in the United States continue to change. Emphasis continues to be placed on maintaining wellness, limiting length of stay in acute care facilities, controlling costs through managed care, providing short- and long-term rehabilitation and restorative care in more cost-effective settings, and increasing home care services. In addition, the population of the United States is aging, with the greatest increase in the number of people over 65. As a result, restorative care and home care services will be major components in health care. Nursing assistants will provide much of this service. It is essential that nursing assistants be prepared to assume these vital responsibilities.

NINTH EDITION

Numerous revisions were made in the 9th edition to keep pace with the evolution of health care. New health care settings, new and improved technology, shorter acute care stays, an aging population, and drug-resistant microorganisms are some of the factors that are changing the ways in which care is provided. These factors also affect the way in which nursing assistants provide care.

The following updated and enhanced content addresses the changing character of nursing assistant responsibilities.

- Text box alerts were added with pertinent information on infection control, OSHA, communication, age-appropriate care, legal implications, safety, culture, difficult situations and patient care, and patient care tips.
- URLS were added to each unit for further information and research.
- Handwashing information was updated in keeping with the CDC handwashing guidelines from October 2002.
- Infection control content was added on *e. coli* 0157:H7, pseudomembranous colitis (*C. difficile*), and hantavirus.
- Information was added on violence in the workplace.
- Many new procedures, guidelines, and information were added, including electronic blood pressure monitoring, using the waterless bath (bag bath), setting up sequential compression therapy, and recognizing compartment syndrome and autonomic dysreflexia.
- Pain content was updated throughout the text.
- A new unit on comfort, rest, and sleep was added.
- Guidelines for computerized documentation were added.
- Therapeutic diet information was expanded, and new information added on calorie counts, food intake studies, and dysphagia.
- Information on working within professional boundaries was added.
- Guidelines for assisting patients with behavior problems, delirium, and wandering were expanded.
- Unit 36 is a new unit reflecting trends in alternative and complementary medicine and integrative approaches to patient care.
- New content is provided regarding personal safety for home health assistants.
- The subacute care unit was expanded to include information on checking capillary refill, using a pulse oximeter, understanding care of patients with implanted medication pumps, care of the patient with a tracheostomy, continuous ambulatory peritoneal

dialysis, and care of patients with central intravenous catheters.

- The respiratory unit was expanded to include care of the patient with a chest tube and continuous positive airway pressure (CPAP). Additional information is provided on oxygen therapy.
- The arthritis and osteoporosis content was expanded, and new information added on fibromyalgia, fracture care, care of the patient with hip surgery, and continuous passive motion (CPM) therapy.
- The procedure for obtaining a fingerstick blood sugar was added.
- Many new conditions were added to the neurologic nursing unit, including content on post polio syndrome, amyotrophic lateral sclerosis (ALS), autonomic dysreflexia, cataract surgery, glaucoma, applying warm and cold eye compresses, seizure care, and flaccid and spastic paralysis.
- Content on care of patients with problems of the lower bowel, prostate cancer, and ovarian cancer was expanded.
- New procedures were added to the advanced skills unit, including removing an indwelling catheter, sterile technique, setting up a sterile field using a sterile drape, adding an item to a sterile field, adding liquids to a sterile field, applying and removing sterile gloves, and using transfer forceps. Caring for an ostomy was expanded in this unit, and content added on the automatic external defibrillator (AED).
- A new unit was added on caring for the patient with cancer.

EXTENSIVE TEACHING/ LEARNING PACKAGE

The complete supplement package was developed to achieve two goals:

1. To assist students in learning essential information to permit them to become certified and function as skilled nursing assistants
2. To assist instructors in planning and implementing their instructional program for the most efficient use of time and other resources

Each supplement has been extensively revised to reflect text changes.

Student Workbook

The comprehensive workbook reinforces the text content. It is recommended that the student complete each workbook unit to confirm understanding of essential content.

The workbook content includes:

- Tips on how to study more effectively
- Organization by units with student activities to increase comprehension. Each unit consists of objectives to

focus the content for the student; a unit summary to point out key topics; nursing assistant alerts that provide key actions, with an explanation of the benefit resulting from the action; and various exercises (review questions, vocabulary exercises and games, and clinical situations).

- Student Performance Record — alphabetical listing of 163 text procedures to monitor student completion of return demonstrations
- Flash cards provide a review of basic medical terms, including combining forms, prefixes, and suffixes.

Instructor's Manual

The Instructor's Manual provides the following support:

- An extensive list of resource materials
- A list of health care and aging-related organizations providing free or low-cost educational materials
- Curriculum syllabus for a typical 75–90 hour nursing assistant program
- Organization by corresponding text unit: instructor objectives, suggested activities, and answers to unit review questions
- Answers to student workbook exercises
- Section tests with answers
- Comprehensive final examination with answers
- Extra bank of test questions (with answers) to simplify preparation of tests or to provide additional testing material for advanced students
- Procedures Evaluation Form that can be duplicated for each student as a checklist of progress in successfully demonstrating procedures; essential OBRA procedure skills are identified as an aid in monitoring student progress
- Transparency masters
- The Manual is available as a separate item or as part of the Instructor's Resource Kit.

Computerized Test Bank

The computerized testbank (Windows) with more than 1,800 questions gives the instructor an expanded capability to create tests. The testbank is available as a separate item or as part of the Instructor's Resource Kit.

Instructor's Resource Kit

This supplement provides the instructor with resources to simplify the planning and implementation of the instructional program. It integrates the use of the text, Student Workbook, Instructor's Manual, and video series to help the instructor develop an efficient instructional plan.

The complete Instructor's Resource Kit includes the following list of sections, plus the complete Instructor's Manual and the computerized testbank.

Section Content

- Section A — Teaching Methods and Strategies provides tips on teaching adult learners, including English as a second language (ESL) students.
- Section B — Teaching Resources includes a listing of *Delmar's Nursing Assisting Video Series*, other audiovisual aids, software resources, reference texts, models and charts, media sources, and a listing of professional health organizations.
- Section C — course syllabi for 70- to 90-hour, 120-hour, 300-hour, and 600-hour programs. Each syllabus outlines the number of hours for didactic work and clinical experience and relates these to the use of *Nursing Assistant, A Nursing Process Approach, 9E.*
- Section D — Lesson Plans in which the supplemental materials and the text are related into a cohesive plan for presenting each topic.
- Section E — Unit Outlines highlight the essential topics for each unit. Suggested activities provide a means of generating student interest and interaction in class to reinforce learning.
- Section F — English-Spanish Flash Cards show common terms and simple phrases in English and Spanish to facilitate communication in the workplace. ESL students can use the flash cards to improve English skills. English-speaking students will find them useful in communicating with Spanish-speaking colleagues, patients, and residents.
- Section G — Computerized testbank.

WebTutor™

WebTutor™ for Web CT or Blackboard is a content-rich, Web-based teaching and learning aid that reinforces and clarifies key concepts. This course management and delivery system accompanies the text and can be used to supplement on-campus course delivery. WebTutor™ provides communication tools to instructors and students, including a course calendar, chat, e-mail, and threaded discussions. Each unit contains the following items:

- Advanced Preparation—details what a student should do before starting each online unit
- Unit Objectives—alert the student to what is expected as outcomes for each unit
- Class Notes—are helpful tips that provide further clarification and expansion of text content
- Frequently Asked Questions (FAQs)—provide answers to questions that students commonly ask
- Glossary of terms—is specific to the unit and is also rolled into a comprehensive glossary for the course

- Discussion Topics—provide interactive classroom discussion by means of a threaded bulletin board
- Learning Links—require students to search the Web for information to reinforce and expand learning; students report back findings to instructors through email
- Online Exercises—provide further reinforcement of learning with immediate feedback

WebTutor™ also includes a midterm test and a final test.

Delmar Learning's Basic Core Skills for Nursing Assistants Video Series

This skill-based video series will help prepare nursing assistants for the certification examination. Each of the 76 core procedures is presented step-by-step for maximum effectiveness. In addition to the procedures, general guidelines are included for lifting and moving, ambulation, handling clean or soiled linen, and observation and reporting. Critical beginning and ending procedure actions are detailed in Module 1 with a concise review introducing subsequent Modules. These steps must be performed for each patient care procedure. Safety and infection control practices are emphasized in each procedure. The series includes the following Modules:

Module 1	Obstructed Airway; Handwashing; Beginning and Completion Procedure Actions; Communication Skills
Module 2	Personal Protective Equipment, Standard Precautions, and Transmission-Based Precautions
Module 3	Positioning, Transfers, and Ambulation
Module 4	Bedmaking and Bathing
Module 5	Bladder, Bowel, and Perineal Care
Module 6	Personal Care
Module 7	Dressing, Meal Care, and Restraints
Module 8	Vital Signs, Height, and Weight
Module 9	Observation/Reporting Guidelines and Postmortem Care
Module 10	Range of Motion and Mechanical Lift

Features

- Each procedure opens with a listing of the equipment and supplies needed for the procedure
- Each step-by-step procedure is followed by a concise review of the steps for reinforcement.
- Where appropriate, the one-glove method is used to minimize contamination of environmental surfaces
- Critical beginning and ending procedure actions are reviewed in each Module

acknowledgments

Each new edition brings with it the pleasant task of acknowledging the contributions of a number of individuals.

The following individuals provided valuable information and resources for new content:

- Pat Carroll RN, C, CEN, RRT, MS, for extensive assistance with the respiratory content
- Janine Anderson, BS, RN, for her prompt response to my many requests for resources and research articles
- Kadel Laxson, OrthoRehab, Inc., for extensive assistance with joint replacement and CPM content
- Marc Hopkins and Linda Jaakobovitch, Cincinnati Eye Clinic, for information and assistance with cataract surgery content
- Sharmila Majumdar, PhD, Professor, UCSF, for information and assistance with osteoporosis content
- Ed Lowry and Gina Bon, Alaris Medical, for assistance with electronic blood pressure monitoring
- Lisa Vallino, RN, BSN, and Betty Rozier, IV House, Inc., for assistance with content related to IV site care
- George Beggs, Tactilics, Inc., for assistance with bed alarms
- Rick Hammesfahr, MD, owner of www.arthroscopy.com, for assistance with CPM content
- Jef Bradshaw, Amdrecor, Inc., for assistance with face shields and personal protective equipment
- Cathy Pelletier, PhD, MS, CCC-SLP, for assistance with dysphagia content
- Pat Ridgely, MD, and Linnea Burman, Medtronic, Inc., for extensive assistance and information on care of the patient with an implanted medication pump
- Donna Wong, PhD, RN, for extensive assistance on pain management and use of the FACES pain scale

A book of this size represents an enormous investment of time and talent by many dedicated individuals. I sincerely appreciate the support and assistance of the following individuals at Delmar Learning: Marge Bruce, developmental editor, whose steadfast support was invaluable in manuscript construction and development; Sherry Gomoll, acquisitions editor, whose vision and tolerance of my idiosyncrasies is sincerely appreciated; Jennifer Conklin, editorial assistant, who coordinated many facets of manuscript review, copying, and shipping. I am always delighted when Brooke Graves lends her many copyediting talents to my projects.

I would also like to recognize the contributions of Dennis Clarkson, CNA, and Shari Allen, CNA. These individuals touched my life deeply, and enhanced my understanding of the trials, tribulations, joys, and pleasures faced by the career nursing assistant in the 21st century. Both of these assistants made many positive, unselfish, and lasting contributions to nursing assistant practice. Their untimely passing at a young age had a profound impact on my life during manuscript development, and their many contributions are sincerely appreciated and will be sorely missed.

Reviewers

The revision was aided by a dedicated group of instructors who reviewed content at different stages of the revision process. For their valuable suggestions and corrections, we thank:

Deana Allison, RN
Glendive, MT

Mary Jo Gerlach, RN, MSNEd
Assistant Professor — Adult Nursing (Retired)
Medical College of Georgia — School of Nursing
Augusta, GA

Marge Konieczny, RN, MSN
Adjunct Faculty — Lead Instructor Nursing Assistant
    Program
Lake Tahoe Community College
South Lake Tahoe, CA

Lori Pfeister, BSN, RN, CRRN
Clinical Educator for Certified Nursing Assistants
Our Lady of the Lake Regional Medical Center
Baton Rouge, LA

Pat Reinhart, RN
Nursing Faculty and Healthcare Representative for
    Customized Training and Continuing Education
Minneapolis Community and Technical College
Minneapolis, MN

Debi Shelman, RN, LPN, EMT-I,
    CNA/Home Health Aide
Instructor — Nursing Assistant and Home Health
    Aide Programs
Tucson College
Tucson, AZ

Lois R. Stotter, RNC, BSN
Clinical Nurse Education
Borgess Medical Center
Kalamazoo, MI

features of this book

The ninth edition of *Nursing Assistant, a Nursing Process Approach* has been carefully designed and updated to make the study of nursing assistant tasks and responsibilities easier and more productive. For best results, you may want to become familiar with the features incorporated into this text and accompanying learning tools.

Table of Contents

For each unit, the table of contents lists the unit title, major topic headings, general guidelines for specific areas of care and topics of importance to the nursing assistant, and patient care procedures.

Unit Opening Page

Each unit opening page contains objectives and vocabulary terms.

The **objectives** help you know what is expected of you as you read the text. Your success in mastering each objective is measured by the review questions at the end of each unit.

The **vocabulary** list alerts you to new terms presented in the unit. When each term is first used in the unit, it is highlighted in boldface and color. Each term is defined at this point in the unit. Read the definition of the term and note the context in which it is used so that you will feel comfortable in using the term. Note that the glossary at the back of the book also defines these highlighted terms.

Text Alerts

The alerts provide important content on infection control, OSHA, communication, age-appropriate care, legal implications, safety, difficult patient care, and general patient care. The information makes the learner aware of best practices in patient care, includes practical tips based on experience, and highlights critical infection control, safety and other OSHA workplace guidelines.

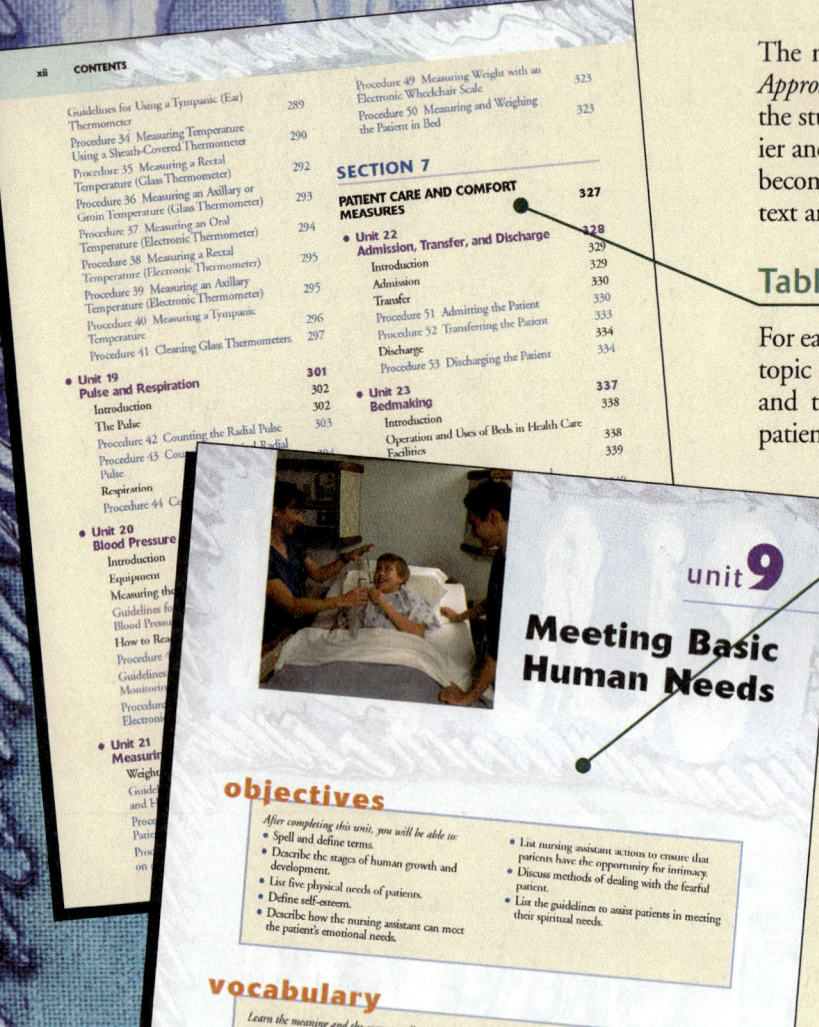

unit **9**

Meeting Basic Human Needs

objectives

After completing this unit, you will be able to:
• Spell and define terms.
• Describe the stages of human growth and development.
• List five physical needs of patients.
• Define self-esteem.
• Describe how the nursing assistant can meet the patient's emotional needs.
• List nursing assistant actions to ensure that patients have the opportunity for intimacy.
• Discuss methods of dealing with the fearful patient.
• List the guidelines to assist patients in meeting their spiritual needs.

vocabulary

Learn the meaning and the correct spelling of the following words and phrases:
adolescence
bisexuality
celibate
growth
heterosexu...
...

UNIT 27 Warm and Cold Applications — 433

SAFETY *Alert*
The nurse will instruct you on the frequency for monitoring vital signs when an aquathermia blanket is being used. The patient's temperature and the blanket temperature are usually monitored and documented every 15 to 30 minutes. Inform the nurse immediately if the patient's temperature drops more than one degree in 15 mi... perature monitoring is necess... removed because the pati... continue to drop as much ... procedure ends.

AGE-APPROPRIATE CARE *Alert*
In children, temperatures tend to rise higher than in adults. This puts children at greater risk for seizures.

... Provide...

using. Turn the unit off. (Some ... in for 30 to 60 minutes to dr... unit.) Dry the patient's skin and ... gown. Position the patient in ... Remove the aquathermia blanke... designated time. Continue chec... and output every 30 minutes ... hourly or as directed by the nur...

Hypothermia

Hypothermia is a drop in core ... 95°F (35°C) rectally. This can o...
• when people are exposed to c... protection.
• in the elderly, when a person... temperatures as warm as 60°F...
• when deliberately induced be... metabolism.
Indications of hypothermia to...
• Drop in body temperature
• Poor coordination and confu...
• Slurred speech
• Decreased respiratory and he...

Nursing Assistant Ac...
• Report observations to the su...
• Check the environmental tem...

364 SECTION 7 Patient Care and Comfort Measures

Perineal Care
The **perineum** is the area between the legs. In females, it is the area between the vagina and the anus. In males, it is the area between the scrotum and the anus. **Perineal care** may be performed as part of general bathing, or as a separate procedure, as needed. **Perineal care** means to wash the area including the genitals and anus (see Procedures 63 and 64). Always wear gloves and use standard precautions when caring for the perineal area.

Tips: If the patient has been incontinent, remove the wet pad or linen and replace with a dry pad before beginning perineal care. Clean excess stool off with toilet tissue before beginning.

COMMUNICATION *Highlight*
Patients who need assistance with perineal care and those who become incontinent may feel guilty and embarrassed. Avoid showing disgust. Be sensitive to the patient's feelings. Communicate with the patient tactfully. Use proper terms when referring to body parts and excretions.

INFECTION CONTROL *Alert*
Providing perineal care is one of the most important procedures you will perform as a nursing assistant. Always apply the principles of standard precautions. Remember that there are mucous membranes in the genital area. If you are wearing gloves, change them before beginning care. Using proper technique is critical because of the high risk of contamination and infection. Avoid scrubbing back and forth. Always wipe from clean to dirty with a single wipe, then turn or discard the cloth, according to facility policy. Guidelines for female perineal care vary with the institution. In some facilities, you will be instructed to clean the center first, then each side. In others, you will clean the sides of the genitalia first, then the center. Know and follow your facility policies. Discard your gloves properly and avoid contaminating environmental surfaces with your used gloves.

PROCEDURE 63

FEMALE PERINEAL CARE
... beginning procedure actions.
4. Remove the bedspread and blanket. Fold and place them on the back of the chair.

Photographs and Line Drawings

Numerous color illustrations and photos, including more than 100 new photos taken for this edition, help to clarify and reinforce the unit content. Many figures are used in the procedures to help you visualize critical steps. Full color anatomy drawings help you to locate body components and understand body organization.

Guidelines

The table of contents identifies guidelines included in units. These guidelines highlight important points that you need to remember for specific situations or types of care. They are presented in an easy-to-use format that you can refer to repeatedly until you know the actions you must take when confronted with the situation.

Procedures

The text contains 163 clinical procedures in a step-by-step format. Each procedure reminds you to perform the beginning procedure actions. A list of equipment and supplies needed for the procedure is provided. Any notes or cautions about performing the procedure are given. The steps take you carefully through the procedure, emphasizing at all times the need to work safely and to protect the patient's privacy. At the end, you are reminded of the procedure completion actions.

Review and Testing Material

Unit Reviews

A variety of review questions at the end of each unit test your understanding of the unit content. Each review contains a **Nursing Assistant Challenge** that presents a typical clinical situation and asks questions about your response to the situation. These questions require you to integrate what you have learned to arrive at an appropriate solution or set of actions.

For additional activities and exercises to reinforce your learning, refer to the Student Workbook. Your instructor may also give you additional questions and tests from the Instructor's Manual, Instructor's Resource Kit or the Computerized Testbank that accompany the text.

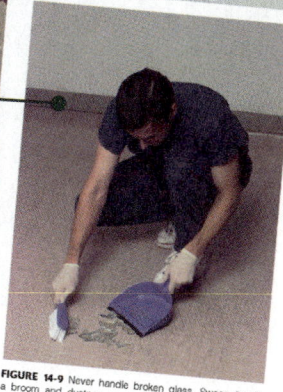

FIGURE 14-8 Unsafe electrical equipment is tagged and locked until it can be repaired.

FIGURE 14-9 Never handle broken glass. Sweep it with a broom and dustpan or use an instrument to pick up large pieces. Wear gloves. Discard the glass in the proper container.

guidelines *for*

Safe Ambulation

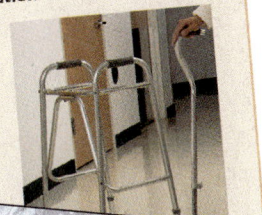

- Encourage independent patients to use the hand rail when walking.
- Always stand on the patient's affected side when walking with her.
- Always use a gait belt (transfer belt) if the patient needs assistance with ambulation. Grasp the belt in the back with an underhand grip (Figure 17-4). Place your other hand on the patient's shoulder if balance is unsteady.
- Make sure the patient is wearing sturdy shoes with nonslip soles and that laces are tied. Clothing should not be too loose or drag on the floor.
- Check floor for clutter or puddles that could cause a fall.
- If you are unsure of the patient's endurance or balance, ask another nursing assistant to follow behind you with the wheelchair. If the patient becomes weak, dizzy, or tired, she can sit in the wheelchair.
- Check rubber tips on bottoms of canes, crutches, and walkers, and also check the rubber handgrips (Figure 17-5). These should be replaced if the rings are cracked, loose, or worn down. If the ridges are filled with debris, use alcohol and cotton swabs to clean them. Replace the handgrip if it is loose or cracked.
- Check screws, nuts, and bolts for tightness. Do not use any device that appears unsafe. Report the problem to the appropriate person.
- Practice good body mechanics for both you and the patient.

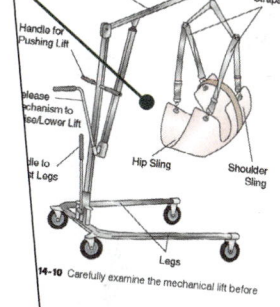

14-10 Carefully examine the mechanical lift before

PROCEDURE 31

ASSISTING THE PATIENT TO WALK WITH A WALKER AND THREE-POINT GAIT

1. Carry out beginning procedure actions.
2. Assemble equipment:
   - Walker as ordered
   - Gait belt
3. Make sure the patient has on sturdy shoes with nonslip soles. Check clothing to be sure it does not hang down over shoes.
4. Place a gait belt on the patient and assist the patient to a standing position. Place the walker in front of the patient and have her grasp the walker with both hands. Stand on the patient's affected side. Place your closest hand in the gait belt, using an underhand grip (Figure 17-11).

   Note: *The walker is not a transfer device and should not be used to help the patient stand up. The patient grasps the walker after she is standing. To sit, the patient releases her grip on the walker while still*

9. This process is repeated while the patient is walking.
10. Note the patient's endurance, balance, and strength while walking. Stop immediately if the patient has trouble and help her to the closest chair. Call the nurse.
11. Assist the patient to sit in the chair or to lie down in bed. Remove the gait belt. Store the walker in an appropriate area.
12. Document the distance the patient ambulated and her tolerance of the procedure.
13. Carry out procedure completion actions.

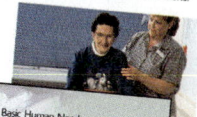

REVIEW

A. True/False.

Mark the following true or false by circling T or F.

1. T F Growth and development go from the simple to the complex.
2. T F Body development proceeds from the head toward the feet.
3. T F All individuals move through the stages of growth.
4. T F Growth and development progression are interdependent.
5. T F Ossification of bones is not complete at birth.
6. T F The Moro reflex occurs when the infant's palm is touched.
7. T F The sucking reflex occurs when the infant is startled.
8. T F The three-month-old infant cries real tears.
9. T F The six-month-old infant can walk if well supported.
10. T F First teeth begin to erupt about the sixth month of life.
11. T F The one-year-old infant has progressed to eating table foods.
12. T F The toddler period finds children interacting freely and playing well with one another.
13. T F Between the ages of three and five years, the child seems to have an endless list of questions.
14. T F The school-age child is interested in and chooses members of the same sex as close friends.
15. T F One of the developmental tasks of old age is to learn to deal successfully with loss.
16. T F Basic human needs are the same at all ages, but different ways must be found to satisfy them.
17. T F Erikson believed that one of the developmental tasks of infancy is learning to trust.
18. T F Erikson states that the developmental task of the middle years is to integrate life's experience.

B. Matching.

Match the appropriate chronologic age to the life time period by matching Column I and Column II.

Column I

22. _____ old age
23. _____ adolescence
24. _____ later maturity
25. _____ school age
26. _____ adulthood

Column II

a. 65 years old
b. 16 years old
c. 7 years old
d. 35 years old
e. 80 years old

C. Multiple Choice.

Select the one best answer for each of the following.

27. Growth and development
   a. move from limbs to torso and feet to head.
   b. involve more complex tasks during growth spurts.
   c. can proceed normally even if tasks are not mastered.
   d. have specific tasks that must be mastered at each stage.
28. The main activity (activities) of the toddler period is (are)
   a. exploration and investigation.
   b. cooperative play.
   c. establishing peer relationships.
   d. showing concern for others.
29. Preschoolers are
   a. less reliant on their mothers.
   b. able to join groups like Scouts.
   c. able to choose sex-differentiated friends.
   d. unable to tolerate brief separation from their mother.
30. The ways in which we react to the events in our lives are called
   a. personality.
   b. self-identity.
   c. tasks of personality development.
   d. hierarchy of needs.

Dedication

This text is dedicated to the memory of Barbara R. Hegner. Barbara was a visionary who saw the need for formalized instructional materials to help educate and develop skilled nursing assistants. She was committed to this unique and important group of health care professionals.

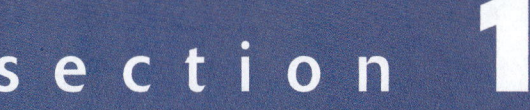
Introduction to Nursing Assisting

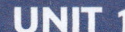

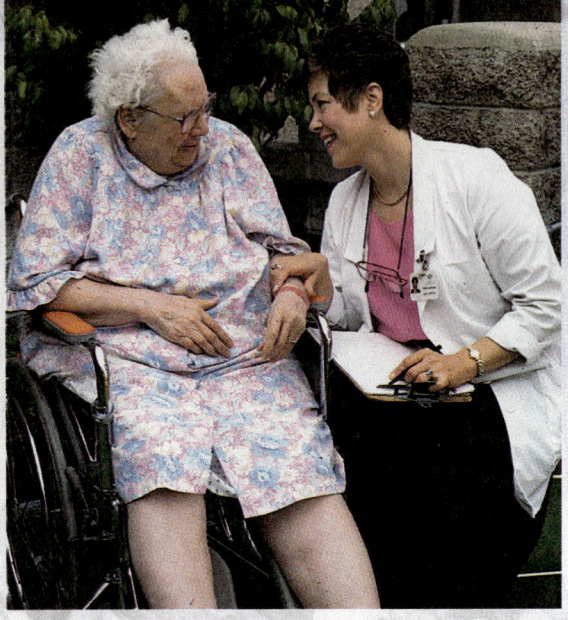

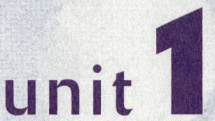

unit 1

Community Health Care

objectives

After completing this unit, you will be able to:

- Spell and define terms.
- List the five basic functions of health care facilities.
- Describe four changes that have taken place in health care in the last few years.
- Describe the differences between acute care and long-term care.

- Name the departments within a hospital.
- Describe the functions of the departments within a hospital.
- Explain three ways by which health care costs are paid.
- State the purpose of health care facility surveys.

vocabulary

Learn the meaning and the correct spelling of the following words and phrases:

acute illness	hospice	Occupational Safety	prenatal
certification	hospital	and Health	psychiatric
chronic illness	Joint Commission	Administration	quality assurance
citation	for Accreditation	(OSHA)	(QA)
client	of Healthcare	occupational therapy	rehabilitation
community	Organizations	orthopedic	resident
diagnosis related	(JCAHO)	pathology	respiratory therapy
groups (DRG)	license	patient	skilled care facility
facility	managed care	patient focused care	speech therapy
health care	Medicaid	pediatric	survey
consumer	Medicare	physical therapy	surveyor
health maintenance	obstetric	post-anesthesia	
organization		recovery (PAR)	
(HMO)		postpartum	

INTRODUCTION

Nursing assistants play an important role in the care of people who are ill or injured. You will give care to these persons under the direction and supervision of licensed, professional health care workers, such as doctors and nurses. Care is provided in various types of health care facilities. The term facility refers to the place in which care is given. A hospital is a complex organization that provides a full range of health care services. Highly sophisticated equipment and treatments are available there. A skilled care facility provides care to persons whose conditions are stable but who need monitoring, nursing care, and treatments. All health care facilities have five basic functions:

1. Providing services for the ill and injured (Figure 1-1).
2. Preventing disease.
3. Promoting individual and community health.
4. Educating health care workers (Figure 1-2).
5. Promoting research in medicine and nursing.

OVERVIEW OF HEALTH CARE

Health care today emphasizes patient focused care. This care focus is based on the fact that each patient is a unique individual and has different needs. Attention must be given to the physical, mental, and emotional aspects of the person's being if that person is to lead a fulfilling and satisfying life.

Because people are living longer, quality of life has become an important consideration in health care delivery. Some

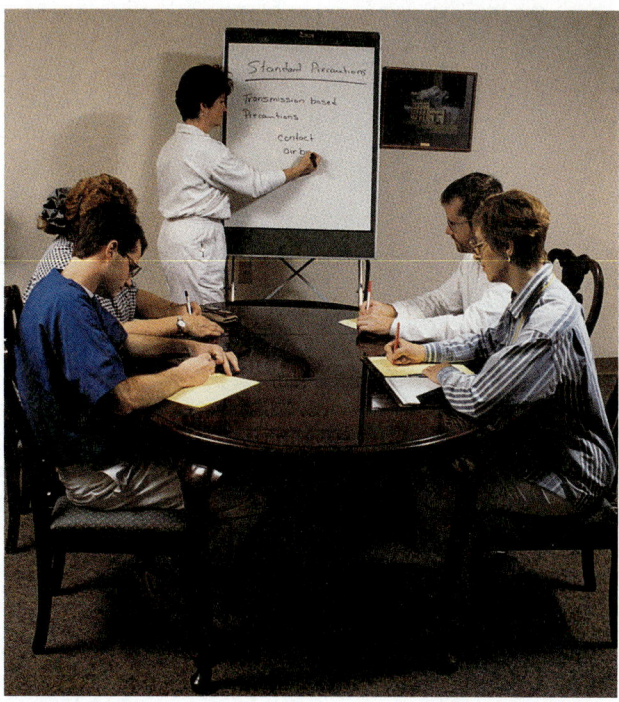

FIGURE 1-2 Education is an important health care objective.

health care decisions are made with the patient's future quality of life in mind. Quality-of-life policies and requirements focus on creating and maintaining an environment that humanizes and individualizes each patient. In some situations, preserving the quality of the patient's life is viewed as more important than increasing the length or duration of life.

Many changes have occurred in health care within the last few years. There are several reasons for these changes:

- People are living longer. As people age, their need for health care increases, so more services are needed (Figure 1-3).

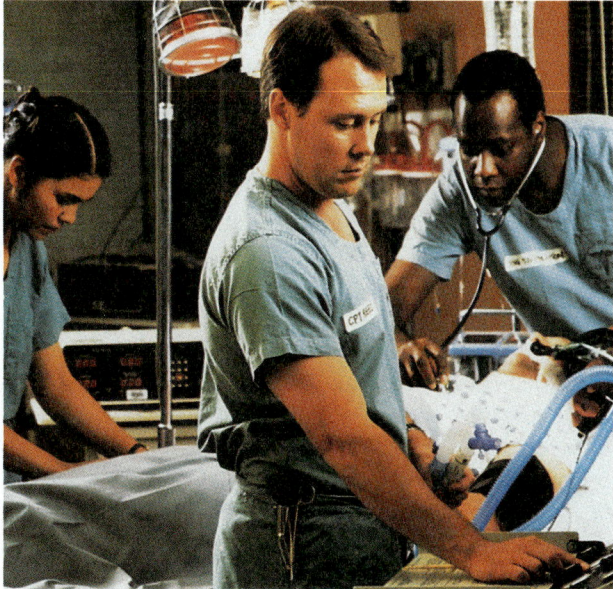

FIGURE 1-1 Health care facilities provide many different services to ill and injured patients. *("Be All You Can Be," Courtesy United States Government, as represented by the Secretary of the Army)*

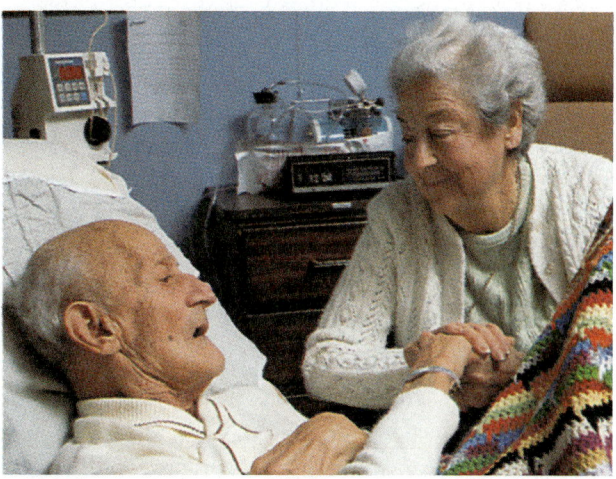

FIGURE 1-3 As the population ages, more health care services are needed to care for patients with illness and disability.

- Advanced technology means that more lives are saved. Although life is maintained, some of these individuals need continuing health care.
- The cost of health care has increased tremendously because of the demand for services and because of advances in technology.
- Science has created many ethical (moral) questions that must be answered by health care providers and health care consumers.

To reduce the cost of health care, patients are discharged earlier from hospitals. These patients may still require health care. This care can be given more economically in skilled care facilities and in the patient's home. More diagnostic tests and procedures are provided in outpatient facilities to further decrease costs. Surgicenters, urgent care centers, and clinics are examples of such facilities. It is less expensive, for example, to receive treatment for a throat infection in an urgent care center than in a hospital emergency room.

Most health care is paid for with insurance. Insurance companies use **managed care** to provide the services in the most efficient manner at the lowest cost. Briefly, this means that the insurance company will:

- Not permit certain procedures or diagnostic tests until they have been approved by the insurer.
- Negotiate with specific physicians, hospitals, pharmacies, and other care providers to render services at a lower cost to the company's members.
- Approve only a certain number of days of hospitalization for specific diagnoses. A woman giving birth, for example, may be allowed up to 48 hours of hospitalization.
- Require that specific procedures be done on an outpatient basis rather than having the patient admitted to the hospital.

NEEDS OF THE COMMUNITY

People who live in a common area and share common health needs form a **community**. Provisions for disposal of wastes, assurance of safe drinking water, availability of healthful foods, protection from disease, and health care are important to every person within a community. Public

health laws regulate these services and are enforced by government agencies.

Health care is needed throughout life. The care may be short-term or long-term and includes:

- Preventive care
  - **Prenatal** care (care of the mother during pregnancy).
  - Well-baby checkups and immunizations.
  - Health education to teach individuals how to avoid disease and injury.
  - Physical examinations throughout life.
- Emergency care
  - Short-term care given for sudden illness or injury.
- Surgery
  - To repair an injured body or remove a diseased organ.
- Rehabilitation (hospital)
  - To help a patient to regain abilities after illness or injury.
- Long-term care
  - For patients who have chronic or incurable conditions.
- **Hospice** care
  - For patients who are dying and their families.

Persons receiving health care are called **health care consumers**. They are also identified by the type of care they need:

- **Patient** is a term used for persons in acute care facilities such as hospitals.
- **Client** is a term used for persons receiving care in their own homes.
- **Resident** is usually a term for people in long-term skilled care facilities.

COMMUNITY HEALTH CARE SERVICES

There are two main types of health care facilities: those that provide short-term care and those that provide long-term care (Table 1-1). Short-term care is given to patients who have a routine or minor problem, such as a urinary tract infection. The care may be given in the physician's office, an outpatient clinic, or an urgent care center. Uncomplicated surgeries, such as hernia repair, require only short-term care and may be done in a surgicenter. Hospitals provide short-term care for acute illnesses. An **acute illness** or injury comes on suddenly and requires intense, immediate treatment. Heart attacks, severe burns, strokes, and uncontrolled diabetes are examples of acute conditions.

Long-term care is necessary for persons who have chronic conditions. A **chronic illness** is one that is treatable but not curable and is expected to require lifelong care. This care may be given in a skilled care facility, adult day-care setting,

TABLE 1-1 TYPES OF HEALTH CARE FACILITIES

Short-Term Care	Long-Term Care
Hospitals	Skilled care facilities
Urgent care facilities	Adult day care
Surgicenters	Assisted living facilities Rehabilitation centers Psychiatric hospitals
Outpatient clinics	Respite care
Psychiatric hospitals	
Physician's offices	Home care

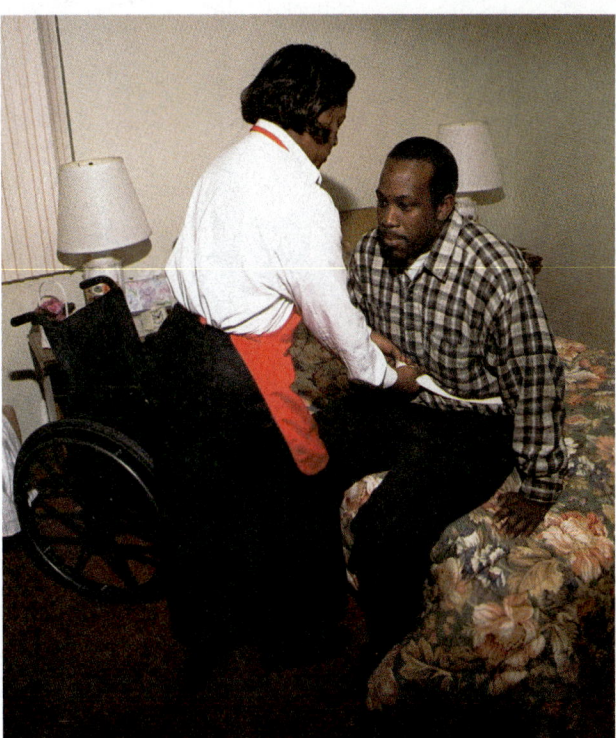

FIGURE 1-4 Health care is often given in the client's home.

respite care facility, assisted living facility, or the patient's home (Figure 1-4). Cardiovascular disease (heart and blood vessels), Alzheimer's disease, multiple sclerosis, Parkinson's disease, and diabetes are examples of chronic illnesses. Additional information about long-term care is given in Section 10.

Hospitals

Most hospitals are licensed to care for patients of all ages and for patients with a variety of problems. Some hospitals take care of patients with special conditions or care for specific age groups:

- **Pediatric** hospitals care only for children from birth to 18 years of age.
- **Psychiatric** hospitals provide care for persons with mental illness.
- **Rehabilitation** hospitals provide restorative services to patients following disease, illness, or injury. These services are designed to help the patient regain the ability to function at the highest level possible, considering the patient's illness or injury.

Hospital Organization

Hospitals are organized in ways that provide the most efficient delivery of service. Major departments are established within each facility to meet the needs of patients with specific conditions (Figure 1-5). These units provide nursing care 24 hours a day, 7 days a week.

- Medical department: cares for patients with medical conditions such as pneumonia or heart disease.
- Surgical department: cares for patients before, during, and after surgery. There may be many operating rooms where surgical procedures are performed, and a **post-anesthesia recovery (PAR)** area where patients are

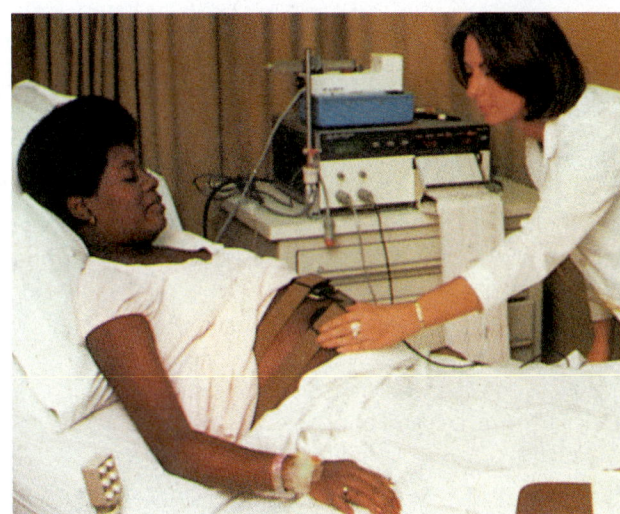

FIGURE 1-5 The various departments within the health care facility are organized to meet the needs of many patients. *(Courtesy of Long Beach Medical Center, Long Beach, CA)*

closely monitored after surgery. Patients remain in this area until they are stable enough to leave the surgical department.

- Pediatric department: cares for sick or injured children.
- **Obstetric** department: cares for newborns and their mothers. This department includes the labor and delivery unit, the **postpartum** unit (for mothers who have given birth), and the nursery for the newborns (Figure 1-6).

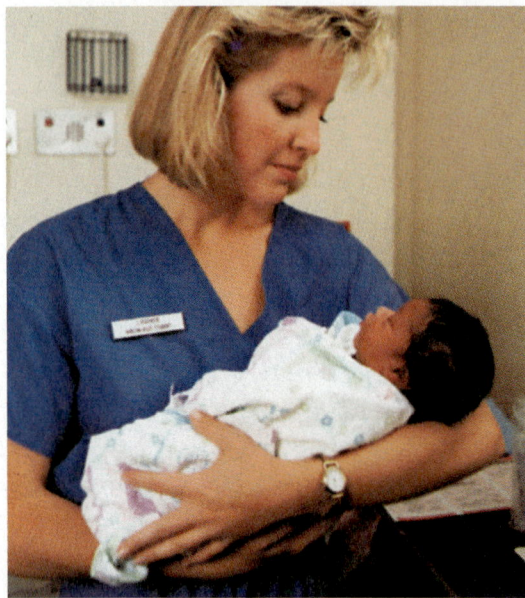

FIGURE 1-6 The obstetric department cares for mothers and newborn infants.

- Emergency department: cares for victims of trauma or of natural disasters (tornadoes, for example), or medical emergencies.
- Critical care department: cares for seriously ill patients who require constant monitoring and care.

Larger hospitals have many specialized units staffed by nurses and therapists who have been trained to care for persons with specific problems such as cancer, cardiovascular disease, or kidney disease, or for those requiring orthopedic (bones and muscles) surgery. Specialized health care workers provide direct or indirect services to the patients in these units. Specialized services include:

- Dietary services. A registered dietitian plans the meals for all patients and provides educational services to patients on special diets. The hospital's food service department prepares meals and delivers them to patients.
- Pharmacy services. Registered pharmacists prepare and provide all medications and intravenous therapy solutions.
- Diagnostic services.
  - Pathology (study of disease). Physicians and technicians perform diagnostic tests on specimens taken from body tissue to help the doctor make a diagnosis.
  - Diagnostic imaging and radiology. Physicians and technicians take x-rays and do other specialized procedures to help make a diagnosis.
  - Laboratory. A department equipped to perform diagnostic tests and investigative procedures. Various specimens are sent to the laboratory for analysis. The results of the tests are used by the physician and other individuals in the care of patients.

- Rehabilitation services.
  - Physical therapy assists patients to regain mobility skills.
  - Occupational therapy helps patients to regain self-care skills.
  - Speech therapy helps patients to regain the ability to communicate and works with patients who have swallowing disorders.
  - Respiratory therapy provides care for patients who have disorders of the cardiopulmonary system, respirations, and sleep disorders that affect the patient's breathing.
- Social services. Staff members provide counseling for patients and their families, help needy families get financial assistance, plan for patient discharge, and arrange for patient transfers from one facility to another (Figure 1-7).
- Environmental services.
  - Housekeeping is responsible for the overall cleaning of the hospital (Figure 1-8).
  - Maintenance cares for and repairs equipment.
  - Laundry services provide and clean all hospital linens.
- Business services are responsible for patient billing, employee payroll, and other financial concerns.
- Medical records department transcribes and catalogs all patient records.
- Volunteers provide services free of charge and perform tasks such as delivering mail and flowers, running the gift shop, directing visitors, and raising funds for the facility (Figure 1-9).
- Pastoral care helps patients meet their religious and spiritual needs and provides counseling.

Patients may be transferred from one unit to another within a hospital. For example, a patient having surgery

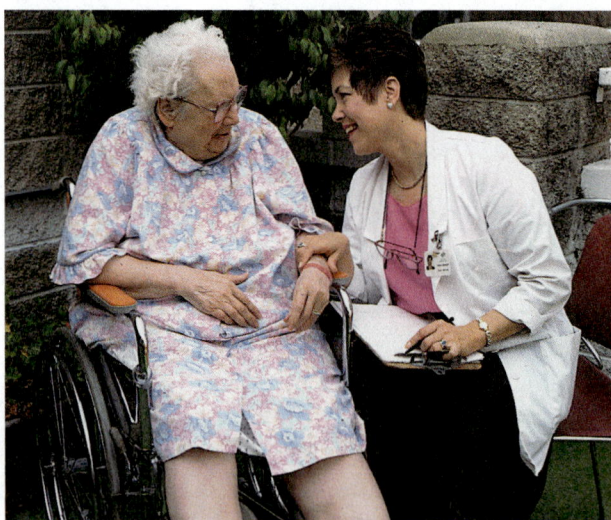

FIGURE 1-7 The social worker is responsible for ensuring that the patient's discharge plans are complete.

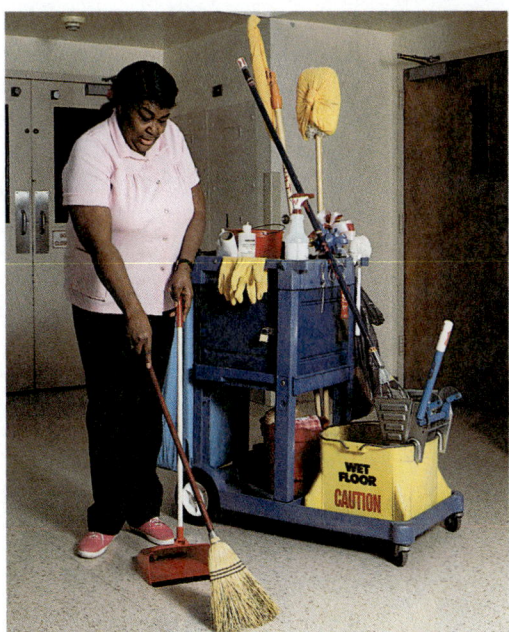

FIGURE 1-8 The housekeeping department keeps the facility clean and sanitary.

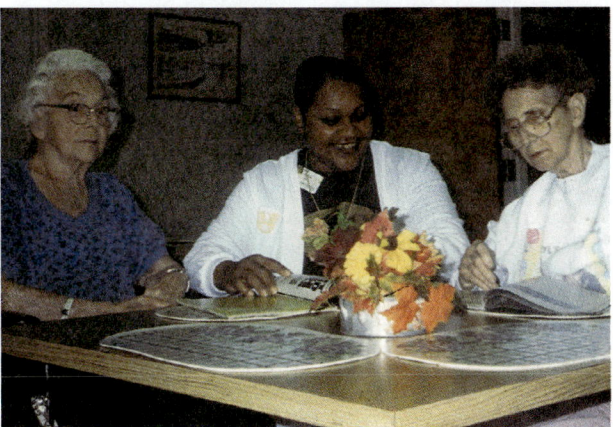

FIGURE 1-9 Volunteers give their time freely to help meet patient needs.

will go from the operating room to the PAR room and then to the surgical nursing unit.

FINANCING HEALTH CARE

Health care is paid for by:
- Insurance. Employers may offer a group insurance plan, or persons may buy individual insurance. Premiums are expensive—employers may pay all or a portion of the cost of a group insurance plan. **Health maintenance organizations (HMO)** are one type of prepaid insurance.
- Out-of-pocket payments by the health care consumer who has no insurance or for expenses not covered by insurance.

- **Medicare** is a federal government program that pays a portion of health care costs for persons 65 years and over and for younger persons who are permanently disabled and who qualify for the benefit.
- Medicare payment is made based on **diagnosis related groups (DRGs)**. The actual cost of care is not considered. Rather, studies were done to determine the average length of stay required for various medical diagnoses, procedures, and treatments. Medicare set the payment rates based on these data. Although a hospital may charge variable rates for patient care, Medicare pays only the fixed amount that it has determined is equitable for care based on the DRG.
- **Medicaid** is a state and federal government program that pays health care costs for persons of any age who do not have financial resources for health care.

Cost containment is a priority, which means that the maximum benefit of health care must be achieved for every dollar spent. Each care provider must do everything possible to avoid waste and to keep expenditures down.

REGULATORY AGENCIES

Many external agencies regulate health care facilities. Some regulatory agencies are branches of the state and federal government, but several are voluntary, private organizations.

Health care facilities must meet certain quality standards to operate. The various agencies inspect the facility periodically to ensure that it meets health and safety regulations and complies with accepted standards. A **survey** is a review and evaluation to ensure that facilities are maintaining acceptable standards of practice. Many different agencies establish quality standards for health care facilities. Different types of facilities must meet different quality standards.

Each facility holds a state **license**, which permits it to conduct business. Some facilities also possess a **certification**. Certification is necessary to collect Medicare and Medicaid payments. Licensure and certification surveys are done by the state health department or human services agency. During a survey, a number of **surveyors** inspect conditions in the facility. Surveyors are representatives of the agency that reviews the facility.

Joint Commission for Accreditation of Healthcare Organizations

The **Joint Commission for Accreditation of Healthcare Organizations (JCAHO)** is an agency that inspects and accredits hospitals, nursing homes, home care providers, medical suppliers, ambulance services, and many other health care agencies. Participation in the accreditation process is voluntary. However, hospitals are not eligible to receive Medicare payment unless they are JCAHO accredited. Medicare is an important source of revenue, and most hospitals could not survive financially without it. JCAHO sets very high standards that the facility must meet to become accredited and to keep that accreditation. To ensure quality care, JCAHO surveyors visit periodically to ensure that the facility meets these standards.

JCAHO requirements state that employees must be assigned to care for patients based on identified patient needs and caregiver qualifications, training, and experience. Caregiver qualifications and training are reviewed. Surveyors review the patient's medical record to evaluate the quality of services provided. Surveyors also review age-related care appropriate for the patients on each unit.

JCAHO standards state that employees must be competent to carry out their responsibilities. The facility is required to periodically evaluate staff competence, and maintain a record of these checks. Staff members must participate in ongoing educational programs. Surveyors may ask staff how their competency was evaluated. They may also ask how you would operate a piece of equipment or perform a specific procedure.

Surveyors review facility policies and procedures and determine whether staff is following them. Emphasis is placed on making sure that employees know and follow facility policies and procedures when caring for patients.

During a JCAHO survey, the survey team evaluates the health care organization's level of compliance with the JCAHO standards. After the survey is completed, a report is issued to the facility detailing areas in which the agency's performance must improve. Accreditation is granted if the survey is acceptable. If significant problems are identified, accreditation will be awarded if the facility's administration agrees to correct the problems promptly. If severe deficiencies are identified, JCAHO will follow up with the facility to check its progress in making corrections.

OSHA Surveys

The **Occupational Safety and Health Administration (OSHA)** also surveys health care facilities. OSHA is a governmental agency that protects the health and safety of employees. OSHA inspectors review infection control, isolation practices, employee tuberculin testing, material safety data sheets, and other policies and facility practices. An OSHA survey involves interviews with employees and a tour of all areas of the facility. The inspector will ask questions about health and safety practices. OSHA inspectors will make recommendations for correcting unsafe conditions. If the inspector notes dangerous or unsafe conditions during the survey, the agency may receive a **citation** or fine. A *citation* is a written notice that informs the facility of the violations of OSHA rules. The employer must post the written report of each citation, at or near the place where the violation occurred, for three days, or until the unsafe condition is corrected.

QUALITY ASSURANCE

All health care facilities have a program called **quality assurance (QA)**. Some facilities call this program Continuous Quality Improvement (CQI). You may be asked to participate on the quality assurance committee. The purpose of quality assurance is to conduct internal reviews to identify problems and find solutions for improvement. The quality assurance committee meets periodically to evaluate care provided and practices in the facility. Restraint use, infections, pressure ulcers, and infection control are some of the areas commonly reviewed. Committee members audit practices related to these topics on each unit and make recommendations to administration to improve care. Patient care should be continuously reevaluated by the facility and adjusted to meet patient needs. The quality assurance program performs this important function.

The quality assurance committee is very important to the operation of the facility and to the facility's success in surveys. The committee identifies problems and corrects them. This self-improvement process prevents problems with regulatory agencies and improves the quality of care delivered.

REVIEW

A. True/False.

Mark the following true or false by circling T or F.

1. (T) F Nursing assistants work under the supervision of licensed professional health care workers.

2. (T) F Hospitals provide a full range of health care services.

3. (T) F Skilled care facilities provide care to persons who require monitoring, nursing care, and treatments.

4. T (F) The only function of a health care facility is to provide services for the ill and injured.

5. (T) F Patient focused care means treating all patients as unique individuals.

6. T (F) Patients can remain in the hospital until they feel well enough to go home.

7. T (F) Persons receiving care in the hospital are called residents.

8. (T) F People who live in a common area and share common health needs form a community.

9. (T) F Many procedures and treatments are done on an outpatient basis in an effort to reduce costs.

10. T (F) A chronic illness comes on suddenly and is usually curable.

B. Multiple Choice.

Select the one best answer for each of the following.

11. The general term for a person needing health care is
    a. patient.
    b. resident.
    (c.) health care consumer.
    d. health care provider.

12. Psychiatric hospitals provide care only to
    a. children.
    (b.) persons with mental illness.
    c. persons with contagious diseases.
    d. dying persons.

13. Health care facilities
    a. treat most patients on an outpatient basis rather than admitting them.
    b. must always obtain approval from the insurer before rendering emergency care.
    (c.) provide a variety of health care services to ill and injured patients.
    d. allow patients to stay as long as they want if they cannot care for themselves.

14. Health care has changed because
    a. there is less demand for services.
    (b.) people are living longer.
    c. the death rate is decreasing.
    d. it is too expensive for most people.

15. Hospice care is provided to patients who
    (a.) are dying.
    b. need rehabilitation.
    c. need surgery.
    d. are pregnant.

16. Managed care means that insurance companies
    a. are more generous than private insurers in approving length of the patient's stay.
    (b.) negotiate with health care providers to render service at a lower cost.
    c. require all surgery to be done on an outpatient basis.
    d. approve only patients with certain medical conditions.

17. The obstetrics department of the hospital cares for patients
    a. with heart disease.
    (b.) before, during, and after childbirth.

c. with conditions of the bones and muscles.
d. who are mentally ill.

18. Social services provides
    a. nursing care 24 hours a day.
    b. diagnostic testing.
    (c.) counseling for patients.
    d. activities to relieve boredom.

19. Environmental services includes
    a. nursing.
    (b.) housekeeping.
    c. therapy.
    d. surgery.

20. One type of prepaid health care insurance is
    a. Medicare.
    b. Medicaid.
    (c.) health maintenance organization.
    d. out-of-pocket payment.

21. The organization that accredits most health care facilities is the
    a. OSHA.
    b. Medicare.
    (c.) JCAHO.
    d. quality assurance committee.

22. Medicare payment is made based on
    (a.) diagnosis related groups.
    b. services needed by the patient.
    c. actual charges billed to the government.
    d. medical supplies used.

23. The purpose of quality assurance is to
    a. guarantee quality to the government.
    (b.) identify and correct problems, thereby improving care.
    c. ensure that the facility receives payment for services.
    d. pass the accreditation inspection.

C. Word Choice.

Choose the correct word from the following list to complete each statement in questions 24–33.

1. hospitals	6. physical therapy
2. Medicare	7. prenatal
3. occupational therapy	8. residents
4. pathology	9. skilled care facility
5. patient focused care	10. surgicenter

24. A __9__ provides care to persons whose conditions are stable but require monitoring, nursing care, and treatments.

25. __1__ are complex organizations that provide a full range of health care services.

26. ___5___ is given when the patient is considered a unique individual with specific needs.

27. ___7___ care is given to a mother during her pregnancy.

28. Persons living in a skilled care facility are usually called ___8___.

29. Uncomplicated surgeries may be performed in a ___10___.

30. ___4___ means the study of disease.

31. ___3___ helps patients regain self-care skills.

32. ___6___ helps patients regain mobility skills.

33. A federal program that pays health care costs for persons 65 years of age and older is called ___2___.

D. Nursing Assistant Challenge.

Mrs. Hernandez is pregnant with her first child. She wants to do everything she can to make sure that she has a safe and uncomplicated pregnancy, labor, and delivery, and that her baby is healthy. Consider how Mrs. Hernandez will move through the health care system to achieve this goal.

34. What is the first type of care that Mrs. Hernandez needs to help her meet the goal of an uncomplicated pregnancy?

35. In your community, where is this type of care provided?

36. What programs are offered to pregnant women in your community?

37. From which hospital departments do you think Mrs. Hernandez will receive services when she delivers her baby?

38. After the baby is born, what health care will the baby need?

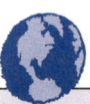

EXPLORING THE WEB

Description	Location
Health care delivery system	http://www.delmarhealthcare.com/olcs/whiteduncan/pnotes.asp (see Chapter 5) http://www.delmarhealthcare.com/olcs/white/pnotes.asp
Wellness concepts	http://www.delmarhealthcare.com/olcs/white/pnotes.asp (see Chapter 15)
American Hospital Association Resources	http://www.hospitalconnect.com
Center to Advance Palliative Care (CAPC) U.S. Hospital Information	http://64.85.16.230/educate/content/elements/ushealthcare.html
Centers for Medicare and Medicaid Services (CMS)	http://www.cms.gov
Department of Health and Human Services	http://www.hhs.gov
Fast Fact Hospital Statistics	http://www.hospitalconnect.com
Healthy People, Healthy Communities	http://www.nnh.org
Joint Commission for Accreditation of Healthcare Organizations (JCAHO)	http://www.jcaho.org
Kaiser Network	http://www.kaisernetwork.org
Seton Hall Gateway to Health Science Resources	http://library.shu.edu

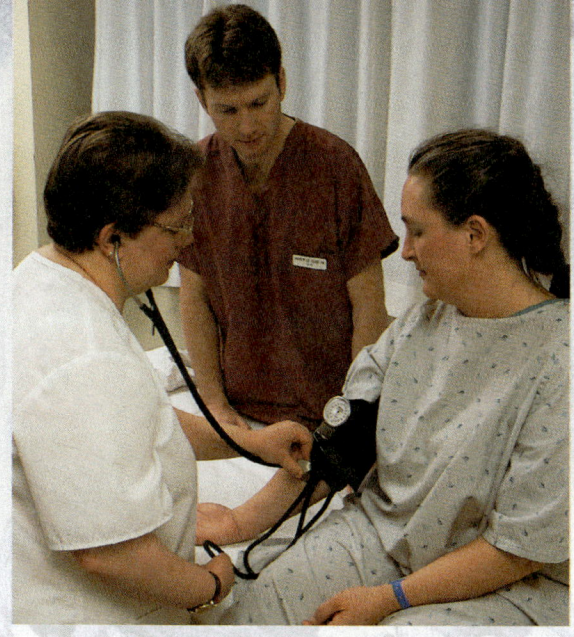

Role of the Nursing Assistant

objectives

After completing this unit, you will be able to:

- Spell and define terms.
- Identify the members of the interdisciplinary health care team.
- Identify the members of the nursing team.
- List the job responsibilities of the nursing assistant.
- Make a chart showing your facility's lines of authority.

- Describe the importance of good human relationships.
- List the ways to build productive working relationships with staff members.
- List the rules of personal hygiene and explain the importance of a healthy mental attitude.
- Describe the appropriate dress for the job.

vocabulary

Learn the meaning and the correct spelling of the following words and phrases:

attitude	interpersonal	Nurse Aide	Omnibus Budget
burnout	relationships	Competency	Reconciliation Act
cross-trained	licensed practical	Evaluation	(OBRA)
empathy	nurse (LPN)	Program (NACEP)	partners in practice
interdisciplinary	licensed vocational	nursing assistant	registered nurse (RN)
health care team	nurse (LVN)	nursing team	scope of practice

THE INTERDISCIPLINARY HEALTH CARE TEAM

The nursing assistant is an important member of the interdisciplinary health care team. This team includes the patient, members of the patient's family, the physician, the nursing team, and other specialists trained to meet both general and specific patient needs (Figure 2-1). The physician names the condition or illness (makes a diagnosis) and prescribes treatment. Physicians frequently specialize in one area of medical practice. Table 2-1 lists common medical specialties, the name for the physician who practices each specialty, and a description of the care provided by each specialist.

The nursing team provides skilled nursing care. The team consists of registered nurses, licensed practical (or vocational) nurses, and nursing assistants. Registered nurses plan and direct the nursing care of patients in cooperation with the physician's orders. All members of the team provide direct patient care.

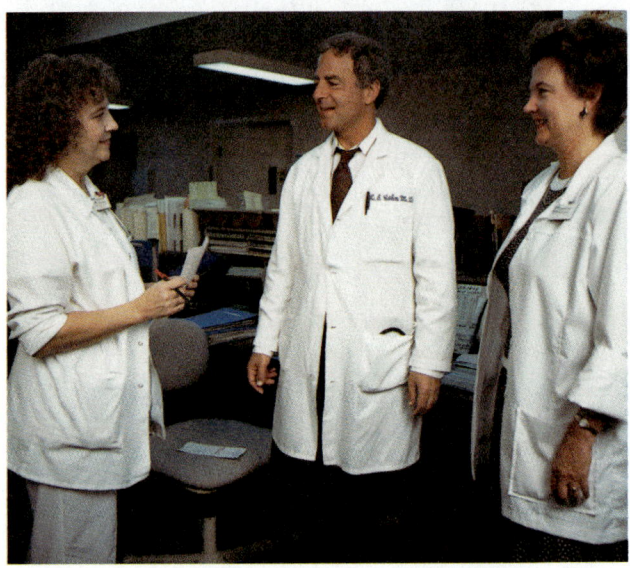

FIGURE 2-1 Each member of the health care team makes an important contribution to the well-being of the patients and overall operation of the facility.

TABLE 2-1 MEDICAL SPECIALTIES

Specialty	Physician	Type of Care
Allergy	Allergist	Diagnoses and treats patients with hypersensitivities
Cardiovascular diseases	Cardiologist	Diagnoses and treats patients with disorders of the heart and blood vessels
Dermatology	Dermatologist	Diagnoses and treats patients with disorders of the skin
Gastroenterology	Gastroenterologist	Diagnoses and treats patients with disorders of the digestive system
Gerontology	Gerontologist	Specializes in diagnosing and treating disorders of the aging person
Gynecology	Gynecologist	Diagnoses and treats disorders related to the female reproductive tract
Hematology	Hematologist	Diagnoses and treats patients with disorders of the blood and blood-forming organs
Internal medicine	Internist	Diagnoses and treats patients with disorders of the internal organs
Neurology	Neurologist	Diagnoses and treats patients with disorders of the nervous system
Obstetrics	Obstetrician	Specializes in providing care to women during pregnancy, childbirth, and immediately thereafter
Oncology	Oncologist	Diagnoses and treats people with cancerous tumors
Ophthalmology	Ophthalmologist	Diagnoses and treats patients with disorders of the eyes
Pediatrics	Pediatrician	Diagnoses, treats, and prevents disorders in children
Psychiatry	Psychiatrist	Diagnoses and treats disorders of the mind
Radiology	Radiologist	Diagnoses and treats disorders with x-rays and other forms of imaging technology
Urology	Urologist	Diagnoses and treats disorders of the urinary tract and male reproductive tract

Care provider specialists who may also be part of the team include the dietitian, physical therapist, occupational therapist, speech therapist, respiratory therapist, and pharmacist. Table 2-2 provides details of the training and certification or licensure requirements for the members of the health care team mentioned here, as well as others.

TABLE 2-2 INTERDISCIPLINARY HEALTH CARE TEAM MEMBERS

Each of these disciplines requires a specified course of study (usually a minimum of a college degree and clinical training). Most require either licensing by a state agency or certification from a professional association. Requirements may vary from state to state for some disciplines.

Patient	The most important member of the interdisciplinary team. The patient has input into the planning and implementation of care. The family may participate with the patient or in place of the patient if the patient is unable to do so.
Physician	Licensed by the state to diagnose and treat disease and to prescribe medications. Many specialty areas within medicine require additional education.
Clinical Nurse Specialist (CNS)	An advanced-practice registered nurse with a master's degree whose care focuses on a very specific patient population (e.g., medical, surgical, diabetic, cardiovascular, operating room, emergency room, critical care, or geriatric, neonatal, etc.).
Nurse Practitioner (NP)	A registered nurse with advanced academic and clinical experience, which enables him or her to diagnose and manage common acute and chronic illnesses, either independently or as part of a health care team. A nurse practitioner provides some care previously offered only by physicians and in most states has the ability to prescribe medications.
Physician Assistant (PA)	A health care professional licensed to practice medicine with physician supervision. PAs conduct physical exams, diagnose and treat illnesses, order and interpret tests, counsel on preventive health care, assist in surgery, and in most states can write prescriptions. Because of the close working relationship the PAs have with physicians, PAs are educated in the medical model designed to complement physician training.
Registered Nurse (RN)	Licensed by the state to make assessments and plan, implement, and evaluate nursing care. Supervises other nursing staff and may coordinate the interdisciplinary health care team. Many specialty areas within nursing require additional education.
Licensed Practical Nurse (LPN or LVN)	Licensed by the state to provide direct patient care under the supervision of a registered nurse. Called *licensed vocational nurse* in Texas and California.
Nursing Assistant	Has completed at least 75 hours of a state-approved course, passed a competency examination, and is certified to provide direct patient care under the supervision of a licensed nurse.
Medication Aide (MA)	A certified nursing assistant who has taken additional classes in medication administration methods and completed a state certification examination. Allowed to pass medications in nursing facilities and home health care in some states under the supervision of a licensed nurse.
Restorative Assistant (RNA)	A certified nursing assistant who has additional education in restorative nursing care. Delivers care designed to assist the patient to attain and maintain his or her highest level of function, and prevent physical deformities.

[handwritten annotation next to Medication Aide (MA): "at nursing home CNA doing medications"]

Specialty Services

Respiratory Therapist (also called respiratory care practitioner)	Licensed to evaluate and treat diseases and problems associated with breathing and the respiratory tract.

continues

TABLE 2-2 *continued*

Specialty Services *continued*

Occupational Therapist	Licensed to provide rehabilitative services to evaluate and treat persons with physical injury or illness, psychosocial problems, or developmental disabilities. Occupational therapy assistants and aides have completed specified courses of study and work under the supervision of a physical occupational therapist. Most care is directed towards improving fine motor skills and activities of daily living.
Orthotist	Licensed by the state to design and fit braces and splints for the extremities.
Physical Therapist	Licensed by the state to provide rehabilitative services to evaluate and treat persons with physical injury or illness, psychosocial problems, or developmental disabilities. Physical therapy assistants and aides have completed specified courses of study and work under the supervision of a physical therapist. Most care is directed towards restoring gross motor skills, mobility, and ambulation.
Speech Therapist	Licensed by the state to provide services to individuals with speech and swallowing disorders caused by acute and chronic illness and trauma.
Social Worker	Licensed by the state to assess and provide services for the nonmedical, psychosocial needs of patients.
Chaplain	Provides services to meet the religious and spiritual needs of patients. Provides emotional support.

Support Services

Pharmacist	Licensed by the state to fill prescriptions for medications as ordered by the physician. Acts as information resource to nurses and physicians for updates on new medications and for maintaining safe drug therapy for patients.
Phlebotomist	Individuals who are trained to use needles to puncture a vein for the purpose of drawing blood.
Laboratory Technician	Laboratory worker who prepares specimens, operates automated analyzers, and performs manual tests.
Laboratory Technologist	Individual who has a bachelor's degree and is trained to perform complex laboratory tests and microscopically examine blood, tissue, and other body substances.
Dietitian	Licensed by the state to assess nutritional needs and provide food services for patients.

In addition to these members of the interdisciplinary health care team, other employees in the health care facility provide services that benefit patients.

- Administrator—Provides general administration and supervision.

- Environmental Services—Maintain a clean and comfortable environment.

- Volunteers—Provide personal services such as delivering mail, doing errands, and providing reading materials.

THE NURSING TEAM

The Registered Nurse

The **registered nurse (RN)** becomes registered by passing a national licensure examination given by the state. The nurse has a four-year college education with a baccalaure-ate degree, or an associate in applied science degree from a two-year community college or technical school program, or a diploma from a hospital school of nursing. Because they have taken and successfully passed a licensing examination and are registered, all these nurses use the initials RN after their names.

Registered nurses have been educated to assess, plan for,

evaluate, and coordinate the many aspects of patient care. Registered nurses teach patients and their families about good health practices. They also provide nursing care and supervise any duties they delegate to others.

Nurses may specialize in a specific area of nursing practice. Some of the common nursing specialties are:

- Maternal and child health
- Anesthesiology
- Gerontology
- Oncology
- Administration
- Public health
- Teaching
- Telemetry
- Surgery
- Home care
- Cardiac care
- Independent practice (nurse practitioner)
- Research
- Infection control

The Licensed Practical/Vocational Nurse

The licensed vocational or licensed practical nurse has generally completed a 1-year to 18-month training program and has passed a national licensure examination administered by the state. She or he is identified by the initials LVN or LPN. This nurse works under the supervision of the registered nurse, a physician, or a dentist. The LPN is able to provide most of the care when the patient's nursing needs are not complex, and also assists the RN in more complicated situations.

The Nursing Assistant

The nursing assistant is trained to assist with the care of patients under the supervision of either an RN or an LPN (Figure 2-2). Because the assistant's responsibilities and skills are not as great as those of the RN or LPN/LVN, the basic training period is shorter. However, growth and learning will continue throughout your career as a caregiver. In the health care facility, the assistant is called by one of the following names:

- Patient care attendant
- Nurse's aide
- Clinical support associate
- Nursing assistant
- Health care assistant
- Personal care assistant
- Patient care technician

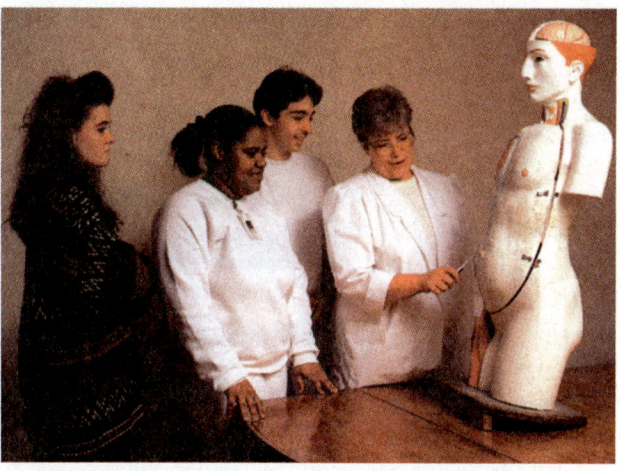

FIGURE 2-2 A professional nurse directs the nursing team and supervises the nursing assistant team members.

ORGANIZATION OF NURSING CARE

Nursing care may be organized in one of four ways:

1. Primary nursing - *given by RN*
2. Functional nursing - *older method*
3. Team nursing
4. Partners in practice

The nursing assistant has a functional role in each.

Primary Nursing

In primary nursing, care is given by a registered nurse. This nurse is responsible for an assigned patient's care for that patient's entire hospitalization. Licensed staff and assistants help with the care when the RN is not actually on duty. The nurse plans and coordinates the nursing care, teaches, carries out treatments, gives direct nursing care, and plans for the patient's discharge. Patients appreciate primary nursing because it enables them to relate directly to one specific nurse. Each RN is assigned to and responsible for six to eight patients in the primary nursing situation.

Functional Nursing

Functional nursing is a task-oriented way to organize care service. It is an older method that is once again being used more frequently. In this method of service organization, the charge nurse is the one person responsible for all patients. All other staff members are assigned specific tasks, such as giving medications, administering treatments, or providing hygienic care.

Patients may find this type of nursing confusing because many people are involved in their care. However, some facilities feel that this method uses available, qualified personnel to best advantage.

Team Nursing

Team nursing is one of the most common methods of delivering nursing care. In this system, a registered nurse team leader determines the nursing needs of all the patients assigned to the team for care. In some work settings, the LPN or LVN is a team leader. He or she is supervised by a registered nurse. Team members receive instructions and assignments from, and report back to, the team leader.

The team approach is successful when:

- Team members understand the philosophy, goals, and purposes of restorative care. Restorative care helps patients reach their highest possible level of functioning.
- Team members understand their responsibilities.
- All team members, including the patient, and family members if the patient desires, attend the care plan conference.

Partners in Practice

In the **partners in practice** method of providing care, a registered nurse or primary nurse is paired with a nursing assistant or other team member. The team members work together to meet the needs of their assigned patients. In some facilities, they work on the same schedule.

PATIENT FOCUSED CARE

In addition to the models of care described here, the trend in health care has moved toward the patient focused method of care delivery. This method of care emphasizes the needs of the patient above the convenience of the various departments involved with patient care. Team members on the unit make decisions jointly, and plan and deliver care promptly to meet patient needs. This is faster and involves fewer individuals than other methods of care that require coordination of service among different departments. Thus, the patient is the focus of the service.

The goals of patient focused care are to:

- Limit the number of people involved in patient care.
- Contain costs.
- Meet patients' needs efficiently.

Staff members are prepared as multiskilled workers by cross-training them to perform special skills. This training allows the staff members to carry out selected duties that are usually performed by other workers, such as drawing blood, giving special treatments, working in specialty departments, and using more sophisticated instruments to perform tests. For example, a multiskilled nursing assistant may be **cross-trained** to draw blood, give respiratory treatments, or perform an electrocardiogram. These tasks can be done without calling a technician from another department or moving the patient out of the unit.

You can be an effective member of the interdisciplinary team by:

- Recognizing the importance of all team members.
- Appreciating each member's contribution to the team.
- Learning as much as possible about the patients and their families, to help you understand their feelings and concerns.
- Attending care plan conferences and giving the team your observations and ideas.
- Attending in-service training sessions to increase your knowledge.
- Becoming cross-trained, if possible, to increase your skills.
- Cooperating with other team members to provide patient focused care.

REGULATION OF NURSING ASSISTANT PRACTICE

Nursing assistants must understand the scope of the specific tasks they will be expected to carry out. They should also know the state regulations that govern their clinical practice. Federal regulations for the training and certification of nursing assistants require that all states spell out the duties and responsibilities of the assistant, as well as the basic education and level of competency required for practice.

In 1987, a federal law was passed that regulates the education and certification of nurse aides. The law is called the **Omnibus Budget Reconciliation Act (OBRA)**. OBRA includes statements from the Department of Health and Human Services and the Center for Medicare and Medicaid Services (CMS, formerly the Health Care Financing Administration) that established the minimum requirements for nurse aide competency evaluation programs.

Effective October 1, 1990, all persons working as nurse aides had to complete a competency evaluation program or approved course. The actual training and education of nursing assistants is under individual state jurisdiction, guided by federal regulations.

The National Council of State Boards of Nursing, Inc., then developed the **Nurse Aide Competency Evaluation Program (NACEP)**. NACEP meets the requirements of OBRA. NACEP is a guide for individual programs that register and award credentials to nurse aides. NACEP specifies the minimum skills to be achieved. Programs may exceed these minimums.

Nursing assistants who wish to be certified must complete a minimum of 75 hours of theory and practice. Some states require a minimum of 80 to 150 program hours in written or oral and clinical skills in several areas. These areas include:

- Basic nursing skills
- Basic restorative services

- Mental health and social service needs
- Personal care skills
- Resident rights
- Safety and emergency care

Other regulations that guide nursing assistant practice require:

- Completion of a competency evaluation program by October 1, 1990, of all persons who were working as nurse aides prior to July 1989.
- At least three opportunities for noncertified nursing assistants to meet requirements.
- Completion of a new training and competency program or retesting by persons who wish to work as nursing assistants but who have not performed nursing or nurse-related services for pay for a continuous 24-month period after completing a training and competency evaluation program.
- Continuing education (12 to 48 hours per year, in some states).

The OBRA regulations are important because they:

- Give nursing assistants recognition through registration.
- Help define the scope of nursing assistant practice.
- Provide better uniformity in the care provided by nursing assistants.
- Promote educational standards for nursing assistants.

Be sure you are familiar with any specific state regulations or laws that relate to your role as an assistant.

LINES OF AUTHORITY

Nursing assistants receive their assignments from the team leader or charge nurse, nurse manager, or unit manager. When they finish their assignments, they report to this same person. This represents the assistant's immediate line of authority and communication.

If the hospital is a large one, the assistant may work with a team whose leader is a licensed practical nurse or a registered nurse. In this case, the assistant's immediate superior is the team leader. The team leaders receive their instructions from the charge nurse. The charge nurse is responsible for the total care of a certain number of patients. Sometimes this includes all the patients on a wing, a unit, or a floor of the facility. Supervisors are responsible for several charge nurse units. They receive their authority and direction from the director of nursing. Health care facilities vary in the complexity of their staffing.

Assistants should learn the lines of authority in their health care facility, as shown in Figure 2-3. As a student, your immediate authority is your teacher or the person designated as your supervisor.

The physician directs the patient's medical care. The registered nurse carries out the physician's orders and plans the patient's nursing care. The authority for nursing care passes

from the registered nurse supervisor to the charge nurse, to the team leader, and then to the nursing assistant. When you accept the responsibility for an assignment, you must fully understand the assignment and be capable of handling it. *If there is any doubt, you should discuss it with the team leader or charge nurse* (Figure 2-4).

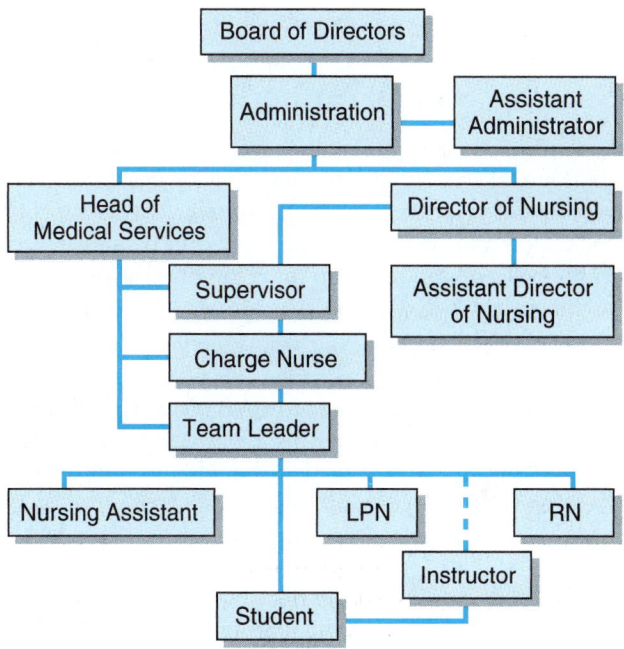

FIGURE 2-3 Typical model of lines of authority for the nursing department. (Each facility's model may vary slightly.)

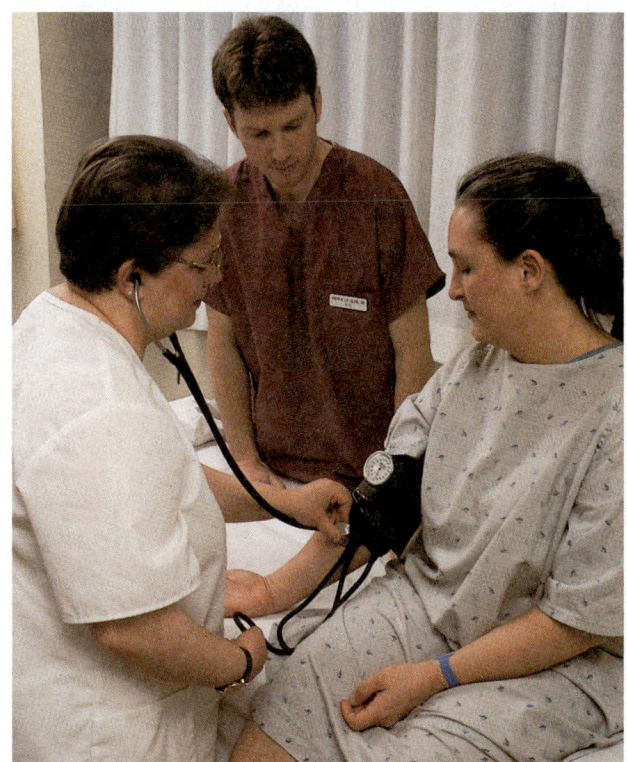

FIGURE 2-4 Clarify directions if you are unsure how to proceed.

GUIDELINES FOR THE NURSING ASSISTANT

Only perform tasks that you have been trained to do. If you are unsure how to carry out a procedure that was part of your training program, inform the nurse. Do not feel embarrassed. It is better to ask for clarification and supervision than to make an error and injure a patient.

Seeking Higher Authority

Sometimes a report you make to your immediate supervisor is not taken seriously. It seems to fall on deaf ears. Make very sure of your facts and try again to make your supervisor understand. If you fail and your information is very important, you can move up the chain of command.

For example, if you report that a person is being harmed by a coworker's inattention, but your supervisor does not listen to your report of the situation, for your patient's safety you must try again. If the second attempt also fails, the next step is to bring the problem to the attention of the next level of authority. This situation should not occur often if there are good staff relations, but it can happen.

Scope of Practice

Scope of practice means the skills the nursing assistant is legally permitted to perform by state regulations. If another health care worker asks you to perform a task that is clearly out of your scope of training, such as giving medications, be prepared to refuse. Explain in a courteous manner that this is a task for which you have not been technically or legally prepared. Report the incident to your charge nurse so that your scope of duties can be clearly understood by all staff members.

For the same reason, nursing assistants do not take orders from doctors or tell families about the contents of patient care plans or records. These actions are not within the scope of nursing assistant practice.

Nevertheless, be willing to learn new skills under the close supervision of your nurse. If the new skill is within the scope of nursing assistant practice, this will increase your

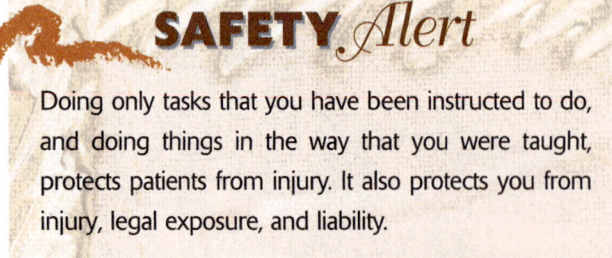

SAFETY *Alert*

Doing only tasks that you have been instructed to do, and doing things in the way that you were taught, protects patients from injury. It also protects you from injury, legal exposure, and liability.

LEGAL *Alert*

Scope of practice is a very important legal concept. Your scope of practice is described in the job description given to you by your employer. Functioning within this scope of practice protects the nursing assistant and the facility.

ability to provide good, safe nursing care. If, for example, your nurse suggests a new way to lift a patient that is different from the way you learned in your program, listen and watch carefully as the instruction is given. Seek supervision as you practice the new technique until both you and your supervisor feel you can do it safely on your own.

THE ROLE AND RESPONSIBILITIES OF THE NURSING ASSISTANT

The nursing assistant works directly with the patient, giving physical care and emotional support. This care is always given under the direction of the registered nurse. The nursing assistant has an important role and can contribute much to the patient's comfort and safety. Observations made during the delivery of care are reported to the nurse and are recorded on the patient's chart.

Tasks commonly assigned to nursing assistants are listed in Table 2-3. Remember that not all health care facilities assign the same tasks to nursing assistants.

Not everyone can be a nursing assistant. Nursing assistants are special people: they are interested in others, they take pride in themselves, and they are willing to learn the skills necessary to care for those who are ill.

This interest in and caring for people can be a valuable asset to the entire nursing team. You are the person the patient sees most often. This means that you have the chance to observe and hear many things that the other team members will not. By transmitting these observations to your charge nurse, you are likely to give the other team members valuable insight into the patient's illness and attitude toward that illness. For example, you may see that the patient's attitude toward the attending doctor or nurse is much less relaxed than it is with you, the nursing assistant. For that same reason, the patient is far more likely to tell you of "minor complaints" that may not be minor at all. Competent, caring nursing assistants make a valuable contribution to the comfort and safety of the patients.

TABLE 2-3 TYPICAL JOB DESCRIPTION FOR A NURSING ASSISTANT

Nursing assistants commonly participate in the nursing process by carrying out the activities listed. **Note:** Use standard precautions while providing care.

1. Assist with patient assessment and care planning.
   a. Check and record vital signs
   b. Measure height and weight
   c. Measure intake and output
   d. Collect specimens
   e. Test urine and feces
   f. Observe patient response to care given
   g. Report and record observations of patients' conditions

2. Assist patients in meeting nutritional and elimination needs.
   a. Check food trays
   b. Pass food trays
   c. Feed patients
   d. Provide fresh drinking water and nourishments
   e. Assist with bedpans, urinals, and commodes
   f. Empty urine collection bags
   g. Assist with colostomy care
   h. Give enemas
   i. Observe feces and urine

3. Assist patients with mobility.
   a. Turn and position
   b. Provide range-of-motion exercises
   c. Transfer to wheelchair or stretcher
   d. Assist with ambulation

4. Assist patients with personal hygiene and grooming.
   a. Bathe patients
   b. Provide nail and hair care
   c. Give oral hygiene
   d. Provide denture care
   e. Shave patients
   f. Assist with dressing and undressing

5. Assist with patient comfort and anxiety relief.
   a. Protect patient privacy and maintain confidentiality
   b. Keep call bell within patient's reach
   c. Answer call bells promptly
   d. Provide orientation to the room or unit and to other patients and visitors
   e. Assist patients with communications
   f. Protect personal possessions
   g. Provide diversional activities
   h. Give backrubs
   i. Prepare hot and cold applications

6. Assist in promoting patient safety and environmental cleanliness.
   a. Use side rails and restraints appropriately
   b. Keep patient unit clean and clutter-free
   c. Make beds
   d. Clean and care for equipment
   e. Carry out isolation precautions
   f. Observe oxygen precautions
   g. Assist in keeping recreational and nonpatient areas clean and free of hazards
   h. Participate in fire drills and patient evacuation procedures

7. Assist with unit management and efficiency.
   a. Transport patients
   b. Take specimens to lab
   c. Assist with special procedures
   d. Do errands as required
   e. Assist with cost-containment measures
   f. Answer the telephone
   g. Document care provided and assist with unit recordkeeping

PERSONAL VOCATIONAL ADJUSTMENTS

You will have to make a certain amount of personal adjustment to your new work situation. Health care facility rules and orders from supervisors must be obeyed promptly, even if you do not agree with them. Rules are written for the protection and welfare of both the patient and the health care provider. You must also learn to accept con-

structive criticism and profit by it. It means you are willing to learn and grow.

You show your maturity in many ways. You demonstrate:

- Dependability and accuracy by reporting for duty on time (Figure 2-5) and completing your assignments carefully.
- Respect for your coworkers and the place you share together on the nursing team when you are ready to help.

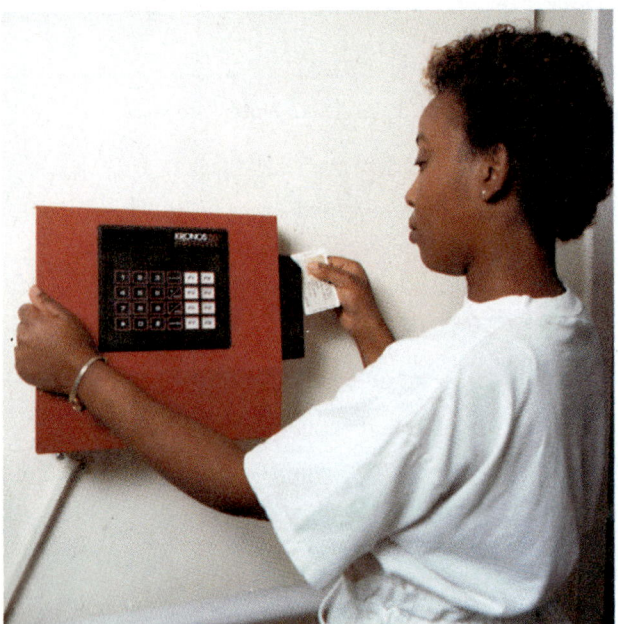

FIGURE 2-5 Reporting for duty on time demonstrates dependability.

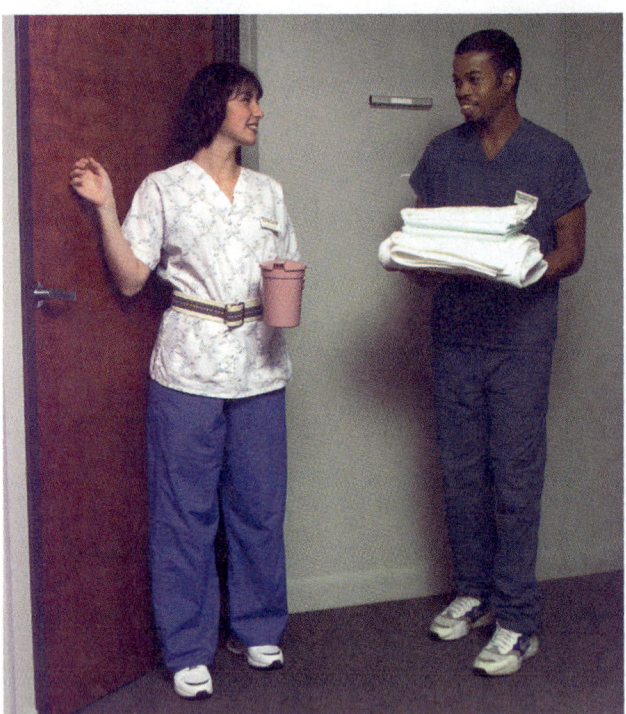

FIGURE 2-6 Maintaining a positive attitude and spirit of cooperation makes the workplace pleasant.

- Understanding of human relationships by being empathetic, patient, and tactful with others.

Interpersonal Relationships

Interpersonal relationships are simply interactions between people. You develop interpersonal relationships with everyone you know. Some relationships are deep and lasting, and some are only casual. But to some degree, you react to others and they react to you. Friendship is a good example of an interpersonal relationship that is satisfactory to two people.

Much of the satisfaction that a nursing assistant gets from work comes from the quality of the relationships that are developed with other staff members and patients. Some people call this the ability to get along with others.

Similarly, good relationships with others begin with your own personality and attitudes. If you are a warm and accepting person with positive attitudes, others will respond in the same way. If you walk down the street and someone smiles at you, without thinking, your reaction is to smile back. Most human relationships are like this.

It is not necessary for you personally to like someone else to be pleasant and cooperative with him or her as you carry out your duties (Figure 2-6).

Attitude

Perhaps the most important single characteristic that you bring to your job is your attitude. Your attitude is developed throughout your lifetime, and it is shaped by the experiences you have had. Some people think having an "attitude" means being negative or opinionated, but all people show attitude through their behavior. Sometimes the attitude demonstrated is good and sometimes it is poor. All the other characteristics described are an outer reflection of your inner feelings—of your attitude toward yourself and others. Your attitude should reflect:

- Caring
- Courtesy
- Cooperation
- Emotional control
- Empathy (understanding)
- Tact
- Patience

Patients have the right and need to be cared for in a calm, unhurried atmosphere by people with a caring attitude.

Patient Relationships

Patients come in all sizes and shapes and ages: young, old, and in between. Some have major, complicated illnesses. Others have physical problems that can be helped with rest and medication. Some patients are in the health facility to begin their lives. Others will end their lives there. A good nursing assistant shows empathy for the patient by being eager to serve and by using a gentle touch.

Every patient entering a health care facility presents a unique set of problems and concerns to the staff. These problems and concerns are important. As you compare the conditions of many patients in your own mind, however, it might seem that one has more serious problems than another. Because patients do not share your knowledge, they will not know this. Never forget that, to the patient, her or his own problems are the most important.

Meeting the Patient's Needs

Patients' personalities are shaped by their life experiences, which are now complicated by illness. Their social, spiritual, and physical needs must continue to be met even though they are in a different, more confined setting. The restrictions imposed by illness limit, to some degree, their ability to satisfy these needs through the normal channels. This is naturally frustrating and puts great strain on the patient's ability to establish and maintain good interpersonal relationships.

Some patients become irritable, complaining, and uncooperative because of:

- Fears about their diagnosis, disfigurement, disability, and death
- Pain
- Unrealistic perceptions of activities around them
- Uncertainties about the future
- Worries about family
- The loss or lack of social support systems
- Dependence on others
- Financial concerns

Offer emotional support (Figure 2-7), listen carefully, and report these concerns to the nurse.

Meeting the Family's Needs

Families and friends are very concerned when one of their loved ones is in a health care facility, especially when that person may have a life-threatening illness. This puts stress in their lives too. They need to be reassured. Their anxiety sometimes makes them demanding and uncooperative.

The nursing assistant who understands human behavior makes allowances for these stresses and realizes that ill people, coworkers, and families under stress may be touchy and not always on their best behavior. This is why sensitivity and awareness of the needs of others are most important at this time (Figure 2-8). It is in these situations that patience and tact are most needed. Sometimes just quietly

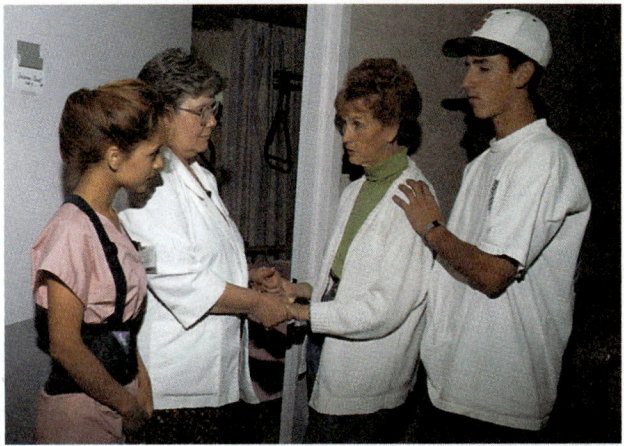

FIGURE 2-8 Concerned family members need the support of staff.

listening to another or rephrasing your sentences can change an entire interaction. Try to be aware not only of the words used but also of the body language. As with words, clues such as the tone of a voice or a hand movement reveal much about the inner feelings of other people. Always keep in mind that people are three-dimensional. They are physical beings, emotional beings, and social beings.

Staff Relationships

You are part of the staff of a health care facility. All workers share a single goal: to help the patient. This single purpose welds you together into a unit that must work smoothly if your goal is to be accomplished. Good interpersonal relationships will make your working hours satisfying and productive. Good relationships can be formed if you:

- Remember that each of you has a specific role to fulfill and jobs to carry out.
- Do not overstep your authority or criticize others.
- Listen to instructions from your supervisor carefully. Phrase questions about your assignment in such a way that your supervisor knows you are looking for clarification—not challenging authority.
- Remember that your tone of voice and body language can change the message you are trying to convey.
- Promptly carry out orders and report any work that you are unable to finish.
- Offer help to others and accept help when you need it. Coworkers can often help one another when a task is particularly difficult or physically taxing (for example, lifting a heavy patient or moving equipment). Simply being available when another member of the team gets behind in his or her work is a great help.
- Have a cheerful, positive attitude. This is as important for staff members' relationships as it is in establishing rapport (sympathetic understanding) with patients.

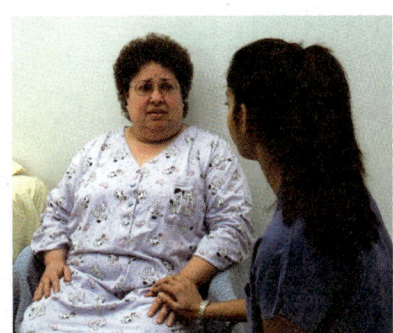

FIGURE 2-7 The worried patient responds to gentle touch and reassurance.

- Extend the same dignity and courtesy to every staff member that you would to patients.
- Always keep your common goal in mind. Recognize coworkers as important members of the total team.

Professional and personal adjustments are made easier if the nursing assistant:

- Understands and follows facility policies and procedures.
- Treats patients, coworkers, and visitors with respect.
- Practices proper hygiene and grooming, good nutrition, and stress reduction.

PERSONAL HEALTH AND HYGIENE

Good personal grooming is essential, because the assistant is in close contact with patients (Figure 2-9). Because the work of the assistant, although rewarding, can be physically challenging, it is important that all body odors be controlled. The nursing assistant is often the last to know that he or she has bad breath or body odor. A daily shower or bath and the use of an antiperspirant/deodorant are essential. The mouth and teeth must be kept clean. The nursing assistant should also recognize that strong perfumes, aftershave lotions, and cigarette odors are often offensive to patients.

Hair should be clean and either short or tied back in a controlled style. Fingernails should be kept short and clean. If nail polish is used, it should be clear, not colored.

Stockings and socks should be freshly laundered. Shoes and shoelaces should be cleaned daily. Fatigue will be lessened if shoes give proper support to the feet and are well-fitted.

Jewelry is not part of the nursing assistant's uniform, as it is a ready medium for bacterial growth. Jewelry may also

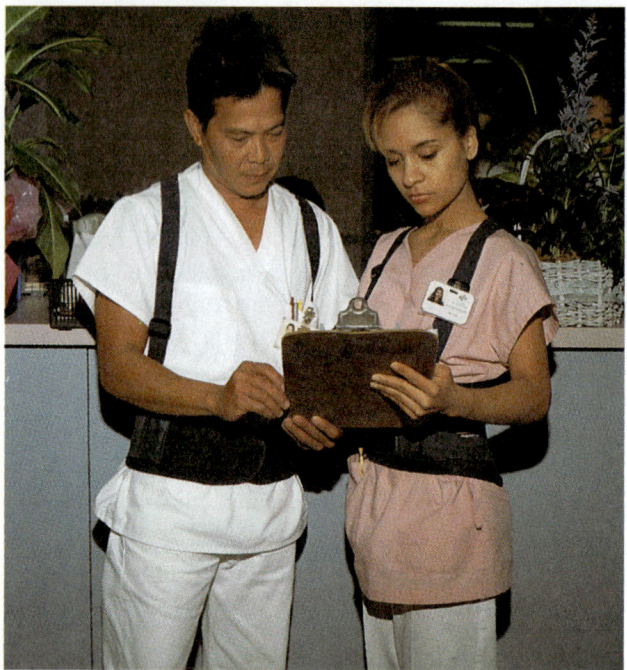

FIGURE 2-9 Well-groomed caregivers instill confidence in patients and families.

SAFETY *Alert*

Keeping long hair pulled back reduces the risk of injury from hair becoming entangled in equipment or being inadvertently pulled by a patient. Small stud-type pierced earrings also reduce your risk of injury from an earring being pulled or caught.

INFECTION CONTROL *Alert*

Your hair is like a magnet for germs. Keeping it short makes it easier to care for. Washing your hair regularly is best. Long fingernails, artificial nails, and chipped nail polish are also good hiding places for germs. Avoid acrylic and artificial nails. Keep your natural nails short and clean. Jewelry also harbors germs. Sharp stones and settings can injure patients and tear gloves. Only simple jewelry, such as a plain wedding band, should be worn when on duty.

injure the patient or the assistant, especially if the patient is confused or is a young child. Long, dangling earrings can be especially dangerous to the assistant, because they are easily caught in linen or pulled out by a combative patient. Most health care agencies permit members of the nursing staff to wear wedding rings and small earrings. Watches with second hands are used to monitor the condition of patients and to measure vital signs.

Uniforms

Many health care facilities allow health care workers great leeway in selecting the type and style of their uniforms. Traditionally, patients were able to identify the various types of health care workers by their uniforms, including caps. Today, it can be very difficult to distinguish between a physical therapist, registered nurse, physician, or social worker. It is no wonder that newly admitted patients are often confused as to whom they should approach for information or help. To help avoid this confusion, some states and many health care facilities require personnel to wear a name badge or photo identification tag at all times while on the job. The name badge may state only your first name and title. Some facilities do not list the last name of a worker on the name badge, as a protective measure.

If your health care facility requires that you wear a uniform, you should wear it only while you are on duty. If your health care agency does not provide facilities for changing your uniform before and after going on duty, be sure to wear a cover-up as you travel to and from work so you will not spread germs. When you get home, remove your uniform, fold it inside out, and put it into the laundry. This helps keep the dirtiest part of your uniform away from the other clothes in the laundry. Wearing a fresh uniform every day should become a habit. It should be clean and in good condition. Torn hems and missing buttons should be repaired and replaced.

Above all, remember that your patients' safety and comfort are your main concerns. Try to keep in mind their needs and feelings. After all, would you feel confident if you were ill and the assistant caring for you had long fingernails that could scratch you, or that could collect dirt and possibly infect your surgical incision? How would you feel if the assistant who was preparing you for surgery kept having to push the hair out of his eyes? Or if the assistant assigned to give you a backrub wore clanking bracelets on her wrists?

Remember, too, that how you look reflects the pride you have in yourself and in your work. Well-groomed nursing assistants who pay attention to the details of their person and appearance show others, especially their patients and coworkers, that they are likely to have the same pride and caring attitude in their work. If you are well groomed and have good personal habits, patients will feel more secure and confident, and other staff members will regard you as mature and reliable. As you develop good health habits, you become a role model for your family, friends, and coworkers.

Reducing Stress

Your work as a nursing assistant is physically and emotionally demanding because you must give so much of yourself to those in your care. To stay healthy and do your best, you will need:

- Sufficient rest
- Good nutrition
- Satisfying leisure activities (Figure 2-10)
- Ways to reduce stress

Burnout is total mental, emotional, and sometimes physical exhaustion. Burnout is common among those working in health care facilities. You can reduce the stress that leads to burnout by balancing your work with rest and recreation. Some facilities offer programs to help employees reduce stress. Group discussions, exercise programs, and special counseling are available for general stress management and

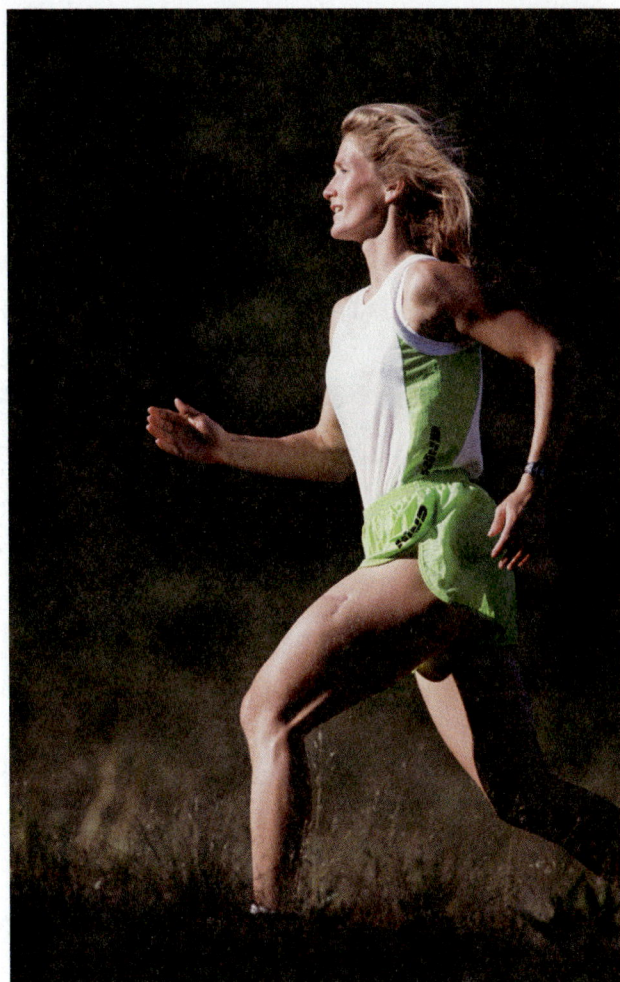

FIGURE 2-10 Work should be balanced with recreational activities.

to meet special circumstances, such as when a patient dies or when individual interstaff conflicts arise. Death is always a possibility, but the staff usually focus on improvement and recovery. The loss of a patient, especially a child, can be very stressful. Caring for an abused child can take a great toll on the staff as they try to work with the child and family.

Occasionally personality conflicts are aggravated by the daily close contact. Stress caused by these situations can often be handled through a stress management group discussion.

Personal Stress Reduction

You can learn personal stress-reducing techniques. Food, alcohol, or other drugs are used by some people to reduce stress, but these substances can cause serious health problems. For example, some people use chemicals or drugs to reduce stress. This is dangerous because chemicals and drugs alter the body's chemistry, causing serious changes to thought and behavior. In some cases, drug use becomes addictive and can cause death.

There are better and safer ways to prevent burnout and relieve stress. To reduce stress:

- Talk to your supervisor; a team conference may help.
- Try sitting for a few moments with your feet up.
- Shut your eyes and take some deep breaths.
- With your eyes shut, picture a special place you like and, in your mind, take yourself there.
- Take a warm, relaxing bath.
- Listen to some quiet music.

- Carry out a specific relaxation exercise.
- Make yourself a cup of herbal tea and drink it slowly.
- Exercise.
- Devote time to hobbies such as sewing, painting, woodworking, or playing a musical instrument.
- Go for a walk.
- Take advantage of available stress reduction programs.

REVIEW

A. True/False.

Mark the following true or false by circling T or F.

1. (T) F   The registered nurse plans and directs the nursing care of patients.
2. (T) F   Interdisciplinary health care providers work as a team.
3. T (F) The LVN has completed a four-year college-based program.
4. (T) F   The nursing assistant gives physical care and emotional support to patients under the direction of the licensed nurse.
5. (T) F   The nursing assistant is an important member of the nursing team.
6. (T) F   Patients enjoy primary nursing because it allows them to relate directly to one specific registered nurse.
7. (T) F   Team nursing is a common way of providing patient care.
8. T (F) It is all right to perform a task even if you are unsure how to do it.
9. (T) F   Nursing assistants are special people.
10. (T) F   Nursing assistants should be willing to learn and practice new skills under the supervision of the nurse.
11. (T) F   Caring about people is a valuable asset for a nursing assistant.
12. T (F) It is not important for the nursing assistant to be well groomed.
13. (T) F   Patients may find strong perfumes or aftershave lotions offensive.
14. (T) (F) Hair and fingernails should be kept short and clean.
15. T (F) It is all right to wear your uniform when you go grocery shopping.
16. (T) F   How you look reflects the pride you feel in yourself.

17. (T) F   Patient safety and comfort are main concerns for all caregivers.
18. (T) F   Being a nursing assistant can be very stressful.
19. T (F) Smoking and eating are the best ways to reduce stress.
20. (T) F   One of the most important characteristics you bring to your job is a positive attitude.

B. Multiple Choice.

Select the one best answer for each of the following.

21. The interdisciplinary team member who writes the medical orders for patient care is the
    a. registered nurse.
    b. social worker.
    c. physician.
    d. dietitian.

22. The nursing care approach that is task-oriented is
    a. primary nursing.
    b. functional nursing.
    c. team nursing.
    d. patient focused care.

23. A nursing assistant who has a question regarding an assignment should properly ask the
    a. physician.
    b. charge nurse.
    c. physiotherapist.
    d. administrator.

24. A patient tells you that he has difficulty making a fist because his hand feels weak. He did not mention the fact to the nurse. You must
    a. ignore it. The patient should have told the nurse.
    b. tell another assistant.
    c. tell the nurse.
    d. tell the physician.

25. You demonstrate maturity by
   a. rushing assignments.
   b. being disrespectful to coworkers.
   c. "bending" the rules.
   d. reporting for duty on time.

C. Matching.

Match the interdisciplinary team member and his or her function.

26. _b_ Licensed to fill prescriptions for medications.

27. _e_ Qualified to test hearing.

28. _c_ Licensed to provide services to meet spiritual needs.

29. _a_ Licensed to fit and design braces and splints for extremities.

30. _d_ Licensed to provide rehabilitative services and to evaluate and treat persons with physical injury or illness, psychosocial problems, or developmental disabilities.

a. orthotist
b. pharmacist
c. chaplain
d. occupational therapist
e. audiologist

D. Completion.

Complete the following.

31. Why is it improper for nursing assistants to take orders directly from the physician? _your not legally qualified._

32. The benefits of a nursing assistant certification are:
   a. _recognition_
   b. _better_
   c. _promote education_
   d. _____

E. Nursing Assistant Challenge.

Read each clinical situation and answer the questions.

33. Enrique is given his assignment and has questions.
   a. He must check his assignment with _charge nurse_
   b. One of his assignments is to bathe patients. Is this appropriate? _yes_
   c. One of his assignments is to give medications. Is this appropriate? _no_

34. Felicia once worked as a part-time assistant to an elderly woman but was never certified as a nursing assistant. What can you tell her about the requirements?
   a. Is a competency evaluation program required? _yes_
   b. How many opportunities are there to meet requirements? _3_
   c. How much continuing education is required once certification is granted? _12_

35. Peggy reported for duty wearing bracelets, long earrings, and pale pink nail polish. Her uniform was clean and crisp but the hem was hanging down on one side. Her shoes were dirty. State ways in which her appearance can be improved.
   start over

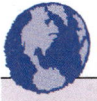

EXPLORING THE WEB

Description	Location
Health care disciplines and education	*http://www-hsl.mcmaster.ca*
Interdisciplinary team issues	*http://eduserv.hscer.washington.edu/bioethics*
Nursing history	*http://www.delmarhealthcare.com/olcs/white/pnotes.asp* (see Chapter 4)
Skills for success	*http://www.delmarhealthcare.com/olcs/white/pnotes.asp* (see Chapter 3)
Stress, adaptation, and anxiety	*http://www.delmarhealthcare.com/olcs/white/pnotes.asp* (see Chapter 6)
Teamwork	*http://www.vta.spcomm.uiuc.edu*

continues

EXPLORING THE WEB   *continued*

Description	Location
"Ten Steps to Better Time Management"	*http://www.advancefornurses.com*
Wellness concepts	*http://www.delmarhealthcare.com/olcs/whiteduncan/pnotes.asp* (see Chapter 7)
You First Health Risk Assessment	*http://www.youfirst.com*
About.com	*http://nursing.about.com*
American Nurses Association	*http://www.nursingworld.org*
Career Nurse Assistants Programs	*http://www.cna-network.org*
Center to Advance Palliative Care (CAPC)	*http://64.85.16.230*
Direct Care Alliance	*http://www.directcarealliance.org*
Iowa Caregivers Association	*http://www.iowacaregivers.org*
NA Resources on the Web	*http://www.nursingassistant.org*
National Clearinghouse on the Direct Care Workforce	*http://www.directcareclearinghouse.org*
National Council State Boards of Nursing	*http://www.ncsbn.org*
Paraprofessional Healthcare Institute	*http://www.paraprofessional.org*

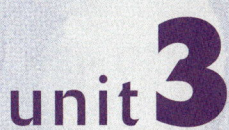

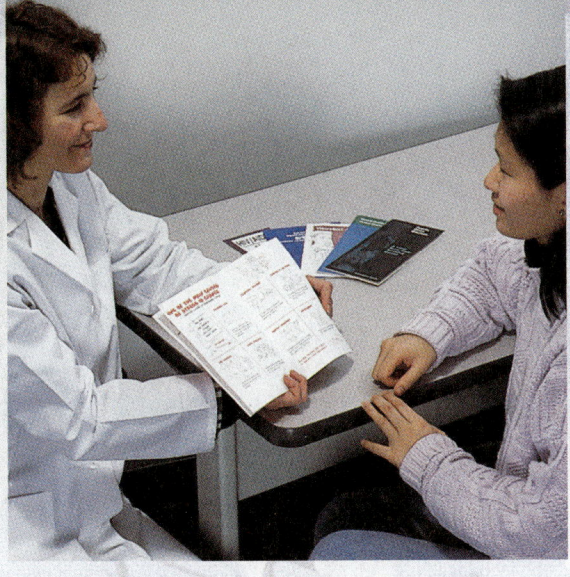

Consumer Rights and Responsibilities in Health Care

objectives

After completing this unit, you will be able to:

- Spell and define terms.
- Explain the purpose of health care consumer rights.
- Describe six items that are common to Resident's Rights, the Patient's Bill of Rights, and the Client's Rights in Home Care.

- List three specific rights from each of the three documents.
- Describe eight responsibilities of health care consumers.

vocabulary

Learn the meaning and the correct spelling of the following words and phrases:

advance directives	corporal punishment	informed consent	Patient's Bill of Rights
Client's Rights	grievance	involuntary seclusion	Resident's Rights

CONSUMER RIGHTS

All citizens in the United States have certain rights (for example, the right to vote) that are guaranteed by law. Health care consumers have rights to ensure that they will receive quality patient care. There are different documents for patient rights, depending on where care is given. In each setting, if the health care consumer is unable to read or understand the document, it is given to the person's family. A copy of the **Resident's Rights** is given to each person before he or she is admitted to a skilled care facility (Figure 3-1). The rights of residents in skilled care facilities were legislated by the federal government in the Omnibus Budget Reconciliation Act (OBRA) of 1987. The resident must sign a form indicating that the resident and/or the resident's family have received the document. The **Patient's Bill of Rights** is given to patients upon admission to a hospital. Persons receiving care in their homes are given a copy of the **Client's Rights** by the nurse on the first visit to the home. The client is asked to sign a form indicating that he or she received the document.

All persons working in health care should be familiar with the document that pertains to the facility they work in. Supporting the rights of the health care consumer contributes to more effective care. Each of these documents is similar and emphasizes the right of the patient, resident, or client to:

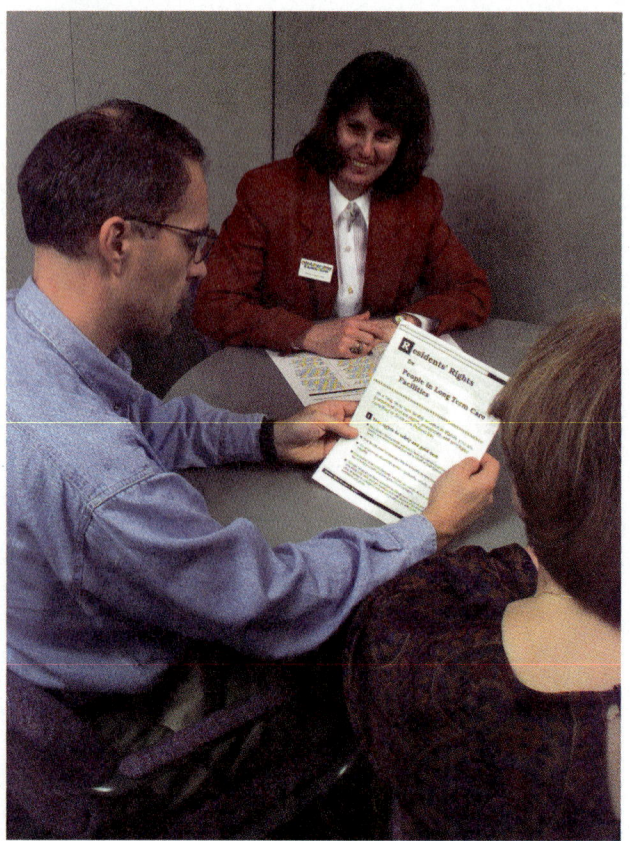

FIGURE 3-1 The Resident's Bill of Rights is presented to each resident upon admission to the long-term care facility.

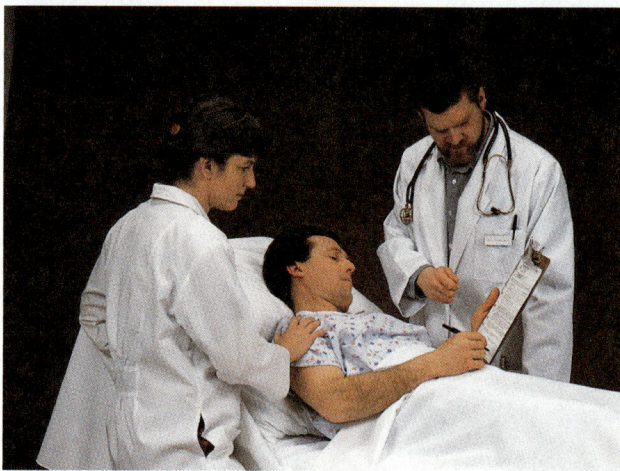

FIGURE 3-2 Informed consent is necessary for certain procedures.

- Be treated in a respectful, dignified manner—this includes the right to privacy and to confidentiality.
- Have the benefit of open and honest communication with caregivers.
- Have a role in decision making for treatment choices and planning of care. **Informed consent** means that the consumer gives permission for care or procedures after full disclosure of the purpose of the care or procedure, the benefits, and any risks involved with the care or procedure (Figure 3-2).
- Be advised of their rights about **advance directives** (documents that give instructions about the consumer's wishes for treatment if the consumer is unable to communicate).
- Receive continuity of care.
- Be informed of resources for resolving conflicts or grievances. A **grievance** is a situation in which the consumer feels there are grounds for complaint.

Each rights document is reproduced in this unit (Figures 3-3, 3-4, and 3-5).

RESPONSIBILITIES OF HEALTH CARE CONSUMERS

Providing for the rights of the consumer will not ensure quality care unless consumers are willing to fulfill certain responsibilities. These responsibilities include:

- Maintaining personal health care records so information is readily available when it is needed.
- Communicating openly and honestly with the physician and other caregivers and being willing to give a complete health and family history.
- Providing information regarding past hospitalizations and medications.

Resident's Rights

This is an abbreviated version of the Resident's Rights as set forth in the Omnibus Budget Reconciliation Act. This document must be given to all residents and/or their families prior to admission to a long-term care facility.

1. The resident has the right to free choice, including the right to:
   - choose an attending physician
   - full advance information about changes in care or treatment
   - participate in the assessment and care planning process
   - self-administer medications if the resident is assessed as being able to do so
   - consent to participate in experimental research
2. The resident has the right to freedom from abuse and restraints, including freedom from:
   - physical, sexual, mental abuse
   - **corporal punishment** (the use of physical force) and **involuntary seclusion** (isolating a resident without a medical reason)
   - physical and chemical restraints
3. The resident has the right to privacy, including privacy for:
   - treatment and nursing care
   - receiving/sending mail
   - telephone calls
   - visitors
4. The resident has the right to confidentiality of personal and clinical records.
5. The resident has the right to accommodation of needs, including:
   - choices about life
   - receiving assistance in maintaining independence
6. The resident has the right to voice grievances.
7. The resident has the right to organize and participate in family and resident groups.
8. The resident has the right to participate in social, religious, and community activities, including the right to:
   - vote
   - keep religious items in the room
   - attend religious services
9. The resident has the right to examine survey results and correction plans.
10. The resident has the right to manage personal funds.
11. The resident has the right to information about eligibility for Medicare/Medicaid funds.
12. The resident has the right to file complaints about abuse, neglect, or misappropriation of property.
13. The resident has the right to information about advocacy groups.
14. The resident has the right to immediate and unlimited access to family or relatives.
15. The resident has the right to share a room with the spouse if they are both residents in the same facility.
16. The resident has the right to perform or not perform work for the facility if it is medically appropriate for the resident to work.
17. The resident has the right to remain in the facility except in certain circumstances.
18. The resident has the right to use personal possessions.
19. The resident has the right to notification of change in condition.

FIGURE 3-3 Resident's Bill of Rights.

A Patient's Bill of Rights

Introduction

Effective health care requires collaboration between patients and physicians and other health care professionals. Open and honest communication, respect for personal and professional values, and sensitivity to differences are integral to optimal patient care. As the setting for the provision of health services, hospitals must provide a foundation for understanding and respecting the rights and responsibilities of patients, their families, physicians, and other caregivers. Hospitals must ensure a health care ethic that respects the role of patients in decision making about treatment choices and other aspects of their care. Hospitals must be sensitive to cultural, racial, linguistic, religious, age, gender, and other differences as well as the needs of persons with disabilities.

The American Hospital Association presents *A Patient's Bill of Rights* with the expectation that it will contribute to more effective patient care and be supported by the hospital on behalf of the institution, its medical staff, employees, and patients. The American Hospital Association encourages health care institutions to tailor this bill of rights to their patient community by translating and/or simplifying the language of this bill of rights as may be necessary to ensure that the patients and their families understand their rights and responsibilities.

Bill of Rights*

1. The patient has the right to considerate and respectful care.

2. The patient has the right to and is encouraged to obtain from physicians and other direct caregivers relevant, current, and understandable information concerning diagnosis, treatment, and prognosis.

   Except in emergencies when the patient lacks decision-making capacity and the need for treatment is urgent, the patient is entitled to the opportunity to discuss and request information related to the specific procedures and/or treatments, the risks involved, the possible length of recuperation, and the medically reasonable alternatives and their accompanying risks and benefits.

   Patients have the right to know the identity of physicians, nurses, and others involved in their care, as well as when those involved are students, residents, or other trainees. The patient also has the right to know the immediate and long-term financial implications of treatment choices, insofar as they are known.

3. The patient has the right to make decisions about the plan of care prior to and during the course of treatment and to refuse a recommended treatment or plan of care to the extent permitted by law and hospital policy and to be informed of the medical consequences of this action. In case of such refusal, the patient is entitled to other appropriate care and services that the hospital provides or transfer to another hospital. The hospital should notify patients of any policy that might affect patient choice within the institution.

4. The patient has the right to have an advance directive (such as a living will, health care proxy, or durable power of attorney for health care) concerning treatment or designating a surrogate decision maker with the expectation that the hospital will honor the intent of that directive to the extent permitted by law and hospital policy.

   Health care institutions must advise patients of their rights under state law and hospital policy to make informed medical choices, ask if the patient has an advance directive, and include that information in patient records. The patient has the right to timely information about hospital policy that may limit its ability to implement fully a legally valid advance directive.

5. The patient has the right to every consideration of privacy. Case discussion, consultation, examination, and treatment should be conducted so as to protect each patient's privacy.

**These rights can be exercised on the patient's behalf by a designated surrogate or proxy decision maker if the patient lacks decision-making capacity, is legally incompetent, or is a minor.*

AHA

A Patient's Bill of Rights was first adopted by the American Hospital Association in 1973. This revision was approved by the AHA Board of Trustees on October 21, 1992.

FIGURE 3-4 A Patient's Bill of Rights. *(Courtesy of American Hospital Association, © copyright 1992)* ***continues***

6. The patient has the right to expect that all communications and records pertaining to his/her care will be treated as confidential by the hospital, except in cases such as suspected abuse and public health hazards when reporting is permitted or required by law. The patient has the right to expect that the hospital will emphasize the confidentiality of this information when it releases it to any other parties entitled to review information in these records.

7. The patient has the right to review the records pertaining to his/her medical care and to have the information explained or interpreted as necessary, except when restricted by law.

8. The patient has the right to expect that, within its capacity and policies, a hospital will make reasonable response to the request of a patient for appropriate and medically indicated care and services. The hospital must provide evaluation, service, and/or referral as indicated by the urgency of the case. When medically appropriate and legally permissible, or when a patient has so requested, a patient may be transferred to another facility. The institution to which the patient is to be transferred must first have accepted the patient for transfer. The patient must also have the benefit of complete information and explanation concerning the need for, risks, benefits, and alternatives to such a transfer.

9. The patient has the right to ask and be informed of the existence of business relationships among the hospital, educational institutions, other health care providers, or payers that may influence the patient's treatment and care.

10. The patient has the right to consent to or decline to participate in proposed research studies or human experimentation affecting care and treatment or requiring direct patient involvement, and to have those studies fully explained prior to consent. A patient who declines to participate in research or experimentation is entitled to the most effective care that the hospital can otherwise provide.

11. The patient has the right to expect reasonable continuity of care when appropriate and to be informed by physicians and other caregivers of available and realistic patient care options when hospital care is no longer appropriate.

12. The patient has the right to be informed of hospital policies and practices that relate to patient care, treatment, and responsibilities. The patient has the right to be informed of available resources for resolving disputes, grievances, and conflicts, such as ethics committees, patient representatives, or other mechanisms available in the institution. The patient has the right to be informed of the hospital's charges for services and available payment methods.

The collaborative nature of health care requires that the patients, or their families/surrogates, participate in their care. The effectiveness of care and patient satisfaction with the course of treatment depend, in part, on the patient fulfilling certain responsibilities. Patients are responsible for providing information about past illnesses, hospitalizations, medications, and other matters related to health status. To participate effectively in decision making, patients must be encouraged to take responsibility for requesting additional information or clarification about their health status or treatment when they do not fully understand information and instructions. Patients are also responsible for ensuring that the health care institution has a copy of their written advance directive if they have one. Patients are responsible for informing their physicians and other caregivers if they anticipate problems in following prescribed treatment.

Patients should also be aware of the hospital's obligation to be reasonably efficient and equitable in providing care to other patients and the community. The hospital's rules and regulations are designed to help the hospital meet this obligation. Patients and their families are responsible for making reasonable accommodations to the needs of the hospital, other patients, medical staff, and hospital employees. Patients are responsible for providing necessary information for insurance claims and for working with the hospital to make payment arrangements, when necessary.

A person's health depends on much more than health care services. Patients are responsible for recognizing the impact of their life-style on their personal health.

Conclusion

Hospitals have many functions to perform, including the enhancement of health status, health promotion, and the prevention and treatment of injury and disease; the immediate and ongoing care and rehabilitation of patients; the education of health professionals, patients, and the community; and research. All these activities must be conducted with an overriding concern for the values and dignity of patients.

FIGURE 3-4 *continued*

Client's Rights in Home Care

The persons receiving home health care services or their families possess basic rights and responsibilities. As the client, you have:

The right to:
1. be treated with dignity, consideration and respect
2. have your property treated with respect
3. receive a timely response from the agency to requests for service
4. be fully informed on admission of the care and treatment that will be provided, how much it will cost, and how payment will be handled
5. know in advance if you will be responsible for any payment
6. be informed in advance of any changes in your care
7. receive care from professionally trained personnel, and to know their names and responsibilities
8. participate in planning care
9. refuse treatment and to be told the consequences of your action
10. expect confidentiality of all information
11. be informed of anticipated termination of service
12. be referred elsewhere if you are denied services solely based on your inability to pay
13. know how to make a complaint or recommend a change in agency policies and services

The responsibility to:
1. remain under a doctor's care while receiving services
2. provide the agency with a complete health history
3. provide the agency all requested insurance and financial information
4. sign the required consents and releases for insurance billing
5. participate in your care by asking questions, expressing concerns, and stating if you do not understand
6. provide a safe home environment in which care can be given
7. cooperate with your doctor, the staff, and other caregivers
8. accept responsibility for any refusal of treatment
9. abide by agency policies that restrict the duties our staff may perform
10. advise agency administration of any dissatisfaction or problems with your care

FIGURE 3-5 Client's Rights in Home Care.

- Informing the physician and other caregivers if they anticipate problems with following prescribed treatment.
- Accepting responsibility for learning how to manage their own health (Figure 3-6).
- Asking for clarification if they do not fully understand instructions or explanations.
- Living a healthy lifestyle and avoiding unnecessary risks of illness or injury.
- Accepting financial responsibility for payment of health care and providing information for insurance claims.

The rights of health care consumers have both a legal and an ethical basis. Legal and ethical aspects are discussed in Unit 4.

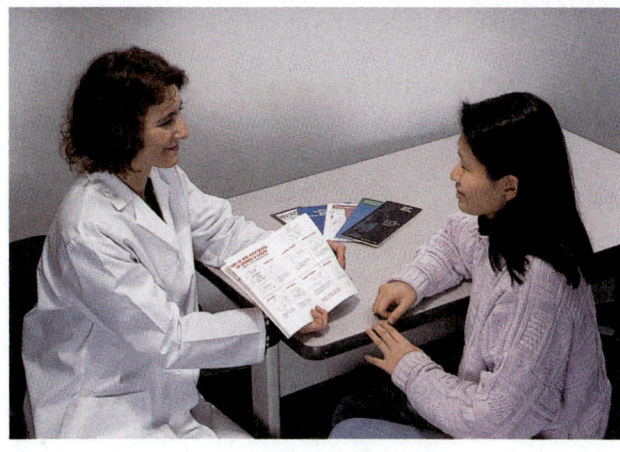

FIGURE 3-6 Nurses teach patients how to manage their own health.

REVIEW

A. True/False.

Mark the following true or false by circling T or F.

1. T (F) The rights of health care consumers are important only to patients in hospitals.
2. (T) F All United States citizens have certain rights that are guaranteed by law.
3. (T) F The Client's Bill of Rights is given to persons receiving home care.
4. T (F) The Patient's Bill of Rights was legislated by the OBRA of 1987.
5. (T) F Health care consumers in any setting have the right to prepare advance directives.

B. Multiple Choice.

Select the one best answer for each of the following.

6. Resident's Rights are given to persons before they are admitted to
   a. home care.
   (b.) a skilled care facility.
   c. the hospital.
   d. hospice services.
7. All types of consumer rights state that the consumer has the right to
   (a.) be treated in a respectful, dignified manner.
   b. select the individuals assigned to provide health care to them.
   c. private-duty nursing care, if desired by the patient or family.
   d. withhold information and records describing their medical condition.

8. The purpose of advance directives is to
   (a.) allow individuals to give instructions about their care should they become unable to do so.
   b. give individuals the right to choose their caregivers.
   c. provide a resource for resolving conflicts.
   d. permit the physician to prescribe treatment without conferring with the individual.
9. Health care consumers are responsible for
   a. leaving their bad habits at home when they are admitted to a health care facility.
   b. reading and studying medical books to learn all there is to know about their conditions.
   c. making treatment decisions in keeping with their physician's wishes.
   (d.) communicating openly and honestly with their physician and caregivers.

C. Completion.

Choose the correct word from the following list to complete each statement in questions 10–15.

1 advance directive	4 involuntary seclusion
2 grievance	5 privacy
3 informed consent	6 respect

10. ___3___ means that the consumer gives permission for care or procedures after full disclosure.
11. A ___2___ exists when the consumer feels there are grounds for complaint.

12. A document that gives instructions about the consumer's wishes for treatment if the consumer is unable to communicate is called a[an] ___1___.

13. Isolating a resident without a medical reason is called ___4___.

14. By not opening and reading the consumer's mail, you are respecting the consumer's right to ___5___.

15. All health care consumers have the right to be treated with ___6___.

D. Nursing Assistant Challenge.

Mr. Delmonico was admitted to General Hospital for surgery to repair a fractured hip. After a few days in the hospital, he will be transferred to Memorial Nursing Center, a skilled care facility, for additional rehabilitation. After discharge from Memorial, it is expected that he will need home care for four to six weeks. Briefly explain how the different rights of each document will affect Mr. Delmonico's care.

16. Consider Mr. Delmonico's diagnosis and the services he will need for recovery. Which aspects of the Patient's Bill of Rights are especially important to his hospital care?

17. Discuss the statements in the Residents' Rights document that pertain specifically to rehabilitation and independence.

18. For which items in the Clients' Rights would the nursing assistant be responsible?

 # EXPLORING THE WEB

Description	Location
Center for Health Care Rights	*http://www.healthcarerights.org*
National Health Law Program	*http://www.healthlaw.org*
Patient's Bill of Rights	*http://www.hospitalconnect.com*
Principles of Patient Rights and Responsibilities	*http://www.nhcouncil.org*

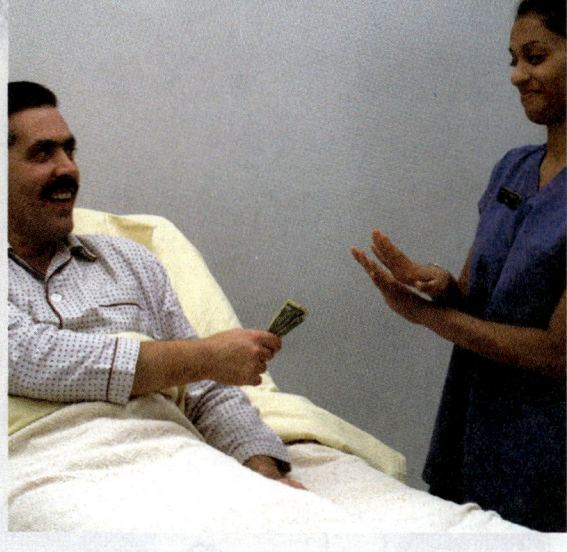

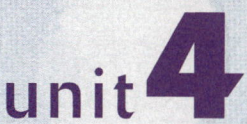

Ethical and Legal Issues Affecting the Nursing Assistant

objectives

After completing this unit, you will be able to:

- Spell and define terms.
- Discuss ethical and legal situations in health care.
- Describe the ethical responsibilities of the nursing assistant concerning patient information.
- Describe tactful ways to refuse a tip offered by a patient.
- Describe the legal responsibilities of a nursing assistant.
- Describe how to protect the patient's right to privacy.

vocabulary

Learn the meaning and the correct spelling of the following words and phrases:

abuse	defamation	legal standards	physical abuse
aiding and abetting	ethical standards	liable	psychological abuse
assault	false imprisonment	libel	sexual abuse
battery	informed consent	malpractice	slander
coercion	invasion of privacy	neglect	theft
confidential	involuntary seclusion	negligence	verbal abuse

ETHICAL STANDARDS AND LEGAL STANDARDS

Each day, as you carry out your work and relate to patients, coworkers, families, and others from the community, you will be faced with decisions to make about your actions. Some of these decisions involve the moral right or wrong of an action. Other decisions involve the legality of your behavior.

Two sets of rules help govern these moral and legal actions you will take. They are:

1. **Ethical standards**. These are guides to moral behavior. People who give health care voluntarily agree to live up to these standards. When these rules are not followed, the nursing assistant fails to live up to the promise to give safe, correct care and to do no harm.

2. **Legal standards**. These are guides to lawful behavior. When laws are not obeyed, the nursing assistant may be prosecuted and found **liable** (held responsible) for injury or damage. Legal guilt can result in the payment of fines or imprisonment.

The ethical standards and legal standards are established to ensure that only safe, quality care is given. Following these standards also protects the caregiver. Sometimes the rules that govern moral actions and the laws that govern legal actions cover the same area.

ETHICS QUESTIONS

Probably at no other time in history have the questions of medical ethics been under such scrutiny. Questions health care providers ask include:

- When is life gone from a person on life support systems?
- How much lifesaving or resuscitation effort should be given in situations of terminal illness?
- When does human life actually begin?
- How much assistance should be given to the conception process?
- Should the body organs of a brain-dead person be harvested for transplants for the living?
- Does an unborn baby have rights?
- Is assisting a patient during or after an abortion right or wrong?
- Is euthanasia (assisted death) ever justified?
- Should animals be used in research of potential value to human life?
- Should food and water be withheld to speed death when the patient has expressed the desire to have this action performed?
- Who makes decisions about removing life support systems when there is no direct expression of the patient's wishes or there is conflict within the family?

- How will a choice be made when two or more people could benefit from an organ transplant but only one organ is available?
- How should the limited money available be spent when many serious disease conditions need to be researched?
- Who has the final authority over whether a woman will carry a pregnancy to term?
- Should marijuana be used for medicinal purposes?

Many facilities have ethics committees that advise the staff on ethical matters. The members of the ethics committees often include staff, clergy, interested community members, and advocates for the sick and elderly.

The committee usually does not make recommendations for specific cases. Instead, the committee reviews the ethical problems and principles involved to help guide the staff and family.

Respect for patients and their wishes is the primary concern. Part of this respect for life is shown by having patients actively involved in decisions about their care and future.

As a nursing assistant, you will take directions from the legal and ethical guidelines established by your facility.

RESPECT FOR LIFE

One of the most basic rules of ethics is that life is precious. Everyone involved in the care of patients has the promotion of health and the quality of life as primary goals (Figure 4-1). Death, however, is a natural progression of life. When death is certain, the objective is to keep the dying person comfortable. Today, there is a greater appreciation of individual wishes and the quality of life expected. One fact remains clear—the major responsibility of medicine and all members of the health care team is to maintain quality of life and make comfortable those whose lives are limited.

LEGAL *Alert*

At some point in your life, you probably learned to "Do unto others as you would have them do unto you." Use this principle to guide your nursing assistant practice. You will find many instances in which personal comfort and convenience could potentially interfere with the care you give. By placing the patient's interests ahead of your own, you fulfill the ethical and legal obligations of your practice, protect patient safety, and reduce your risk of legal exposure.

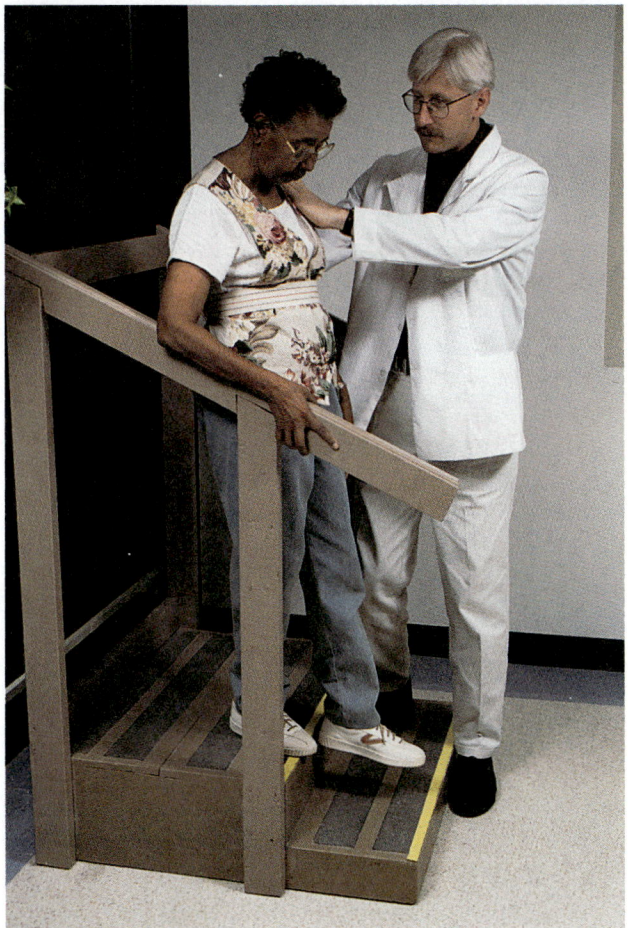

FIGURE 4-1 Promoting good health and quality of life is a primary goal.

RESPECT FOR THE INDIVIDUAL

Respect for each patient as a unique individual is another ethical principle. This uniqueness is demonstrated by differences in:

- age
- race
- religion
- gender
- sexual preference
- culture
- attitudes
- background
- response to illness

You may find the differences that make the patient so special also make dealing with the patient challenging or difficult. If you respect each patient as a valuable person, you can learn to accept and work with each one in the best possible way.

PATIENT INFORMATION

The ethical code asserts that information about patients is privileged and must not be shared with others (Figure 4-2).

1. Discuss patient information only in appropriate places.
   a. It is unwise to discuss a patient's condition while in the patient's room, even if the patient is unresponsive. The patient may be able to hear everything that is said. This could cause the patient unnecessary worry.
   b. Never discuss the patients in your care with your family or in the community.
   c. Never discuss the patients during lunch or coffee breaks, even with your coworkers.
2. Discuss information only with the proper people.
   a. At times you will be approached by others requesting information about a patient. For example, you might be asked for such information by other patients, family members, or members of the public, such as news reporters.
   b. Discuss patients and their personal concerns only with your supervisor during conference or report. Make sure you will not be overheard by visitors or other patients.
   c. You will learn to evade inquiries tactfully by:
      – Stating that you do not know all the details of the treatment or the patient's condition.

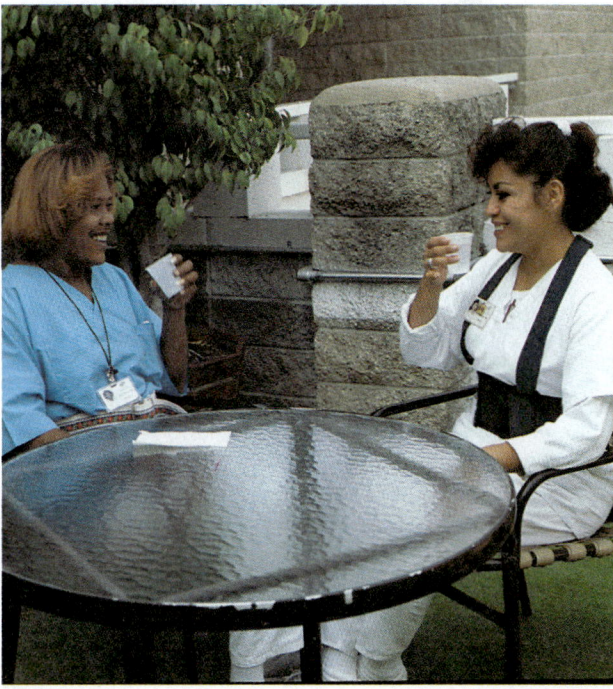

FIGURE 4-2 Information about patients is confidential and must not be discussed casually.

– Redirecting inquirers to the proper authority.

– Firmly, but politely, indicating that you do not have the authority to provide the answers they seek.

3. Refer patient requests for information about laboratory results, the patient's condition, or course of the illness to the nurse or doctor.

4. Let the nurse or doctor relay information about a patient's death. Never give information concerning the death of a patient to the patient's family. When done with tact, a refusal of this kind is rarely resented by the family.

5. Follow the ethical code to ensure respect of the patient's personal religious beliefs. People of all faiths or beliefs and those with no proclaimed faith are admitted for care. These differences must be respected. You show your respect when you:

   a. Inform the nurse of requests for clergy visits.

   b. Know correct information about the type of chaplain services available in your facility.

   c. Know if a chapel is open for use by patients and families.

   d. Respectfully treat the patient's religious articles, such as a Bible, crucifix, Koran, or holy pictures.

   e. Avoid imposing your own religious beliefs on patients.

   f. Assist patients to practice their religious beliefs and rituals, if requested.

When the clergy visits (Figure 4-3), you should:

   a. Be helpful and courteous.

   b. Escort the clergyperson to the patient's bedside.

c. Draw the curtains or close the door for privacy.

d. Leave the room.

TIPPING

If you follow the ethical code, the service you give will depend on need. It will *not* depend on the patient's race, creed, color, or ability to pay. There is no place for tipping within the health care system (Figure 4-4).

Patients are charged for the services they receive while in the hospital. The salary you are paid is included in that charge.

Sometimes patients will offer a "little something" to you. A firm but courteous refusal of the money is usually all that is necessary to assure the patient of your meaning.

As you can see, the ethical code ensures that the patient is treated with dignity and respect in ways that always promote safe care.

LEGAL ISSUES

Laws are passed by governments (local, state, and federal) and are to be obeyed by citizens. Anyone who fails to obey a law may be liable (responsible) for fines or imprisonment.

You need not fear breaking these laws if you are careful to:

- Stay within your scope of practice and do not overstep your authority.
- Do only those things that you have been taught and that are within the scope of your training.
- Carry out procedures carefully and as you were taught.
- Keep your skills and knowledge up to date.
- Request guidance from the proper person before you take action in a questionable situation.
- Always keep the safety and well-being of the patient foremost in your mind, and act accordingly.

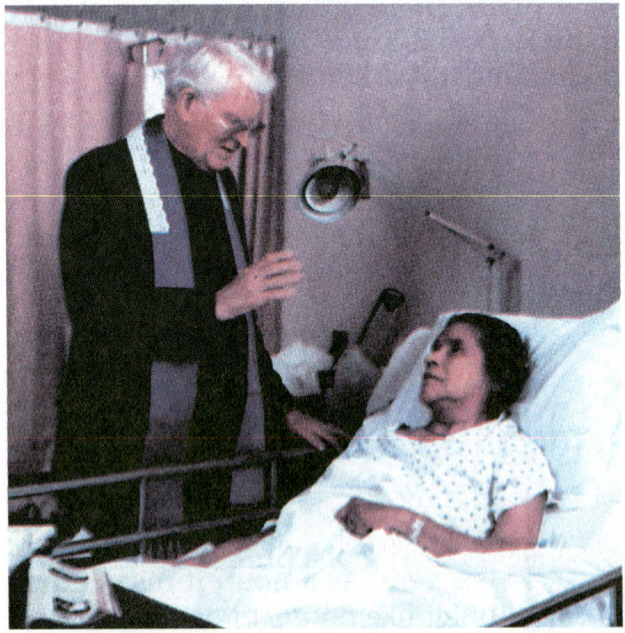

FIGURE 4-3 A private visit from the clergy can be very comforting and reassuring.

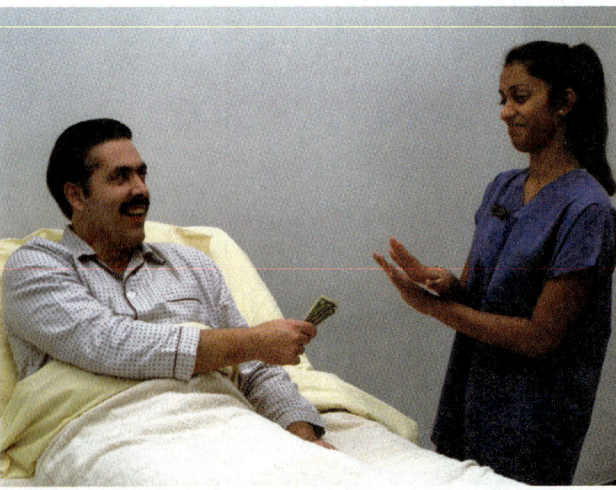

FIGURE 4-4 Tips must be courteously refused.

- Make sure you thoroughly understand directions for the care you are to give.
- Perform your job according to facility policy.
- Stay within OBRA guidelines.
- Maintain in-service requirements of OBRA.
- Do no harm to the patient.
- Respect the patient's belongings (property).

Situations you must avoid are negligence, theft, defamation, false imprisonment, assault and battery, abuse, and invasion of privacy.

Negligence

Negligence is the failure to exercise the degree of care considered reasonable under the circumstances, when that failure results in an unintended injury to a patient. Simply put, negligence is carelessness, which is often caused by hurrying or not focusing on the task at hand.

Nursing assistants are trained care providers and are expected to perform in certain ways. You would be guilty of negligence if you injured a patient by:

- Not performing your work as taught. For example, a patient is burned by an enema solution that you prepared and was too hot.
- Not carrying out your job in a conscientious manner. For example, your facility has a policy that two workers are necessary to transfer a patient with the mechanical lift, but you fail to ask another worker to assist you in moving a patient. The lift tips and the patient is injured.

Malpractice is improper, negligent, or unethical conduct that results in harm, injury, or loss to a patient. Practicing within your scope of practice, following facility policies and procedures, and doing things in the way you were taught will help protect your patients from injury. Being discreet, respecting confidentiality, and avoiding gossip will help protect you from inadvertently harming a patient emotionally. Be kind and polite to patients. If a patient complains about something you have done, apologize and promptly correct the problem without becoming defensive.

Theft

Taking anything that does not belong to you makes you guilty of theft. If you are caught, you will be liable. The article taken need not be expensive to be considered stolen.

If you see someone stealing something and do not report it, you are guilty of aiding and abetting the crime.

Because of the nature of their work, people working in facilities must be honest and dependable. Despite careful screening, dishonest people are sometimes hired and things do disappear. These range from washcloths, money, and patients' personal belongings to drugs.

Sometimes workers are reluctant to report things that they see other people doing. Remember, however, that you are responsible for your own actions and must take the proper actions. For a nursing assistant, opportunities for poor practice, illegal activities, and neglect are always present. Resist the temptation to lower your standards. Honesty and integrity are the hallmarks of the sincere and conscientious nursing assistant.

Defamation

If you make false statements about someone to a third person and the character of the first person is injured, you are guilty of defamation. This is true if you make the statement verbally (slander) or in writing (libel). For example, if you inaccurately tell a coworker that a patient has AIDS, you have slandered that patient. If you write the same untrue information in a note, you are guilty of libel.

False Imprisonment

Restraining a person's movements or actions without proper authorization constitutes unlawful or false imprisonment. For example, patients have the right to leave the hospital *with or without* the physician's permission. You may not interfere with this right. If you do interfere, you will be guilty of false imprisonment.

If you learn of a patient's intention to leave the hospital without permission, inform your supervisor. The supervisor will handle the situation.

Using physical restraints, or even threatening to do so, in order to make a patient cooperate can also constitute false imprisonment. Restraints may be in the form of physical devices or chemical agents. A physical restraint is any manual method or physical or mechanical device, material, or equipment attached or adjacent to the resident's body that:

- A patient cannot easily remove.
- Restricts a patient's movement.
- Does not allow the patient normal access to his or her own body.

Examples of physical restraints include:

- Wrist/arm and ankle/leg restraints
- Vests
- Jackets
- Hand mitts
- Geriatric and cardiac chairs
- Wheelchair safety belts and bars
- Bed rails, which are considered physical restraints if they meet the definition listed

In general, many devices and practices meet the definition of physical restraints if the patient does not have the physical or mental ability to remove the device. Examples of other practices that constitute restraint are:

- Tucking in, tying, or using Velcro to hold a sheet, fabric, or clothing tightly so that a patient's movement is restricted.

- Using devices in conjunction with a chair (such as trays, tables, bars, or belts) that the patient cannot remove easily and that keep the patient from rising.
- Placing a patient in a chair that prevents the patient from rising.
- Placing a chair or bed so close to a wall that the wall prevents the patient from rising out of the chair or voluntarily getting out of bed.

Psychoactive medications are considered chemical restraints because they affect the patient's mobility. The use of restraints is discussed further in Unit 14 on safety.

Sometimes it is necessary to support and restrain the movement of patients. Supports and restraints cannot be used without a physician's order. This order indicates the extent of restraint or support to be used, when it is to be used, and the reason for it.

Assault and Battery

Assault and battery are serious legal matters. **Assault** means intentionally attempting to touch the body of a person or even threatening to do so. **Battery** means actually touching a person without that person's permission.

The care we provide is given with the patient's permission or **informed consent**. This means the patient must know and agree to what we plan to do before we start. Consent may be withdrawn at any time. For example, you are assigned to give a patient a warm foot soak. Despite your explanation of the reasons for the order, the patient refuses. You may not force the patient to submit. Doing so would make you guilty of battery. You commit assault if you threaten the patient by telling her or him that you will get others to assist you if she or he refuses.

Either situation could make you liable for legal charges. You can avoid this legal pitfall by:

- Informing the patient of what you plan to do.
- Making sure the patient understands.
- Pausing before starting, to give the patient an opportunity to refuse.
- Reporting refusal of care to your supervisor and documenting the facts.
- Never carrying out a treatment on your own against the patient's wishes.

Coercion means forcing the patient to do something against his or her wishes. Refusal of treatment creates a dilemma for the nursing assistant when the patient is mentally confused. In general, a family member or other responsible person consents to treatment and hospital care for patients who are confused. In this situation, we presume that the patient would agree to the care if he or she were mentally able to do so. The patient may refuse a procedure, such as a bath, but the legally responsible person has already consented to the procedure, so you may perform it. Gaining the patient's cooperation and trust is always best. You may be able to perform the procedure if you wait awhile, then

return. Avoid forcing the patient. If in doubt about how to handle refusals of care, consult your supervisor.

Abuse

Abuse of a patient (doing harm to a patient) violates ethical principles and makes you liable for legal prosecution. Ethical standards require that you do no harm to patients. Legal standards enforce this through laws, with subsequent penalties if you are found guilty.

Abuse is defined as any act or failure to act that is non-accidental and causes or could cause harm or death to the patient. Some forms of abuse are subtle but nevertheless cause the patient physical harm or mental anguish. Abuse can occur in several forms, including verbal, sexual, physical, and mental abuse and involuntary seclusion.

Verbal abuse may be directed toward the patient or expressed about the patient. You are guilty of verbally abusing a patient if you:

- Use profanity (swearing) in dealing with the patient.
- Raise your voice in anger at the patient.
- Call the patient unpleasant names.
- Tease or embarrass the patient.
- Use threatening or obscene gestures.
- Make written threats or abusive statements.
- Use inappropriate words to describe a person's race or nationality.

Sexual abuse is the use of physical means or verbal threats to force a patient to perform sexual acts. In many states,

LEGAL *Alert*

Most states have laws prohibiting abuse of children and elderly adults. These laws often require mandatory reporting of suspected patient abuse to police and state agencies. The penalties for abusing a patient can be severe, and may include imprisonment. Caregiver stress is frequently the cause of patient abuse. Learning and practicing methods of reducing stress is best for your mental, emotional, and physical health. Recognize signs of stress, including difficulty sleeping, irritability, feelings of sadness, anxiety, guilt, indecisiveness, loss of appetite, loss of interest in sexual activity, isolation, loss of interest in work, hopelessness, drug or alcohol misuse, and inability to concentrate. If a combination of these symptoms is present, seek help in managing your stress.

sexual abuse is any behavior that is seductive, sexually demeaning, harassing, or reasonably interpreted as sexual by the patient. Examples of sexual abuse include:

- Tormenting or teasing a patient with sexual gestures or words.
- Touching a patient in a sexual way.
- Suggesting that the patient engage in sexual acts with you.

Physical abuse does actual physical harm to the patient. Examples of physical abuse include:

- Handling a patient roughly (Figure 4-5).
- Hitting, slapping, pushing, kicking, or pinching the patient.
- Performing the wrong treatment on the patient, such as ambulating a patient who should remain in bed.

Psychological abuse includes:

- Making the patient fearful of you, such as threatening not to respond when the patient calls.
- Threatening the patient with harm.
- Threatening to tell something to others that the patient does not want known.
- Threatening to withhold care.
- Making fun of or belittling the patient in any way (Figure 4-6). Calling the patient by names such as "honey" and "grandma" is another way of belittling the patient.
- Calling the attention of others to a patient's behavior.

Involuntary seclusion is the separation of a patient from

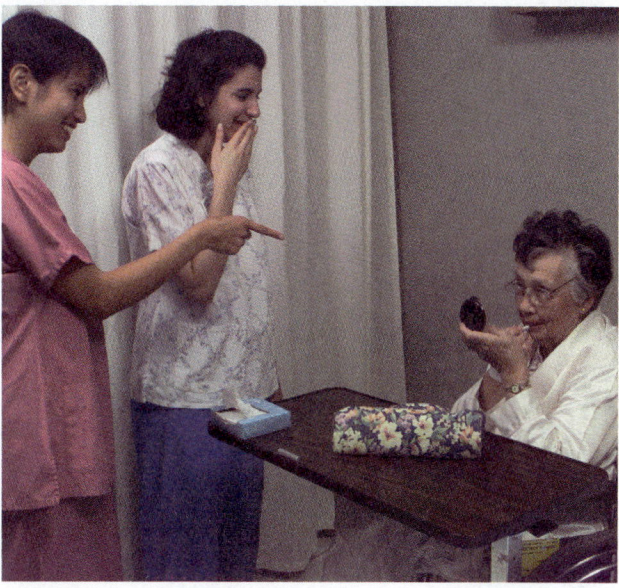

FIGURE 4-6 Making fun of a patient is psychological abuse.

other patients against the patient's will. Examples of involuntary seclusion are:

- Shutting the door to the patient's room when the patient is confined to bed and wants the door open.
- Continually placing a patient's gerichair far from others.
- Leaving a patient without a form of communication, such as a signal cord or call bell.

Separation may be permitted if it is part of a therapeutic plan to reduce agitation. The decision to use seclusion must be made by the nurse. This form of seclusion requires accurate documentation and a plan of care. The seclusion must be effective. Note: When describing a patient's behavior, avoid the use of words such as *uncooperative*, *belligerent*, or *hostile*. Instead, describe the exact actions that you observed. Often, so-called uncooperative behavior is a problem caused by faulty communication on the part of the health care provider. People should not be unfairly labeled.

Abuse by Others

If you suspect that a person in your care is being abused by others, discuss this matter with your supervisor. Laws require a health care provider who suspects abuse to report the situation so the patient can be protected. In some states, a person who does not report the abuse is held as guilty as the abusing person.

It may be difficult to understand why anyone would abuse a person who is weak or infirm, but it happens. A few people may take satisfaction out of feeling that they have control of others. Most abuse, however, probably originates in feelings of frustration or fatigue.

Anyone can be abused, but the old and the young are the most vulnerable. Usually, the caregiver or a family member is the abuser.

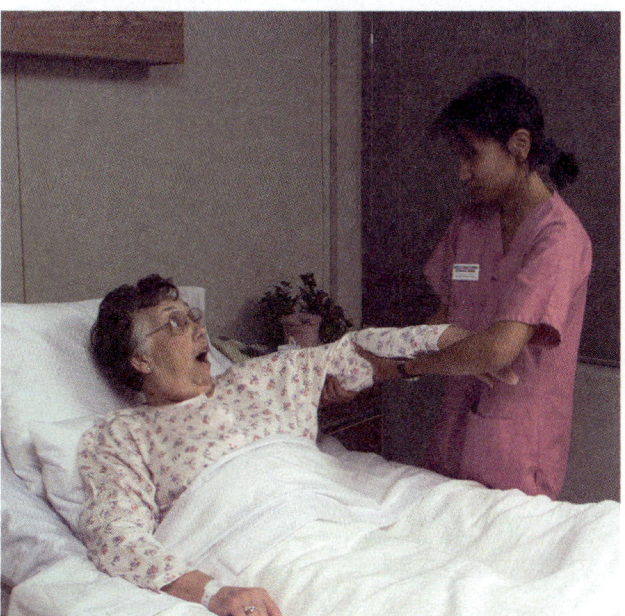

FIGURE 4-5 Handling a patient roughly constitutes physical abuse.

- Some families provide loving, capable care for older, dependent relatives for many years without assistance. After providing care for a long period, they may be physically and emotionally exhausted and may also have depleted their financial resources.
- In some cases, one spouse has abused the other for a long time.
- Self-abuse may occur when a disabled person is unable to adequately carry out activities of daily living and is unwilling to accept help.

It is not the responsibility of the nursing assistant to determine if an individual has been abused or what type of abuse has been inflicted. It *is* the nursing assistant's responsibility to report to the nursing supervisor any signs or symptoms that might be the result of abuse. This includes:

- Statements by the patient that reflect neglect or abuse.
- Unexplained bruises or wounds.
- Signs of neglect such as poor personal hygiene.
- A change in personality.

Remember, these do not necessarily indicate that the person is being abused. However, they may indicate a need for further investigation by your supervisor. Any observed abusive behavior toward patients, whether inside or outside a facility, must be reported to the appropriate authority.

When Your Patience Is Stressed

If you feel that your own tolerance level is being tested, you need to find ways to safeguard the patient and release your own stress. You might:

- Try to identify the exact cause of your irritation.
- Talk with your supervisor about your feelings.
- Consider asking to be assigned to another patient.
- Try to reduce your overall stress and fatigue so you bring a more positive, patient attitude to your job.
- Request counseling through an employee assistance program.

Neglect

Neglect is the failure to provide the services or care necessary to avoid physical harm, mental anguish, or mental illness. Neglect can be deliberate or accidental, such as forgetting an assignment and not providing care. Neglect is also a violation of the law. The nursing assistant is not expected to determine if neglect has occurred. You *are* responsible for reporting signs of neglect to your supervisor, who will investigate the situation. Examples of neglect include:

- Failing to turn the patient as often as needed, causing impaired circulation and pressure ulcers.
- Failing to perform regular exercises so that the patient experiences pain when unused joints are finally moved.
- Failing to carry out proper hygiene, such as not shaving the patient regularly.
- Failing to provide mealtime assistance to a patient who cannot eat independently.
- Failing to provide water to a patient who is on bedrest and has an order to encourage fluids.

Invasion of Privacy

Patients have a right to have their person and personal affairs kept **confidential**. To do otherwise is an **invasion of privacy**. Invading the privacy of another is against the law. You can protect the patient's privacy by:

- Protecting the patient from exposure of the body.
- Knocking and pausing before entering a room.
- Drawing curtains when providing care.
- Leaving while visitors are with the patient.
- Not listening as patients make telephone calls.
- Abiding by the rules of confidentiality.
- Not trying to force a patient to accept your personal beliefs or views.
- Not discussing the patient's condition with anyone outside of work.

REVIEW

A. Multiple Choice.

Select the one best answer for each of the following.

1. You overhear another assistant raise his voice when speaking to Mrs. Ryan. The assistant is guilty of
   a. negligence.
   b. theft.
   c. abuse.
   d. invasion of privacy.
2. Mr. Deonne offers you two dollars for picking up a newspaper for him. Your response should be to
   a. ignore the money and pretend not to see it.
   b. take the money—you earned it.
   c. report the matter to the supervisor.
   d. politely refuse because tipping is not allowed.
3. Mr. Chan's daughter is visiting and wants to know what her father's blood pressure reading is. Your best response is to
   a. tell her.
   b. say you don't know.
   c. refer her to the nurse.

d. refer her to another assistant who measured blood pressure this morning.

4. You observe another assistant slipping a patient's rosary into her pocket. Your response is to
  a. know you are not required to do anything.
  b. report the matter to your supervisor.
  c. tell the patient.
  d. tell the patient's family.

5. You notice that every time a patient makes a telephone call, one nursing assistant stands so that she can hear the conversation. That assistant is guilty of
  a. invasion of privacy.
  b. defamation.
  c. negligence.
  d. libel.

6. An assistant forgets that she is assigned to care for Mr. Huynh, a mentally confused patient. The nurse discovers that Mr. Huynh has developed a pressure ulcer. This is an example of
  a. abuse.
  b. libel.
  c. involuntary seclusion.
  d. neglect.

7. Mrs. Rosario has very fragile skin that tears and bruises easily. The nurse instructed Tony, a nursing assistant, to handle the patient gently to prevent injury. Tony is in a hurry and bumps Mrs. Rosario's leg against the side rail, causing a large skin tear. This is an example of
  a. slander.
  b. invasion of privacy.
  c. libel.
  d. negligence.

8. Mr. McNally tells you he is tired and does not want his bath right now. You should
  a. tell him you will not have time to bathe him later.
  b. ask him when he would like you to return to assist him.
  c. advise him that the doctor insists that he bathe.
  d. forget the bath for today.

9. Mr. Strong, a mentally confused patient, has a visitor. After he leaves, you discover a large bruise on the patient's arm that was not there previously. You should
  a. notify the charge nurse of your observations.
  b. call the police.
  c. do nothing, as this is not your responsibility.
  d. inform the nurse that the visitor abused Mr. Strong.

10. A patient with cancer tells you that she no longer wants to live. She confides that she is collecting her medicine so she can take an overdose and die. You should
  a. respect the patient's right to confidentiality and tell no one.
  b. notify the patient's husband when he visits.
  c. inform your supervisor immediately.
  d. ask a more experienced assistant to reason with the patient.

B. True/False.

Mark the following true or false by circling T or F.

11. T **F** A patient may not refuse any treatment prescribed by the physician.

12. **T** F You may learn much about a patient's personal life as you provide care.

13. T **F** Lunchtime is the best time to discuss your patients with others.

14. T **F** If you accept a tip, you are guilty of abuse.

15. **T** F Your patient has an order to encourage fluid intake, and you fail to do this. You are guilty of neglect.

16. **T** F You forget to put side rails up when ordered, and a patient falls. You are guilty of negligence.

17. **T** F Failure to report your observation of an illegal act makes you guilty of aiding and abetting the action.

18. **T** F Leaving a patient unnecessarily exposed is an invasion of the patient's privacy.

19. **T** F Jackets, belts, vests, and straps can be considered unlawful restraints.

20. **T** F Ethics relates to moral rights and wrongs of behavior.

21. **T** F Anxiety can sometimes make a person very demanding.

22. T **F** People give up their right to privacy when they are admitted to health care facilities.

23. **T** F If an error occurs as you give care, it is important to report it immediately.

24. T **F** Patients should not question the cost of care.

25. **T** F Every patient has the right to considerate, respectful care.

26. **T** F Honesty and integrity are the hallmarks of a conscientious nursing assistant.

27. T **F** You should report all requests for clergy visits to the doctor.

28. T **F** If a patient resists you, you may apply restraints to make sure the treatment is given.

29. **T** F Patients may not be subjected to either verbal or physical abuse.

C. Nursing Assistant Challenge.

In each of the following situations, describe the correct nursing assistant action.

30. Ms. Harvey is dying. Her doctors believe that she will live only a few days. What is your responsibility to this patient? _____

31. Mrs. Wybok insists on saying her prayers every morning just as breakfast is ready. _____

32. Mr. Bishop's daughter asks you what medicine the doctor ordered for her father's heart condition.

_____

 EXPLORING THE WEB

Description	Location
Elder abuse and neglect	*http://www.webster.edu*
Ethical responsibilities	*http://www.delmarhealthcare.com/olcs/white/pnotes.asp* (see Chapter 4)
Ethical responsibilities	*http://www.delmarhealthcare.com/olcs/whiteduncan/pnotes.asp* (see Chapter 7)
Legal responsibilities	*http://www.delmarhealthcare.com/olcs/white/pnotes.asp* (see Chapter 6)
Legal responsibilities	*http://www.delmarhealthcare.com/olcs/whiteduncan/pnotes.asp* (see Chapter 3)
"The Top Ten Things You Can Do to Get Sued"	*http://www.advancefornurses.com* (see past articles for 8/20/01)
All Health Net	*http://www.allhealthnet.com*
American Association of Nurse Attorneys	*http://www.taana.org*
Center for Clinical Ethics	*http://wings.buffalo.edu*
Center for Health Care Ethics	*http://www.slu.edu*
Centre for Applied Ethics	*http://www.ethics.ubc.ca*
Ethical Conduct for Health Care Institutions	*http://www.hospitalconnect.com*
Journal of Nursing Risk Management	*http://www.afip.org*
Kennedy Institute of Ethics	*http://www.georgetown.edu*
National Clearinghouse on Child Abuse and Neglect Information	*http://www.calib.com*
Risk Management Sourcebook	*http://www.thedoctors.com*

Scientific Principles

UNIT 5
Medical Terminology and Body Organization

UNIT 6
Classification of Disease

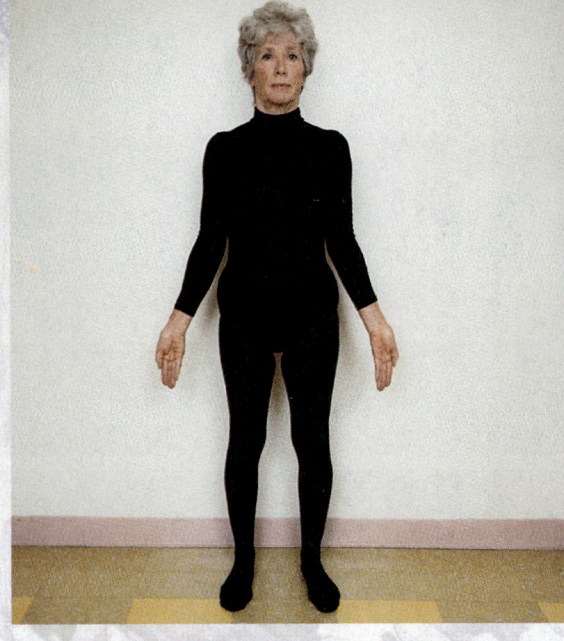

Medical Terminology and Body Organization

objectives

After completing this unit, you will be able to:

- Spell and define terms.
- Recognize the meanings of common prefixes, suffixes, and root words.
- Build medical terms from word parts.
- Write the abbreviations commonly used in health care facilities.
- Describe the simple to complex organization of the body.
- Name four types of tissues and their characteristics.
- Name and locate major organs as parts of body systems, using proper anatomic terms.

vocabulary

Learn the meaning and the correct spelling of the following words and phrases:

abbreviation	distal	muscle tissue	skeletal (voluntary)
anatomic position	dorsal	nerve cell	muscle
anatomy	epithelial cell	nervous tissue	smooth (involuntary)
anterior	epithelial tissue	organ	muscle
cardiac muscle	health	pericardium	suffix
cavity	inferior	peritoneum	superior
cell	lateral	physiology	synovial membranes
combining form	medial	pleura	system
connective tissue	membranes	posterior	tissue
connective tissue cell	meninges	prefix	umbilicus
cutaneous	mucous membrane	proximal	ventral
membrane	mucus	quadrant	word root
disease	muscle cell	serous membrane	

MEDICAL TERMINOLOGY

Medical science and health care have a special language called *medical terminology* or the language of health care. In this language, the terms are formed by building on common word parts (Figure 5-1). Terms are developed by combining:

- **Word root**—the foundation of a medical term. A word root usually, but not always, refers to the part of the body or condition that is being treated, studied, or named by the term.
- **Combining form**—a vowel may be added to the end of the word root to make it easier to form medical words. This combination of the word root and vowel is called a combining form.
- **Prefix**—word part added to the beginning of a word to change or add to its meaning.
- **Suffix**—word part added to the end of a word to change or add to its meaning.
- **Abbreviation**—shortened form of a word (often letters). You already know the abbreviation RN (registered nurse). You will soon become familiar with additional abbreviations that are common to the world of medicine and health care.

Each health care facility also has special abbreviations that it uses (Figure 5-2). Check with the procedure or policy manual of your facility to determine which abbreviations have been approved for use. A good medical dictionary is also a helpful tool.

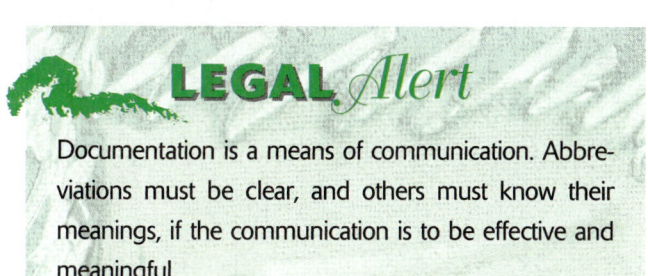

LEGAL *Alert*

Documentation is a means of communication. Abbreviations must be clear, and others must know their meanings, if the communication is to be effective and meaningful.

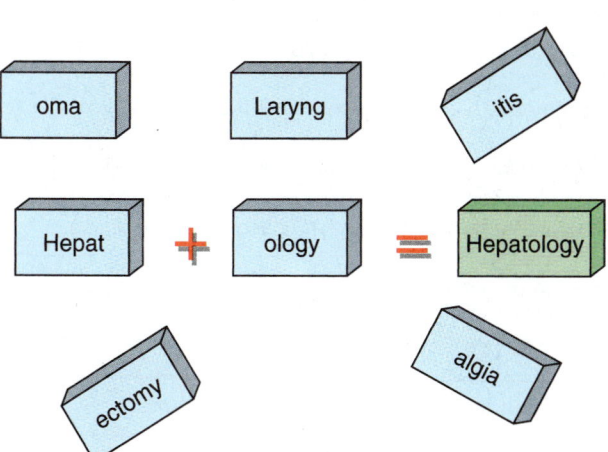

FIGURE 5-1 New words can be formed by combining prefixes and suffixes.

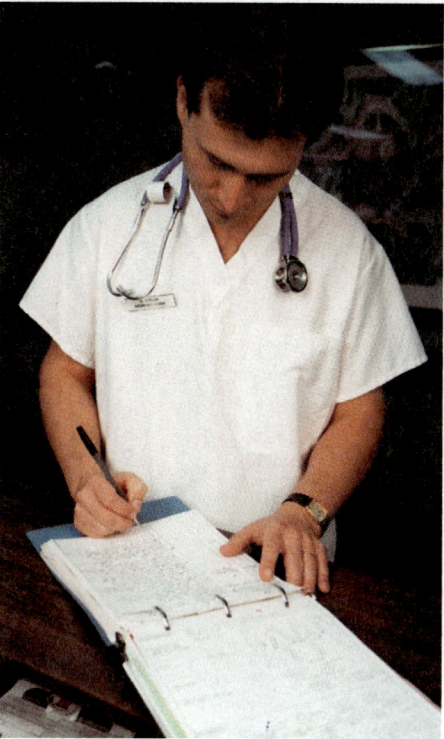

FIGURE 5-2 A sound foundation in medical terminology makes charting easier.

MEDICAL WORD PARTS

Word Roots

Familiarity with the important word parts comes from study and repeated usage. You will gain experience with the word parts as you practice reporting and charting, and by communicating with your coworkers.

A single medical word root can sometimes be placed in different parts of a word and still have a specific meaning. For example, the root *cyte* means cell:

- *cyt*ology—the study of cells
- a leuko*cyte*—a white blood cell
- poly*cyt*osis—an illness in which there are too many red and white blood cells

No matter where the form *cyte* occurs in a medical word, it refers to cells. It may be a prefix, a suffix, or a word root.

Word roots are often derived from Greek or Latin. For example, the word root *nephro* is derived from the word for kidney. This root may be used to form a variety of medical terms. For example:

- Nephroma—a tumor of the kidney
- Nephrectomy—surgical excision of the kidney
- Nephrolithiasis—presence of kidney stones

Give special attention to the exercises and activities in this unit. Learning the new words and parts of words in this unit will make it easier for you to recognize meanings of medical terms.

Table 5-1 lists combining forms (word roots plus vowel).

TABLE 5-1 COMBINING FORMS

Combining Form	Meaning	Example	Meaning
abdomin (o)	abdomen	abdominal	portion of body between the thorax and pelvis
aden (o)	gland	adenoma	a glandular tumor
angi (o)	vessel	angioedema	recurrent large areas of subcutaneous edema of sudden onset, commonly an allergic reaction to foods or drugs
arteri (o)	artery	arteriogram	x-ray of an artery after injection of contrast medium (dye)
arthr (o)	joint	arthritis	inflammation of a joint
bronch (i) (o)	bronchus bronchi	bronchiectasis	one of the larger passages conveying air to and within the lungs becomes abnormally enlarged
cardi (o)	heart	cardialgia	pain in the region of the heart
cephal (o)	head	cephaloma	soft or encephaloid tumor
cerebr (o)	brain	cerebrovascular accident	another name for a stroke
chol (e)	bile	cholecystitis	inflammation of the gallbladder
col (o)	colon, large intestine	colectomy	excision of the colon
crani (o)	skull	craniotomy	opening of the skull
cyst (o)	bladder, cyst	cystitis	inflammation of the bladder
cyt (o)	cell	cytology	study of cells
dent (i) (o)	tooth	dentist	person licensed to practice dentistry
dermat (o)	skin	dermatitis	inflammation of the skin
encephal (o)	brain	encephaloma	herniation of brain substance
enter (o)	small intestine	enteritis	inflammation of the intestines
erythr (o)	red	erythroblastosis	presence of many red blood cells
fibr (o)	fiber	fibroadenoma	benign growth commonly occurring in breast tissue
gastr (o)	stomach	gastritis	inflammation of the lining of the stomach
geront (o)	elderly	gerontology	scientific study of process and problems related to aging
gloss (o)	tongue	glossodynia	burning or painful tongue
glyc (o)	sugar	glycosuria	urinary excretion of sugar
gynec (o)	female	gynecomastia	excessive development of male mammary glands
hem (o)	blood	hematuria	discharge of blood in urine

continues

TABLE 5-1 *continued*

Combining Form	Meaning	Example	Meaning
hepat (o)	liver	hepatitis	inflammation of the liver
hydr (o)	water	hydrocephalus	enlargement of the cranium caused by abnormal accumulation of fluid
hyster (o)	uterus	hysterectomy	surgical removal of the uterus
lapar (o)	abdomen, flank, loin	laparoscopy	examination of the contents of the abdomen through a scope passed through the abdominal wall
laryng (o)	larynx	laryngectomy	partial or total removal of the larynx by surgery
lith (o)	stone	lithiasis	formation of stones in any hollow structure of the body
mamm (o)	breast	mammography	imaging examination of the breasts
mast (o)	breast	mastitis	inflammation of the breast
men (o)	menstruation	menorrhagia	excessive menstrual flow
my (o)	muscle	myalgia	muscular pain
myel (o)	bone marrow, spinal cord	myelocele	protrusion of the spinal cord
nephr (o)	kidney	nephrolithiasis	presence of renal calculi (kidney stones)
neur (o)	nerve	neuropathy	any disease of the nervous system
ocul (o)	eye	oculodynia	pain in the eyeball
opthalm (o)	eye	ophthalmoscope	instrument used to view the inside of the eye
oste (o)	bone	osteitis	inflammation of the bone
ot (o)	ear	otitis media	inflammation of the middle ear
ped (i) (o)	child	pedodontics	dental care of children
pharyng (o)	throat, pharynx	pharyngitis	inflammation of the pharynx
phleb (o)	vein	phlebitis	inflammation of a vein
pneum (o)	lung, air, gas	pneumonectomy	resection of lung tissue
proct (o)	rectum	proctoscopy	rectal exam with a proctoscope
psych (o)	mind	psychology	study of human behavior
pulm (o)	lung	pulmonary	pertaining to the lungs
py (o)	pus	pyogenic	producing pus
rect (o)	rectum	rectocele	hernial protrusion of part of the rectum into the vagina
rhin (o)	nose	rhinorrhea	discharge from nasal mucous membrane

continues

TABLE 5-1 *continued*

Combining Form	Meaning	Example	Meaning
splen (o)	spleen	splenoma	enlarged spleen
stern (o)	sternum	sternotomy	incision into or through the sternum
thorac (o)	chest	thoracotomy	opening of the chest
thromb (o)	clot	thrombocytopenia	abnormally small number of platelets in the circulating blood
tox (o)	poison	toxoplasmosis	disease produced by a parasite; can cause birth defects if acquired during pregnancy
trache (i) (o)	trachea	tracheotomy	incision of the trachea for exploration
ur (o)	urine, urinary tract, urination	urinalysis	analysis of the urine
urethr (o)	urethra	urethralgia	pain in the urethra
urin (o)	urine	urinometer	an instrument for determining the specific gravity of urine
uter (i) (o)	uterus	uterotonic	drugs that give tone to uterine muscle
ven (o)	vein	venostat	any instrument used to suppress venous bleeding

Prefixes and Suffixes

Many medical words have common beginnings (prefixes) or common endings (suffixes). By learning some of the more common prefixes (Table 5-2) and suffixes (Table 5-3), you can put together many new words.

Common Abbreviations

Table 5-4 lists abbreviations and their meanings. They have been grouped according to most common usage for easier learning. Other abbreviations will be presented in following units, with the circumstances where they are most often used.

TABLE 5-2 COMMON PREFIXES

Prefix	Meaning	Example	Meaning	Prefix	Meaning	Example	Meaning
a-	without	asepsis	without infection	poly-	many	polyuria	excessive urine
brady-	slow	bradycardia	slow heart rate	post-	after	postoperative	after surgery
dys-	pain or difficulty	dysuria	painful urination	pre-	before	premenstrual	before the menses
hyper-	above, excessive	hypertension	high blood pressure	retro-	behind, backward	retrograde	moving backward, degenerating
hypo-	low, deficient	hypotension	low blood pressure	tachy-	fast	tachycardia	pulse rate above normal
pan-	all	pandemic	widespread epidemic				

TABLE 5-3 COMMON SUFFIXES

Suffix	Meaning	Example	Meaning	Suffix	Meaning	Example	Meaning
-algia	pain	arthralgia	pain in the joints	-oma	tumor	fibroma	a tumor containing fibrous tissue
-ectomy	removal of	appendectomy	removal of the appendix	-otomy	incision	tracheotomy	incision of trachea
-emia	blood	anemia	lacking sufficient quality or quantity of blood	-plegia	paralysis	hemiplegia	paralysis of one side of the body
-gram	record	electro-cardiogram	record produced by electrocardiography	-pnea	breathing, respiration	apnea	temporary cessation of breathing
-itis	inflammation	appendicitis	inflammation of the appendix	-scope	examination instrument	otoscope	instrument for inspecting or auscultating the ear
-logy	study of	hematology	study of blood	-scopy	examination using a scope	proctoscopy	rectal exam with a proctoscope

TABLE 5-4 COMMON ABBREVIATIONS

Body Parts

abd	abdomen
ant	anterior
ax	axillary
bld	blood
GI	gastrointestinal
GU	genitourinary
int	internal
lt	left
rt	right
quad	quadrant
sh	shoulder
vag	vagina, vaginal

Diagnosis

AFB	acid fast bacillus
AIDS	acquired immune deficiency syndrome
AKA	above knee amputation
AMI	acute myocardial infarction
ASHD	arteriosclerotic heart disease
BKA	below knee amputation
CA	cancer
CAD	coronary artery disease
CBC	complete blood count
CHD	coronary heart disease
CHF	congestive heart failure
COPD	chronic obstructive pulmonary disease
CVA	cerebrovascular accident; stroke

DJD	degenerative joint disease
DVT	deep vein thrombosis
FUO	fever of unknown origin
Fx	fracture
HBV	hepatitis B virus (infection)
HCV	hepatitis C virus (infection)
HIV	human immunodeficiency virus (infection)
IDDM	insulin-dependent diabetes mellitus
IH	infectious hepatitis
KS	Kaposi's sarcoma
LBP	low back pain
MD	muscular dystrophy
MI	myocardial infarction (refers to the death of tissues due to loss of blood supply)
MRSA	methicillin resistant *Staphylococcus aureus*

continues

TABLE 5-4 *continued*

Diagnosis *continued*

MS	multiple sclerosis
NB	newborn
NIDDM	non–insulin-dependent diabetes mellitus
NSU	nonspecific urethritis
OA	osteoarthritis
OBS	organic brain syndrome
PID	pelvic inflammatory disease
PUD	peptic ulcer disease
PVD	peripheral vascular disease
RF	renal failure
RO, R/O	rule out
SDAT	senile dementia of Alzheimer's type
STD	sexually transmitted disease
TIA	transient ischemic attack
URI	upper respiratory infection
UTI	urinary tract infection
VRE	vancomycin resistant *enterococcus*

Patient Orders and Charting

@	at
$\bar{a}$	before
AAROM	active assistive (assisted) range of motion
abd.	abduction; abdomen
ACT	active, actively, activities
add.	adduction
ADL	activities of daily living
ad lib.	as desired
adm	admission; administer; administrator
ADT	admission, discharge, transfer
AEB	as evidenced by
AFO	ankle foot orthosis
aka	also known as
AMA	against medical advice
amb	ambulate, ambulatory

AROM	active range of motion
ASAP	as soon as possible
assist	assistance
as tol	as tolerated
B, (B), Ⓑ	bilateral, both
BB	bed bath
bil, bilat	bilateral
BLE	both lower extremities
B.M., bm	bowel movement
B/P	blood pressure
BPM	beats per minute
B.R.	bedrest; bathroom
BRP	bathroom privileges
BS	blood sugar
BSC	bedside commode
BSE	breast self-examination
BUE	both upper extremities
$\bar{c}$	with
cal	calorie
cath	catheterize, catheter
CBB	complete bed bath
CBR	complete bed rest
ck or √	check
ck or √ freq	check frequently
cl liq	clear liquid
C/O	complains of
CP	care plan; chest pain
CPM	continuous passive motion
CPR	cardiopulmonary resuscitation
DAT	diet as tolerated
dep	dependent
disch	discharge
DNR	do not resuscitate
DOA	dead on arrival
Dr	doctor
drsg	dressing
DSD	dry sterile dressing
Dx	diagnosis
E	enema
et	and

ETOH	ethanol (often used to refer to alcoholic beverages)
Eval	evaluation
ex.	exercise
exam	examination
ext.	extension; extremity; external
F	fair
FB	foreign body
FE	Fleet's enema
flex	flexion
FM	flow meter
FU, f/u	follow-up
FUO	fever of unknown origin
FWB	full weight bearing
G	good
g/c, GC	geriatric chair
GT	gastrostomy tube
H	hydrogen
H_2O	water
H_2O_2	hydrogen peroxide
HOB	head of bed
HOH	hard of hearing
ht	height
Hx	history
Ⓘ, ind.	independent
I&O	intake and output
IM	intramuscular
irrig	irrigation
isol	isolation
IV	intravenous
K^+	potassium
L	left
lat	lateral
LBP	low back pain
lg, lge, L	large
liq	liquid
L/min, LPM	liters per minute
LOC	loss of consciousness
max	maximum
min	minimum

continues

TABLE 5-4 *continued*

meds	medications	Rx	treatment; prescription	PMH	past medical history
mmHg	millimeters of mercury	s̄	without	R/O	rule out
mod	moderate	s/s, S & S	signs and symptoms	SOB	short(ness) of breath
NA, N/A	not applicable; nurse aide; nursing assistant	sm	small	UCD	usual childhood diseases
		SOB	short(ness) of breath	UK	unknown
N/C, no c/o	no complaints	SBA	standby assistance	WDWN	well-developed, well-nourished
neg, -	negative	SSE	soapsuds enema		
NG	nasogastric	stat	at once; immediately	WFL	within functional limits
NKA	no known allergies	std prec	standard precautions	WNL	within normal limits
NN	nurses' notes	Sx	symptoms	Y/O	years old
NPO	nothing by mouth	T, temp	temperature	YOB	year of birth
N/S, NSS	normal saline solution	TIAN	toilet in advance of need		
N & V	nausea and vomiting	TKO	to keep open	**Tests**	
NVD	nausea, vomiting, diarrhea	TLC	tender loving care		
NWB	no weight bearing	TPN	total parenteral nutrition	ABG	arterial blood gas study
O₂	oxygen	TPR	temperature, pulse, respiration	C & S	culture and sensitivity
occ	occasional			CBC	complete blood count
OOB	out of bed	trach	tracheostomy	CXR	chest x-ray
O, OS	oral; mouth	TWE	tap water enema	FBS	fasting blood sugar
P	poor, pulse	Tx	treatment	FSBS	fingerstick blood sugar
PB, PBB	partial bath, partial bed bath	ung	ointment (oint)	H & H	hemoglobin and hematocrit
per	by	vc	verbal cues	MRI	magnetic resonance imaging
p.o., PO	by mouth	V.S.	vital signs		
postop	postoperative	w/c	wheelchair	spec	specimen
preop	preoperative	WB	weight bearing	UA, U/A	urinalysis
prep	prepare	WBAT	weight bearing as tolerated		
p.r.n.	whenever necessary	wt	weight	**Places or Departments**	
prog	progress; prognosis				
PROM	passive range of motion	**Physical and History**		CS	central supply
PWB	partial weight bearing			DR, D/R	delivery room; dining room
Px	prognosis (prog)	CC	chief complaint		
q̄	each, every	DOB	date of birth	ED/ER	emergency department/ emergency room
q.s.	sufficient quantity	EENT	eye, ear, nose, throat		
qt	quiet	ENT	ear, nose, throat	ECG, EKG	electrocardiogram
R	rectal; respiration; right	FH	family history	EEG	electroencephalogram
re:	regarding	H & P	history and physical	EENT	eye, ear, nose, throat
rehab	rehabilitation	LMP	last menstrual period	GYN	gynecology
resp	respiration	L & W	living and well	ICCU	intensive coronary care unit
rot	rotated, rotation	M & F	mother and father		
rt (R)	right; routine	MH	marital history	IDT	interdisciplinary team
r/t	related to	NB	newborn	Lab	laboratory
RT	respiratory therapy	PE	physical examination	LTC	long-term care
		PI	present illness	MRD	medical record department

continues

TABLE 5-4 *continued*

Places or Departments *continued*

OPD	outpatient department
OR	operating room
OT	occupational therapy
PAR	post-anesthesia recovery
Peds, pedi	pediatrics
PT	physical therapy
RR	recovery room
RT	respiratory therapy
SNU	skilled nursing unit
ST	speech therapy
XR, X/R	x-ray

Time Abbreviations

a.c.	before meals
AM	morning
b.i.d.	twice a day
h	hour
noc, noct	night
p̄	after
p.c.	after meals
PM	evening or afternoon
q̄h	every hour
q̄4h	every four hours
q.i.d.	four times a day
q̄m (q̄AM)	every morning
t.i.d.	three times a day
WA, W/A	while awake

x, X	times
x2, x3 …	two times, three times, …

Roman Numerals

I	1
II	2
III	3
IV	4
V	5
VI	6
VII	7
VIII	8
IX	9
X	10

Other Common Numbers

1°	first; primary; first degree
2°	second; secondary to; second degree
3°	third; tertiary; third degree
1x, 2x, …	one time, one person; two times, two people, …

Measurements and Volume

amt.	amount
gtt	drop
mL	milliliter

L	liter
oz, ℥	ounce

Weight/Height

cm	centimeter
ft	feet
kg	kilogram
lb	pounds
in	inches
oz	ounce

Temperature

F	Fahrenheit
C	Celsius
°	degree

Symbols

♂	male
♀	female
↑	up, increase
↓	down, decrease
//	parallel
−, ⊖	minus, negative
+, ⊕	plus, positive
±, +/-	plus or minus
Δ	change to
°	degrees
∅	zero, none, nothing
✳	important

BODY ORGANIZATION

All nursing care is directed toward helping patients reach optimum health and independence. **Health** is a state of well-being in which all parts of the body and mind are functioning properly. **Disease** is any change from the healthy state. Disease takes many forms. Medical science is the study of disease and its effects on the human body. These effects are easier to understand when you have a clear picture in your mind of a normal and properly functioning body. The first step is to understand the organization of the body.

ANATOMIC TERMS

The **anatomy** (structure) and **physiology** (function) of the body are most easily understood and learned if they are studied in an orderly manner. Special terms are used to describe the relationship of one body part to another.

Whenever we describe the relationship of the body parts, keep in mind the **anatomic position** (Figure 5-3), which is:

- Standing erect with feet together or slightly separated
- Facing the observer
- Arms at the sides with the palms forward

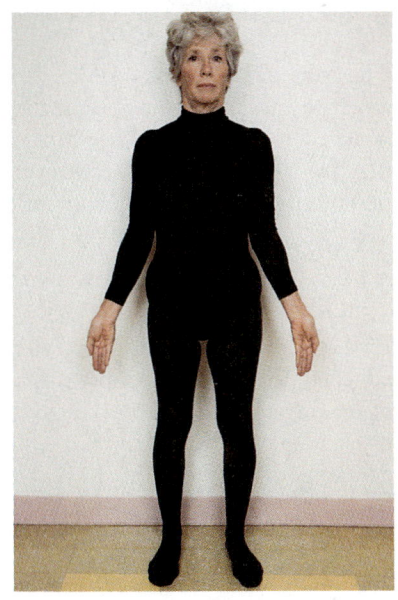

FIGURE 5-3 All references to body parts are made in relationship to the anatomic position.

In our own minds, we should always position the body in this way before describing any body part or area. This gives everyone the same frame of reference.

Notice as you look at a patient's body or the pictures in the book that you are seeing a mirror image of yourself. The patient's right side is opposite to your left and your left is opposite to the right of the patient or the picture.

Descriptive Terms

Imaginary lines drawn through the body (Figure 5-4) provide us with other reference terms.

- A line drawn down the center of the body from head to foot (the *midline*) divides the body into equal right and left sides. Note that the body has the same parts on either side. For example, there is an arm, a leg, an eye, and half of a nose on each side of the line.

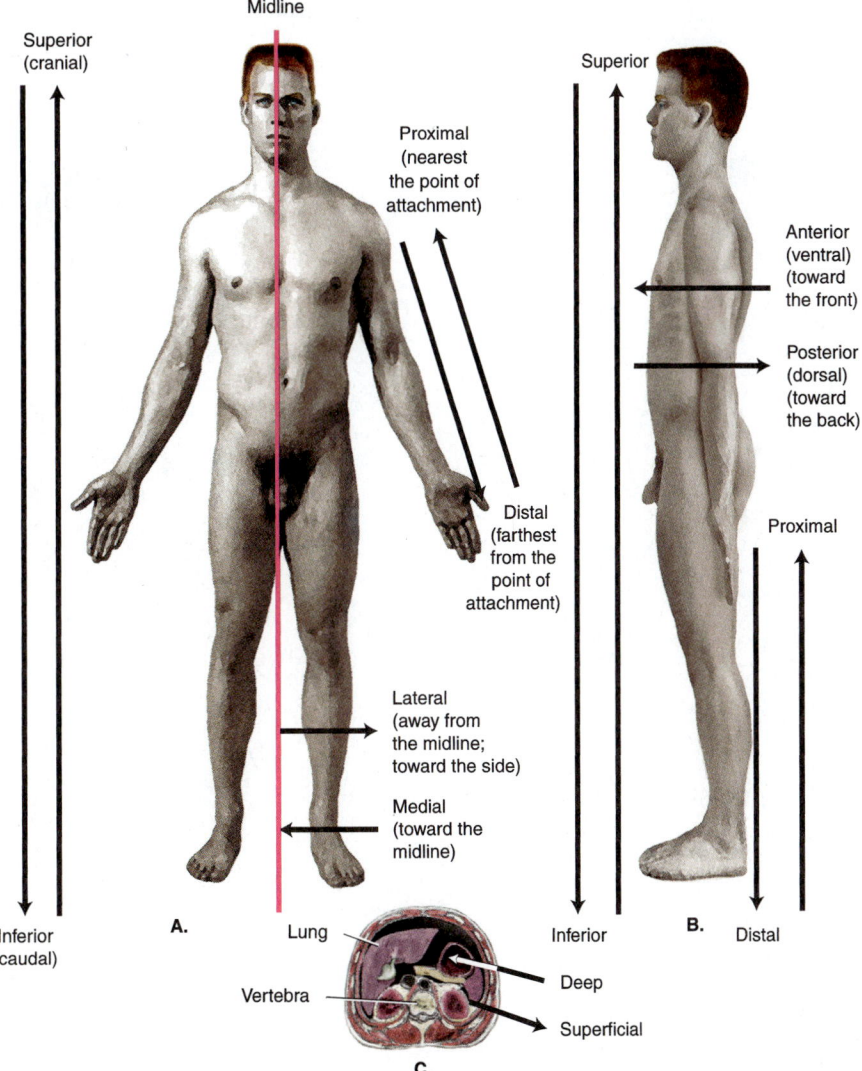

FIGURE 5-4 Imaginary lines are used to section the body to make it easier to locate parts. Directional terms relating to the anatomic position: (A) anatomic position; (B) lateral views of the body; (C) directional terms *deep* and *superficial*.

- Parts close to this line are **medial** to the line.
- Parts farther away from the line are **lateral** to the line.

For example, in the anatomic position, the thumbs are more lateral to the line and the little fingers are more medial to the line.

Another line drawn parallel to the floor divides the body into upper and lower parts. This line can be drawn at any level on the body as long as it is parallel to the floor.

- Parts located above this line are **superior** to the line.
- Parts located below this line are **inferior** to the line.

For example, if the line is drawn between the knees and ankles, the knees are superior to the ankles and the ankles are inferior to the knees.

A third line can be drawn to divide the body into front and back.

- Parts in front of this line are **anterior** or **ventral** to the line.
- Parts in back of this line are **posterior** or **dorsal** to the line.

Points of Attachment

The arms and legs are called the *extremities* of the body. The arms are attached to the body at the shoulders. The legs are attached to the body at the hips. Two terms are used to describe the relationship between the parts of the extremities and their points of attachment to the body.

- **Proximal**—means closest to the point of attachment
- **Distal**—means farthest away from the point of attachment

Because the upper arm is closest to the shoulder, where it is attached, this part is described as *proximal* when compared to the fingers, which are farthest away. The fingers are *distal* or farthest away from the point of attachment of the upper extremity.

Abdominal Regions

The abdomen is divided into four **quadrants**, with the **umbilicus** (navel) at the central point (Figure 5-5A). The abdomen can also be divided into nine regions (Figure 5-5B). Knowing these regions will be important as you report and document your observations.

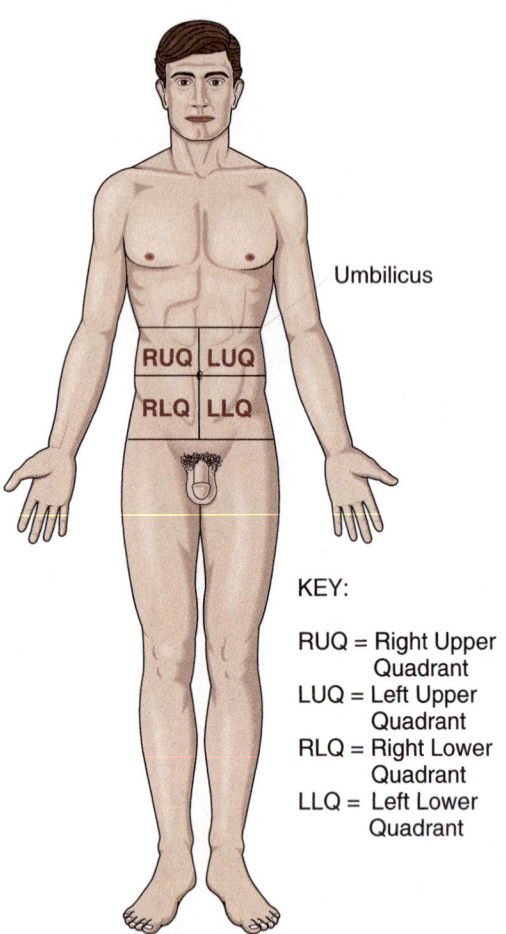

FIGURE 5-5A The abdominal quadrants.

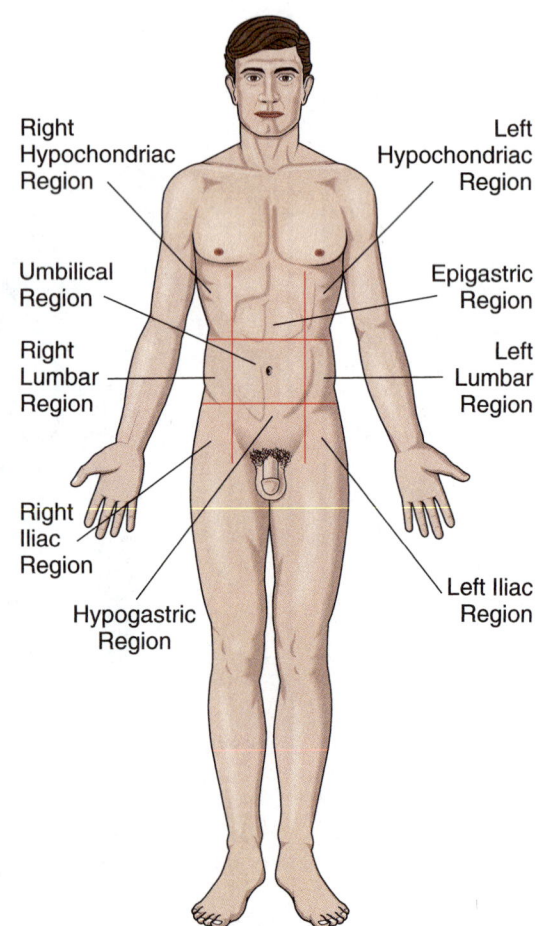

FIGURE 5-5B The abdomen can also be divided into nine regions.

ORGANIZATION OF THE BODY

All parts of the body are interdependent. The basic unit of the body is the **cell**. Groups of similar cells are organized into **tissues**. Different tissues form **organs**. The organs are organized into systems that perform the body functions.

Cells

Each cell performs the same basic functions that the total body performs, but on a smaller scale. These functions are breathing (respiration), reproduction, nutrition, and excretion (eliminating wastes). Some cells perform different kinds of work necessary for the body as a whole to function. Some of the various specialized types of cells are:

- Epithelial cells
- Nerve cells
- Muscle cells
- Connective tissue cells

Epithelial cells, which are very close together, form protective coverings and sometimes produce body fluids.

Nerve cells carry electrical messages to and from the different parts of the body, coordinating activities and making us aware of changes in the environment.

Muscle cells are special in their ability to shorten or lengthen, changing their shape and the position of parts to which they are attached. They also surround body openings, such as the mouth, to control the size of these openings.

Connective tissue cells are present throughout the body in many different types. They support and connect body parts.

Tissues

Groups of similar cells are organized into tissues. The basic tissue types are:

- Epithelial tissue
- Connective tissue
- Nervous tissue
- Muscle tissue

Epithelial tissue is specialized in its ability to absorb, secrete (produce) fluids, excrete (eliminate) waste products, and protect.

Nervous tissue forms the brain and spinal cord and the nerves throughout the body. This tissue is also found in the special sense organs such as the eyes, ears, and tastebuds. The activities of the rest of the body are directed and coordinated through the nervous tissues.

Three kinds of **muscle tissue** are found in the body:

- **Skeletal (voluntary) muscle** is attached to bones for movement.
- **Cardiac muscle** forms the heart wall.
- **Smooth (involuntary) muscle** (visceral) forms the walls of body organs such as the stomach and intestines.

Connective tissue forms blood, bone, and fibrous and elastic tissues to hold the skin on the body, attach muscles to bones, and support delicate cells throughout the body. Generally, connective tissues support and form connections for other tissue types.

Organs

Each organ is made up of more than one kind of tissue and performs special functions that contribute to the function of the body systems. Some organs, like the kidneys, are found in pairs. Some single organs contribute to more than one system. For example, the pancreas contributes secretions to both the endocrine and digestive systems.

Systems

The body has 10 major body systems. Table 5-5 lists the organs that contribute to the function of each system. Notice that some organs are included with more than one system. For example, the ovaries contribute to the endocrine system by producing female hormones and to the reproductive system by producing the egg.

Membranes

Membranes are sheets of epithelial tissues supported by connective tissues. Membranes:

- Cover the body
- Line body cavities
- Produce some body fluids

Important membranes include:

- **Mucous membranes**
  - Produce a fluid called **mucus**
  - Line body cavities that open to the outside

Because the respiratory, digestive, and genitourinary systems all open to the outside, they are lined with mucous membranes. The eyelids are also lined with a mucous membrane; a mucous membrane covers the eyeballs.

- **Synovial membranes**
  - Produce synovial fluid
  - Line joint cavities

The synovial fluid is a clear fluid resembling the white of an egg. It reduces the friction between the bones of active joints and the tendons.

- **Serous membranes**
  - Produce serous fluid
  - Cover the organs and line the closed cavities of the body

Serous fluid reduces friction as the organs work and move. Important serous membranes are the:

- **Pericardium**—surrounds the heart
- **Pleura**—surrounds the lungs and lines the thoracic cavity
- **Meninges**—cover the brain and spinal cord and line the dorsal cavity
- **Peritoneum**—covers the digestive organs and lines the abdominal cavity

TABLE 5-5 SYSTEMS OF THE BODY

System	Function	Structures
Cardiovascular	Transports materials around the body; carries oxygen and nutrients to the cells and carries waste products away; part of the immune system that provides protective cells and chemicals to fight current infections and protect against future infections	Heart, arteries, capillaries, veins, spleen, lymph nodes, lymphatic vessels, blood, lymph
Endocrine	Produces hormones that regulate body processes	Pituitary gland, thyroid gland, parathyroid glands, thymus gland, adrenal glands, testes, ovaries, pineal body, islets of Langerhans in pancreas
Gastrointestinal (Digestive)	Digests, transports food, absorbs nutrients, and eliminates wastes	Mouth, esophagus, pharynx, stomach, small intestine, large intestine, salivary glands, teeth, tongue, liver, gallbladder, pancreas
Integumentary	Protects the body from injury and against infection, regulates body temperature, eliminates some wastes	Skin, hair, nails, sweat and oil glands
Skeletal	Supports and protects body parts, produces blood cells, acts as lever in movement	Bones, joints
Muscular	Protects organs by forming body walls, forms walls of some organs, assists in movement by changing position of bones at joints	*Smooth* muscles—form walls of organs *Skeletal* muscles—attached to bones *Cardiac* muscles—form wall of heart
Nervous	Coordinates body functions	Brain, spinal cord, spinal nerves, cranial nerves, special sense organs such as eyes and ears
Reproductive	Reproduces the species, fulfills sexual needs, develops sexual identity	*Male:* Testes, epididymis, urethra, seminal vesicles, ejaculatory duct, prostate gland, bulbourethral glands, penis, spermatic cord *Female:* Breasts, ovaries, oviducts, uterus, vagina, Bartholin glands, vulva
Respiratory	Brings in oxygen and eliminates carbon dioxide	Sinuses, nose, pharynx, larynx, trachea, bronchi, lungs
Urinary	Manages fluids and electrolytes of body, eliminates liquid wastes	Kidneys, ureters, urinary bladder, urethra

- **Cutaneous membrane** (skin)
  - Protects the body
  - Covers the entire body
  - Helps to control body temperature
  - Eliminates wastes through sweat glands
  - Produces vitamin D when exposed to sunlight

Special epithelial cells in this membrane, called glands, secrete perspiration and oils.

Cavities

The body seems like a solid structure, but **cavities** (spaces) within it contain the organs. Table 5-6 lists the two main cavities, the dorsal cavity and the ventral cavity. Each of these cavities is lined by and divided into other cavities by serous membranes. These other cavities are also listed in the table, as are the organs contained in each.

Figure 5-6 is a simple drawing of the location of these cavities.

TABLE 5-6 BODY CAVITIES AND THE ORGANS CONTAINED WITHIN EACH CAVITY

	Cavity	Organs	
Dorsal Cavity			
	Cranial	Brain, pineal body, pituitary gland	
	Spinal	Nerves, spinal cord	
Ventral Cavity			
	Thoracic	Lungs, heart, great blood vessels, thymus gland	
	Abdominal Peritoneal	Stomach, small intestine, most of large intestine, liver, gallbladder, pancreas, spleen	
	Pelvic	*Male*	*Female*
		Seminal vesicles, prostate gland, ejaculatory ducts, urinary bladder, urethra, rectum	Uterus, oviducts, ovaries, urinary bladder, urethra, rectum
	Retroperitoneal space	Kidneys, adrenal glands, ureters	

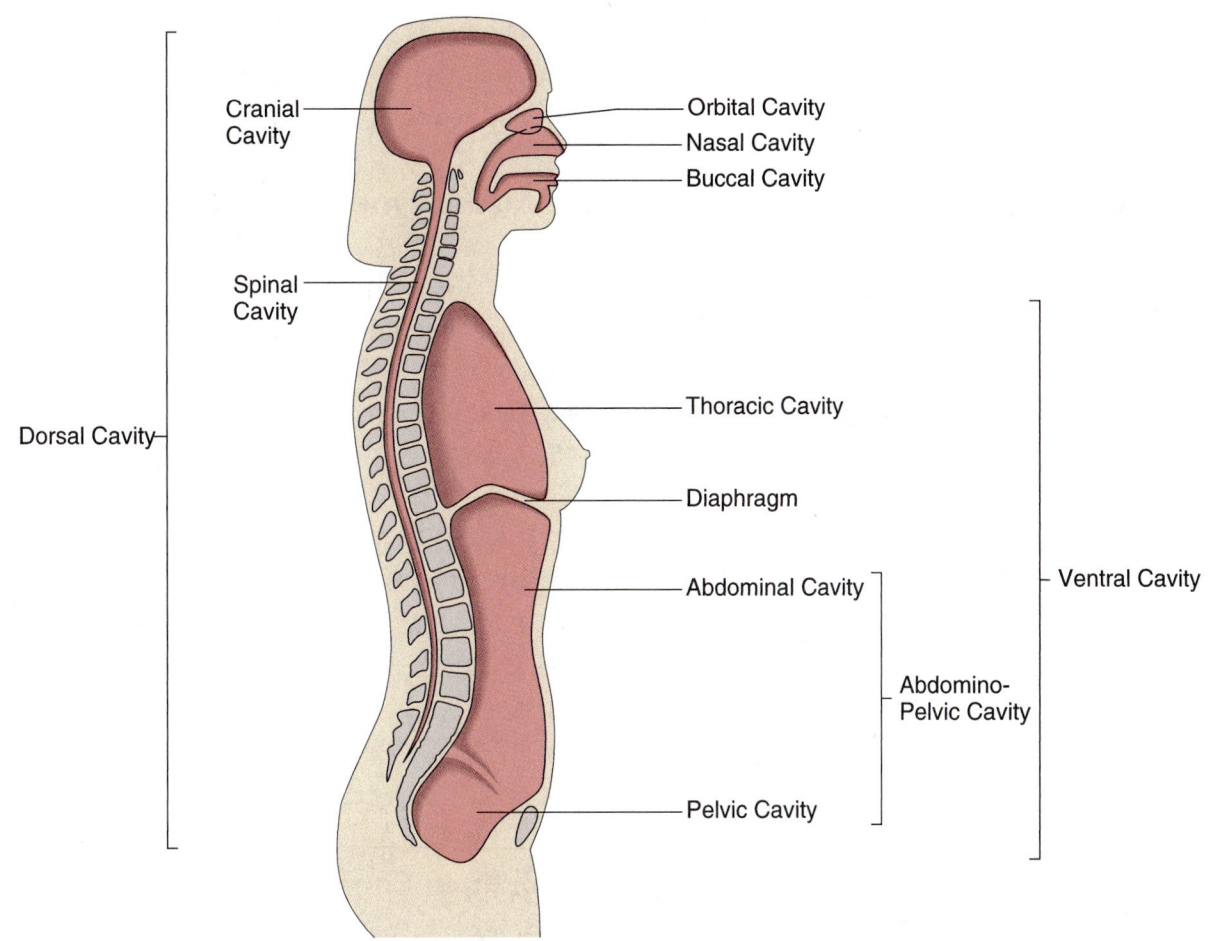

FIGURE 5-6 Lateral (side) view of the body cavities.

REVIEW

A. Matching.

Match the abbreviations in Column I with their meanings in Column II.

Column I

1. _d_ a.c. before
2. _i_ b.i.d.
3. _e_ OR
4. _b_ p.r.n.
5. _f_ p.o.
6. _j_ stat
7. _c_ h₂o
8. _l_ c̄
9. _k_ ung.
10. _h_ s̄
11. hs - sleep   hours
12. p̄ - after

Column II

a. three times a day
b. whenever necessary
c. water
d. before meals
e. operating room
f. by mouth
g. after meals
h. without
i. twice a day
j. at once
k. ointment
l. with

B. Matching.

Match the prefixes in Column I with their meanings in Column II.

Column I

11. _____ ur (o)
12. _____ cardi (o)
13. _____ chol (e)
14. _____ dermat (o)
15. _____ gastr (o)
16. _____ ot (o)
17. _____ ped (o)
18. _____ pneum (o)
19. _____ my (o)
20. _____ pharyng (o)

Column II

a. bile
b. ear
c. lung
d. child
e. muscle
f. pharynx
g. stomach
h. larynx
i. heart
j. urine
k. chest
l. skin

C. Define the following medical terms.

Then circle the prefix that you have learned.

21. dysuria _____
22. apnea _____
23. craniotomy _____
24. hypertension _____
25. tachycardia _____

D. Define the following medical terms.

Then circle the suffix that you have learned.

26. neuralgia _____
27. apnea _____
28. appendectomy _____
29. hematology _____
30. fibroma _____

E. Write the medical term that means the following.

31. kidney stones _____
32. examination of the rectum using an instrument _____
33. incision into thorax _____
34. inflammation of the stomach _____
35. white blood cell _____

F. In each of the following, circle the prefix and underline the suffix.

36. anemia
37. neuritis
38. pharyngitis
39. pandemic
40. tracheotomy

G. Measurements.

Print the abbreviations for the following.

41. milliliter   ml
42. kilogram   Kg
43. pound   lb.
44. Fahrenheit   F
45. inches   in

H. Print the Roman numerals for each of the following.

46. 2 _____
47. 5 _____
48. 6 _____
49. 9 _____
50. 10 _____

I. Multiple Choice.

Select the one best answer for each of the following.

51. When describing the relationship of the hand to the elbow, you should refer to the hand as being

a. proximal.
b. posterior.
c. distal.
d. anterior.

52. The appendix is located in which quadrant of the abdomen?
    a. URQ
    b. RLQ
    c. ULQ
    d. LLQ

53. Which membrane covers the lungs?
    a. Pleura
    b. Pericardium
    c. Peritoneum
    d. Meninges

54. Which organs are located in the dorsal cavity?
    a. Heart and liver
    b. Kidney and spleen
    c. Brain and spinal cord
    d. Uterus and testes

55. Which organ pumps blood throughout the body?
    a. Lungs
    b. Heart
    c. Liver
    d. Adrenal glands

56. Which organ is part of the skeletal system?
    a. Ureters
    b. Sternum
    c. Gallbladder
    d. Testes

57. The breasts are part of which system?
    a. Muscular
    b. Urinary

c. Cardiovascular
d. Reproductive

58. Membranes that line body cavities that open to the outside are called
    a. mucous membranes.
    b. basilar membranes.
    c. serous membranes.
    d. fibrous membranes.

59. The eye and ear are part of which system?
    a. Endocrine
    b. Nervous
    c. Cardiovascular
    d. Digestive

60. The endocrine system
    a. reproduces the species.
    b. brings in oxygen.
    c. transports blood.
    d. produces hormones.

(handwritten margin notes) benign — not cancerous; malignant — cancerous; inflammation — red hot; emetasicise — growing

J. True/False.

Mark the following true or false by circling T or F.

61. T F The urinary bladder and gallbladder are the same structure.

62. T F The pancreas functions in both the digestive and endocrine systems.

63. T F Muscular tissue enables the body to move.

64. T F Structures of different tissues acting together to carry out a specific function are called organs.

K. Nursing Assistant Challenge.

Examine the sample care plan and use your understanding of medical science and terminology to define each medical term and abbreviation used on the plan.

1.	**Patient Name** Bruce Tratt	**Age** 47	**Rel** Prot	#876-3291-7	
2.	**Physician** R. Morgan M.D.	**Dx** Splenomegaly—Diabetes Mellitus			
3.	**Orders**				
4.	**Preop orders** 3/18	on call for OR @ 8 am 3/19			
5.	Stat CBC, ABG, FBS				
6.	UA				
7.	NG Tube @ 6 am 3/19				
8.	Foley cath this pm.				
9.	Surg Prep.				
10.	NPO p̄ midnight				
11.	SSE @ HS.				
12.	Amb ad lib. this pm.				
13.					
14.	Anesthesiologist will call preop meds.				
15.					

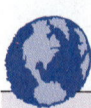 ## EXPLORING THE WEB

Description	Location
Converting common abbreviations to English terms	http://www.delmarhealthcare.com/olcs/jones/djappendices/glossaryc.pdf
Converting English terms to common abbreviations	http://www.delmarhealthcare.com/olcs/jones/djappendices/glossaryd.pdf
Converting English terms to medical word elements	http://www.delmarhealthcare.com/olcs/jones/djappendices/glossaryb.pdf
Converting medical word elements to English terms	http://www.delmarhealthcare.com/olcs/jones/djappendices/glossarya.pdf
Whole body terminology	http://www.delmarhealthcare.com/pdf/0766804933_04.pdf
Anat Line	http://anatline.nlm.nih.gov/Anatline/index.html
Focus on Medterms.com	http://www.medterms.com
Free-ed.net	http://www.free-ed.net
Gray's Anatomy	http://www.bartleby.com
Harvey Project	http://harveyproject.org
Med Term Web	http://ec.hku.hk/mt
MT Desk	http://mtdesk.com
National Institutes of Health (NIH)	http://health.nih.gov
Online Medical Dictionary	http://cancerweb.ncl.ac.uk
Online Tutorials	http://medi-smart.com
Patient's Guide to Med Term	http://www3.bc.sympatico.ca
Science Web	http://www.scienceteacherprogram.org
Stedman's Online Medical Dictionary	http://www.stedmans.com

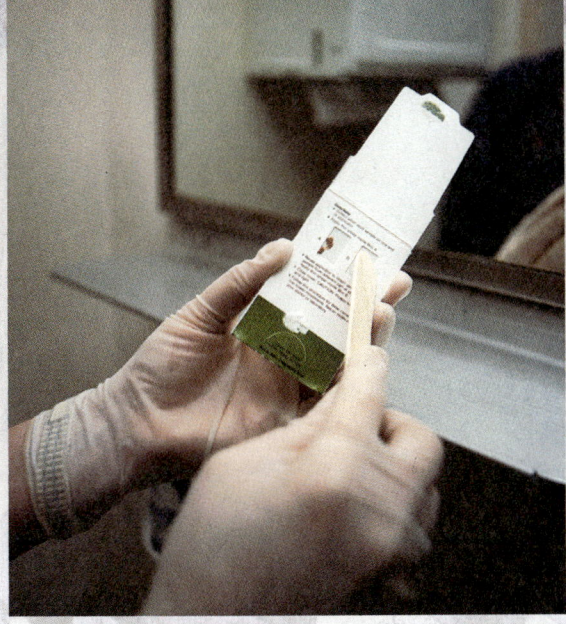

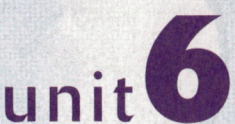

Classification of Disease

objectives

After completing this unit, you will be able to:
- Spell and define terms.
- Define disease and list some possible causes.
- Distinguish between signs and symptoms.
- List six major health problems.
- Identify disease-related terms.
- List ways in which a diagnosis is made.
- Describe malignant and benign tumors.

vocabulary

Learn the meaning and the correct spelling of the following words and phrases:

acute disease	congenital	malignant	risk factors
acute exacerbation	etiology	medical diagnosis	sarcoma
antibodies	genetic	metastasize	signs
autoimmune	hypersensitivity	neoplasm	symptoms
benign	immune response	noninvasive	therapy
cachexia	infection	obstruction	trauma
carcinoma	inflammation	predisposing factor	tumor
chronic disease	invasive	prognosis	vaccine
complication	ischemia	protocol	

INTRODUCTION

The nurse values your observations and uses them when making evaluations and planning nursing care for patients, as part of the nursing process. The better you understand the basic principles of disease, the more accurate information you can provide.

DISEASE

The body is a complex chemical factory that depends upon all of its parts to perform efficiently. It is subject to external and internal forces and stress that can threaten its ability to function properly (Figure 6-1).

Disease is any change from a healthy state. The disease (illness) may be a change in structure or function, or it may be the failure of a part of the body to develop properly. Each illness has

- An **etiology**—cause of the illness or abnormality.
- A usual set of indications that the illness is in progress. These are called signs and symptoms.
- A usual course or disease progression.
- A **prognosis** or probable outcome of the process.

Predisposing factors to disease are general conditions, such as malnutrition, that may contribute to the development of illness. Some diseases have related risk factors. **Risk factors** are specific behaviors or conditions that tend to

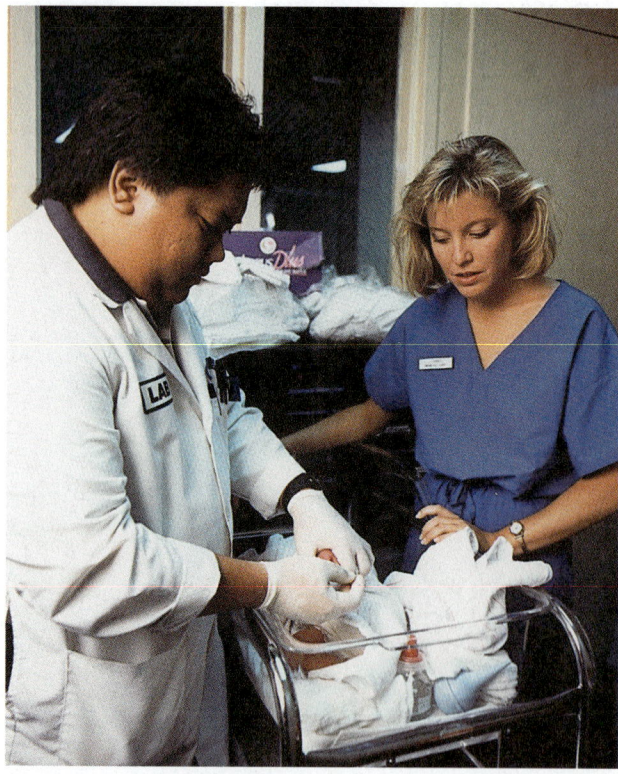

FIGURE 6-1 The laboratory technician draws blood from the heel of this newborn.

promote certain diseases (Figure 6-2). For example, smoking is a risk factor that increases the likelihood that the person will develop lung disease. Other risk factors and associated diseases include:

- Excess weight—high blood pressure, strokes, heart attack
- Poor nutrition—infections, skin breakdown
- Lack of exercise—osteoporosis
- High-fat, low-fiber diet—cancer of the colon
- Unprotected sex—hepatitis, AIDS, gonorrhea
- Family history—breast cancer, heart disease, diabetes mellitus

A young child who is malnourished and underweight is much more likely to develop an infection than one who is well nourished. The germs causing the infection are the actual cause of the illness, but the age and nutritional state of the child contribute to the development of the infectious process. Table 6-1 lists common causes of disease (both external and internal) and a number of risk factors for disease.

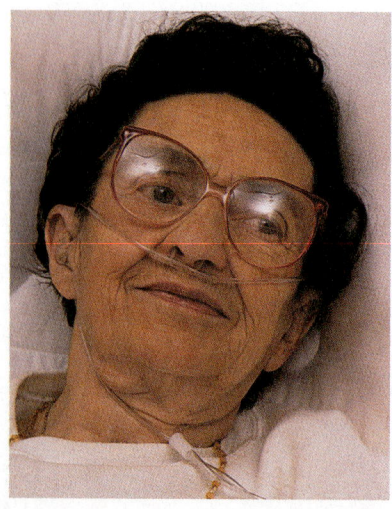

FIGURE 6-2 Advanced age is a factor that predisposes the person to the development of some diseases.

TABLE 6-1	COMMON CAUSES OF DISEASE AND PREDISPOSING FACTORS	
External Etiology	**Internal Etiology**	**Predisposing Factors**
traumas	metabolic disorders	age
radiation	congenital abnormalities	malnutrition
microorganisms	tumors	heredity
chemical agents		previous illness

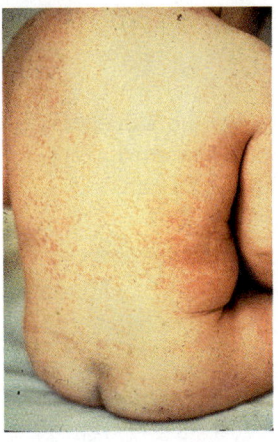

FIGURE 6-3 A maculopapular rash is characteristic of skin changes in measles (rubeola). *(Photo courtesy of the Centers for Disease Control and Prevention, Atlanta, Georgia)*

Signs and Symptoms

Signs of a disease can be seen by others. The color or condition of the skin is an example of a sign of disease (Figure 6-3). **Symptoms** are felt by the patient, who tells us about them. Pain is a symptom common to many illnesses (Figure 6-4).

The Course (Pattern) of Disease

The development and course of different illnesses vary greatly. **Acute disease** develops suddenly, progresses rapidly, and lasts for a predictable period, and then the person recovers (or dies). For example, the signs and symptoms of an infected finger may develop rapidly and last a relatively short period. Then, as the body controls the process, recovery is seen.

With a **chronic disease**, there are often periods when the patient experiences the signs and symptoms and periods when evidence of the disease is less pronounced or disappears altogether. Rheumatoid arthritis is such a disease. At times the affected joints are red, hot to the touch, swollen, and painful. At other times, the signs and symptoms seem

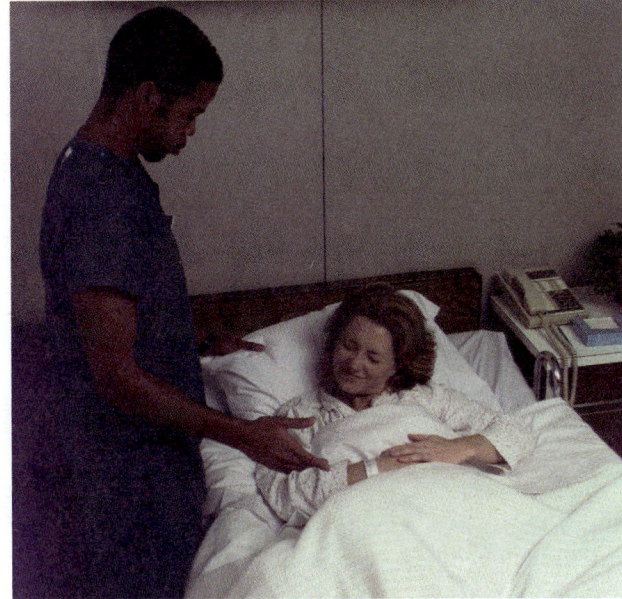

FIGURE 6-4 Sometimes patients communicate pain through their body language.

to go away. An **acute exacerbation** of a chronic disease is when the severity of signs and symptoms increases.

Complications

A **complication** makes the original condition more serious. For example, if a child has measles and develops pneumonia (a serious lung condition), the pneumonia is a complication that makes it more difficult for the child to recover.

MAJOR CONDITIONS

Some of the major conditions or illnesses that can affect the body's ability to function are:

- **Ischemia**—the lack of adequate blood supply to a body tissue, which prevents delivery of the essential

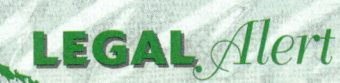

LEGAL *Alert*

Reporting and recording your observations of patients are key nursing assistant responsibilities. Pay attention to details. Practice good communication skills. You will learn which observations must be reported immediately, and which can wait until the end of the shift. An alert, observant nursing assistant is invaluable in protecting patients' safety and well-being.

oxygen and nutrients. For example, a blood clot (thrombus) that has formed within a blood vessel wall can block the blood vessel.

- **Congenital** abnormalities—abnormalities that are present at birth (Figure 6-5). Some abnormalities occur while the baby is growing in the mother's uterus. Examples include:
  - Spina bifida—a defect in the formation of the vertebral column
  - Cleft lip—an imperfection in the formation of the upper lip
  - Agenesis of a kidney—one kidney fails to develop, so the baby is born with only one functioning kidney
  - Talipes (club foot)—the child's foot is turned or twisted out of its normal position

Some abnormalities are due to defects in the **genetic** information passed from the parents to the child. Examples include:

- Sickle cell anemia—the red blood cells are improperly formed so they do not maintain their normal disc shape
- Color blindness—the person is unable to distinguish between certain colors
- Hemophilia—there is a lack of an important blood component needed for proper blood clotting.

- **Infection**—Infectious organisms or their products cause infection, including pneumonias, scarlet fever, and abscesses. Inflammation is usually part of the infectious process.

- **Inflammation** is a localized protective reaction of tissue to irritation, injury, or infection. It is characterized by pain, redness, swelling, a feeling of heat on the skin, and loss of function. Inflammations that develop for reasons other than infection include:
  - **Autoimmune** reactions—Mechanisms that are designed to protect the body turn against the body and cause damage, resulting in conditions such as rheumatoid arthritis (RA), systemic lupus erythematosus (SLE), and multiple sclerosis (MS).
  - **Hypersensitivity** reactions—Allergic types of reactions such as hay fever, skin rashes, and asthma.
  - Irritations—May be caused by seeds in the intestinal tract, stones in the gallbladder or kidney, or redness of the skin due to chemical exposure.

- Metabolic imbalances—Conditions of fluid and electrolyte imbalance include malnutrition, edema, scurvy, alcoholism, and diabetes mellitus.

- **Obstruction**—Tubes throughout the body carry a variety of materials that must continue to flow. Obstructions impede the flow. Examples of obstructions include blood clots in blood vessels, stones in the bile ducts or the kidneys, and blockages that occur when the tube structures become twisted, as in an intestinal obstruction.

- **Trauma**—Injuries that cause tissue damage resulting from a blow to the body, such as an auto accident. Exposure to unusual pressure or extremes of temperature also causes trauma.

- Neoplasm—The word **neoplasm** means new growth. It is another term for **tumor**. Neoplasms are an important kind of disease. There are two types of neoplasms: benign or nonmalignant tumors and malignant tumors. Sometimes benign tumors can change and become malignant. People with a malignant tumor or a malignancy are said to have cancer. Neoplasms are discussed further later in this unit.

DIAGNOSIS

The **medical diagnosis** (the process of identifying and naming the disease) is made by the physician. To do this, the patient is examined, a history of previous illness is taken and reviewed, and various laboratory and diagnostic tests are performed. The physician compiles the information, matches it to possible diseases, and then names the process to establish the medical diagnosis.

Diagnostic Studies

Laboratory tests (Figure 6-6) and diagnostic studies give the physician valuable information for naming the disease process and for planning the proper treatment for the patient. The nursing staff prepares the patient for the ordered tests and cares for the patient after the tests are completed. The nursing assistant helps give this care and may be assigned to collect certain specimens.

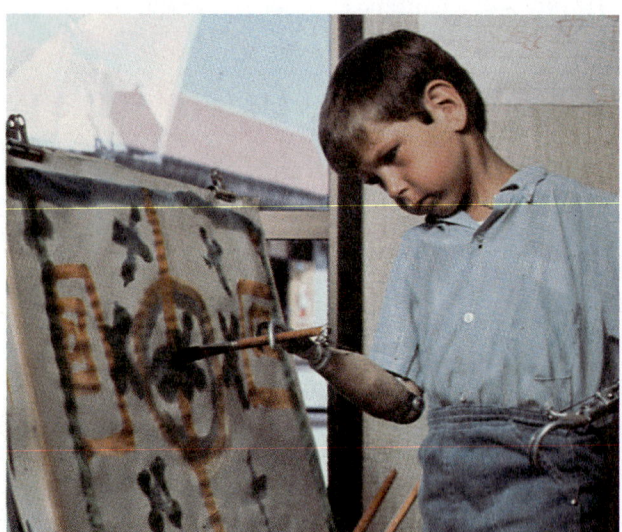

FIGURE 6-5 This child has phocomelia. His hands did not develop before birth because a drug taken by the mother during early pregnancy interfered with limb development. *(Photo courtesy of the March of Dimes—Birth Defects Foundation)*

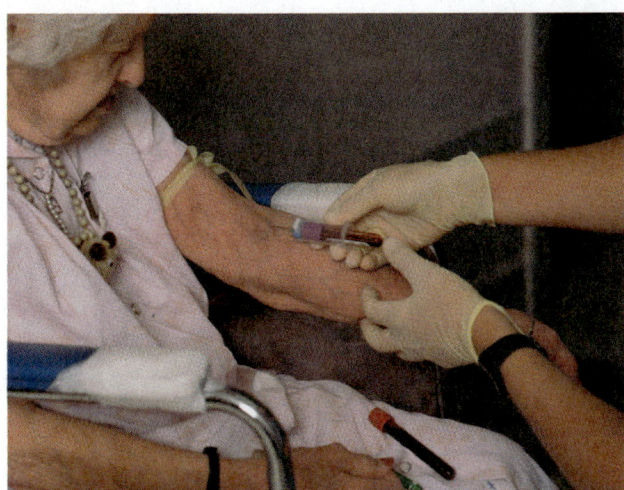

FIGURE 6-6 Blood tests provide information about the chemistry of the body and contribute to a correct medical diagnosis.

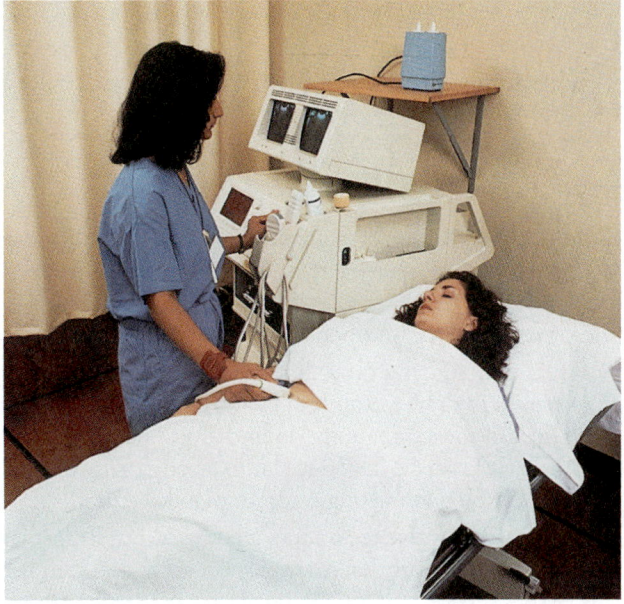

FIGURE 6-7 The sonogram of the uterus provides useful information about the developing fetus.

Protocols are standards of procedure and care developed for the preparation and care of the patient for each test or study. Protocols must be followed carefully to achieve satisfactory results. Improper patient preparation can result in:

- Inability to perform the test
- Inaccurate test results
- Delayed diagnosis
- Increased costs
- Increased patient anxiety
- Slower recovery

Noninvasive Tests

Some tests and studies are **noninvasive**. This means that the techniques used do not break the skin or damage body tissues. For example, x-rays do not break the skin, but do give information about internal body structures. Commonly ordered noninvasive tests include:

- Ultrasound—sound waves are bounced against the body to measure variations in tissue density (Figure 6-7). For example, the Doppler ultrasound probe measures the blood flow in blood vessels. Sonograms of a pregnant woman's uterus give information about the growing fetus.
- Thermography—measures the temperature in different body tissues. Thermograms of the breast indicate increased temperature in tumorous tissue.
- X-ray and fluoroscopy—use short-wavelength electromagnetic radiation to examine internal tissues. X-ray techniques are sophisticated. One of the newest techniques is computerized axial tomography (CT scan or CAT scan). This procedure gives a three-dimensional view of the internal structures of the body. A computer records and prints out information.
- Magnetic resonance imaging (MRI)—an imaging technique that provides excellent pictures (images) with

minimal risk to the patient (Figure 6-8). The body is placed in a strong magnetic field. Radio frequency pulses cause certain chemicals (ions) in body tissues to change position. When the radio waves are discontinued, the ions return to their original positions. As they go back to normal, the energy given off is recorded. All of this occurs without the patient feeling any of it.

- Recording of the electrical activity occurring in different body organs. A recording of this activity is made on paper or on a screen for viewing. Such examinations include:
  - Electrocardiogram (EKG or ECG) to record electrical activity of the cardiac cycle

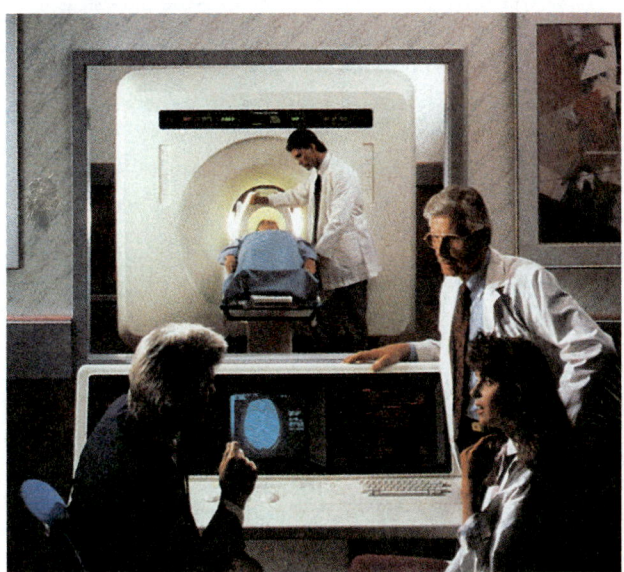

FIGURE 6-8 An MRI provides much detail during scans of portions of the body. *(Courtesy of GE Medical Systems)*

– Electroencephalogram (EEG) to record electrical activity of the brain
– Electromyogram (EMG) to record electrical activity of muscles

Invasive Tests

Some tests and studies actually penetrate body surfaces and thus are known as **invasive** tests. Examples of invasive tests include taking tissue samples, introducing contrast media, and probing deeply into body cavities.

A sternal puncture is a procedure in which a needle pierces the sternum to draw a sample of blood-producing cells. For some invasive examinations, iodine dyes, barium compounds, or air may be introduced into a body cavity to produce contrast when making recordings and pictures.

Most of these invasive techniques are carried out in special areas, such as laboratories, that are specifically designed for this purpose. Also, patient specimens usually are examined in laboratories.

Some special invasive procedures include:

• Direct visualization procedures—to examine body parts with instruments (scopes) introduced into the body. For example, the proctoscope, inserted in the anus, allows direct observation of the interior rectum. Other direct visualization procedures are:
  – Cystoscopy to observe the bladder
  – Laryngoscopy to observe the larynx
  – Sigmoidoscopy to observe the colon
• Dye studies—dyes are introduced into the body to outline body parts so that they will show up on x-rays. Some examples are:
  – Upper GI series (barium swallow)—the patient swallows a barium solution and then x-rays or fluoroscopy show the structures highlighted.
  – Lower GI series (barium enema)—the patient is given the barium rectally. The patient holds the solution while x-rays are taken.
  – Myelogram—dye is introduced into the spinal canal and then x-rays are taken.
• Cardiac catheterization—a catheter (small sterile tube) is introduced into the vascular system and delivers a dye. As the catheter is moved through the blood vessels and heart chambers, a monitor shows the dye flowing through this system.

Other Techniques

Chemical and microscopic studies examine samples of various body tissues and secretions. Getting some samples requires invasive procedures. Other sampling requires non-invasive procedures. The most common samples are:

• Blood
• Urine

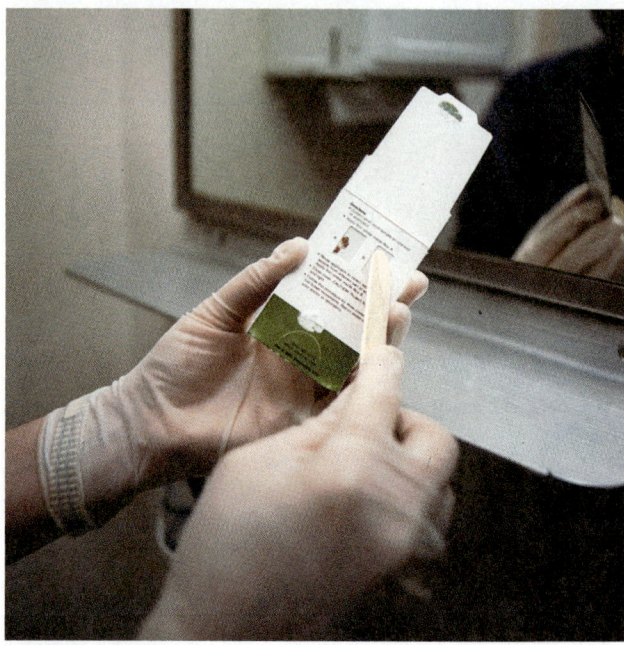

FIGURE 6-9 Stool specimens may be examined for occult (hidden) blood.

• Sputum from the lungs
• Cultures from infected tissues
• Gastric secretions
• Feces (Figure 6-9)

THERAPY

Once the medical diagnosis is confirmed, it is possible to predict the course of the disease and a probable prognosis (likely outcome or course of the disease process). Then the most appropriate **therapy** (treatment) is determined.

There are four basic approaches to therapy. They may be used alone or in different combinations.

1. Surgery: This form of therapy may remove unhealthy tissue (Figure 6-10), replace unhealthy parts, or repair injured, malformed, or congenitally defective areas. Prostatectomies remove unhealthy prostate glands. Coronary bypasses replace blocked arteries with other arteries. Herniorrhaphies repair weakened muscle walls.

2. Chemotherapy: This form of therapy uses drugs and chemicals to promote and improve body functions and to control pain (Figure 6-11). For example, the patient with a fever is given an antipyretic, such as acetaminophen (Tylenol), to reduce the temperature.

3. Radiation: This form of therapy uses controlled radioactivity or x-rays to destroy tumor cells.

4. Supportive (palliative) care: This form of therapy is designed to support the patient's body in its attempt

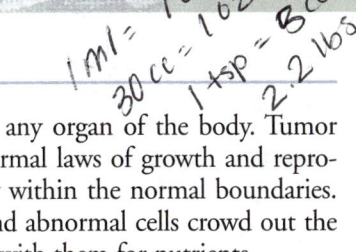

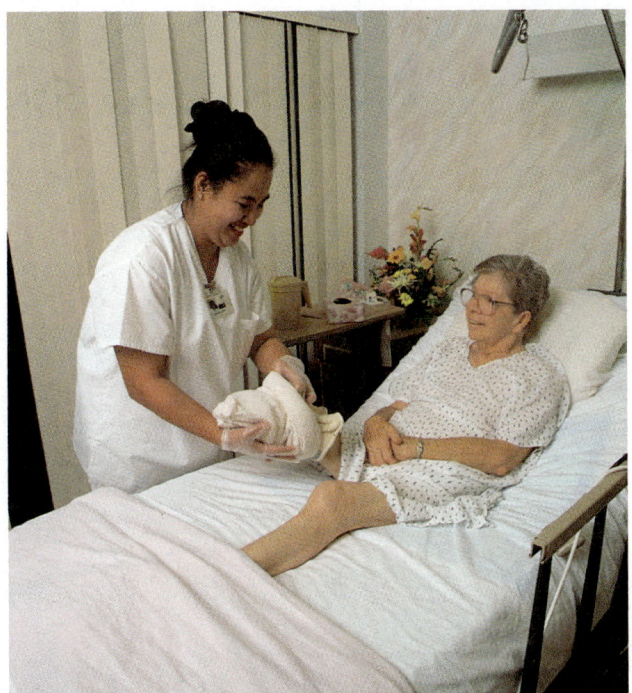

FIGURE 6-10 This patient's leg was amputated because of peripheral vascular disease.

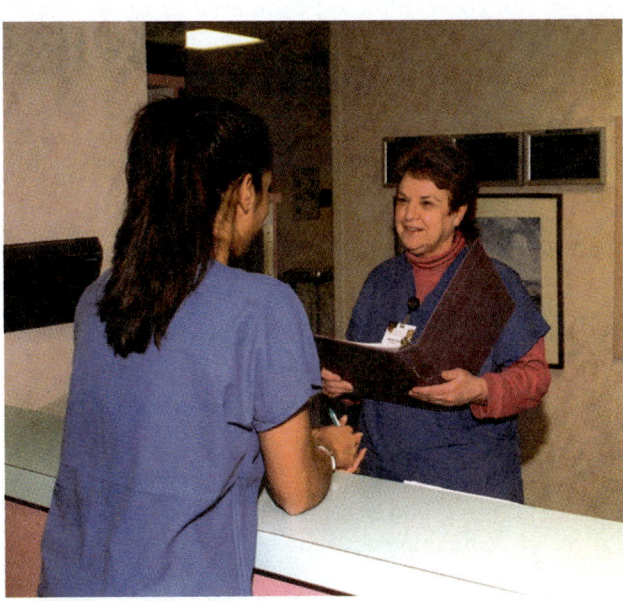

FIGURE 6-11 The nursing assistant reports the patient's complaint of the pain to the registered nurse, who will administer pain medication ordered by the physician.

to stay healthy or return to health. For example, positioning a person upright makes it easier for him to breathe when he is having an asthmatic attack. Pain control, rest, proper nutrition, fluid intake, and good hygiene all aid the body's own attempt to control the effects of illness.

NEOPLASMS

Tumors can affect almost any organ of the body. Tumor cells do not follow the normal laws of growth and reproduction and may not stay within the normal boundaries. Excess numbers of cells and abnormal cells crowd out the normal cells and compete with them for nutrients.

Types of Tumors

Different types of tumors are more common among certain groups of people. Children have more tumors of the nervous system, urinary system, and hematopoietic (blood-forming) system. Adults have more tumors of the reproductive organs, lungs, and colon.

The two major types of tumors are classified as benign or malignant. Each type has its own characteristics.

Benign or nonmalignant tumors:

- Usually grow slowly
- Do not spread
- Are usually encapsulated (surrounded by a capsule)
- Do not cause death unless located in a vital area such as the brain
- Are usually named by stating the part of the body involved and adding the suffix -oma. For example, *osteoma* names a benign bone tumor.

Malignant tumors or cancerous growths:

- Grow relatively rapidly
- Spread to other body parts (**metastasize**)
- If untreated, cause death
- May be named sarcoma or carcinoma or have special names like leukemia.
  - **Carcinomas** are spread primarily by way of the lymph system to the lymph nodes. They occur more commonly in people over 40 years of age.
  - **Sarcomas** are spread primarily by way of the bloodstream. They occur more commonly in people under 40 years of age.

Early Detection

Early detection of cancer can often result in a cure. The sooner the cancer is found, the higher the rate of cure. Pain is usually a late symptom.

Early Signs and Symptoms. Early signs and symptoms of malignancies include:

Change in bowel or bladder habits

A sore that does not heal

Unusual bleeding or discharge

Thickening or lump in breast or elsewhere

Indigestion or difficulty in swallowing

Obvious change in wart or mole

Nagging cough or hoarseness

Note: The first letters of these early signs and symptoms spell **CAUTION**.

Late Signs and Symptoms. Late signs and symptoms of malignancies include:

Fever of unknown origin

Cachexia or general wasting of the body tissues with loss of weight

Anemia

Pain due to pressure, obstruction, and ischemia

Hormonal irregularities

Inflammations of the skin

BODY DEFENSES

The body has a natural line of defense against disease. These defenses include:

- Unbroken skin and mucous membranes, which act as mechanical barriers
- Mucus, which traps foreign particles, and cilia (small hairlike structures), which propel them out of the body
- The acidity of certain body secretions such as perspiration, saliva, and stomach juices, which slows the growth of microorganisms
- White blood cells, which surround and destroy anything foreign that enters the body
- Inflammation
- The immune response

Inflammation

The process of inflammation, which we often associate with infections such as boils and abscesses, is really an important part of the body's natural defenses. When anything foreign enters the body, small blood vessels (capillaries) in the area get bigger (dilate), bringing more blood to the infected part. In the blood are white blood cells and other protective substances. Fluid (serum) and white blood cells pass through the capillary walls into the area and a wall is gradually built up around the foreign object. As the white blood cells try to destroy the invader, pressure builds up to force the material to the surface of the body. The inflammatory process takes place to some extent in the body whenever injury occurs. The signs and symptoms of acute inflammation are:

- Redness
- Swelling
- Heat
- Loss of function
- Pain

Immune Response

Immune response (immunity) protects the body against specific infections by producing special chemicals called **antibodies**. For example, a person exposed to the measles virus may become ill with the disease. After recovery, the antibodies formed by the person against the measles virus will protect him from becoming sick again with the same disease.

Vaccines (altered germs or their products) may be given before exposure to a disease. The body can then produce antibodies before actual exposure occurs.

REVIEW

A. Matching.

Match the statements in questions 1–10 with the correct terms in the list a–j.

1. __g__ Probable outcome
2. __e h__ Color of the skin
3. __d__ Cause of disease
4. __b__ Noncancerous tumor
5. __i__ Pain as reported by the patient
6. __a__ Illness with sudden onset and short course
7. __j__ Injury
8. __c__ Inflammation

a. acute
b. benign
c. a natural body defense
d. etiology
e. genetic
f. malignancy
g. prognosis
h. sign

9. __e__ Condition transmitted from one generation to another

10. __f__ Cancer

i. symptom
j. trauma

B. Fill-In.

For each of the items in questions 11–15, mark which is a sign and which is a symptom.

11. sign dry, flushed skin
12. sym nausea
13. sym dizziness
14. sym sign rapid pulse
15. sym elevated temperature
sign

C. Matching.

Match the abnormality with its classification by matching Column I with Column II.

Column I	Column II
16. _d_ abscessed tooth	a. ischemia
17. _g_ adenosarcoma	b. congenital
18. _h_ renal stones	c. infectious
19. _a,h_ thrombosis	d. inflammation
20. _c_ strep throat	e. metabolic imbalance
21. _f_ frostbite	f. trauma
22. _g_ osteoma	g. neoplasm
23. _d_ rheumatoid arthritis	h. obstruction
24. _b_ spina bifida	
25. _b_ sickle cell anemia	

D. True/False.

Mark the following true or false by circling T or F.

26. T (F) The medical diagnosis is made by the supervising nurse.

27. (T) F Nursing assistants may be assigned to collect certain specimens.

28. T (F) Protocols are drugs given in diagnostic testing.

29. (T) F Proper patient preparation contributes to the success of diagnostic testing.

30. (T) F Improper patient preparation may cause faulty results.

31. (T) F Ultrasound is used to give information about a growing fetus.

32. T (F) Thermography uses radio waves to test the electrical current of tissues.

33. T (F) An upper GI series is an x-ray of the gallbladder. *stomach*

34. (T) F Nursing assistants may be asked to deliver specimens.

35. (T) F Nursing assistants may contribute to the diagnostic testing process by offering emotional support to the patient.

E. Completion.

Write out the early signs of possible malignancies.

36. C *hange in bowel*

37. A *sore that doesn't heal*

38. U *nusual bleeding*

39. T *hickening /lump in breast*

40. I *ndigestion*

41. O *bvious change in wart/mole*

42. N *agging cough*

F. Nursing Assistant Challenge.

Read each clinical situation and answer the questions.

43. Your patient is 82 years old, poorly nourished, and has a diagnosis of pneumonia.

   a. Name two factors that might predispose your patient to pneumonia. _____

   _____

   b. Will these factors make recovery more or less difficult? _____

   c. How would you classify the illness pneumonia?

   _____

44. Your patient is six years old and has a broken leg. He also has a condition that he inherited from his parents. This condition makes his bones brittle so they break more easily.

   a. What word would you use to describe his inherited condition? _____

   b. What term would you use to classify his inability to make strong bones? _____

   c. Do you think this kind of injury might occur often? _____

45. Your patient is 45 years old, 40 pounds overweight, and gets little exercise. Her diagnosis is high blood pressure. She is scheduled for an ECG.

   a. What factors might contribute to her diagnosis?

   _____ _____

   b. For what conditions is she at risk? _____

   c. What information will the ECG provide?

   _____

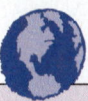
EXPLORING THE WEB

Description	Location
ADAM Medical Encyclopedia	*http://www.nlm.nih.gov/medlineplus/encyclopedia.htm*
Combined Health Information Database	*http://chid.nih.gov*
Discovery Health	*http://health.discovery.com*
Health on the Net	*http://www.hon.ch*
Merlot Health Science	*http://www.merlot.org*
National Health Information Center	*http://www.health.gov/nhic*
National Institutes of Health (NIH)	*http://health.nih.gov*
National Library of Medicine	*http://www.nlm.nih.gov*
Virtual Hospital	*http://www.vh.org*

Basic Human Needs and Communication

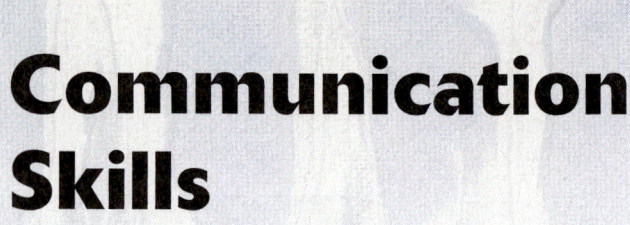

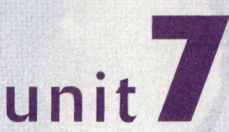

Communication Skills

objectives

After completing this unit, you will be able to:

- Spell and define terms.
- Explain the types of verbal and nonverbal communication.
- Describe and demonstrate how to answer the telephone while on duty.

- Describe four tools of communication for staff members.
- Describe the guidelines for communicating with patients with impaired hearing, impaired vision, aphasia, and disorientation.

vocabulary

Learn the meaning and the correct spelling of the following words and phrases:

aphasia	communication	nonverbal	staff development
assignment	disorientation	communication	symbols
body language	ethnic	organizational chart	verbal
braille	medical chart	shift report	communication
care plan	memo	sign language	

INTRODUCTION

Communication is a two-way process. It is the way in which information—whether facts or feelings—is shared. For communication to happen, both a "sender" and a "receiver" of the information are needed. Information can be sent orally, in writing, and through body language. Nursing assistants communicate with their patients (Figure 7-1), with visitors, with their coworkers, and with their supervisors when they are working. As a nursing assistant, you will need to receive and send information about your:

- Observations and care of patients
- Interactions with patients and visitors
- Patients' feelings

This information is received and sent through the process of communication.

COMMUNICATION IN HEALTH CARE

Communication between staff members must be effective if the patients are to receive the safest and best care. Communication with your patients and their visitors is also important. You and your patients must understand each other. Three things are needed for successful communication: (1) a sender, (2) a clear message, and (3) a receiver.

Verbal Communication

Verbal communication uses words. They may be spoken or written. Written communication also depends on the use of **symbols**. Traffic signs are an example of symbols. You will use words to explain to patients what you plan to do in carrying out a procedure and how they can help. Your nurse or team leader will use words to explain your assignment. You will use words to report your observations (Figure 7-2), as well as written communication in your charting. You will use words to answer visitors' questions.

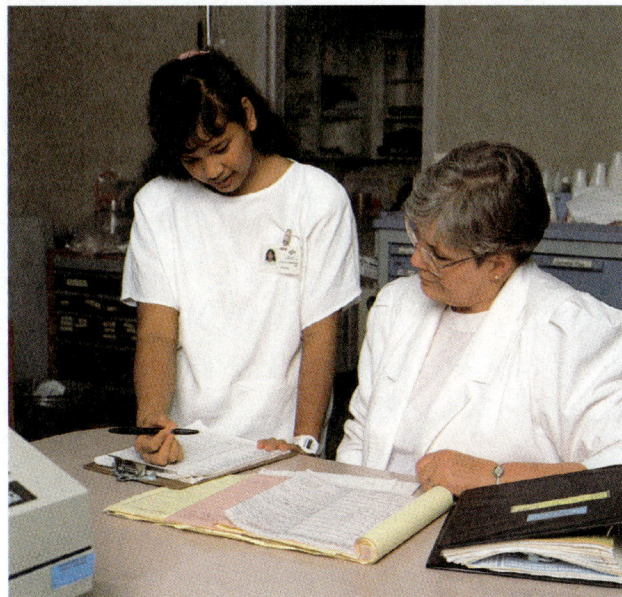

FIGURE 7-2 Verbal communication is used to report your observations to the nurse.

Choose words carefully so that your message is clear. Tone of voice, choice of words, and hand movements give clues to the real meaning of the message. Listen carefully to the message and watch the sender's facial expressions and body language.

Nonverbal Communication

Nonverbal communication is a message that is sent through the use of one's body, rather than through speech or writing. This kind of communication, called **body language**, can tell you a great deal (Figure 7-3). Often nonverbal messages send even stronger signals than verbal messages. A patient who is in pain may protect the affected area. Tears or an unwillingness to make eye contact with you may be a sign of depression. Some of the other ways

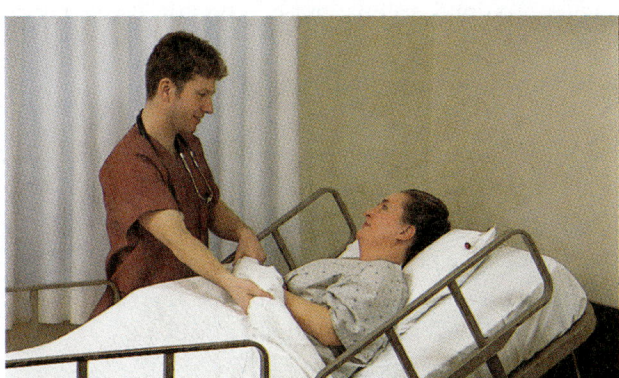

FIGURE 7-1 Nursing assistants communicate with patients in many different ways.

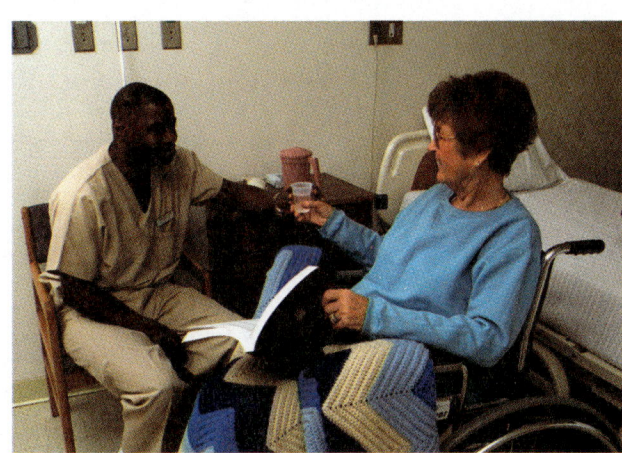

FIGURE 7-3 This patient's body language sends a positive message.

your patients may "talk" to you through their body language include:

- posture
- hand and body movements
- activity level
- facial expressions
- overall appearance
- body position

COMMUNICATING WITH STAFF MEMBERS

In Unit 2 you learned that each health care facility has a line of authority and communication. The organizational chart is a guide for communication and spells out the line of authority. Each facility has an organizational chart that illustrates how a department relates to other departments. Some of the larger departments, such as nursing, have their own charts that indicate the line of authority within the department (Figure 7-4). As a nursing assistant, you will need to learn methods to communicate with other staff members in nursing and with members of other departments.

Oral Communications

Oral reports are used frequently to communicate information about patients. When you first come on duty, you will listen to the shift report. The nurse who worked the previous shift will report to oncoming staff. This report will include:

- changes in patients' conditions
- information about new patients

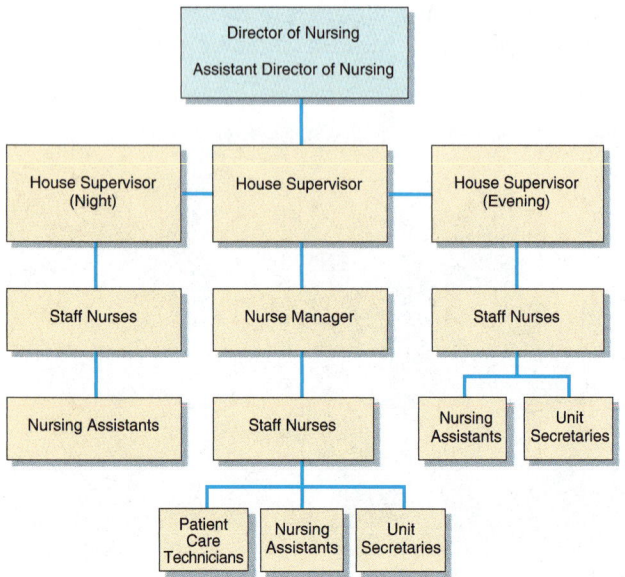

FIGURE 7-4 Nursing department organizational chart.

- names of patients who were discharged or died
- any incidents that occurred to patients
- new physicians' orders
- special events for the patients that will occur during your shift

Listen carefully to the report because it will help you plan your assignment (Figure 7-5). Your assignment tells you:

- which patients you will care for during your shift
- the procedures you will need to do for these patients

Your supervising nurse will then give you additional information about your assignment based on the shift report. This information may include orders to complete procedures for specific patients:

- take temperature, pulse, respirations, and blood pressures on designated patients
- obtain weights on designated patients
- allow a patient to remain in bed because of a change in condition
- make observations of a patient who has had a recent change in condition

During your shift, you will give oral reports to the nurse about procedures you have completed and observations you have made. At the end of the shift, you will summarize your assignment to the nurse so that the information can be included in the shift report to the employees coming on duty after you. When you leave the nursing unit for any reason during your shift, always report to the nurse before you go. Unit 8 gives additional information about oral reports.

Answering the Telephone

Many telephone calls come into a health care facility. Families call to inquire about the condition of a loved one. Physicians call frequently to leave new medical orders. The laboratory may call to give test results. Remember that nursing assistants are not allowed to take physicians' orders, to take results of diagnostic tests, or to give information to families. You must call the nurse to do this. If you answer the telephone:

- Identify the nursing unit: "third floor, north" for example.
- Identify yourself and your position: "Mary Smith, nursing assistant."
- Ask the caller's name and ask the caller to wait while you locate the person called.
- If the person is unavailable, take a message (Figure 7-6) and write down the following information:
  - date and time of call
  - caller's name and telephone number
  - message left by caller

CNA ASSIGNMENT SHEET   DATE ___4-18-XX___

Rm.	Resident	Bath	Pos. Sched.	ROM	V.S.	WT.	B+B	ADL Prog.	Transfer	Safety
101ᴬ	J. Damski	X	X	X			X	X	2+TB	X
101ᴮ	G. Jones		X	X	X	X			Mech Lift	
102ᴬ	C. Hernandez	X				X			Indep.	
102ᴮ	R. Lattini	X	X	X			X		2+ TB	X
103	N. Goldberg	X			X	X	X		SBA	
104ᴬ	M. Welch		X	X					Mech Lift	
104ᴮ	L. Ordoni		X	X			X	X	1+TB	X
105	B. Brinzoski	X			X		X		Indep.	
106ᴬ	A. Feinstein	X				X		X	1+TB	
106ᴮ	D. Farmell		X	X	X		X	X	2+TB	
107	T. Green	X	X	X		X	X		2+TB	
108ᴬ	H. Johnson	X	X	X	X			X	2+TB	
108ᴮ	B. Miller		X	X		X			1+TB	X

FIGURE 7-5 The assignment sheet provides an overview of patient needs and activities.

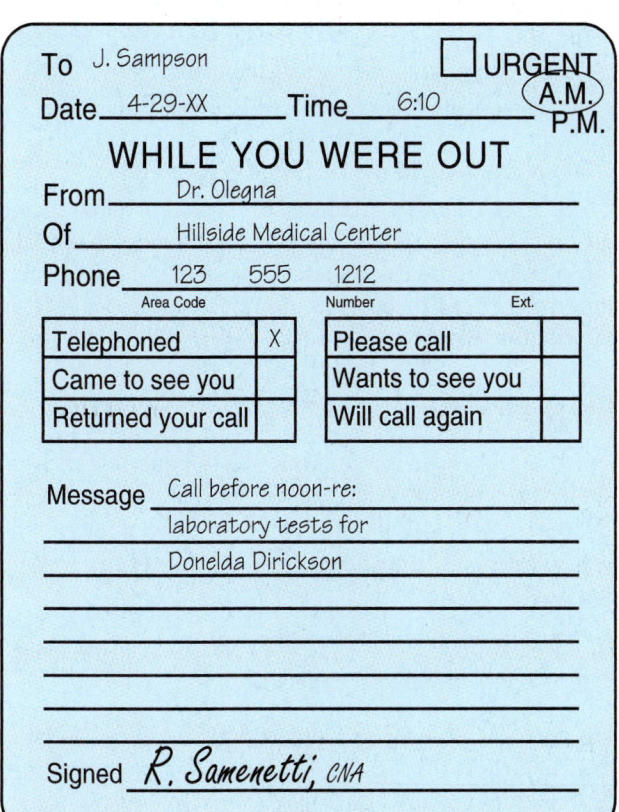

FIGURE 7-6 Telephone message.

– whether the person is to return the call or whether the caller will telephone again later

– your signature

Some facilities have more complex telephone systems. You will be taught how to transfer calls or to voice-page. Most facilities do not allow employees to make or receive personal telephone calls while they are on duty, except in an emergency.

Written Communications Among Staff Members

In many situations, you and other staff members must rely on written communications. The ability to accurately read the communication is essential to your patient care.

Memos

A **memo** (Figure 7-7) is a brief communication that informs or reminds employees of:

- changes in policies or procedures
- upcoming meetings or staff development programs
- admission of new patients
- promotions of staff members

Be sure you know where memos are posted so that you will be aware of the facility activities.

MEMO

Date: April 21, XXXX
From: Jane Sowalski, RN Director of Nursing
To: All nursing staff

Please note that the Nursing Procedure Manual has been updated and revised. The list of changes is attached. Please read the indicated procedures and sign the attached page.

Thank you.

FIGURE 7-7 Memos provide important information.

Manuals

All facilities have several manuals that provide information about policies and procedures (Figure 7-8). These may include:

- Employee Personnel Handbook—Describes all personnel policies and benefits.

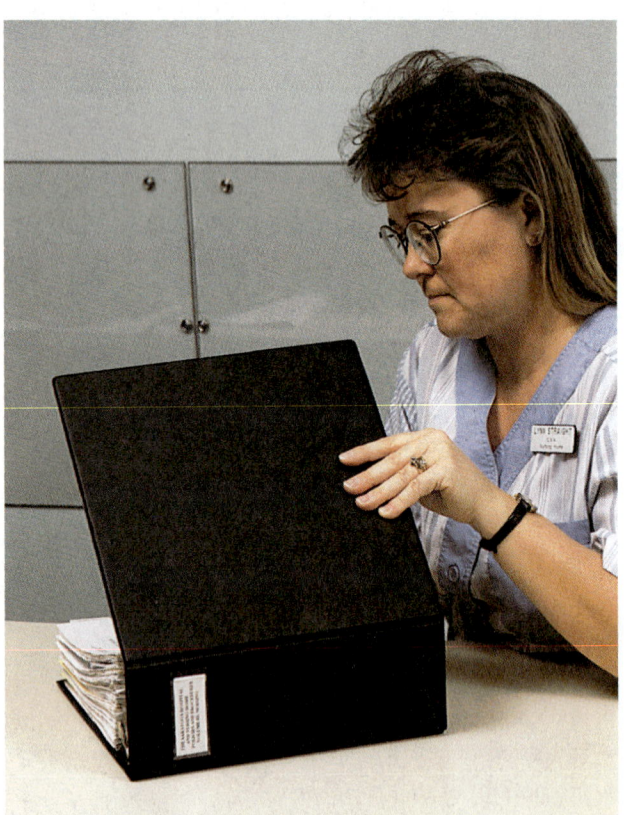

FIGURE 7-8 Manuals are an excellent source of information.

LEGAL *Alert*

Becoming familiar with the location and contents of facility policy and procedure manuals will help you do your job and practice within your scope of responsibility. The golden rule implies your intent to provide adequate care. However, your intentions are effective only when combined with action. You have the ethical responsibility to maintain competence in your practice. Health care is always changing, and attending educational classes is necessary to stay abreast of current information. As a nursing assistant, you must attend 12 or more hours of continuing education each year to maintain your certification. Look forward to this as a means of learning new things that will benefit both you and the patients.

- Safety and Disaster Manual—Gives directions for actions to take in case of fire or other disasters.
- Procedure Manual—Gives directions on how all procedures should be performed for patients.
- Nursing Policy Manual—Describes rules and regulations pertaining to the care of the patients.
- Material Safety Data Sheet (MSDS) Manual—Contains information on safe use and handling of substances used in the facility.

There may be other manuals for infection control and quality assurance. You are not expected to memorize all the information in these manuals, but you should know where they are kept on the nursing unit and be able to look up information when you need to.

Staff Development   *inservice*

Staff development is a process used to educate staff from all departments in the facility (Figure 7-9). Classes may be given to inform staff of:

- new rules and regulations
- new procedures
- recent health findings from research
- how to use new equipment

The Patient Care Plan

The interdisciplinary health care team develops an individualized **care plan** for each patient. Unit 8 presents more information on the patient care plan.

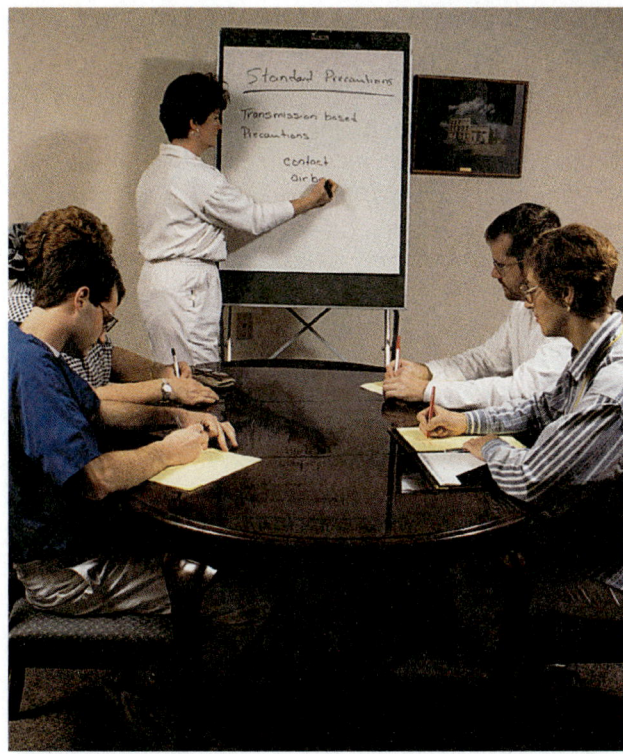

FIGURE 7-9 Health care changes rapidly. Nursing assistants must participate in regular staff development, information sharing, and educational programs.

The Patient's Medical Chart

Each patient has a **medical chart** or record. The medical chart contains:

- the physician's medical orders for that patient: medications, treatments, diagnostic tests
- the medical history of the patient: summary of all past illnesses and surgeries
- results of physical examinations
- results of all diagnostic tests: blood tests and x-rays
- progress notes from the physician and from all disciplines involved in the patient's care: brief, periodic descriptions of the patient's condition and response to treatment
- assessments from all disciplines: the assessment identifies the patient's problems
- nursing notes: information that describes the patient's condition, nursing care that has been given, and the patient's response to the care

The information entered into the chart is called *documentation*. The chart is a legal document. It may be used to:

- determine payments by insurance companies
- determine settlement of lawsuits

Unit 8 gives instructions for documenting (making notations) on the patient's chart.

Other Methods of Communication

Modern technology has increased opportunities for communication. You will see computers at the nurses' station and throughout the building. Computers have many uses within health care facilities. They are used for:

- Writing letters, memos, policies, and procedures. Performing these tasks is called *word processing*.
- Compiling databases. A *database* may be developed that includes every patient and every employee within the facility. The database contains information such as name, address, telephone numbers, and social security number. The database allows the storage, retrieval, and manipulation of large amounts of information and simplifies procedures such as maintaining patient and personnel records.
- Doing mathematical calculations, which are performed with *spreadsheet programs*. These programs are used for budgeting and financial analysis.
- Communicating, using programs that allow computers to "talk" to each other over telephone lines, using special equipment called *modems*. Persons using this feature may be able to communicate with other computers within the facility or anywhere in the world. Messages can be sent via electronic mail (e-mail), equipment and supplies can be ordered, and information can be retrieved on just about any topic.

Most facilities will have at least one desktop computer in each department. In the nursing department, computers are used to document patient care, to maintain databases, to communicate with physicians' offices, and to maintain records of supplies and equipment. Some facilities have computers in every patient room. Nursing staff can then document appropriate information before they leave the bedside.

If you will be expected to use a computer and have had very little experience doing so, remember:

- Do not be intimidated by the computer. You have the ability to learn how to use one. You do not have to be a computer expert to use a computer.
- Learn from classes, from manuals, and from other users. Be creative and try to figure out some things on your own.
- Be patient, be determined, and do not panic. Do not be afraid to ask questions. You will not learn everything right away, but your confidence will grow by leaps and bounds as you master new tasks.

You will be given special training if you will be expected to use a computer (Figure 7-10).

Fax machines are common in health care facilities (Figure 7-11). They are used to send and receive information from physicians and laboratories.

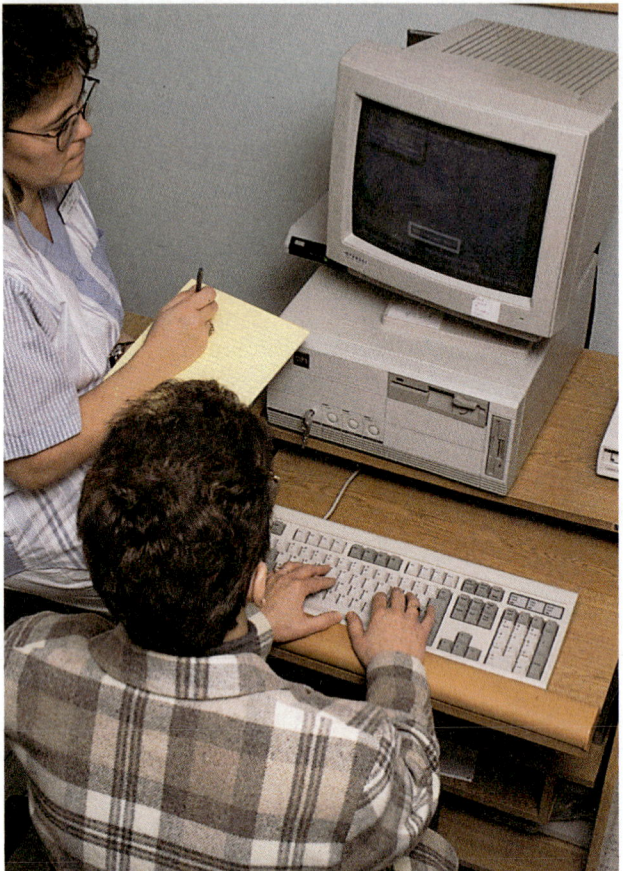

FIGURE 7-10 The use of computers in health care is increasing.

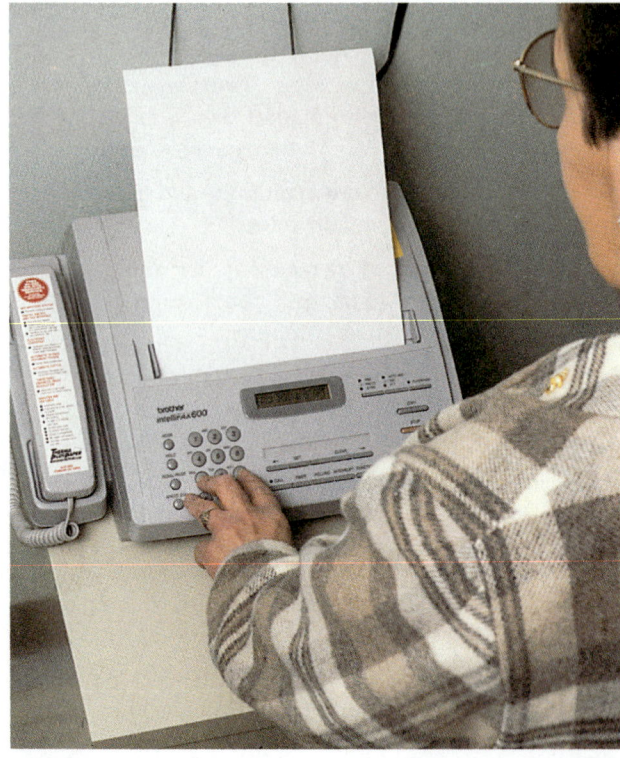

FIGURE 7-11 Fax machines are a convenient means of communication.

COMMUNICATING WITH PATIENTS

Your skill in communicating with patients will develop with experience. It is not always the words we choose that are important, but the way in which we say them. Tone of voice, facial expression, and even the way you touch a patient all communicate a sense of honest caring to the patient. Looking directly at the patient as you speak and addressing him or her respectfully by name are also indications of caring.

Listening actively is a special skill requiring more than just being physically present. When you listen actively, all your attention is focused on the speaker. You maintain eye contact and do not interrupt while the other person is speaking. You ask questions that encourage the speaker to continue and respond to specific questions that he or she asks. Follow these guidelines to communicate effectively with patients.

Communicating with Patients with Special Needs

There are many reasons why communication with patients may be impaired. The patient may:

- be hearing impaired
- be vision impaired
- have aphasia
- be disoriented
- be from a culture different from the nursing assistant's

These patients have special communication needs that should be addressed on the care plan. Always check the care plan before attempting to communicate with a patient who has special communication needs. Specific approaches may be established for all staff members to use with the patient. Lack of consistency in use of these approaches is confusing and frustrating to the patient.

COMMUNICATION *Highlight*

Remember that one of the most important and powerful messages you send to patients is that you care about them. You do this in many ways, including your demeanor when you enter the room, your body language, your tone of voice, and your touch. Verbal communication with some patients will be very limited. Use nonverbal communication to send the message that you care to all patients.

guidelines *for*

Communicating with Patients

1. Be sure you have the patient's attention.
2. Avoid chewing gum, eating, or covering your mouth with your hand when you speak.
3. Use nonthreatening words and gestures.
4. Speak clearly and courteously.
5. Use a pleasant tone of voice.
6. Use appropriate body language.
7. Be alert to the patient's needs to communicate with you—allow time for the patient to talk and respond. Show interest and concern (Figure 7-12).
8. Do not speak about the patient in front of the patient or other patients.
9. Do not interrupt the patient.
10. Reflect the patient's feelings and thoughts by rewording his or her statements into questions.
11. Ask for clarification if you are unsure of what the patient is saying.
12. Give the patient only factual information—not your personal feelings, opinions, or beliefs.
13. Information concerning the patient's condition, medications, and treatments should be given by the physician or nurse.
14. Do not argue with patients.

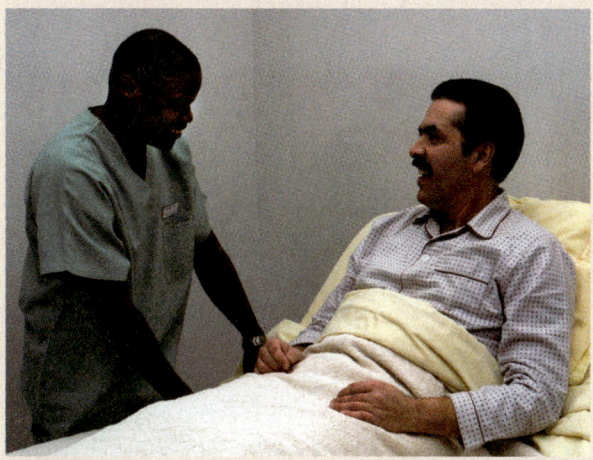

FIGURE 7-12 Recognize the patient's need to communicate with you.

Communicating with Patients Who Have Hearing Impairments

1. Get the patient's attention first.
   - Make sure the patient sees you.
   - Touch the patient lightly to indicate that you wish to speak.
   - Recognize that individuals who are hard of hearing hear less well when they are tired or ill.
2. If the patient uses a hearing aid, be sure that the patient is wearing it and that the hearing aid is on.
3. If the patient has a "good" ear, stand or sit on that side.
4. Do not chew gum, eat, or cover your mouth while talking.
5. Keep the light behind the patient, so your face can be clearly seen (Figure 7-13).
6. Face the patient; many people with hearing impairments can read lips or interpret your facial expressions.
7. Reduce outside distractions. Speak in a quiet, calm manner.
8. Start conversations with a key word or phrase so the patient has some clues as to what you are saying (context).

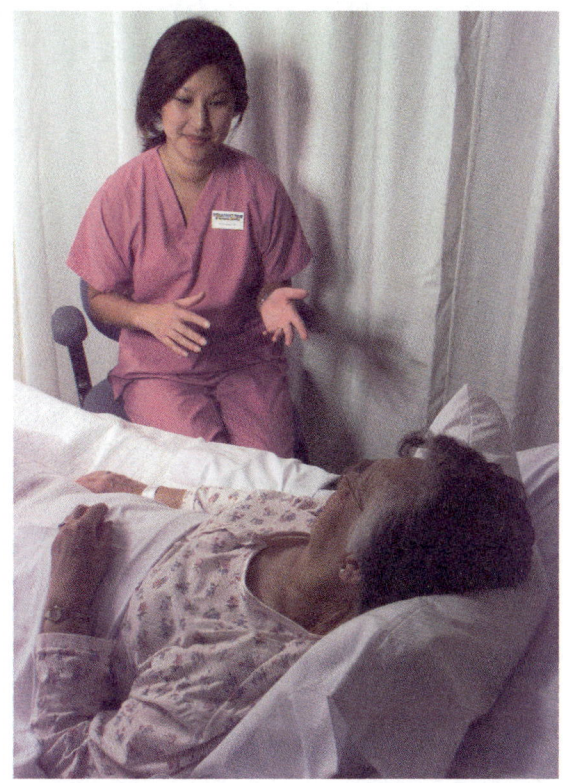

FIGURE 7-13 The light source should be behind the patient if she is hearing impaired.

9. Avoid abrupt changes of subject, because your hard-of-hearing listener depends heavily on context to understand what you are saying. Also, do not interrupt your conversation with "small talk."

10. Keep your voice pitch low.

11. Speak slowly, distinctly, and naturally.

12. Form words carefully, use familiar words, and keep sentences short.

13. Pronounce words clearly. If the patient who has a hearing impairment has difficulty with letters and numbers, say: "M as in Mary," "2 as in twins," "B as in boy." Say each number separately: "five six" instead of fifty-six. Remember that *m, n* and *2, 3, 56, 66* and *b, c, d, e, t,* and *v* sound alike.

14. Rephrase words as needed.

15. Avoid shouting, mouthing, or exaggerating words, or speaking very slowly. This only makes it harder for the patient to understand you.

16. Keep a notepad handy and write your words if the patient does not understand.

17. Use facial expressions, gestures, and body language to help express your meanings.

18. Some patients with hearing impairment use **sign language**.
    - Signing depends upon hand and finger movements and facial expressions.
    - This is a skill that requires learning and practice (Figure 7-14).
    - There are different forms of sign language, just as there are different spoken languages.
    - There are some basic signs that may be helpful (Figure 7-15).

19. Patients who have been hearing impaired for several years may have speech that is difficult to understand.

20. Some hearing-impaired people are embarrassed to tell you when they do not understand you.

21. People who cannot hear may appear confused when they are not.

22. Never walk away leaving a patient with a hearing impairment puzzling over what you said and thinking that you do not care.

Communicating with Patients Who Have Visual Impairments

Patients who have visual impairments may have problems communicating because they are unable to see the sender or the sender's facial expressions and body language.

1. When approaching a person who is visually impaired, address the person by name and then touch lightly on the hand or arm to avoid startling.

2. After you speak to the patient, identify yourself and explain why you are there. "Hello, Mr. Smith. My name is Mary Jones and I would like to take your blood pressure."

3. Be specific when giving directions. "I am putting your call light on the right side of your bed."

4. When giving directions on how to find an area in the building, tell the patient how many doors he or she will pass and when to turn right or left.

5. When you leave the patient, make sure you announce your departure. "I am leaving your room now. Can I get you anything else?"

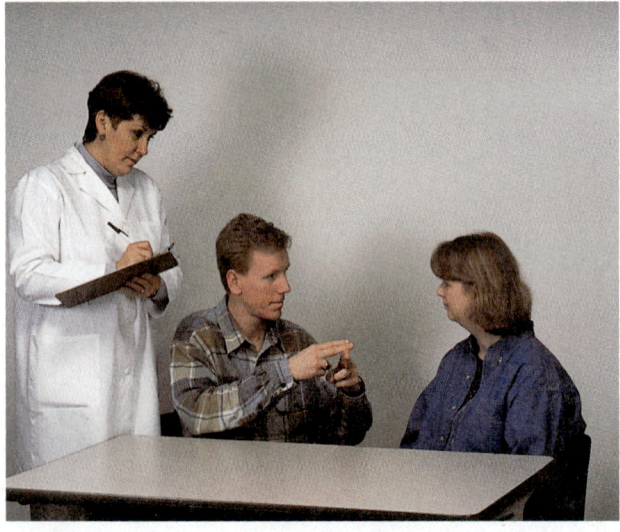

FIGURE 7-14 Learning sign language takes special skill and training.

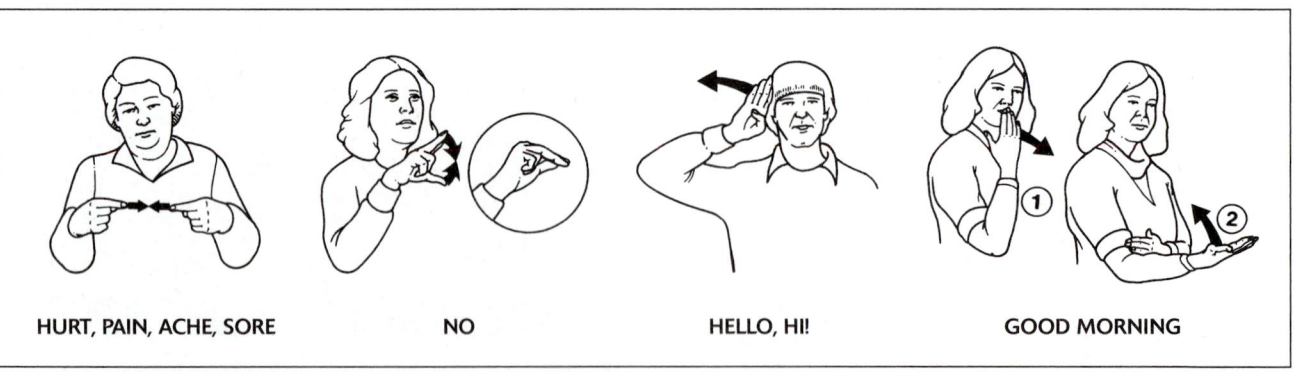

HURT, PAIN, ACHE, SORE   NO   HELLO, HI!   GOOD MORNING

FIGURE 7-15 Basic signs.

6. Offer to read mail to visually impaired patients.

7. If the patient has a telephone, make sure he or she can use it. The patient can count the numbers on the dial to make calls.

8. Tactfully inform a person who has visual impairment if clothing is soiled, mismatched, or in need of repair.

9. Encourage the patient to listen to the radio or television to keep up with news and current events.

10. Make sure the patient is aware of talking book machines. Inform Social Services if the patient wishes to use one.

11. Describe the environment and objects around the patient so a frame of reference is established. This helps avoid disorientation related to vision impairment. Never change the location of items or furniture without discussing it with the patient.

12. Some patients may read **braille**, a system that uses a series of raised dots to represent letters and words (Figure 7-16). The patient reads the letters and words by moving his or her fingertips over them.

Communicating with Patients Who Have Aphasia

Patients who have had a stroke or brain damage due to an injury may have aphasia. **Aphasia** means that the patient cannot understand spoken or written language, or cannot express spoken or written language, or both. Trying to communicate with patients who have aphasia can be frustrating to both the patient and the caregiver.

1. Face the patient and make eye contact before speaking.

2. Say the patient's name and give a social greeting before asking questions or giving instructions.

3. Speak slowly and clearly. Use short, complete sentences.

4. Pause between sentences to allow the patient time to comprehend and interpret what you said.

5. Check the patient's comprehension before you proceed. Ask a question based on information you just gave the patient.

6. Use nonverbal cues to augment spoken communication. Use gestures, facial expressions, or pictures.

7. Ask questions that require only short responses or ones that can be answered nonverbally.

8. Repeat what the patient just said to help him or her keep focused on the conversation.

9. Find out if the speech therapist has devised methods of nonverbal communication, such as communication boards or picture books (Figure 7-17).

10. Do not avoid talking to a person with aphasia. Speak in a normal tone of voice. Do not shout to try to make him understand.

11. If you sense frustration, let the patient know that you are aware of the frustration. Suggest that you talk about something else for a while and then try again.

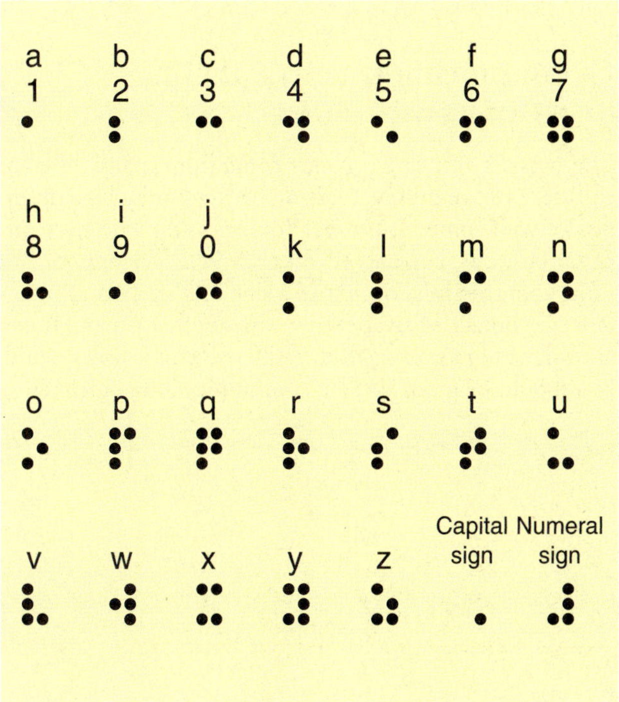

FIGURE 7-16 Many persons with visual impairments use braille.

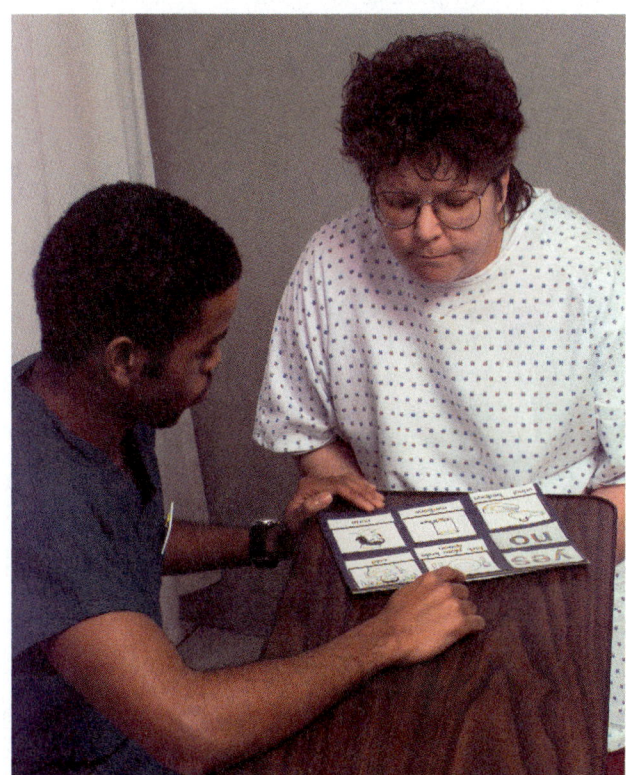

FIGURE 7-17 Patients with aphasia may use communication boards to make their needs known.

Communicating with Disoriented Patients

Some patients you care for may be disoriented. **Disorientation** means that the patient is confused about time, place (his physical location), or person (who he is). Disorientation can be caused by Alzheimer's disease, stroke, or other disorders or injuries of the brain.

1. Begin conversation by identifying yourself and calling the patient by name. Do not ask the patient if she remembers you or if she knows who you are.
2. Talk to the patient at eye level and maintain eye contact.
3. Maintain a pleasant facial expression while you are talking and listening.
4. Place a hand on the patient's arm or hand, unless this causes agitation (Figure 7-18).
5. Make sure the patient can hear you. Avoid distractions of noise and activity.
6. Use a lower tone of voice.
7. Use short, common words and short, simple sentences.
8. Give the patient time to respond.
9. Ask only one simple question at a time. If you must repeat it, say it exactly the same.
10. Ask the patient to do only one task at a time.
11. Patients with dementia will eventually be unable to comprehend verbal communication.
    - Use pictures, and point, touch, or hand her things.
    - Demonstrate an action when you want her to complete a task.
12. The patient may use word substitutes. If these are consistent, find out what they mean. Use them yourself to see if the patient understands you better.
13. Avoid abstract, common expressions. For example, "You can hop into bed now" means just that to the patient.
14. Repeat the patient's last words to help him stay on track during conversation.
15. Do not try to "make" the patient understand. Avoid lengthy explanations and excessive verbal communication. This tends to agitate most people with dementia.

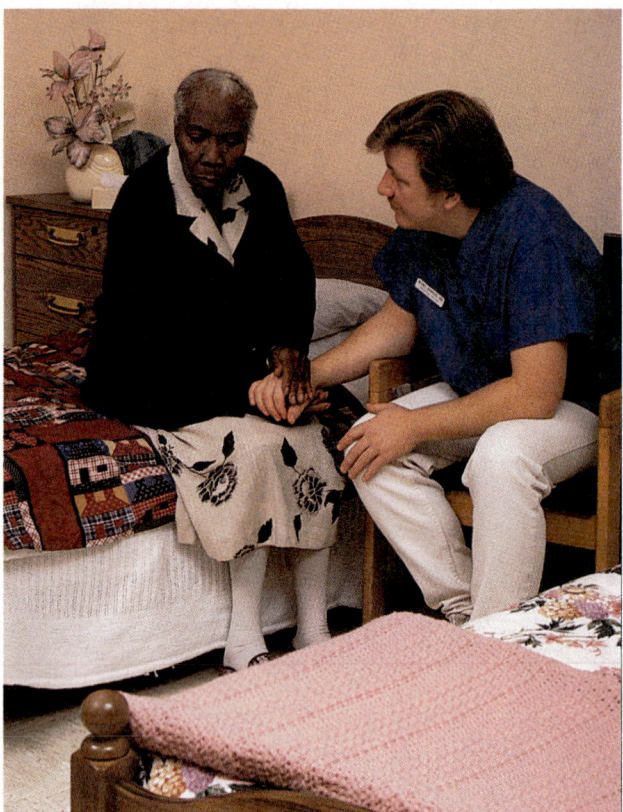

FIGURE 7-18 Gently touching a patient's hand or arm may be comforting.

16. Use nonverbal praise freely and always respect the patient's feelings.

Communicating with Patients of a Different Culture

The persons you care for may come from many different cultures or have different **ethnic** backgrounds. This means people who come from other countries and who have different customs, languages, and traditions. For example, in some countries it is considered a sign of disrespect to maintain eye contact when speaking with another person. If you are assigned to someone from a different ethnic background, you should be given specific communication guidelines.

REVIEW

A. Multiple Choice.

Select the one best answer for each of the following.

1. Successful communication is essential for
   a. body language to be meaningful.
   b. patient only.
   c. staff only.
   d. safe care.

2. Verbal communication includes
   a. talking and listening.
   b. facial expressions.
   c. writing reports.
   d. using a fax machine.

3. Verbal communication is
   a. written words only.
   b. spoken or written words.
   c. spoken words only.
   d. a combination of words and facial expressions.

4. Examples of nonverbal communication include
   a. reading and using the patient's care plan.
   b. answering the telephone.
   c. listening to shift report.
   d. conversing with patients.

5. A nursing assistant may give or take which information over the telephone?
   a. Report of a patient's condition
   b. Physician's orders
   c. Results of laboratory tests
   d. Name of person leaving the message

6. The shift report is given by the
   a. administrator.
   b. physician.
   c. nurse who worked the previous shift.
   d. director of nursing.

7. The purpose of the shift report is to
   a. give information about all the patients on the nursing unit.
   b. discuss the social activities of the staff.
   c. tell the nursing assistants when they are scheduled for days off.
   d. rest before starting work.

8. You must report to the nurse when you
   a. prepare to take vital signs.
   b. complete each patient's care.
   c. begin your documentation.
   d. leave the unit for any reason.

9. One purpose of a memo is to inform staff of
   a. meetings or educational programs.
   b. patients' conditions.
   c. new physician's orders for specific patients.
   d. weather conditions.

10. Examples of manuals that are found on nursing units include
    a. computer manual, laboratory manual, quality assurance manual.
    b. procedure manual, infection control manual, disaster manual.
    c. employee assistance program manual, personnel manual, benefits manual.
    d. isolation manual, x-ray manual, nuclear medicine manual.

11. The patient's care plan provides information for
    a. the nursing assistant assignments.
    b. employee benefits.
    c. the procedure for fire drills.
    d. licensed personnel only.

12. The patient's medical record or chart is
    a. used only by the physician.
    b. used by all members of the interdisciplinary health care team.
    c. a temporary record.
    d. a report of the nursing assistant's competencies.

13. The patient grimaces and holds his right arm close to his body when he moves. You suspect he may
    a. be right-handed.
    b. not want to get out of bed.
    c. be tired.
    d. be having pain.

14. If a patient is disoriented, it means that the patient is
    a. mentally ill.
    b. unaware of the environment and the time.
    c. unable to communicate with you.
    d. unable to hear.

15. Aphasia means that the patient
    a. has an infection of the respiratory tract.
    b. is hearing impaired.
    c. is disoriented.
    d. is unable to speak or to understand the spoken language of others.

16. When working with patients who have hearing impairments, you should

a. speak in a calm, quiet manner.

b. talk louder.

c. avoid speaking if possible.

d. speak very slowly.

17. When working with patients who have aphasia, it is best to

a. use only hand gestures to communicate.

b. speak louder.

c. avoid communication if at all possible.

d. face the patient and make eye contact before speaking.

18. Persons with visual impairment should

a. stay in their rooms to avoid getting lost in the facility.

b. have identification on their clothing so everyone realizes they are visually impaired.

c. learn to use sign language.

d. be given directions for locating various areas in the building.

19. When working with disoriented patients, you should

a. ask the patient if he or she remembers you or knows who you are.

b. try to make the patient understand you.

c. avoid distractions of noise and activity when communicating with them.

d. get as close as possible to the patient when talking or giving care.

20. Touching the patient can be a successful method of communication if you

a. ask the family's permission.

b. are not offended by touch.

c. are gentle and caring.

d. always grasp the patient firmly.

B. Completion.

Choose the correct word from the following list to complete each statement in questions 21–30.

1 aphasia	6 medical chart
2 body language	7 memo
3 braille	8 nonverbal communication
4 care plan	9 shift report
5 disorientation	10 verbal communication

21. Persons who cannot express themselves verbally or understand verbal communication have ___1___.

22. Loss of recognition of time, place, location, or person is called ___5___.

23. The exchange of information given by the nurse going off duty to those coming on duty is called the ___9___.

24. The ___6___ is a legal document.

25. A brief, written message that provides information is a ___7___.

26. ___2___ is an example of nonverbal communication.

27. The record that contains a description of the patient's problems, the goals for resolving the problems, and the approaches used is the ___4___.

28. Sign language is an example of ___8___.

29. Talking orally is ___10___.

30. ___3___ is used by persons with visual impairment.

C. Nursing Assistant Challenge.

Miss Johnson is one of your patients. She is in the hospital because she has a heart problem and is visually impaired. Miss Johnson can feed herself and can give herself a bath, brush her teeth, and comb her own hair if she has adequate assistance. Think about suggestions presented in this unit for communicating with persons with visual impairment.

31. What can you do to set up meal trays so that Miss Johnson can feed herself?

32. How can you prepare bath items so that she can give herself her bath?

33. What can you do to enable her to comb her own hair and brush her teeth?

34. What other actions can you take to help this patient maintain as much independence as possible?

Thur. 18, 19, 20.

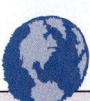

EXPLORING THE WEB

Description	Location
Communication	*http://www.delmarhealthcare.com/olcs/white/pnotes.asp* (see Chapter 5)
Communication	*http://www.delmarhealthcare.com/olcs/whiteduncan/pnotes.asp* (see Chapter 8)
Communication in nursing	*http://www06.homepage.villanova.edu*
—Cooperative communication skills	*http://www.coopcomm.org*
—Transcultural communication stumbling blocks	*http://www.delmarhealthcare.com/pdf/0766802566_04.pdf*
—Virtual communication assistants	*http://www.ku.edu*
Communication skills	*http://www.mapnp.org*
—Adjusting to Fluency Problems	*http://www.advancefornurses.com* (see past articles 1/8/01)
—Communicating with Respect	*http://www.advancefornurses.com* (see past articles 2/5/01)
—Developing Professional Language	*http://www.advancefornurses.com* (see past articles 11/20/00)
—Listening Skills	*http://www.advancefornurses.com* (see past articles 1/22/01)
—The Professional Voice	*http://www.advancefornurses.com* (see past articles 12/4/00)
—Suite 101	*http://www.suite101.com*
—Think Before You Speak	*http://www.advancefornurses.com* (see past articles 2/19/01)
—Your Rate of Speech	*http://www.advancefornurses.com* (see past articles 1/8/01)

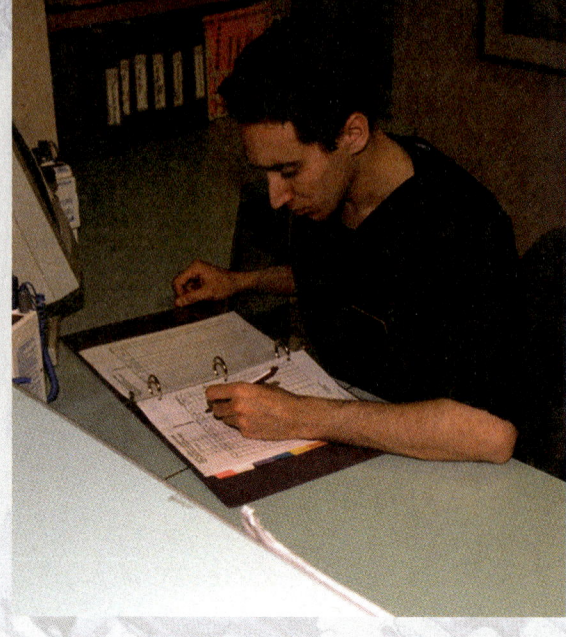

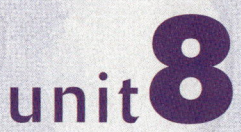

unit 8

Observation, Reporting, and Documentation

objectives

After completing this unit, you will be able to:

- Spell and define terms.
- List the four components of the nursing process.
- Explain the responsibilities of the nursing assistant for each component of the nursing process.
- Describe two observations to make for each body system.

- Describe the purpose of the care plan.
- List three times when oral reports are given.
- Describe the information given when reporting.
- Describe the purpose of the patient's medical record.
- Explain the rules for documentation.

vocabulary

Learn the meaning and the correct spelling of the following words and phrases:

analgesic	critical (clinical)	implementation	objective observation
approaches	pathways	intervention	observation
assessment	document	Kardex	oral report
care plan	evaluation	nurse's notes	planning
conference	flow sheet	nursing diagnosis	subjective
charting	goal	nursing process	observation

INTRODUCTION

One of the responsibilities of the nursing assistant is to collect and communicate information about the patients. Information is collected by making observations of the patient. Information is communicated to other team members by reporting and documenting. The mechanism used to carry out these actions is called the **nursing process**.

NURSING PROCESS

The registered nurse is responsible for achieving patient focused care by using the nursing process. The nurse coordinates care and delegates responsibilities to other caregivers in an effort to achieve this goal. The nursing process consists of five steps:

- Assessment
- Problem identification
- Planning
- Implementation
- Evaluation

Assessment involves the collection of data (information) about the patient. The nurse coordinates assessment with other members of the interdisciplinary team. The data are entered on a special form contained in the patient's medical record (Figure 8-1). Information is obtained from:

- interviewing the patient
- the medical record
- the patient's family if the patient is unable to communicate
- physical examination (Figure 8-2 on page 93)

The nursing assistant is responsible for collection of data by making and reporting observations. This is explained later in the unit. After the assessment is finished, the nurse analyzes the data, identifies the patient's problems, and formulates nursing diagnoses. A **nursing diagnosis** is the statement of a patient problem and the cause of the problem. For example, the nursing diagnosis may be impaired physical mobility (the problem) related to hemiplegia due to stroke (the cause of the problem). Nursing diagnoses may reflect actual clinical problems, the risk that certain problems will develop, or wellness objectives. The nursing diagnoses provide the foundation for nursing care to achieve outcomes for which nurses are accountable. Table 8-1 gives a few examples of nursing diagnoses and what they mean.

Planning the care of the patient (developing a care plan) is done after the nursing diagnoses are made. The purpose of planning is to:

- identify possible solutions to the problems (nursing diagnoses).
- develop **approaches** (what team members are going to do) that will help the patient solve the problems. Approaches may also be called **interventions**.
- establish **goals** for the patient (a goal is an outcome) so that caregivers will know whether the approaches are successful and whether the problems are being resolved.

Planning may be done at a **care plan conference** (Figure 8-3 on page 93). This is a meeting of the members of the interdisciplinary team who are directly involved with the care of the patient. The patient and/or the family (if the patient consents) should be invited to attend the conference. The care plan developed at the conference contains a list of the nursing diagnoses, the approaches, and the patient's goals (Figure 8-4 on page 94). The care plan may be kept in the patient's medical record or in a file called a **Kardex** (Figure 8-5A on page 95 and Figure 8-5B on page 96) at the nurses' station. The nursing assistant is responsible for contributing information (observations) that will help the team develop a workable care plan. Some facilities invite nursing assistants to attend the care plan conference.

Implementation is the activation of the care plan. It means carrying out the approaches listed on the care plan in an effort to resolve the problems (nursing diagnoses) and to help the patient reach the goals (Figure 8-6 on page 98). The approach states:

- who is to carry out the approach
- when the approach is carried out
- how the approach is carried out

See Figure 8-4 for examples of approaches. The nursing assistant is responsible for knowing when and how the approach is to be carried out and for implementing the approach correctly.

Evaluation is the final step of the nursing process, but it is an ongoing procedure. The evaluation determines:

- whether the patient is reaching the goals on the care plan
- why the goals are not being reached, if the patient is not successful in obtaining the goals
- what should be done to assist the patient to reach the goals
- when goals are reached, they may be extended; for example if the patient reaches the goal of walking 200 feet, it may be increased to 250 feet

The nursing assistant is responsible for reporting to the nurse when the:

- approach cannot be carried out for any reason
- patient is having problems with the approach

Critical (Clinical) Pathways

The DRG method of payment has affected many health care practices and shortened hospital stays. Many hospitals are using **critical (clinical) pathways** to direct care. The pathways are written documents that detail the expected course of treatment and expected outcomes for a DRG. New goals are set each day during the patient's stay. The pathway lists nursing actions to help the patient achieve the goal. The nursing assistant is responsible for many of these interventions. Review the Kardex containing the patient's care plan or critical pathway at the beginning of each shift to help plan your day.

NURSING ASSESSMENT   Patient Label

Instructions: Check mark indicates YES, no check mark indicates NO.
Check ONLY appropriate box, unless otherwise indicated.

Informant: Family _____ Patient _____ Other _____

SECTION I NEUROLOGICAL / COGNITIVE

#1 Oriented to
___ Person
___ Place
___ Time
___ None of the above

#2 Level of Consciousness
___ Alert ___ Lethargic
___ Responds appropriately
___ Unresponsive
___ Comatose

#3 Communication
___ Aphasic
___ Can read
___ Can write
___ Speaks clearly
___ Uses gestures
___ Attention span deficit
___ Hemianopsia

#4 Memory / Recall
___ Short term
___ Long term
___ Follows directions

#5 Eyes / Vision
___ Vision deficit
___ Macular degeneration
___ Glaucoma
___ Cataracts
___ Glasses
___ Contact lenses
___ Other

Pupil Reaction
              Right   Left
Brisk   ____   ____
Slow   ____   ____
None   ____   ____
___ Pupils equal round
___ Inflamed
___ Eye conditions (explain)
___ Cloudy iris
___ Date of last eye exam

#6 Hearing
___ Hearing deficit
___ Hearing aid: R ___ L ___
___ Ear drainage: R ___ L ___
___ Wax: R ___ L ___
___ Date of last hearing exam

#7 Behavior
___ Combative
___ Anxious
___ Depressed (Dx or Sx)
___ Angry
___ Insomnia
___ Alcohol use
___ Hx drug habits
___ Hx poor health maintenance / poor hygiene

#8 Miscellaneous
___ Headache
___ Numbness
___ Tingling
___ Tremors
___ Dizziness
___ Ear(s) ringing
___ Asymptomatic

Explain if checks:
_____
_____
_____

Comments:

SECTION II INTEGUMENTARY / WOUND

#1 Appearance
___ Pale
___ Flushed
___ Mottled
___ Cyanotic
___ Jaundiced

___ Normal
___ Good skin turgor
___ Tenting present
___ Other

#2 Temperature
Lower extremities:
___ Hot ___ Warm ___ Cold
Upper extremities:
___ Hot ___ Warm ___ Cold

#3 Pain
___ Yes ___ No
* If YES complete pain assessment form
Pain meds ordered ___ Yes ___ No

** Complete Pressure Ulcer Risk Assessment
** Complete Wound Assessment (if applicable)

Comments:

SECTION III CIRCULATORY

#1 Vitals
Pulse
P – Palpable
N – Nonpalpable
Radial R ___ L ___
Pedal R ___ L ___
Radial pulse (record)
_____ Right _____ Left
Blood Pressure (Record)
_____ Right _____ Left
Temperature (Record) _____
Respirations (Record) _____

#2 Cardiac Rhythm
___ Regular ___ Irregular
___ Strong ___ Weak
___ Palpitations

#3 Edema (Use Key)
___ Right Upper Extremity
___ Left Upper Extremity
___ Right Lower Extremity
___ Left Lower Extremity
___ Sacral
___ Ascites

#4 History of:
___ Chest pain
___ Syncope
___ Epistaxis

___ Pacemaker

KEY: 0 = Absent   2+ = Mild (< 1/2")   4+ = Severe (> 1")
        1+ = Slight (< 1/4")   3+ = Moderate (1/2" – 1")

Comments:

SECTION IV RESPIRATORY

#1 Breath Sounds
___ Clear all lobes R ___ L ___
___ Wheeze R ___ L ___
___ Crackles R ___ L ___
___ Diminished R ___ L ___
___ Equal bilaterally R ___ L ___
___ Abnormal R ___ L ___

#2 Breathing effort:
___ Easy
___ Labored
___ Uses accessory muscles

#3 Cough
___ Nonproductive
___ Productive (explain)
_____

#4 History of:
___ Dyspnea
___ On exertion
___ Without exertion
___ Orthopnea
___ Smoking ___ # packs / day
___ Chews (explain)
_____

#5 Miscellaneous
___ Trach
___ Oxygen Rx
___ Nebulizer
___ Respiratory therapy

Comments: *continues*

FIGURE 8-1 The nursing assessment form is used to collect data about the patient on admission.

SECTION V   ELIMINATION GASTROINTESTINAL

#1 Mouth
___ Normal ___ Abnormal
Glands
___ Normal ___ Abnormal
___ Own teeth
___ Broken teeth
___ Dentures
Upper ___ Full ___ Partial
Lower ___ Full ___ Partial

Comments:

#2 Bowels _____
___ Bowel sounds present
___ Colostomy
___ Hemorrhoids
___ Rectal bleeding
___ Rectal prolapse
___ Hernia
___ Continent
___ Incontinent ___ Total ___ Occasional
___ Smears
___ Diarrhea
___ Constipated

#3 Bowel Program
___ Maintenance
___ Training
___ Uses incontinent garments
    ___ Dri–pride
    ___ Dri–pride pad
    ___ Other
___ Ostomy (type)

#4 Miscellaneous
___ Laxative / Freq _____
___ Suppository / Freq _____
___ Enema / Freq _____
___ Abdominal distension
___ Abdomen soft
___ Abdomen hard
___ Abdominal tenderness
___ G–tube
___ N / G tube
___ Other (explain)
_____

SECTION VI   URINARY

#1 Urine Appearance
___ Clear ___ Cloudy
___ Yellow
___ Amber
___ Hematuria

Comments:

#2 Symptoms
___ Frequency
___ Burning
___ Urgency
___ Dribbling
___ Nocturia
___ Hx UTI

#3 Elimination
___ Continent
___ Incontinent
Night
___ Occasional
___ Total
Day
___ Occasional
___ Total
Evening
___ Occasional
___ Total
___ Cath / size _____
___ Ostomy / type _____

#4 Bladder Program
___ Maintenance
___ Training
___ Uses incontinent garment
    ___ Dri–pride
    ___ Dri–pride pad
    ___ Other

SECTION VII   REPRODUCTIVE

#1 Male (Genitalia)
___ Urethral discharge / drainage
___ Swelling
___ Abnormalities

Prosthesis: _____

Comments:

#2 Female (Breast)
___ Discharge / drainage
___ Breast masses
___ Nipples
___ Mastectomy
    R ___ L ___
___ Menopausal
___ Menses

#3 Female (Genitalia)
___ Itching
___ Redness
___ Abnormal bleeding
___ Discharge / drainage
___ Atrophy
___ Prolapse
___ None

SECTION VIII   MUSCULOSKELETAL

Indicate: RUE, LUE, BUE, RLE, LLE, BLE
___ Joint stiffness
___ Swelling
___ Tremors
___ Contractures
___ Amputation
___ Internal rotation
___ External rotation
___ Shortening
___ Asymptomatic

Comments:

Miscellaneous
___ Quadriplegia
___ Hemiplegia
___ Paraplegia
___ Hand grasps equal
___ Hand grasps unequal
___ Weakness R ___ L ___
___ Generalized left sided weakness
___ Generalized right sided weakness

Signature & Date

_____
_____
_____
_____
_____

Signature & Date

_____
_____
_____
_____
_____

continues

FIGURE 8-1 *continued*

BODY CHECK

Complete Upon Admission / Significant Change of Condition / Per Policy

Height _____   Allergies: _____

Weight _____   _____

_____

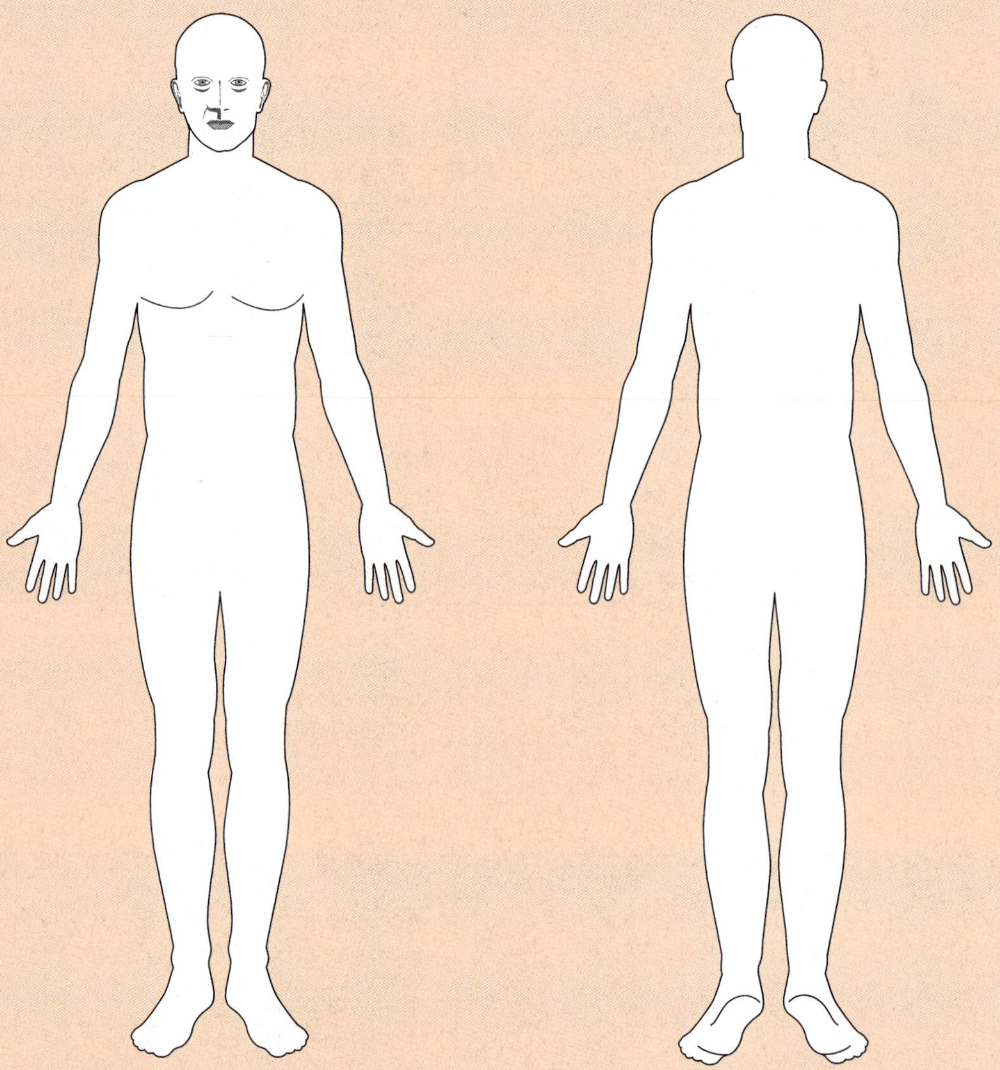

Initial body check completed by: _____   Date: _____

Note on body check:

Scars	**Feet / Ankles**
Moles	Corns
Petechiae	Callouses
Incision (s) (suture line)	Bunions
Bruises	Other
Rash	If yes or if diabetic, complete foot assessment
Skin tear (s)	
Pressure ulcer (s)	
Stasis ulcer (s)	
Surgical site (s)	
Surgical drain site (s)	

FIGURE 8-1 *continued*

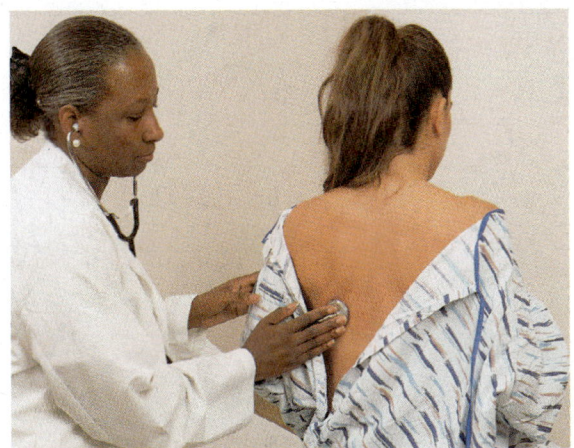

FIGURE 8-2 Part of the nursing assessment process involves physical examination. The nurse is auscultating (listening to) the patient's lungs. These data are used as a basis of comparison for future assessments.

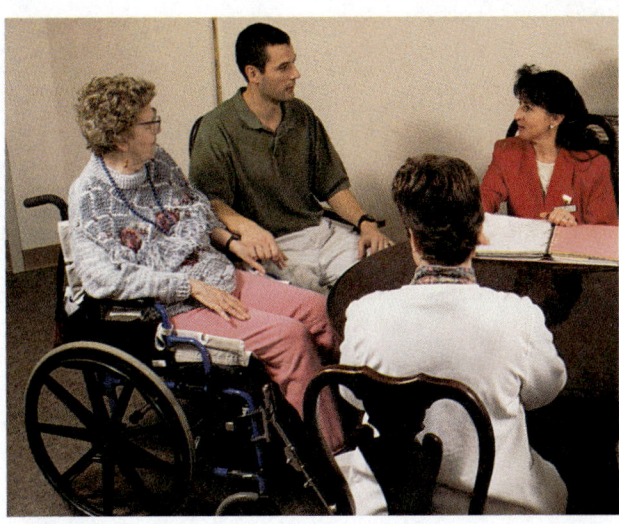

FIGURE 8-3 The patient's care plan is developed in a care conference.

TABLE 8-1 EXAMPLES OF NURSING DIAGNOSES AND OBSERVATIONS TO MAKE

Nursing Diagnosis	Observations to Make
Altered nutrition; less than body requirements	• Food/fluid intake • Weight loss • Inability to eat • Pain in abdomen or mouth • Sores in mouth
Constipation	• Lack of bowel movement or hard, dry stools • c/o feeling full • Abdomen distended and firm
Urge urinary incontinence	• Incontinence, urgency, painful urination
Decreased cardiac output	• Changes in B/P, irregular pulse, fatigue, difficulty breathing
Risk of aspiration	• Difficulty in swallowing, depressed cough and gag reflex, reduced level of consciousness
Impaired skin integrity	• Redness or destruction of skin
Impaired verbal communication	• Inability or difficulty with speaking, difficulty breathing, disorientation
Ineffective coping	• Change in usual communication patterns • c/o inability to cope or meet basic needs • Change in behavior
Impaired adjustment	• Disbelief, anger, inability to solve problems
Impaired physical mobility	• Ability to move in bed, range of motion, balance, coordination, endurance
Activity intolerance	• Fatigue, weakness, shortness of breath • Irregular pulse
Disturbed sleep pattern	• c/o not sleeping • Changes in behavior or speech
Anxiety	• Shakiness, quivering voice, increased movements • Poor eye contact, helplessness

NURSING DIAGNOSIS	NURSING INTERVENTIONS	EVALUATION
Ineffective breathing pattern R/T operative site/incisional pain.	1. Auscultate breath sounds q̄ 4h. & PRN. 2. Assist pt. tr turn, cough, and deep breathe q̄ 2h while awake.	1. Lungs clear on auscultation. 2. "It doesn't hurt as much to cough today."
Risk for infection R/T surgical incision & indwelling catheter.	Asses for s/s of infection q̄ 4h	T-100.2°, incision site warm & pink, non-edematous. "It really hurts under the bandage."
Risk for constipation R/T abdominal surgery.	1. Restart oral fluids gradually. Offer clear liquids frequently. 2. Observe for abd. distension & evaluate tolerance when pt. begins taking fluid/foods.	Unable to tolerate oral fluids — vomited p̄ taking ice chips.

FIGURE 8-4A Handwritten care plan.

PLAN OF CARE

PC: ABDOMINAL SURGERY

PB: TD:____/____Ineffective breathing pattern r/t: op site/incision pain.

EO: Respiratory rate & effort WNL with good chest expansion.

  1: Auscultate breath sounds Q4H & PRN. Note diminished/absent sounds, rales wheezing, crackles, rhonchi. DOCUMENT IN NURSES' NOTES.

  2: Assist pt to turn, cough, and deep breathe Q2H while awake. Support incision. DOCUMENT RESPONSE & EFFORT.

PB: TD:____/____Risk for infection r/t surgical incision/indwelling cath.

EO: Surgical incision healing w/out s/s of infection.

  1: Assess for s/s of infection Q4H: (fever, chills, swelling, redness, pain, drainage, increased WBC, etc) DOCUMENT IN NURSES' NOTES.

PB: TD:____/____Acute pain r/t_____ surgical incision/operative site.

EO: Pt reports pain relieved/ controlled.

  1: Implement Patient Controlled Analgesia (PCA) Protocol and PCA Teaching Protocol.

PB: TD:____/____Risk for constipation r/t_____surgery.

EO: Pt's bowel elimination is normal within limits of surgical procedure.

  1: Restart oral fluids gradually. Offer clear liquids frequently.

  2: Observe for abdominal distention & evaluate tolerance when pt begins taking fluid/foods post-op. DOCUMENT IN NURSES' NOTES.

                 INT   SIGNATURE

FIGURE 8-4B Computerized care plan. *(Courtesy of St. Tammany Parish Hospital, Covington, LA)*

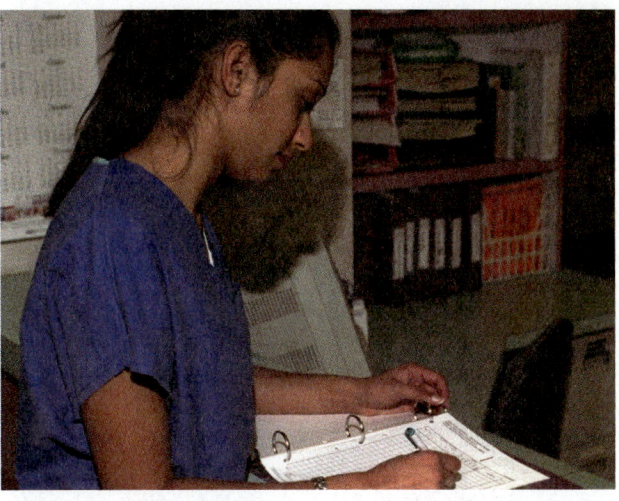

FIGURE 8-5A Care plans are often kept in the Kardex at the nurse's station.

MAKING OBSERVATIONS

An **observation** is information that is obtained by using one's senses: seeing, hearing, smelling, or feeling. This information can help the care team determine:

- A change in the patient's physical condition. *Example:* a patient with diabetes may be having an insulin reaction.
- A new condition that is developing. *Example:* a pressure ulcer may be noted.
- A change in the patient's mental condition. *Example:* a patient who has shown no signs of disorientation is now wandering about, saying he does not know where he is.
- A change in the patient's emotional condition. *Example:* a patient is crying and says she "does not want to continue living."
- The effectiveness of a medication or treatment. *Example:* a patient may be taking an antibiotic for a urinary tract infection. If the signs and symptoms of the infection are not going away, then the medication may not be effective and the physician will need to change the order.

There are two types of observations: subjective and objective. An **objective observation** is one that is factual or measurable in some way. For example, blood in the urine is factual. Blood pressure, temperature, pulse, and respirations are measurable. A **subjective observation** is a statement or complaint made by the patient. For example, "I have a headache," or "I feel sick to my stomach" are subjective observations.

You make observations by using your senses.

- You use your *eyes* to *see* observations:
  - blood in the urine
  - bruises or breaks in the skin (Figure 8-7)
  - the patient crying
  - a change in the way the patient walks

Case Presentation

Mrs. White is admitted with medical diagnoses of hyperglycemia, ketoacidosis, and a history of diabetes mellitus (DM), all diagnostic indicators of diabetic ketoacidosis (DKA). Mrs. White is having labored breathing, vomiting, and weakness. Mr. White states that his wife takes insulin for her diabetes, she doesn't follow her diet, and she has been complaining of thirst and frequent urination. On examination, the client complains of weakness and abdominal pain, and she has an acetone breath.

White, Mary	F 56
MR#: 000135039	ACCT#: 9710144268
Dr: J. Smith	2/W 402–XX
DX: Diabetic Ketoacidosis (DKA)	DATE: 12/14/XX

SUMMARY: 12/14　　　　0701 to 1501

CILIENT INFORMATION

10/14	ADVANCE DIRECTIVES: No. Advance directive does not exist
10/14	ORGAN DONOR: Unknown
10/14	ADMIT DX: Diabetic Ketoacidosis (DKA)
10/14	ALLERGIES: None Known
10/14	ISOLATION: Not at this time

MISC. CLIENT DATA

10/14　　History of Diabetes Mellitus (DM): Insulin-Dependent Diabetic

MEDICAL DIAGNOSES

10/14	PROBLEM # 1: Hyperglycemia
10/14	PROBLEM # 2: Ketoacidosis
10/14	PROBLEM # 3: Hyperventilation
10/14	PROBLEM # 4: Hypovolemia, Hypernatremia
10/14	PROBLEM # 5: Hypotension
10/14	PROBLEM # 6: Hypokalemia

NURSING DIAGNOSES

10/14	PROBLEM 1: Deficient fluid volume r/t osmotic diuresis associated with hyperglycemia
10/14	PROBLEM 2: Ineffective breathing pattern: Kussmaul respirations/air hunger r/t metabolic acidosis associated with DKA
10/14	PROBLEM 3: Decreased cardiac output r/t hypokalemia associated with metabolic acidosis
10/14	PROBLEM 4: Risk for injury: circulatory collapse, renal shutdown, and coma r/t persistent, untreated hyperglycemia
10/14	PROBLEM 5: Risk for injury: seizure susceptibility if hyperglycemia is corrected too abruptly
10/14	PROBLEM 6: Ineffective airway clearance: aspiration r/t presence of vomiting and altered level of conciousness
10/14	PROBLEM 7: Risk for infection r/t invasive procedures
10/14	PROBLEM 8: Altered nutrition: less than body requirements r/t anorexia, nausea, or vomiting associated with ketoacidosis and hypokalemia
10/14	PROBLEM 9: Deficient knowledge: prevention of DKA r/t proper management of DM
10/14	PROBLEM 10: Ineffective therapeutic regimen management r/t inadequate motivation for incorporating strategies for prevention of DKA into daily living

FIGURE 8-5B Sample computer-generated Kardex, based in part on information from the case presentation. *(From Springhouse. [2001]. Mastering documentation. Springhouse, PA; Springhouse. Reiner, A. [Ed.] [2001]. Manual of patient care standards. Gaithersburg, MD; Aspen and Williams [2001]. Decision making in critical care nursing. Philadelphia, PA; Decker)*

ALL CURRENT MEDICAL ORDERS

NURSING ORDERS:

10/14	Activity: Bedrest
	VS: Q15" first 2 Hours, then Q30" until within normal limits, then Q1H
10/14	Telemetry
10/14	Daily Weight: 0600
10/14	Intake & Output: Q 15 min. first 2 Hours, then Q 30 min. until output stable at 30 ml/H, then Q1H
10/14	Urine: Specific Gravity Q1H
10/14	Measure blood glucose levels: Q1H, notify physician when serum glucose is less than 300 mg percent
10/14	Oral Hygiene Q1H
10/14	Monitor for s/s of infection: IV site, Triple-lumen, central line, right subclavian and indwelling foley catheter
10/14	Institute fall precautions

SUMMARY: 10/14   0701 to 1501

DIET:

10/14	NPO; Diabetic: 1600 cal., start with breakfast tomorrow

IVS:

10/14	Central line #1....0.9 percent normal saline, 1000 ml @ rate of 1 L/H for first 2 H, infusion pump; then decrease infusion of 0.9 percent normal saline, 500 ml @ rate of 500 ml/H for the next 2 H; then decrease infusion of 0.9 percent normal saline, 250 ml @ rate of 250 ml/H
10/14	Central line #2...50 U of regular insulin to 500 ml normal saline to produce a concentration of 0.1 U/ml, infuse @ 7 U/kg per hour, infusion pump
10/14	Administer KCL IV: If serum K^+ is <3.5 give 40 mEq/H; 3.5–5.5 give 20 mEq/H; >5.5 give no K^+

SCHEDULED MEDICATIONS:

10/14	None

STAT/NOW MEDICATIONS:

10/14	IV bolus of regular insulin of 0.2 U/kg

PRN MEDICATIONS:

10/14	None

LABORATORY:

10/14	Stat Chem Profile 23
	Blood Glucose Q1H
	Stat Arterial Blood Gases
	Urinalysis Now

ANCILLARY:

10/14	Stat EKG
10/14	FSBS prn s/s hypo/hyperglycemia

Last Page

FIGURE 8-5B *continued*

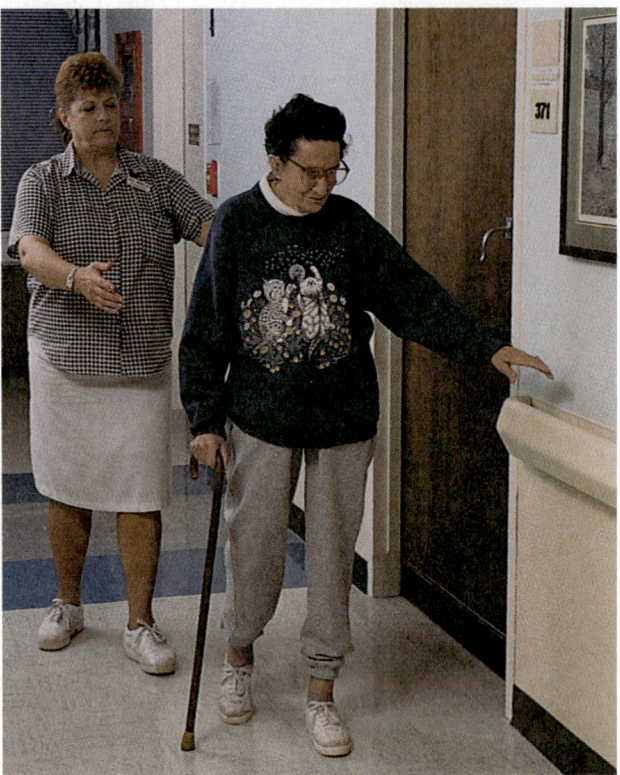

FIGURE 8-6 Nursing assistants are responsible for implementing many of the care plan approaches.

- Your *ears* to *hear* observations:
  - wheezing when the patient breathes
  - pulse or blood pressure with a stethoscope
  - comments from the patient, such as "I am very tired today"
- Your *nose* to *smell* observations:
  - body odor

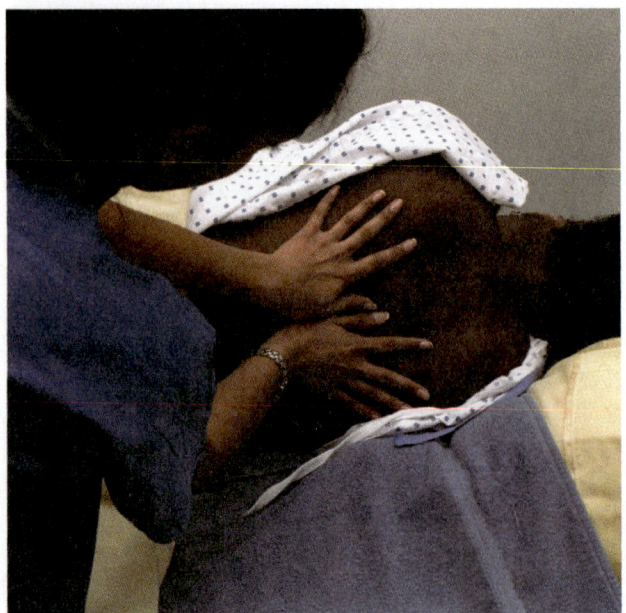

FIGURE 8-7 The nursing assistant observes the skin for bruised, red, or open areas while giving a backrub.

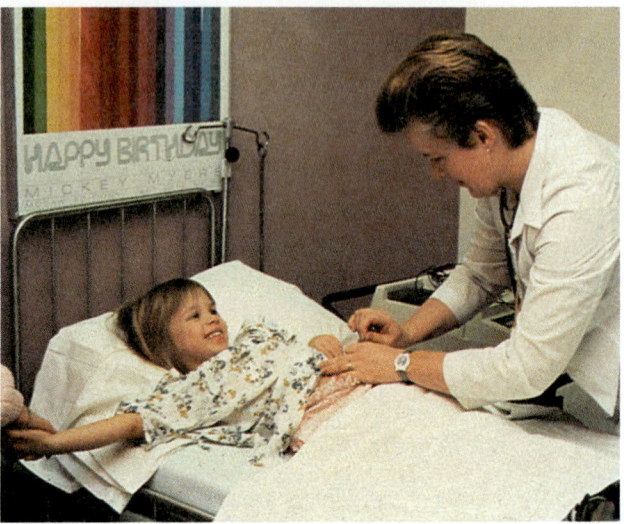

FIGURE 8-8 Lumps under the skin may be felt using the sense of touch. *(Photo courtesy of Henrietta Egleston Hospital for Children, Atlanta, GA. Photograph by Ginger Lovering)*

  - stool or urine when the patient is incontinent
- Your *hands and fingers* to *feel* observations:
  - a lump under the patient's skin (Figure 8-8)
  - radial pulse
  - warmth or coolness of the patient's skin

Remember that observations must be:

- accurate and timely
- reported to the nurse in a timely manner
- documented in the patient's record, either by you or the nurse

Making Initial Observations

To make accurate observations, you must first know what is expected or normal for an individual. For this reason, baseline information is collected when the patient is admitted to the facility. If you help admit a patient, make observations while you are completing your assignment. It is especially important to note any possible signs of injury or skin breakdown. Think of the body systems as described in the following list. This information will give you a basis for making future comparisons. For example, one patient may have a blood pressure of 110/68 on admission. If you take the patient's blood pressure later and it is 140/88, you should report this to the nurse, because this is not the usual blood pressure for this person. Try to establish a routine way of making observations. Keep in mind the age and known illnesses of the patients. It may be helpful to think of each body system and note the following:

- Integumentary system (skin, nails)
  - Color: flushed, pale, jaundiced (yellow color), or cyanotic (bluish, ashen, gray color); nails pale, pink, or cyanotic.
  - Temperature: warm, hot, cool.
  - Moisture: dry, moist, perspiring.

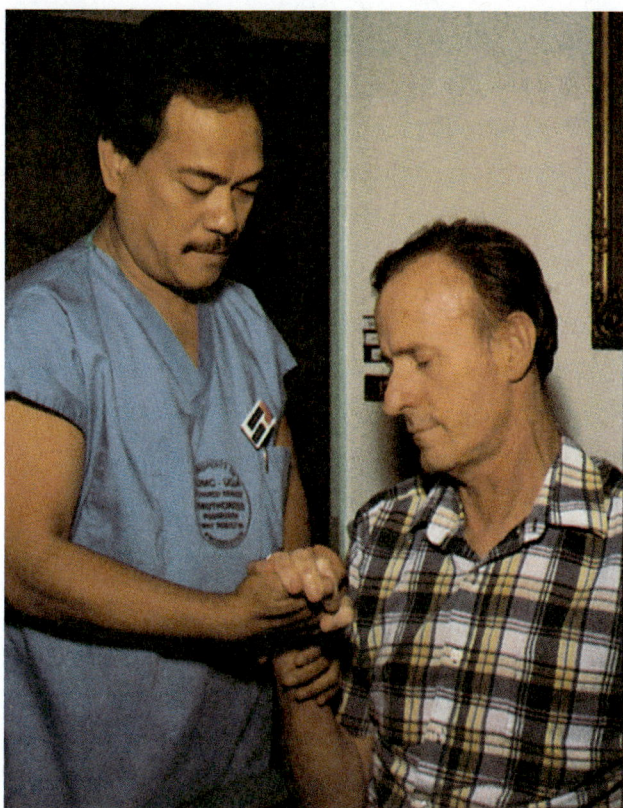

FIGURE 8-9 Report to the nurse if there is a change in the patient's ability to move the joints.

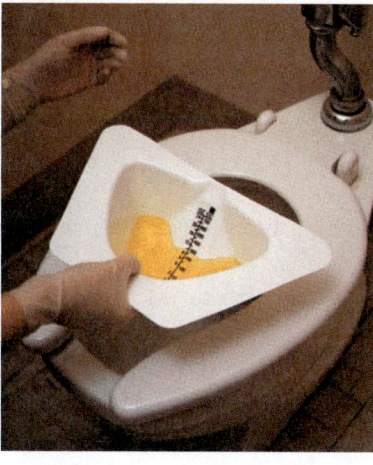

FIGURE 8-10 Examine the urine before discarding it. If you observe abnormalities, save it for the nurse to view.

- Nose: drainage, bleeding.
- Sense of touch: ability to feel pressure and pain.
- Urinary system (kidneys, ureters, bladder, urethra)
  - Urination: frequency, amount, color, clarity, odor, presence of blood or sediment (Figure 8-10); ability to hold urine, incontinence.
  - Pain on urination (dysuria).
- Digestive system (mouth, teeth, throat, esophagus, stomach, large and small intestines, gall bladder, liver, pancreas)
  - Full or partial dentures
  - Dental caries (cavities)
  - Appetite: amount of fluids and food consumed (Figure 8-11), tolerance to foods, belching or burping.

- Abnormalities: rashes, bruises, scars, pressure ulcers, areas of redness.
- Musculoskeletal system (muscles, bones, joints)
  - Posture: stooped, curled up in bed, straight.
  - Mobility: ability to move in bed, to get out of bed, to stand, to walk, and to maintain balance.
  - Range of motion: ability to move all joints (Figure 8-9).
- Circulatory system (heart, blood vessels, blood)
  - Pulse: strength, regularity, rate.
  - Skin: (see integumentary system).
  - Nails: (see integumentary system).
  - Blood pressure.
- Respiratory system (nose, throat, trachea, bronchi, lungs)
  - Respirations (breathing): rate, regularity, depth, difficulty in breathing, shortness of breath upon exertion or while still, wheezing or crackling heard.
  - Cough: frequency; dry, loose, productive. Color and consistency of sputum (if any).
- Nervous system (brain, spinal cord, nerves)
  - Mental status: orientation to time, place, person. Ability to make verbal or nonverbal responses.
- Senses (eyes, ears, nose, sense of touch)
  - Eyes: reddened, drainage, pupils equal in size.
  - Ears: drainage.

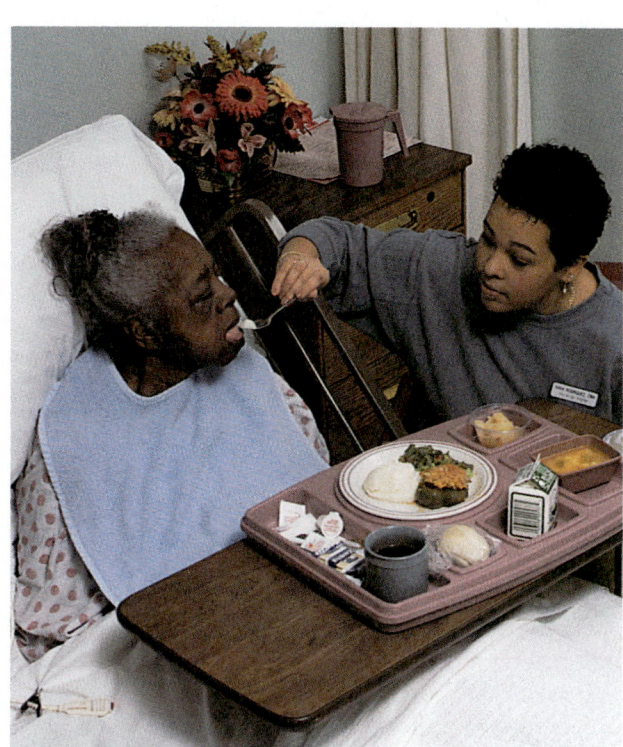

FIGURE 8-11 Monitor and record the amount of food and fluid consumed.

- – Eating: difficulty chewing or swallowing.
- – Nausea and/or vomiting.
- – Bowel elimination: Frequency, amount, consistency, color of stools; diarrhea, constipation, incontinence, flatus; difficulty in passing stool.
- Endocrine system (glands)
  - – Signs and symptoms of diabetes (hypoglycemia, hyperglycemia).
- Reproductive system (male and female internal and external sex organs)

  Female

  - – Breasts: condition of nipples, presence of lumps, discolorations.
  - – Menstrual periods: frequency, amount, and character of bleeding; cramping.
  - – Vaginal drainage: amount, odor, and character.

  Male

  - – Testes: lumps.
  - – Penis: amount and character of drainage.

In addition to the body systems observations, you also need to note facts related to pain, behavior, and function.

- Pain: location, type of pain (sharp, dull, aching), constant or intermittent or related to specific activities, time pain started
- Behavior: actions, conduct
- Function: ability to move about and complete tasks such as bathing

When reporting behavior, avoid using "labels" based on your judgment of the patient. Report only what you see and hear.

You may make additional observations related to the patient's medical diagnoses. For example, if a patient has a kidney condition, you would look for edema (swelling) of the face, hands, and ankles (Figure 8-12). You would also monitor the person's fluid intake and output. You will learn more about observations related to medical diagnoses as you study these conditions.

In some situations, you may be expected to report "normal" observations. This information tells the nurse and physician whether the patient's condition is improving. For example, if a patient has had a respiratory tract infection and the signs and symptoms have diminished, it is important to report "no coughing or respiratory distress is noted." Abnormal observations that should be reported to the nurse are listed in Table 8-2.

PAIN

It is important that you be very factual in reporting observations of pain and behavior. Never try to judge whether a patient really has pain or how severe the pain is. Some individuals are very expressive about pain and others are very stoical (they try not to show their discomfort). A person's

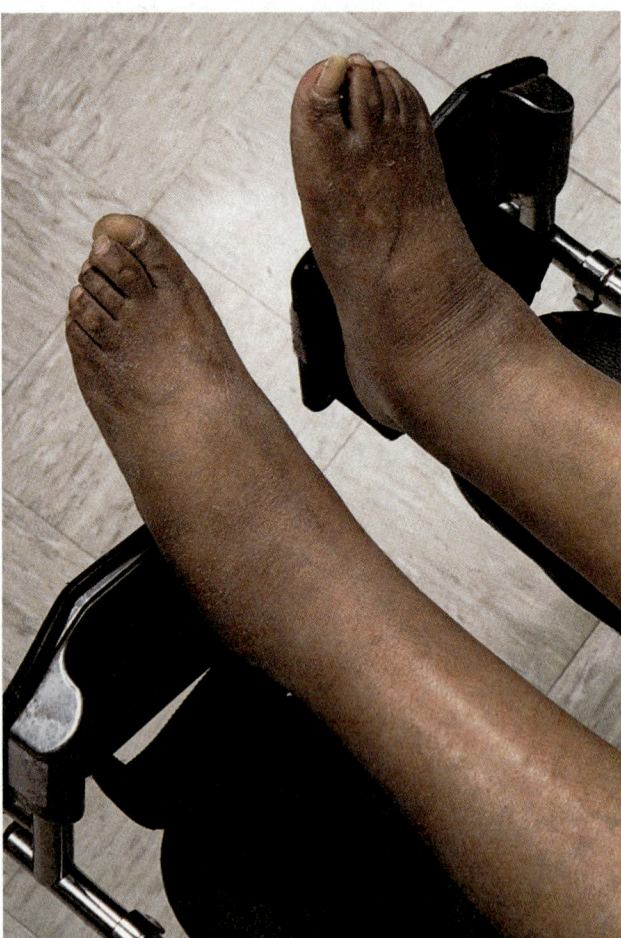

FIGURE 8-12 Patients with heart, circulatory, or kidney problems may develop edema of the lower extremities.

culture may also affect his or her response to pain. Never compare patients. One person may seem to have more pain than another person with the same diagnosis. It is not appropriate to think that they should both respond in the same way.

Pain is never normal. Always report patient complaints of pain to the nurse. Determining whether pediatric or cognitively impaired patients are in pain may be difficult because they may be unable to describe the nature of the problem. Patients from other cultures may have varying reactions to pain. In some cultures, displaying outward signs of pain is considered to be a weakness, and is unacceptable.

Body language is often the first clue that a patient is having pain. This may be the only clue in some pediatric and cognitively impaired patients, those from other cultures, and patients who are comatose. Look for pain upon movement, facial expressions, crying, moaning, rigid posture, and guarded positioning. The patient may withdraw when he or she is touched or repositioned. Watch for restlessness, irregular or erratic respirations, intermittent breath holding, dilated pupils, and sweating. The patient may favor one extremity. He or she may become irritable, fatigued, or withdrawn. The patient may refuse to eat for no apparent

TABLE 8-2 OBSERVATION AND REPORTING GUIDELINES

General signs and symptoms of illness that should be reported to the nurse

Chest pain	Nausea or vomiting	Lethargy
Shortness of breath	Diarrhea	Unusual drainage from a wound or body cavity
Difficulty breathing	Cough	Changes in vital signs
Weakness or dizziness	Cyanosis or change in color	Profuse sweating
Headache	Change in mental status	
Pain	Excessive thirst	

System or Problem	Observation to Report	System or Problem	Observation to Report
Signs/symptoms of infection	Elevated temperature Sweating Chills Skin hot or cold to touch Skin flushed, red, gray, or blue Inflammation of skin as evidenced by redness, edema, heat, or pain Drainage from wounds or body cavities Any unusual body discharge, such as mucus or pus	Respiratory System	Respiratory rate below 12 or above 20 Irregular respirations Noisy, labored respirations Dyspnea Shortness of breath Gasping for breath Wheezing Coughing Retractions Blue color of lips, nail beds, or mucous membranes
Evidence of pain	Chest pain Pain that radiates Pain upon movement Pain during urination Pain when having a bowel movement (Pain is not normal; all complaints of pain should be reported to the nurse)	Integumentary system	Rash Redness in the skin that does not go away within 30 minutes after pressure is relieved New, abnormally dark areas in patients with dark skin Pressure sores, blisters Irritation Bruises Skin discoloration Swelling Lumps Abnormal sweating Excessive heat or coolness to touch Open areas/skin breakdown Drainage Foul odor Complaints such as numbness, burning, tingling, itching Signs of infection Unusual skin color, such as blue or gray color of the skin, lips, nail beds, roof of mouth, or mucous membranes Abrasions, skin tears, lacerations
Cardiovascular system	Abnormal pulse below 60 or above 100 Blood pressure below 100/60 or above 140/90 Unable to palpate pulse or hear blood pressure Chest pain Chest pain that radiates to neck, jaw, or arm Shortness of breath Headache, dizziness, weakness, vomiting Cold, blue, or gray appearance Cold, blue, painful feet or hands Shortness of breath, dyspnea, or abnormal respirations Feeling faint or lightheaded		

continues

TABLE 8-2 *continued*

System or Problem	Observation to Report	System or Problem	Observation to Report
Integumentary system *continued*	Skin growths Poor skin turgor/tenting of skin Sunken, dark appearance around eyes	Nervous system	Change in level of consciousness, orientation, awareness, or alertness Feeling faint or lightheaded Increasing mental confusion Progressive lethargy Loss of sensation Numbness, tingling Change in pupil size; unequal pupils Abnormal or involuntary motor function Loss of ability to move a body part Loss or lack of coordination
Gastrointestinal system	Sores or ulcers inside the mouth Difficulty chewing or swallowing food Unusual or abnormal appearance of bowel movement Blood, mucus, or other unusual substances in stool Unusual color of bowel movement Hard stool, difficulty passing stool Complaints of pain, constipation, diarrhea, bleeding Frequent belching Changes in appetite Excessive thirst Fruity smell to breath Complaints of indigestion or excessive gas Nausea, vomiting Choking Abdominal pain Abdominal distention Coffee-ground appearance of emesis or stool		
		Musculoskeletal system	Pain Obvious deformity Edema Immobility Inability to move arms and legs Inability to move one or more joints Limited/abnormal range of motion Jerking or shaky movements Weakness Sensory changes Changes in ability to sit, stand, move, or walk Pain upon movement
Genitourinary system	Urinary output too low Oral intake too low Fluid intake and output not balanced Abnormal appearance of urine: dark, concentrated, red, cloudy Unusual material in urine: blood, pus, particles, mucus Complaints of difficulty urinating Complaints of pain, burning, urgency, frequency, pain in lower back Urinating frequently in small amounts Sudden-onset incontinence Edema, signs of fluid retention Sudden weight loss or gain Respiratory distress Change in mental status	Mental status	Change in level of consciousness, awareness, or alertness Changes in mood or behavior Change in ability to express self or communicate Mental confusion Excessive drowsiness Sleepiness for no apparent reason Sudden onset of mental confusion Threats of harm to self or others

reason. Often, the patient acts opposite of normal. For example:

- A cognitively impaired geriatric patient who is normally very quiet may become noisy.
- A pediatric patient may cry for no apparent reason.
- A patient with garbled speech may accurately describe his or her pain.
- The agitated and combative patient may become quiet and nonverbal.
- A friendly and outgoing patient may begin to cry easily and withdraw.
- The patient who is normally active may become still and quiet.

Always suspect pain if the patient's behavior changes. Although the patient may not display an outward appearance of pain, asking if he or she is having pain is the best way to find out. Report your observations to the nurse compared with the normal behavior for the patient. If the behavior changes back to normal after the nurse administers an *analgesic* (pain) medication, this confirms that the change in body language or behavior was caused by pain.

Although many patients with pain display outward signs through their body language and behavior, avoid making assumptions about the presence or absence of pain if the patient is laughing, talking, or sleeping. For example, some health care workers assume that patients who are smiling or laughing cannot be in pain. These workers believe that patients who are having pain should be grimacing, frowning, or crying. This is untrue. Some patients may appear comfortable even while they are having severe pain. Once again, avoid judging the patient. His or her own report of pain is the most accurate and reliable indicator of pain, and should be believed and respected. Simply notify the nurse of the patient's complaint of pain.

Pain management is an important part of patient care. Take complaints of pain very seriously. Respect and support the patients' right to pain assessment and management without judgment or disbelief. You are responsible for reporting the information to the nurse, who will assess the patient and take the appropriate action. Avoid passing judgment on patients who take narcotic medications to control their pain. Many health care workers try to discourage patients from taking these drugs because of the potential for addiction. Studies have shown that very few patients with severe pain become addicted to the drugs.

Pain Assessment Scales

The nurse may use a pain scale to help assess and manage the patient's pain. The scale is a tool for communication. The patient selects the scale that best helps him or her describe the pain. Most facilities have several different pain scales available. Different scales may be used for children and adults. Using a pain scale prevents subjective opinions, and keeps everyone informed as to the level and intensity of the patient's pain. The patient and nurse may have established a pain management goal using the scale. The patient may refer to the goal in conversation with you, so you should become familiar with the scales used at your facility.

Many different pain scales are used in health care (Figure 8-13A and Figure 8-13B). The scales shown in Figure 8-13 are for example only. Your facility may use similar or different tools for evaluating pain. Pain scales use pictures, words, or numbers to help the patient describe pain intensity. Most scales range from no pain to very severe pain. Picture scales use a range from smiling faces and neutral faces to frowns and tears.

Some patients may not complain of pain and may appear to be comfortable. Asking them if they are having pain is not offensive. Always ask instead of assuming. Likewise, if a patient has been medicated for pain, but continues to complain, inform the nurse. Do not assume that the pain has been relieved after a medication has been given, even if the patient is laughing or talking. Ask the patient. If he or she admits to continued pain, the nurse must assess the patient further.

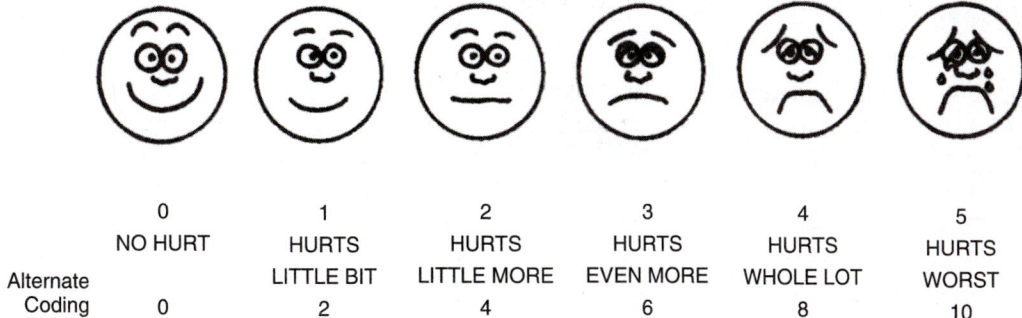

	0	1	2	3	4	5
	NO HURT	HURTS LITTLE BIT	HURTS LITTLE MORE	HURTS EVEN MORE	HURTS WHOLE LOT	HURTS WORST
Alternate Coding	0	2	4	6	8	10

FIGURE 8-13A Each patient will select the pain scale that best helps him or her describe the level and intensity of pain. The FACES pain rating scale is an excellent tool for children and adults. *(From Wong D. L., Hockenberry-Eaton M., Wilson D., Winkelstein M. L., Schwartz P.: Wong's essentials of pediatric nursing, ed. 6, St. Louis, 2001, p. 1301. Copyrighted by Mosby, Inc. Reprinted by permission.)*

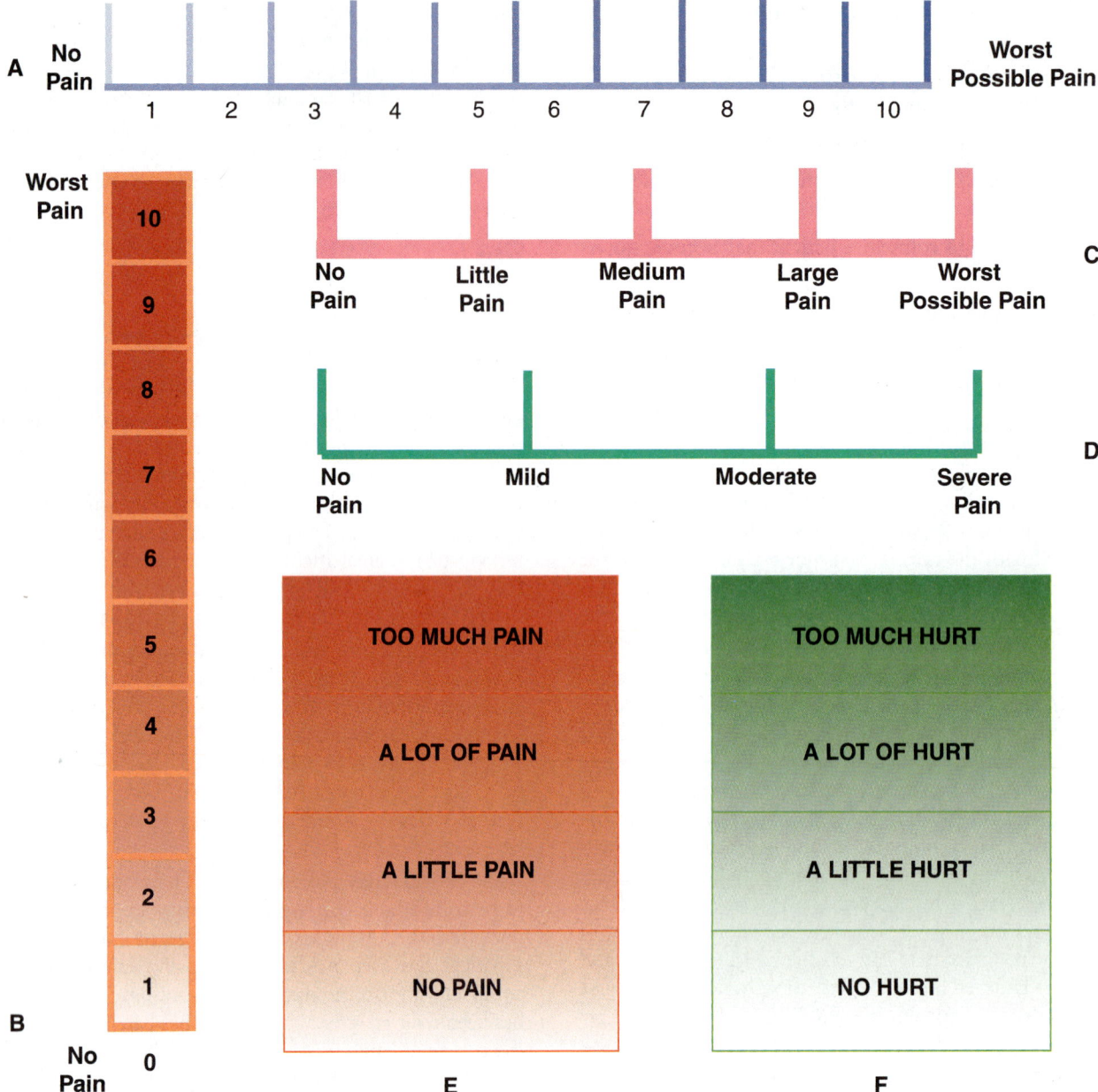

FIGURE 8-13B (A) Horizontal numeric pain scale. (B) Vertical numeric pain scale. (C) Verbal descriptor pain scale. (D) Verbal pain scale. (E) Verbal pain scale. (F) Verbal pain scale.

REPORTING

Giving an **oral report** is one method used to relay information from one person to another. The nursing assistant may participate in oral reports several times on a shift. Oral reports are given by the:

- nurse going off duty to the staff coming on duty (Figure 8-14) (in some facilities the nurse may give a report only to the charge nurse of the oncoming shift)—this is called a shift report. Some facilities leave a taped report for the next shift.
- nursing assistant to the nurse when leaving the nursing unit for any reason (such as lunch break).

- nursing assistant to the nurse at the end of the shift.
- nursing assistant to the nurse if any unusual or new observations are made.

Be specific when you report your observations. If you are relaying a subjective observation (something the patient has told you), repeat it exactly the way the patient told it to you. Here are some examples:

- Mr. Jones in 249 says it hurts every time he urinates.
- Mrs. Goldberg was wandering around in the hall and said she did not know where she was.

To report objective observations, state your measurement or fact:

- Mrs. Dominick's blood pressure is 142/86.

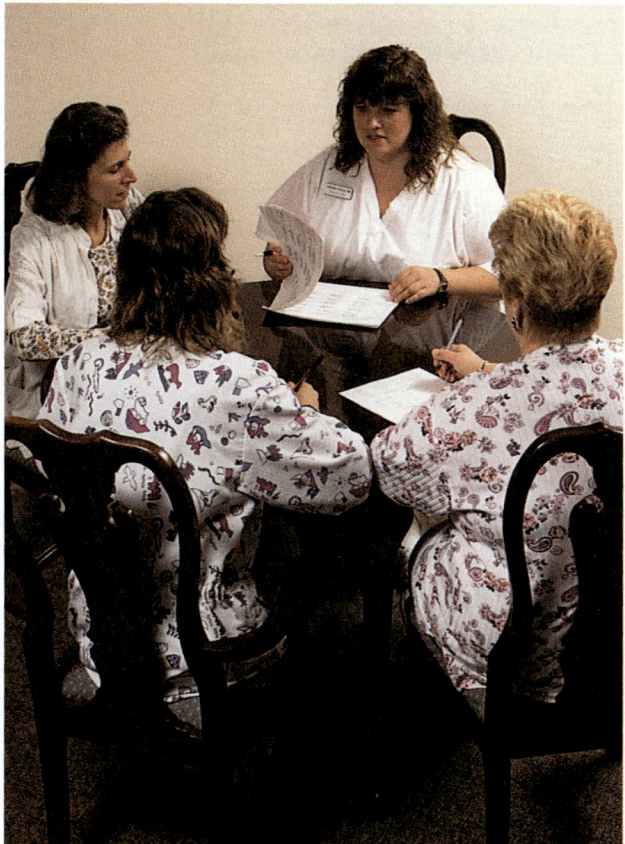

FIGURE 8-14 Report is given to the oncoming shift by the nurse who worked the previous shift.

- Mr. Hernandez ate 50 percent of his meal at lunch time.

When you report off duty at the end of your shift, report to the nurse:

- the condition of each of the patients you were assigned to
- the care you gave each patient
- observations you made while giving care

COMMUNICATION
Highlight

You will learn when to report your observations about patients as you gain experience. In general, high-priority items for reporting include abnormal vital signs, chest pain, difficulty breathing, change in color, change in mental status, bleeding, and pain. If you are in doubt about the urgency of reporting to the nurse, report your observation immediately. If the patient's condition changes after you have reported your observations, inform the nurse again.

DOCUMENTATION

In some facilities you may be expected to record your observations on the patient's medical record (chart) (Figure 8-15). The medical record is a **document**. A document is a legal record. The process of recording the patient's care, response to treatment, and progress in the patient's chart is called **charting** or *documentation*. Nursing assistants may document on **flow sheets** (Figure 8-16) in the chart or on the **nurse's notes** (Figure 8-17) (sometimes called nurse's progress notes). The charting must:

- address the problems listed in the patient's care plan or critical pathway
- describe the approaches (interventions) listed in the care plan or critical pathway and note whether the interventions are effective
- indicate the progress the patient is making toward meeting the goals on the care plan or critical pathway

Charting Guidelines

A patient's medical record (chart) is a legal document and may be used in court as evidence. It is important that everything be correct and legible. All charting and records must be in clear, simple, and accurate language. Entries must be printed or written carefully so that there can be no misunderstanding of the meaning. If you follow the established rules of charting, there will be no problem.

Each chart relates only to one patient, so it is unnecessary to use the term *patient* or to use the patient's name. Use phrases rather than full sentences, and do not make erasures or leave empty spaces on the record. All entries are made in black ink because the chart is a permanent record; no erasable ink or correction fluid is allowed.

If you use medical terms in your charting, make sure you are using the correct words and that spelling is correct. Use a medical dictionary if you are not sure. Abbreviations are allowed, but they must be on your facility's approved list. Do not make up your own abbreviations. You must chart only for yourself and only when the procedure or assignment has been completed.

The time of entry must be noted when the entry is made. Most health care facilities use international time (Table 8-3)

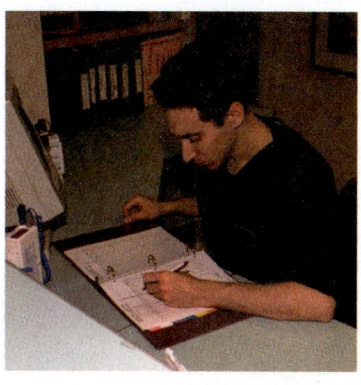

FIGURE 8-15
Observations are recorded in the patient's medical record.

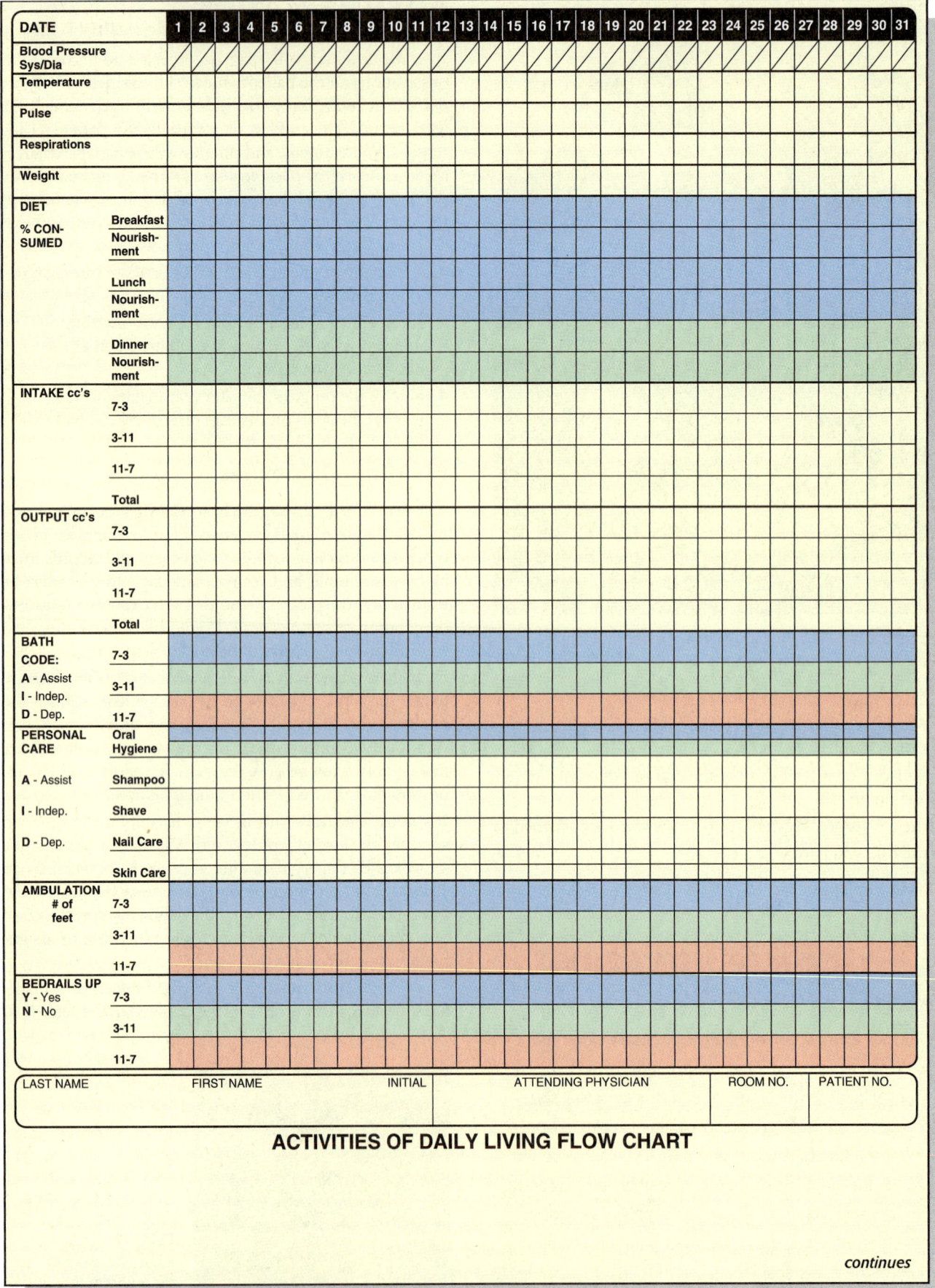

DATE		1	2	3	4	5	6	7	8	9	10	11	12	13	14	15	16	17	18	19	20	21	22	23	24	25	26	27	28	29	30	31
Blood Pressure Sys/Dia																																
Temperature																																
Pulse																																
Respirations																																
Weight																																
DIET % CON-SUMED	Breakfast																															
	Nourish-ment																															
	Lunch																															
	Nourish-ment																															
	Dinner																															
	Nourish-ment																															
INTAKE cc's	7-3																															
	3-11																															
	11-7																															
	Total																															
OUTPUT cc's	7-3																															
	3-11																															
	11-7																															
	Total																															
BATH CODE: A - Assist I - Indep. D - Dep.	7-3																															
	3-11																															
	11-7																															
PERSONAL CARE A - Assist I - Indep. D - Dep.	Oral Hygiene																															
	Shampoo																															
	Shave																															
	Nail Care																															
	Skin Care																															
AMBULATION # of feet	7-3																															
	3-11																															
	11-7																															
BEDRAILS UP Y - Yes N - No	7-3																															
	3-11																															
	11-7																															

LAST NAME	FIRST NAME	INITIAL	ATTENDING PHYSICIAN	ROOM NO.	PATIENT NO.

ACTIVITIES OF DAILY LIVING FLOW CHART

continues

FIGURE 8-16 You may be expected to document your care and observations on a flow sheet.

DATE		1	2	3	4	5	6	7	8	9	10	11	12	13	14	15	16	17	18	19	20	21	22	23	24	25	26	27	28	29	30	31
UP IN CHAIR	7-3																															
A - Assist	3-11																															
I - Indep. D - Dep.	11-7																															
ROM Exercises	7-3																															
A - Active P - Passive	3-11																															
POSITION changed	7-3																															
A - Assist I - Indep.	3-11																															
D - Dep.	11-7																															
BLADDER ACTION	7-3																															
C - Continent I - Incontinent	3-11																															
F - Foley # x's	11-7																															
BOWEL ACTION	7-3																															
C - Continent I - Incontinent	3-11																															
# x's	11-7																															
CONSISTENCY	7-3																															
L - Liquid S - Soft formed	3-11																															
H - Hard formed	11-7																															
PERI CARE	7-3																															
A - Assist I - Indep.	3-11																															
D - Dep.	11-7																															
RESTRAINT P - Pelvic W - Waist	7-3																															
B - Belt G - Geri Chair	3-11																															
Check q 1/2 Hr. Release q 2 hrs.	11-7																															
Nursing Assistant's Initials	A.M.																															
	P.M.																															
	NOC.																															
Licensed Nurse Initials	A.M.																															
	P.M.																															
	NOC.																															

Nursing Assistant's Initials and Signature

Licensed Nurse Initials and Signature

LAST NAME	FIRST NAME	INITIAL	ATTENDING PHYSICIAN	ROOM NO.	PATIENT NO.

FIGURE 8-16 *continued*

NURSE'S PROGRESS NOTES

DATE AND TIME	NURSING CARE NOTES	SIGNATURE
3-16-XX	2200 Found lying on floor beside bed. Responds verbally. States was "trying to get to the bathroom." Nurse notified immediately	C. Simmons CNA
	2205 ROM satisfactory. Denies having pain. No injuries noted. ROM wnl. No obvious deformities. Assisted back to bed. Call light within reach. Instructed to use call light when having to go to B.R. Pulse 86, strong and regular. B/P 136/84. Oriented to time, place, person. Incontinent after fall. Pajamas chgd. Dr. Stone & responsible party notified.	
	2300 Sleeping s̄ distress	B. Selici RN
3-17-XX	2400-0200 Sleeping soundly. Respirations regular. Pulse 78 strong and regular.	
	0230 Awake. c/o "arthritis pain" in both hips. Acetaminophen 500 mg tabs ī̄ given with water. Assisted to bathroom. Voided large amt. clear urine.	
	0230-0630 Slept soundly. Pulse 72 strong and regular. B/P 128/80. T 98⁶(O). Denies pain anywhere. No	
3-17-XX	other c/o distress.	P. Hernandez RN
	0710 Up to B.R. c̄ assistance ——— Error ES	E. Seldes LPN

FIGURE 8-17 The nurse's notes are a narrative record of patient care and observations.

to avoid confusion between A.M. and P.M. With international time, the 24 hours of each day are identified by the numbers 0100 (1:00 A.M.) through 2400 (12:00 A.M., midnight). The last two digits indicate the minutes of each hour (from 01 to 59). Thus, 0101 would be one minute after 1:00 A.M.; 1210 would be ten minutes after 12 P.M. (noon); 1658 would be 4:58 P.M., and so on.

Many health care facilities are using flow sheets for documenting patient care. Flow sheets save nursing time and simplify the documentation process. However, there are some things you should be aware of to avoid problems:

- Understand what you are supposed to be documenting. Read the flow sheet carefully.
- Never initial any procedure or observation that you did not do.
- Initial for the right procedure, on the right day, on the right shift.
- Put your complete signature on each flow sheet (usually at the bottom of the page).
- Remember that flow sheets are legal records just like the other forms in the medical record.

guidelines *for*

Documentation on the Computerized Medical Record

- Do not be afraid of computerized charting. When documenting on a specific patient, double-check to make sure you have entered the correct identification code.
- Do not give your identification code or password to others.
- Access only information you are authorized to obtain.
- Document only in areas you are authorized to use.
- Many computer programs place expert reminders

or error codes on the screen. Read and follow the directions.

- The procedure for late entry and addendum documentation will be different than it is in a narrative system. Know and follow your facility policies for this type of charting.
- Stay current. Attend continuing education programs to learn how to maximize the use of computerized charting and information systems.

TABLE 8-3 INTERNATIONAL TIME

Standard Clock	Int'l. Time	Standard Clock	Int'l. Time
AM 12 midnight	2400	PM 12 noon	1200
1	0100	1	1300
2	0200	2	1400
3	0300	3	1500
4	0400	4	1600
5	0500	5	1700
6	0600	6	1800
7	0700	7	1900
8	0800	8	2000
9	0900	9	2100
10	1000	10	2200
11	1100	11	2300

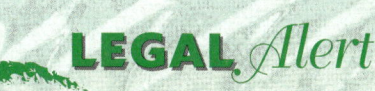

LEGAL *Alert*

In health care, there is a saying, "If it's not charted, it wasn't done." Although some facilities use a system called "charting by exception," most adhere to the time-tested maxim and chart all care given. The purpose of documentation is to communicate care given and the patient's response. Documentation is a true record of patient care, and is the first line of defense in proving accountability for excellent care. Never chart care that you did not provide. For example, some assistants will chart that a patient was "turned every two hours" because they know that this is the care that is supposed to be given. Document only the facts. If you are unable to turn the patient every two hours, inform the nurse early in the shift. Always chart after giving care. Never document on the medical record in advance. If you forget to document, follow your facility policy for making a late entry. Specify the exact date and time the entry was recorded, as well as the exact date and time the event occurred. Clearly mark your documentation as a late entry.

guidelines *for*

Charting

- Check for: right patient, right chart, right form, right room
- Fill out new headings completely
- Use correct color of ink
- Date and time each entry
- Chart entries in correct sequence
- Make entries brief, objective, and accurate
- Print or write clearly
- Spell each word correctly
- Leave no blank spaces or lines between entries
- Do not use the term *patient*
- Do not use ditto marks
- Sign each entry with your first initial, last name, and job title
- Make corrections by drawing one line through the entry; then print the word "error" on the line and your initials above

REVIEW

A. True/False.

Mark the following true or false by circling T or F.

1. T (F) The nursing process is a method used by the nurse to supervise the work of others.
2. T (F) The nursing assistant is responsible for completing an assessment on all patients.
3. (T) F Assessment involves the collection of data.
4. T (F) A statement of a patient's medical condition is called a nursing diagnosis.
5. (T) F An approach is sometimes called an intervention.
6. (T) F The patient's goal is called an outcome.
7. (T) F The care plan is developed at the care plan conference.
8. T (F) Nursing assistants are not responsible for the development or implementation of the care plan.
9. (T/F) Taking a patient's weight is an example of an objective observation.
10. (T) F The patient's chart is a legal document.

B. Multiple Choice.

Select the one best answer for each of the following.

11. The purpose of the nursing process is to
    a. make a medical diagnosis.
    (b.) achieve patient focused care.
    c. make assignments.
    d. cure illness.
12. The nursing assistant contributes to the nurse's assessment of the patient by
    a. listening to the heart and lungs.
    b. keeping the environment neat and tidy.
    c. establishing goals for the patient.
    (d.) reporting observations and vital signs.
13. The statement of a patient's problem and its cause is called
    a. a medical diagnosis.
    b. an approach.
    c. an assessment.
    (d.) a nursing diagnosis.
14. The purpose of evaluation is to determine whether the
    (a.) patient is reaching the goals on the care plan.
    b. laboratory tests are accurate.
    c. patient agrees with the critical pathway.
    d. family understands the patient's condition.

15. The purpose of making observations is to
    a. make sure the nurse gets along with the patient.
    b. inform the doctor of how the patient's family is doing.
    (c.) note changes in condition or new problems developing.
    d. see if the medical diagnosis is accurate.
16. An example of an objective observation is that the patient
    a. complains of abdominal pain.
    b. says she is feeling sad.
    (c.) has a pulse of 72.
    d. says she is not hungry.
17. When you offer to give Mrs. Jones a bath, she says, "Get out of here and don't come back." You report this to the nurse and say
    (a.) "Mrs. Jones told me to leave her room and not come back."
    b. "Mrs. Jones is angry today."
    c. "Mrs. Jones is not cooperating with me."
    d. "Mrs. Jones does not want a bath today."
18. The form on which nurses enter daily information about the patient is called the
    a. progress notes.
    (b.) nurse's notes.
    c. nurse's daily flow log.
    d. document.
19. Charting should always be
    a. done in pencil.
    (b.) done after the procedure is completed.
    c. signed at least once each day.
    d. done before care is given.
20. In international time, midnight would be called
    a. 12:00 A.M.
    (b.) 2400
    c. 1200
    d. 12:00 P.M.

C. Nursing Assistant Challenge.

Mr. Fensten is a 47-year-old patient on the medical floor. He has had a stroke. These events occur while you are taking care of him:

- He has trouble walking because of hemiplegia (paralysis) on the right side of his body and almost falls while you are walking him to the bathroom.

- He refuses to eat his breakfast.
- He throws the washcloth across the room when you help him with his bath.
- His B/P is 146/88.
- He smiles and hugs his wife when she comes to visit.
- You do range-of-motion exercises on all joints without any problem.

- You notice a persistent reddened area on his coccyx (tailbone).

For each of these observations, write out the documentation exactly as you would on the patient's medical record.

Think about these observations and consider how many examples of verbal and nonverbal communication are given.

Do any of these situations involve Mr. Fensten's rights as a patient? If so, describe them.

EXPLORING THE WEB

Description	Location
Assessment	*http://www.delmarhealthcare.com/olcs/white/pnotes.asp* (see Chapter 25)
Critical thinking	*http://www.delmarhealthcare.com/olcs/white/pnotes.asp* (see Chapter 2)
Critical thinking	*http://www.delmarhealthcare.com/olcs/whiteduncan/pnotes.asp* (see Chapter 2)
Critical thinking and the nursing process	*http://www.delmarhealthcare.com/pdf/0766824101_01.pdf*
Documentation	*http://www.delmarhealthcare.com/olcs/white/pnotes.asp* (see Chapter 10)
Nursing process	*http://www.delmarhealthcare.com/olcs/white/ppts/chapter%2009.ppt*
Nursing process	*http://www.delmarhealthcare.com/olcs/white/pnotes.asp* (see Chapter 9)
Nursing process and the CNA	*http://www.nursingassistant.org/nursprocess.html*
Care Plan Problem Statements	*http://www.careplans.com*
Change of Shift in the Computer Age	*http://www.advancefornurses.com* (see past articles 8/28/00)
Hospital Soup	*http://www.hospitalsoup.com*
Nurse Scribe	*http://www.enursescribe.com*
Nurses in Training	*http://nursesintraining.8m.com*
Nursing Documentation in the Medical Record	*http://www.utmb.edu*
Nursing process PowerPoint slides	*http://www.rsu.edu*
Physical Exam Study Guides	*http://www.medinfo.ufl.edu*
Problem Oriented Care Plans	*http://www.cnsonline.org*
RN Central	*http://www.rncentral.com*
Student Nurse	*http://studentnurse.hypermart.net*

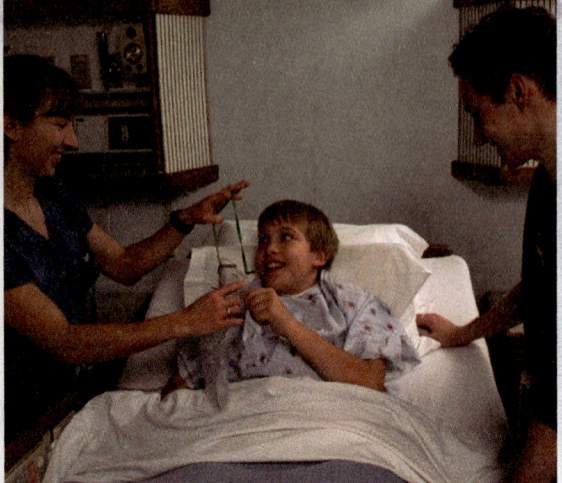

Meeting Basic Human Needs

objectives

After completing this unit, you will be able to:
- Spell and define terms.
- Describe the stages of human growth and development.
- List five physical needs of patients.
- Define self-esteem.
- Describe how the nursing assistant can meet the patient's emotional needs.

- List nursing assistant actions to ensure that patients have the opportunity for intimacy.
- Discuss methods of dealing with the fearful patient.
- List the guidelines to assist patients in meeting their spiritual needs.

vocabulary

Learn the meaning and the correct spelling of the following words and phrases:

adolescence	growth	personality	tasks
bisexuality	heterosexuality	preadolescence	tasks of personality
celibate	homosexuality	reflex	development
coitus	intimacy	self-esteem	toddler
continuum	masturbation	self-identity	
development	neonate	sexuality	

INTRODUCTION

Each of us has things that we need to live successfully. These are called *needs* simply because we cannot get along without them. When a patient is admitted to the hospital, his or her needs come too. The difference now is in the way those needs are expressed and fulfilled. Expression and fulfillment have to be different because of the hospital environment and the illness. Remember that the basic needs remain the same, regardless of how they are expressed or how they have to be met because of an individual's level of development or state of health.

HUMAN GROWTH AND DEVELOPMENT

Human beings change as they age, through the processes of growth and development. Growth involves the changes that take place in the body. It is usually measured by height and weight and degree of system maturation. Development involves the changes that take place on a social, emotional, and psychological level. Developmental levels are shown in behavior and interpersonal skills.

People move from one level of development to the next (Table 9-1). At each level, they change in both the way they look and the way they think and act (Figure 9-1). Each level presents tasks that must be mastered before the person can move on to the next level.

The tasks to be mastered are those things that lead to healthy and satisfactory participation in society. The tasks are defined by the needs of the individual and the pressures of society.

Sometimes growth spurts occur and developmental skills must catch up. Both growth and development progress from simple to complex. Each depends on the other to

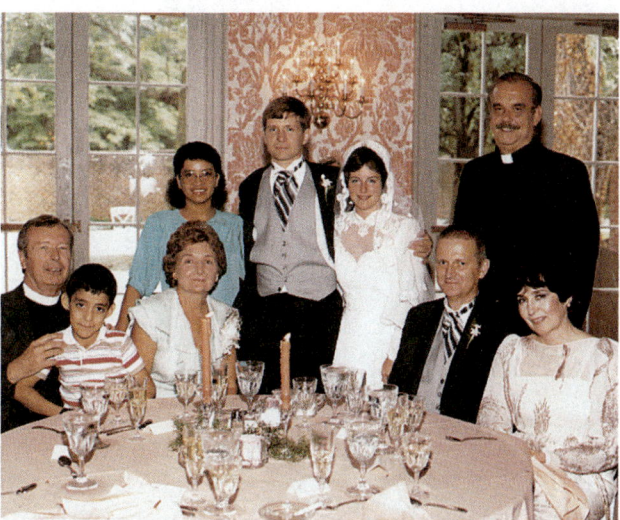

FIGURE 9-1 The characteristics of different age groups are reflected in this family picture.

TABLE 9-1 STAGES OF GROWTH AND DEVELOPMENT

Neonate	Birth to 1 month
Infancy	1 month to 2 years
Toddler	2 years to 3 years
Preschool	3 years to 5 years
School Age	5 years to 12 years
Preadolescence	12 years to 14 years
Adolescence	14 years to 20 years
Adulthood	20 years to 50 years
Middle Age	50 years to 65 years
Later Maturity	65 years to 75 years
Old Age	75 years and beyond

achieve the orderly progression. For example, a child cannot be toilet trained until the nerve pathways have matured. Growth and development follow a set of basic principles of progression.

- There is a continuous movement from simple to more complex. For example, baby sounds progress to speech patterns.
- Development and growth move from head to feet and from torso to limbs. The infant first raises the head, then sits, stands, and finally walks.
- Each stage of development has a specific set of tasks that the person must master before he or she can successfully move on to the next level. For example, the child learns to catch big balls before she can catch a baseball.
- Progression moves forward in an orderly manner, but the rate varies for each person. There are growth spurts in the preschool and teen years, but not all children grow to the same extent or at the same rate.
- Growth patterns progress at their own individual rate.

Neonatal and Infant Period
(Birth to Two Years)

The neonatal and infant period extends through the first two years of life. It is a time of rapid physical growth and development (Table 9-2). The infant gradually learns to:

- Sit
- Crawl
- Stand
- Take first steps

Other changes also occur during this period:

- Emotional attachments move from self-awareness and parental or caregiver attachment toward ties with other family members.
- Systems that are relatively immature at birth become more stabilized.
- Alertness and activity increase.
- Teeth appear (erupt).
- Food intake progresses from milk to solid food.
- Verbal skills begin to develop.

The mother or primary caregiver of the infant is the central figure of emotional attachment. Growth and development progress so rapidly that changes can be seen each month. The **neonate** (newborn) (Figure 9-2):

- Weighs 7–8 pounds
- Is approximately 20–21 inches long
- Has a head that seems disproportionately large compared to the body
- Has skin that is wrinkled, thin, and red
- Has an abdomen that seems to stick out (protrude)
- Has dark blue eyes

In the newborn, the:

- Conversion of cartilage to bone (ossification) is not complete. This can be seen in the soft spots (fontanels) and suture lines (joints) of the skull.
- The nervous system is not fully developed, so muscular activities are uncoordinated.

TABLE 9-2	HEIGHT/WEIGHT FOR THE FIRST YEAR OF LIFE (BOYS)	
Age (Months)	**Height (Inches)**	**Weight (Pounds)**
Birth	20	7–8
1 month	21¼	7½
2 months	22½	10
3 months	23¾	11½
4 months	24¾	12½
5 months	25½	14
6 months	26	15
7 months	26¾	16¾
8 months	27½	18
9 months	28	19
10 months	28½	20
11 months	29	20¾
12 months	29½	21½

Remember that the figures are averages only.

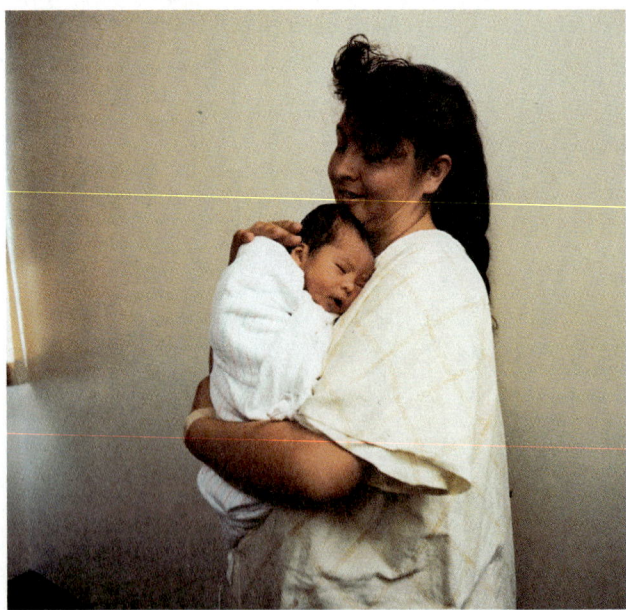

FIGURE 9-2 Newborn infant (neonate).

- Vision is not clear, but hearing and taste are developed. Certain **reflexes** (automatic responses) are also developed. They are the:
  - Moro reflex—when a loud noise startles the infant, the arms are spread across the chest, the legs are extended, and the head is thrust back. This response is also called the *startle reflex*.
  - Grasp reflex—touching the infant's palm causes the fingers to flex in a grasping motion.
  - Rooting (sucking) reflex—stroking the cheek or side of the lips stimulates the infant to turn its head in the direction of the stroking. This is important in finding the nipple to suck the milk.
- Diet is milk or milk substitute.
- Routine is largely sleeping, eating, and eliminating.

The neonate is completely dependent on the caregiver for all needs. The infant is unable to support her head, so the newborn must be handled carefully and be well supported when held.

The three-month-old infant:

- Has gained enough muscular coordination to hold her head up and raise her shoulders.
- Has lost the Moro, rooting, and grasp reflexes.
- Produces real tears.
- Can follow objects with his eyes.
- Can smile and coo at the caregiver.

The six-month-old infant:

- Has learned to roll over.
- Can sit for short periods of time.
- Holds things with both hands and directs them toward his mouth.
- Responds with verbal sounds when a caregiver speaks.
- Is beginning to cut front teeth.
- Eats finger foods and strained fruits and vegetables.
- Recognizes family members.
- Develops fear of strangers.

The nine-month-old infant:

- Crawls and may begin to stand when supported.
- Has more teeth erupt.
- Can respond to her name.
- Says one- and two-syllable words such as "mama."
- Shows a preference for right- or left-hand control.
- Eats junior baby foods.

The one-year-old infant:

- Understands simple commands such as "No."
- Begins to take steps—supported at first, then independently.
- Eats table foods and can hold her own cup.
- Weighs three times what he weighed at birth (refer to Table 9-2).

AGE-APPROPRIATE CARE *Alert*

When caring for the one- to three-year-old, tell the child who you are. Call him or her by name. Introduce yourself to the parents and explain procedures to the parents. Have them explain the procedure to the child, or do so yourself using simple terms. Allow the child to handle equipment with supervision. Communicate by using simple words and commands. Smile, be gentle, and speak to the child during care. Avoid prolonged separation from the parents, if possible. Allow the child to be as independent as possible.

Toddler Period (Two to Three Years)

The **toddler** period is a busy, active phase. It is a time when exploration and investigation are the main activities. It is also a period in which motor abilities develop (Figure 9-3) and vocabulary and comprehension increase.

During this period, the toddler:

- Learns to control elimination.
- Begins to become aware of right and wrong.
- Often reacts with frustration and negative responses to attempts at socialization and discipline as she becomes more aware of herself as a separate person.

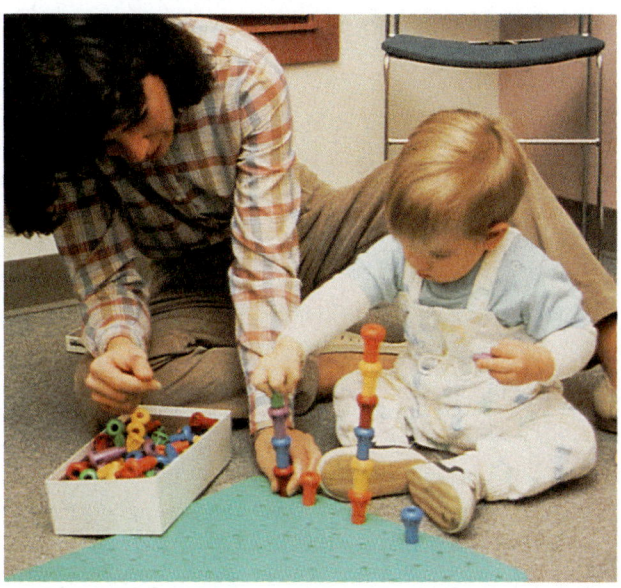

FIGURE 9-3 The toddler begins to develop gross motor skills. *(Photo courtesy of Henrietta Egleston Hospital for Children, Atlanta, GA. Photograph by Ginger Lovering)*

- Tolerates brief periods of separation from the mother, but the mother still remains the source of security and comfort.
- May play in the company of other children but with no interaction. This age group is very possessive. "No" and "mine" are a major part of their vocabularies.

Reaching the end of this period, the toddler is able to:

- Walk and run.
- Display motor (manual) skills that include feeding himself and riding toys.
- Put words together and speak more clearly. The average vocabulary of a two-year-old is about 300 words.
- Play near others, but is not able to interact in play with children of the same age (peers).

Preschool Years (Three to Five Years)

The three- to five-year-old (Figure 9-4) builds on the motor and verbal skills developed as a toddler. During this period, the preschooler:

- Grows less reliant on the mother. Children in this age group begin to recognize their position as members of the family unit and their uniqueness from other members.
- Develops rivalries with siblings and develops greater attachments to the father or alternate caregiver.
- Gradually increases cooperative play.
- Improves language skills and asks many questions.
- Develops a more active imagination.
- Becomes more sexually curious.

By the end of this period, children have become far more socialized than they were as toddlers. They are more cooperative. They seem almost eager to follow established rules within limits. They enjoy interacting with family members and peers.

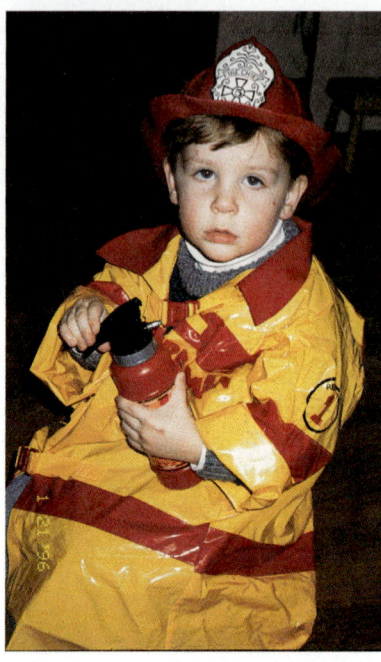

FIGURE 9-4 The preschooler expands his awareness of the world around him.

School-Age Children (6 to 12 Years)

The school-age child (Figure 9-5):

- Is able to communicate.
- Has developed small (fine) motor skills. With these skills, the child is able to master tasks such as writing.
- Develops an increased sense of self.
- Establishes peer relationships.
- Reinforces proper social behavior through games, simple tasks, and play.
- Chooses sex-differentiated friends.
- Joins groups like Scouts. This serves to further identify the individual as a person of a particular gender.
- Begins to show concern for other living things (Figure 9-6).

AGE-APPROPRIATE CARE *Alert*

Communicate with the three- to five-year-old child by calling him or her by name. Tell the child who you are. Explain procedures to the child in simple language. Tell him what you will do each time. Do not expect him to remember. Demonstrate procedures on a doll or stuffed animal, whenever possible. Use simple words and short sentences. Smile often. Use familiar times, such as "before lunch" or "after dinner," rather than stating the time. Reward the child for positive behavior with attention and special treats, as allowed. Allow her to be as independent as possible.

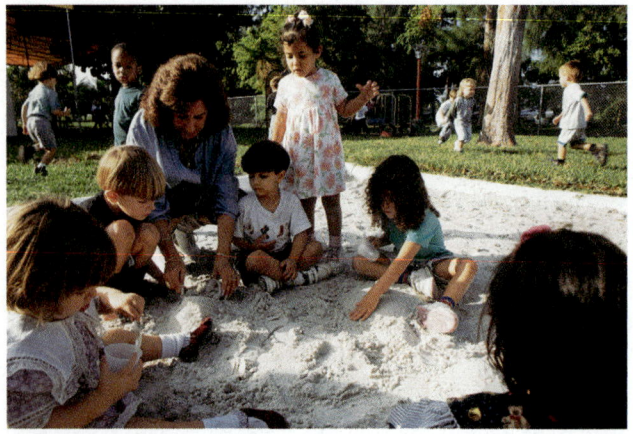

FIGURE 9-5 School-age children like to play in peer groups.

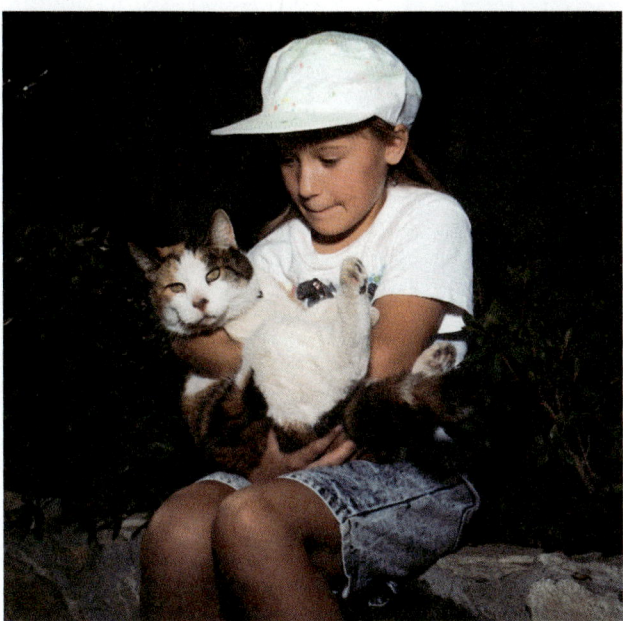

FIGURE 9-6 Young children learn to reach out and have concern for others.

- Arms and legs seem out of proportion to the rest of the body.

Adolescence (14 to 20 Years)

Adolescence is marked by:

- The gradual development of sexual maturity.
- A greater appreciation of the individual's own identity as a male or a female person.
- Conflicting desires for the freedom of independence and the security of dependence. Because of these conflicting desires, this is often a troublesome period.
- The establishment of personal coping systems and the ability to make independent judgments and decisions.
- Gradual success in mastering the developmental tasks of the age. The adolescent is able to make comparisons between the values she has been taught and reality.

Preadolescence (12 to 14 Years)

Preadolescence is a transitional stage. It is a period of great uncertainty. During this period:

- Hormonal changes stimulate the secondary sex characteristics.
- The individual feels on the threshold of tremendous change, though not yet in a period of sexual functioning.
- Mood swings and feelings of insecurity are common.
- There is a growing awareness of and interest in the opposite sex.

Adulthood (20 to 50 Years)

Early adulthood is marked by:

- Independence and personal decision making.
- The choice of a mate.
- Establishment of a career and family life.
- Optimal health.
- The choice of friends to form a support group.

Middle Age (50 to 65 Years)

Middle age is associated with:

- Final career advancement, ending in retirement.
- Children who were reared during the period of adulthood leaving home to enter their own adult period.
- Health that is usually still at good levels, though some slowing may be seen.
- More time that can be spent on leisure activities.
- More time and money to pursue personal interests.
- Revitalizing one's relationship with a mate.
- Enjoying grandchildren.
- For some middle-aged persons, being a member of the "sandwich" generation—caring for both their own parents and their children or grandchildren.

Later Maturity (65 to 75 Years)

Later maturity is marked by:

- A gradual loss of vitality and stamina.
- Physical changes that signal the aging process. For example, sight and hearing diminish.
- Chronic conditions that develop and persist.
- A period of gradual losses: loss of mate, friends, self-esteem, some independence.
- Examination of a lifetime.
- More time to pursue personal interests.
- Fewer responsibilities related to raising a family and holding a job.
- Increased wisdom.

Old Age (75 Years and Beyond)

Old age is frequently characterized by:

- Failing physical health and growing dependency (Figure 9-7).
- The need to deal with illness, loneliness, loss of friends and loved ones, and the realization of mortality.

Success in this final period depends on the mechanisms of coping that the older adult has developed over the years. The extent of available emotional and physical support is also important.

Aging is a gradual process that begins at birth. Old age can be a period of development and enjoyment.

AGE-APPROPRIATE CARE *Alert*

When caring for elderly adults (age 65 and older), introduce yourself. Address the patient by title and last name unless he or she instructs you otherwise. Avoid demeaning names, such as "honey" and "dear." Speak slowly and clearly, making good eye contact. Be alert to vision and hearing problems. Do not assume that the patient is mentally impaired. Make adaptations for impaired vision and hearing as necessary, such as cleaning glasses and providing a pad and pen for written communication. Allow adequate time for the patient to respond to you. Be sensitive to the patient's need to communicate and allow time to talk. Be a good listener. Explain procedures honestly. Treat the patient with respect. Allow the patient to set her own routine, as much as possible. Adjust room temperature to the patient's preference. Control environmental noise. Inform the patient about policies, services, and routines, as appropriate. Avoid rapid changes in position. Allow the patient to dangle at the bedside prior to transfer and ambulation. Maintain a well-lighted, safe environment.

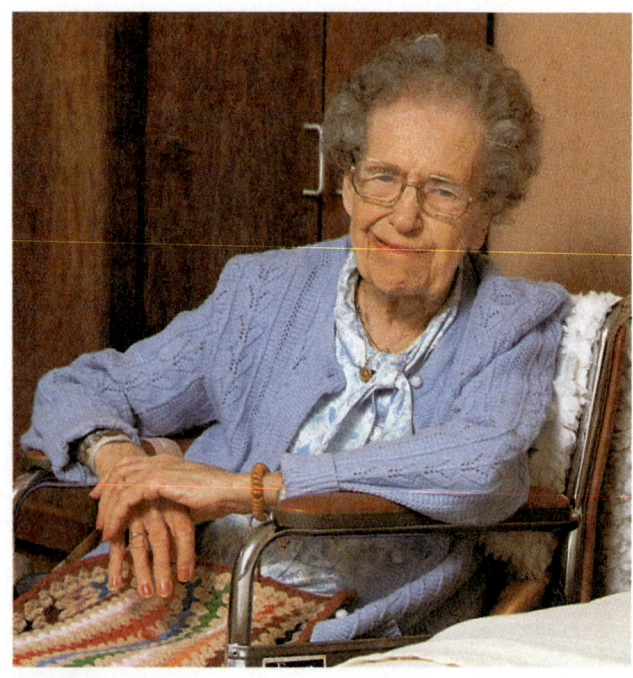

FIGURE 9-7 Physical status often declines in old age.

BASIC HUMAN NEEDS

Developmental skills and physical growth may vary during the life span. The basic human needs, however, are much the same for every individual.

Basic human needs are the things and activities required by all persons to successfully and satisfactorily live their lives. The needs are the same for all people at all ages. Cultural backgrounds influence the way in which individuals express these basic needs. *Culture* refers to those customs and practices that are common to groups of people that become ingrained beliefs, habits, and responses. Culture embraces language, dietary habits, health practices, expressions of spirituality, and ways of celebrating. These cultural patterns are part of the uniqueness of each individual and must be considered when providing the person's care.

Abraham Maslow and Erik Erikson are two leaders in the field of human behavior. They have helped us understand the basic needs and how people go about satisfying them.

Personality

Exactly how each person goes about satisfying personal psychological needs reflects his personality. **Personality** is the sum of ways we react to the events in our lives. It is gradually formed through experience and molded by cultural heritage.

Erikson suggested that our personalities are formed as we mature from infancy to old age. He believed that we pass through eight growing stages in search of who we really are (**self-identity**). During each stage, there are choices to be made before moving on to the next task. He called these the **tasks of personality development** (Table 9-3).

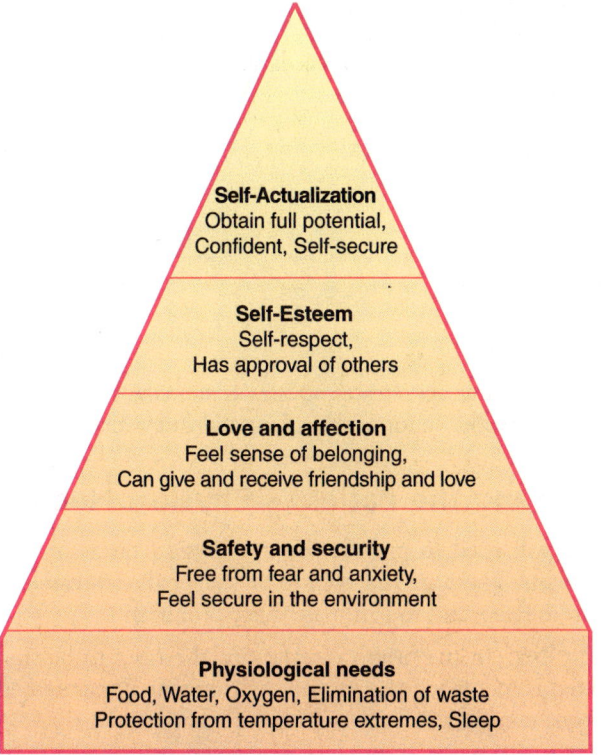

FIGURE 9-8 Maslow's hierarchy of needs.

Maslow described human needs as physical, psychological, and sociological. He placed the needs on a **continuum** in which physical needs had to be satisfied first. The psychological or sociological needs can be met only after the physical needs have been satisfied (Figure 9-8). The progression of needs is called a *hierarchy of needs*.

TABLE 9-3 TASKS OF PERSONALITY DEVELOPMENT ACCORDING TO THE STAGES DEFINED BY ERIKSON		
Physical Stage	**Year of Occurrence**	**Tasks to Be Mastered**
Oral-sensory	Birth–1 year (infant)	To learn to trust (Trust)
Muscular-anal	1–3 years (toddler)	To recognize self as an independent being from mother (Autonomy)
Locomotor	3–5 years (preschool years)	To recognize self as a family member (Initiative)
Latency	6–11 years (school-age years)	To demonstrate physical and mental skills/abilities (Industry)
Adolescence	12–18 years	To develop a sense of individuality as a sexual human being (Identity)
Young Adulthood	19–35 years	To establish intimate personal relationships with a mate (Intimacy)
Adulthood	35–50 years	To live a satisfying and productive life
Maturity	50+ years	To review life's events and examine how they have influenced the development of a unique individual (Ego integrity)

Physical Needs

The most basic human needs are physical needs. They include:

- Nutrition
- Rest
- Oxygen
- Shelter
- Elimination
- Activity
- Sexuality

Illness at any age creates stresses that make meeting the needs a challenge for both patient and caregivers.

Meeting the Patient's Physical Needs

You will need to provide for the physical needs of your patients. These are the need to be sheltered, to breathe, to eat, to sleep, and to eliminate waste products.

Shelter. In the health care facility, the need to be sheltered is met when the proper environment is maintained. Some examples include making sure that:

- A comfortable room temperature is maintained.
- Needed repairs are reported, such as a leaking faucet.

Oxygen. Most of us take breathing for granted. We hardly give it more than a passing thought until it becomes difficult. There are many reasons why people have trouble breathing. When they do have difficulty, though, the need is always the same. The body cannot live without oxygen, which is found in the air. It may be necessary, therefore, to give the patient extra oxygen and moisture to ensure that body tissues receive enough oxygen. Oxygen delivered by cannula, mask, or another device may be used for this purpose (Figure 9-9). Sometimes this need can be met by adjusting the overbed table in such a way that the patient, supported by pillows, is able to lean on it, making breathing easier.

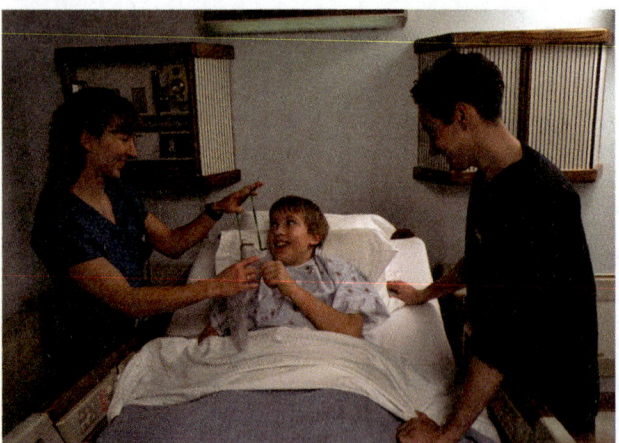

FIGURE 9-9 Some patients may need additional oxygen.

Food. Patients may lose their appetites when they are in the hospital. Decreased appetite and intake of fluids may be due to:

- Inactivity
- Hospital odors
- Pain
- Fear and anxiety
- Types of food served
- Illness itself
- Age of the patient

Some patients have to be fed because of their condition. Some may be given only special foods. Some are unable to take food in the usual way. Some patients are given liquid nourishment through a feeding tube. Fluid replacement may also be given through a sterile tube into the veins.

Because patients receive nourishment in such a variety of ways, you need to meet the special needs of each individual. There are, however, some general points to keep in mind:

- Patients will eat better and will be more comfortable if allowed or assisted to use the bathroom before meals.
- Appetites improve when food is served at the proper temperature in pleasant surroundings.
- Bathroom doors should be closed and room deodorants used to get rid of unpleasant odors.
- Unneeded equipment should be removed from sight.
- Cultural preferences should be considered.
- Patients should be prepared by allowing them to wash hands and face. Help them sit up in bed or get out of bed, if permitted.
- The tray should be offered in a calm, pleasant manner, even if the food is not what you like. Even a bland diet offered in this way is more acceptable.
- Patients should be allowed to do as much as they are able for themselves. Be available, however, to assist if needed.

Sleep. See Unit 10 for a discussion of patient's sleep and rest needs.

Elimination. To stay healthy, the body must be able to rid itself of perspiration, urine, and feces. Elimination is promoted by:

- Bathing, which helps get rid of perspiration and keeps the skin healthy.
- Encouraging the patient to drink six to eight glasses of fluids and, if possible, to eat foods high in fiber.
- Providing additional help, if needed, to relieve the patient's body of waste. A sterile tube (catheter) can be inserted into the urinary bladder to drain the urine out. The sterile catheter may be left in the bladder to provide constant drainage. The tube is then attached to a bag that collects the urine. Enemas, laxatives, and suppositories help the bowels get rid of solid wastes in the form of feces.

- Helping patients who are unable to use the usual toilet facilities, by providing them with bedpans, urinals, and bedside commodes.

Physical Activity. People, by nature, are active beings. When illness occurs, it often limits activity. Sometimes the patient must stay in bed for a long time. The staff must find ways to promote appropriate activity for these individuals. The capability of the patient and the goals of treatment must be kept in mind when the activity level of any patient is established.

The complications resulting from inactivity and actions to take to avoid these complications are presented in Units 40 and 47.

Activity promotes improved functioning of all systems. Circulation and respiration are increased. Muscles, bones, and joints function more efficiently. The body as a whole responds in a positive way to activity.

When patients are unable to carry out activity, such as walking, getting into and out of bed, and using the bedpan or commode independently, you may have to help them (Figure 9-10). Be sure you are aware of the patient's limitations, as well as the degree and type of activity allowed. Encourage patients to do as much as possible, but do not allow them to become either overstressed or tired.

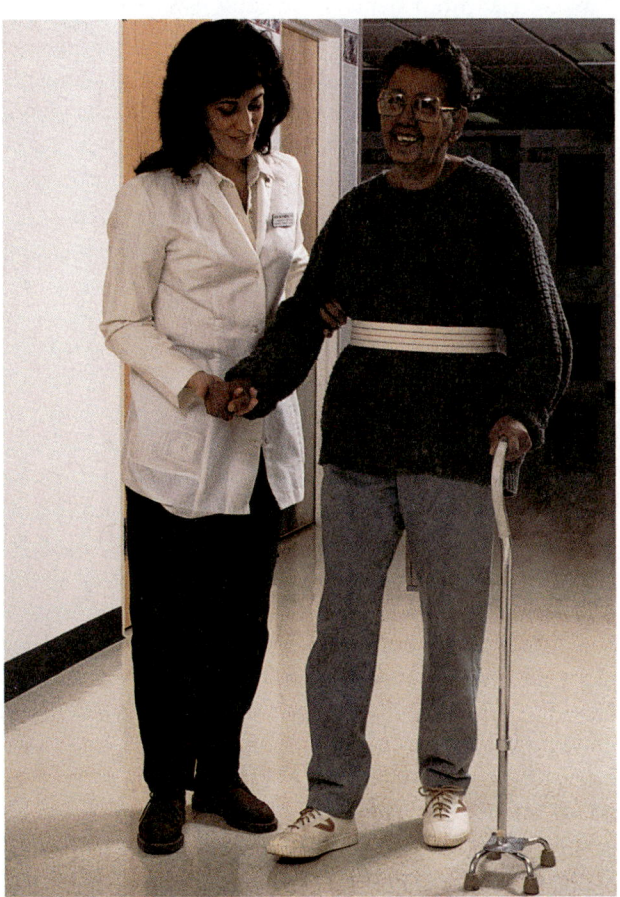

FIGURE 9-10 This patient may need assistance with ambulation.

Security and Safety Needs

If physical needs are not being met, the individual has no energy to be concerned about safety. For example, a mother whose children are starving may risk her life to provide food. Once physical needs are provided for, safety and security become priorities. Security and safety for patients are provided by:

- Maintaining a safe environment (see Units 14 and 15)
- Knowing how to respond to medical emergencies, such as patient falls
- Knowing how to respond to facility emergencies, such as fire
- Implementing the patient's care plan as indicated

Emotional Needs

The third and fourth levels of Maslow's hierarchy are related to emotional needs, including the need for love and belonging and the need for esteem. There is a need:

- To give love
- To feel love
- To be loved
- To be treated with respect and dignity
- To feel that self-esteem (our opinion of ourselves) is protected

All individuals—you, your coworkers, and your patients—have in their own minds an idea of how they appear and wish to appear to others. This idea is referred to as self-esteem. A person's self-esteem must be protected at all costs.

For example, a person might visualize and project to others the image of a very self-reliant person, capable of making important decisions and able to care for self and family. Suddenly that same person is scantily dressed in a hospital bed. A stranger is taking care of her most intimate physical functions. Even the times to eat and bathe are decided for her. This set of circumstances threatens even the most secure person's self-esteem.

A patient's response to this threat to self-esteem depends on two things. First, it depends on how often the patient has had these feelings of helplessness before, and how well he has dealt with them. Second, it depends on you and your ability to appreciate those feelings.

One patient may feel frustrated and angry. He may not even know that these feelings are based on fear. The patient may act out these feelings by complaining about the hospital, the staff, roommates, you, or the food. In fact, every aspect of the care may be cause for complaint. Be open and receptive to these actions, recognizing the underlying feelings.

Still another patient may react quite differently to the same emotional stress. That person may be quiet and withdrawn. She may be completely cooperative and noncomplaining (Figure 9-11). The behavior shown is a false front. It hides

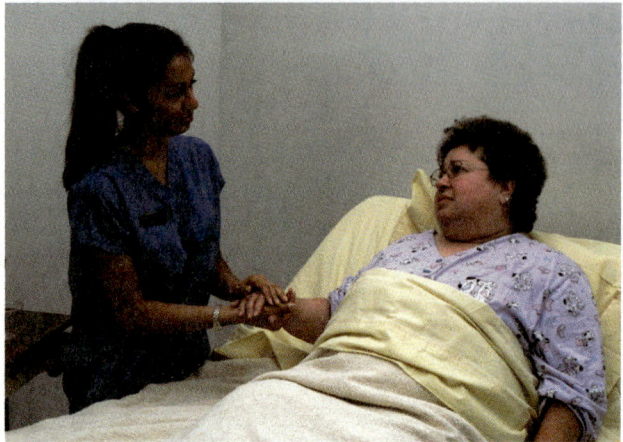

FIGURE 9-11 Patience may be necessary to break through a wall of fear and frustration.

the patient's feelings of not being able to cope with the situation. The nursing assistant must be aware of these feelings and the need for caring support.

Intimacy and Sexuality

Intimacy is a feeling of closeness with another human (Figure 9-12). It is a relationship marked by feelings of love and affection. It is an integral part of human response.

Sexuality is a lifelong characteristic that defines the maleness or femaleness of each person. This definition may be different for each person. All individuals are sexual, whether or not they have physical sexual relations. Sexuality has to do with the ability to develop relationships, to give of oneself to others, and to appreciate the giving by others. Intimacy is one aspect of sexuality.

Intimacy may be shared between friends or lovers. Also, a degree of intimacy is established when patient and caregiver learn they can trust and have confidence in each other.

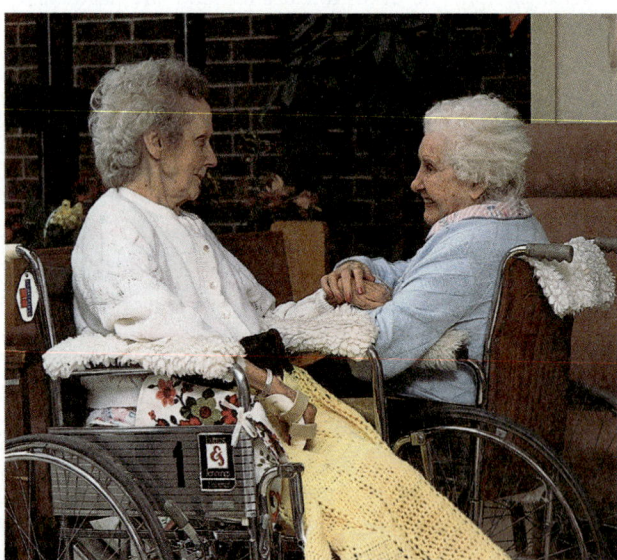

FIGURE 9-12 Most persons have a need for intimacy.

Intimate relationships may be sexual and expressed in different ways. Humans express sexual intimacy depending on orientation, preference, opportunity, and moral standards. Sexual behavior is a personal choice, but intimacy is an important aspect of the human sexual experience.

Each intimate relationship has an element of commitment. Sometimes this commitment includes a sexual aspect and sometimes it does not. For example, a loving couple may choose not to have sexual intercourse. Despite remaining **celibate** (no sexual intercourse), they still share an intimacy and commitment that is natural and fulfilling.

Being old, ill, or disabled does not diminish human sexuality. However, our society tends to associate youth, beauty, and physical agility with sexuality. By these standards, persons who are old or disabled are not considered to be sexual beings. It is important to remember that the person within a human being does not change. Although the hair is gray, or the body is not so agile, the person inside still has feelings and longing for love, affection, and intimacy. As a nursing assistant, there are several actions you can take to help patients maintain their sexuality:

- Give attention to the patient's grooming and appearance.
- Give sincere compliments on their appearance.
- Converse with patients on an adult level.

It is important to recognize that not everyone has the same orientation, preference, opportunities, or moral standards. This does not mean that differences make one person wrong and another right. As a caregiver, you must be understanding of others who do not share your personal views.

Some terms related to human sexual expression are:

- **Heterosexuality**—sexual attraction between opposite sexes.
- **Homosexuality**—sexual attraction between persons of the same sex. Female partners are called lesbians. Male partners are often referred to as being gay.
- **Bisexuality**—sexual attraction to members of both sexes.
- **Masturbation**—self-stimulation for sexual pleasure.

The range of ways to express love is enormous. Genital and nongenital caressing, exchange of loving gestures, talking, hugging, and touching are all ways love is expressed between people. **Coitus** (intercourse), although an enjoyable part of many relationships, is not always necessary for satisfaction.

Providing opportunities for patients to meet sexual and intimate needs in a health care setting is not always easy. However, there are some actions that nursing assistants can do to help patients meet these needs:

- Respect patients' privacy. Always knock and wait before opening a closed door.
- Speak before opening curtains drawn around the bed.
- Do not judge behaviors and preferences that are different from yours as wrong.

- Do not discuss personal sexual information about a patient with others.
- Provide privacy if a patient is masturbating.
- Discourage patients who make sexual advances to you. State in a calm, matter-of-fact way that you are not interested and move on to other work. If a patient persists, report the matter to the nurse.
- Recognize that the need for intimacy is a basic human need that is expressed in many ways.

Human Touch

The need for human touch should not be overlooked. Pleasure and satisfaction are felt by a parent and child as they touch one another. The same human feelings are also experienced by adults.

As people grow older, they tend to reserve touching for intimate friends and family members. When circumstances change and opportunities for touching become fewer, people often feel deprived and lonely. This is especially true when one lives alone or is a resident in long-term care.

A friendly hug and smile, a pat on the shoulder, a clasp of a hand, and a backrub are ways that nursing assistants can satisfy the patient's need for human contact. Never force your attentions on a patient, but be open to nonsexual touching. It can mean much to the lives of those in your care.

Dealing with the Fearful Patient

The experienced nursing assistant does not take remarks personally. The assistant realizes that the patient's complaints and refusal to cooperate may be a way of saying, "I need to be reassured and protected." Give the patient an opportunity to talk. Listen carefully to everything that is said (Figure 9-13). You may be able to convince the fearful patient to assume some personal care whenever possible. If help in feeding, shaving, elimination, or other such personal matters is needed, act in a very gentle, efficient manner and assure the patient's privacy at all times.

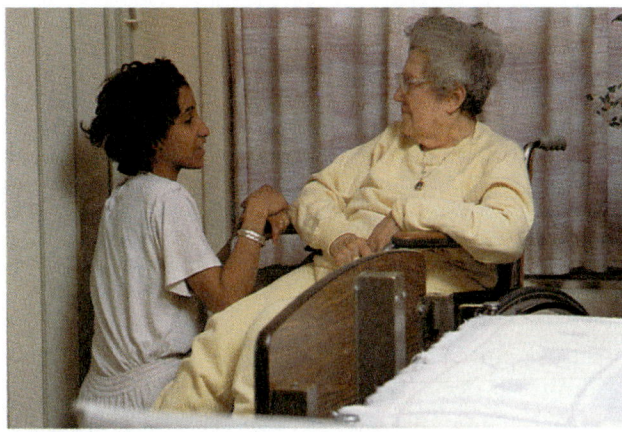

FIGURE 9-13 Successful communication is a two-way exchange.

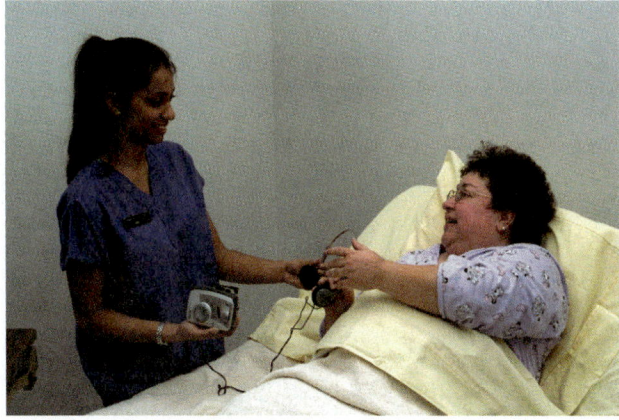

FIGURE 9-14 Activities help pass the time during convalescence.

To handle these situations successfully, the nursing assistant must:

- Recognize that this patient is a person with individual likes and dislikes.
- Give the quality of care that considers these likes and dislikes.
- Help the patient find ways to fill the time while in the hospital (Figure 9-14). Boredom alone can lead to irritability. Some hospitals have volunteers who bring books and other activities directly to the bedside.

Patient Privacy

Patients in the hospital give up a good bit of control over their lives. They put their lives and well-being into the hands of caregivers. In exchange, patients assume that certain of their rights will be assured. These rights include the right to privacy.

Patients must feel certain that their privacy will be protected. Even though you perform the most intimate procedures for them, you must do so in a way that neither exposes them unnecessarily nor embarrasses them. Privacy may be provided by means of:

- Curtains or screens placed around the bed.
- Knocking and saying the patient's name before entering a room.
- Speaking to the patient before entering a screened area. Privacy must be provided for the patient who is:
  - bathing
  - using the bedpan
  - receiving treatments
  - being visited by clergy.

Be prompt at other times to recognize a patient's need for privacy and to provide it.

Patients must also be secure in knowing that personal information they share with you will not be told to others. You add to patients' sense of security if you always treat them with the courtesy you would extend to a guest in your home.

Understanding what patients are really trying to tell us is one of the most difficult parts of giving nursing care. When we are successful, it is probably the most rewarding. With this in mind, always remember to treat the patient as a unique individual.

Spiritual Needs

Spiritual beliefs are deeply held by some patients and disregarded by others. When beliefs are strongly held, they are apt to guide a patient's actions and responses in direct ways such as praying, reading religious writings, and participating in ceremonies and celebrations. Some personal items may have special religious significance and must be treated with respect.

Patients' spiritual needs are often greater when they are fearful and ill (Figure 9-15). Be prepared to act on requests for clergy visits and spiritual support. Do not impose your beliefs on the patient.

There is always the temptation to share your personal religious faith with others. This is especially true when the patient directly asks your opinion. To handle such a situation appropriately is a challenge. Here are some guidelines to assist you.

- Remember that each person has a right to believe in any faith system or to deny the existence of any beliefs.
- Listen to the patient's thoughts and keep them confidential.
- Your role is to reflect the patient's ideas. Do not try to convince the patient of your ideas. For example, if the patient asks you if you believe in God, reflect the

patient's thinking with a statement such as "You have been thinking about God," or "Would you like to talk?"

The patient may want to visit with a familiar clergy member, or may ask about the chaplain or clergy service available at the health care facility.

Some health care facilities ask clergy from the community to make visits to patients who want such a visit but who do not know a particular minister, priest, or rabbi. Larger facilities have chaplain educational residencies for people preparing for careers in the clergy. The residencies serve patients' spiritual needs while offering training for the chaplains.

Chapels are open in some facilities. Both visitors and ambulatory patients often find comfort in visiting them. Religious services are sometimes broadcast to patients' rooms from these chapels.

Know what services are available to your patients. When asked, share this information, but do not recommend any particular service. Patients should be free to make their own choices. You should always be ready and willing to support the choice.

Social Needs

When primary physical, psychological, and spiritual needs have been met, the person is free to pursue the third level of social needs and activities that are unique to the individual. These activities make one feel good as a person and increase self-esteem. They give a sense of accomplishment. Sociological needs are met by interactions with others and opportunities for free personal expression.

One of the most basic needs of all people is the need to understand others and to be understood. We achieve this sense of understanding when we communicate successfully with others. We usually try to communicate verbally. Sometimes we do this also by the:

- Words we choose
- Way we say the words
- Tone of voice
- Facial expression
- Form of touch

Even the way we stand or reach out says a lot. We know it is not always easy to find the right words to express our thoughts and feelings. Thus, caregivers must be constantly aware of the patient's need to communicate effectively, too.

Volunteers and visitors, as well as television and reading, can provide entertainment and diversion for the patient who is confined. Try to find out about your patients' special interests. Look for ways to support them in these interests.

If all care providers are interested and unhurried in talking with their patients, they make it easier for patients to say what they need. This approach also makes it easier for the staff to find proper ways to fulfill these needs.

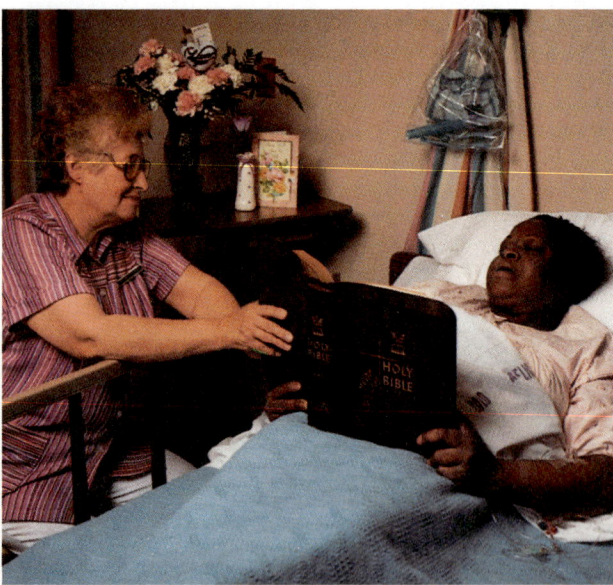

FIGURE 9-15 Spiritual needs may be greater during illness.

REVIEW

A. True/False.

Mark the following true or false by circling T or F.

1. T F Growth and development go from the simple to the complex.

2. T F Body development proceeds from the head toward the feet.

3. T F All individuals move through the stages of growth.

4. T F Growth and development progression are interdependent.

5. T F Ossification of bones is not complete at birth.

6. T F The Moro reflex occurs when the infant's palm is touched.

7. T F The sucking reflex occurs when the infant is startled.

8. T F The three-month-old infant cries real tears.

9. T F The six-month-old infant can walk if well supported.

10. T F First teeth begin to erupt about the sixth month of life.

11. T F The one-year-old infant has progressed to eating table foods.

12. T F The toddler period finds children interacting freely and playing well with one another.

13. T F Between the ages of three and five years, the child seems to have an endless list of questions.

14. T F The school-age child is interested in and chooses members of the same sex as close friends.

15. T F One of the developmental tasks of old age is to learn to deal successfully with loss.

16. T F Basic human needs are the same at all ages, but different ways must be found to satisfy them.

17. T F Erikson believed that one of the developmental tasks of infancy is learning to trust.

18. T F Erikson states that the developmental task of the middle years is to integrate life's experiences.

19. T F Patients who are fearful often behave in angry or frustrated ways.

20. T F Spiritual needs are part of basic human needs.

21. T F Culture has no influence over how basic human needs are met.

B. Matching.

Match the appropriate chronologic age to the life time period by matching Column I and Column II.

Column I	Column II
22. _____ old age	**a.** 65 years old
23. _____ adolescence	**b.** 16 years old
24. _____ later maturity	**c.** 7 years old
25. _____ school age	**d.** 35 years old
26. _____ adulthood	**e.** 80 years old

C. Multiple Choice.

Select the one best answer for each of the following.

27. Growth and development
    a. move from limbs to torso and feet to head.
    b. involve more complex tasks during growth spurts.
    c. can proceed normally even if tasks are not mastered.
    d. have specific tasks that must be mastered at each stage.

28. The main activity (activities) of the toddler period is (are)
    a. exploration and investigation.
    b. cooperative play.
    c. establishing peer relationships.
    d. showing concern for others.

29. Preschoolers are
    a. less reliant on their mothers.
    b. able to join groups like Scouts.
    c. able to choose sex-differentiated friends.
    d. unable to tolerate brief separation from the mother.

30. The ways in which we react to the events in our lives are called
    a. personality.
    b. self-identity.
    c. tasks of personality development.
    d. hierarchy of needs.

D. Nursing Assistant Challenge.

Mrs. McClendon is a 35-year-old patient with a diagnosis of breast cancer. She has lost most of her hair and has no appetite as a result of chemotherapy. Mrs. McClendon has lost weight and has occasional severe pain. She has a husband and three young children. Consider the needs that all people have and think about Mrs. McClendon.

31. Which physical needs may be difficult to meet? What can the nursing staff do to help Mrs. McClendon meet these needs?

32. Do you think her need for safety and security will be met? What information do you have indicating that she has reason to feel fear and anxiety?

33. How might Mrs. McClendon's condition affect her relationship with her husband and children?

34. How do you think her sexuality may be affected?

35. Maslow states that human needs are on a hierarchy. Describe how this hierarchy may change throughout the day for Mrs. McClendon.

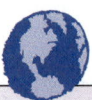 **EXPLORING THE WEB**

Description	Location
The life cycle	*http://www.delmarhealthcare.com/olcs/white/pnotes.asp* (see Chapter 14)
Biology Online	*http://www.biology-online.org*
Center for Human Growth and Development	*http://www.umich.edu*
Child Growth and Development	*http://kidshealth.org*
Human Growth and Development	*http://www.webster.edu*
Institute for Human Development Life Course and Aging	*http://www.utoronto.ca*
Meeting Religious and Spiritual Needs of Elder Residents	*http://www.nursinghome.org*

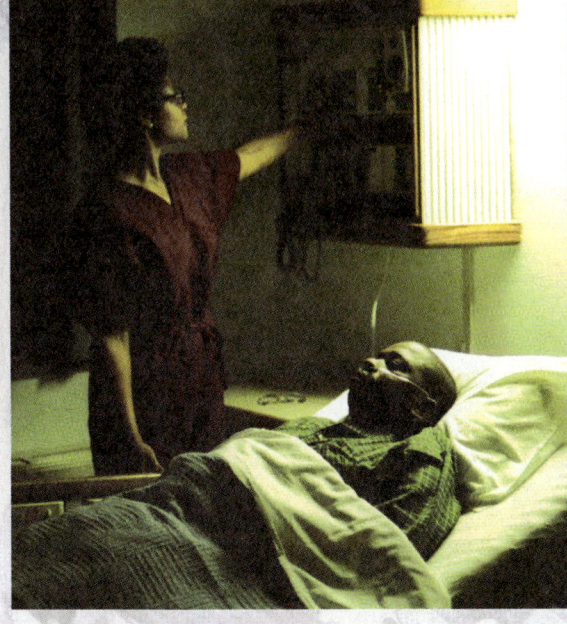

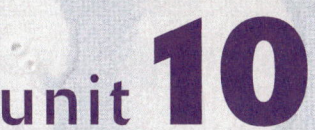

Comfort, Pain, Rest, and Sleep

objectives

After completing this unit, you will be able to:
- Spell and define terms.
- Explain why nursing comfort measures are important to patients' well-being.
- List six observations to make and report for patients having pain.
- Describe nursing assistant measures to increase comfort and relieve pain.

- List nursing comfort measures that promote rest.
- Describe the phases of the sleep cycle and the importance of each.
- List nursing measures to promote sleep.

vocabulary

Learn the meaning and the correct spelling of the following words and phrases:

bruxism	narcolepsy	rapid eye movement	sleep deprivation
comfort	nonrapid eye	(REM) sleep	somnambulism
enuresis	movement	rest	
hypersomnia	(NREM) sleep	sleep	
insomnia	pain	sleep apnea	

PATIENT COMFORT

All humans need comfort, rest, and sleep for physical and emotional well-being, health, and wellness. **Comfort** is a state of physical and emotional well-being. The patient is calm and relaxed, and is not in pain or upset. Assisting patients with their comfort needs is a major nursing assistant responsibility. In fact, assisting patients with physical or emotional comfort needs is at the heart of nursing care.

Many factors affect patients' comfort. Environmental factors that interfere with comfort are unfamiliar environment, lack of privacy, noise, odor, temperature, lighting, and ventilation. Personal and uncontrollable factors that may increase or contribute to discomfort include age, activity, injury, illness, surgery, stress, and pain.

As a rule, patients are uncomfortable when their physical and emotional needs are not met. Unmet needs cause tension and anxiety, and interfere with comfort and rest (Figure 10-1). Using basic nursing measures to meet patients' needs promotes comfort, aids in relaxation, and provides a sense of well-being.

PAIN

Pain (Figure 10-2) is a state of discomfort that is unpleasant for the patient. Pain is always a warning that something is wrong. It interferes with the patient's optimal level of function and self-care. Patients may limit movement when they are having pain. Unrelieved pain contributes to complications of immobility, increasing the risk of pneumonia, skin breakdown, and other problems. Pain decreases quality of life, and may cause hopelessness, anxiety, depression, and a feeling of helplessness. Pain may cause acting out, crying, and other strange, belligerent, or combative behavior

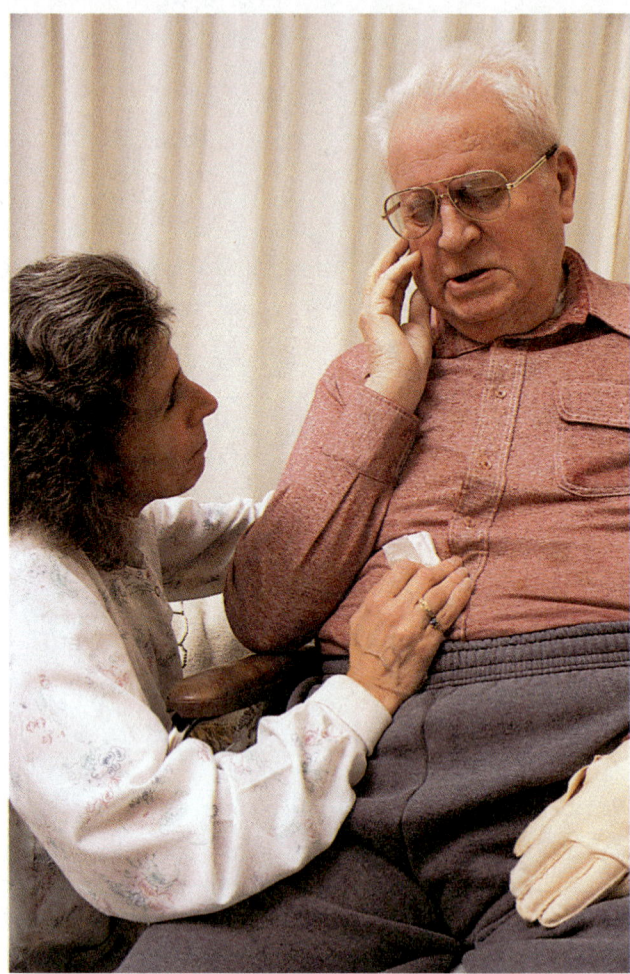

FIGURE 10-2 This patient is having severe pain.

in children and adults. Pain is a major preventable public health problem that slows recovery in individuals with acute illness and increases health care costs.

Relieving pain has always been an important nursing responsibility. Nursing staff must identify patients who are having pain, and those who are at risk for pain, then take the appropriate action to ensure that all patients are made as comfortable as possible.

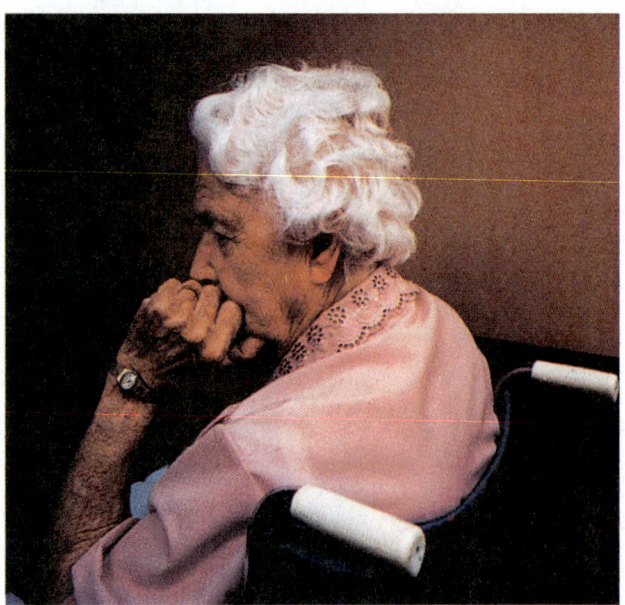

FIGURE 10-1 This patient's body language betrays the tension and anxiety she is feeling.

AGE-APPROPRIATE CARE *Alert*

The golden rule for pain relief is that whatever is painful to adults is painful to children unless proven otherwise. Pain control should be based on scientific facts, not personal beliefs or opinions. Never lie to a child when asked if a procedure will hurt. Admit that it will, but assure the child that you will be there and that the child will be made as comfortable as possible.

Patients' Responses to Pain

Patients' responses to pain vary widely. Some individuals do not feel pain as acutely as others. Some try to ignore pain. Other patients may try to deny pain because they are afraid of what it means. Ignoring or denying pain increases the risk of injury because the normal warning that pain provides goes unrecognized or unheeded.

Never ignore body language or other signs of pain in patients. Use nursing measures to make the patient comfortable. Always report pain to the nurse. Your observations are a valuable contribution to the nursing assessment and patients' comfort.

Patients' responses to pain may be related to culture. People from some cultures are very emotional when they are in pain. Others are very stoic. Some think that showing pain is a sign of weakness. Some believe that pain is a punishment from a deity or higher power.

Pain causes stress and anxiety, interfering with comfort, rest, and sleep (Figure 10-3). Rest and sleep are necessary for the body to repair itself and to restore strength and energy. Insomnia (inability to sleep), restlessness, and disturbed sleep may be caused by pain.

Identifying Patients in Pain and at Risk for Pain

Pain is a serious condition that affects well-being and quality of life. Patients have the right to timely pain assessment and management. Many factors affect patients' reactions to pain. The reactions may be different from one moment to the next and from one patient to another. Four types of pain are listed in Table 10-1. Monitor the patients' body language for signs of pain.

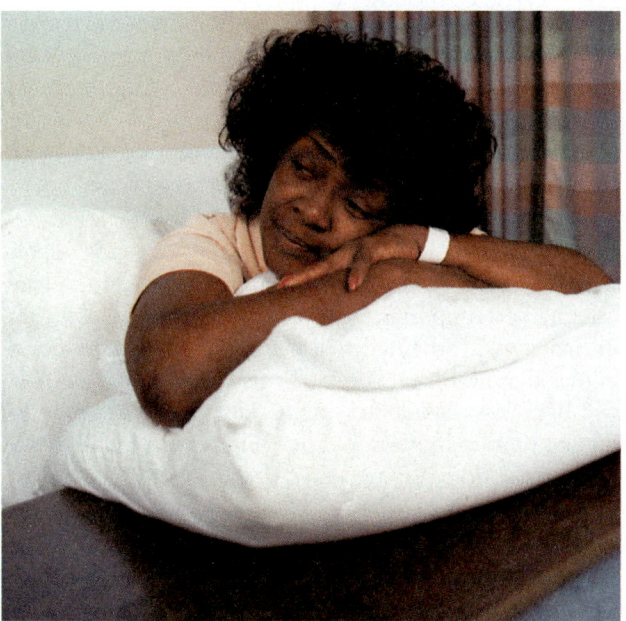

FIGURE 10-3 Although her expression is stoic, this patient cannot sleep because of pain and anxiety.

TABLE 10-1	**TYPES OF PAIN**
Type of Pain	**Description**
Acute pain	Occurs suddenly and without warning. Acute pain is usually the result of tissue damage, caused by conditions such as injury or surgery. Typically, acute pain decreases over time, as healing takes place.
Chronic pain (persistent pain)	Chronic pain lasts longer than six months. It may be intermittent or constant. Chronic pain may be caused by multiple medical conditions.
Phantom pain	Phantom pain occurs as a result of an amputation. For example, the patient has had a leg removed, but complains of pain in the toes. The pain is real, not imaginary.
Radiating pain	Radiating pain moves from the site of origin to other areas. For example, when a patient is having a heart attack, the pain may radiate from the chest to the jaw or arm.

Regularly ask patients if they are in pain. Some will not volunteer this information if not asked directly. *The patient's self-report of pain is the most accurate indicator of the existence and intensity of pain, and should be respected and believed.* Never question the validity of the patient's complaints. Patients may be smiling, talking, or sleeping and still be having pain. Vital signs may be normal. Avoid making assumptions about a patient's pain.

When asking patients about pain, make sure the patient can see and hear you. Allow enough time for the patient to process your questions and respond. Be patient. Use language that is appropriate for the patient's age and mental status. Remember that patients may use different words for pain, such as "hurt," "sore," or "tender." Children and patients who are mentally confused may surprise you. Some can describe their pain accurately. Some will admit to having pain only if you ask them directly, so do not omit this important step. Always ask patients who are crying, who display body language suggesting pain, or whose behavior suggests pain.

Observing and Reporting Signs and Symptoms of Pain

Pain always requires further intervention. It should never be ignored. Always report verbal complaints of pain, describing the pain in the patient's exact words. Be aware of signs and symptoms of pain in patients who have difficulty communicating, such as infants, children, patients who cannot speak, and patients with cognitive impairments. Clues that the patient is having pain include:

- facial expressions
- grimacing
- refusing to move
- stiff, rigid, or limited movements
- moaning, crying, yelling, or screaming

Report your observations to the nurse.

A nursing assessment of pain involves many different factors. Your observations contribute to this assessment and the patient's well-being. Other important information you may see, hear, and observe that should be reported to the nurse includes:

- Vital signs
- Skin color
- Location of pain (specific site of pain on the body)
- Radiation (movement of pain to other areas)
- Time of onset (when the pain began)
- Duration (how long the pain lasts)
- Frequency (how often it occurs)
- Pain quality (nature and type of pain)
- Pain intensity (strength and description of pain, in the patient's own words)
- Aggravating and alleviating factors (things that improve or worsen the pain)
- Character (properties, features, characteristics)
- Variation or patterns of pain (changes in pain or cycles of pain)
- Pain management history, if any (things the patient tells you about past history of pain and things that make it better or worse)
- Present pain management regimen, if any, and its effectiveness (things the patient does to relieve pain, including response to comfort measures and medications)
- Effect of pain on activities of daily living, sleep, appetite, relationships, emotions, concentration, and the like
- Direct observation of abnormalities at the site of the pain
- Other observations, such as facial expressions, body language, movements, nausea or vomiting
- Side effects of analgesic (pain-relieving) medications, if applicable
- Response to pain medications and other forms of treatment, if applicable

Using a Pain Rating Scale. Your facility will have policies and procedures for pain management. Most facilities have adopted several different pain rating scales (see Unit 8) to evaluate the level of patients' pain. In fact, many facilities now consider pain the "fifth vital sign." In these facilities, pain is regularly and frequently evaluated.

Because pain is personal and subjective, consistent pain evaluation by the various health care workers involved in care of a patient is a concern. Using a pain rating (assessment) scale helps nurses assess the patient and keeps caregivers from forming their own opinions about the level of the patient's pain. Using a pain scale prevents subjective opinions, provides consistency, eliminates some barriers to pain management, and gives the patient a means of describing the pain accurately. Pain scales are an important tool for communication to help the patient best describe his or her pain. Pain rating scales can be used to evaluate pain in patients of all ages and cultures.

Although you will not directly assess patients' pain, you must understand the purpose of the scales used in your facility and how they are interpreted. Many facilities use a 0 to 10 scale, with 0 meaning no pain and 10 meaning intolerable pain. If the patient tells you that she is having pain at "level 5," for example, you must know what this means and report the problem to the nurse. Likewise, if the patient complains of pain at "level 9" an hour after receiving pain medication, this suggests a potentially serious problem and must be reported immediately.

Managing Pain

Unrelieved pain has a negative effect on the patient's health and functional status. Notify the nurse as soon as the patient complains, before pain becomes severe or out of control. Report your observations objectively. Observe the patient carefully after pain medications have been given, and report your observations to the nurse.

Sometimes the physician orders several different medications for a patient's pain. The nurse will select which drug to use based on an assessment of the patient. Your observations, the patient's self-report of pain intensity, and physical assessment findings are all considered when the nurse determines which medication to administer, when more than one is ordered. If the first drug does not relieve the pain, the nurse may have the option of administering another, so always report unrelieved pain. The quality of pain control is influenced by the education, experience, and attitude of the health care providers who are caring for the patient.

Although you as a nursing assistant are not directly responsible for pain management, your observations and nursing care are very important, because you work so closely and intimately with the patients. Understanding the responsibilities that health care providers have regarding pain relief will help you provide nursing comfort measures, monitor for signs and symptoms of pain, and report your observations to the nurse.

Nursing Assistant Comfort Measures. Relieving discomfort helps reduce pain and anxiety. Nursing assistants can use many basic nursing measures to make a patient more comfortable. These include:

- Telling patients what you plan to do and how you will do it

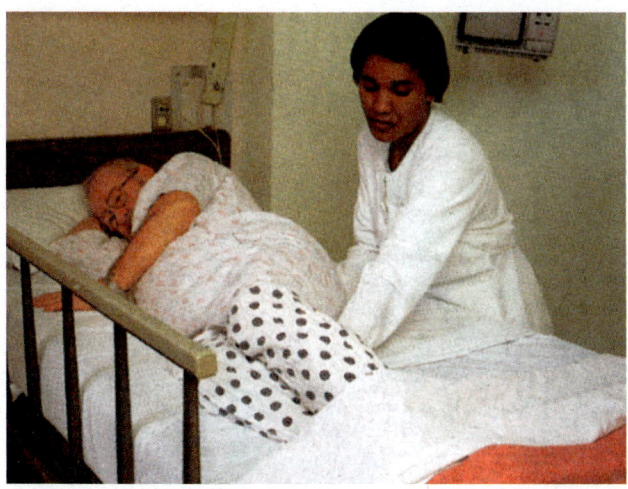

FIGURE 10-4 Assisting the patient into a comfortable position will enable him to relax and rest.

- Providing privacy
- Assisting the patient to assume a comfortable position (Figure 10-4)
- Repositioning the patient to relieve pain and muscle spasms
- Changing the angle of the bed to relieve tension on surgical sites or injured areas
- Avoiding sudden, jerking movements when moving or positioning the patient
- Performing passive range-of-motion exercises to reduce stiffness and maintain mobility
- Using pillows to support the affected body part(s) (Figure 10-5)
- Providing extra pillows and blankets for comfort and support
- Straightening the bed and linen
- Giving a backrub
- Washing the patient's face and hands

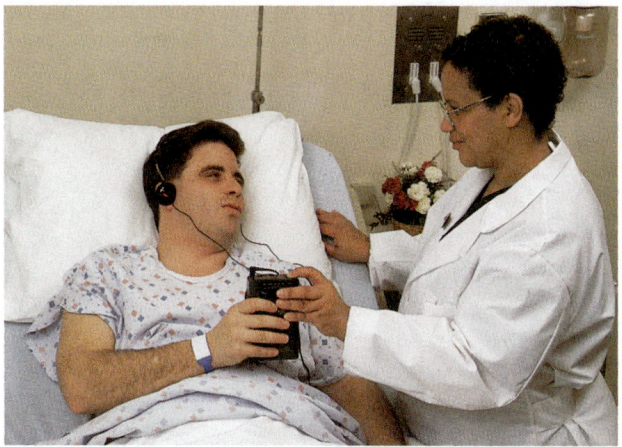

FIGURE 10-6 Playing music is pleasant and relaxing.

- Placing a cool, damp washcloth on the patient's forehead
- Providing oral hygiene
- Providing fresh water, food, or beverages as permitted
- Playing soft music to distract the patient (Figure 10-6)
- Listening to patients' concerns
- Providing emotional support (Figure 10-7)
- Maintaining a comfortable environmental temperature
- Providing a quiet, dark environment
- Eliminating unpleasant sights, sounds, and odors from the environment
- Waiting at least 30 minutes after the nurse administers pain medication before moving the patient, performing procedures, or undertaking activities
- Timing patient care to coincide with pain medication

Regularly incorporate these steps into your patient care. Follow the directions on the individual patient's care plan. The nurse may also direct you to apply warm or cold applications (see Unit 27) to make the patient more comfortable.

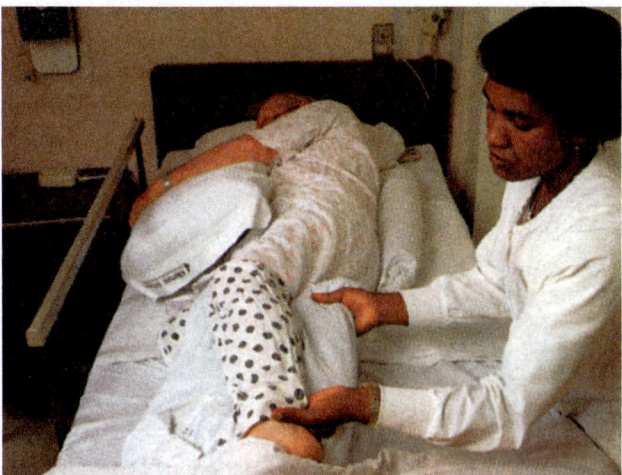

FIGURE 10-5 Support the arm and leg with pillows to relieve discomfort.

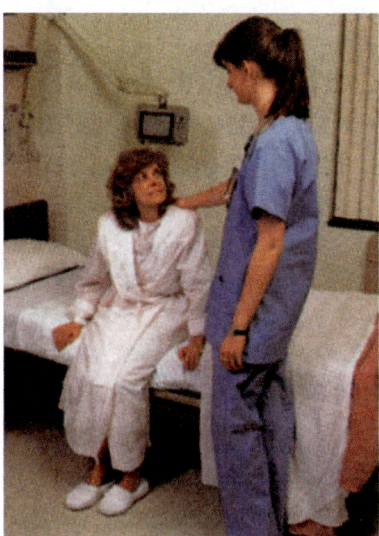

FIGURE 10-7 Providing emotional support will reduce anxiety and make the patient feel better.

REST

Rest is a state of mental and physical comfort, calmness, and relaxation. The patient's basic needs of hunger, thirst, elimination, and pain must be met before effective rest is possible. He or she should be dressed comfortably, and feel fresh and clean. The patient may sit or lie down, or may do things that are pleasant and relaxing (Figure 10-8). Some patients have rituals, such as reciting the rosary.

The environment should be calm and quiet to promote rest. If basic care is tiring for the patient, allow him or her to rest before continuing. Some patients feel refreshed after 15 minutes of rest. Others need more time. Some patients must rest frequently throughout the day. Plan your schedule and activities to allow for rest periods. Providing a backrub, nursing comfort measures, or other relaxation activities may assist the patient to rest. Follow the care plan and the nurse's instructions.

AGE-APPROPRIATE CARE *Alert*

Children will often rest better if they have a personal comfort or security item with them, such as a special blanket, stuffed animal, doll, or toy. Treat this item with respect. Avoid making fun of the item, and do not make fun of the child for using it.

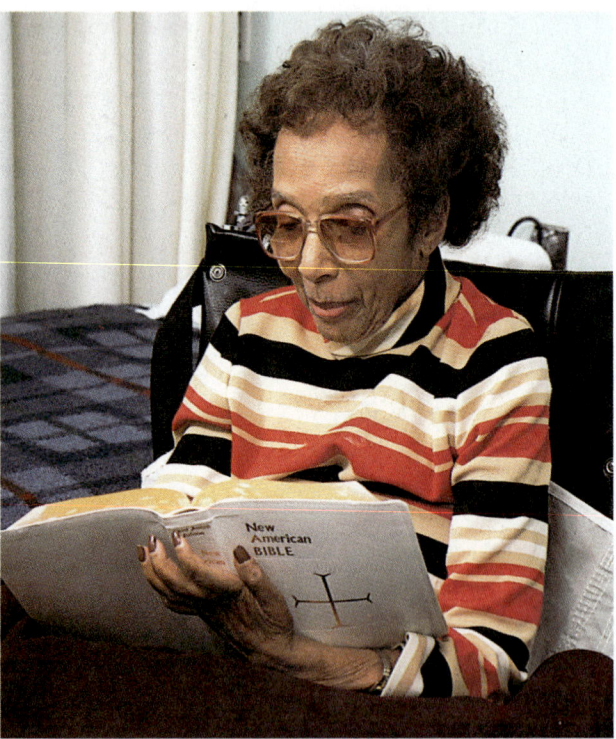

FIGURE 10-8 Reading the Bible is relaxing for this patient.

SLEEP

Sleep is a period of continuous or intermittent unconsciousness in which physical movements are decreased. Sleep is a basic need of all humans, as it allows the mind and body to rest. Adequate sleep is necessary for the body and mind to function properly.

Sleep occurs in a cycle that lasts for several hours at a time. The body repairs itself during sleep. Because movement and activity are limited, the body's metabolic needs are reduced. The patient may become cold and need a blanket because he or she is not moving. It is common for vital signs to decrease during sleep.

The need for sleep decreases as a person ages. Elderly patients require less sleep than younger adults or middle-aged patients. Infants and children require more sleep than adults. In fact, newborns may sleep as much as 20 hours a day. Sleep needs by age group are listed in Table 10-2. Weight loss may decrease the need for sleep, whereas weight gain often increases the need for sleep.

Many factors affect sleep. Sleep problems often result from a combination of several factors. Obvious problems that may interfere with the quality and quantity of sleep are:

- pain
- hunger
- thirst
- need to eliminate
- illness
- exercise

TABLE 10-2 SLEEP NEEDS THROUGHOUT THE LIFE CYCLE
• Newborn infants sleep in 3- to 4-hour intervals for a total of 16–20 hours of sleep a day
• Infants require 12 to 16 hours of sleep a day
• Toddlers require 12 to 14 hours of sleep a day, usually broken into 10 to 12 hours of sleep at night, with one or more daytime naps
• Preschool children require 10 to 12 hours per day
• Elementary-school children require 10 to 12 hours a day
• Adolescents require 8 to 10 hours per day
• Young adults aged 18 to 40 require about 7 to 8 hours a day
• Middle-aged adults aged 40 to 65 require about 7 hours a day
• Elderly adults over the age of 65 require about 5 to 7 hours per day

- noise
- temperature
- ventilation
- light intensity
- physical discomfort
- some medications
- caffeine intake
- alcohol and/or drug use
- some foods and beverages
- lifestyle changes
- anxiety, stress, fear, emotional problems
- changes in the environment, unfamiliar environment
- treatments and therapies
- staff providing routine care

Worry is another factor that interferes with comfort, rest, and sleep. Patients worry about many things, such as:

- What the future will bring
- How much the hospitalization will cost
- Who is taking care of their home and work responsibilities

You will not have the answers to all these pressing concerns. You can listen, however. Share these concerns with the nurse. This is not gossiping. The nurse and the other members of the staff may be able to help the patient solve the problems. With worries reduced, the patient will rest better.

The Sleep Cycle

Each person has a sleep–wake cycle. An internal biological clock tells the person when it is time to sleep and wake up. The sleep cycle (Figure 10-9) includes two types of sleep:

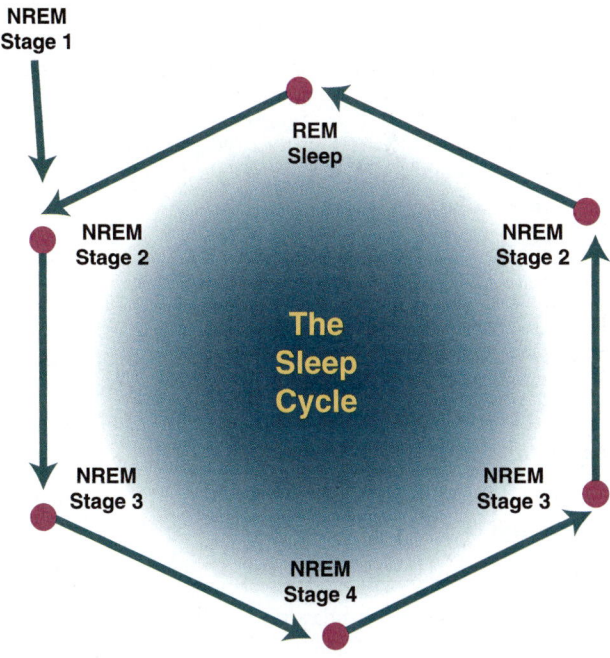

FIGURE 10-9 The sleep cycle.

- **Nonrapid eye movement (NREM) sleep** has four phases, progressing from light to very deep. This part of the sleep cycle begins when the patient first falls asleep. In the first two phases, the patient is easily aroused. As he or she progresses through the cycle, arousal becomes more difficult and sleep becomes deeper.
- **Rapid eye movement (REM) sleep** restores mental function. If you look closely, you will see the patient's eyes moving behind closed lids during this phase. Avoid awakening a patient who is in REM sleep, whenever possible. This is the part of the cycle in which dreams occur. The patient passes into REM sleep within approximately 60 to 90 minutes after falling asleep. Hospitalized patients may not experience prolonged periods of sleep time, so total REM time is less than normal. They awaken feeling less rested and may be more tired during the day.

The stages of the sleep cycle are further described in Table 10-3.

Sleep is important to prevent feelings of fatigue, and for healing of medical and surgical problems. Getting enough sleep and rest allows patients to function at their highest level. Moving through the stages of the sleep cycle uninterrupted is important. Some patients become irritable if they do not have enough sleep. Elderly patients who do not sleep well may become disoriented (Figure 10-10). This correctable problem may be mistaken for confusion! It is easily corrected by allowing uninterrupted sleep. Other signs and symptoms of inadequate sleep are:

- slow mental and physical responses
- decreased attention span
- forgetfulness or difficulty remembering things
- reduced reasoning and judgment
- puffy, red, swollen eyes
- dark circles under eyes
- disorientation
- mood swings, moodiness
- lethargy, sleepiness, fatigue
- agitation, restlessness
- clumsiness or lack of coordination
- difficulty finding the right word
- slurred speech
- hallucinations in severe sleep deprivation

Sleep Disorders

Sleep has been studied extensively. Some facilities have units and clinics specializing in the diagnosis and treatment of sleep disorders. The most common sleep disorders are:

- **Insomnia**, a chronic deprivation of quality or quantity of sleep because sleep is ended or interrupted prematurely.
- **Hypersomnia**, a disorder characterized by sleeping very late in the morning and napping during the day. Causes can be physical or psychological.

TABLE 10-3 THE SLEEP CYCLE

Stage I: NREM Sleep

- Lasts a brief time; a few minutes
- Lightest sleep; patient is easily awakened
- Vital signs decrease progressively
- Body metabolism gradually slows
- Patient feels relaxed and drowsy
- If aroused during this phase, patient may feel as if he or she had been daydreaming

Stage II: NREM Sleep

- Relaxation progresses, but patient remains easy to arouse
- Progresses into sound sleep
- Body functions and vital signs continue to decrease
- Lasts 10 to 20 minutes

Stage III: NREM Sleep

- First stage of deep sleep
- Patient is difficult to arouse
- Little to no body movement
- Muscles are completely relaxed
- Vital signs continue to decrease
- Lasts 15 to 30 minutes

Stage IV: NREM Sleep

- Patient is very difficult to arouse
- Deepest stage of sleep cycle
- Body rest and restoration occur
- Vital signs significantly reduced compared with waking values
- Sleepwalking and enuresis (bedwetting)/incontinence may occur during this stage
- Lasts about 15 to 30 minutes

REM Sleep

- Rapid eye movements may be seen through closed eyelids
- Begins about 50 to 90 minutes after first falling asleep
- Full-color dreaming
- Blood pressure, pulse, respirations vary
- Limited or no voluntary movement
- Patient is very difficult to arouse
- Mental restoration occurs
- Lasts about 20 minutes

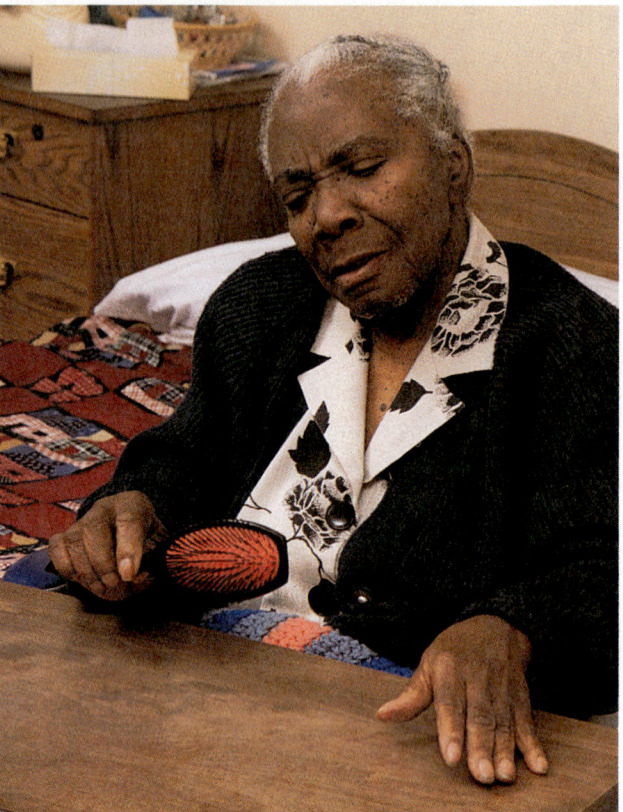

FIGURE 10-10 Lack of sleep can increase confusion and disorientation in elderly adults.

- **Narcolepsy**, a condition in which patients have sudden, uncontrollable, unpredictable urges to fall asleep during the daytime hours. These individuals also get adequate sleep at night.
- **Sleep apnea**, a potentially serious condition in which air flow stops for 10 seconds or more. Untreated, this condition leads to severe medical problems.
- **Sleep deprivation**, which is prolonged sleep loss (inadequate quality or quantity of REM or NREM sleep).

High-Risk Conditions. Abnormal physiological problems cause several complications of the sleep cycle in some patients. These are:

- **bruxism** (grinding of the teeth)
- **enuresis** (bedwetting)
- **somnambulism** (sleepwalking)

Patients with these problems are at high risk of injury when they are asleep. Special monitoring and safety measures will be listed on care plans of patients with these conditions, to reduce the risk of incidents and injuries.

Nursing Assistant Measures to Promote Comfort, Rest, and Sleep

Basic nursing comfort measures, such as those used to relieve pain, are also effective in helping patients to rest and sleep. Specific measures for each patient will be listed in the care plan. Measures that promote comfort, rest, and sleep are the following:

- Help the patient into loose-fitting, comfortable clothing or nightwear.
- Assist with toileting, cleanliness, oral care, and personal hygiene needs.
- Providing a warm bath or shower, if permitted.
- Avoid serving beverages containing caffeine after the evening meal.
- Provide a snack, if desired.
- Straighten the bed.
- Assist the patient into a comfortable position and provide pillows and props as needed for comfort.
- Provide a comfortable environmental temperature and ventilation.
- Provide an extra blanket, if desired.
- Eliminate unpleasant odors.
- Eliminate noise.
- Adjust the lighting to a comfortable level, darkening the room as much as possible for sleep, and provide a nightlight if desired (Figure 10-11)
- Provide nursing comfort measures, such as a backrub or repositioning the patient into a more comfortable position.
- Report pain to the nurse.
- If the patient is having pain, wait at least 30 minutes after pain medication is administered before performing procedures.
- If the patient is anxious, listen to what he or she says. Eliminate the cause of the anxiety, if possible (Figure 10-12).
- Avoid startling the patient.
- Handle the patient gently during care.
- Organize routine care to allow the patient uninterrupted sleep or rest.
- Avoid physical activity or activities that may upset the patient before bedtime.
- Assist with personal bedtime rituals, if any.
- Allow the patient to select his or her own bedtime.
- Allow the patient to read, watch television, or listen to the radio, if desired.
- Read to the patient from a favorite book.
- Assist with relaxation exercises and activities, as directed.
- If the patient receives a sleeping medication, make sure the patient is ready for sleep before the nurse administers the medication.
- Close the door to the patient's room.

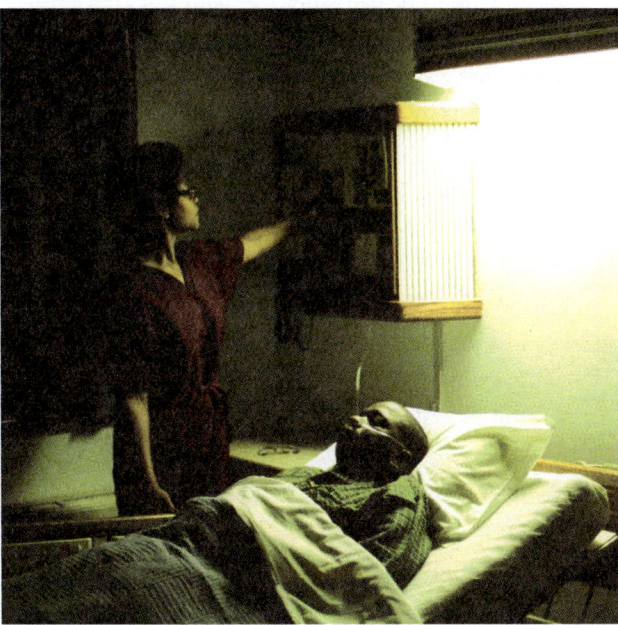

FIGURE 10-11 After the patient is comfortable and settled, turn the light off.

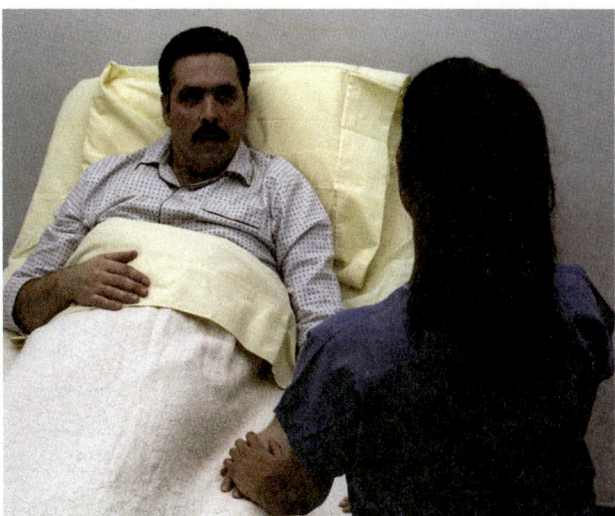

FIGURE 10-12 Listening to the patient's concerns provides emotional support and relieves anxiety.

REVIEW

A. True/False.

Mark the following true or false by circling T or F.

1. T F Comfort is a state of self-actualization.
2. T F Lack of privacy can affect a patient's comfort.
3. T F Unrelieved pain can lead to complications of immobility.
4. T F Chronic pain never lasts longer than one month.
5. T F Acute pain results from tissue damage.
6. T F Phantom pain is imaginary pain.
7. T F Radiating pain always encircles the area in which the pain originates.
8. T F You can assume that the patient is not in pain if he does not complain.
9. T F Rest and sleep are necessary for the body to repair itself and restore strength and energy.
10. T F Pain always indicates that something is wrong.
11. T F Culture has no effect on patients' responses to pain.
12. T F The patient's self-report of pain is the most accurate indicator of the existence and intensity of pain.

B. Matching.

Choose the correct word from Column II to match the phrases in Column I.

Column I

13. _____ sleeping all morning
14. _____ air flow stops for 10 seconds or more
15. _____ teeth grinding
16. _____ restores mental function
17. _____ bedwetting
18. _____ uncontrolled daytime sleeping
19. _____ chronic sleep deprivation
20. _____ state of discomfort

Column II

a. insomnia
b. narcolepsy
c. REM sleep
d. sleep apnea
e. hypersomnia
f. bruxism
g. pain
h. enuresis

C. Completion

Complete the statements in questions 21 to 26 by writing in the correct word from the following list.

comfort	REM
hypersomnia	sleep apnea
NREM	somnambulism

21. Full-color dreaming occurs during the _____ phase of the sleep cycle.
22. _____ is a state of well-being.
23. A patient with _____ sleeps very late in the morning.
24. _____ sleep restores mental function.
25. A patient with _____ stops breathing for 10 seconds or more.
26. The medical term for sleepwalking is _____ .

D. Multiple Choice.

Select the one best answer for each of the following.

27. Pain is
    a. not the nursing assistant's responsibility.
    b. a sign of something wrong.
    c. an objective sign.
    d. a normal part of illness.

28. Pain
    a. does not normally interfere with rest and sleep.
    b. is not stressful or worrisome.
    c. negatively affects well-being.
    d. can usually be ignored.

29. If a patient expresses her problems and worries, the nursing assistant should
    a. stay out of the patient's business.
    b. not tell the nurse about the patient's concerns.
    c. allow her to talk about it and be a good listener.
    d. provide answers to the problems.

30. Aggravating and alleviating factors are
    a. things that worsen or improve pain.
    b. the strength and intensity of pain.
    c. the areas to which pain radiates.
    d. properties and characteristics of all pain.

31. Pain assessment is considered to be the
    a. first vital sign.
    b. frequency at which pain is evaluated.
    c. measurement of the "fifth vital sign."
    d. effectiveness of pain medication.

32. A state of mental calmness, comfort, and relaxation is
    a. comfort.
    b. sleep.
    c. leisure.
    d. rest.

33. A period of continuous or intermittent unconsciousness in which physical movements are decreased is
   a. relaxation.
   b. comfort.
   c. sleep.
   d. diversion.

34. When a patient is sleeping
   a. vital signs may be lower than usual.
   b. temperature increases.
   c. movement increases.
   d. the pulse decreases and respirations increase.

35. During the REM sleep cycle, the patient
   a. dreams.
   b. awakens readily.
   c. progresses through four sleep phases.
   d. may feel hot to the touch.

E. Nursing Assistant Challenge.

Mr. Huynh is grimacing and supporting his right side with his hands when you enter the room. He smiles and nods at you. Complete the following statements regarding this patient.

36. Can Mr. Huynh smile if he is having pain?

37. If Mr. Huynh's right side hurts, you may be able to position him for comfort and support by using _____.

38. Should Mr. Huynh's body language be reported to the nurse?

39. Should you ask Mr. Huynh if he is having pain?

40. List six nursing assistant measures you can take to make Mr. Huynh more comfortable.

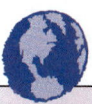

EXPLORING THE WEB

Description	Location
Rest and sleep	*http://www.delmarhealthcare.com/olcs/white/pnotes.asp* (see Chapter 19)
Pain in children and adults	*http://www.nursing.uiowa.edu*
Pain management assessment	*http://www.delmarhealthcare.com/olcs/white/pnotes.asp* (see Chapter 26)
American Academy of Pain Medicine	*http://www.painmed.org*
City of Hope Mayday Resource Center	*http://www.cityofhope.org/prc/web*
Comfort Theory	*http://www3.uakron.edu*
The Fifth Vital Sign	*http://www.advancefornurses.com* (see past articles 2/4/02)
General Comfort Questionnaire	*http://www.uakron.edu*
Hospice Comfort Questionnaire	*http://www.uakron.edu*
Intelihealth Pain Scales	*http://www.intelihealth.com*
Management of Chronic Pain in Older Persons (American Geriatrics Society)	*http://www.americangeriatrics.org*
Pain.com	*http://www.pain.com*
Trouble Sleeping?	*http://www.advancefornurses.com* (see past articles 8/28/00)

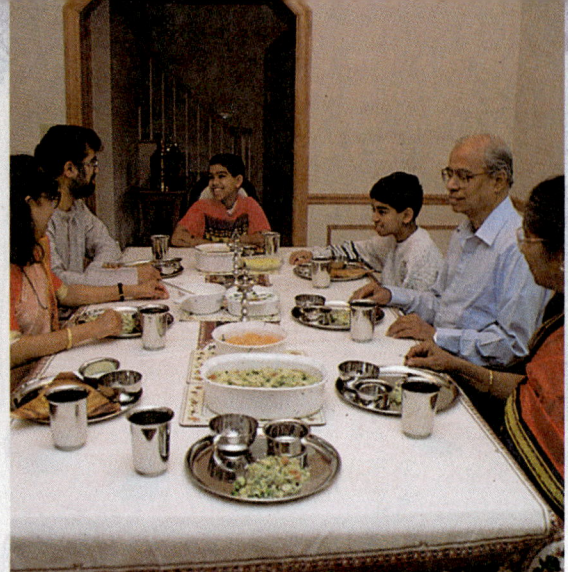

Developing Cultural Sensitivity

objectives

After completing this unit, you will be able to:

- Spell and define terms.
- Name six major cultural groups in the United States.
- Describe ways the major cultures differ in their family organization, communication, need for personal space, health practices, religion, and traditions.

- List ways nursing assistants can develop sensitivity about cultures other than their own.
- List ways the nursing assistant can help patients in practicing rituals appropriate to their cultures.
- State ways the nursing assistant can demonstrate appreciation of and sensitivity to other cultures.

vocabulary

Learn the meaning and the correct spelling of the following words and phrases:

acupuncture	dialect	race	standard
amulet	ethnicity	ritual	stereotype
belief	mores	sensitivity	talisman
culture	personal space	spirituality	tradition

INTRODUCTION

America is a nation of people whose ancestors came primarily from other countries. Each group brought its own cultural heritage with its language, beliefs, and customs. These people are your patients. Each one is a unique individual whose development is the result of his or her own culture, current lifestyle and community participation, and personal experiences. As a health care provider, you are expected to show sensitivity to the individuality and cultural heritage of each patient. **Sensitivity** is the ability to be aware of and to appreciate the personal characteristics of others.

When members of different groups must live and work together in a community, it is easy for members of each group to form specific beliefs about the other groups. When these beliefs are rigid and are based on generalizations, they are called **stereotypes**. For example, others may view people of Asian heritage as present-focused (thinking about immediate rather than long-term goals), not self-expressive, and reluctant to make eye contact. These traits are stereotypes when applied to an entire group without consideration of the traditions of the group and individual characteristics. In contrast to these stereotypes, Van (whose heritage is Vietnamese) (Figure 11-1) is outgoing, looks directly at a person speaking to her, has a quick smile, and is future-oriented as she studies to become a health care provider.

Health care providers must be careful not to make assumptions about their patients based on stereotypes of the group of which the patient is a part. The longer a group is associated with the American culture, the less its members rely on the cultural values and traditions of the country of origin. Young immigrants and second- or third-generation residents of the United States are much closer to American culture than to their original culture. Older people and new immigrants tend to cling more closely to the customs of their homeland.

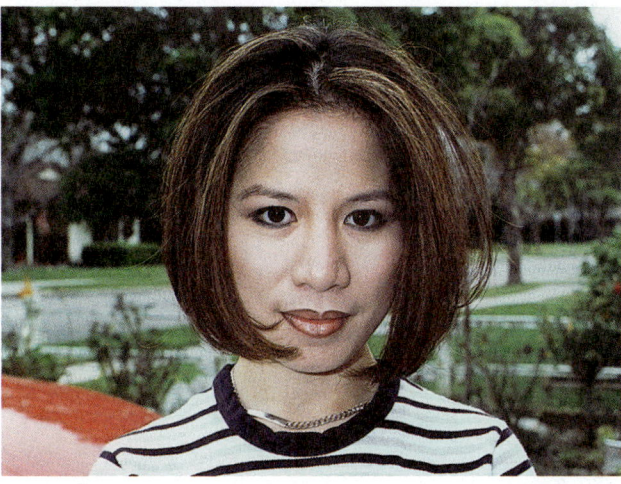

FIGURE 11-1 This young woman, whose parents were Vietnamese immigrants, has absorbed aspects of her parents' culture and the American culture in which she lives.

RACE, ETHNICITY, AND CULTURE

The terms *race*, *ethnicity*, and *culture* are used to describe groups of people. **Race** is the classification of people according to shared physical characteristics such as skin color, bone structure, facial features, hair texture, and blood type.

Ethnicity

Ethnicity refers to special groups within a race as defined by national origin and/or culture. Members of an ethnic group share common:

- heritage
- national origin
- social customs
- language

Six ethnic groups predominate in the United States (see Table 11-1):

- Caucasians—those of European and Scandinavian descent
- African Americans—those of African, Haitian, or Dominican Republic descent
- Hispanics—those whose ancestors came from Spanish-speaking countries
- Asians/Pacific—those whose ancestors came from the islands and countries of the Pacific Rim
- Native Americans—those descended from one of the more than 600 tribes of North America
- Middle Easterners/Arabs—those whose ancestors came from Middle Eastern countries

TABLE 11-1 MAJOR ETHNIC GROUPS IN AMERICA

Group	Some Countries and Areas of Origin
Caucasian	England, Scotland, Ireland, Poland, Scandinavia, Italy, Russia
African American	Africa, Haiti, Jamaica, Dominican Republic
Hispanic	Cuba, Puerto Rico, Mexico, Latin and South America
Asian/Pacific	China, Japan, Philippines, Vietnam, Cambodia, Korea, Hawaii, Samoa
Native American	Hundreds of tribes, such as Cherokee, Apache, Navajo, Blackfoot, Inuit (Alaskan)
Middle Eastern	Egypt, Iran, Yemen, Palestine, Lebanon, Jordan, Saudi Arabia, Kuwait

Culture

Culture refers to the way a particular group views the world and the set of traditions that are passed on from generation to generation. Culture enforces the **standards** (rules) established by the group based on the values and beliefs of the group. Cultural differences among ethnic groups include:

- family organization
- personal space needs
- communication
- beliefs about health/illness and health care practices
- religions
- traditions

Cultural **mores** (customs) influence the way people will interact. Ethnicity and culture contribute to an individual's sense of self-identity as he or she relates to the group and to other cultures. Cross-cultural nursing recognizes the individual within an ethnic and cultural group and provides nursing care that assures cultural as well as individual acceptance and comfort.

Family Organization. Families form the basic cultural social groups, but their structure varies from culture to culture. The family organization determines who will be the decision makers and who is responsible for providing health care. In some families, the father or oldest male is the authority figure. In others, both the mother and father make decisions. In Hispanic and Middle Eastern families, the father is the dominant person, whereas in many African American households the mother has the strongest influence. In Caucasian families, the highest wage earner is often given the greatest respect and authority.

Health care may be a family responsibility. Figure 11-2 shows an extended family and Figure 11-3 a nuclear family. For example, in Asian families the elderly are given great respect, and caring for them is considered a duty and privilege by all family members. In Asian, Hispanic, and Native American cultures, extended families are common, and may include grandparents, aunts, and uncles. In these cases, caregiving is personal and shared by family members. Caucasian families tend to be structured as more independent units consisting of mother, father, and children. In

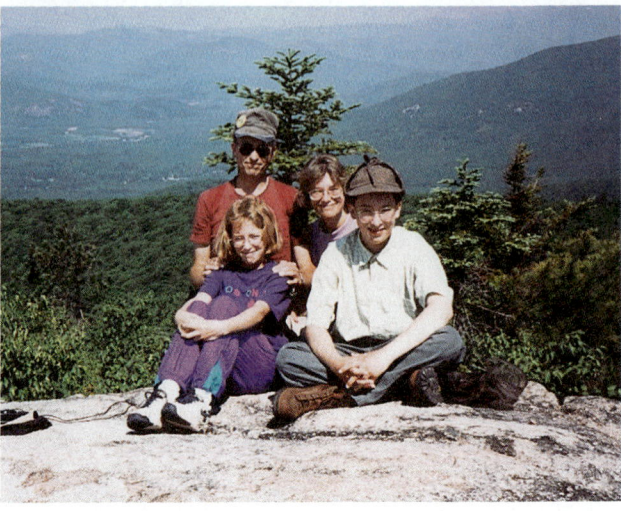

FIGURE 11-3 A nuclear family.

this case, care of the elderly is more likely to be given over to others.

Personal Space Needs. **Personal space** refers to the actual physical closeness that one person is comfortable with during social interaction with others. Personal space can be invaded by standing too close to another person, patterns of eye contact, and touching.

Caucasians prefer to stand and speak at a distance of about 18 to 36 inches from one another. African Americans are comfortable standing closer to another person (5 to 10 inches). Space is important to Native Americans but has no specific boundaries. Asians tend to be uncomfortable if standing too close to another person.

Eye contact travels through the visual personal space and is interpreted differently by different cultures (Table 11-2).

CULTURE *Alert*

Culture affects the type of care the patient expects to receive in the hospital. In some cultures, patients are comfortable doing self-care, if able. However, patients from other cultures may expect you to provide total care, even if they are physically able to do some things. Their feeling is that if they are sick, they should not expend their energy in caring for themselves. In some cultures, family members are expected to care for the patient. In other cultures, only caregivers of the same gender may care for the patient. The care plan should guide you in culturally sensitive care. Consult the nurse if necessary.

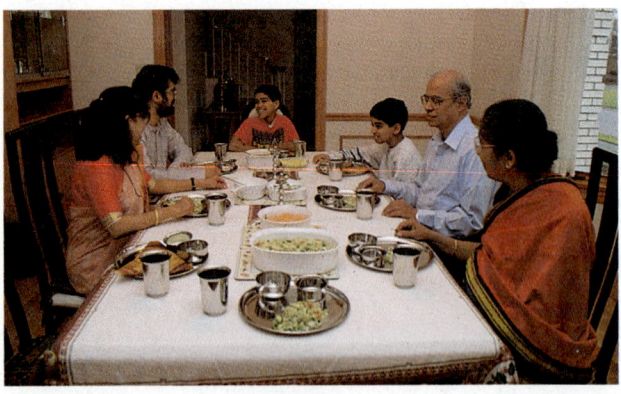

FIGURE 11-2 An extended family.

TABLE 11-2 CULTURAL INTERPRETATION OF NONVERBAL COMMUNICATION AND PERSONAL SPACE

Culture	Nonverbal Communication
American (U.S.)	Personal space 18 to 36 inches. Eye contact is acceptable. Lack of eye contact may be interpreted as lack of self-esteem or not telling the truth.
African American	Eye contact is acceptable; close personal space.
American Indian	*See* Native American.
Arab American	Women usually avoid eye contact with males and others whom they do not know well. Close personal space.
Asian	Eye contact is acceptable; close personal space, but avoid touching.
Brazilian	Lack of eye contact is viewed by some as a sign of respect. Close personal space.
Cambodian	Eye contact is acceptable; close personal space.
Chinese American	Avoid eye contact with authority figures as a sign of respect; will make eye contact with family and friends. Distant personal space.
Columbian	May avoid eye contact in presence of an authority figure. Close personal space.
Cuban	Eye contact expected during conversation. Close personal space with friends and family.
Ethiopian	Avoid eye contact with those perceived to be in authority. Close personal space with family and friends.
European	Eye contact acceptable; distant personal space.
Filipino	May avoid eye contact with authority figures. Close personal space.
Gypsy (Romany)	Facial expressions reflect mood. Close personal space with family members. Generally avoid contact with non-Gypsies. Also avoid surfaces considered unclean (areas that lower body has touched).
Haitian	Avoid eye contact with those perceived to be in authority.
Hmong	Avoid prolonged eye contact, which is considered rude.
Iranian	Make eye contact only with equals and close family and friends. Close personal space.
Japanese American	Little eye contact. Touching may be considered offensive.
Korean	Little direct eye contact. Touching is considered offensive. Although Koreans maintain close personal space with family, invading their personal space is a sign of disrespect.
Mexican American	Avoid eye contact with those perceived to be in authority. Some may believe touch by strangers is disrespectful or offensive.
Native American	Eye contact avoided as a sign of respect. Distant personal space is considered respectful.
Puerto Rican	Personal space varies with age group; generally closer with younger women, more distant with older women.
Russian	Close personal space with family and friends. Direct eye contact acceptable during conversation.
South Asian	May consider direct eye contact with elderly individuals offensive or rude. Close personal space with family members.
Vietnamese	Avoid eye contact with those perceived to be in authority. Distant personal space.
West Indian	Eye contact is avoided. Distant personal space.

Asians consider eye contact inappropriate. The averted eyes and shifting gaze perceived as respectful in Asian cultures may be interpreted by Americans as inattention or insincerity. The direct eye contact of Caucasians and African Americans may be considered an invasion of visual space by an Asian patient. Members of Hispanic cultures make direct eye contact when speaking but consider prolonged contact disrespectful.

Touching a person is considered an invasion of personal space in some cultures. A handshake is traditional in the United States for both men and women. In Middle Eastern countries, however, only men may greet other men in this manner. Greeting with handshakes and hugs is common in Hispanic cultures. Persons from Asian cultures are less likely to shake hands, especially with women.

Touching the body of another person may be even more restricted than the touching of hands in greeting. In Middle Eastern countries, men may not touch females who are not members of their immediate family. Uncovering the body is considered disrespectful in some cultures and is forbidden for women in others. For example, Muslim women may be completely veiled (Figure 11-4). Uncovering the shoulders of a person from India may be considered disrespectful. The mode of dress and body covering is very important to an individual's modesty. In some cultures, caregivers cannot care for members of the opposite sex.

As you care for patients from cultures other than your own, remember that the customs of the individual's culture greatly influence the acceptance of the person giving care and how the care is given, the amount of disrobing that is permitted, and the degree of touch that is comfortable for and accepted by the patient. Ask the nurse for guidance. You can also learn much about the patient's desires by watching the interactions of the patient with his or her family and with other staff members.

Communication. Touching and eye contact are nonverbal forms of communication. A common verbal language

COMMUNICATION *Highlight*

Sickness, medication, anesthesia, pain, aging, culture, and disease can affect the patient's ability to communicate. Some patients may have trouble seeing, hearing, or speaking. Some have language barriers and do not speak English. Practice empathy with patients who have difficulty communicating by putting yourself in the patient's shoes and understanding how it feels. Imagine how frustrating it would be if you were unable to make your needs known and communicate with others! Be patient when communicating with patients who do not speak English. Do not assume that patients who are unable to speak are mentally confused. Patients who cannot speak often understand what is said to them. Some have limited writing skills or dictionaries to assist them in making their needs known. Communicate caring through your body language and demeanor. Treat all patients with dignity and respect.

is one characteristic of an ethnic group. Silence may be an important part of the language. For example, some Native American groups consider silence to be essential to understanding. Silence does not always mean that the listener has not heard or is inattentive to the speaker.

An ethnic group may share a common language, but local terminology and usage may vary (a **dialect**). For example, Hispanic Americans may have originated in Puerto Rico, Mexico, Cuba, or Central or South America. The basic language of all of these people is Spanish, but there are many dialects depending on the country of origin or even a portion of a country. The Spanish you speak may differ in certain ways from the Spanish your patients speak.

Patients may be bilingual and speak both their native language and English. Some of your patients, however, may have only a minimal understanding of English. Older people and the newest immigrants will be most comfortable communicating in their own language. The desire to return to that which is familiar and most comfortable is especially important when people are ill or frightened. Communicating in a patient's own language adds greatly to his or her sense of security. It is helpful to have an interpreter present, but if this is not possible, some form of communication is required if good nursing care is to be given.

Patients are pleased when a caregiver can speak even a few words in the patient's own language. If many of your patients share a common language, it would be helpful for

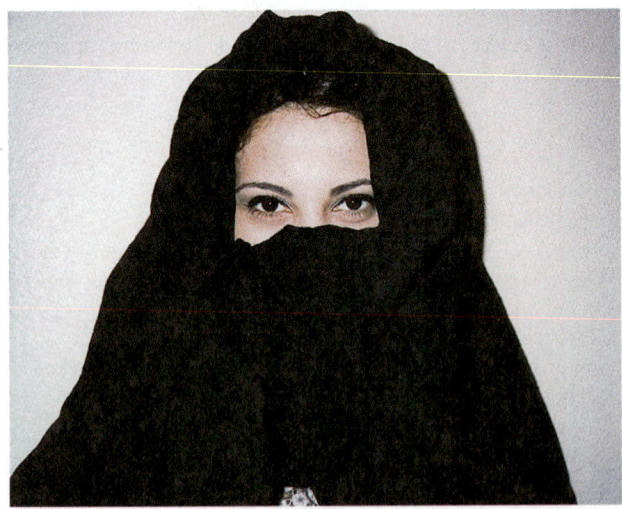

FIGURE 11-4 Traditional Muslim culture requires women to be completely veiled from head to toe.

you to learn some common words and phrases. Remember, too, that body language, gestures, and facial expression can be used to express thoughts and words when verbal language is inadequate.

When communicating:

- Use a normal tone.
- Speak slowly.
- Use simple words.
- Look directly at the listener even if someone is interpreting (be sensitive to any discomfort this may cause the patient because of cultural variations).
- Try to obtain feedback from the patient to determine the level of understanding.

You may wish to go back to Unit 7 to review other ways to communicate.

Beliefs About Health, Illness, and Health Care Practices. Beliefs are based on commonly held opinions, knowledge, and attitudes about the world and life. These beliefs will influence the person's feelings about illness and the kind of health care he will choose. Members of a culture share beliefs about:

- the nature and cause of illness
- types of health care practices
- their relationship to a higher power

People tend to view the causes of health and illness in one of three ways, or in a combination of these ways. Some people hold magical beliefs, in which the causes of illness are supernatural forces. Others hold scientific beliefs, relating health and illness to causes such as infectious agents, the wear and tear on the body caused by daily living and stress, environmental agents, or injury. Still others have holistic beliefs that view the person and the environment as continuously exchanging energy and matter with one another. In this belief system, the mind and body must be in harmony to ensure health.

Those who believe that illness and pain are a penance from a higher power, as punishment for wrongdoing, will be less willing to complain of suffering and to seek relief through medication and scientific medicine. They rely more on the use of charms, chants or holy words, and rituals. Some cultures turn to folk healers or shamans to help bring their bodies back into balance with nature. They believe that the imbalance is the cause of their discomfort. The balance is achieved by eating certain foods, taking natural medicines, or through the power of healing ceremonies.

Those who see illness as the result of environmental factors, infectious agents, or injury are more likely to seek scientifically based medical help. Asian cultures, which have traditional health and illness beliefs, use traditional medications such as herbs, acupuncture (placement of metal needles in the body), and mind-body practices such as tai chi and meditation to achieve balance and wellness.

Arabs who believe that some illnesses are the "Will of Allah" use amulets (charms against evil) and verses from the Koran (a holy book) written on turquoise stones to help them. Native Americans believe illness develops when the harmony between body, mind, and spirit is disrupted. Sand paintings are used in healing rituals to diagnose conditions and prescribe treatment. Hispanics believe that illness is caused when an imbalance exists in the four body fluids. They may use native healers, candles, prayers, and the wearing of medals as methods of treatment and to restore balance. Hot and cold conditions (illnesses) are identified and "hot" and "cold" foods and medicines, similar to those recognized in Asian cultures, are used in treatment. Cold remedies are given to balance a hot condition and vice versa. See Table 11-3 for hot and cold conditions and remedies. Table 11-4 lists some of the common belief systems related to health and illness.

TABLE 11-3 HOT AND COLD CONDITIONS AND REMEDIES

Hot Conditions	Cold Conditions
Constipation	Cancer
Fever	Colds
Infections	Headache
Sore throat	Pneumonia
Ulcers	Tuberculosis

Cold Food Remedies	Hot Food Remedies
Dairy products	Cereals
Milk	Eggs
Lima beans	Beef
Vegetables	Oils
Honey	Spicy foods
Chicken	Wine
Raisins	

Cold Medical Remedies	Hot Medical Remedies
Bicarbonate of soda	Aspirin
Milk of magnesia	Cinnamon
Orange flower water	Cod liver oil
Sage	Garlic
	Penicillin

TABLE 11-4 BELIEF SYSTEMS RELATED TO HEALTH/ILLNESS

Culture	Related Concepts	Health Care Provider	Cause of Illness	Methods of Treatment
European Americans	Illness is not superficial, but can be influenced by poor health practices; disease is treatable and sometimes curable	Physician	• Punishment for sins • Self-abuse; outside forces such as germs	Diet, exercise, home remedies, medication, surgery, religious rituals, wearing amulets
Asian Americans	Body has two energy forces: *yang*, which is cold, and *yin*, which is hot (hot and cold do not refer to temperature); hot conditions are treated with cold foods and treatments; cold conditions are treated with hot foods and treatments	Traditional healers	• Imbalance between the positive (yang) energy and the negative (yin) energy found in the body • Overexertion	Herbs, hot foods for conditions associated with yin conditions and cold foods for conditions associated with yang conditions; home remedies and folk medicines
Hispanic Americans	Body contains four humors (fluids) that must be balanced. Illness develops from imbalance. Humors are blood (hot, moist), phlegm (cold, moist), black bile (cold, dry), yellow bile (hot, dry)	Native healers (jerbero, curandera)	• Punishment from God for sins	Candles, prayers, wearing medals, hot and cold foods to restore balance of humors
Native Americans	Spiritual powers control body's energy; harmony must exist between body, mind, and spirit; illness results when harmony is disrupted	Medicine man, shaman	• Violation of taboo • Attack by witch or evil spirits • Do not believe in germ theory	Sandpainting to diagnose condition and determine treatment; elaborate rituals; carrying medicine bundles; wearing masks to hide from evil spirits
African Americans	Body, mind, and spirit must be in harmony for health; life is a process rather than a state; illness can occur if self-care is not taken	Folk practitioners, root workers	• Punishment from God • Spirits and demons	Prayer, diet, home remedies, wearing copper and silver bracelets, wearing talismans and amulets
Islamic Americans	Magico-religious; emotional distress; expressed as "heart disease"; feel responsible to visit and help ill; the individual has no control over life events, as good and evil usually are result of "Will of Allah"; male-dominated society with male children more highly valued than female children; may use female circumcision to ensure faithfulness and be accepted by the women; may resist medical direction	Traditional healers; physicians	Will of Allah; punishment for sins; various beliefs in causes such as imbalance of hot and cold; influence of an "evil eye"	Magico-religious; prayer; self-care and medical science; use amulets inscribed with verses from the Koran; turquoise stones; charm of a hand with five fingers to protect against the evil eye; male health professionals prohibited from touching or examining females; males may refuse health care from females

Religious Practices. Spirituality is the part of a person that gives a sense of wholeness by fulfilling the human need to feel connected with the world around one and to a power greater than oneself. For many, spirituality is expressed in religious practice. *Religion* is an organized system of belief in a deity (higher power). Spirituality and religion are products of an individual's cultural background and experience. Spiritual values and religious beliefs form the rules of what a person considers to be right or wrong.

Religious beliefs provide a person with guidelines for moral behavior. Religious preferences are highly personal and can vary within a given culture. For example, Hispanics are traditionally Roman Catholic. However, it is not unusual to find a Protestant church of Hispanics in the same community. The major religions of the United States include:

- Protestantism (various denominations)
- Roman Catholicism
- Judaism
- Islam
- Hinduism

Religious items and rituals (solemn and ceremonial acts that reinforce faith) are especially meaningful to practitioners. They must be treated with respect. For example, the crucifix, Bible, and religious medals are important to Roman Catholics. The prayer rug is significant to the Islamic, who pray five times each day in the direction of their holy city, Mecca. Amulets and special charms are important to the religious beliefs of Native Americans and to some peoples in the Middle East. Talismans are engraved stones, rings, or other objects that are used to ward off evil. Copper or silver bracelets and religious medals are important and sacred to some cultures.

If a patient requests a visit from clergy, be sure the request is promptly relayed to the nurse. When the clergy visits, be sure to provide privacy. It is also important to provide privacy when the patient is engaged in a religious act such as praying. Table 11-5 lists five religious faiths common in the United States and some of their beliefs and religious items. Special religious rituals and practices related to dying, death, and care of the body after death are discussed in Unit 1.

Foods are important in some religions. For example, those of the Orthodox Jewish faith may not be served milk and meat products at the same time. Roman Catholics restrict food intake on specific dates and some Baptists, Muslims, and others are not permitted to drink alcohol. Other food restrictions are discussed in Unit 26.

An understanding of some of the major belief systems will help you be more sensitive to your patient's needs. You can support your patient's spirituality and religious practices by:

- Being a willing listener
- Respecting the patient's belief system
- Never trying to convert the patient to your belief system
- Respecting religious symbols
- Not interrupting during religious rituals
- Reading aloud the patient's favorite passages from religious books such as the Bible, Talmud, Koran, or Book of Mormon
- Providing privacy during prayers and meditation or when clergy visits

TABLE 11-5 SOME COMMON BELIEF SYSTEMS (RELIGIOUS)

Religion	Belief in a Deity	Value of Prayer	Belief in Hereafter	Special Practices or Symbols
Protestant	Yes	Important	Yes	Baptism, Holy Communion, cross, Bible
Roman Catholic	Yes	Important	Yes	Baptism, Holy Communion, Anointing the Sick, Reconciliation, Bible, medals, pictures and statues of saints, rosaries, crucifix
Orthodox Judaism	Yes	Important	Yes	Torah, yarmulke (cap), tallith, menorah
Hinduism	Yes (many forms)	Important	Yes	No sacraments
Buddhism	Yes	Important	Yes	No sacraments
Islam (Moslems)	Yes	Important	Yes	Koran, prayer rug

Within the framework of each belief system, there are individual differences in the depth of belief and extent of practice.

TRADITIONS

Traditions are customs and practices followed by members of a culture and passed from generation to generation. Often traditions are related to religious rituals and holiday celebrations. Foods are particularly traditional at holidays. Think about ham at Easter, corned beef and cabbage on St. Patrick's Day, and traditional tacos, tamales, and enchiladas on Cinco de Mayo.

Families carry out traditions from generation to generation. For example, it is a Chinese tradition to have a celebration accompanied by a colorful procession with a dragon to welcome in the Chinese New Year. People all over America watch fireworks to celebrate the Fourth of July. Holidays specific to cultures are celebrated each year.

Many traditions involve the coming to maturity of young people and are related to religious practice. For example, young Jewish boys have a bar mitzvah as they reach puberty. Many Protestant churches present Bibles to children when they are in the third grade of school and are able to read on their own.

Honoring and practicing traditions gives people a sense of stability and continuity. Traditions help to bind the people of a culture closer together.

Nursing assistants have a unique opportunity to learn about other cultures directly from their patients. There are ways to make this process easier for yourself and your patient (see the following guidelines). Always remember that even though a person is part of an identifiable culture, he or she must always be recognized as an individual within the culture.

guidelines *for*

Developing Cultural Sensitivity

- Review your own belief systems.
- Consider how your own culture influences your behavior.
- Always view patients as individuals within a culture.
- Recognize that patients are a combination of heritage, culture, and community.
- Understand that culture influences how people behave and interact with others.
- Remember that personal space needs, eye contact, and ways of communicating are often culturally related.
- Recognize that some cultures have beliefs about health, wellness, and illness that are different from your own.
- Be willing to modify care according to the patient's cultural background and practices.
- Do not expect all members of a cultural group to behave in exactly the same manner.

- Remember that patients' health practices related to culture, values, and belief system are deeply ingrained and not easily changed.
- Avoid stereotyping people within a culture.
- Check with the supervisor to learn special ways to deal with patients of different cultural backgrounds.
- Care for religious articles with respect.
- Provide privacy when a spiritual advisor is visiting the patient or the patient is practicing a devotional act.
- Try to learn about the practices, beliefs, and cultural heritage of the people who are most likely to be your patients. A library and the Internet are good sources.
- Ask patients politely about practices that are unfamiliar.
- Attend staff development classes designed to promote cultural sensitivity.

REVIEW

A. Matching.

Match each word with its definition.

1. _b_ amulet
2. _e_ mores
3. _d_ sensitivity
4. _a_ standard
5. _c_ tradition

a. rules of conduct
b. charms against evil
c. passed from generation to generation
d. awareness and appreciation of
e. customs

B. Completion.

Complete the following sentences by choosing the correct word.

6. Rigid, biased ideas about people are called stereotypes.
   (stereotypes) (characteristics)

7. Classification by shared physical characteristics is based on race.
   (ethnicity) (race)

8. The way a group views the world, and the group's traditions, are the foundation of a culture.
   (race) (culture)

9. Commonly held opinions, knowledge, and attitudes about life are called beliefs.
   (standards) (beliefs)

10. Solemn and ceremonial acts that reinforce faith are called rituals.
    (rituals) (traditions)

C. Multiple Choice.

Select the one best answer for each of the following.

11. The cultural language common to most Hispanics is
    a. English.
    b. French.
    c. Spanish.
    d. German.

12. You may expect that a new black immigrant was born in
    a. Egypt.
    b. Russia.
    c. China.
    d. Poland.

13. The nuclear family is most commonly seen in
    a. African American culture.
    b. Asian culture.
    c. Hispanic culture.
    d. Caucasian culture.

14. Caucasians prefer to stand and speak about
    a. six inches apart.
    b. eighteen inches apart.
    c. four feet apart.
    d. five feet apart.

15. A Middle Eastern man may greet another man by
    a. nodding.
    b. shaking hands.
    c. kissing on either cheek.
    d. hugging.

16. Your patient has a prayer rug and prays five times a day. You believe he is from which culture?
    a. Middle Eastern
    b. African American
    c. Asian
    d. Native American

17. Your Asian patient looks down and says little when you speak. This is
    a. rude in his culture.
    b. respectful in his culture.
    c. his way of showing his anger.
    d. his way of showing fear.

18. Your patient makes direct and prolonged eye contact as you speak. He probably is of what culture?
    a. Asian
    b. Native American
    c. Hispanic
    d. Caucasian

19. Your patient speaks only a few words of English. When you speak to him, you should
    a. raise your voice.
    b. speak slowly.
    c. use slang.
    d. look away.

20. People from this culture believe that illness develops when harmony between the mind, body, and spirit is disrupted.
    a. Asian
    b. Hispanic
    c. Native American
    d. African American

D. Short Answer.

21. You have a Catholic patient. Briefly explain how you can show sensitivity to her religious beliefs.

22. Name your own culture. List two traditions that are common to your culture.

23. List two ways you can improve your cultural sensitivity to a new patient who has a culture different from your own.

E. Nursing Assistant Challenge.

You have a patient who is a new immigrant from Iran. He is Islamic and 60 years old. Mark the following true or false.

24. T **F** The Torah is his holy book.

25. T **F** He will wish to pray once daily.

26. T **F** He will be the person most likely to make his own medical decisions.

27. **T** F He probably feels his condition is due to the "Will of Allah."

28. T **F** He would celebrate Easter and Christmas if he were at home.

EXPLORING THE WEB

Description	Location
Cultural diversity and nursing	http://www.delmarhealthcare.com/olcs/whiteduncan/pnotes.asp (see Chapter 6)
Cultural diversity in nursing	http://www.delmarhealthcare.com/olcs/white/pnotes.asp (see Chapter 12)
Minority health	http://healthweb.org
Minority health care	http://www.omhrc.gov
Transcultural communication stumbling blocks	http://www.delmarhealthcare.com/pdf/0766802566_04.pdf
Transcultural and multicultural health care	http://www.iun.edu
About.com	http://nursing.about.com
Cultural Profiles Project	http://cwr.utoronto.ca/cultural
Culture Diversity	http://www.culturediversity.org
CulturedMed	http://www.sunyit.edu
Disparities in Minority Health	http://www.advancefornurses.com (see past articles 2/5/01)
Diversity Rx	http://www.diversityrx.org
EthnoMed	http://ethnomed.org
The Many Faces of Aging: Resources to Effectively Serve Minority Older Persons	http://www.aoa.gov
Native American Elders Health Care Series	http://learn.sdstate.edu/share
Transcultural C.A.R.E. Associates	http://www.transculturalcare.net
Transcultural Nursing Society	http://www.tcns.org
Racial Disparities in Health Care	http://www.advancefornurses.com (see past articles 9/17/01)

Infection and Infection Control

UNIT 12
Infection

UNIT 13
Infection Control

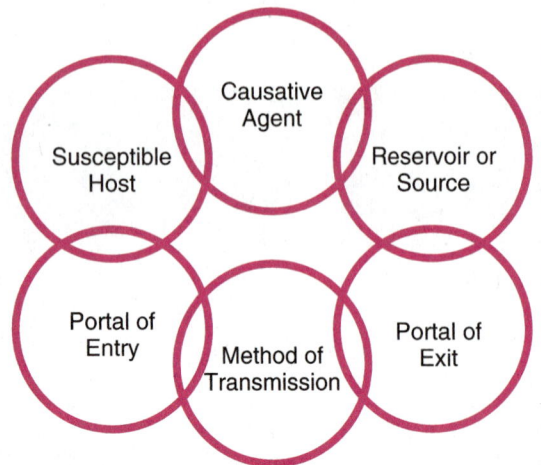

Infection

See Appendix B (page 897) for additional information.

objectives

After completing this unit, you will be able to:
- Spell and define terms.
- Identify the most common microbes and describe some of their characteristics.
- List the links in the chain of infection.
- List the ways that infectious diseases are spread.

- Name five serious infectious diseases.
- Identify the causes of several important infectious diseases.
- Describe common treatments for infectious disease.
- List natural body defenses against infections.
- Explain why patients are at risk for infections.

vocabulary

Learn the meaning and the correct spelling of the following words and phrases:

acquired immune
  deficiency
  syndrome (AIDS)
airborne transmission
allergy
antibiotic
antibody
antigen
bacillus, bacilli
bacteremia
bacteria, bacterium
bioterrorism
carrier
causative agent
chain of infection
coccus, cocci
colony
contact transmission
contagious
contaminated
culture and sensitivity

diplo-
distended
droplet transmission
dysentery
Escherichia coli
  (E. coli) **O157:H7**
flora
fomites
fungi, fungus
hantavirus
hemoptysis
hepatitis
host
human
  immunodeficiency
  virus (HIV)
immune response
immunity
immunization
immunosuppression
incubation

infection
infectious
inflammation
methicillin-resistant
  Staphylococcus
  aureus (MRSA)
microbe
microorganism
mold
nonpathogen
organism
parasite
pathogen
petechiae
phagocyte
portal of entry
portal of exit
protozoa, protozoan
pseudomembranous
  colitis
reservoir

risk factor
seizure
seropositive
source
spirillum, spirilla
staphylo-
strepto-
toxin
transmission
tubercle
tuberculosis disease
tuberculosis infection
vaccine
vancomycin-resistant
  enterococci (VRE)
vector
virus
yeast

INTRODUCTION

Humans are surrounded by a world of tiny **organisms** (living beings). These beings cannot be seen with the naked eye. They make their presence known only by their effect, in much the same way we become aware of the wind. We cannot see the wind, but we do see its effect on the trees, which bend and sway.

These organisms can be seen only with a microscope. They are everywhere—in us, on us, and around us. They are:

- On our skin
- In our mouths
- Within our bodies
- In and on the food we eat
- On what we touch or handle

Micro means small. Because these organisms (agents) are so tiny, they are called **microorganisms** or **microbes**. The organisms live in relationship to us and to each other.

Many of these microbes are useful to us. They are called **nonpathogens** because they do not produce disease. They help in the

- Processing of cheese, beer, and yogurt
- Curing of leather
- Baking of bread

Other microbes are not useful. Microbes that cause disease in humans are called **pathogens** or pathogenic organisms. Pathogens grow best:

- At body temperature
- Where light is limited
- Where there is moisture
- Where there is a food supply
- Where oxygen needs can be met

Infections occur when the pathogens invade the body and cause disease.

MICROBES

There are many different types of microbes, many of which are pathogenic to human beings. Microbes are classified as:

- Bacteria
- Viruses
- Fungi
- Protozoa

Bacteria

Bacteria (singular: **bacterium**) are simple one-celled microbes. They are named according to their shapes and arrangement. They cause infections in the skin, respiratory tract, urinary tract, and bloodstream.

Shapes. In the following list, the first term is the singular form of the word. The word in parentheses is the plural form.

- **Coccus** (**cocci**)—round or spherical (Figure 12-1)
- **Bacillus** (**bacilli**)—straight rod (Figure 12-2)
- **Spirillum** (**spirilla**)—spiral, corkscrew, or slightly curved (Figure 12-3)

Arrangements. Bacteria grow in groups called **colonies**. If we look at a small part of a colony under a microscope, we see that the bacteria typically are arranged in pairs, clusters, or chains.

- Single
- Pairs (**diplo-**)
- Chains (**strepto-**)
- Clusters (**staphylo-**)

The shape and group arrangement of bacteria are important factors in their identification. For example, round microorganisms grouped in chains are called streptococci. A very important member of this family is the *Streptococcus hemolyticus*. It causes septic sore throat and rheumatic fever.

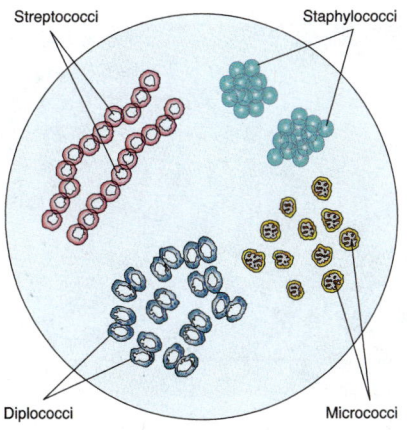

Streptococci

Staphylococci

Diplococci

Micrococci

FIGURE 12-1 Forms of cocci.

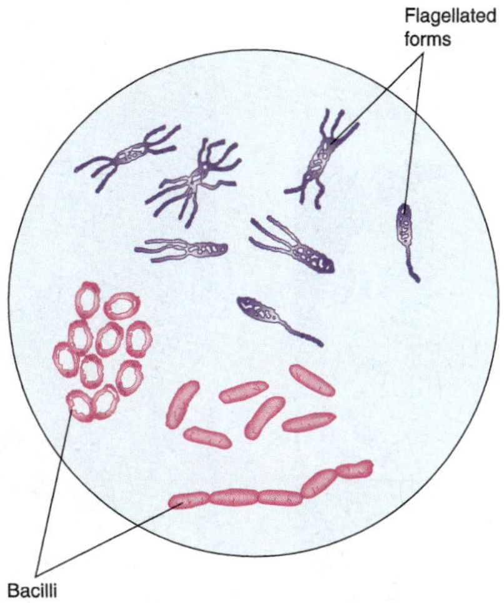

Flagellated forms

Bacilli

FIGURE 12-2 Forms of bacilli.

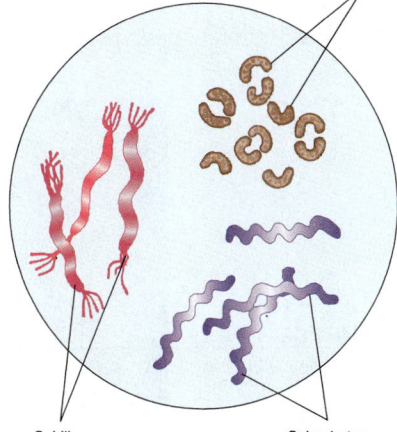

Vibrios

Spirilla

Spirochetes

FIGURE 12-3 Spiral forms of bacteria.

Round organisms grouped in a cluster are called staphylococci. An example of this family is *Staphylococcus aureus*. Staphylococci cause many infections, such as:

- Surgical wound infections
- Abscesses
- Boils
- Toxic shock

Round organisms in pairs are called diplococci. A diplococcus, the *Neisseria gonorrhoeae* (Figure 12-4), causes gonorrhea.

Fungi

Two groups of **fungi** (singular: **fungus**) are most commonly associated with infection in humans:

- **Yeasts**—single-celled budding forms of a fungus. Yeast can infect areas of the body such as:
  - Mouth/vagina: *Candida albicans*
  - Skin: *Tinea capitis* (ringworm)
  - Feet: *Tinea pedis* (athlete's foot)
- **Molds**—A common mold that can cause infection in the lungs of humans is *Aspergillus*

Yeasts and molds are known as opportunistic parasites. (A **parasite** is an organism that lives in or on another organism without benefiting the host organism.) Under normal conditions, the organisms are harmless. However, when the human immune system is impaired and unable to protect the body, these organisms can invade the body and cause severe infections. For example, a patient with AIDS is very susceptible to fungal infections because the immune system is not working properly.

Viruses

A **virus** is the smallest microbe and has a variety of shapes. Ways viruses are classified include:

- Type of nucleic acid core (DNA or RNA)
- Clinical properties

Common viral infections include:

- Hepatitis (Figure 12-5)
- Herpes
- Acquired immune deficiency syndrome (AIDS)

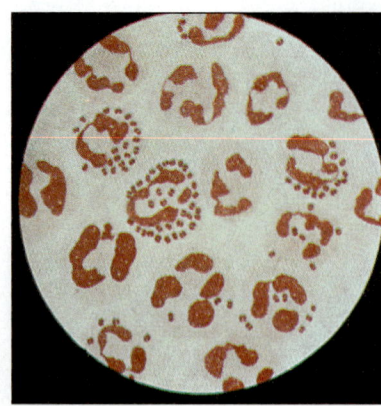

FIGURE 12-4 *Neisseria gonorrhoeae. (Courtesy of the Centers for Disease Control and Prevention, Atlanta, GA)*

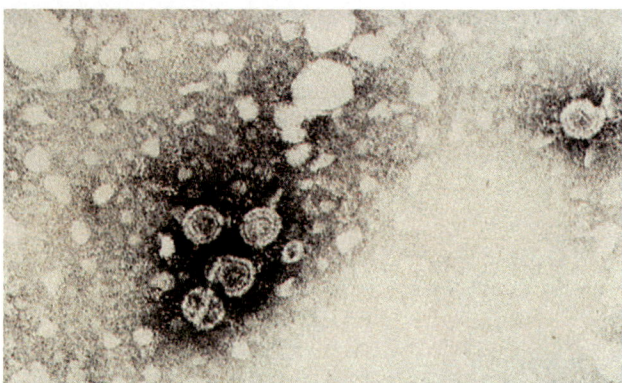

FIGURE 12-5 Electron micrograph of the hepatitis B virus. *(Courtesy of the Centers for Disease Control and Prevention, Atlanta, GA)*

- Chickenpox
- Influenza (Figure 12-6)
- Common cold
- Measles
- Mumps

Protozoa

Protozoa (singular: **protozoan**) are simple one-celled organisms that live on living matter (Figure 12-7). These organisms have a true nucleus. They are classified by the way in which they move. For example, some move by whiplike tails, others by hairlike projections. They cause diseases such as:

- Malaria
- Toxoplasmosis
- African sleeping sickness
- Amebiasis

Some signs and symptoms of diseases caused by protozoa include:

- Diarrhea
- **Dysentery** (infection in the lower bowel)
- Inflammation of the brain (encephalitis)

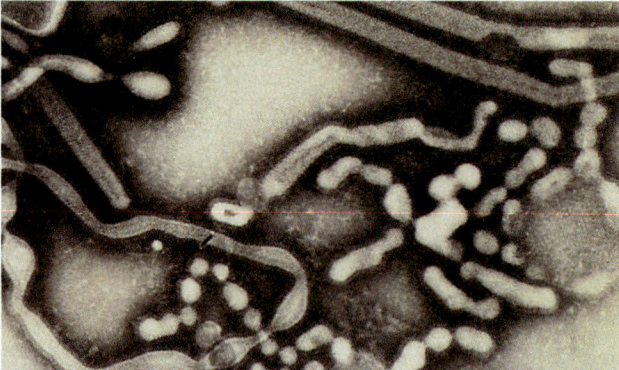

FIGURE 12-6 Electron micrograph of the influenza A virus. *(Courtesy of the Centers for Disease Control and Prevention, Atlanta, GA)*

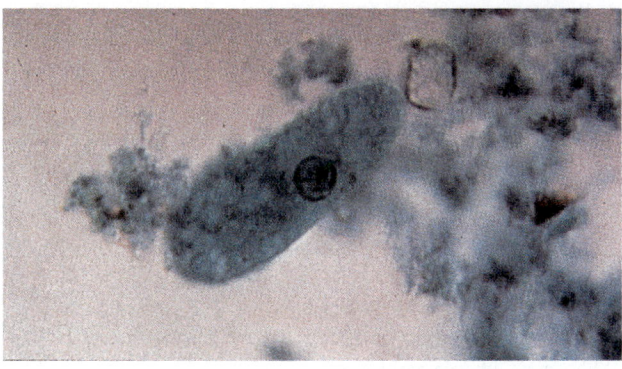

FIGURE 12-7 Intestinal protozoan *Entamoeba coli. (Courtesy of the Centers for Disease Control and Prevention, Atlanta, GA)*

THE CHAIN OF INFECTION

Infections occur when certain conditions exist. These conditions are called the chain of infection (Figure 12-8) and include:

- Causative agent (pathogens) that causes the disease
- Reservoir or source (human body in which the pathogen can live)
- Portal of exit (manner in which the pathogen leaves the body)
- Method or mode of transmission (manner in which the pathogen is carried to another person)
- Portal of entry (manner in which the pathogen enters another person)
- Susceptible host (a person who will become ill from the entry of pathogens into the body)

Pathogens cause disease by entering the body through a portal of entry. They spread disease to others by leaving the body through a portal of exit and being transmitted to another person. They enter that person's body and can again cause disease.

Pathogens enter and leave the body through body openings such as:

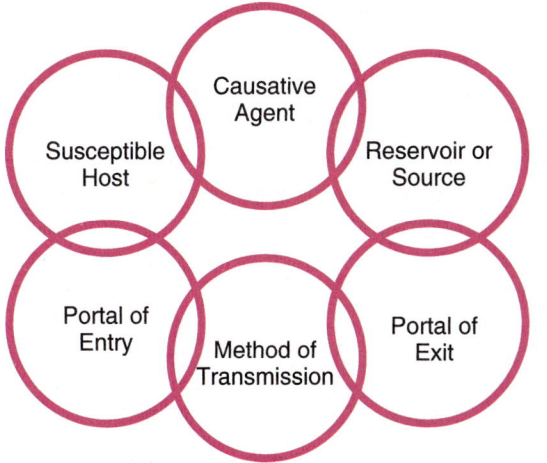

FIGURE 12-8 The chain of infection. If one link in the chain is broken, infection cannot be transmitted.

- Eyes, ears, nose, or mouth
- Breaks in the skin
- Penis, vagina, urinary meatus (bladder opening), or rectum

Causative Agent

The causative agent is the microorganism that can produce the disease process in humans. The most common biological agents of infectious disease are:

- Bacteria
- Viruses
- Fungi
- Protozoa

Reservoir

The reservoir or source is where the pathogens can survive. They may or may not multiply in the reservoir. The four most common reservoirs are:

1. Humans—active cases and carriers
2. Animals
3. Environment
4. Fomites—objects that become contaminated with infectious material that contains the microbe. Fomites are anything that comes in direct contact with the excretions or secretions of an infected person. This includes:
   - Bedpans and urinals
   - Doorknobs, faucet handles
   - Linens
   - Instruments
   - Containers with specimens for laboratory analysis

In the health care setting, the reservoirs include the:

- Patient
- Health care workers
- Environment
- Equipment

Human Reservoirs. The two major human reservoirs are cases and carriers.

- Cases—people with acute illness including obvious signs and symptoms. An example is a person with chickenpox.

- Carriers—those who have and transmit the disease organisms but do not have symptoms and do not display evidence of the disease. Chronic (sustained or intermittent) carriers can spread the disease without being recognized because the illness is not apparent. Another type of carrier is one in whom the organisms are multiplying (incubating) before signs and symptoms develop.

Specific diseases can persist in humans for an indefinite period of time, such as salmonella, hepatitis B, hepatitis C, HIV disease, and typhoid.

Portals of Entry or Exit

Portals of Entry. Organisms enter the body through the following portals of entry:

- Breaks in the skin or mucous membranes—Many organisms that are part of the normal flora, such as staphylococci, enter through breaks in the skin.
- Respiratory tract—Organisms that cause the common cold and many childhood communicable diseases (such as mumps and measles) may enter this way.
- Genitourinary tract—Organisms that cause syphilis, AIDS, gonorrhea, and other sexually transmitted diseases enter this way.
- Gastrointestinal tract—Salmonellosis, typhoid fever, and hepatitis A are examples of diseases caused by organisms that enter the digestive tract.
- Circulatory system—Malaria, yellow fever, and meningitis are diseases that can enter the body directly into the blood through the bite of insects.
- Transplacental (mother to fetus) (AIDS and hepatitis B).

Portals of Exit. Infectious organisms leave the reservoir of the host through body secretions (portals of exit), including:

- Excretions of the respiratory tract (sputum) or genital tract (semen or vaginal excretions)
- Draining wounds
- Urine
- Feces
- Blood
- Saliva
- Tears

In infected persons, these products must be considered infectious or capable of transmitting the disease agent.

Transmission of Disease

Transmission (spread) of infectious organisms may happen in one of three ways (Table 12-1):

- **Airborne transmission.** Small particles remain suspended in the air and move with air currents, or become trapped in dust, which is also carried in air

---

TABLE 12-1	**WAYS IN WHICH MICROBES ARE SPREAD FROM ONE PERSON TO OTHERS**

Airborne Transmission

- Pathogens carried by moisture or dust particles in air; can be carried long distances

Droplet Transmission

- Droplet spread within approximately 3 feet (no personal contact) or infected person by:
  - Coughing
  - Sneezing
  - Talking
  - Laughing
  - Singing

Contact Transmission

- Direct contact with infected person:
  - Touching
  - Sexual contact
  - Blood
  - Body fluids (drainage, urine, feces, sputum, saliva, vomitus)

- Indirect contact with infected person:
  - Clothing
  - Dressings
  - Equipment used in care and treatment
  - Bed linens
  - Personal belongings
  - Specimen containers
  - Instruments used in treatment
  - Food
  - Water

Note that pathogens can also be carried by insects and animals (vectors) and passed to humans.

---

currents. The patient breathes in pathogens carried in this manner.

- **Droplet transmission.** Droplets are moist particles produced by people coughing, sneezing, talking, laughing, or singing. Pathogens are transmitted into the air with the droplets. Droplets usually travel only three feet from the source.
- **Contact transmission.** Direct contact occurs with a person who is the source of the pathogens. Indirect contact occurs when a person touches an item contaminated with pathogens, such as soiled linen.

Not all organisms are transmitted in the same way, and some organisms may be transmitted in more than one way.

Host

The person who harbors infectious organisms is called a host. This person does not have enough resistance to the infectious agent. An infection develops in the host when infectious organisms:

- Penetrate the body
- Begin to multiply
- Cause damage to the host

Risk Factors. Specific characteristics about a person make him or her more or less likely to develop an infection. These characteristics are called risk factors and include:

- Number and strength of the infectious organisms
- General health of the individual
- Age, sex, and heredity of the individual
- Condition of the person's immune system

Emotional stress and fatigue also play a role in the progress of an infectious disease.

TYPES OF INFECTIONS

Infections can be:

- Local (confined to one area)—such as a boil or skin abscess
- Generalized—such as pneumonia (in the lungs)
- Systemic—widespread through the bloodstream (bacteremia)

People who have pathogens in their bodies, but do not show signs of disease, are called *carriers*. Carriers can transmit diseases to others. The pathogens in these persons' bodies are not harmful to the carriers, but they may be harmful to other people. The carrier may not know that he or she is infected.

BODY FLORA

Different microbes live on our body surfaces. These microbes are called the normal body flora. The flora are not the same in all body areas. For example, the organisms making up the flora of the intestinal tract are different from those of the respiratory tract. Healthy individuals live in harmony with the normal body flora. However, the balance may be disturbed by:

- Pathogenic organisms
- Normal flora organisms that become pathogenic
- Flora from one area that are transferred into a different body area
- Drugs such as antibiotics that upset the normal balance of organisms within a flora, allowing one group to flourish

When the organisms of one normal flora, such as those in the intestinal tract, remain within their normal environment, the body functions properly. However, when microbes from the intestines are transferred into the urinary tract, a serious urinary tract infection can result. Organisms that are nonpathogenic in their own environment may become pathogenic when they enter a different environment.

HOW PATHOGENS AFFECT THE BODY

The potential for infection depends on the risk factors listed previously. Two major factors are the susceptibility of the host and the amount of infectious agent that finds a portal of entry into the host. Even then an infection may not occur unless all elements of the chain of infection are present.

Microbes act in different ways to produce disease in the human body. Some pathogens:

- Attack and destroy the cells they invade. For example, the microscopic protozoan that causes malaria invades the red blood cells and eventually causes them to split. The person experiences chills and fever.
- Produce poisons called toxins that harm the body. For example, the tetanus organism produces toxins that travel to and damage the nervous system.
- Cause sensitivity responses called allergies. For example, the person may have a runny nose and watery eyes but no rise in temperature. This same response occurs when pollens or dust irritate the respiratory membranes.

BODY DEFENSES

The body has some natural defenses to protect it from infections. There are several natural external defenses. The most important of these is the skin. Intact skin acts as a mechanical barrier against the entry of pathogens. Other defenses include:

- Mucous membranes lining the respiratory, reproductive, gastrointestinal, and urinary tracts. The mucus is sticky and traps foreign materials before they can cause damage.
- Cilia (fine microscopic hairs) lining the respiratory tract propel the mucus and trapped microbes out of the body.
- Coughing and sneezing remove foreign materials from the respiratory tract.
- Hydrochloric acid, a strong chemical that is produced in the stomach, destroys many microbes.
- Eyes are protected by tears that provide a flushing action to remove most microbes that enter the eyes.

The body also has a number of internal defenses against infectious agents, including:

- Fever.

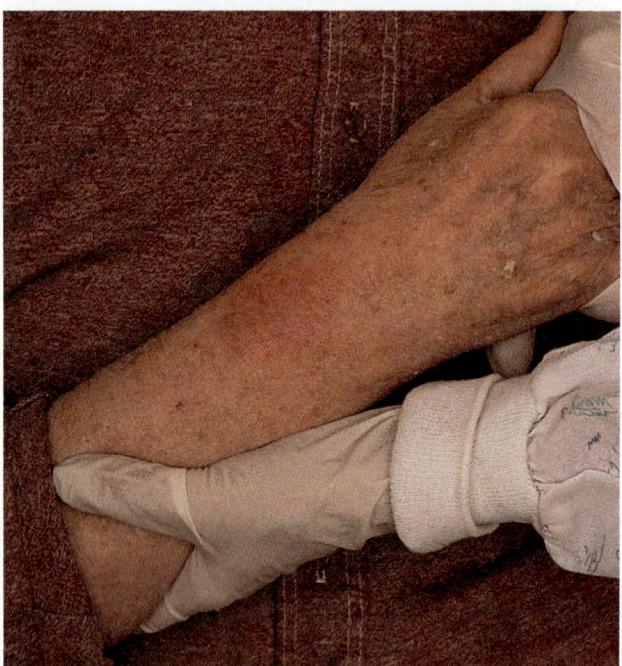

FIGURE 12-9 Redness, swelling, heat, pain, and loss of function are signs of the inflammatory process.

- Special cells in the blood called **phagocytes** that destroy microbes.
- **Inflammation**—a process that brings blood and phagocytes to the area of infection (Figure 12-9). A skin infection, for example, generally causes the skin area to become swollen, hot, and painful, signs that inflammation is occurring.
- Temperature—an elevated temperature is believed to increase the body's ability to fight infection.
- **Immune response**—the body develops protective proteins after having an infectious disease.

IMMUNITY

Immunity is the ability to fight off disease caused by microbes. A pathogenic microbe that enters the body is an **antigen**. In response to this, the blood develops substances called **antibodies**. These antibodies provide immunity (resistance) to the disease caused by that particular antigen. For example, if an individual has had antigens in the bloodstream from measles, he or she will form antibodies in the blood that prevent the occurrence of measles a second time.

IMMUNIZATIONS

Artificial defenses called **immunizations** protect against specific pathogens. Immunization is provided by **vaccines**. These are artificial or weakened antigens that help the body develop protective antibodies before the need arises. Vaccines are available to prevent most childhood diseases, such as measles, rubella (German measles), meningitis, mumps, polio, diphtheria, chickenpox, whooping cough, and tetanus. Pneumonia vaccine and influenza vaccine are frequently given to elderly people. Health workers who have direct contact with patients are advised to take hepatitis B vaccine. Federal legislation requires that employers provide this vaccine without charge to employees who are considered at risk.

Table 12-2 shows the immunizations for health care providers as recommended by the U.S. Public Health Services Advisory Committee in Immunization Practices.

IMMUNOSUPPRESSION

Immunosuppression occurs when the body's immune system is inadequate and fails to respond to the challenge of infectious disease organisms that it normally would fight successfully. The individual becomes more likely to develop a variety of infections. A number of factors can lead to this condition, including:

- Advanced age
- Frailty
- Drug therapy
- Infection with human immunodeficiency virus (HIV)
- Injury or removal of the spleen
- Radiation therapy

SERIOUS INFECTIONS IN HEALTH CARE FACILITIES

Serious bacterial and viral infections are increasing in health care facilities as well as in the general public. Ill patients, especially those who are elderly or frail, are particularly susceptible to infectious diseases, as are the very young and those with compromised (poorly functioning) immune systems.

BACTERIAL INFECTIONS

Bacteria are often the cause of serious skin, respiratory, urinary, and gastrointestinal infections in patients. If the physician suspects that a patient has a bacterial infection, a **culture and sensitivity** test may be ordered. This test can be done on urine, drainage from a wound, blood, or other body fluid. The culture tells the physician what type of microbe is causing the infection. The sensitivity tells the physician which **antibiotic** (antibacterial drug) should be used to treat the infection.

When an antibiotic is prescribed, it is important for the patient to take all the medication prescribed for the stated length of time. If the patient stops taking the antibiotic too soon, some of the microbes may remain and develop a resistance to the antibiotic.

TABLE 12-2 IMMUNIZATIONS

Vaccine Name	Primary Booster Dose Schedule	Indications	Major Precautions	Special Considerations
Hepatitis B (recombinant vaccine)	Two doses 4 weeks apart. Third dose 5 months after second dose. No booster necessary.	Health care personnel who may be exposed to blood and body fluids.	Warning: may cause shock in individuals allergic to baker's yeast.	No apparent adverse effects on developing fetuses. Not contra-indicated by pregnancy.
Influenza vaccine (inactivated whole or split virus vaccine)	Annual single dose vaccine with current virus strain	Health care personnel who have contact with high-risk residents in long-term care facilities; individuals with high-risk medical conditions.	Warning: may cause shock in individuals with allergy to eggs.	No evidence of maternal or fetal risk when given to pregnant women with underlying medical conditions that cause high risk for serious influenza complications.
Measles (live virus vaccine)	One dose immediately, second dose one month later	Health care workers born after or in 1957 without documentation of previous vaccine, physician-diagnosed measles, or laboratory evidence of immunity. Vaccine should be considered for all workers born before 1957 who have no proof of immunity.	Do not give during pregnancy; immuno-compromised state,* history of shock following gelatin ingestion or receipt of neomycin. Do not use if recent recipient of immune globulin.	MMR is the vaccine of choice if the health care worker is also susceptible to rubella and/or mumps. Persons vaccinated between 1963 and 1967, or vaccine of unknown type, should consider being revaccinated.
Mumps (live virus vaccine)	One dose, no booster	Health care workers believed to be susceptible should be vaccinated. Adults born before 1957 can be considered to be immune.	Do not use during pregnancy, immuno-compromised state,* history of shock following gelatin ingestion or receipt of neomycin.	MMR is the vaccine of choice if the health care worker is also susceptible to rubella and/or measles.
Rubella (live virus vaccine)	One dose, no booster	Health care personnel who lack documenta-tion of live vaccine on or after their first birth-day, or of laboratory evidence of immunity. Adults born before 1957 can be considered immune except women of childbearing age.	Do not use during pregnancy, immuno-compromised state,* history of shock following receipt of neomycin.	Risks to fetus if pregnant when vaccinated or women who become pregnant within 3 months of vaccination. MMR is the vaccine of choice if the health care worker is also susceptible to mumps and/or measles.
Varicella zoster (live virus vaccine)	Two doses, 4–8 weeks apart	Health care workers without reliable history of chickenpox or laboratory evidence of immunity.	Do not use during pregnancy, immuno-compromised state,* history of shock follow-ing gelatin ingestion or receipt of neomycin. Salicylate use should be avoided for 6 weeks after vaccination.	Many individuals without a history of chickenpox are immune. Serologic testing may be cost effective.

*Persons immunocompromised because of immune deficiency diseases, HIV infection (who should primarily not receive BCG, OPV, and yellow fever vaccines), leukemia, lymphoma, or generalized malignancy, or immunosuppressed as a result of therapy with corticosteroids, alkylating drugs, antimetabolites, or radiation.

Certain infectious microbes have become resistant to the antibiotics most commonly used against them. This is a serious problem in controlling infections in health care facilities. The antibiotics that are still effective often are more expensive and may have serious side effects compared to the previously preferred antibiotics. It is possible that, in time, these infectious microbes may become resistant to these newer antibiotics as well.

MRSA and VRE

Two groups of organisms have become resistant to two powerful antibiotics, methicillin and vancomycin. These organisms are:

- Methicillin-resistant *Staphylococcus aureus* (MRSA). Staphylococci are normally found on skin and mucous membranes. Figure 12-10 shows *Staphylococcus aureus* organisms. (See Appendix.)
- Vancomycin-resistant enterococci (VRE). Enterococci are found in the gastrointestinal tract. They are a major cause of hospital-acquired infections in health care facilities. Most strains are highly resistant to many antibiotics. Newer strains are resistant to vancomycin.

Other Bacterial Pathogens

Serious infections are also caused by the following types of bacteria:

- *Pseudomonas aeruginosa*—this organism is found in water and on other environmental surfaces. It causes urinary tract infections.
- *Escherichia coli*—bacterium commonly found in the intestinal tract, where it is normally nonpathogenic. Outside the intestinal tract, however, it can cause urinary tract infections or infections in pressure ulcers.
- Streptococcus A—a bacterium that produces powerful enzymes that destroy tissue and blood cells.
- Salmonella—a group of bacteria that cause mild to life-threatening intestinal infections, including "food poisoning."
- *Mycobacterium tuberculosis*—the bacterium that causes tuberculosis.

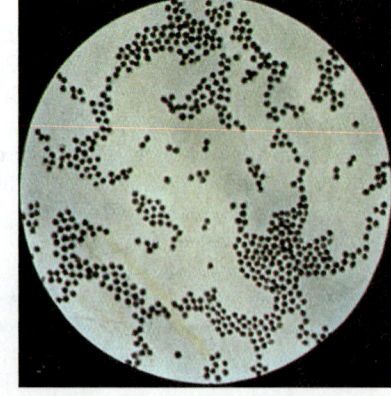

FIGURE 12-10
Methicillin-resistant *Staphylococcus aureus* (MRSA) has developed a resistance to the antibiotics of choice for treating the infection. *(Courtesy of the Centers for Disease Control and Prevention, Atlanta, GA)*

Tuberculosis

Before the development of antibiotics, tuberculosis was a widespread disease with a high fatality rate. In the 1950s, the use of antibiotics effective against tuberculosis caused the numbers of cases and deaths to drop sharply. Since 1985, the number of people infected with tuberculosis has increased, in part because new strains of *Mycobacterium tuberculosis* are resistant to several antibiotics used to treat tuberculosis. There has also been an increase in the number of people who are at risk for infection, including those who:

- Are HIV positive
- Are infected but fail to take their medication for the full treatment period
- Live in poverty and are malnourished
- Have immigrated to the United States from countries where tuberculosis is still common
- Have inactive tuberculosis and have grown older and experience increased disability

Tuberculosis Infection. Tuberculosis infection occurs when the bacterium that causes the disease enters the body. The lungs are the most common site of infection. The body usually responds to the infection by creating a barrier that prevents the spread of pathogens to other parts of the body. This barrier is called a tubercle. As long as the tubercle remains intact and no other tuberculosis bacteria enter the body, the infection is called inactive or controlled. In this state the person is not contagious (capable of passing the infection to others). If the person is immunocompromised, the tubercle may not form and the person develops active tuberculosis disease.

Tuberculosis Disease. Tuberculosis disease develops if the tubercle breaks down or more tuberculosis bacteria enter the body. The bacteria multiply, tissue damage increases, and the bacteria may spread to other parts of the body. As the disease progresses, the person will show one or more of the following signs and symptoms:

- Fatigue
- Loss of appetite and weight
- Weakness
- Elevated temperature in the afternoon and evening
- Night sweats
- Spitting up blood (hemoptysis)
- Coughing

The person with tuberculosis in the lungs can spread it to others through droplets in respiratory secretions.

Diagnosis. The presence of tuberculosis bacterium in the body can be shown by:

- A sputum culture—grows the organisms from a specimen of secretions from the person's lungs
- Chest x-rays—show the extent of the disease process in the lungs
- A positive skin test (Mantoux test)—shows the presence of antibodies to the tuberculosis organisms in the body (Figure 12-11)

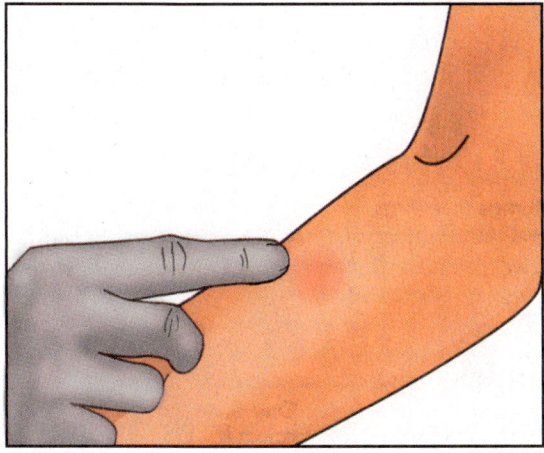

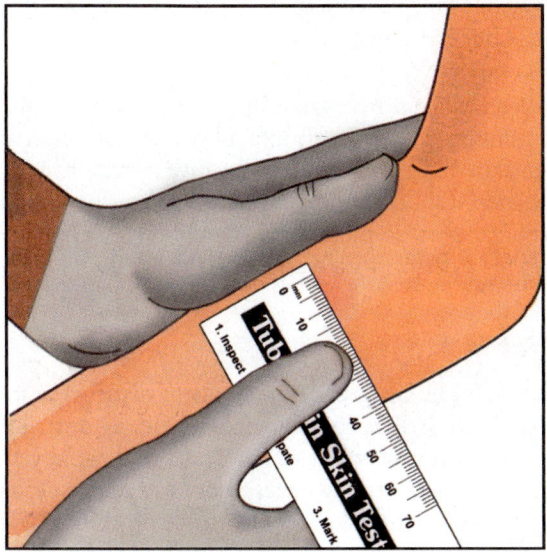

FIGURE 12-11 A positive Mantoux test shows redness and induration (swelling) 48 to 72 hours after the test.

Health care providers in long-term care must undergo a skin test for tuberculosis before employment.

Treatment. A person with tuberculosis is treated with a selected antibiotic or combination of antibiotics. Because many disease organisms have become resistant to specific drugs, a combination of drugs must be used to control them. Once antitubercular drug therapy starts, the patient usually becomes noncontagious (cannot spread the disease organism) within two to three weeks. The therapy, however, continues for six months to two years.

Escherichia coli O157:H7

You have learned that *Escherichia coli* (*E. coli*) can cause serious problems outside the intestinal tract. Another strain, *E. coli O157:H7*, has caused outbreaks resulting in serious illness and death. This form of the bacterium is found in the intestines of some cattle. A small amount of these bacteria can contaminate a large amount of meat,

particularly ground beef. It is transmitted in contaminated and undercooked meat, produce that has been rinsed in water contaminated with feces, or by a person who has been handling contaminated food. It has been found on cutting boards and utensils. The bacteria have been found in unpasteurized milk and apple juice, as well as pools and lakes contaminated with fecal matter. The best way to prevent its spread is to use good handwashing and food preparation practices. Ground beef (hamburger) should be cooked until it is well done in the center. The high temperature required to cook meat to well done will kill the pathogen.

Signs and Symptoms. When *E. coli O157:H7* enters the human intestinal tract (for example, when a person eats contaminated food), the bacterium multiplies rapidly, producing large amounts of toxins. One to two days later, the person develops watery diarrhea, nausea, vomiting, and cramping. In another day or two, the diarrhea becomes bloody. The abdomen becomes **distended** (enlarged) and very tender. The patient may show signs of dehydration, swelling, and **petechiae**, small purplish spots on the body surface, caused by minute hemorrhages. The diarrhea may subside in five to seven days, but the condition injures the mucous membranes, allowing the pathogen to escape into the bloodstream. This creates a situation in which blood flow to the brain, kidneys, and other organs is endangered. The patient develops signs and symptoms of serious illness, such as:

- Decreased urine output that may progress to complete renal failure
- Mental confusion
- **Seizures** (convulsions)
- Muscle weakness
- Pain and numbness of the feet and legs

Treatment. In some conditions, the risk of transmitting infection is highest before the diagnosis is made. Because of this, many facilities place patients in contact precautions (see Unit 13) until the condition is diagnosed. Diapered and incontinent patients remain in contact precautions for the duration of illness. Standard precautions (see Unit 13) may safely be used for other patients.

E. coli O157:H7 can be deadly, particularly to infants, children, and others with conditions that weaken the immune system. Care for this condition is supportive, and the patient requires careful monitoring. Unfortunately, many drugs increase the risk of kidney damage. Water intake is very important, but liquid intake will require very close observation because of the potential for kidney damage. Careful monitoring of the patient's vital signs is required.

Pseudomembranous Colitis

Many bacteria live in the bowel of a healthy person. Most of them are harmless, and some friendly bacteria help with digestion. A few of these have the potential to be troublemakers if they get out of control. Most of the time, the bad bacteria are outnumbered by the good bacteria, and no harm comes to the person. Taking antibiotics can upset the balance in the colon. Many people develop a brief bout of diarrhea because the balance is upset, but the condition resolves quickly on its own.

Pseudomembranous colitis is a very serious condition in which diarrhea is caused by a bacterium called *Clostridium difficile* (*C. difficile*). It is often called by its nickname, "C. Diff." This condition develops in patients who have been on antibiotic therapy. The friendly (good) bacteria die as a result of the antibiotic, and the harmful (bad) bacteria grow out of control. Pseudomembranous colitis occurs because the antibiotics destroy the normal bowel flora except for *C. difficile*, which is particularly resistant. Without the other friendly bacteria to keep it in check, it breeds rapidly, producing toxins that cause serious illness.

C. difficile is very common in health care facilities. It is picked up on the hands, on bedpans, bedside commodes, toilets, sinks, countertops, bed rails, doorknobs, and other surfaces that have been contaminated by stool. It most commonly enters the body through the mouth by contact with unwashed hands.

Signs and Symptoms. Pseudomembranous colitis may occur several weeks or months after a course of antibiotic therapy is completed, so it can be difficult to diagnose. *C. difficile* produces a toxin that affects the lining of the intestine, causing inflammation. This results in sudden, severe, foul-smelling, watery diarrhea. Stopping the antibiotic will not stop the diarrhea. The diarrhea may be so frequent and severe that the patient becomes dehydrated rapidly and develops other serious imbalances within the body. Other signs and symptoms are:

- Cramping and pain in the lower abdomen; sometimes this begins several days before the diarrhea starts
- Fever
- Mucus, pus, or blood in the stool
- Abdomen very tender to touch
- In severe cases, low blood pressure and signs of shock

If the condition is not promptly treated, it can cause ruptured bowel and a condition in which the bowel becomes severely distended and retains stool.

Diagnosis and Treatment. If pseudomembranous colitis is suspected, the doctor will order laboratory analysis on one or more stool cultures. The laboratory will identify the bacteria that are causing the illness. The antibiotic suspected of causing the problem is stopped, if possible. Another antimicrobial drug is used to eliminate the harmful bacteria in the colon. The patient may be given yogurt to eat and several other medications to increase the balance of healthy flora in the bowel. Although drug therapy usually eliminates the condition, it sometimes recurs, making a second course of therapy necessary. The patient is placed in contact precautions (see Unit 13) until 72 hours after the appearance and frequency of stools return to normal, or as ordered by the physician. Use good handwashing with antibacterial soap and water. *Do not use alcohol-based hand cleaners. This disease is spread by spores, and alcohol will not eliminate them.* The friction and running water will remove them from your hands during handwashing.

VIRAL INFECTIONS

Several viral infections are listed in this section. One additional viral infection, genital herpes, is described in Unit 45.

Shingles

Shingles (herpes zoster) occurs in people who were infected by the virus that causes chickenpox. Although the person recovered from chickenpox, the organisms did not leave the body. They remained in the body's nervous system in a nonactive state.

Years later, when the person is in a weakened condition, the organisms become active. Painful blister-like lesions develop in the skin along the paths of sensitive nerves. Eventually the lesions heal on their own. However, they contain infectious organisms, so precautions should be used by anyone caring for a person with shingles.

Influenza

Influenza (or flu) is caused by a family of viruses. The infection can have serious consequences for elderly or frail people. Each year new types of viruses spread rapidly from person to person by way of respiratory secretions, causing many to become ill. Vaccines offer some protection against influenza viruses and are often given to residents in long-term care.

Someone with the flu may experience:

- Malaise (general unwell feeling)
- Chills
- Fever
- Muscle aches and pains
- Coldlike symptoms

In addition to making the person feel ill, the viruses may lower the patient's resistance to other infectious organisms. These other organisms can cause pneumonia and other life-threatening infections. Medicines may be given to limit the effects of the viruses and antibiotics are given to combat bacterial infections that may develop.

You can help protect the patients in your care by:

- Staying healthy
- Not reporting for duty when you are ill
- Carrying out standard precautions faithfully
- Following the facility's policies regarding special precautions when a patient has a respiratory infection
- Encouraging the patient to drink fluids
- Reporting to the charge nurse when a visitor seems to be ill

Hepatitis

Hepatitis is an inflammation of the liver caused by several viruses, including:

- Hepatitis A virus
- Hepatitis B virus
- Hepatitis C virus
- Hepatitis D virus
- Hepatitis E virus
- Hepatitis G virus

Characteristics of these viruses are:

- Hepatitis A virus (HAV)
  - Most common
  - Transmitted by feces, saliva, and contaminated food
  - Vaccine available
  - Rarely fatal
  - Treated with bedrest and avoidance of alcoholic beverages
- Hepatitis B virus (HBV)
  - Can cause liver cancer and death
  - Transmitted by blood, sexual secretions, feces, and saliva
  - Signs and symptoms may mimic the flu; they include fever, aches and pains, nausea, fatigue, and urine that may turn a dark color
  - Infectious for life, even after the patient recovers from acute illness
  - Some patients have no symptoms at all but are still infectious
  - Vaccine available for protection
- Hepatitis C virus (HCV)
  - 50% of people infected develop chronic hepatitis
  - Transmitted mainly through blood and blood products
  - May be mistaken for the flu
  - Common signs and symptoms are extreme fatigue, depression, fever, mood changes, weakness, pain, loss of appetite
  - May cause liver cancer and liver failure
  - Disease may be present for years before patient becomes aware of it; during this time it silently destroys the liver
  - Leading cause of need for liver transplants in the United States
  - Treated with alpha interferon; treatment is not always successful

Any infection of the liver is serious because the liver is a vital organ. Health care workers must take hepatitis very seriously because many individuals have no signs and symptoms of illness, yet are able to transmit the infection to others. You can best protect yourself by:

- Using standard precautions (discussed in Unit 13)
- Taking the vaccine, if available
- Practicing safe sex (using condoms)
- Not using illegal drugs
- Giving your full attention to the handling of sharps, such as needles or razors

Acquired Immune Deficiency Syndrome (AIDS)

Acquired immune deficiency syndrome (**AIDS**) is a viral disease. It is transmitted primarily through direct contact with the bodily secretions of an infected person. The virus that causes AIDS is the **human immunodeficiency virus** (**HIV**).

The ways in which HIV is transmitted include:

- Blood to blood through:
  - Transfusion of infected blood. Note that federal regulations prohibit the use of untested and unregulated blood in the United States.
  - Treatment of hemophilia with clotting factor from infected blood
  - Needle sharing among drug users
  - Prick from a contaminated needle or sharp
  - Unsterile instruments used for procedures such as ear piercing or tattooing
- Unprotected vaginal, oral, or anal intercourse when one partner is infected

INFECTION CONTROL *Alert*

Hepatitis B is much more contagious than HIV. Imagine that a quarter-teaspoon of hepatitis B virus is mixed into a 24,000-gallon swimming pool full of water. Someone draws a quarter-teaspoon of that water into a syringe and injects you with it. Despite the amount of dilution, everyone who receives such an injection will become HBV positive. By comparison, imagine that 10 people are in the room. Someone takes a quarter-teaspoon of HIV and mixes it into one quart of water. A quarter teaspoon of that water is then injected into each person in the room. Statistically, only one person in the room will become HIV positive. Hepatitis B, then, is a much greater threat to health care workers than HIV. Proper use of standard precautions (see Unit 13) will prevent the spread of both infections. Because a vaccine is available to protect workers from hepatitis B, the threat can be eliminated completely.

- Infected mother to infant during:
  - Pregnancy
  - Birth process
  - Nursing

The AIDS Virus. The AIDS virus (HIV):

- Has many variants
- Does not live for long outside the body
- Is affected by common chemicals such as bleach
- Depresses the body's immune system
- Makes the infected person more susceptible to infections
- Makes the infected person more likely to experience complications such as:
  - *Pneumocystis carinii* pneumonia—a serious lung infection
  - Kaposi's sarcoma—a serious malignancy affecting many body organs
  - Brain involvement leading to dementia
  - Eye involvement leading to blindness
  - Tuberculosis
  - Other opportunistic infections

Incubation Period. Not everyone who comes in contact with the HIV virus becomes infected. For those who are infected, there is always a period of time between contact and the start of the signs and symptoms of the infection.

- During this period the virus is in infected cells but is not active. The body does not make antibodies to the virus.
- Most people become **seropositive** or HIV positive (show antibodies to HIV in the bloodstream) approximately three to six months after infection. The person has HIV disease, which may progress to AIDS.
- The asymptomatic period (when no signs and symptoms are present) following infection may last months to years. AIDS does not always develop, but the person is an HIV carrier for life.

Disease Progression. Progression of the disease process is determined by the effect of the viruses on special protective white blood cells known as CD4 cells (T cells). Over time, the number of these protective white blood cells drops. As a result, the immune system of the infected person becomes more suppressed (weaker) and less able to fight infection. When the number of CD4 cells drops to a critical level (below 200 cells/mm^3), the person is diagnosed with AIDS.

Symptoms of HIV infection, when they do appear, consist of:

- Acute flulike symptoms
- Fever
- Night sweats
- Fatigue
- Swollen lymph nodes
- Sore throat
- Gastrointestinal problems
- Headache

One-fourth to one-half of people exposed to HIV show evidence of disease within 5 to 10 years of antibody development (becoming seropositive).

Testing. Several tests have been developed to confirm the presence of antibodies to HIV (positive for HIV infection), to test the level of viral activity, and to confirm the presence of AIDS.

The test for antibodies is also used to check the national blood supply. When people donate blood, it is tested to be sure that it is free of HIV antibodies, to protect the people who receive blood transfusions and other blood products.

Treatment. No specific treatment is able to cure AIDS at the present time. A combination of drugs currently in use reduces both the symptoms and viral activity.

- No vaccine prevents the infection from developing. However, millions of dollars are being spent on research to develop a vaccine.
- Therapy is directed toward vigorously treating each infection as it appears.
- Nutritional and other forms of preventive therapy are aimed at maintaining a person with AIDS in the best health possible.
- The drug industry continues to develop drugs that slow down the disease process or reinforce the immune system. Patients treated with combinations of drugs show decreased viral loads and improved CD4 counts. Every dose must be taken properly. When patients fail to follow the protocol exactly, the disease state returns quickly and more strongly than before. These drugs, however, do not cure the disease.
- At present there is no evidence that AIDS is transmitted:
  - Through kissing, touching, or hugging an HIV-infected person
  - By eating at the same table with an infected person
  - By using the same toilet seat
  - Through insect bites

Hantavirus

In May 1993, a cluster of unexplained deaths occurred among young Native Americans in the southwestern United States. An investigation revealed a new virus that was previously unknown. This situation attracted a great deal of media attention. Several additional outbreaks have been reported since 1993. This strange disease is called **hantavirus**. It is spread by contact with rodents (rats and mice) or their excretions, including urine and stool. Once disturbed, viral particles in the excretions become airborne and are inhaled by the susceptible host. Signs and symptoms appear one to five weeks later and include high fever, chills, muscle aches, cough, nausea, vomiting, diarrhea, dizziness, and feeling very tired. As the disease progresses,

guidelines *for*

Preventing Infections

- Assist patients to maintain adequate fluid intake. This helps prevent urinary tract and respiratory tract infections and keeps the skin healthier.
- Assist patients to maintain adequate nutritional intake. Report to the nurse when patients eat less or refuse food.
- Assist patients to carry out exercise programs established by the nurse or physical therapist. Follow positioning schedules and orders for range-of-motion exercises and ambulation. Exercise improves breathing and circulation.
- Toilet patients who need assistance. This keeps the bladder empty and also assures patients that they will receive help when they need to urinate.
- When cleaning the perineal area of patients, be sure to wipe women from front to back. This prevents contaminating the urethra (bladder opening) with stool or vaginal excretions.
- Perform catheter care as directed. Avoid opening the drainage system.
- Observe patients carefully and report any unusual signs or changes, such as:
  - Changes in frequency of urination or amount of urine voided
  - Complaints of pain or burning on urination
  - Changes in character of urine
  - Coughing or respiratory problems
  - Confusion or disorientation that was not present before or that has increased
  - Drainage or discharge from any body opening or skin wound
  - Changes in skin color
  - Complaints of pain, discomfort, or nausea
  - Elevated temperature
  - Red, swollen areas on body
- Keep patients clean.
- Staff members who have an infectious disease should not be on duty. Caring for your own health is vital in preventing illness in patients. Friends and family of patients should be advised not to visit when they do not feel well. If you notice a visitor coughing and sneezing, or otherwise obviously sick, inform your supervisor.
- Follow your facility policies and procedure for prevention of infection and injury. If you identify health risks, take the proper precautions. It is your responsibility to learn and follow these practices. Cooperate with your infection control nurse or department during audits, education, investigation of outbreaks and exposure, and review of infection control practices. Sometimes recommendations to prevent infection change. It is your responsibility to learn new techniques and make changes in the way you practice.

the patient becomes very short of breath. When this occurs, the disease progresses rapidly, and the patient becomes seriously ill. Respiratory support may be necessary. Hantavirus is not transmitted from person to person. Spread of this condition can be reduced by taking steps to prevent rodents from entering the home or eliminating them if they are present.

OTHER IMPORTANT INFECTIONS

Infection Caused by Fungi

Coccidioidomycosis (valley fever) is caused by *Coccidioides immitis*. It occurs primarily as a respiratory infection. It is treated with antibiotics and is seldom fatal in otherwise healthy people. In people with immunosuppression, however, the death rate is high. It is treated with antibiotics.

Infection Caused by Protozoa

Two diseases caused by protozoa are becoming more common in the general public and in health facilities. Giardiasis is caused by *Giardia lamblia*, which is found in the water supplies of many communities. It causes severe diarrhea but responds to medication. Cryptosporidiosis is caused by the *Cryptosporidium* protozoan, which is found in the digestive tracts of domestic animals and is transferred by contact. It causes severe diarrhea, especially in immunosuppressed people. There is no specific treatment.

BIOTERRORISM

Bioterrorism is the use of biological agents, such as pathogenic organisms or agricultural pests, for terrorist purposes. Since October 2001, state, local, and governmental public health authorities have been investigating cases of bioterrorism-related illness. Specifically, some individuals died from inhalation anthrax, a condition that was spread by a powdery substance containing anthrax spores that was sent through the mail. A number of other individuals developed the cutaneous (skin) version of this disease. Cutaneous anthrax is not fatal. Anthrax cannot be passed from one person to the next. It is transmitted only through contact with spores. Fortunately, the number of workplaces and individuals contaminated was small, but it raised concerns regarding future terrorist attacks. Many individuals could be infected by a biological weapon before the exposure is detected and diagnosed. Some of the diseases that can potentially be used as biological weapons have been considered eradicated for years, and today's health care professionals have never seen or treated them. Thus, bioterrorism is a significant threat.

Many health care facilities have developed disaster plans to address bioterrorism. The plans outline the steps necessary for responding to bioterrorism with the most common agents, including smallpox, botulism toxin, anthrax, and plague. The disaster plan includes information for patients, employees, and visitors, and specifies public health precautions and protocols to follow in the event of an emergency. Sadly, given the state of world affairs, health care facilities must be prepared for potential terrorist actions in the future.

Smallpox

Smallpox is a serious viral infection that is sometimes fatal. The disease emerged thousands of years ago, but was eliminated during the twentieth century. Unfortunately, laboratory stockpiles of the virus that causes smallpox still exist, and there is concern that these samples might be used for terrorist purposes.

Mode of Transmission. Smallpox is caused by the variola virus. It usually spreads through direct face-to-face contact with an infected person. It may also be spread by:

- Direct contact with infected bodily fluids
- Direct contact with contaminated objects, such as linen or clothing
- The air in buildings, buses, and trains, although this is less common

The virus does not live long in the air, and 90% of the virus dies within 24 hours after airborne release. Ultraviolet light eliminates even more of the virus.

Signs and Symptoms. After exposure to the smallpox virus, the newly infected person goes through a 7- to 17-day incubation period in which there are no symptoms of illness. The first symptoms of smallpox include:

- High fever ranging from 101°F to 104°F
- Feeling very tired
- Headache
- Body aches
- Vomiting

Infected persons are usually too sick to carry on their normal activities. This phase lasts for about two to four days.

A rash emerges about four days after the onset of fever. At first, small red spots appear in the mouth and on the tongue. The spots become sores that break open, spreading large amounts of virus into the mouth and throat. The patient is extremely contagious during this time. A rash also develops on the skin, beginning on the face and spreading to the arms, legs, hands, and feet. Within 24 hours, the rash spreads to all parts of the body. When the rash appears, the fever drops and the person begins to feel better.

By the third day of the rash, raised bumps appear. By day four, the bumps fill with a thick, cloudy fluid. The bumps develop a depression in the center. Their appearance has been compared to the appearance of a navel, and is a distinguishing feature of smallpox. During this time, the patient's fever rises again and remains high until scabs develop. The bumps become round and firm to the touch; they may feel like pellets from a BB gun. After approximately five days, the bumps develop scabs. The scabs fall off, leaving scars on the skin. This occurs about three weeks after the rash appears. The person is contagious until the last scab falls off.

Vaccination. A vaccine is available to prevent smallpox, but it has not been routinely given since the 1970s, when the disease was eradicated worldwide. Presently, there is no treatment for smallpox, although this is an area of current research. Receiving the vaccine within three days of exposure will completely prevent or significantly reduce the severity of the illness. Vaccination four to seven days after exposure likely offers some protection from disease or may modify the severity of disease.

In 2002, the United States began recommending that hospitals immunize certain key personnel against smallpox. In case of an outbreak, these individuals would be able to care for patients without contracting the disease. Not everyone can receive the vaccine. For example, health care workers who are HIV positive, pregnant, or have had certain skin and other health conditions should not receive the vaccine.

The smallpox vaccine contains a weakened live virus that stimulates the body into developing immunity. A normal reaction to the vaccine is to develop a blister, which fills with pus, drains, then crusts over. The crust falls off, leaving a scar. Because the vaccine contains a live virus, the injection site must be kept covered.

An individual who has just been immunized can work, but may be under work restrictions for some time after the smallpox immunization. Personnel who have been immunized should not care for newborn infants or patients who are immunocompromised for at least three weeks. The virus is not transmitted in the air, but can be spread by contact with the injection site and dressings or clothing covering the area.

If your facility offers the smallpox vaccine, become familiar with the actions, use, conditions in which the vaccine is not given, and potential side effects and risks. The vaccine provides high-level immunity for three to five years, but then immunity progressively decreases. Individuals who were immunized previously may have longer immunity.

OUTBREAK OF INFECTIOUS DISEASE IN A HEALTH CARE FACILITY

An outbreak of an infection in the facility can be serious for all patients. Unless steps are taken immediately, the infection can spread rapidly. Examples of outbreaks include:

- Influenza
- Gastroenteritis
- Hepatitis
- MRSA
- Scabies (parasites that invade the skin)

Most facilities have an action plan for responding to an outbreak of infection. Nursing assistants will receive instructions from the nurse.

SELF-CARE

You can take steps to stay healthy and free from infections:

- Eat a healthy diet
- Get enough sleep each day
- Keep your body clean
- Live in a clean environment
- Avoid unhealthy habits such as smoking and substance abuse
- Learn how to cope with stress

REVIEW

A. Matching.

Match Column I with Column II.

Column I

1. _____ spiral-shaped bacterium
2. _____ organism that causes ringworm
3. _____ bacteria that grow in pairs
4. _____ organism that causes AIDS
5. _____ bacteria that grow as clusters

Column II

a. staphylococci
b. protozoan
c. diplococci
d. streptococci
e. virus
f. fungus
g. spirillum

B. Word Choice.

Fill in the blanks with the correct word or phrase from the following list.

insects
method of transmission
portal of entry
portal of exit
reservoir
sexual contact
sneezing
susceptible host
water

6. Complete the chain of infection by naming the parts missing from the following figure.

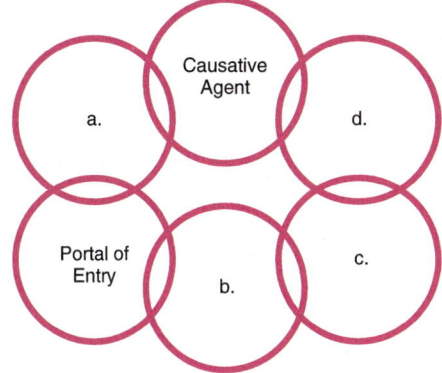

a. _____   c. _____
b. _____   d. _____

7. An example of transmission by direct contact is _____.

8. An example of transmission by indirect contact is _____.

9. A common vehicle for the transmission of microbes is _____.

10. Vectors, such as animals and _____, also transmit disease organisms.

C. True/False.

Mark the following true or false by circling T or F.

11. T F Normal body flora are the same in each part of the body.

12. T F The rectum is a common portal of exit for some infectious organisms.

13. T F The general health of an individual is an important factor in determining if infectious disease will occur.

14. T F Unbroken skin is a mechanical defense against infection.

15. T F A boil is an example of a generalized infection.

16. T F Allergies are known as sensitivity reactions.

17. T F The term *reservoir* may refer to a human body in which the organisms live.

18. T F An immunizing vaccine causes the body to produce antibodies that protect the person against certain infectious diseases.

19. T F MRSA infections are easy to control.

20. T F Bedpans and urinals can act as fomites.

D. Multiple Choice.

Select the one best answer for each of the following.

21. White blood cells that multiply and attempt to destroy pathogens are
   a. antigens.
   b. phagocytes.
   c. antibodies.
   d. red blood cells.

22. Which of the following is not a natural body defense?
   a. Antibiotic
   b. Hydrochloric acid in the stomach
   c. Hair in the nose
   d. Tears

23. Which is an example of a local infection?
   a. Pneumonia
   b. Septicemia
   c. Boil
   d. AIDS

24. One patient's visitor is coughing and looks flushed. Your best action is to
   a. ask the visitor to leave.
   b. put a mask on the visitor.
   c. put a mask on the patient.
   d. refer the matter to the nurse.

25. You woke up not feeling well this morning. You have an elevated temperature. Your best action is to
   a. call in sick.
   b. go to work.
   c. stay home without notifying the facility.
   d. call a friend to go to work for you.

26. Infection with *Escherichia coli O157:H7*
   a. is mildly uncomfortable.
   b. can cause renal failure and death.
   c. is caused by inhaling spores.
   d. is highly infectious to health care workers.

27. Hantavirus is spread by
   a. rodent excretions.
   b. indirect contact with fomites.
   c. contact with an infected person.
   d. inhalation of droplets from an infected patient.

28. Bioterrorism is
   a. not a concern in the United States.
   b. the use of chemicals to cause illness.
   c. the use of biological agents for terrorist purposes.
   d. easily detected and treated.

29. Hepatitis B
   a. is spread by oral–fecal transmission.
   b. can be readily cured with antibiotics.
   c. causes visible signs of serious illness.
   d. can be prevented by vaccination.

E. Nursing Assistant Challenge.

30. Your patient, Mrs. Wallace, has a cold.
   a. What organism is responsible? _____
   b. Could Mrs. Wallace be immunized against this condition? _____
   c. How is the condition most likely transmitted?
   _____

31. Mr. Reynolds has a staphylococcal infection in his finger.
   a. What class of organisms are staphylococci?
   _____
   b. What shape are these organisms? _____
   c. How might Mr. Reynolds have acquired this infection? _____

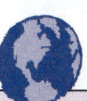 # EXPLORING THE WEB

Description	Location
Categories of Acquired Immunity	*http://www.wisc-online.com*
Infection Control/Asepsis	*http://www.delmarhealthcare.com/olcs/white/pnotes.asp* (see Chapter 21)
Recommendations for Immunization of Health Care Workers	*http://www.cdc.gov/epo/mmwr/preview/mmwrhtml/ 00050577.htm*
Bad Bug Book	*http://vm.cfsan.fda.gov/~mow/intro.html*
Centers for Disease Control and Prevention (CDC)	*http://www.cdc.gov*
Infectious Diseases Syllabi	*http://www.kcom.edu*
National Foundation on Infectious Diseases	*http://www.nfid.org*
National Institutes of Health (NIH)	*http://health.nih.gov*
100% Immunization Campaign	*http://www.immunizeseniors.org*
A Primer on Bioterrorism	*http://www.advancefornurses.com* (see past articles Oct. 29, 2001)
Supercourse	*http://www.pitt.edu*

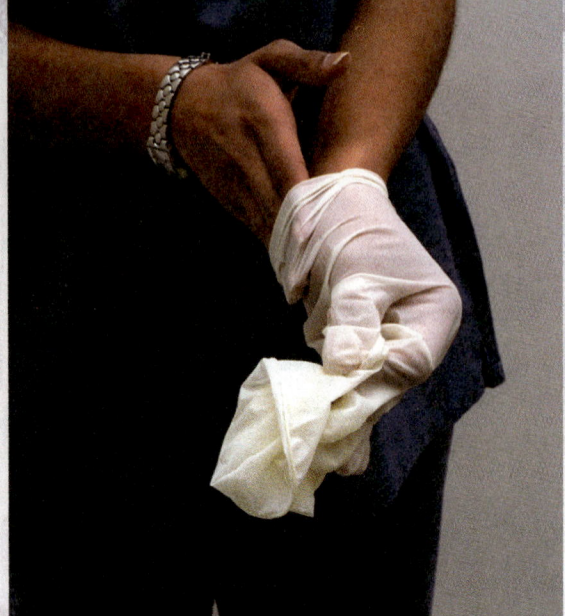

Infection Control

objectives

After completing this unit, you will be able to:

- Define and spell all vocabulary words and terms.
- Explain the principles of medical asepsis.
- Explain the components of standard precautions.
- List the types of personal protective equipment.
- Describe nursing assistant actions related to standard precautions.
- Describe airborne precautions.
- Describe droplet precautions.
- Describe contact precautions.
- Demonstrate the following:
  - Procedure 1 Handwashing
  - Procedure 2 Putting on a Mask
  - Procedure 3 Putting on a Gown
  - Procedure 4 Putting on Gloves

- Procedure 5 Removing Contaminated Gloves
- Procedure 6 Removing Contaminated Gloves, Mask, and Gown
- Procedure 7 Serving a Meal in an Isolation Unit
- Procedure 8 Measuring Vital Signs in an Isolation Unit
- Procedure 9 Transferring Nondisposable Equipment Outside of Isolation Unit
- Procedure 10 Specimen Collection from Patient in an Isolation Unit
- Procedure 11 Caring for Linens in an Isolation Unit
- Procedure 12 Transporting Patient to and from Isolation Unit
- Procedure 13 Opening a Sterile Package

vocabulary

Learn the meaning and the correct spelling of the following words and phrases:

airborne precautions	disinfection	medical asepsis	potentially infectious
airborne transmission	droplet precautions	N95 respirator	material
asepsis	droplet transmission	National Institute of	sharps
autoclave	exposure incident	Occupational Safety	standard precautions
biohazard	face shield	and Health	sterile
communicable disease	goggles	(NIOSH)	sterile field
contact precautions	high-efficiency	nosocomial infection	sterilization
contact transmission	particulate air	occupational exposure	surgical mask
contagious disease	(HEPA) filter mask	personal protective	transmission-based
contaminated	isolation	equipment (PPE)	precautions
dirty	isolation technique	PFR95 respirator	work practice controls
disposable	isolation unit		

DISEASE PREVENTION

In the last unit you learned what infections are and some of their causes. In this unit, you will be introduced to actions and procedures that can help prevent the transmission (spread) of infection to protect yourself, your coworkers, and those in your care.

MEDICAL ASEPSIS

Asepsis is defined as the absence of disease-producing microorganisms. Two ways of achieving asepsis are by medical aseptic technique and surgical aseptic technique. **Medical asepsis** refers to medical practices that reduce the numbers of microorganisms or interrupt transmission from

guidelines *for*

Maintaining Medical Asepsis

To maintain medical asepsis, the nursing assistant should follow these guidelines:

- Wash hands thoroughly and at appropriate times. Protect the skin on the hands by using warm water, drying thoroughly, then applying lotion if needed.

- Treat breaks in the skin immediately by washing thoroughly, cleaning with an antiseptic, and covering. Report any breaks in the skin to your supervisor.

- Use gloves when required.

- Bathe or shower daily. Daily changes of clothing are necessary. Keep your hair clean and away from your face and shoulders. Avoid artificial nails. Keep fingernails short and clean. Do not wear rings, other than a plain wedding band.

- Assist patients with their personal hygiene.

- *Never* use one patient's items for another patient.

- Keep patient personal care items in the proper areas.

  In the top two drawers of the patient's bedside stand, place:

  - toothbrush and toothpaste

  - comb and hairbrush

  - denture cup if patient wears dentures

  Items such as a toothbrush, denture cup, wash basin, and emesis basin should always be placed on a different shelf from items such as a bedpan and a urinal.

  In the second drawer or on the shelf of the bedside stand, or in the bathroom, place:

  - emesis basin

  - wash basin

  - soap and soap dish

  Store on the lower shelf:

  - bedpan

  - urinal for male patients

- Disinfect bathtubs and shower chairs after each use according to facility policy.

- Disinfect equipment that is used by more than one health care provider or patient, such as a stethoscope, before and after each use.

- Disinfect personal care equipment, such as bedpans, urinals, and commodes, according to facility policy.

- Be careful when handling bedpans and urinals after use to prevent spills and splashes. Use a cover when transporting.

- Avoid contaminating environmental surfaces when wearing used gloves.

- Use the overbed table only for clean items, such as food trays, water pitcher, and clean supplies.

- The water pitcher should always be covered at the bedside.

- Keep food and water supplies clean. Food trays are to remain covered until they reach their destination. Remove food dishes immediately after use. Do not place used trays on a cart until all clean trays have been delivered to patients.

- Do not allow patients to keep puddings or custards from meal trays. Bacteria multiply rapidly in these foods when they are not refrigerated.

- Carry soiled equipment, supplies, and linens away from your uniform so that you do not spread microorganisms from patient to patient. Dispose of items according to facility policy.

- Do not use anything that has touched the floor without recleaning or sterilizing it first. If you are in doubt about whether an item is clean, do not use it. Any personal items that touch the floor should be disinfected before use. The floor is heavily contaminated with pathogens.

- Avoid raising dust.

continues

guidelines *continued*

- Do not shake linens. This scatters contaminated dust and lint. Gather or fold linens inward with the dirtiest area toward the center. Keep soiled linen hampers covered. Keep linens (even if soiled) off the floor.
- The soiled linen hamper and housekeeping cart must be separated from the clean linen cart and food cart by at least one room's width.
- Clean from least soiled areas toward the most soiled.
- Keep work areas such as utility rooms clean. Return clean equipment to the proper storage areas after use.

one person to another person or from person to place or object. These practices are often referred to as *medical aseptic technique (clean technique)*.

You will hear the terms *clean* and *dirty* applied to equipment and supplies used in the facility. For example, the linen you take from the linen cart is "clean." After it is carried into the patient's room, it is considered "dirty." If it is not used, it cannot be returned to the clean linen cart; it must be placed in the laundry hamper. Once linen is in the patient's room, it is exposed to the patient's pathogens. To prevent the spread of these pathogens to other patients, the linen must be laundered. Keeping each patient's equipment and supplies separate from those for other patients is part of medical aseptic technique. Articles that have come into contact with known pathogens or have been exposed to potential pathogens are called **dirty** or **contaminated**. Articles that are free of pathogens are considered clean or uncontaminated.

It is not possible to eliminate all microorganisms from our bodies or the environment. However, microbes can be reduced by always using the essential practices of medical aseptic technique:

- Handwashing
- Using nonsterile gloves when contact with blood, moist body fluids (except sweat), mucous membranes, or nonintact skin is likely
- Cleaning and/or disinfecting equipment

See Appendix.

HANDWASHING

Handwashing is the single most important health procedure any individual can perform to prevent the spread of microbes. Handwashing is a vigorous, short rubbing together of all the surfaces of soap-lathered hands. It is followed by rinsing under a stream of running warm water. Warm water is used because it makes a good lather. It is also less damaging to the skin than hot water. In health care facilities, soap is provided in a dispenser. Bar soap is easily contaminated because microbes can grow in the wet soap dish and on the surface of the soap.

Sinks in health care facilities vary in design. In most, you turn the water on by using faucets. Most people wash their hands when their hands are soiled or contaminated, so it stands to reason that the faucets are a potential source of contamination. Always use a paper towel to turn the water on. The water flow in some sinks is controlled by using a knee pedal or foot pedal, reducing the risk of inadvertent contamination. These are operated by stepping on the foot pedal or pushing the knee lever to the right to turn the water on. Push the knee lever to the left to turn the water off.

When washing your hands, always keep your fingertips pointed down. Never lean against the sink with your uniform or touch the inside of the sink with your hands.

The most important aspect of handwashing is the friction created by rubbing the hands together. This friction mechanically removes microbes from the hands. Routine handwashing with soap, running water, and friction by all health care providers:

- Is the most significant control measure for the prevention of a **nosocomial infection** (infection acquired by a patient while being cared for in a health care facility)
- Is the single most important control measure to break the chain of infection

The recommended handwashing technique depends on the purpose of the handwashing. Hands can usually be washed effectively in 15 to 20 seconds. More time will be needed, however, if hands are visibly soiled (refer to Procedure 1).

Handwashing should be done:

- At the beginning of your shift
- After picking up any item from the floor
- Before handling food
- After personal use of the bathroom
- After using a tissue
- After you cough or sneeze
- Before handling a patient's food and drink
- After handling a patient's belongings
- After touching any item or environmental surface that is soiled or in the immediate vicinity of patients
- Before handling any supply considered clean
- Immediately before touching mucous membranes or nonintact skin; if you are already wearing gloves, change them

PROCEDURE 1

HANDWASHING

1. Check that there is an adequate supply of soap and paper towels. A waste container lined with a plastic bag should be in the area near you.

2. Remove rings, if possible, or be sure to lather soap underneath.

3. Remove watch, or push up over wrist.

4. Turn on the faucet with a dry paper towel held between your hand and the faucet (Figure 13-1).

5. Adjust water to a warm temperature. Drop the towel in the waste container. Stand back from the sink so you do not contaminate your uniform. Wet your hands, keeping your fingertips pointed downward (Figure 13-2).

6. Apply soap and lather over your hands and wrists, between fingers, and under rings. Use friction and interlace your fingers (Figure 13-3). Work lather over every part of your hands and wrists. Clean your fingernails by rubbing them against the palm of the other hand to force soap under the nails for 15 to 20 seconds (Figure 13-4).

7. Rinse hands with your fingertips pointed down. Do not shake water from hands.

8. Dry hands thoroughly with a clean paper towel.

9. Turn off the faucet with another paper towel; drop the towel in the waste container.

10. Apply lotion to your hands.

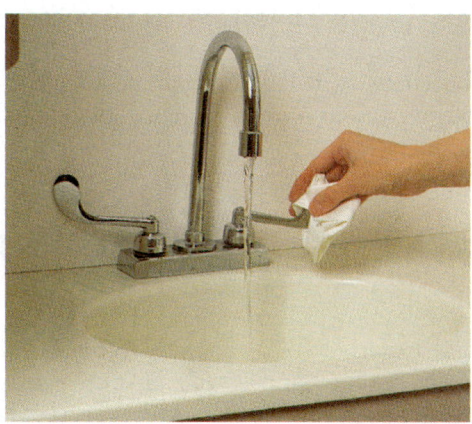

FIGURE 13-1 Use a clean, dry paper towel to turn faucets on and off.

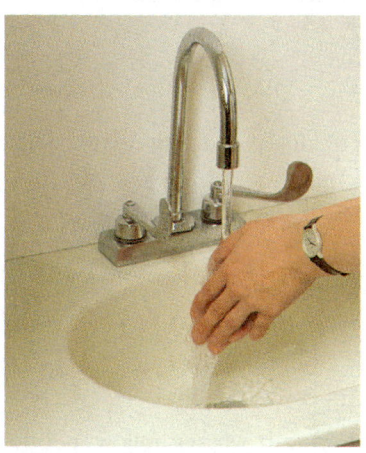

FIGURE 13-2 Keep your fingertips pointed down when washing hands.

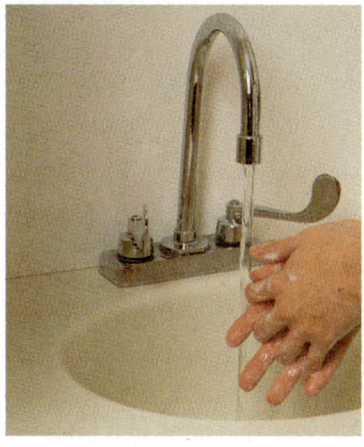

FIGURE 13-3 Interlace the fingers to clean between them.

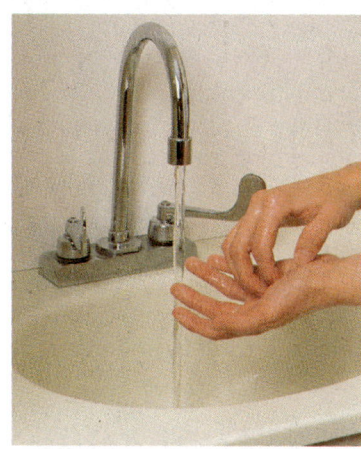

FIGURE 13-4 Rub nails against the palms of the hands to clean under the nails.

- Immediately after accidental contact with blood, moist body fluids, mucous membranes, or nonintact skin
- Before and after any contact with your mouth or mucous membranes, such as touching, eating, drinking, smoking, using lip balm, or manipulating contact lenses
- Before and after every patient contact
- Before applying and after removing gloves
- Whenever your hands are visibly soiled
- Any time your gloves become torn
- At the end of your shift before going home

Most health care facilities do not permit caregivers to wear artificial fingernails of any type, including nail tips, overlays, silk wraps, gels, sculptured, or acrylic nails. Long nails (beyond the fingertips) are also not usually permitted. This is because the long and artificial nails have been proven to harbor bacteria and increase the risk of infection to both the patient and the worker. They are difficult to clean properly and increase the risk of tearing gloves. Facilities may also have restrictions on the types of rings worn when on duty. Rings with many stones and elaborate settings can also hold harmful bacteria, and are difficult to clean. Rings may also tear gloves. Rings other than flat bands are better left at home when you are on duty.

Waterless Hand Cleaners

Many facilities provide dispensers containing waterless hand cleaners in various locations in the facility. The hand cleaners contain an alcohol-based gel, lotion, or foam that is dispensed in small dime- to quarter-sized portions (approximately 2 to 3 ml). In addition to the alcohol, most solutions contain moisturizers that prevent drying of the skin. Each facility has directions for using the product and policies and procedures for when the waterless hand cleaners may be used. In many, the waterless cleaner may be used instead of handwashing during routine patient care. However, washing at the sink may still be required in certain areas, such as the nursery, operating room, and others. Washing at the sink should also be done any time the hands are visibly soiled. To use the waterless cleaning product, dispense the proper amount into the palm of your hand. Rub the product into the hands until it dries, making sure to rub all areas and surfaces, including the nail beds and between the fingers. This takes about 15 seconds. Become familiar with the products used by your facility and their applications. They are very effective in reducing infection and eliminating pathogens from the hands.

PROTECTING YOURSELF

As you perform your duties, you may contact **potentially infectious material** such as blood or other body fluids that may contain pathogens. This is called **occupational exposure**.

OSHA *Alert*

Health care facilities are required to have an *exposure control plan* that describes what to do if you contact blood or body fluid. Immediately wash the area well. Report accidental contact with blood or body fluid to your charge nurse immediately. You will be treated according to the established plan, have blood samples taken, and may begin drug therapy to prevent a bloodborne disease. Medical care and monitoring may continue over a long period of time.

Using proper medical asepsis technique and following standard precautions according to your facility policy are the best ways to limit the potential for being infected.

An **exposure incident** means that your eyes, mouth, or nonintact skin had contact with blood or other potentially infectious material. Rinse immediately with clear water. Report this at once to your supervisor and follow facility procedure.

STANDARD PRECAUTIONS

Standard precautions (Figure 13-5) are the infection control actions used for all people receiving care, regardless of their condition or diagnosis. Standard precautions apply to situations in which care providers may contact:

- Blood, body fluids (except sweat), secretions, and excretions
- Mucous membranes
- Nonintact skin

Some examples of secretions and excretions are:

- Respiratory mucus (phlegm)
- Cerebrospinal fluid
- Urine
- Feces
- Vaginal secretions
- Semen
- Vomitus

This means that all health care workers follow specific procedures, called **work practice controls**, to prevent the spread of infections.

Standard precautions stress handwashing and the use of **personal protective equipment (PPE)**: gloves, gown, mask, and goggles or face shield.

STANDARD PRECAUTIONS FOR INFECTION CONTROL

Wash Hands (Plain soap)
Wash after touching blood, body fluids, secretions, excretions, and contaminated items. Wash immediately after gloves are removed and between patient contacts. Avoid transfer of microorganisms to other patients or environments.

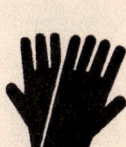

Wear Gloves
Wear when touching blood, body fluids, secretions, excretions, and contaminated items. Put on clean gloves just before touching mucous membranes and nonintact skin. Change gloves between tasks and procedures on the same patient after contact with material that may contain high concentrations of microorganisms. Remove gloves promptly after use, before touching noncontaminated items and environmental surfaces, and before going to another patient, and wash hands immediately to avoid transfer of microorganisms to other patients or environments.

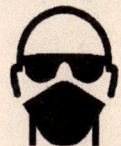

Wear Mask and Eye Protection or Face Shield
Protect mucous membranes of the eyes, nose and mouth during procedures and patient-care activities that are likely to generate splashes or sprays of blood, body fluids, secretions, or excretions.

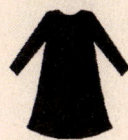

Wear Gown
Protect skin and prevent soiling of clothing during procedures that are likely to generate splashes or sprays of blood, body fluids, secretions, or excretions. Remove a soiled gown as promptly as possible and wash hands to avoid transfer of microorganisms to other patients or environments.

Patient-Care Equipment
Handle used patient-care equipment soiled with blood, body fluids, secretions, or excretions in a manner that prevents skin and mucous membrane exposures, contamination of clothing, and transfer of microorganisms to other patients and environments. Ensure that reusable equipment is not used for the care of another patient until it has been appropriately cleaned and reprocessed. Ensure that single-use items are properly discarded.

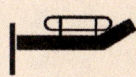

Environmental Control
Follow hospital procedures for routine care, cleaning, and disinfection of environmental surfaces, beds, bed rails, bedside equipment, and other frequently touched surfaces.

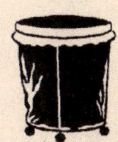

Linen
Handle, transport, and process used linen soiled with blood, body fluids, secretions, or excretions in a manner that prevents exposure and contamination of clothing, and avoids transfer of microorganisms to other patients and environments.

Occupational Health and Bloodborne Pathogens
Prevent injuries when using needles, scalpels, and other sharp instruments or devices; when handling sharp instruments after procedures; when cleaning used instruments; and when disposing of used needles.

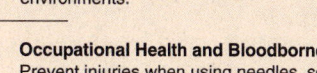

Never recap used needles using both hands or any other technique that involves directing the point of a needle towards any part of the body; rather, use either a one-handed "scoop" technique or a mechanical device designed for holding the needle sheath.

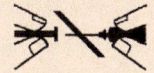

Do not remove used needles from disposable syringes by hand, and do not bend, break, or otherwise manipulate used needles by hand. Place used disposable syringes and needles, scalpels, blades, and other sharp items in puncture-resistant sharps containers located as close as practical to the area in which the items were used, and place reusable syringes and needles in a puncture-resistant container for transport to the reprocessing area.

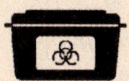

Use resuscitation devices as an alternative to mouth-to-mouth resuscitation.

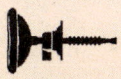

Patient Placement
Use a private room for a patient who contaminates the environment or who does not (or cannot be expected to) assist in maintaining appropriate hygiene or environmental control. Consult Infection Control if a private room is not available.

FIGURE 13-5 Standard precautions. *(Courtesy of BREVIS Corporation, Salt Lake City, UT)*

guidelines *for*

Standard Precautions

1. Wash hands in the situations listed under "Handwashing."

2. Wear gloves for any contact with blood, body fluids, mucous membranes, or nonintact skin, such as when:
   - Hands are cut, scratched, chapped, or have a rash
   - Cleaning up body fluid spills
   - Cleaning potentially contaminated equipment

3. Gloves are provided in patient rooms on supply carts, or in wall-mounted dispensers.

4. Carry gloves with you so they will always be available as you need them.

5. If you have an allergy to latex gloves, follow your physician's advice. Three possible options are:
   - Change to nonlatex gloves (facilities must supply them because latex allergies are common).
   - Apply a skin barrier cream to your hands before putting on latex gloves; the cream protects hands against most irritants, including latex.
   - Put on glove liners that prevent direct contact between the skin of the hands and the latex gloves.

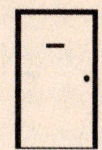

continues

guidelines *continued*

6. Change gloves:
   - After contacting each patient
   - Before touching noncontaminated articles or environmental surfaces
   - Between tasks with the same patient if there is contact with infectious materials
7. Dispose of gloves according to facility policy.
8. Wear a waterproof gown for procedures likely to produce splashes of blood or other body fluids.
   - Remove soiled gown as soon as possible and dispose of it properly according to facility policy.
   - Wash your hands.
9. Wear a mask and protective eyewear or face shield for procedures likely to produce splashes of blood or other moist body fluids. This is to prevent contact with pathogens by your mucous membranes.
   The surgical mask covers both the nose and mouth. The mask is used once and discarded. When a mask is required, a new one is put on for each patient receiving care. If the mask becomes wet, a new one must be put on because the mask loses its effectiveness when moist.
10. Goggles or a face shield help protect the mucous membranes of the eyes from splashes or sprays of blood and other body fluids. A surgical mask must be worn with goggles and with a face shield to protect the nose and mouth.
11. When using PPE, you should:
    - Know where to obtain these items in your work area.
    - Always remove the items before leaving the work area, whether the patient's room, an isolation unit, or the utility room.
    - Place these items in the proper container for laundering, decontamination, or disposal, according to facility policy.

guidelines *for*

Environmental Procedures

1. Handle all patient care items so that infectious organisms will not be transferred to skin, mucous membranes, clothing, or the environment. Reusable equipment must be cleaned and decontaminated according to facility policy before it can be used with another patient. Dispose of single-use items according to facility policy.
2. Follow facility procedures for routine care and cleaning of environmental surfaces, such as beds, bedside equipment, and other frequently touched surfaces.
3. Dispose of sharps—needles, razors, and other sharp items—in a puncture-resistant, leakproof container near the point of use (Figure 13-6). The container should be labeled with the biohazard symbol (Figure 13-7) and color-coded red.
4. Do not recap needles or otherwise handle them before disposal.
5. Mouthpieces or resuscitator bags should be available to minimize the need for mouth-to-mouth resuscitation. Remember that you must be trained to use them.

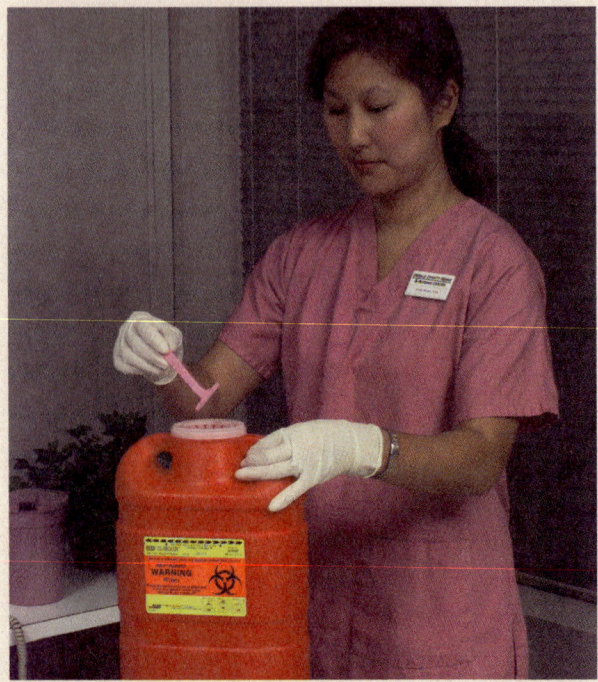

FIGURE 13-6 Carefully discard sharps in a safety container specifically designated for this use.

continues

guidelines *continued*

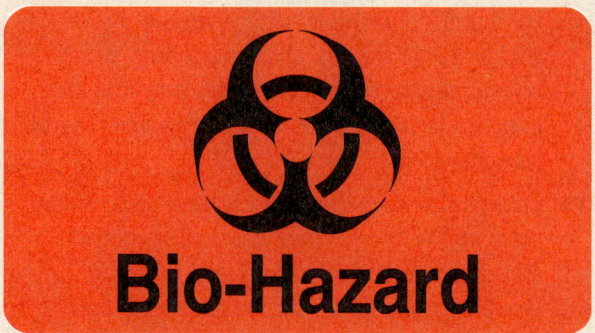

FIGURE 13-7 Containers for contaminated items are identified with the biohazard label. The symbol is black with a red or orange background.

6. Waste and soiled linen should be placed in plastic bags and handled according to facility policy. There are separate containers for regular waste and for biohazardous waste (waste that has contacted blood or body fluids). Containers for biohazardous waste should have the biohazard symbol, or be color-coded in red (Figure 13-8). Learn your facility policy for what is biohazardous waste and follow the guidelines.

7. Wipe up blood spills immediately. Disinfect the floor according to facility policy.
   – Use disposable gloves.
   – For small spills, use 1:100 dilution of bleach or disinfectant required by facility policy.

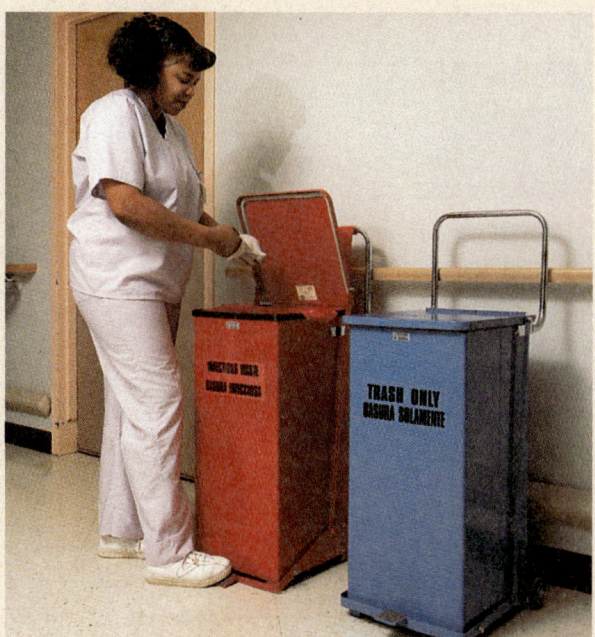

FIGURE 13-8 Discard all potentially infectious materials in the proper container.

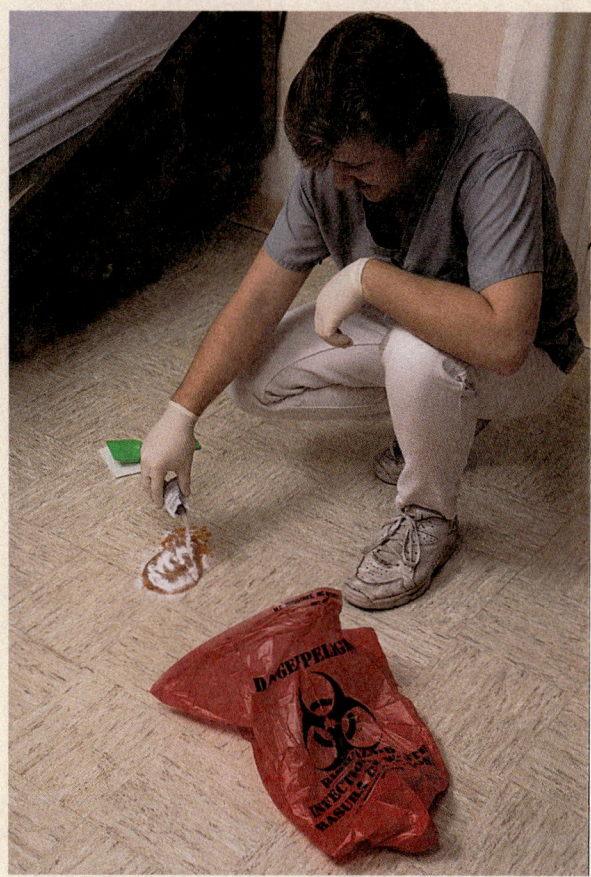

FIGURE 13-9 Clean blood spills immediately then apply 1:100 bleach solution or facility-approved disinfectant. For larger spills, a blood spill kit can be used. The powder in the kit solidifies the blood so it can be easily scooped into a plastic biohazard bag.

   – For larger spills, use a commercial blood cleanup kit. This contains an absorbent powder that is sprinkled over the blood to absorb the spill. The blood and powder are then scooped up with the scoop provided in the kit. The material and scoop are placed in a biohazard bag for disposal (Figure 13-9).
   – Use disposable cleaning cloths.
   – Dispose of gloves and cleaning cloths in appropriate infectious waste receptacles.

8. Dispose of body fluids and contaminated articles according to facility policy. This includes the contents of:
   – Urinary drainage bags
   – Bedpans
   – Urinals
   – Emesis basins

continues

guidelines *continued*

- – Drainage receptacles from tracheal and gastric suction
- – Solutions returned from vaginal douches, enemas, and bladder irrigations
- – Soiled dressings
- – Incontinence pads (Chux®)
- – Vaginal pads
- – Incontinent briefs

9. Eating, drinking, chewing gum, smoking, applying cosmetics or lip balm, and handling contact lenses are prohibited in work areas where there may be exposure to infectious material.

10. Food and drink should not be kept in refrigerators, freezers, shelves, cabinets, or on countertops or benchtops where they may be exposed to blood or other materials that may be contaminated.

11. Do not pick up potentially contaminated broken glassware with your bare hands. Use a brush and dust pan, tongs, or forceps. Clean and disinfect properly. Discard according to facility policy.

12. Consider laboratory specimens and specimen containers to be potentially infectious materials.

INFECTION CONTROL *Alert*

Items that have contacted blood or body fluids are biohazardous waste. Dispose of linen and trash contaminated with blood or body fluids according to your facility policy. These items must always be disposed of in leakproof, tightly closed containers. Biohazardous waste is stored in special areas until it is removed, and requires special handling during removal. This type of handling is very expensive, and storage space is often limited, so do not place non-biohazardous materials in the biohazard disposal containers.

TRANSMISSION-BASED PRECAUTIONS

Standard precautions do not eliminate the need for other isolation precautions. A second set of precautions is used with certain highly transmissible diseases. This second tier of precautions is called transmission-based precautions. Transmission-based precautions are designed to interrupt the mode of transmission so that the disease cannot spread to others. *Standard precautions are always used in addition to transmission-based precautions.*

Diseases may be transferred from one person to another either directly or indirectly. Such diseases are called communicable or contagious diseases. Some diseases are transmitted more easily than others. Specific precautions must be taken to control their spread.

Communicable diseases may be spread:

- Through upper respiratory secretions by airborne transmission and droplet transmission
- By contact transmission (direct contact or indirect contact) with feces or other body secretions and excretions
- Through draining wounds or infective material such as blood on needles

Each mode of transmission requires special precautions to interrupt the movement of microbes from the infected person to others.

If a disease is transmitted by more than one mode, all methods of transmission must be considered when selecting precautions for a specific patient. Table 13-1 lists transmission-based precautions and common diseases in each category.

TABLE 13-1	**TRANSMISSION-BASED PRECAUTIONS FOR COMMON DISEASES**
Transmission-Based Precautions Category	**Disease or Condition**
Airborne	Tuberculosis Measles
Airborne and Contact	Chickenpox Widespread shingles
Droplet	German measles Mumps Influenza
Contact	Head or body lice, scabies Impetigo Infected pressure ulcer with with heavy drainage

Isolation

Isolation means being separated or set apart. The purpose of isolation is to separate the patient with a communicable or contagious disease, to help prevent the spread of the infectious pathogens.

When a patient is in isolation precautions, a private room is used. Two patients with the same disease may share a room. (This practice is called *cohorting*.) For patients in isolation, the proper use of precautions requires extra effort by all care providers, but especially nursing assistants, and is more time-consuming. The fear of infection also makes working with these precautions more stressful for the care providers. Patients in isolation and their families and other visitors also feel stress.

Psychological Aspects of Isolation

The patient in isolation fears both the disease condition that makes the isolation precautions necessary and the practices that must be followed for these precautions to be effective. These include:

- PPE worn by all who enter the isolation unit
- Special procedures for handling waste, specimens, food, linens, and personal effects of the patient
- Restrictions on the patient's movement in the facility
- Procedures to be followed when patient is moved outside of the isolation unit
- Possible restrictions on visiting hours or number of visitors
- Need for visitors to use PPE
- Likelihood that close personal contact, such as kissing of family members, will not be permitted

The patient may be afraid of passing the infection to family and friends. If the patient does not understand the infectious process, this fear is increased. If the patient is confused, he or she may be very fearful of the PPE.

Because of the patient's fears and the need for decreased contact with other patients, family, and friends, the patient in isolation requires more emotional support and care. The extra time required to follow the isolation precautions, such as putting on PPE, could easily lessen the time the care providers spend with the patient at a time when emotional attention is most needed. Nursing assistants should be mindful of the patient's needs and plan their schedules to spend the necessary time with a patient in isolation.

Transmission-Based Isolation Precautions

Standard precautions are used with all patients regardless of their condition. When patients are known to have or are suspected of having an infectious disease, isolation precautions are used *in addition to* standard precautions. The isolation precautions used depend on the way in which the infectious pathogens are transmitted. Guidelines from the Centers for Disease Control and Prevention (CDC) indicate the specific precautions and personal protective equipment to be used based on how the disease is transmitted. The three transmission precautions are:

- Airborne precautions
- Droplet precautions
- Contact precautions

Airborne Precautions. **Airborne precautions** are used for diseases that are transmitted by air currents. The pathogens are small and light and are suspended in the air or on dust particles in the air. They can travel a long distance from the source by natural air currents and through ventilation systems. Tuberculosis is a disease that requires airborne precautions. Figure 13-10 shows the required precautions.

- The patient must be in a private room with negative air pressure. This means that air is drawn into the room and leaves the room through a special exhaust system to the outside. Air from the room does not circulate directly into the facility.
- The door to the room is kept closed.
- All care providers who enter the room must wear a **high-efficiency particulate air (HEPA) filter mask** (Figure 13-11). The special filters in this mask protect the care provider from the very small disease-causing pathogens. A surgical mask does not provide protection. Each care provider must be fitted with a HEPA filter mask. This ensures that air entering the mask comes through the filters only. Follow all facility policies for the use of HEPA filter masks.

The HEPA mask may be disposable or reusable. Men with facial hair cannot wear a HEPA mask because the beard

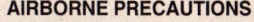

AIRBORNE PRECAUTIONS
(in addition to Standard Precautions)

VISITORS: Report to nurse before entering.

Patient Placement
Use **private room** that has:
Monitored negative air pressure,
6 to 12 air changes per hour,
Discharge of air outdoors or HEPA filtration if recirculated.
Keep room door closed and patient in room.

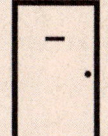

Respiratory Protection
Wear an N95 respirator when entering the room of a patient with known or suspected infectious pulmonary **tuberculosis.**
Susceptible persons should not enter the room of patients known or suspected to have **measles** (rubeola) or **varicella** (chickenpox) if other immune caregivers are available. If susceptible persons must enter, they should wear an N95 respirator. (Respirator or surgical mask not required if immune to measles and varicella.)

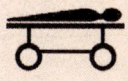

Patient Transport
Limit transport of patient from room to essential purposes only. Use **surgical mask** on patient during transport.

FIGURE 13-10 Airborne precautions. *(Courtesy of BREVIS Corporation, Salt Lake City, UT)*

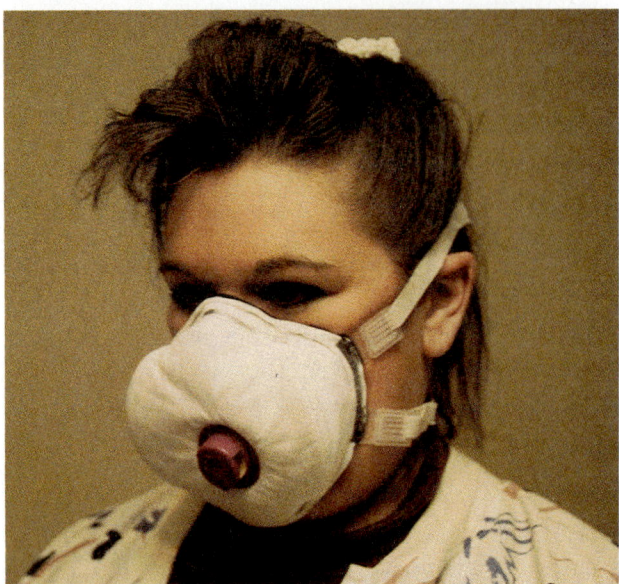

FIGURE 13-11 The HEPA respirator filter is individually fitted to the worker. The respirator is reusable. Store it according to facility policy.

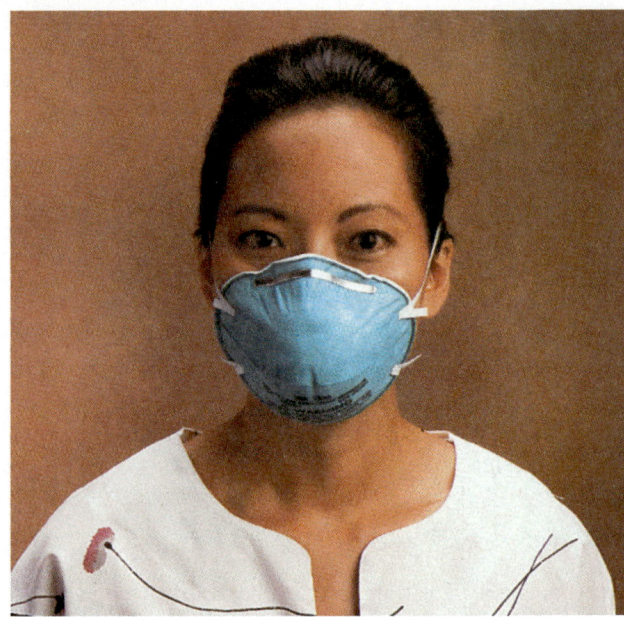

FIGURE 13-13 The N95 respirator is disposable. Some facilities store it for one shift, then discard it.

prevents an airtight seal. In this case, a special HEPA-filtered hood can be worn. The HEPA mask is not the only mask that can be used in an isolation room. Masks that are worn in an airborne precautions room must be approved by the National Institute of Occupational Safety and Health (NIOSH). This agency is part of the CDC, and is responsible for conducting research and making recommendations for the prevention of work-related disease and injury. The PFR95 respirator (Figure 13-12) and the N95 respirator (Figure 13-13) are approved alternatives. Some

workers prefer these masks because they are lighter in weight and more comfortable to wear. Fit-testing of a HEPA mask or respirator is required each time one is put on. Figure 13-14 shows the procedure for fit-testing the N95 respirator.

- People who are not immune to measles (rubeola) or chickenpox (varicella) should not enter the room of a patient known or suspected to have either of these infections. People who have not had chickenpox should not enter the room of a patient in isolation for shingles.
- If transport from the room is necessary, the patient must wear a surgical mask.
- Remember: these precautions are in addition to standard precautions.
- Some facilities do not have the special ventilation required for airborne precautions rooms. These facilities use portable units that are placed in the room to filter the air, creating a negative pressure environment. They are slightly noisier than a ventilation system, but are effective in eliminating pathogens.

Droplet Precautions. Droplet precautions are used for diseases that can be spread by means of large droplets in the air. A person can spread droplets containing infectious pathogens by sneezing, coughing, talking, singing, or laughing. The droplets generally do not travel more than three feet from the source. Influenza is an example of a disease spread by droplets.

Figure 13-15 shows the requirements for droplet precautions.

- If a patient cannot be placed in a private room, then residents requiring the same precautions can be placed together.
- The caregivers should wear surgical masks if they expect to be working within three feet of the patient.

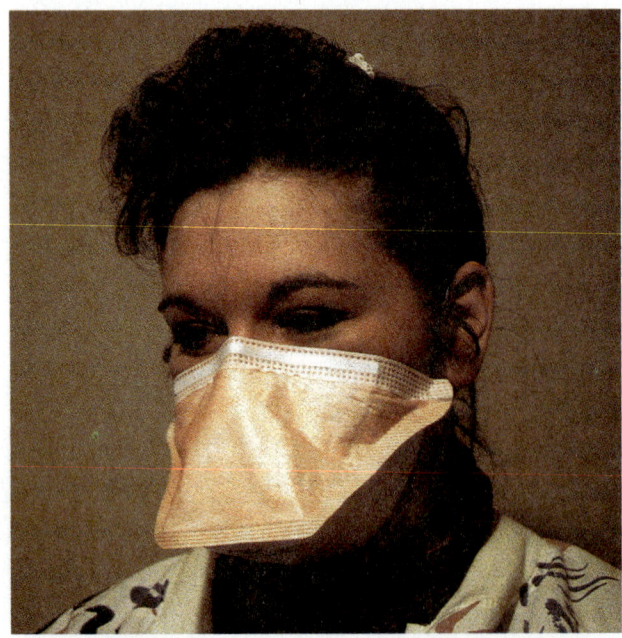

FIGURE 13-12 The PFR95 respirator filter is preferred by many health care workers because it is lightweight and comfortable.

Donning instructions (to be followed each time product is worn):

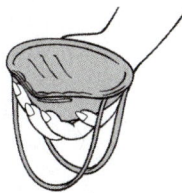 **1** Cup the respirator in your hand with the nosepiece at fingertips, allowing the headbands to hang freely below hands.

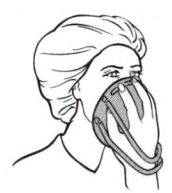 **2** Position the respirator under your chin with the nosepiece up.

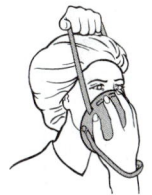 **3** Pull the top strap over your head so it rests high on the back of head.

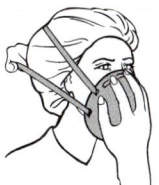 **4** Pull the bottom strap over your head and position it around neck below ears.

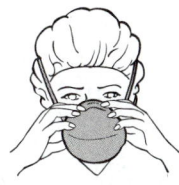 **5** Using two hands, mold the nosepiece to the shape of your nose by pushing inward while moving fingertips down both sides of the nosepiece. Pinching the nosepiece using one hand may result in less effective respirator performance.

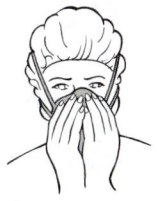 **6** FACE FIT CHECK
The respirator seal should be checked before each use. To check fit, place both hands completely over the respirator and exhale. If air leaks around your nose, adjust the nosepiece as described in step 5. If air leaks at respirator edges, adjust the straps back along the sides of your head. Recheck.

NOTE: If you cannot achieve proper fit, do not enter the isolation or treatment area. See your supervisor.

Removal instructions:

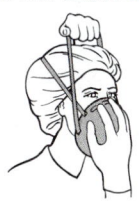 **1** Cup the respirator in your hand to maintain position on face. Pull bottom strap over head.

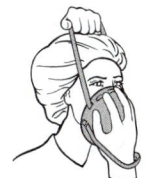 **2** Still holding respirator in position, pull top strap over head.

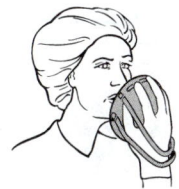 **3** Remove respirator from face and discard or store according to your facility's policy.

FIGURE 13-14 Fit-test the respirator each time you wear it. *(Courtesy of 3M Health Care, St. Paul, MN)*

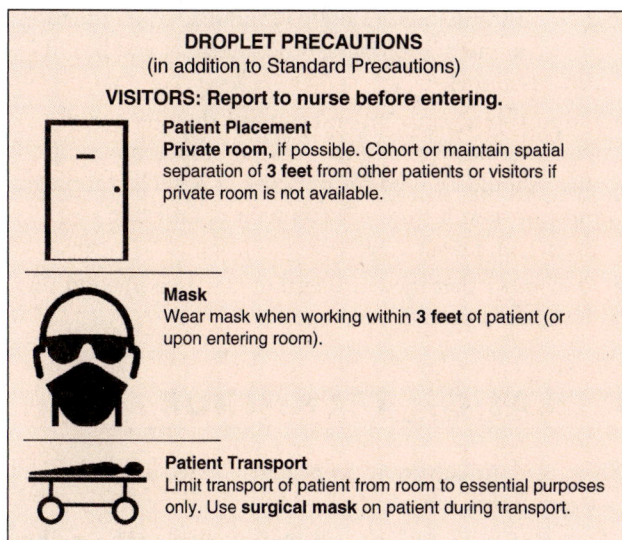

DROPLET PRECAUTIONS
(in addition to Standard Precautions)

VISITORS: Report to nurse before entering.

Patient Placement
Private room, if possible. Cohort or maintain spatial separation of **3 feet** from other patients or visitors if private room is not available.

Mask
Wear mask when working within **3 feet** of patient (or upon entering room).

Patient Transport
Limit transport of patient from room to essential purposes only. Use **surgical mask** on patient during transport.

FIGURE 13-15 Droplet precautions. *(Courtesy of BREVIS Corporation, Salt Lake City, UT)*

The door can be open if the bed is more than three feet from the door.

- If transport from the room is necessary, the patient must wear a surgical mask.
- Remember that these precautions are in addition to standard precautions.

Contact Precautions. Contact precautions are used when the infectious pathogen is spread by direct or indirect contact. *Direct contact* occurs when the caregiver touches a contaminated area on the patient's skin or blood or body fluids containing the infectious pathogen. *Indirect contact* occurs when the caregiver touches items contaminated with the infectious material, such as the patient's personal belongings, equipment or supplies used in the care of the patient, contaminated linens, and so on. Examples of infections requiring contact precautions are scabies, infected pressure ulcers, and gastroenteritis.

Figure 13-16 shows the requirements for contact precautions.

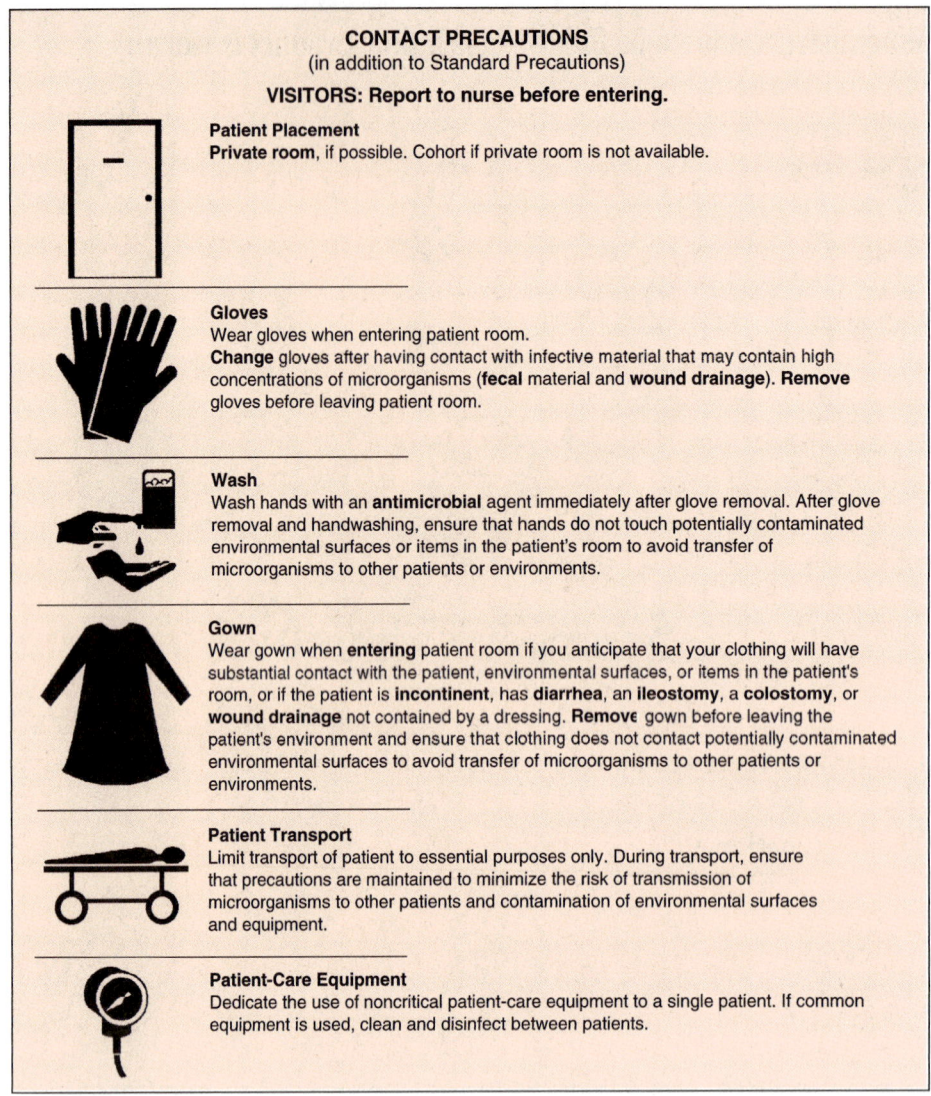

CONTACT PRECAUTIONS
(in addition to Standard Precautions)
VISITORS: Report to nurse before entering.

Patient Placement
Private room, if possible. Cohort if private room is not available.

Gloves
Wear gloves when entering patient room.
Change gloves after having contact with infective material that may contain high concentrations of microorganisms (**fecal** material and **wound drainage**). **Remove** gloves before leaving patient room.

Wash
Wash hands with an **antimicrobial** agent immediately after glove removal. After glove removal and handwashing, ensure that hands do not touch potentially contaminated environmental surfaces or items in the patient's room to avoid transfer of microorganisms to other patients or environments.

Gown
Wear gown when **entering** patient room if you anticipate that your clothing will have substantial contact with the patient, environmental surfaces, or items in the patient's room, or if the patient is **incontinent,** has **diarrhea,** an **ileostomy,** a **colostomy,** or **wound drainage** not contained by a dressing. **Remove** gown before leaving the patient's environment and ensure that clothing does not contact potentially contaminated environmental surfaces to avoid transfer of microorganisms to other patients or environments.

Patient Transport
Limit transport of patient to essential purposes only. During transport, ensure that precautions are maintained to minimize the risk of transmission of microorganisms to other patients and contamination of environmental surfaces and equipment.

Patient-Care Equipment
Dedicate the use of noncritical patient-care equipment to a single patient. If common equipment is used, clean and disinfect between patients.

FIGURE 13-16 Contact precautions. *(Courtesy of BREVIS Corporation, Salt Lake City, UT)*

- The patient should be in a private room. If this is not possible, then patients requiring the same type of isolation precautions can be placed in the same room. The door can be open.

- Gloves are put on before the caregiver enters the patient's room. Gloves are changed whenever there is contact with highly contaminated matter in the room. After removing gloves, always wash your hands before putting on a new pair of gloves. After care is completed, remove gloves and wash hands. Use a paper towel to open the door to leave the room and discard the towel in the trash container inside the room.

- Wear a gown when entering the patient's room if your uniform may contact the patient, blood or body fluids, environmental surfaces, or other items in the room. Remove the gown before leaving the room and dispose of it according to facility policy for biohazardous waste. Be careful not to touch environmental surfaces or other items with your uniform as you leave the room.

- Transport the patient from the room only when necessary. Continue precautions to minimize contamination of environmental surfaces, other patients, and health care personnel.

- Disposable equipment and supplies should be used whenever possible. Noncritical, nondisposable equipment should be used for one patient only. If equipment must be used for more than one patient, it must be cleaned and disinfected between patients.

- Remember that these precautions are used in addition to standard precautions.

ISOLATION TECHNIQUE

There are four key points to be remembered at all times for isolation technique:

1. **Isolation technique** is the name given to the method of caring for patients with easily transmitted diseases.

2. It is essential that every person take responsibility and use the proper isolation techniques to prevent the spread of disease to others.

3. All items that come into contact with the patient's excretions, secretions, blood, body fluids, mucous membranes, or nonintact skin are considered contaminated. This potentially infective material must be treated in a special way.

4. Standard precautions are always used in addition to transmission-based precautions.

Isolation Unit

The isolation unit may be an area or a private room. Patients with the same disease may share a room. A room with handwashing facilities and an adjoining room with bathing and toilet facilities is best. A private room is indicated for patients who:

- Are highly infectious
- Have poor personal hygiene
- Require special air control procedures within the room

Preparing for Isolation

To prepare a patient room for isolation, do the following:

1. Place a card indicating the type of isolation precaution on the door to the patient's room.

2. Place an isolation cart outside the room, next to the door. Place in it quantities of personal protective equipment as needed:
   - Gowns
   - Masks
   - Gloves
   - Goggles or face shields
   - Plastic bags marked for biohazardous waste
   - Plastic bags for soiled linen

3. Line the wastepaper basket inside the room with a plastic bag labeled or color-coded for infectious waste.

4. Place a laundry hamper in the room and line it with a yellow biohazard laundry bag.

5. At the sink, check the supply of paper towels and soap. Soap should be in a wall dispenser or foot-operated dispenser.

PERSONAL PROTECTIVE EQUIPMENT

Personal protective equipment includes gloves, gown, mask, and goggles or face shield. The following sections describe the correct use of this equipment (see Procedures 2 through 6).

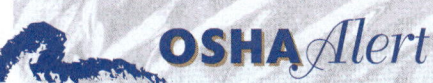

OSHA *Alert*

Personal protective equipment will protect you only if it fits properly, is free from defects, and is used regularly in the way you were taught. Never use equipment that is torn or has defects. Personal protective equipment is also worn during cleaning procedures when contact with blood, body fluids, secretions, or excretions is likely. Personal protective equipment is discarded, laundered, or decontaminated according to facility policy after use. Be sure to replace what you have used so it is available the next time it is needed.

Cover Gown

A gown made of a moisture-resistant material is used when soiling or splashing with blood, body fluids, secretions, or excretions is likely (Figure 13-17). The gown prevents contamination of the health care provider's uniform. A gown should be worn only once. Discard gowns according to facility policy after use.

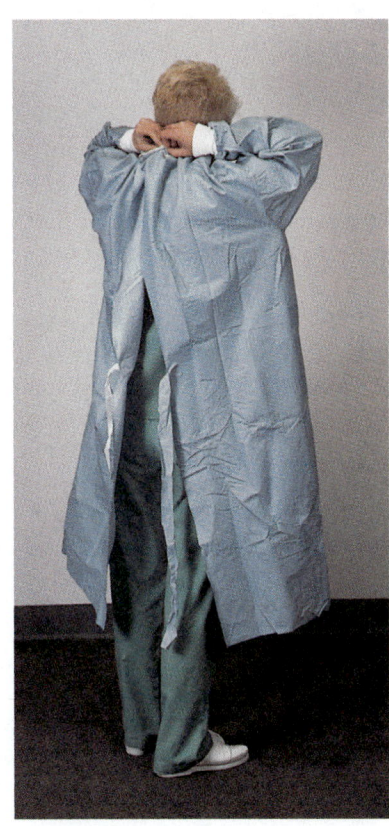

FIGURE 13-17 Put on a gown if your uniform may have contact with blood or moist body fluids.

Gloves

The use of gloves prevents the spread of disease. Usually the nursing assistant will wear nonsterile latex or vinyl disposable gloves, but there are also times when other types of gloves are worn. Gloves should be worn for most health care procedures, and they are always worn when contact with blood, body fluids (except sweat), secretions, excretions, mucous membranes, or nonintact skin is expected. You should also wear gloves if you have cuts or open sores on your hands. Gloves are also used during many routine cleaning procedures that the nursing assistant performs. In this case, utility gloves may be worn. The use of gloves does not replace the need for handwashing. Always wash your hands before and after glove use. If you accidentally touch a potentially contaminated environmental surface after removing your gloves, wash your hands again.

Gloves are used for three main purposes:

1. To prevent the nursing assistant from picking up a pathogen from the patient
2. To avoid giving the patient a pathogen that the nursing assistant has picked up on the hands
3. To avoid picking up a pathogen on a patient or the environment and carrying it to another patient on the hands

For gloves to be effective, they must be intact and have no visible cuts, tears, or cracks. They must fit your hands well. Gloves come in different sizes. Select the size that most comfortably fits your hand. If the glove is too large or too small, a measure of protection is lost. Do not wash your hands while wearing gloves. Handwashing damages the pores of the gloves and may allow microbes to enter. If your hands need to be washed, remove the gloves, wash your hands, then reapply new gloves. Table 13-2 lists times when gloves should be changed. Remember to wash your hands every time you remove gloves. Table 13-3 lists common nursing assistant tasks and the correct personal protective equipment to use for each job.

Gloves are for single patient use only. Do not wear them to care for more than one patient. Take care that you do not contaminate environmental surfaces with your gloves. Some facilities use the "one-glove technique" (Figure 13-18). This

TABLE 13-2 SUGGESTED TIMES TO CHANGE GLOVES

Remember to wash your hands before applying and after removing gloves. Never touch environmental surfaces with a contaminated glove.

Change gloves:

- Before giving any patient care
- After giving patient care
- Immediately before touching mucous membranes
- Immediately before touching nonintact skin
- Immediately after touching secretions or excretions
- Immediately after touching blood or body fluids
- After touching equipment or environmental surfaces that are potentially contaminated
- Any time your gloves are torn
- If your gloves become visibly soiled

involves carrying a contaminated item in a gloved hand. The glove on the other hand is removed to open doors, turn on faucets, and touch other environmental surfaces and supplies.

Health care facilities have many different policies regarding how and where gloves are discarded. Many facilities require

TABLE 13-3 PERSONAL PROTECTIVE EQUIPMENT IN COMMON NURSING ASSISTANT TASKS

Note: Use this chart as a general guideline only. Add protective equipment if special circumstances exist. Know and follow your facility policies for using personal protective equipment.

Nursing Assistant Task	Gloves	Gown	Goggles/ Face Shield	Surgical Mask
Washing/rinsing utensils in the soiled utility room	Yes	Yes, if splashing is likely	Yes, if splashing is likely	Yes, if splashing is likely
Holding pressure on a bleeding wound	Yes	Yes	Yes	Yes
Wiping the shower chair with disinfectant	Yes	No	No	No
Emptying a catheter bag	Yes	Yes, if facility policy	Yes, if facility policy	Yes, if facility policy
Passing meal trays	No	No	No	No
Passing ice	No	No	No	No
Giving a backrub to a patient with a rash	Yes	No	No	No
Giving special mouth care to an unconscious patient	Yes	Yes, if facility policy	Yes, if facility policy	Yes, if facility policy
Assisting with a dental procedure	Yes	Yes	Yes	Yes
Changing the bed after an incontinent patient has an episode of diarrhea	Yes	Yes	No	No
Taking an oral temperature with a glass thermometer (gloves are not necessary with an electronic thermometer unless this is your facility policy)	Yes	No	No	No
Taking a rectal temperature	Yes	No	No	No
Taking an axillary temperature	No	No	No	No
Taking a blood pressure	No	No	No	No
Assisting an alert patient to brush teeth	Yes	Yes, if facility policy	Yes, if facility policy	Yes, if facility policy
Washing a patient's eyes	Yes	No	No	No
Giving perineal care	Yes	No	No	No
Washing the patient's abdomen when the skin is not broken	No	No	No	No
Washing the patient's arms when skin tears are present	Yes	No	No	No
Brushing a patient's dentures	Yes	No	No	No
Assisting the nurse while he or she suctions an unconscious patient with a tracheostomy	Yes	Yes	Yes	Yes

continues

TABLE 13-3 *continued*

Nursing Assistant Task	Gloves	Gown	Goggles/ Face Shield	Surgical Mask
Turning an incontinent patient who weighs 85 pounds	Yes, if linen is soiled	Yes, if your uniform will have substantial contact with the linen	No	No
Shaving a patient with a disposable razor	Yes, because this is a high-risk procedure	No	No	No
Shaving a patient with an electric razor	No	No	No	No
Cleaning the soiled utility room at the end of your shift	Yes	No	No	No

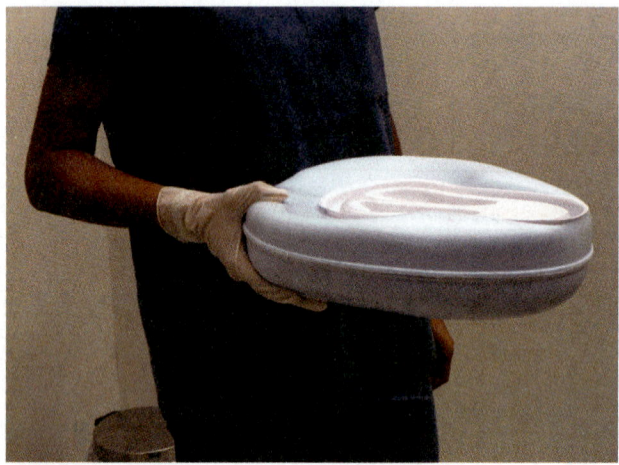

FIGURE 13-18 The one-glove technique is used to carry contaminated items.

the staff to discard gloves in sealed or covered containers and prohibit you from discarding gloves in open wastebaskets in the room. Know and follow your facility policy.

Face Mask

Surgical masks should be worn when exposure to droplet secretions may occur. The mask should cover the nursing assistant's nose and mouth. For example, a mask would be worn when caring for a patient with influenza who is coughing and releasing droplets containing the flu pathogen into the environment. The mask protects you when you are working within three feet of the patient. It is also used whenever protective eyewear is worn. When a surgical mask is needed, it is:

- Used only once and discarded
- Changed if it becomes moist

COMMUNICATION *Highlight*

Remember that one way to communicate is through touch. Do not carry glove use to the extreme. Use gloves when necessary, but avoid using them for all patient contact. Using gloves at all times sends a negative message. It says that the patient is untouchable. Touching is very important to all human beings. Use gloves only when contact with blood, body fluids, secretions, excretions, mucous membranes, or nonintact skin is likely. Also, wear gloves if the skin on your hands is cut, cracked, or chapped. Be very careful not to contaminate clean equipment, supplies, or environmental surfaces with used gloves.

- Handled only by the ties
- Never left secured around the neck, because it can contaminate the uniform and the environment

Protective Eyewear

A full face shield (Figure 13-19), or goggles (Figure 13-20), are worn any time splashing of blood, body fluid, secretions, or excretions may occur. The eyewear does not protect the mucous membranes of the nose and mouth, so a surgical mask is always worn with eyewear. A good rule to follow is that a surgical mask may be worn without protective eyewear, but protective eyewear is never worn without

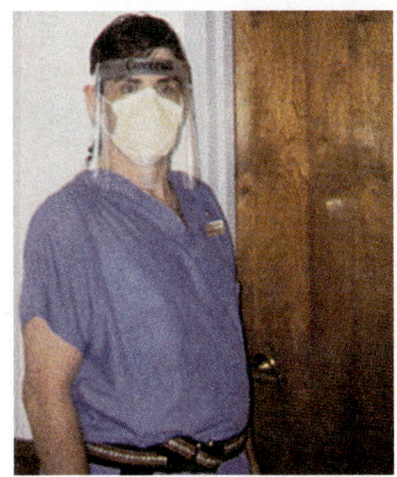

FIGURE 13-19
A surgical mask is always worn under a face shield.

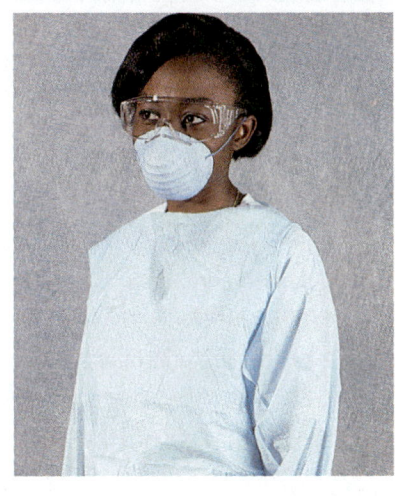

FIGURE 13-20
Always protect your nose and mouth with a surgical mask when wearing goggles.

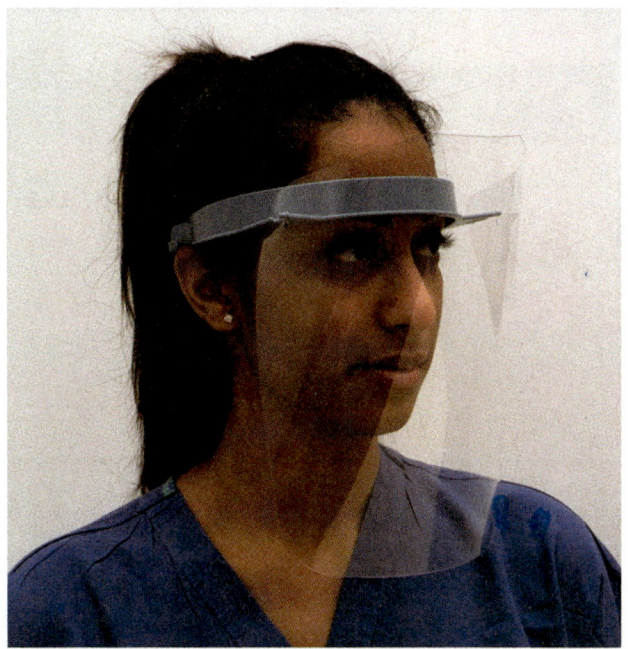

FIGURE 13-21 The large face shield is used for some tasks without a mask. The design of the face shield covers a larger area than most face protectors. *(Face shield courtesy of Amdrecor, Inc., Houston, TX [800] 356-2938)*

3. Goggles or face shield
4. Mask
5. Gown
6. Wash hands

Equipment

Disposable (used once and discarded) patient care equipment is used by many facilities. It is ideal for patients on isolation precautions. Frequently used equipment remains in the patient's unit. Most articles will not require special handling unless they are contaminated (or likely to be contaminated) with infective material.

Special precautions are not necessary for dishes unless they are visibly contaminated with infective material. An example of this is dishes that have blood, drainage, or secretions on them. Disposable dishes contaminated with infective material can be handled as disposable patient care equipment.

Containment of Contaminated Articles

Contaminated articles leaving the patient's room must be handled so that pathogens will not be spread. It is important that contaminated equipment be bagged, labeled, and disposed of according to the health care facility's policy for the disposal of infectious waste. Used articles are placed in an impenetrable bag (such as plastic) before they are removed from the room or unit of the patient. A single bag may be used if it is waterproof and sturdy enough to confine and contain the article without contaminating the outside of the bag. (Refer to Procedures 7 through 10.)

a surgical mask. Some masks have a protective eyeshield attached to them. The mask is put on before the protective eyewear. When removing the mask and eyewear, wash your hands, remove the eyewear, then the mask.

Large face shields are now available that cover the entire face, neck, and chin (Figure 13-21). Because of the shield design, some facilities permit employees to wear this face shield without a mask, depending on the task. Follow facility policies for the equipment you are using and procedure being done.

Sequence for Applying Personal Protective Equipment

1. Wash hands
2. Mask
3. Gown
4. Goggles or face shield
5. Gloves

Sequence for Removing Personal Protective Equipment

1. Gloves
2. Wash hands

PROCEDURE 2

PUTTING ON A MASK

1. Assemble equipment:
   - mask
2. If gown and gloves are needed, the mask goes on first. (If a face shield is used, it is put on next.)
3. Adjust mask over nose and mouth.
4. Tie top strings of mask first, then bottom strings.
5. Replace your mask if it becomes moist during procedures.
6. Do not reuse a mask and do not let the mask hang around your neck.

PROCEDURE 3

PUTTING ON A GOWN

To be effective, a gown should have long sleeves, be long enough to cover the uniform, and be big enough to overlap in the back. Gowns should be waterproof.

1. Assemble equipment:
   - Clean gown
   - Paper towel
2. Remove wristwatch; place it on a paper towel.
3. Wash hands.
4. If a mask and goggles or face shield are required, put them on first.
5. After tying on the mask, put on the gown outside the patient's room. Put on gown by slipping your arms into the sleeves (Figure 13-22A).
6. Slip the fingers of both hands under the inside neckband and grasp the ties in back. Secure the neckband (Figure 13-22B).
7. Reach behind and overlap the edges of the gown. Secure the waist ties (Figure 13-22C).
8. Take your watch into the isolation unit, leaving it on the paper towel.
9. Remember when using gowns:
   - A disposable gown is worn only once and then is discarded as infectious waste.
   - A reusable cloth gown is worn only once and then is handled as contaminated linen.
   - Carry out all procedures in the unit at one time, to avoid unnecessary waste of gowns.

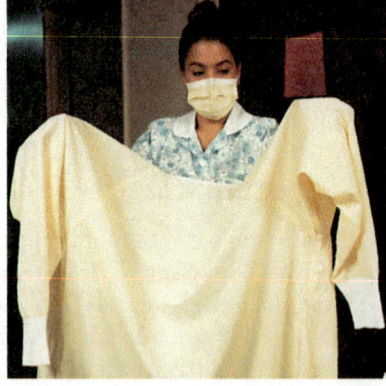

FIGURE 13-22A Apply the clean cover gown before entering the patient's room. After putting on the mask, apply gloves.

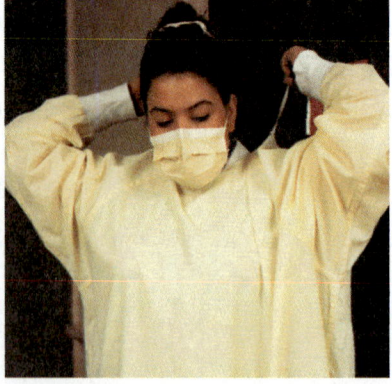

FIGURE 13-22B Slip fingers inside the neckband and tie the gown.

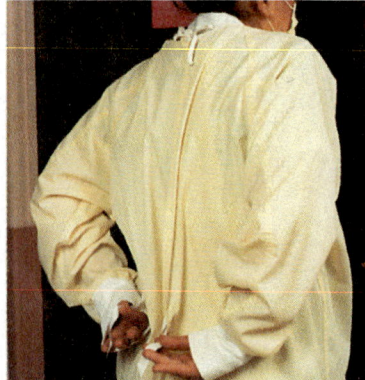

FIGURE 13-22C Reach behind, overlapping the edges of the gown so your uniform is completely covered, then tie the waist ties.

PROCEDURE 4

PUTTING ON GLOVES

1. Assemble equipment:
   - Disposable gloves in correct size
2. Wash your hands.
3. If a gown is required, put gloves on after the gown is put on.
4. Pick up a glove by the cuff and place it on the other hand.
5. Repeat with a glove for the other hand.
6. Interlace fingers to adjust the gloves on your hands.
7. Remember when using gloves:
   - Wash hands before and after using gloves.

- Remove gloves if they tear or become heavily soiled. Wash hands and put on a new pair.
- Gloves are used whenever there is the possibility of contacting body fluids, blood, secretions, excretions, mucous membranes, or nonintact skin.
- Change gloves between patients and wash hands.
- Discard gloves immediately after removing, in biohazardous waste receptacle.
- Avoid contaminating environmental surfaces with used gloves.

PROCEDURE 5

REMOVING CONTAMINATED GLOVES

1. Grasp the cuff of one glove on the outside with the fingers of the other hand (Figure 13-23A).

2. Pull cuff of glove down, drawing it over the glove and turning the glove inside out (Figure 13-23B). Pull that glove off your hand.

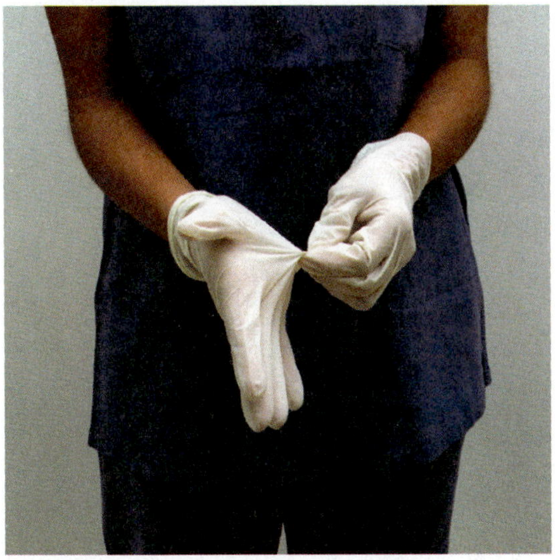

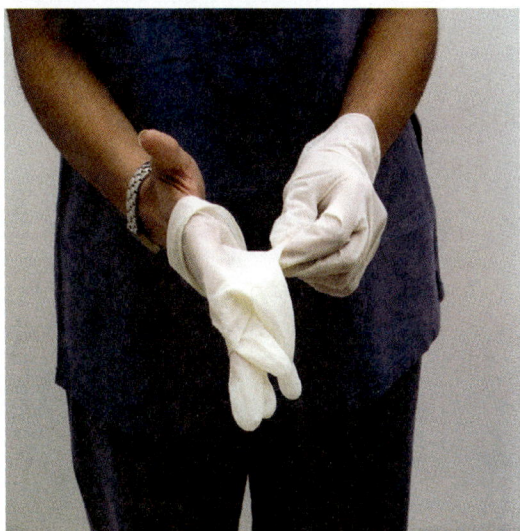

FIGURE 13-23A With the fingers of one gloved hand, grasp the glove on the other hand.

FIGURE 13-23B Pull the glove down over the hand and fingers and remove it. The glove is inside out with the contaminated side inside.

continues

PROCEDURE 5

continued

3. Hold the glove with the still-gloved hand.

4. Insert the fingers of the ungloved hand under the cuff of the glove on the other hand (Figure 13-23C).

5. Pull the glove off inside out, drawing it over the first glove.

6. Drop both gloves together into the biohazardous waste receptacle (Figure 13-23D).

7. Wash your hands. Dry with a paper towel and discard the towel in the proper container. Use a dry towel to turn off the water faucet. Discard the towel.

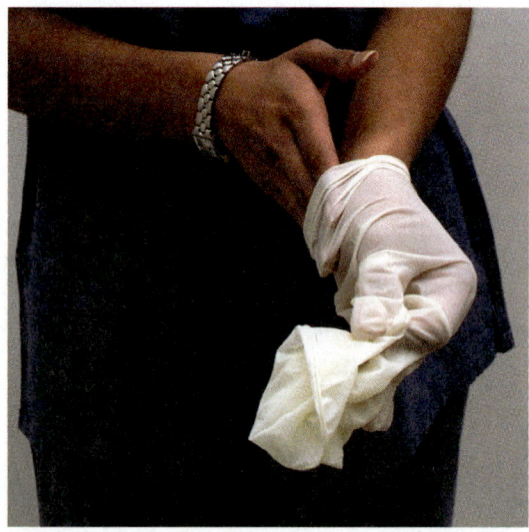

FIGURE 13-23C Hold the glove just removed in the gloved hand. Insert fingers of the ungloved hand inside the cuff of the other glove.

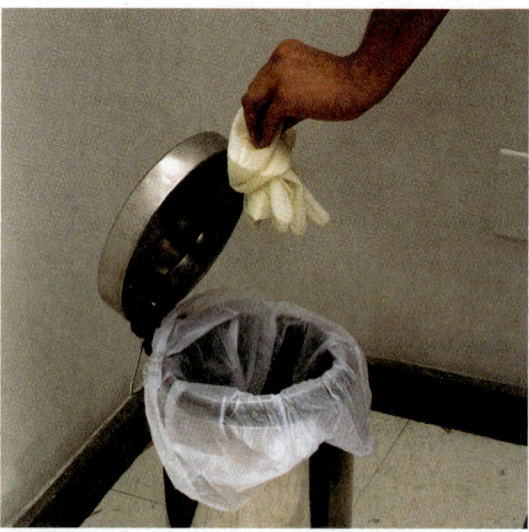

FIGURE 13-23D Pull the glove down over the hand and then pull both gloves off, holding the inside (noncontaminated side of glove). Discard the gloves in the proper container.

PROCEDURE 6

REMOVING CONTAMINATED GLOVES, MASK, AND GOWN

1. Assemble equipment:
   - Biohazardous waste receptacle for disposable items
   - Waste receptacle for gown if it is not disposable
   - Paper towels

2. Follow Procedure 5 for removing contaminated gloves.

3. Undo waist ties of gown (Figure 13-24A).

4. Turn faucets on with a clean paper towel. Discard the towel.

5. Wash your hands and dry them with a clean paper towel.

6. Use a clean, dry paper towel to turn off the faucet.

7. Remove goggles if used. Dispose of goggles according to facility policy.

continues

PROCEDURE 6

continued

8. Remove mask:
   - Undo the bottom ties first, then the top ties (Figure 13-24B).
   - Holding top ties, dispose of mask in appropriate waste receptacle.

9. Undo the neck ties and loosen gown at shoulders (Figure 13-24C).

10. Slip the fingers of your dominant hand inside the cuff of the other hand without touching the outside of the gown (Figure 13-24D).

11. Using the gown-covered hand, pull the gown down over the dominant hand (Figure 13-24E) and then off both arms.

12. As the gown is removed, fold it away from the body with the contaminated side inward and then roll it up (Figure 13-24F). Dispose of the contaminated gown in the appropriate receptacle.

13. Wash your hands.

14. If you brought a watch into the area (see Procedure 3), remove the watch from the paper towel. Hold the clean side of the paper towel and dispose of the towel in a wastepaper receptacle.

15. Use a paper towel to grasp the door handle as you leave the patient's room. Discard the paper towel in an appropriate receptacle before you leave the unit.

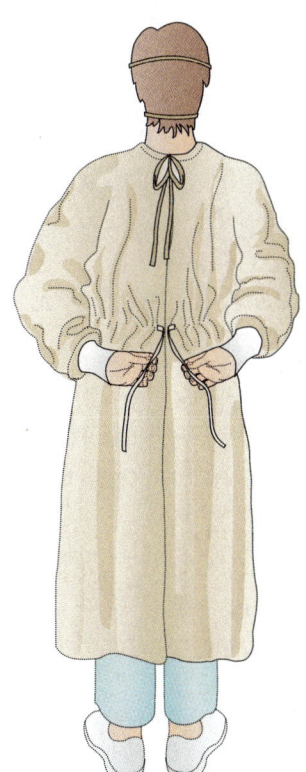

FIGURE 13-24A Remove gloves. Wash hands and then untie waist tie of gown.

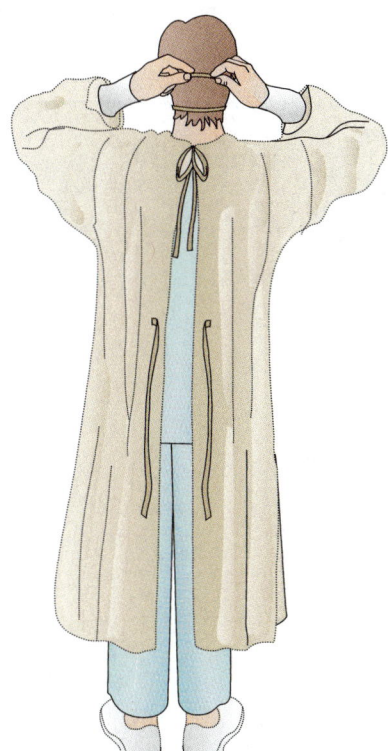

FIGURE 13-24B Remove mask by untying top ties first, then bottom ties. Holding mask by ties, place in contaminated trash.

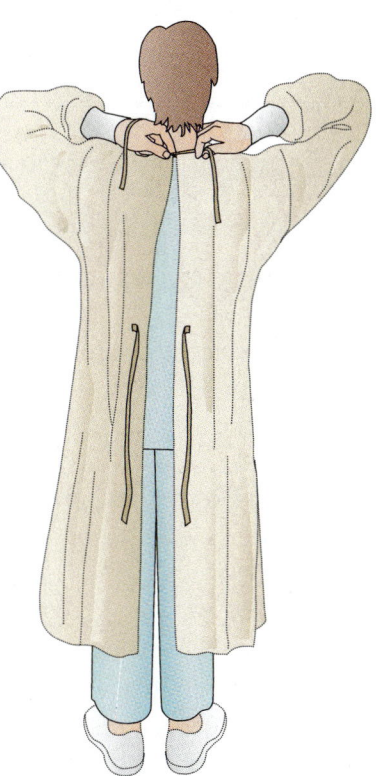

FIGURE 13-24C Untie neck ties of gown.

continues

PROCEDURE 6

continued

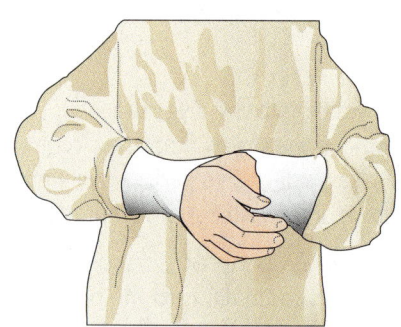

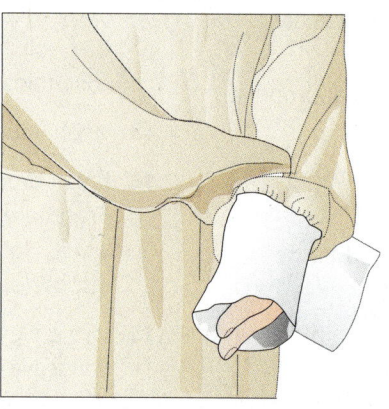

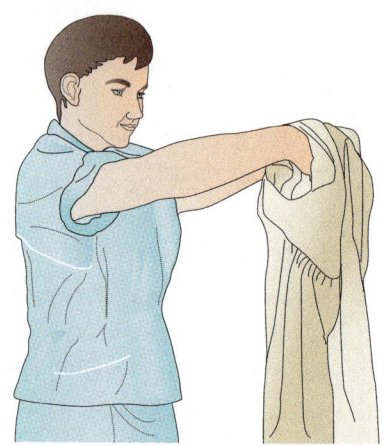

FIGURE 13-24D Slip fingers of one hand inside the cuff of the other hand. Pull gown down over the hand. Do not touch the outside of the gown with either hand.

FIGURE 13-24E Using the gown-covered hand, pull the gown down over the other hand.

FIGURE 13-24F Pull the gown down off the arms, being careful not to touch the outside of the gown. Hold the gown away from your uniform and roll it with the contaminated side in.

PROCEDURE 7

SERVING A MEAL IN AN ISOLATION UNIT

1. Before entering the isolation unit:
   - Wash your hands.
   - Obtain the meal tray for the patient. Check the meal card on the tray and check that the correct menu was provided.
   - Ask for the assistance of another member of the team.
   - Place the tray on the isolation cart.
   - Put on PPE as required by the type of isolation precautions used.

2. Enter the isolation room and identify the patient.

3. Explain what you plan to do.

4. Provide privacy.

5. Allow the patient to help as much as possible.

6. Raise the bed to a comfortable working height.

7. Pick up the meal tray that remains in the room. Make sure the tray is clean.

8. Return to the door and open it. The team member assisting holds the meal tray while you carefully transfer items to the isolation tray.

9. Place the isolation meal tray on the overbed table. Prepare the patient for the meal.

10. Check the patient's identification band against the meal tray card.

11. Assist the patient with food preparation and feeding as needed.

12. When the patient finishes, note how much food and liquid have been eaten. Uneaten food (except bones) is flushed down the toilet.

13. All disposable items (bones, dishes, eating utensils, covers, plastic wrap, foil, napkins, cups, cartons) are placed in the appropriate waste receptacle.

continues

PROCEDURE 7

continued

14. Reusable dishes may be handled as follows:
- Use a paper towel to open the door to the isolation unit.
- Prop the door open with your foot. Transfer dishes to a tray held by another assistant outside the door.
- Assistant outside the room covers the dishes and returns the tray to the food cart.

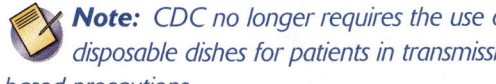 **Note:** *CDC no longer requires the use of disposable dishes for patients in transmission-based precautions.*

15. Clean the isolation meal tray and store it in the isolation unit.

16. Carry out all procedure completion actions.

17. Remove PPE and discard in the appropriate receptacle.

18. Wash your hands.

19. Use a paper towel to open the door to leave the isolation unit. Discard the towel before leaving the unit.

PROCEDURE 8

MEASURING VITAL SIGNS IN AN ISOLATION UNIT

Note: *Equipment to measure vital signs in isolation should be dedicated to the patient. (This means that the equipment will remain in the room with the patient.) If the equipment must be shared with other patients, it must be cleaned and disinfected before use with another patient.*

1. Before entering the isolation unit:
- Wash your hands.
- Remove your wristwatch and place it on a clean paper towel.
- Put on PPE as required by the type of transmission-based precautions used.

2. Pick up the paper towel with the watch. Enter the isolation unit.

3. With the watch still on the paper towel, place it where you can see it during the procedures.

4. Identify the patient and explain what you plan to do.

5. Provide privacy.

6. Allow the patient to help as much as possible.

7. Raise the bed to comfortable working height.

8. Using the equipment dedicated to the patient, measure vital signs.

9. Note the readings so you do not forget them.

10. Clean and store the equipment used according to facility policy.

11. Carry out all procedure completion actions (see Unit 15).

12. Remove and discard PPE according to facility policy.

13. Wash your hands, dry them, and pick up your watch.

14. Handling only the clean side of the paper towel, discard it in the appropriate receptacle.

15. Pick up your notes. Use a clean paper towel to open the door and leave the isolation unit. Discard the paper towel before you leave the unit.

Soiled linen is a source of pathogens and should be handled with care. (Refer to Procedure 11.) Some facilities place dirty linen in water-soluble bags that melt in the washer. If these bags are used, they must be placed inside a second plastic bag, because the water-soluble bag will begin to melt if it touches wet linen.

- Handle linen as little as possible.

- Fold the dirtiest side inward.
- Do not shake.
- Do not place soiled linen on the floor or tabletop.
- Bag linen before leaving the room.
- Keep soiled linen separate from general linen.
- Transport soiled, wet linen in a leakproof bag.

PROCEDURE 9

TRANSFERRING NONDISPOSABLE EQUIPMENT OUTSIDE OF ISOLATION UNIT

1. Nondisposable equipment used with a patient in transmission-based precautions may be dedicated to that patient. This means that the equipment remains in the isolation unit and is used only by that patient. Cleaning as required is done in the room by the nursing assistant or the housekeeping staff according to facility policy.

2. If the equipment must be used for other patients, it must be removed from the isolation unit and disinfected or sterilized before use with another patient.

3. Before leaving the isolation unit, clean the equipment with a disinfectant.

4. Place the equipment in a biohazard plastic bag.

5. Follow Procedure 6 for removing contaminated gloves, mask, and gown.

6. Pick up the bag containing the equipment and leave the isolation unit.

7. Once outside the unit, follow facility policy for disinfection or sterilization of the equipment.

8. Some equipment may be terminally (finally and completely) cleaned with disinfectant in the patient's unit when isolation is discontinued.

PROCEDURE 10

SPECIMEN COLLECTION FROM PATIENT IN AN ISOLATION UNIT

1. Outside the isolation unit, assemble equipment:
   - Clean specimen container and cover
   - Paper towel
   - Biohazard bag for specimen container (Figure 13-25)
   - Two completed labels, one for the specimen container and one for the specimen bag

   Note: The specimen bag may have a preprinted block on the bag that can be completed with the required information. In this case, a second label is not needed.

2. Place the equipment on the isolation cart while you put on PPE.

3. The biohazard bag for specimen transport remains outside the isolation unit.

continues

PROCEDURE 10

continued

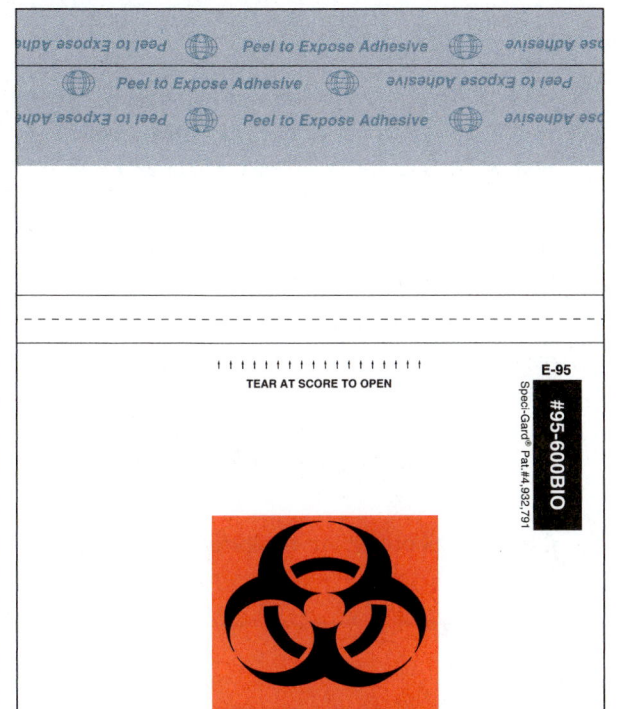

1) **Insert Specimen in Longer Pouch.**

2) **Pull Off Liner, Press to Close.**

3) **Insert Requisition into Outside Pocket.**

4) **Tuck Top of Requisition Under Flap.**

SPECI-GARD®
PAT.#4,932,791

FIGURE 13-25 Transport specimens in the sealed, labeled transport bag.

4. Carry the specimen equipment into the isolation unit. Place the container and cover on a paper towel.

5. Identify the patient and explain what you plan to do.

6. Provide privacy.

7. Allow the patient to help as much as possible.

8. Raise the bed to comfortable working height.

9. Place the specimen into the container without touching the outside of the container.

10. Cover the container and apply a label.

11. Clean the equipment used to obtain the specimen according to facility policy.

12. Carry out all procedure completion actions (see Unit 15).

13. Remove personal protective equipment as described in Procedures 5 and 6.

14. Wash your hands.

15. Use a paper towel to pick up the specimen container. Use another paper towel to open the door to leave the isolation unit.

16. Outside the unit, gather the towel in your hands so the edges do not hang loosely. Place the specimen container in the biohazard transport bag, being careful not to allow the paper towel to touch the outside of the transport bag.

17. Discard the paper towels in the appropriate receptacle.

18. Follow facility policy for transporting the specimen.

19. Wash your hands.

PROCEDURE 11

CARING FOR LINENS IN AN ISOLATION UNIT

1. Assemble any linen required and place on a chair or stand outside isolation unit.

2. Wash and dry your hands.

3. Outside the isolation unit, put on PPE as required by type of transmission-based precautions.

continues

PROCEDURE 11

continued

4. Once inside the isolation unit, place the clean linen on a chair.

5. Identify the patient and explain what you plan to do.

6. Provide privacy.

7. Allow the patient to help as much as possible.

8. Raise the bed to comfortable working height.

9. Remove the soiled linen from the bed by starting at the edges and working toward the center. Roll the linen toward the center with the soiled side inside.

10. Handle soiled linen as little as possible. Pick up the linen from the bed and hold it away from your uniform and gown (if used).

11. Place soiled linen in a meltaway laundry bag (a bag that dissolves in the wash water in the laundry), or follow facility policy.

12. Place the meltaway bag in a laundry hamper lined with a biohazard plastic bag, or follow facility policy. Bag should be labeled as biohazardous material for laundry.

13. Secure the bag and route soiled linen to the laundry according to facility policy.

14. If gloves are heavily contaminated from the soiled linens, remove gloves and dispose of them in the appropriate receptacle. Wash your hands, dry them, and put on a clean pair of gloves. Then remake the patient's bed with the clean linens.

15. Carry out all procedure completion actions (see Unit 15).

Transporting the Patient in Isolation

Sometimes a patient in isolation has to be transported to another area of the health care facility for treatment or testing. Notify the receiving unit of your intention to transport the patient and describe the type of transmission-based precautions being used. If the patient is on airborne or droplet precautions, the patient should wear a surgical mask while out of the isolation room. (HEPA masks are not used on patients.) If the patient is on contact precautions, the infectious area of the skin should be covered while the patient is out of the room. The nursing assistant wears personal protective equipment when picking up and returning the patient to the isolation room, but does not wear the personal protective equipment while transporting the patient in the hallway. (Refer to Procedure 12.)

You may remove your PPE after you have finished all tasks in the patient's room. Follow the instructions in Procedures 5 and 6.

Table 13-4 summarizes some rules for nursing assistants in the practice of infection control.

PROCEDURE 12

TRANSPORTING PATIENT TO AND FROM ISOLATION UNIT

1. Wash your hands.

2. Assemble equipment:
   - Transport vehicle (wheelchair or stretcher)
   - Clean sheet
   - Mask for patient, if isolation precautions require it

3. Notify the department to which patient is to be transported that a patient from an isolation unit is being transported.

4. If the patient is to be transported by stretcher, ask for assistance in moving the patient to the stretcher. Two other care providers will be needed.

continues

PROCEDURE 12

continued

5. Cover the transport vehicle with a clean sheet. Do not let the sheet touch the floor.

6. Wash your hands.

7. Put on PPE as required by type of precautions being used. If other care providers are needed to move the patient onto a stretcher, they also must put on PPE.

8. Wheel the transport vehicle into the isolation unit.

9. Identify the patient. Explain what you plan to do.

10. Provide privacy.

11. Allow the patient to help as much as possible.

12. If the patient is to be transported by wheelchair, the bed must be in the lowest horizontal position. For transport by stretcher, raise the bed to the same height as the stretcher.

13. Assist the patient into the wheelchair or onto the stretcher.

14. Put mask on the patient, if required.

15. Wrap the patient in a sheet, if required. Make sure the sheet does not touch the floor.

16. Remove PPE and wash your hands. Open the door and take the patient out of the isolation unit (Figure 13-26).

17. To return a patient to an isolation unit, place a wheelchair or stretcher near the wall of the room as you put on PPE.

18. Enter the isolation unit, unwrap the patient from the sheet and remove the patient's mask, if used.

19. Assist the patient from the wheelchair or stretcher (with help of other caregivers) and return the patient to bed.

20. Carry out procedure completion actions (see Unit 15).

21. Place the sheet in the laundry hamper for contaminated linens and discard the patient's mask in the receptacle for biohazardous trash.

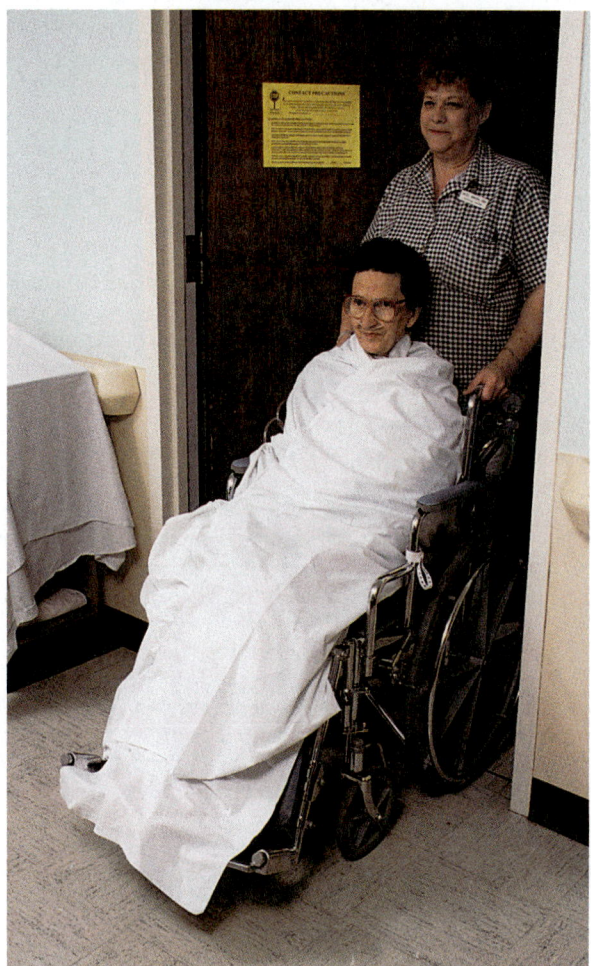

FIGURE 13-26 This patient is leaving her room, where contact precautions are in effect. The receiving area has been notified of her arrival.

22. Remove PPE and wash your hands.

23. Remove the transport vehicle from the isolation unit. Follow facility procedure for cleaning and storing the vehicle used for the patient in isolation.

24. Report completion of procedure: transport of patient in isolation to another department and back to isolation unit.

TABLE 13-4 RULES OF INFECTION CONTROL

Do

- Observe standard precautions and use barrier equipment (PPE) any time contact with blood, body fluids, secretions, excretions, mucous membranes, or nonintact skin is likely. Contact may be with a patient or an environmental surface.

- Clean up dishes immediately after use.

- Damp-dust daily and be conscientious about cleaning while you carry out a task.

- Provide a bag for the disposal of used tissues.

- Turn the face to one side so that the assistant and the patient are not breathing directly on each other.

- Cover your nose and mouth when coughing or sneezing.

- Protect the skin on your hands by using warm water, drying thoroughly, and applying lotion if needed.

- Treat breaks in the skin immediately by washing thoroughly, cleaning with an antiseptic, and covering. Report any breaks in the skin to the nurse.

- Disinfect equipment that is used by more than one staff member or patient, such as a stethoscope, before and after each use.

- Gather or fold linen inward, with the dirtiest area toward the center.

- Clean reusable equipment immediately after use.

- Handle and dispose of soiled material according to facility policy.

- Practice good personal hygiene.

- Wash your hands frequently.

- Keep clean and dirty items separate in patient rooms and storage areas.

- Bring only needed items into the patient's room.

- Keep soiled linen and trash covered in closed containers.

- Perform procedures in the manner in which you were taught.

- Empty wastebaskets frequently, if this is your responsibility.

Do Not

- Shake bed linens, because any microbes present could be released into the air.

- Allow dirty linen to touch your uniform.

- Eat or share food from a patient's tray.

- Borrow personal care items from another patient or employee, or use such items for another patient.

- Permit the contents of bedpans or urinals to splash when being emptied.

- Report for duty if you have an infectious disease.

- Permit linen to touch the floor, which is always considered dirty.

- Carry clean linen against your uniform or bring more linen than necessary into the patient's room.

- Store lab specimens in the refrigerator with food.

DISINFECTION AND STERILIZATION

Disinfection is the process of eliminating harmful pathogens from equipment and instruments. A chemical called a *disinfectant* is used for this procedure. You may be required to disinfect personal care items such as wash basins, bedpans, and urinals. You may also use disinfectants to clean wheelchairs and other furniture items. Items are usually washed before they are disinfected. The procedure for disinfection depends on the chemicals used. Follow the directions of your facility for use of disinfectants. Wear gloves and a gown for completing these procedures. You may also need a face shield. Wear PPE that is appropriate to the procedure.

Sterilization removes all microorganisms from an item. This process can be completed in an autoclave, which uses steam and pressure to kill organisms. Gas sterilization is also used in some health care facilities. Sterilization procedures are used for all nondisposable equipment that is exposed to potentially infectious materials. Equipment to be sterilized is wrapped in special material. Strips on the packaging material turn a particular color when the package is sterilized (Figure 13-27). Do not use the package if the strip has not turned the appropriate color. Do not use a sterilized package that has been accidentally opened.

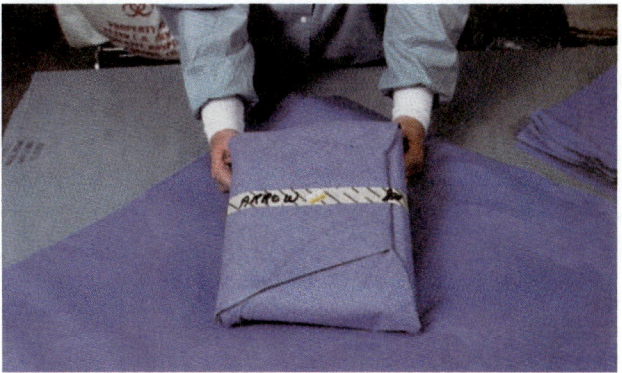

FIGURE 13-27 Indicator tape after exposure to sterilization process. Tape would not show stripes prior to sterilization.

STERILE PROCEDURES

Surgical asepsis is the means by which the environment is kept free of microorganisms, both pathogens and nonpathogens. In procedures where surgical asepsis is used, equipment and supplies must be sterile. In other words, items used in the procedure must go through a sterilization process.

In most facilities, nursing assistants are not expected to carry out procedures requiring sterile techniques. If you are responsible for sterile procedures, you should first be given thorough training. Your responsibilities may include opening sterile packages such as gloves. (See Procedure 13.)

PROCEDURE 13

OPENING A STERILE PACKAGE

1. Wash your hands.

2. Assemble equipment:
   - Sterile package

3. If color code has not changed, or seal does not look intact, do not consider article sterile. *If you have any doubt about sterility, consider item unsterile and inform the nurse.*

4. Touch only outside of package. Only sterile surfaces contact other sterile surfaces. Never reach over a sterile field.

5. Commercially prepared products will be sealed. If package is in poor condition or discolored, do not consider item sterile. Discard item.

6. Place package with fold side up on a flat, clean surface.

7. Remove tape.

8. Unfold flap farthest away from you by grasping outer surface only between thumb and forefinger (Figure 13-28A).

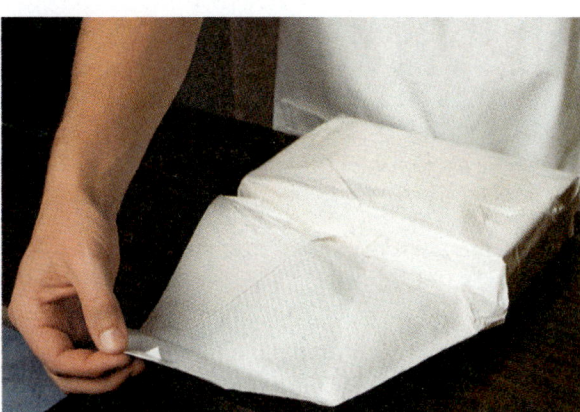

FIGURE 13-28A Touching only the corner, open the distal (top) flap away from your body.

continues

PROCEDURE 13

continued

9. Open right flap with right hand using same technique (Figure 13-28B).

10. Open left flap with left hand using same technique (Figure 13-28C).

11. Open final flap (nearest you) (Figure 13-28D). Touch only the outside of flap. Be careful not to stand too close. Do not allow your uniform to touch the flap as it is lifted free. Be sure the flaps are pulled open completely to prevent them from folding back over sterile items.

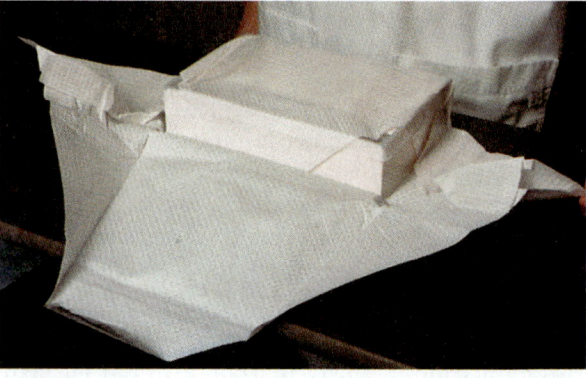

FIGURE 13-28C Carefully grasp the wrapper, opening the left side of the package.

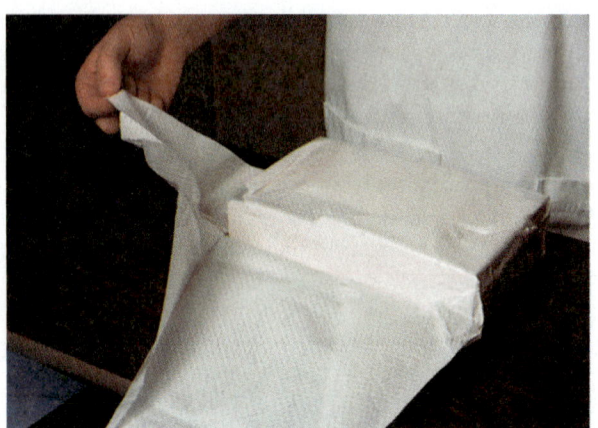

FIGURE 13-28B Open the right side. Avoid touching or crossing over the center of the package.

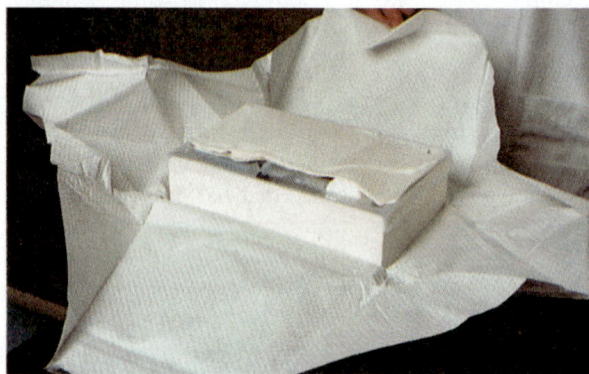

FIGURE 13-28D Open the proximal (closest) flap toward you. Avoid touching the flap or inside of the package with your hands or clothing.

Sterile Field

The term **sterile field** refers to an area of sterile equipment and materials. When working with a sterile field and sterile equipment, keep the following points in mind:

- The sterile field may be a table covered with a sterilized sheet or a sterile towel placed on an overbed table.
- Only the center of the towel is actually used.
- Equipment is kept two inches in from the edges all around, as an added precaution.
- Never reach for or pass anything that is unsterile over a sterile field. You might drop the unsterile article onto the field or touch the field. Instead, carry the unsterile object around the sterile field or hold it away from the sterile field.

- If there is even a suspicion that anything unsterile has touched any part of the sterile field, the field must be considered contaminated. The entire setup must be discarded.
- Coughing or sneezing while preparing a sterile field, or after the field has been set up, contaminates the field.
- Moisture means contamination. If a sterile towel is placed on an unsterile surface, any wetness on the towel means that the towel is contaminated. The towel and anything on the towel must be replaced.

REVIEW

A. True/False.

Mark the following true or false by circling T or F.

1. T/F When working in the droplet precautions room, always wear a HEPA mask.

2. T (F) Surgical masks may be reused.

3. T (F) It is permitted for two patients in the same room to share equipment.

4. (T) F Food and drink should not be kept where they may be exposed to contaminated materials.

5. T (F) When a patient is placed in transmission-based precautions, only licensed nurses are responsible for carrying out proper isolation technique.

6. (T) F Disposable patient care equipment is preferred when caring for a patient in isolation.

7. (T) F Droplet precautions do not require the use of a covering gown.

8. T (F) Handwashing should be done in cold water.

9. T (F) Always hold fingertips up when rinsing hands during handwashing.

10. T (F) Handling sterile equipment is a routine procedure for the nursing assistant.

11. T (F) A mask need not be worn if protective eye equipment is in place.

12. (T) F Asepsis is the absence of pathogens.

13. T (F) If an article is "clean," that means it is sterile.

B. Completion.

Complete the statements by writing in the correct word(s).

14. The single most important health procedure a nursing assistant can carry out is _handwashing_.

15. Accidental contact with infectious or potentially infectious materials is known as a/an _exposure incident_

16. Gloves, gown, masks, goggles, and face masks are part of _PPE_.

17. Small blood spills may be cleaned up by using _1/100 bleach_.

18. Sharps and needles should be disposed of by placing them in the _designated container_.

C. Complete the Chart.

In addition to standard precautions, indicate the transmission-based precautions required by each disease condition. Place an x to make your choice.

Disease	Airborne	Droplet	Contact
19. Draining infected pressure ulcer			✔
20. Tuberculosis	✔		
21. Mumps		✔	
22. Infected surgical wound			✔
23. Influenza		✔	

D. Multiple Choice.

Select the one best answer for each of the following.

24. Housing and caring for a person with an infection is known as
    a. segregation.
    (b.) isolation.
    c. sequestration.
    d. separation.

25. To remove PPE after caring for a resident on isolation precautions, you should
    a. remove the gown first.
    (b.) remove the gloves first.
    c. remove the mask first.
    d. remove PPE in any order.

26. If a nursing assistant is sensitive to latex gloves, he or she
    a. need not wear gloves.
    b. should wear the latex gloves anyway.
    (c.) should ask the supervisor for nonlatex gloves.
    d. should put powder in the gloves.

27. The basic foundation of medical asepsis is
    (a.) handwashing.
    b. wearing goggles.
    c. wearing a mask.
    d. wearing a gown.

28. If there is an exposure incident, you should
    a. ignore the situation.
    (b.) report it at once to the supervisor.
    c. call the doctor.
    d. tell other nursing assistants.

E. Nursing Assistant Challenge.

29. Mrs. Minion has just been placed on isolation. Your assignment is to set up the room.
    a. What equipment should be assembled and where is each item placed? _____
    b. What effect might being placed on isolation have on Mrs. Minion? _____
    c. What might you do to make her adjustment easier? _____
    d. How might her visitors feel? _____

30. You are reporting on duty. Some of your responsibilities will be handling food trays, making beds, straightening out your patients' overbed tables, and helping to change a patient who is wet with urine. During your shift you will use a facial tissue and visit the rest room.

List six times you will need to wash your hands.
    a. after bathroom
    b. enter room
    c. after changing patient
    d. before handling food tray
    e. after sneezing
    f. after leaving room

EXPLORING THE WEB

Description	Location
Infection control, medical asepsis, and sterilization	http://www.delmarhealthcare.com/pdf/0766824187_22.pdf
Infection control skills checklists	http://www.delmarhealthcare.com/olcs/acello/03checklists.pdf
Standard precautions	http://www.delmarhealthcare.com/olcs/white/pnotes.asp (see Chapter 22)
All the Virology on the WWW	http://www.tulane.edu
American Academy of Pediatrics Head Lice in Children	http://www.medem.com
Association of Professionals in Infection Control (APIC)	http://www.apic.org
Centers for Disease Control and Prevention (CDC)	http://www.cdc.gov
—CDC Evolution of Isolation Practices	http://www.cdc.gov/ncidod/hip/isolat/isopart1.htm
—CDC Guidelines and Recommendations	http://www.cdc.gov/ncidod/hip/Guide/guide.htm
—CDC Guidelines for Handwashing	http://www.cdc.gov/ncidod/hip/GUIDE/handwash_pre.htm
—CDC Guidelines for Long Term Care	http://www.cdc.gov/ncidod/hip/GUIDE/longterm.htm
—CDC Issues in Healthcare Settings	http://www.cdc.gov/ncidod/hip/DEFAULT.HTM
—CDC National Prevention Information Network	http://www.cdcnpin.org
—Guideline for Handwashing and Hospital Environmental Control	http://www.cdc.gov/ncidod/hip/guide/handwash.htm
—Guideline for Isolation Precautions in Hospitals	http://www.cdc.gov/ncidod/hip/isolat/isolat.htm
—Guidelines for Prevention of Tuberculosis in Healthcare Settings	http://www.cdc.gov/mmwr/preview/mmwrhtml/00001897.htm
—Overview of the Seven CDC Guidelines on Prevention of Healthcare Associated Infections	http://www.cdc.gov/ncidod/hip/guide/overview.htm
Clean Hands Campaign	http://www.washup.org
National Pediculosis Association	http://www.headlice.org
National Tuberculosis Center	http://www.umdnj.edu
OSHA Bloodorne Pathogen Fact Sheets	http://www.osha.gov/OshDoc/data_BloodborneFacts/index.html
Hidden Killers: Deadly Viruses	http://library.advanced.org
HIV InSite	http://hivinsite.ucsf.edu

Safety and Mobility

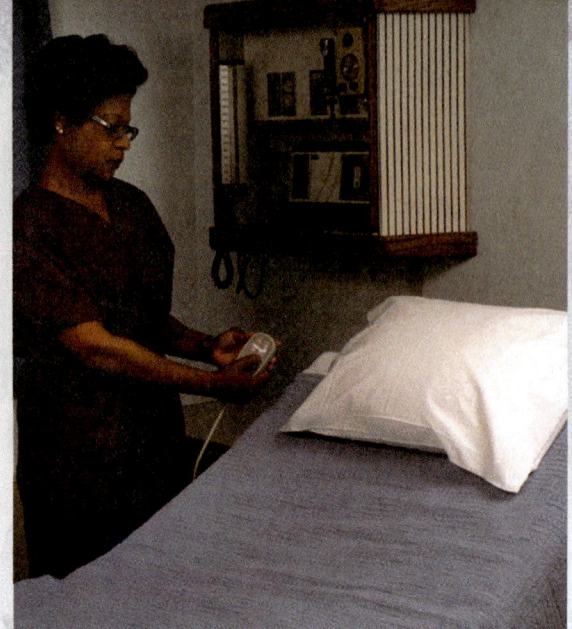

Environmental and Nursing Assistant Safety

objectives

After completing this unit, you will be able to:

- Spell and define terms.
- Describe the health care facility environment.
- Identify measures to promote environmental safety.
- List situations when equipment must be repaired.
- Describe the elements required for fire.
- List five measures to prevent fire.
- Describe the procedure to follow if a fire occurs.
- Demonstrate the use of a fire extinguisher.
- List techniques for using ergonomics on the job.
- Demonstrate appropriate body mechanics.
- List at least 10 guidelines for dealing with a violent individual.
- Describe the types of information contained in Material Safety Data Sheets (MSDS).

vocabulary

Learn the meaning and the correct spelling of the following words and phrases:

concurrent cleaning	incident report	private room	ward
environmental safety	Material Safety Data	RACE	workplace violence
ergonomics	Sheet (MSDS)	semiprivate room	
incident	PASS	side rails	

INTRODUCTION

The hospital room is the patient's home while he or she is hospitalized (Figure 14-1). The room becomes the patient's world. Cheerful and pleasant surroundings give the patient a better sense of well-being. Consistent attention to safety helps foster feelings of security in this strange environment. *Both* aid in speeding recovery.

The nursing assistant helps keep the patient's unit safe and clean. All health care providers share the task of keeping the entire nursing unit safe and clean.

Environmental safety refers to the condition of an entire facility—patient rooms, hallways, and all departments. The environment includes:

- Temperature (heating and air conditioning)
- Air circulation
- Light
- Cleanliness
- Noise control
- Walls, ceilings, and floors
- Plumbing
- Electricity
- Equipment and furniture

Prevention of injuries to patients, visitors, volunteers, and staff members is of primary concern.

THE PATIENT ENVIRONMENT

In a health care facility, the basic patient unit consists of a/an:

- Hospital bed with rails (Figure 14-2)
- Bedside table
- Chair
- Reading lamp

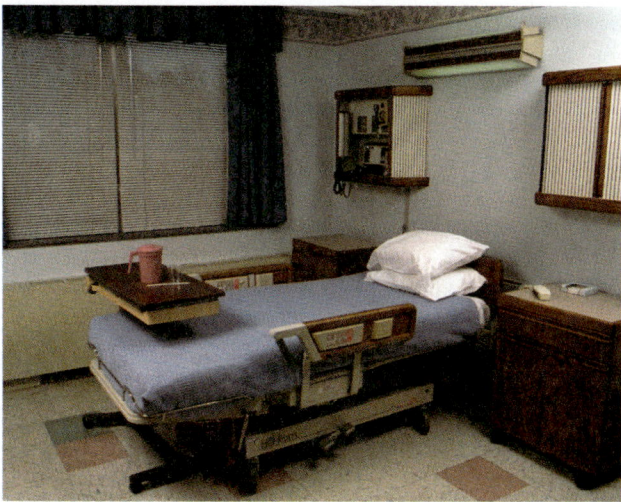

FIGURE 14-1 The patient's unit is his home during his stay in the hospital.

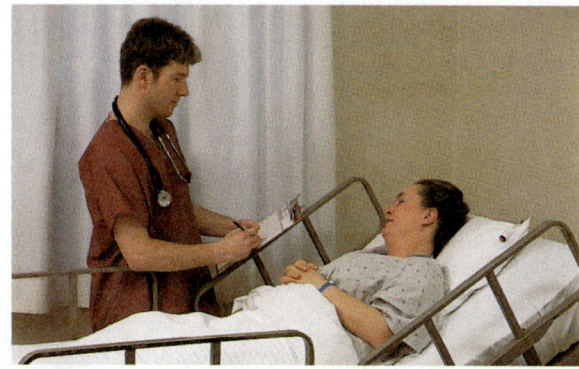

FIGURE 14-2 All hospital beds are equipped with side rails. These are split rails that can be raised and lowered in any combination.

- Waste basket
- Overbed table
- Signal cord

This equipment may be located in a single-, double-, or multiple-bed room. A **private room** contains only one bed. **Semiprivate rooms** contain two beds. **Wards** are multiple-bed rooms.

Each room is numbered. The beds are marked by letters or numbers. For example, Room 871 in a large medical center may be a four-unit ward. The beds are labeled A, B, C, D (or 1, 2, 3, 4). The patient in the fourth bed is in Unit 871–D or Unit 871–4.

The equipment from one unit should not be used by other patients. For home care, the same unit elements will be present, but they will be modified. For example, there may not be an adjustable hospital bed or an overbed table.

Hospital Beds

Hospital beds mostly have the same features, but there may be some differences. Hospital beds:

- Differ in the ways in which they operate. Some are controlled electrically (Figure 14-3). Others are operated by the turning of cranks or gatch handles (Figure 14-4).

OSHA*Alert*

Elevating the bed to a proper working height is one of the most important measures to use for protecting your back. If a gatch handle is used to elevate the bed, use good body mechanics by squatting down when you turn the handle. For patient safety, make sure you lower the bed when you leave the room.

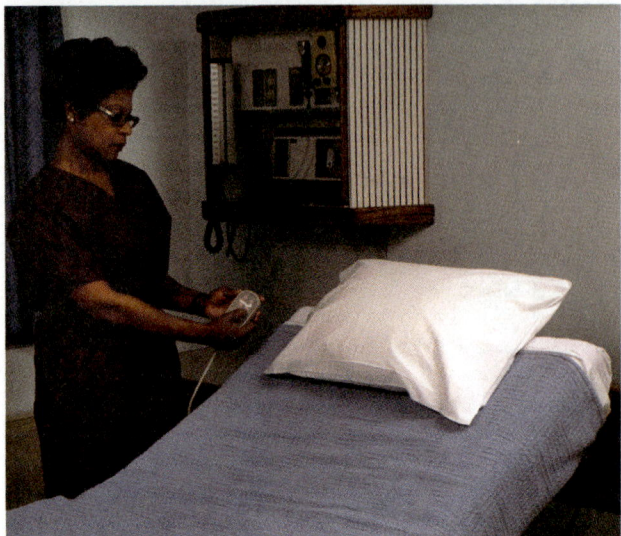

FIGURE 14-3 Electrically operated hospital beds may have foot controls, handheld controls, or controls mounted on the side to control the position of the bed.

- May be raised to a high horizontal position. In this position, there is less strain for those giving care. Beds must be returned to the lowest horizontal position when you leave the room.
- Are on wheels, to make it easy to move beds from one place to another. The wheels should always be locked unless the bed is being moved.
- Break in the middle so that the head may be raised.
- Break behind the knees to increase physical comfort for the bedridden patient.

Side rails are attached to the hospital bed. They protect the patient from falling. Side rails are considered to be restraints in some circumstances. Most health care facilities have policies, procedures, and guidelines describing their use. Potential benefits of side rails are that they:

- Provide support and a "handle" for the patient to use for turning and repositioning in bed.
- Provide a "handle" for getting into and out of bed.
- Give the patient a feeling of security.
- Reduce the risk of the patient falling out of bed when he or she is being transported in the bed.
- Provide access to bed and television controls that are part of the bed rail design.

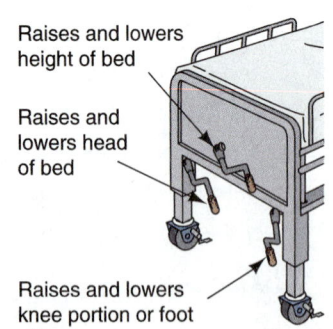

Raises and lowers height of bed

Raises and lowers head of bed

FIGURE 14-4 Gatch handles are used to change the position of nonelectric beds.

Raises and lowers knee portion or foot of bed

The potential risks of side rails include:

- Strangulation, suffocation, bodily injury, or death when the patient or part of the patient's body becomes entrapped between the bars of the side rails or between the side rails and the mattress.
- Serious injuries if the patient climbs over the rails and falls from this height.
- Skin tears, bruises, cuts, scrapes.
- Agitation caused by a feeling of being trapped or caged in.
- Feelings of isolation or restriction.
- Sadness because of loss of independence and having to call for help.
- Actual loss of independence, such as the ability to get up to use the bathroom or to retrieve an item dropped on the floor.

Several types of side rails are used on hospital beds. One type is a single rail that runs the length of the bed. Split rails are more common in acute care hospitals. Each side of the bed has two half-rails. One or both can be raised, depending on the patient's needs and plan of care. When side rails are used, they:

- Should be checked and attached securely before you leave the bedside, unless ordered otherwise.
- Should be down only when beds are in the lowest horizontal position, or if a release form has been signed by the patient.
- Should never be used for the attachment of tubes such as IV lines or catheters. Raising and lowering the side rails could put undue stress on such tubes and even pull them out.
- Should never be used for the attachment of restraints.

The use of side rails may upset some patients. Sometimes it may be necessary to reassure the patient that her condition is not becoming worse. The patient should be told that the raising of side rails is hospital policy or is being done as a reminder of a new environment.

Temperature, Air Circulation, and Light

As you adjust and maintain the temperature, light, and ventilation, keep in mind the patient's condition, the patient's personal preference, and the needs of the other patients in the room.

- The best temperature is about 70 degrees. A lower temperature may cause chilling and a higher one may make the patient uncomfortable.
- Movement of air and the temperature may be controlled by opening windows at the top and bottom if air conditioning is not being used. (In some facilities the windows are sealed shut.)
- Patients can be shielded from drafts by screens or curtains.

In most hospitals and health facilities, rooms are automatically air-conditioned. The thermostat may be set from a central location, or set individually in each patient's room.

Lighting comes from several sources. There will be times when less light is desired. At other times, more light will be needed (Figure 14-5). Use as much light as needed to safely carry out your job. Be careful to shield other patients as much as possible.

Patients often find it difficult to sleep if lights are too bright. There should be only enough light at night to enable the staff to work safely.

- Rooms are equipped with lights above each bed. These illuminate a single patient bed.
- There may also be a ceiling light.
- Additional spotlights can be brought from the utility room when needed to provide extra light for delicate procedures.
- The best lighting is indirect; glare causes fatigue.
- Be sure to return extra lights as soon as you are finished, because added clutter in a room is hazardous.
- Be sure to turn ceiling lights off when leaving the room.

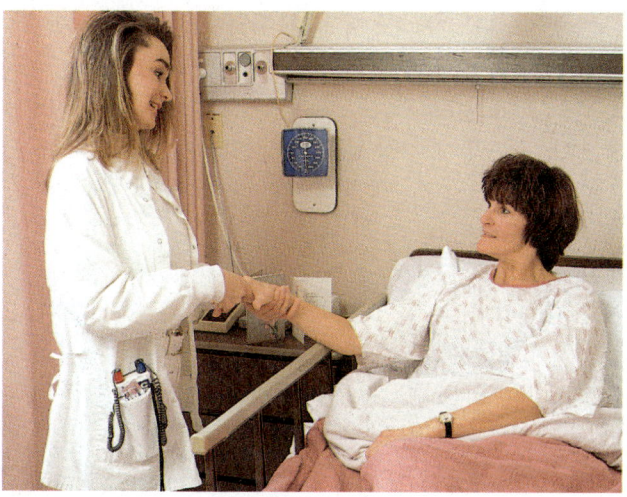

FIGURE 14-5 The overbed light can be adjusted to several different lighting levels.

INFECTION CONTROL *Alert*

Make sure clean and soiled items are separated in patient rooms and storage areas. Keep the lids tightly closed on trash cans and linen hampers. Avoid putting biohazard contaminated trash into open wastebaskets. Discard soiled items in a plastic bag or a covered trash can.

- Night lights are often left on for very ill or elderly patients.

Cleanliness and Noise Reduction

You are responsible for the cleanliness, quiet, and order of the patient units to which you are assigned. To contribute to the comfort of the patient:

- Speak quietly.
- Report squeaky equipment wheels that should be oiled.
- Avoid banging equipment and trays against other surfaces.
- Keep the area neat as you work. Check its overall appearance before you leave.
- Return equipment to its proper location after completing patient care.
- Do not turn the TV on or up while giving care to patients unless the patient asks you to do so.

You are responsible for keeping the patient supplied with fresh water, ice, disposable drinking cups, tissues, and straws. Make sure that all necessary pieces of equipment, such as the wash basin, emesis basin, bedpan, urinal, soap, and towels, are always available, clean, and in good condition (Figure 14-6). These items should always be stored in the bedside table.

INFECTION CONTROL *Alert*

When two or more patients share a room, make sure that all personal care items are labeled with each patient's name. Keep personal care items in the appropriate area. Store grooming supplies in a clean area. Avoid storing personal care equipment and supplies in community areas, such as bathrooms; storage in these areas increases the risk that personal care items will be used for the wrong patient(s).

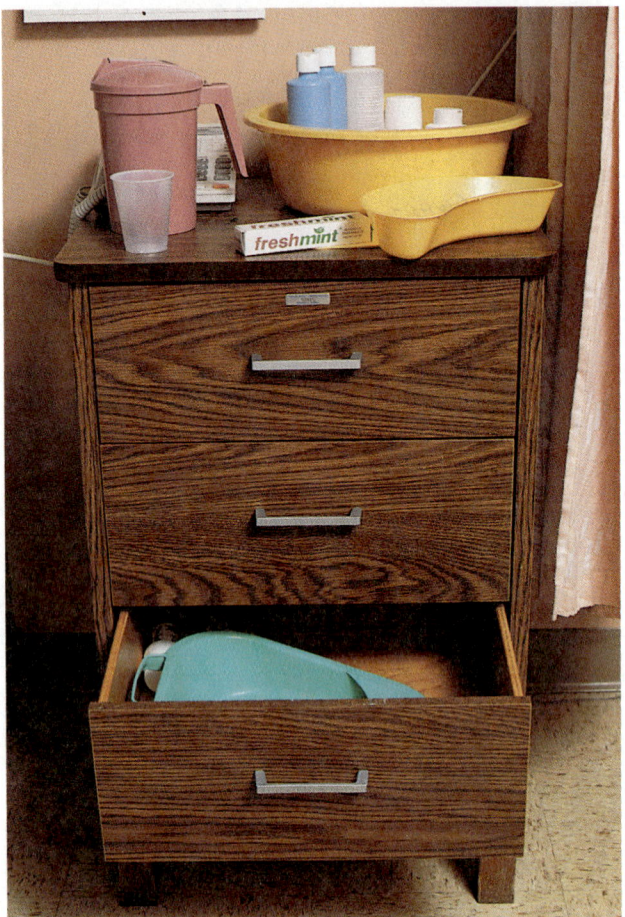

FIGURE 14-6 Personal care supplies are stored in the bedside stand. Items considered clean and dirty are stored in separate drawers.

SAFETY MEASURES

Safety is the responsibility of everyone. A safe environment is essential for both the patients and the staff. Safety must be a part of everything you do. This concern extends to the safety of the unit and the entire environment. The number of accidents involving patients and staff can be greatly reduced if simple measures are followed.

When an accident occurs in the health care facility, it is referred to as an **incident**. An incident is any unexpected occurrence or event that interrupts normal procedures or causes a crisis. Incidents can cause harm to a patient, employee, or any other person. If you see an incident or are involved in one, you need to report it to your charge nurse. The nurse fills out an **incident report** (Figure 14-7) after obtaining information from the persons involved. Prevention of incidents depends on employees:

- Knowing their jobs and following all policies and procedures related to safety
- Maintaining a safe environment
- Knowing the patients and implementing safety measures to decrease their risk of injury

Environmental Safety Conditions

Incidents can be prevented by keeping hallways and other walkways free of equipment and clutter. Most facilities require that all equipment that must be in the hall be kept on the same side of the hall. Report these situations promptly:

- Burnt-out light bulbs and light switches or electric plugs that do not work.
- Water leaks from faucets or pipes.
- Faucets or water fountains that do not flow properly.
- Loose or missing floor tiles.
- Windows that do not close tightly or are cracked or broken.
- Temperatures that are too hot or too cold and cannot be controlled within the room. (State licensing agencies have strict regulations regarding environmental temperatures.)
- Loose or missing ceiling tiles or leaks from the ceiling.
- Toilets that do not flush properly.

INCIDENT REPORT

Family Name	First Name	M.I.	Room No.	Hosp. No.

Address	City	State	Zip Code	Age	Sex M F

Date of Incident	Time ___ a.m. p.m.	Place	Attending Physician

Status of person involved: Patient _____   Employee _____   Visitor _____   Other _____

Diagnosis: _____

_____

Describe condition before incident: Disoriented ____ Senile ___ Sedated ___ Normal ___Other ___

_____

Was height of bed adjustable? Yes ___ No ___ Was bed up? Yes ___No ___ Was bed down? Yes ___ No ___
Were bed rails ordered? Yes___ No___ Were they present? Yes___ No ___ Were they up? Yes___No ___
Were they down? Yes ___ No ___ Other _____

Describe incident entirely, include part of body injured and treatment:

_____
_____
_____
_____
_____
_____
_____
_____
_____
_____
_____

Vital Signs: Temp _____   Pulse _____   Resp _____   Blood Pressure _____

Indicate on diagram location of injury

– over –

FIGURE 14-7 A special report is completed any time an incident occurs. *continues*

Was physician called? Yes_____ No_____ Time_____ a.m. p.m.

Who responded?_____ Time_____ a.m. p.m.
Attending physician_____ On-call physician_____

Statement of physician_____

_____

_____

_____

_____

Was family called? Yes_____ No_____ Time_____ a.m. p.m. Who:_____

Give names, addresses, and phone numbers of any who witnessed incident_____

_____

_____

A copy of this report will be sent to Patient's physician.

Date of Report_____ Signed_____
Signature and title of person preparing report

Nursing Office Review of Incident: Date_____ Signed_____

Comments:_____

_____

_____

_____

_____

FIGURE 14-7 *continued*

Equipment and Its Care

The daily or **concurrent cleaning** of equipment is an important part of your job. It contributes to the safety of your patient. The housekeeping department maintains environmental cleanliness. However, spills must be mopped up immediately to avoid falls.

In most health care facilities, equipment is tagged when it needs repair (Figure 14-8). That equipment is not to be used again until the tag is removed. Facility policy differs as to who is responsible for applying and removing the tag. Reporting broken or nonfunctioning equipment is the responsibility of everyone.

You can prevent accidents related to equipment by:

1. Reporting needed repairs promptly. Possible hazards include:
   - lost screws
   - frayed straps
   - loose wheels
   - broken control knobs
   - latches that do not hook
   - side rails that do not fasten correctly
   - faulty brakes on wheelchairs and stretchers
   - frayed electrical cords

2. Reporting immediately if call lights (signal cords) are not working.

3. Disposing of equipment in proper containers. Facilities must dispose of sharps, such as needles and blades, in special containers.

4. Never handling broken bits of glass with your hands. Put on gloves. Large pieces can be picked up with forceps. Broken glass can also be cleaned up using a brush or broom and a dustpan (Figure 14-9).

5. Always knowing what you are handling and the proper method for its disposal.

6. Inspecting mechanical lifts (Figure 14-10) carefully before using. Check:
   - Handle, to make sure legs open and close safely

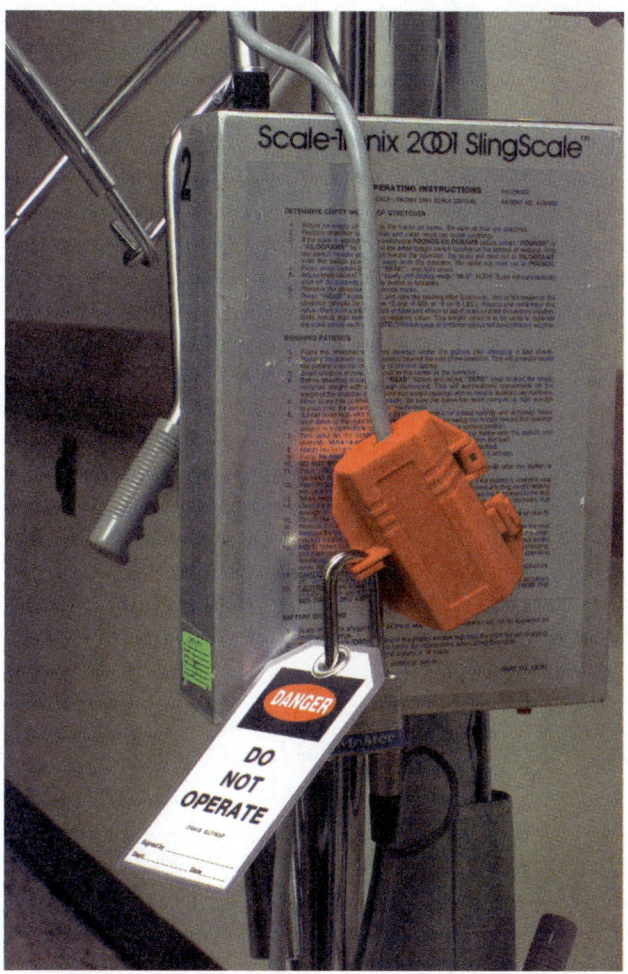

FIGURE 14-8 Unsafe electrical equipment is tagged and locked until it can be repaired.

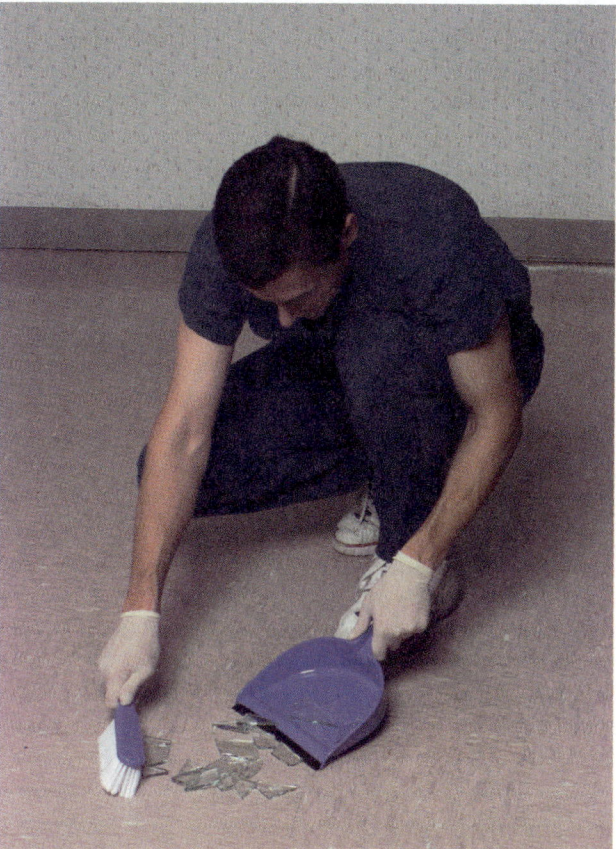

FIGURE 14-9 Never handle broken glass. Sweep it with a broom and dustpan or use an instrument to pick up large pieces. Wear gloves. Discard the glass in the proper container.

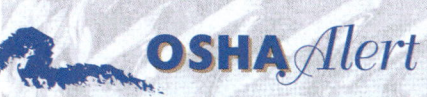

OSHA *Alert*

Handle needles, razors, and other sharp objects with care. Needles are never cut, bent, broken, or recapped by hand. After using a sharp object, dispose of it in a puncture-resistant "sharps" container. Avoid overfilling the sharps container. Seal the cap when it is three-quarters full. The cap is designed so it cannot be snapped back off after it is closed. The sealed sharps container is stored until it can be picked up with the biohazardous waste. The biohazardous waste disposal area is used for discarding items contaminated with blood or body fluids. Special precautions are taken to contain waste in this area.

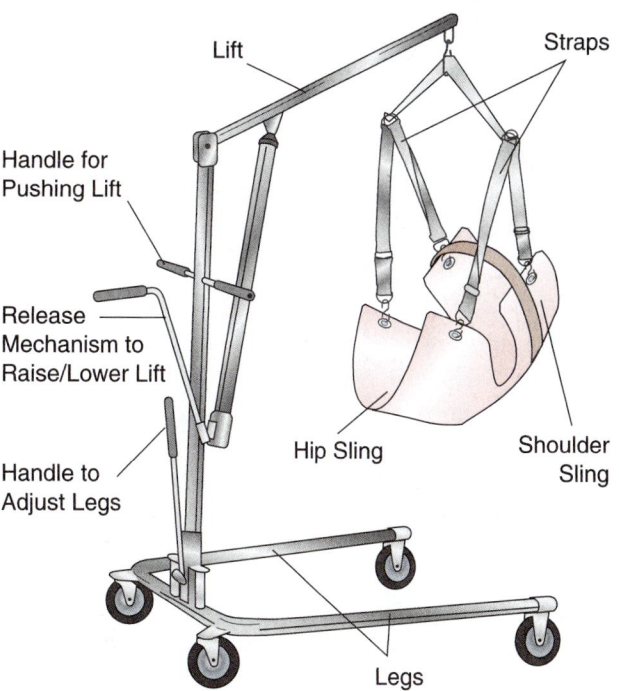

Lift

Straps

Handle for Pushing Lift

Release Mechanism to Raise/Lower Lift

Handle to Adjust Legs

Hip Sling

Shoulder Sling

Legs

FIGURE 14-10 Carefully examine the mechanical lift before using it.

- Release mechanism for raising and lowering lift
- All straps and chains for frayed areas or clasps that do not close correctly
- Sling, to be sure it is the right sling to use with that lift and that there are no frays or tears
- For hydraulic fluid on the floor—do not use the lift if fluid is present

7. Making sure that equipment and supplies are stored properly. Never block a doorway with equipment. Items in boxes should not be stored on the floor.

FIRE SAFETY

It is a scientific fact that if three elements are present in the right proportions (Figure 14-11), there will be a fire. The three elements are heat, fuel, and oxygen.

It is the responsibility of every staff member to know and regularly practice the fire and evacuation plans for the facility.

- Role-play the emergency procedures until you are completely secure. Remember that in any emergency the welfare and safety of the patients are most important.

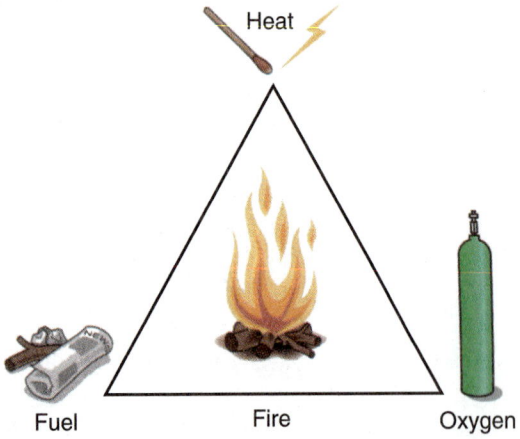

FIGURE 14-11 The fire triangle shows the elements needed to start a fire.

- Learn the location of escape routes and the location and operation of all fire control equipment (Figure 14-12), such as:
  - Fire alarms
  - Extinguishers
  - Sprinklers
  - Fire doors
  - Fire escapes
- Know and practice fire drill procedures. These are conducted on a regular basis by each facility. Many patients could be injured during a fire because of the confusion and their inability to help themselves.
- Keep alert to all possible fire hazards. Report them immediately to the proper authorities.

Fire Hazards

Some possible fire hazards include:

- Frayed electrical wires
- Overloaded circuits
- Plugs that are not properly grounded
- Accumulated clutter such as papers and rags
- Improper protection during oxygen therapy
- Uncontrolled smoking; most health care facilities prohibit smoking throughout the facility
- Matches left where children or others have unauthorized access to them
- Smoking in rooms where oxygen is in use

Fire Prevention

You and every staff member can do a great deal to prevent the disaster of fire. In general:

- Check for frayed electrical wires.
- Do not overload circuits with too many electrical cords.
- Do not use a lightweight electrical cord with equipment that draws a heavy power load.
- Use three-prong grounded plugs.
- Do not allow clutter to accumulate in doorways or traffic lanes.
- Empty wastepaper cans in proper receptacles.

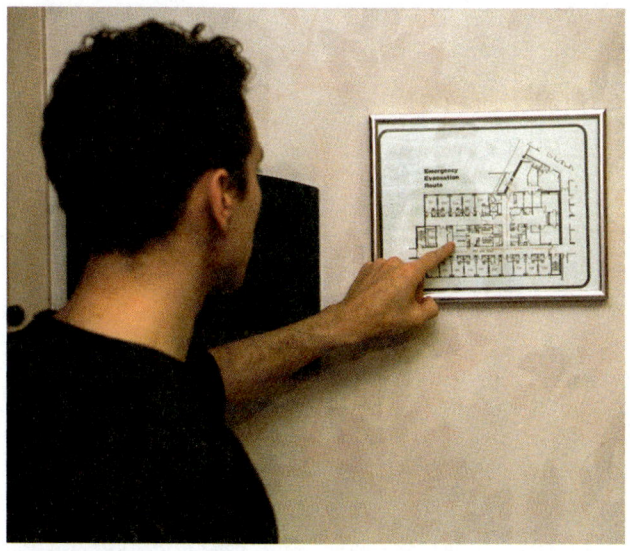 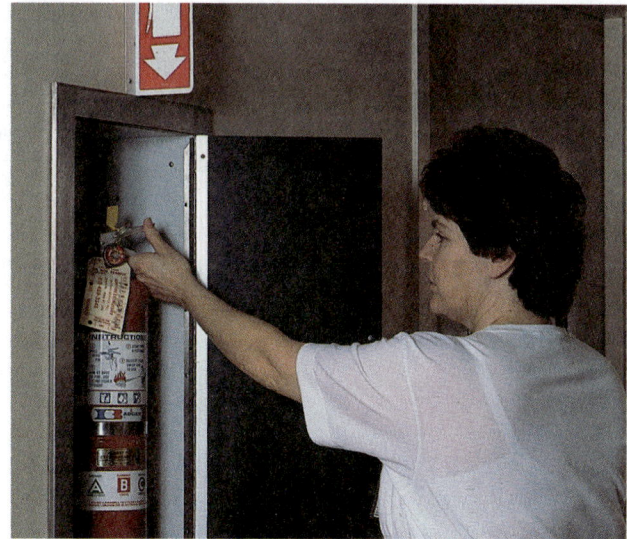

FIGURE 14-12 All personnel must be familiar with the evacuation plan, the location of fire extinguishers, and how to use them.

- Do not store oily rags or paint rags.
- Report any possible hazards right away.
- Report smoke and/or burning smells.
- Keep all fire exits clear of equipment and debris.
- Know and practice fire drill safety.
- Do not let visitors give cigarettes to patients.

Smoking

Smoking in bed should never be permitted. Smoking should be strictly limited to specific areas, if it is permitted at all. Most health care facilities do not permit smoking by anyone in any area.

This applies to patients, visitors, and staff alike. Ashtrays should be large. The use of matches should be watched. Smoking materials are usually stored at the nurse's station. Patients who do not have smoking privileges should not have smoking materials. If you notice that a patient who is not allowed to smoke has smoking materials, collect the materials and inform the nurse. Some patients may need direct supervision whenever they smoke.

Oxygen Precautions

The use of oxygen presents a specific hazard. When oxygen is in use:

- Never permit smoking, lighted matches, or open flames in the area.
- Do not use flammable liquids such as oils, alcohol, nail polish, aftershave, lotions, perfume, or hair spray.
- Do not use electrical equipment such as radios, hair dryers, electric razors, heating pads, or toys.
- Post a sign indicating that oxygen is in use.
- Use cotton blankets and gowns for the patient.

SAFETY *Alert*

Oxygen is a prescription item, like a medication. Using oxygen is safe as long as you follow facility policies and safety guidelines. Never change the fittings from one type of oxygen bottle to another. Make sure you use the correct adaptor and plug for the unit. Make sure the oxygen cylinder is secure in an upright position. If it is accidentally knocked over, it has the potential to turn into a missile and cause great damage. If you have reason to believe that an oxygen tank or liquid oxygen canister is leaking, remove the patient from the room and close the door. Report the problem to the proper person. Never attempt to carry or move an oxygen cylinder or canister if it is leaking.

SAFETY *Alert*

Bed linen can absorb oxygen. Any time oxygen is in use, avoid sparks. Static electricity can start a fire.

- Wear cotton uniforms and nonwool sweaters when providing care.
- Be certain there are no cigarettes, matches, or lighters in the room.
- Do not adjust the liter flow.

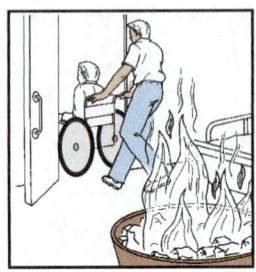 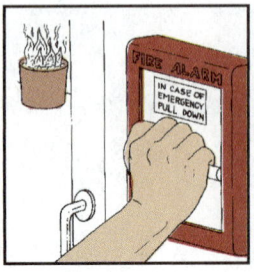 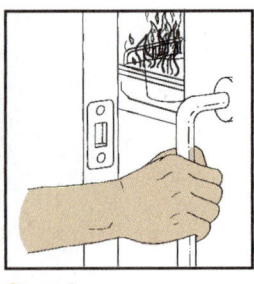 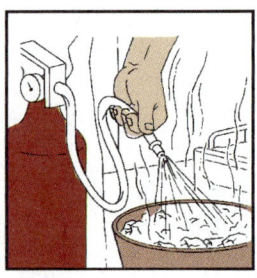 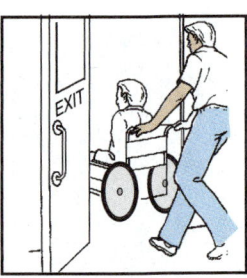

Remove   **A**ctivate   **C**ontain or   **E**xtinguish or   **E**vacuate

FIGURE 14-13 Remember the sequence of critical actions in case of fire.

In Case of Fire

You must be familiar with the fire policies and procedures for your facility. In case of fire, keep calm. Be sure those in immediate danger are moved to safety, then sound the alarm according to facility policy. Follow the evacuation plan as you have practiced. The patients may be confused and frightened. Therefore, the staff must be calm and in control. In a fire emergency, remember **RACE** as defined here (Figure 14-13):

- **R** = Remove patients. Move patients to safety. Patients who can walk can be escorted. In some cases, they may be called upon to assist others to escape routes. Patients may need to be moved in their beds out of the danger areas. If a person is unable to walk and the bed cannot be moved, bedsheets may be used as cradles and the patient pulled to safety.
- **A** = Alarm. Sound the alarm. Use the intercom, emergency signal bell, telephone, or fire alarm as directed by facility policy. Give the location and type of fire.
- **C** = Contain fire. Close windows and doors (Figure 14-14) to prevent drafts, which cause the fire to spread more rapidly.
- **E** = Extinguish fire or evacuate the area.

Follow the fire emergency plan for your facility:

- Keep calm. Be prepared to follow directions when a person in authority takes charge.
- Shut off air conditioning and other electrical equipment.
- Shut off oxygen.
- Do not use elevators.

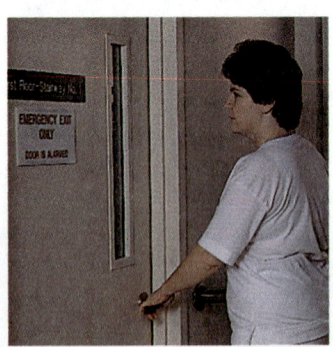

FIGURE 14-14 Fire doors slow the spread of fire when closed.

SAFETY *Alert*

Health facilities are built with safety features that prevent fires from spreading. These safety features include doors that close automatically when the fire alarm sounds, an automatic sprinkler system, smoke detectors, and fire exits. Many materials used on the floors, doors, walls, and furnishings are fire-rated. This means that they will take longer to burn. Nevertheless, fire prevention is an important responsibility. Despite the built-in safety features, health care facilities catch on fire. Many lives can be lost.

SAFETY *Alert*

When a fire occurs, patients are removed from immediate danger. After the alarm is sounded, the fire is contained by closing doors and windows. Patients are moved behind closed doors to keep them safe. Closing doors and windows slows the spread of fire. The hallways are cleared of patients and pieces of equipment that will burn. If the fire is large and spreading rapidly, patients may be evacuated from the building.

Use of a Fire Extinguisher

If you have been trained in the use of a fire extinguisher, you may use it on small fires.

- Fire extinguishers should be carried upright.
- Remove the safety pin.

SAFETY *Alert*

Smoke from a fire is very dangerous. If you are in a smoke-filled area, stay as close to the floor as possible. If you can crawl to an exit, cover your mouth and stay on your knees. The floor has the most oxygen available, because smoke rises. Before entering a room, touch the door with the *back* of your hand. *If the door is hot to the touch, do not open it.* If you are trapped in a room and the door is hot to the touch, stay in the room and place wet blankets or towels under the door to keep the smoke out. Opening the door could cause the fire to enter explosively.

- Push the top handle down.
- Direct the hose at the base of the fire.

Remember the letters **PASS**.

P—PULL the pin
A—AIM the nozzle at the base of the fire
S—SQUEEZE the handle
S—SWEEP back and forth along the base of the fire

OTHER EMERGENCIES

There may be other disasters for which you and your facility must be prepared. Tornadoes, hurricanes, floods, earthquakes, and bomb threats are examples of such disasters. Each facility has its own policies. Be sure you are familiar with them.

In all emergency situations, get patients to safety, follow your facility's policy, and keep calm.

VIOLENCE IN THE WORKPLACE

Episodes of violence in the workplace are increasing in our society. Hospitals and other health care facilities are not exempt from violence incidents. Serious violence has occurred in both rural and urban communities. Many facilities have violence prevention training programs. The goal of this training is to eliminate or reduce worker exposure to conditions that can lead to injury. OSHA has developed guidelines for preventing violence in the health care facility and many employers use these guidelines to implement safety programs and train their employees.

Workplace violence is any physical assault, threatening behavior, or verbal abuse that occurs in the workplace. The

SAFETY *Alert*

Although rare in some parts of the country, a tornado can occur anywhere. A *tornado watch* means that conditions are favorable for a tornado to develop. A *tornado warning* means that a tornado is actually in the area. Patients are not evacuated during a tornado watch. Someone is designated to monitor the weather in case the situation changes. During a tornado warning, you will help with the evacuation of patients. This means that all patients will be moved to the basement, if the facility has one. In multiple-story buildings, patients are moved to the lowest level. Frequently patients are moved to a strong area in the center of the building. Patients should not be moved to areas where there are windows, as flying glass may cause serious injuries. Evacuation must be done very quickly, as tornadoes strike with little warning. If patients cannot walk, they are moved in wheelchairs or beds. You may be instructed to cover patients with blankets to protect them from flying debris. You may also be required to close the room doors, fire doors, windows, and curtains facing the direction of the oncoming tornado. Do not go near the windows during the storm.

workplace includes, but is not limited to, the facility buildings and the surrounding perimeters, including parking lots, field locations, clients' homes, and traveling to and from work assignments. Workplace violence includes:

- Beatings
- Stabbings
- Suicides and attempted suicides
- Shootings
- Rapes
- Psychological traumas
- Threats or obscene telephone calls
- Intimidation
- Verbal or physical harassment
- Being followed, sworn at, or shouted at

Violence in the workplace can be committed by strangers, patients, coworkers, or personal acquaintances. Some of the potential causes of health care facility violence are:

- The prevalence of handguns and other weapons
- Use of hospitals by the criminal justice system for criminal holds and the care of disturbed, violent individuals

- Acute and chronically mentally ill patients
- Individuals who abuse alcohol and drugs
- The availability of controlled substances in the facility, making it a likely target of robbery
- The increasing number of gangs and gang members in many communities
- Unrestricted movement of the public in health care facilities
- Drug and alcohol abuse

- Distraught family members and other individuals who become angry and frustrated
- Low staffing levels, particularly during meals and at other times when staff is busy caring for patients and unable to observe activity in the hallways
- Poorly lit parking lots, garages, and ramps
- Lack of staff awareness of risk factors
- Failure to use safety precautions, such as locking doors and reporting suspicious individuals

guidelines *for*

Violence Prevention

Follow all facility policies and procedures involving safety and security. Other things you can do to prevent potential incidents are:

- Participate in continuing education programs to learn how to recognize and manage escalating agitation, assaultive behavior, or criminal intent.
- Attend classes on cultural diversity that offer sensitivity training on racial and ethnic issues and differences.
- If you are responsible for a secured area, control access to the area and keep it locked. Avoid propping locked doors and windows open. Never disable a door alarm.
- Do not leave keys unattended. Never share security alarm codes with unauthorized persons.
- Close shades or curtains at night.
- Report assaults or threats of assaults to the nurse manager immediately.
- Avoid wearing scarves, necklaces, earrings, and other jewelry that could cause injury if a patient or other individual attacks you.
- Do not carry valuables or large sums of cash to work.
- Avoid remote, dark areas when you are alone.

- Report lights that are burned out and locks that are not working.
- Exercise caution in elevators, stairwells, and unfamiliar areas. Immediately leave the area if you believe a hazard exists.
- Use the "buddy system" if personal safety may be threatened.
- If a patient or other person is "acting out," or you believe you may be assaulted, do not let the person come between you and the exit.
- Keep your head up, look ahead, and be aware of your surroundings.
- If your facility has security personnel, request that they escort you in dark or potentially dangerous areas. If no security personnel are on duty, ask other staff members to accompany you.
- Park in well-lighted areas. Always lock your car after parking. Look in the car before getting in, then lock the doors after you get in. Do not roll windows down to speak with individuals approaching your car.
- Report suspicious individuals or other potential safety hazards to the proper person. Never approach a suspicious person by yourself.

guidelines *for*

Dealing with a Violent Individual

- Remain calm and avoid raising your voice, which may further agitate the person.
- Speak slowly, softly, and clearly.
- Call for help, if possible, or send someone to get help.
- Move away from heavy or sharp objects that may be used as weapons.

- Monitor your body language and avoid movements that could be challenging, such as placing your hands on your hips, moving toward the person, pointing your finger, or staring directly at the person. However, focus your attention on the person so you know what he or she is doing at all times.

continues

guidelines *continued*

- Position yourself at right angles to the person. Avoid standing directly in front of him or her. Maintain a distance of 3 to 6 feet.
- Position yourself so that an exit is accessible. Never let the person come between you and the exit.
- Avoid making sudden movements.
- Listen to what the person is saying. Encourage the person to talk, and communicate that you genuinely care and will try to help. Acknowledge that you understand that he or she is upset. Break big problems into smaller, manageable ones.
- Avoid arguing and defensive statements. Accept criticism in a positive way. If you sincerely feel criticism is unwarranted, ask clarifying questions.
- Ask the person to leave and return when he or she is calmer.
- Ask questions to help regain control of the conversation.
- Avoid challenging, bargaining, or making promises you cannot keep.
- Describe the consequences of abusive behavior.
- Avoid touching an angry person.
- If a weapon is involved, ask the person to place it in a neutral location while you continue talking. Avoid trying to disarm the person, which may put you in danger.

NURSING ASSISTANT SAFETY

The work performed by nursing assistants requires a great deal of lifting and moving of patients, objects, and equipment. It is important that you use your body correctly to avoid injury.

Ergonomics

The word **ergonomics** means adapting the environment and using techniques and equipment to prevent injury to the body. If certain risk factors are present, it is more likely that an ergonomic (work-related) problem will occur. These risk factors include:

1. Performing the same motion or motion pattern every few seconds for more than two to four hours at a time.
2. Being in a fixed or awkward posture for more than a total of two to four hours.
3. Using forceful hand exertions for more than two to four hours at a time.
4. Doing heavy lifting, unassisted, for more than one to two hours.

Here are several ergonomic techniques you can use to reduce the risk of having an incident:

1. Use correct body mechanics at all times, both at work and when you are off duty.
2. Raise beds to a comfortable working height (remember to lower the beds when you finish your task).
3. Use mechanical lifts when you need to transfer very heavy and/or dependent patients from the bed or chair and back.
4. Use back supports if your employer requires them or if this is your preference. The use of back supports is controversial, but many nursing assistants find them helpful (Figure 14-15).

5. Get another person to help when you need to transfer a patient who cannot bear his own weight fully.
6. Use a cart to move heavy items.

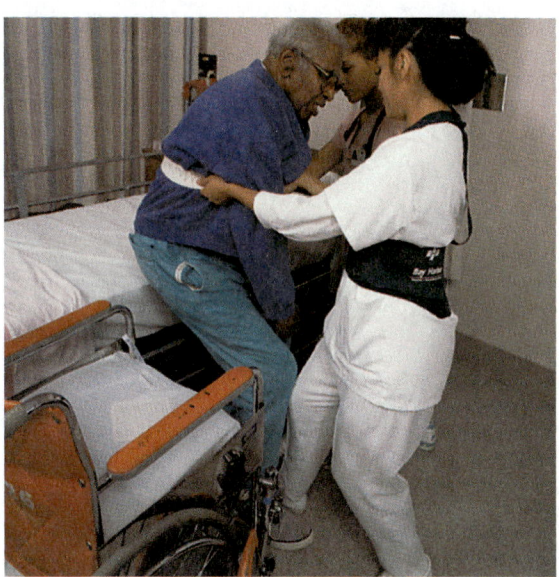

FIGURE 14-15 Some employers require employees to wear back support belts when lifting and moving patients.

OSHA *Alert*

The back support belt works by keeping your spine in good alignment. You are less likely to be injured if your spine is straight and you are using good body mechanics. Do not lift more than you would if you were not wearing the belt. Using a back support belt does not make you stronger.

If you follow these eight commandments for lifting, you will greatly decrease the risk of injuring yourself.

1. Plan your lift and test the load (Figure 14-16A).
2. Ask for help (Figure 14-16B).
3. Get a firm footing (Figure 14-16C).
4. Bend your knees (Figure 14-16D).
5. Tighten your abdominal muscles (Figure 14-16E).
6. Lift with your legs (Figure 14-16F).
7. Keep the load close (Figure 14-16G).
8. Keep your back upright (Figure 14-16H).

Warming up before working is another way to maintain a healthy body. The exercises shown in Figures 14-17A through 14-17J can be performed before each work shift. Check with your physician before beginning any exercise program.

Remember that you can avoid many problems if you also:

- Exercise every day.
- Eat a nourishing, well-balanced diet.
- Get adequate sleep.
- Avoid alcohol, cigarettes, drug use, and too much caffeine.
- Wear comfortable shoes with good support.

SAFETY *Alert*

Have you ever heard the expression, "When your feet hurt, you hurt all over"? Most experienced health care workers will tell you this old adage is true. Buying a sturdy pair of athletic shoes or duty shoes is one of the best investments you will make in your uniform. Make sure that the shoe soles are appropriate for the floor surface in your facility. In most cases, this means having a nonslip sole. Having proper footwear will make you feel better and reduce your risk of falls and injuries.

Hazards in the Work Environment

All health care facilities have hazards in the work environment that can potentially cause injury to employees. Many of these items are chemicals that you may have in your own home (chlorine bleach, for example). On a nursing unit you might find cleaning supplies, disinfectants, and other

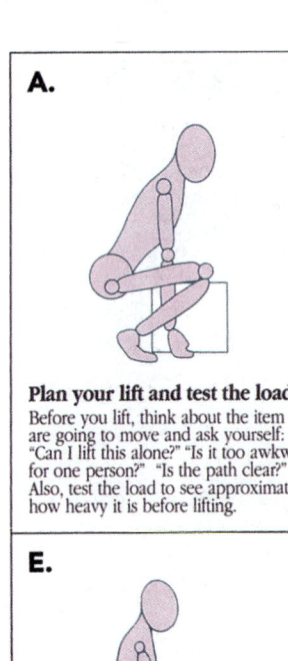

A.

Plan your lift and test the load.
Before you lift, think about the item you are going to move and ask yourself: "Can I lift this alone?" "Is it too awkward for one person?" "Is the path clear?" Also, test the load to see approximately how heavy it is before lifting.

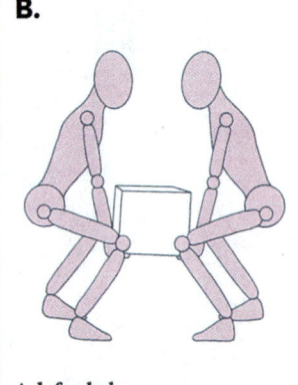
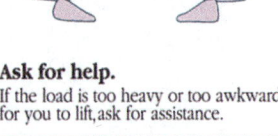

B.

Ask for help.
If the load is too heavy or too awkward for you to lift, ask for assistance.

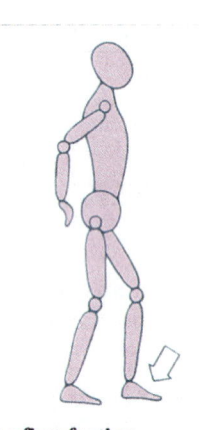

C.

Get a firm footing.
Keep your feet apart for a stable base and point your toes out.

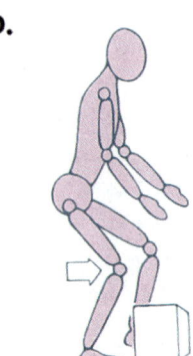

D.

Bend your knees.
Don't bend at the waist. Keep the principles of leverage in mind at all times. Don't do more work than you have to.

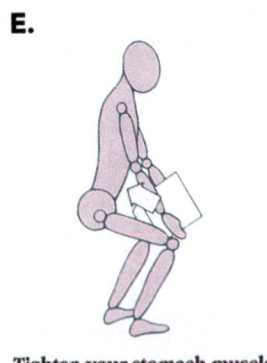

E.

Tighten your stomach muscles.
Use intra-abdominal pressure to support your spine when you lift, offsetting the force of the load. Train your muscles to work together.

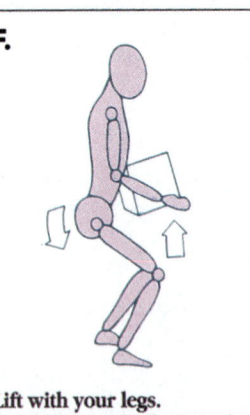

F.

Lift with your legs.
Let your leg muscles do the work of lifting. Don't rely on your weaker back muscles.

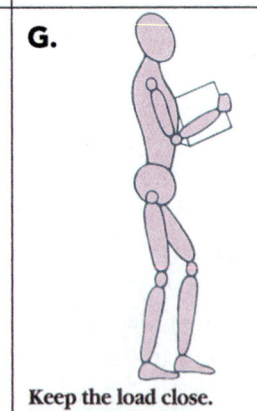

G.

Keep the load close.
Don't hold the load away from your body. The closer it is to your spine, the less force it exerts on your back.

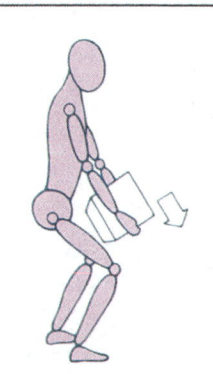

H.

Keep your back upright.
Whether lifting or putting down the load, don't add the weight of your body to the load. Avoid twisting.

FIGURE 14-16 Eight rules for lifting. *(Reprinted with permission from Ergodyne Corporation, St. Paul, MN)*

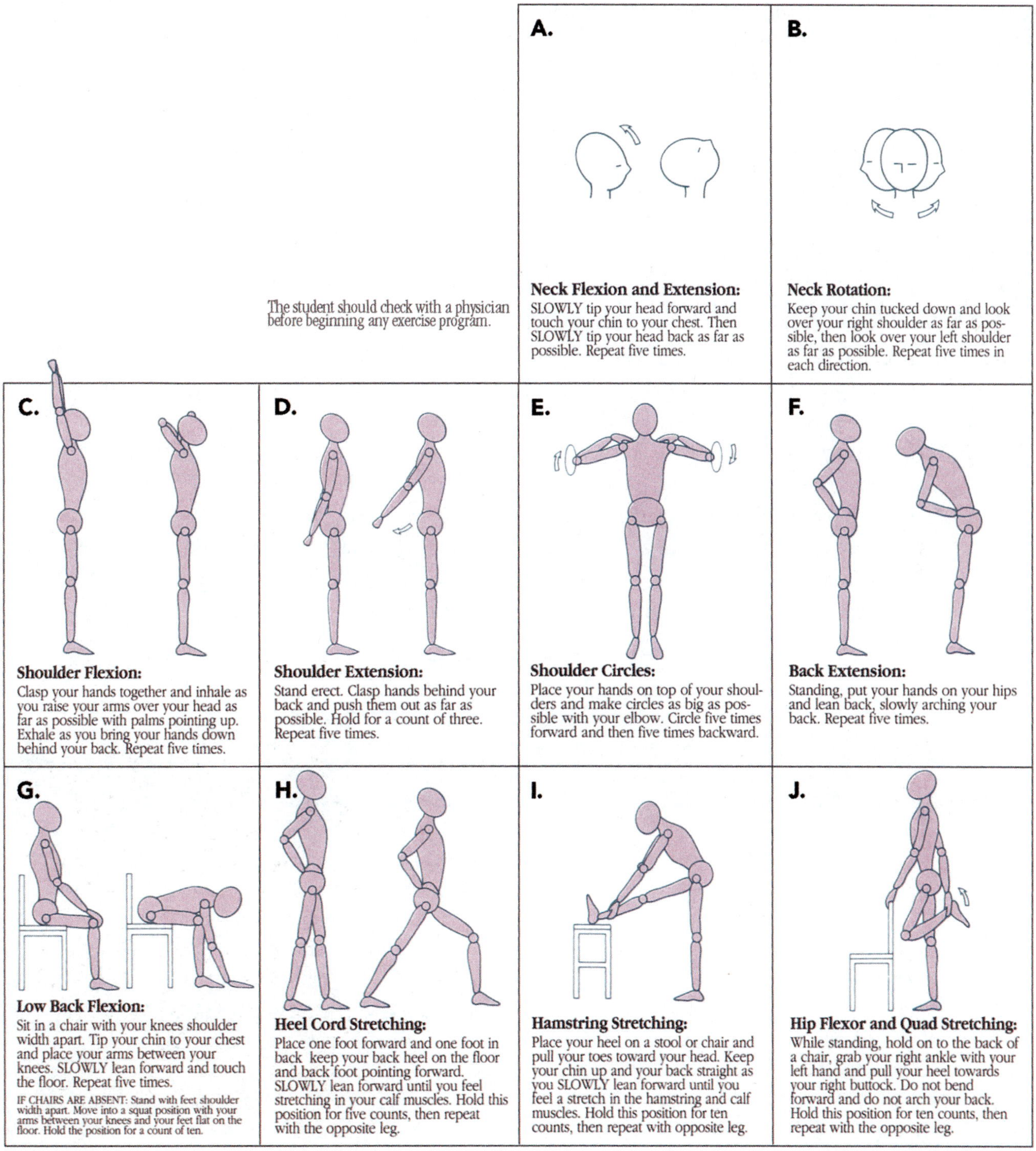

The student should check with a physician before beginning any exercise program.

A.

Neck Flexion and Extension:
SLOWLY tip your head forward and touch your chin to your chest. Then SLOWLY tip your head back as far as possible. Repeat five times.

B.

Neck Rotation:
Keep your chin tucked down and look over your right shoulder as far as possible, then look over your left shoulder as far as possible. Repeat five times in each direction.

C.

Shoulder Flexion:
Clasp your hands together and inhale as you raise your arms over your head as far as possible with palms pointing up. Exhale as you bring your hands down behind your back. Repeat five times.

D.

Shoulder Extension:
Stand erect. Clasp hands behind your back and push them out as far as possible. Hold for a count of three. Repeat five times.

E.

Shoulder Circles:
Place your hands on top of your shoulders and make circles as big as possible with your elbow. Circle five times forward and then five times backward.

F.

Back Extension:
Standing, put your hands on your hips and lean back, slowly arching your back. Repeat five times.

G.

Low Back Flexion:
Sit in a chair with your knees shoulder width apart. Tip your chin to your chest and place your arms between your knees. SLOWLY lean forward and touch the floor. Repeat five times.
IF CHAIRS ARE ABSENT: Stand with feet shoulder width apart. Move into a squat position with your arms between your knees and your feet flat on the floor. Hold the position for a count of ten.

H.

Heel Cord Stretching:
Place one foot forward and one foot in back keep your back heel on the floor and back foot pointing forward. SLOWLY lean forward until you feel stretching in your calf muscles. Hold this position for five counts, then repeat with the opposite leg.

I.

Hamstring Stretching:
Place your heel on a stool or chair and pull your toes toward your head. Keep your chin up and your back straight as you SLOWLY lean forward until you feel a stretch in the hamstring and calf muscles. Hold this position for ten counts, then repeat with opposite leg.

J.

Hip Flexor and Quad Stretching:
While standing, hold on to the back of a chair, grab your right ankle with your left hand and pull your heel towards your right buttock. Do not bend forward and do not arch your back. Hold this position for ten counts, then repeat with the opposite leg.

FIGURE 14-17 Warming up before work can help prevent injuries. *(Reprinted with permission from Ergodyne Corporation, St. Paul, MN)*

products that are considered hazardous. Injuries can be prevented if you know what the hazards are and how to protect yourself and others. The Occupational Safety and Health Administration (OSHA) is a section of the Department of Labor under the federal government. OSHA is responsible for employee safety. OSHA requires that all manufacturers of these items supply **Material Safety Data Sheets** (**MSDS**) with any hazardous products they sell. The MSDS provide hazard communications that explain:

- What precautions to take in the presence of a hazard (for example, wearing personal protective equipment)

- Instructions for safe use of the potentially dangerous substance

- How to clean up and dispose of the hazardous product

- First aid measures to use if exposure occurs

OSHA has also established other rules for a safe environment. Employers are required to inform employees of:

- The location of the MSDS
- The hazards that exist in the work environment and where they are in the building
- The location of information related to the hazards
- How to read and understand chemical labels and hazard signs

- What type of personal protective equipment should be worn while working with these chemicals, and where the personal protective equipment is stored
- How to manage spills and where cleaning equipment is stored

All hazardous products must be kept in their original containers with the original labels intact and legible. Health care facilities must keep all chemicals in locked cupboards.

OSHA *Alert*

Many chemicals can be hazardous to both patients and nursing assistants. Always use chemicals according to the directions on the label. Make sure they are properly diluted and that containers and surfaces are properly rinsed. Never repackage chemicals into unmarked containers. Use only the original container or special, small containers provided by the manufacturer. Chemicals should always be under your visual control, meaning you can see them. If you cannot see a chemical, it should be stored in a locked area. Wear utility gloves when using chemicals for cleaning procedures. Many chemicals will cause defects in the examination gloves used for patient care. This can irritate your hands, and the chemicals may be absorbed through your skin. Wear eye protection if there is a possibility of splashing or spraying chemicals during a cleaning procedure. Learn the locations of your facility's MSDS sheets, eye wash station, and body wash station.

REVIEW

A. Multiple Choice.

Select the one best answer for each of the following.

1. The patient's name is Phe Quan. She is in Room 116-D. From this information, you know that she is occupying a bed in a
   a. private room.
   b. rehabilitation department.
   c. semiprivate room.
   d. ward.

2. Side rails should be up and secure when
   a. the bed is at the lowest horizontal height.
   b. the patient has a catheter.
   c. leaving the patient after care, unless there is a signed release.
   d. the patient does not have an order for restraints.

3. The best room temperature is approximately
   a. 45°F.
   b. 65°F.
   c. 70°F.
   d. 78°F.

4. Which of the following represents a fire hazard?
   a. Frayed electrical wire
   b. Using three-prong plugs
   c. Supervised smoking
   d. Using UL-approved items

5. Ashtrays should be emptied into
   a. a plastic container.
   b. a metal container.
   c. a paper sack.
   d. the open wastebasket.

6. Which of the following contributes to unsafe conditions in the facility?
   a. Equipment sitting in the halls
   b. Chemicals in locked cupboards
   c. Allowing patients to smoke with supervision
   d. Teaching patients how to use assistive devices such as canes and walkers

7. When oxygen is in use, you should not
   a. use cotton blankets on the patient's bed.
   b. remove cigarettes from the room.

c. adjust the liter flow.

d. post a sign on the door.

8. Every staff member should know

   a. the facility fire procedure.

   b. the RACE procedure.

   c. the distance from the fire department to the facility.

   d. how to extinguish a fire by aiming the extinguisher at the top of the flames.

9. The word that means adapting the environment to prevent body injury is

   a. body mechanics.

   b. incident.

   c. ergonomics.

   d. RACE.

10. One principle of good body mechanics is to

   a. bend from the waist when lifting.

   b. keep your feet close together when lifting.

   c. use the strong muscles of your arms for lifting.

   d. keep the load as far from your body as possible.

11. Material Safety Data Sheets (MSDS) are required to include information that

   a. describes how to repackage the product.

   b. explains first aid measures to use if exposure occurs.

   c. describes how to use the product.

   d. lists other approved uses of the product.

12. When dealing with a potentially violent individual, the nursing assistant should

   a. speak loudly and clearly.

   b. maintain a distance of 2 feet.

   c. listen to what the person is saying.

   d. attempt to touch the person gently.

B. Completion.

Choose the correct word from the following list to complete each statement in questions 12–20.

1 body mechanics	4 mechanical lift
2 call light	7 Material Safety Data
3 ergonomics	8 Sheets (MSDS)
4 hips and knees	8 OSHA
5 incident	9 RACE

13. Using your body correctly while you are working is called ___1___.

14. Basic rules for lifting include bend from the ___4___ and not from the waist.

15. An unexpected situation that can cause harm to an employee, a patient, or a visitor is called (a, an) ___5___.

16. Adapting the environment and using techniques and equipment to prevent body injury is called ___3___.

17. You should use a ___6___ when you need to transfer very heavy or dependent patients.

18. All patients must have access to a ___2___ because it may be the only way they have to summon help.

19. All manufacturers must supply ___7___ with the hazardous products they sell.

20. The section of the federal government that oversees employee safety is called ___8___.

21. The acronym used to remember the sequence of critical actions in case of fire is ___9___.

C. True/False.

Mark the following true or false by circling T or F.

22. **T** F The bed should be left in the lowest horizontal position when the patient is sleeping.

23. **T** F Side rails are restraints in certain circumstances.

24. **T** F There should always be enough light to enable staff to work safely.

25. **T** F Noise and clutter are very disturbing to most people.

26. **T** F Needed repairs should be reported immediately.

27. **T** F The signal cord is the patient's way of letting the staff know that he is in need.

28. T **F** It is all right to play while at work as long as no one gets hurt.

29. **T** F You are responsible for knowing and practicing fire drill procedures.

30. T **F** In case of a fire, follow your own plan of action.

31. T **F** It is wise to use an elevator during a fire emergency.

D. Nursing Assistant Challenge.

Mary Hernandez is a new nursing assistant at Community Memorial Hospital. She has just completed her CNA course. Consider the information she needs to receive in orientation in order to be a safe and efficient worker.

32. What information does Mary need to learn about the facility to prevent fires and to follow correct procedure in the event of a fire?

33. Mary will need information on equipment she will be working with. What items of equipment is she likely to be using on her job?

34. Discuss everything Mary can do to prevent work-related injuries.

35. What chemicals is she likely to be using?

EXPLORING THE WEB

Description	Location
Ergonomics articles	*http://www.hill-rom.com*
Safety/hygiene	*http://www.delmarhealthcare.com/olcs/white/pnotes.asp* (see Chapter 20)
Back Belts: Do They Prevent Injury?	*http://www.cdc.gov/niosh/backbelt.htm*
Back Care for Nurses	*http://www.phil-e-slide.com* *http://www.spineuniverse.com*
Back Injury Prevention	*http://www.twcc.state.tx.us*
Back Injury Prevention Guide for Health Care Providers	*http://165.235.90.100/DOSH/dosh_publications/backinj.pdf*
Back Safety	*http://www.mmhospital.org*
Example Safety Program and Policies	*http://www.costaffing.com*
Fire Safety	*http://www.nfpa.org*
Health and Safety Info	*http://www.healthsafetyinfo.com*
Hospital Linx	*http://www.hospitaladminlinx.com*
International Association for Healthcare Safety and Security	*http://www.iahss.org*
Material Safety Data Sheets	*http://www.phys.ksu.edu*
Occupational Safety and Health Administration (OSHA)	*http://www.osha.gov*
—Ergonomics for the Prevention of Musculoskeletal Disorders: Guidelines for Nursing Homes	*http://www.osha.gov/ergonomics/guidelines/nursinghome/index.html*
—OSHA Ergonomics Recommendations	*http://www.osha.gov/ergonomics/index.html*
Risk Management Foundation	*http://www.rmf.harvard.edu*
Safe Patient Movement and Handling	*http://www.va.gov*
Safety Alerts	*http://www.safetyalerts.com*
Safety Info	*http://www.safetyinfo.com*
University of Michigan Risk Management	*http://www.umich.edu*

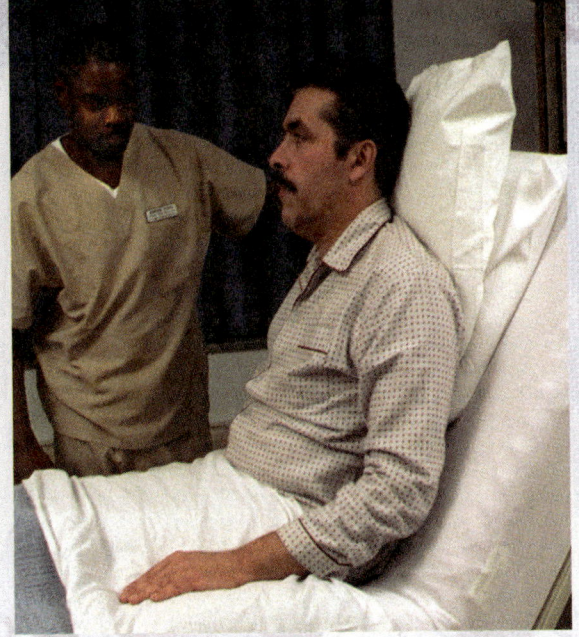

Patient Safety and Positioning

objectives

After completing this unit, you will be able to:
- Spell and define terms.
- Identify patients who are at risk for having incidents.
- List alternatives to the use of physical restraints.
- Describe the guidelines for the use of restraints.
- Demonstrate the correct application of restraints.
- Describe two measures for preventing these types of incidents: accidental poisoning, thermal injuries, skin injuries, and choking.
- List the elements that are common to all procedures.

- Describe correct body alignment for the patient.
- List the purposes of repositioning patients.
- Demonstrate these positions using the correct supportive devices: supine, semisupine, prone, semiprone, lateral, Fowler's, and orthopneic.
- Demonstrate the following procedures:
  - Procedure 14 Turning the Patient Toward You
  - Procedure 15 Turning the Patient Away from You
  - Procedure 16 Moving a Patient to the Head of the Bed
  - Procedure 17 Logrolling the Patient

vocabulary

Learn the meaning and the correct spelling of the following words and phrases:

ambulate	high Fowler's	postural support	spasticity
aspiration	laceration	pressure ulcer	splint
body alignment	lateral	procedure	supine
chemical restraint	mobility	prone	supportive device
contracture	orthopneic position	semi-Fowler's	transfer
draw sheet	orthotic devices	semiprone	trochanter roll
enabler	(orthoses)	semisupine	turning (moving)
Fowler's position	physical restraint	Sims' position	sheet

PATIENT SAFETY

In Unit 14, you learned how to maintain a safe environment and how to avoid personal injuries. The prevention of patient injuries is another very important part of your job as a nursing assistant. Patients in health care facilities are at risk for incidents, because they may:

- Have impaired **mobility** (ability to move about) due to an injury, disease, or surgery
- Be receiving medications that affect mental status, balance, and coordination
- Be disoriented because of the change in environment or because of a medical disorder
- Have impaired hearing or impaired vision

Because of these risk factors, most incidents involving patients in any health care setting are falls. Falls may occur because the patient:

- Misjudges the distance from the bed to the floor
- Feels weak or dizzy when trying to get up
- Changes position too rapidly and loses balance when trying to stand up
- Encounters hazards when walking
- Is walking in a poorly lit area

USE OF PHYSICAL RESTRAINTS

In the past, restraints were often used routinely as a preventive measure to avoid falls. Research has shown that side rails and restraints do not necessarily accomplish this purpose. In fact, many falls occur with side rails up and restraints intact. This can result in serious injury and even death. There are two types of restraints: physical restraints and chemical restraints. **Chemical restraints** are medications that affect the patient's mood and behavior. As a nursing assistant, you will be more concerned with the use of physical restraints. **Physical restraints** are defined as any technique or device that is attached or next to the patient's body that the patient cannot easily remove and that restricts freedom of movement and normal access to the body. OBRA (1987) clearly states when and how chemical and physical restraints may be used in a long-term care facility. The Residents' Rights state that "residents have the right to be free from physical and chemical restraints." According to this definition, many devices qualify as restraints if the patient does not have the physical or mental ability to remove the device readily. These guidelines have been implemented in acute care facilities as well. Physical restraints are to be used only when the safety of the

guidelines *for*

Preventing Patient Falls

- Always leave the bed in its lowest horizontal position when you have finished giving care.
- Keep brakes locked on bed wheels at all times except when the bed is being moved.
- Check to see whether the side rails are to be raised. Make sure they are attached securely.
- Check and adjust protruding objects such as bed wheels or gatch handles.
- Do not block or clutter open areas with supplies and equipment.
- Wipe up spills immediately.
- Encourage patients to use the rails along corridor walls when walking (Figure 15-1).
- Monitor patients for signs of weakness, fatigue, dizziness, and loss of balance.
- Monitor patients for safe practice if they independently:
  - propel their wheelchairs
  - **transfer** (get out of bed)
  - **ambulate** (walk)

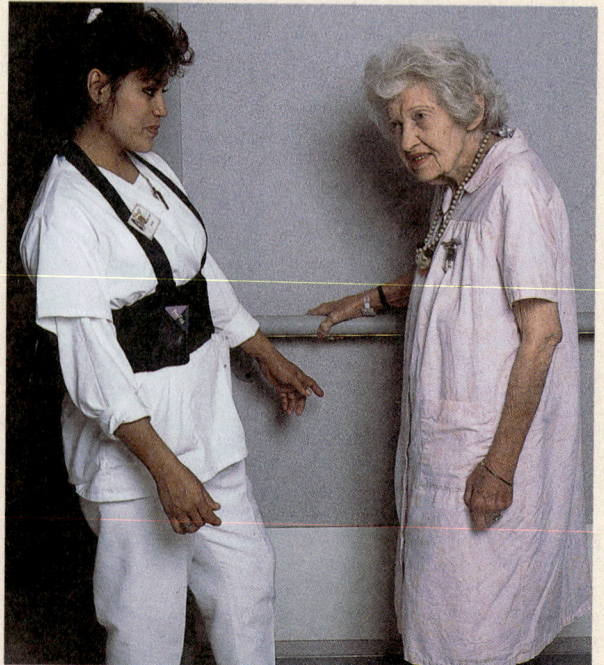

FIGURE 15-1 Encourage patients to hold rails on corridor walls when walking.

continues

guidelines *continued*

- Provide adequate lighting.
- Eliminate noise and other distractions that may increase confusion and create anxiety.
- Avoid leaving patients alone in the tub or shower unless you are given specific permission to do so.
- Check patients' clothing for fit and safety. Loose shoes and laces, long robes, and slacks increase the risk of falling. Footwear should be appropriate for the floor surface. In general, this means using nonskid shoes (Figure 15-2) on tile floor surfaces. For carpeted floors, consult the physical therapist if there is a question about appropriate footwear for the patient. Nonskid shoes may stick to the carpeting, causing falls. A leather or synthetic shoe sole may be more appropriate for a carpeted surface.
- Care for the patient's physical needs promptly. Many incidents occur when patients attempt to get out of bed to go to the bathroom.
- Always use the correct techniques for transferring and walking patients.
- Use a gait belt when assisting patients to transfer

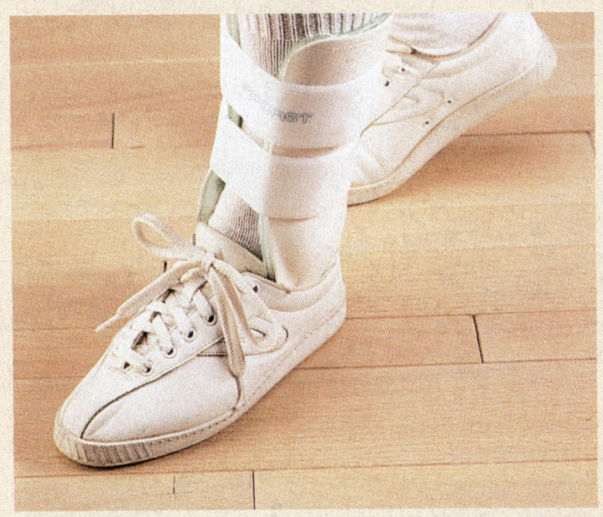

FIGURE 15-2 Patients should wear nonskid shoes for transfers and walking on tile floors. (*Aircast® ankle stirrup is provided by Sammons Preston, Inc., a Bissell® HealthCare Company. Reprinted with permission.*)

or ambulate.
- Follow the care plan when assisting patients with transfers and ambulation.

---

patient or other persons is at risk. Before a restraint is used, the staff must:

- Document all patient behavior indicating the need for a restraint.

- Document all actions that were taken as an alternative to restraints.
- Consult with the patient and the family or legal guardian when alternatives are unsuccessful and obtain their approval and consent to apply a restraint (Figure 15-3).

Examples of physical restraints include:

- Wrist/arm (Figure 15-4) and ankle/leg restraints
- Vests (Figure 15-5)
- Jackets (Figure 15-6)
- Hand mitts (Figure 15-7)
- Geriatric and cardiac chairs (Figure 15-8)
- Wheelchair safety belts, bars, and tables (Figure 15-9)
- Bed rails (if they meet the definition of a restraint)

Restraints are medical devices. They should never be used as a form of punishment, or for the convenience of the nursing staff. Patients have been seriously injured and died as a result of restraint use, so restraint application must be considered very seriously and avoided whenever possible. Other potential complications of restraints are listed in Table 15-1.

Before restraints are used, the staff must assess the patient's capabilities and the reasons for use of the restraint. If the cause of the patient's problem can be identified and corrected, the need for a restraint may be eliminated. For example, if restraints are being considered to prevent falls,

Physical Restraint Informed Consent

Patient's name _____

Method of physical restraint used _____

The reason the physical restraint is needed _____

_____

Times when restraint will be applied _____

Alternatives tried _____

In compliance with federal and state regulations, this facility is committed to limiting of the use of physical restraints only to situations necessary to maximize a patient's physical, mental, and psychological well-being. It is the policy of this facility that, if physical restraints are deemed necessary, the least restrictive method will be applied for the shortest amount of time possible.

Physical restraints will be used by this facility only when it has been determined that they are required to treat a patient's medical symptoms or a therapeutic intervention, as ordered by a physician, and based on (1) a documented assessment, by an appropriate health professional, of the patient's capabilities; the physical condition or mental treatment that requires the use of physical restraints; the less restrictive measures or therapeutic interventions that have proved ineffective; and the specific physical restraint most effective for the patient's condition; and (2) demonstration by the care planning process that using a physical restraint as a therapeutic intervention will promote the care and services necessary for the patient to attain or maintain the highest practicable physical, mental, or psychosocial well-being.

This patient has been assessed regarding his or her need for appro-priate physical restraint. He or she will be reassessed at least quarterly or as his or her needs change throughout the stay at this facility. A report will be made each quarter as to the effectiveness of the physical restraint in maximizing the patient's physical, mental, or psychosocial well-being. Ongoing assessments help to further this goal. The duration of consent for the use of this physical restraint is good only until the next annual assessment of the patient's needs, or if there is a need for more restrictive physical restraints. At those times, a new informed consent will be required.

The benefits of physical restraints include the prevention of injuries to oneself or to others, enhancement of functional abilities, reduced potential for falling, and continued provision of medically necessary procedures. Potential complications associated with physical restraints include incontinence, decreased range of motion, decreased ability to ambulate, symptoms of withdrawal or depression, or reduced social contact. This facility will monitor the use of physical restraints daily and respond to any developing complications to physical restraint use.

By virtue of my signature, I state that I received, read, and had an opportunity to discuss any questions I may have regarding the application of physical restraints in this facility. I give consent for the use of physical restraints when the benefits outweigh the identified risks in accordance with this informed consent. I understand that I can revoke consent for this physical restraint at any time. I further consent to physical restraint reduction as soon as feasible.

_____
(Signature of Patient or Authorized Individual)   (Date)

_____
(Signature of Witness)   (Date)

[   ] Patient unable to sign.

FIGURE 15-3 Many facilities obtain written consent from the patient or responsible party before applying a restraint.

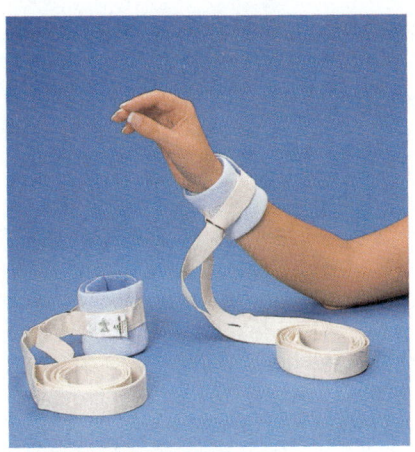

FIGURE 15-4 Wrist restraints may be used to prevent the patient from pulling on IVs and other tubes.

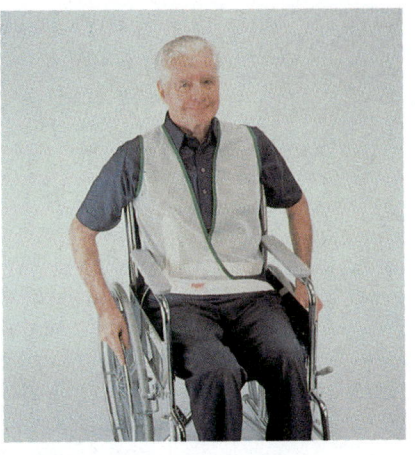

FIGURE 15-5 Vest restraints must be applied as pictured here, with the straps crossed over in front of the patient.

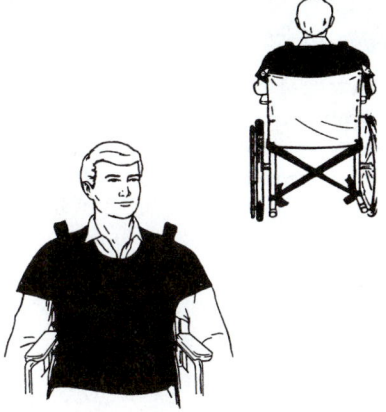

FIGURE 15-6 Jacket restraint.

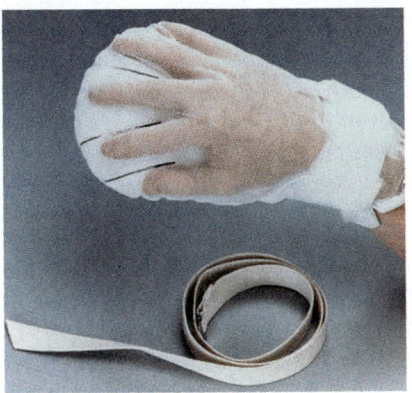

FIGURE 15-7 Hand mitts may be applied to keep the patient from injuring himself or pulling on tubes.

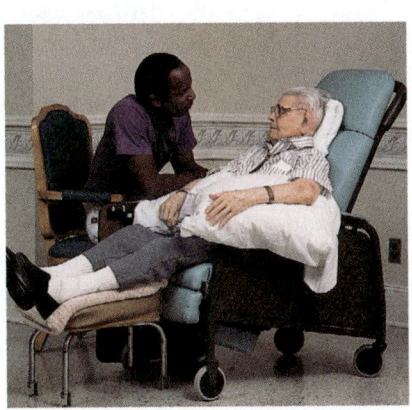

FIGURE 15-8 Geriatric chairs are restraints in some circumstances.

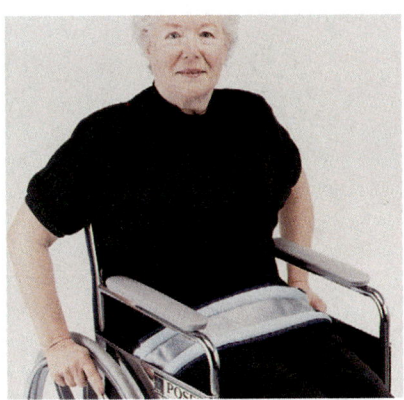

FIGURE 15-9 Wheelchair safety belts, bars, and tables are considered restraints if the patient does not have the physical or mental ability to remove them.

(Figures 15–4, 15–5, 15–6, 15–7, and 15–9 are all courtesy of J.T. Posey Co., Inc., Arcadia, CA.)

the patient's individual risk factors associated with falls are assessed. If some risk factors can be eliminated or modified, this reduces the risk of falls, and restraints may not be necessary. For example, an unsteady male patient gets up to use the bathroom at night, but does not call for help. His risk of falls can be modified by making sure a urinal is within reach and emptied regularly.

If a patient is a danger to himself or others, or requires emergency medical treatment, restraints may be appropriate. However, less restrictive alternatives to restraints must be considered first. Many alternative devices are available to use instead of restraints. If a restraint is determined to be the best approach, it is applied. However, an ongoing assessment of the factors creating the need for restraints is necessary, and personnel must work to reduce or eliminate the need for the restraint.

If restraints are indicated, the least restrictive restraint required to keep the patient safe should be selected. The restraint should be used as infrequently as possible. Using restraints requires careful assessment, planning, and monitoring. Studies have proven that it takes more time to care for patients in restraints than to care for patients who are not restrained. The physician must agree to the use of restraints and write an order before they can be used. The care plan will provide information about the type of restraint to use, the time the restraint is to be applied, and other special information and instructions.

Enablers. Enablers are devices that empower patients and assist them to function at their highest possible level. For example, a patient in a wheelchair is unable to sit up straight to feed herself, so she is fed by staff. If a supportive

TABLE 15-1 COMPLICATIONS OF RESTRAINTS

Potential Physical Problems	Potential Psychosocial Problems
Decreased independence	Worsening of behavior problems
Pressure ulcers	
Weakness	Withdrawal, loss of social contact
Decreased range of motion	
Muscle wasting	Depression
Contractures (frozen, deformed joints)	Forgetfulness
	Fear
Loss of ability to ambulate	Anger
Edema of ankles, lower legs, feet, fingers	Shame
	Agitation
Decreased appetite, weight loss	Mental confusion
Dehydration	Combativeness
Acute mental confusion	Restlessness
Distended abdomen	Sense of abandonment
Urge to void frequently, dribbling	Frustration
	Loss of self-esteem
Incontinence	Depression
Urinary tract infection	Screaming, yelling, calling out
Constipation	
Fecal impaction	
Lethargy	
Shortness of breath	
Pneumonia	
Bruising, redness, cuts, skin tears	
Falls	
Impaired circulation	
Blood clots	
Choking	
Death	

device is applied to correct her posture and allow her to feed herself, the device is an enabler. Devices used as enablers that maintain body position and alignment are commonly called **postural supports**. Used correctly, they give patients a higher degree of independence and enable them to perform tasks they were previously unable to do. In this case, using the restraint improves the patient's self-esteem.

The wheelchair lap tray (Figure 15-10) is a restraint alternative that is also used as an enabler. The tray is simple to use: it is attached to the back of the wheelchair with Velcro® straps. Patients can lean on it, and its surface can hold personal items or reading and writing supplies. A tray may enable the patient to feed himself by moving the food closer so he can reach it. The tray also reminds the patient not to stand up. If the tray allows the patient to perform a task, it is an enabler. If it is used strictly to keep the patient in the chair, and he does not have the physical or mental ability to remove the tray, it is considered a restraint. If the tray can be removed by the patient, it is a restraint alternative.

Side Rails as Restraints. By definition, side rails are restraints. They can also be an enabler. Many patients pull on them to position and turn themselves in bed. Some patients may feel more secure if the rails are up. Side rails must always be up for patients who are restrained in vests, belts, and extremity restraints in bed.

Studies have shown that serious injuries can occur if patients attempt to climb over side rails and fall. This is a common cause of hip fractures in confused elderly patients. Leaving the rails down may be a much safer alternative. Alarms are available that sound if the patient attempts to get up. If side rails are used, monitor the patient frequently. When side rails are used, it is important to check the space between the rail and the mattress. Hospital beds are permanent pieces of equipment that are used for years. Mattresses wear out and are replaced. There have been cases of injury and death in which patients became trapped between the mattress and side rails because the replacement mattress was not the same size as the original. Patients at high risk for entrapment include those with conditions such as confusion, restlessness, lack of muscle control, or a combination of these factors. Make sure that the gap between the mattress and the side rail is not large enough to cause injury. Figure 15-11 shows areas of potential entrapment.

Facilities and commercial manufacturers have developed many excellent alternatives to the use of side rails. Each patient's care plan or critical pathway will provide instructions regarding use of restraints, side rails, or alternative devices. Before applying restraints or raising the rails, ask yourself if the risks associated with their use presents less danger than other available options, including making the environment as safe and user-friendly as possible. Other possible alternatives to the use of side rails are:

- Keeping the bed in the lowest possible position with the wheels locked.
- Beds that can be raised and lowered close to the floor.
- Placing mats on the floor next to the bed, so that if a fall occurs, the patient will fall on a padded surface instead of the hard floor.
- Anticipate reasons why the patient might get up, including need to use the bathroom, hunger, thirst, restlessness, and pain. Meet these needs promptly and provide calm interventions when you are in the room.
- Using side rail bolster cushions (Figure 15-12).
- Pressure-sensitive bed and chair alarms that sound when a patient attempts to get up (Figures 15-13A, 15-13B, 15-13C).

Each health care facility has policies addressing when side rails may be used. Know and follow your facility policies.

The Vail Bed. A Vail bed (Figure 15-13D) is a useful alternative for confused adult patients who try to climb over the side rails. It is not used for mentally alert patients. This bed looks somewhat like a canopy bed or adult crib.

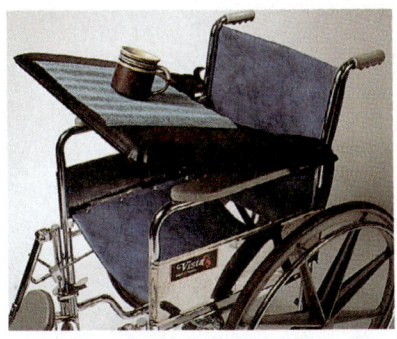

FIGURE 15-10 The lap tray is an enabler if it improves function, permitting the patient to eat independently. This tray is lined with gripper, a non-slip surface that holds the dishes in place. The tray is a restraint if it is used to keep the patient in the chair and he cannot remove it by himself. *(Courtesy of Skil-Care Corporation, Yonkers, NY, (800) 431-2972.)*

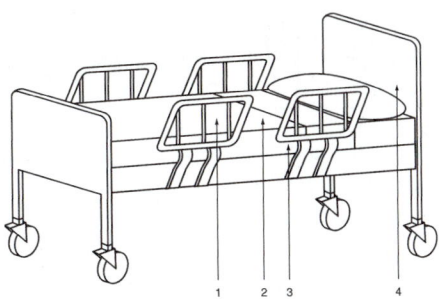

FIGURE 15-11 Entrapment between the mattress and side rails occurs in one of the following ways (numbers 1–4 in the diagram): (1) through the bars of an individual side rail; (2) through the space between split side rails; (3) between the side rail and mattress; or (4) between the headboard or footboard, side rail, and mattress.

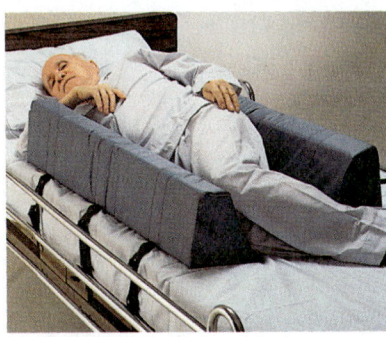

FIGURE 15-12 Bed control bolsters are a good option to use in place of side rails. *(Courtesy of Skil-Care Corporation, Yonkers, NY, (800) 431-2972.)*

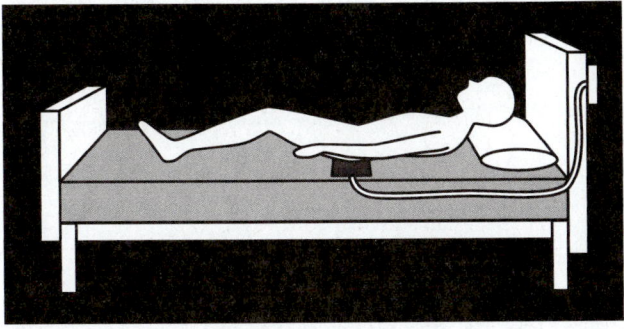

FIGURE 15-13A The pressure-sensitive pad is placed under the sheet. When the patient attempts to stand, an alarm sounds. *(Courtesy of RN+ Systems, Boulder, CO, (800) 727-1868.)*

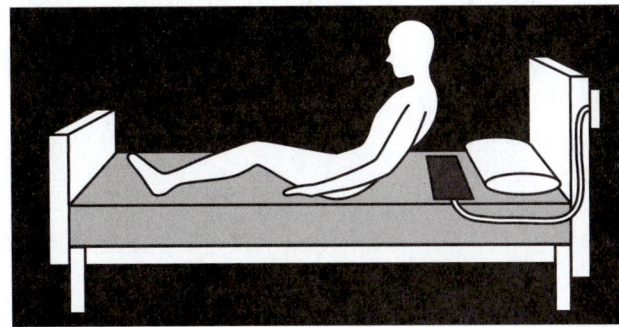

FIGURE 15-13B This pressure-sensitive pad is placed under the sheet beneath the patient's shoulders. When he lifts his upper body off the pad, the alarm will sound. *(Courtesy of RN+ Systems, Boulder, CO, (800) 727-1868.)*

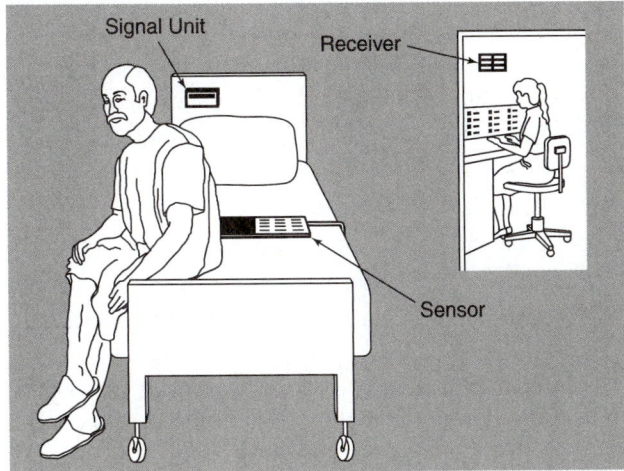

FIGURE 15-13C The pressure-sensitive pad is placed under the sheet. The signal unit is placed in the room. When the patient relieves pressure from the pad, a distinctive alarm sounds at the desk. The alarm sound is optional in the patient's room. *(Courtesy of RN+ Systems, Boulder, CO, (800) 727-1868.)*

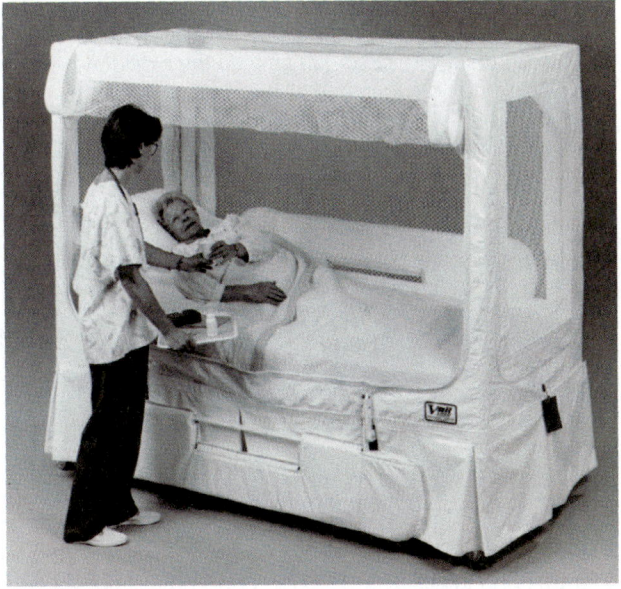

FIGURE 15-13D The Vail bed keeps patients safe without restricting mobility. *(Photo courtesy of Vail Products, Inc.)*

The top and sides are surrounded by netting. From the inside, the netting seems to fade out and is not perceived as a barrier. The patient views the room as though looking through a screen door. The patient can move about in the bed without becoming entangled or falling out of bed. The netting protects the caregiver if the patient becomes aggressive. The bed is accessible from all sides through special zippers in the netting that open only from the outside. Patients should not be left unattended with the covers unzipped. Pediatric versions of this bed are also available for infant and child patients.

Alternatives to the Use of Restraints

Alternatives to restraints should be tried before restraints are applied. Restraints are used only as a last resort in situations where the patient may harm himself or others. Nursing assistants can take a number of actions to help reduce the need to use restraints.

1. Care for patients' personal needs promptly.
   - Take patients to the bathroom regularly.
   - Provide adequate food and fluids to prevent hunger and thirst.
   - Report signs and symptoms of pain or illness promptly.
   - Follow all instructions for positioning and for assisting patients with exercise.
   - Be sure that patients have their eyeglasses and hearing aids if they need them.

   - Answer call signals promptly.
   - Check patients often to see if they need anything.
   - Provide appropriate exercise and activities.
2. Know which patients are at risk for falling. Monitor these patients regularly during your shift.
3. Observe patients who walk and transfer independently. Sometimes falls occur because patients use incorrect and unsafe methods. Report these situations and learn how to teach patients the correct way.
4. Report immediately any physical or mental change that could increase the risk of an incident, such as:
   - Disorientation (patient does not know time, place, or self)
   - Complaints of dizziness
   - Problems with balance and coordination
5. Maintain a safe, quiet, calm, environment.
6. Provide comfortable chairs. Use supportive devices as necessary.
7. A number of security devices are available that are designed to prevent falls and eliminate the need for restraints. These devices include:
   - Special sensors attached to a patient's wrist, leg, or wheelchair. The sensor will set off an alarm if the patient tries to leave the unit or building.
   - Special sensors (a pad) placed in the patient's bed or chair that will set off an alarm if the patient attempts to rise.

guidelines *for*

The Use of Restraints

There are a few situations in which a patient may need a restraint, no matter how many alternatives are tried. When restraints are necessary, these guidelines must be followed:

1. A physician's order must be obtained by the nurse before restraints may be used. The order must indicate the type of restraint to use and the reason for its use. Try the least restrictive device first.

2. Use the right type and size of restraint. All restraints must be applied according to manufacturer's directions.

   Check the device before use—do not use if it is frayed, torn, has parts missing, or is soiled. Restraints are put on over clothing, never next to bare skin. When applying a restraint to a female patient, make sure the breasts are not under the strap to the restraint.

3. Even if the patient does not seem to understand, always explain what you are doing. After application, check the fit of the device. You should be able to slip the width of three fingers between the restraint and the patient's body. The device should never restrict breathing.

4. The straps should be positioned so the patient is unable to reach them. The restraint straps should be smooth. Avoid twisting. Pad the restraint if necessary to prevent irritation to the skin.

5. Tie restraint straps with slip knots for quick release in an emergency.

6. The patient should always have access to the signal light. Check every 15 minutes for the patient's comfort and safety. Make changes as needed.

7. When the patient is restrained in a wheelchair, the brakes should be locked when the chair is parked. The large part of the small front wheels of the chair should face forward. This changes the center of gravity of the chair, making the chair more stable and preventing tipping.

8. Release the restraint at least every 2 hours for at least 10 minutes to:
   - Check for irritation or poor circulation
   - Change the patient's position

   - Exercise—ambulate the patient or do passive range-of-motion exercises
   - Take the patient to the bathroom
   - Change incontinent patients and cleanse their skin
   - Provide fluid or nourishment
   - Attend to any other needs

   Document each of these actions.

9. Maintain good body alignment whether the patient is in bed or a chair.

10. When restraints are used in bed:
    - There must be full side rails on the bed, and they must be raised
    - The patient should always be positioned in the middle of the mattress
    - Always secure the restraint to the movable part of the bed frame (Figure 15-14)

11. Do not use restraints in moving vehicles or on toilets unless you are sure the device is intended for that use by the manufacturer.

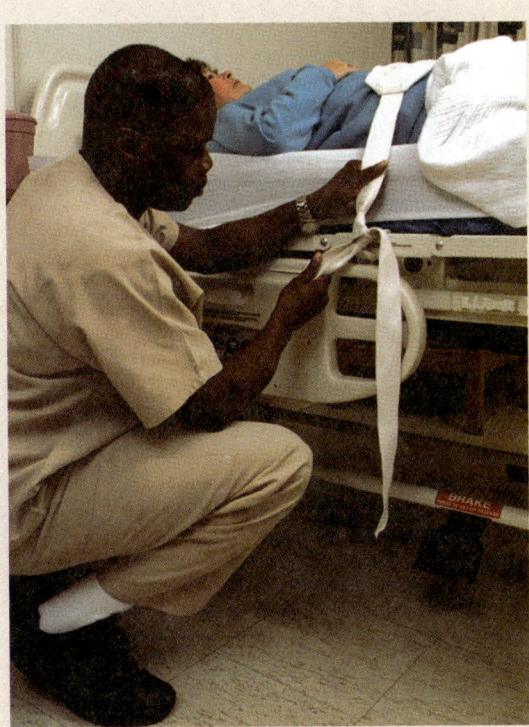

FIGURE 15-14 Always tie restraints to the movable part of the bed frame.

Many commercial devices are available to use in place of restraints. Sometimes clothing or other items can be used as restraint alternatives. For example, a male patient who pulls at his urinary catheter can be fitted with boxer shorts. A patient with a feeding tube in the abdomen can be covered with a t-shirt or abdominal binder. A patient with an intravenous infusion (IV) in the arm can wear a long-sleeved shirt. Covering the medical device may be all that is necessary to keep the patient from pulling on it. Previously, wrist restraints would have been used to keep the patient from dislodging tubes. Giving the patient something to hold, such as a Nerf® ball, will occupy the hands and serve as a distraction.

The nursing assistant plays an important role in knowing the patients' needs and making recommendations for restraint alternatives. Making sure the patient is in touch with his or her environment reduces agitation and confusion. Simply ensuring that she can see or hear well may improve mental orientation. Other observations that will help eliminate the need for restraints are:

- Does the patient see and hear well? Does the patient normally wear glasses? Is she wearing them now? Are they clean? Does the hearing aid work? Are the patient's ears plugged with wax? Sometimes behavior problems, balance problems, and other safety concerns arise because the patient is out of touch with the environment. Applying these simple corrective devices may eliminate the need for a restraint.

- Is the patient able to make her needs known? Sometimes unsafe behavior is caused by an unmet need, such as hunger, thirst, or need to use the bathroom. Discovering the unmet need and meeting it may help you avoid using a restraint.

- Does noise or confusion in the environment cause the patient to become agitated? Noise can be caused by other patients or staff, the public address system, radios, or television. Eliminating the noise may stop the behavior.

- Does the behavior occur during a certain time of day, during a certain activity, or when a specific person is providing care?

- Does the patient seem uncomfortable? Physical pain, hunger, thirst, or need to use the bathroom can cause unsafe behavior.

- Does the patient seem lonely or isolated? Bored? Boredom, loneliness, or looking for a misplaced item can cause unsafe behavior.

- Does the patient try to get out of bed or chair without help? Is the patient steady on her feet? Does she normally use a cane or walker? Is she using it now? Is the call signal available, and does the patient know how to use it? Would the patient benefit from use of an alarm that sounds when she stands up? Would use of an alarm remind the patient to sit down, alert the staff, and eliminate the need for a restraint?

If you observe a condition that causes confusion or agitation, or discover an approach that is effective in eliminating or reducing the need for restraints, inform your nurse manager. Other common restraint alternatives are pictured in Figure 15-15 through Figure 15-21.

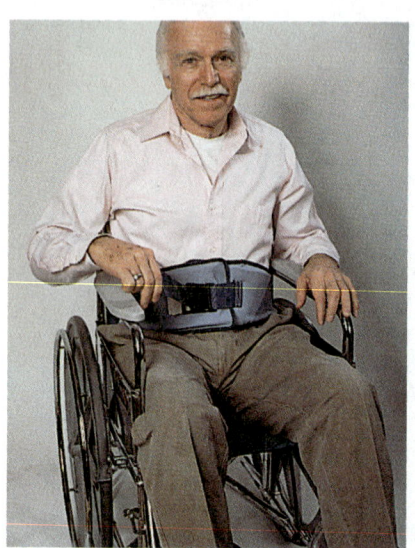

FIGURE 15-15 The self-release belt serves as a reminder to call for help before rising. It is not a restraint if the patient has the physical and mental ability to release the Velcro® fastener. *(Courtesy of Skil-Care Corporation, Yonkers, NY, (800) 431-2972.)*

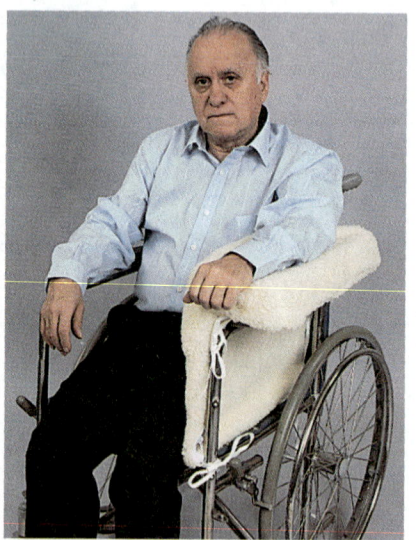

FIGURE 15-16 Some patients lean to the side, necessitating restraint to keep them upright in the chair. The lateral armrest supports and keeps the patient upright, making restraint unnecessary. *(Courtesy of Skil-Care Corporation, Yonkers, NY, (800) 431-2972.)*

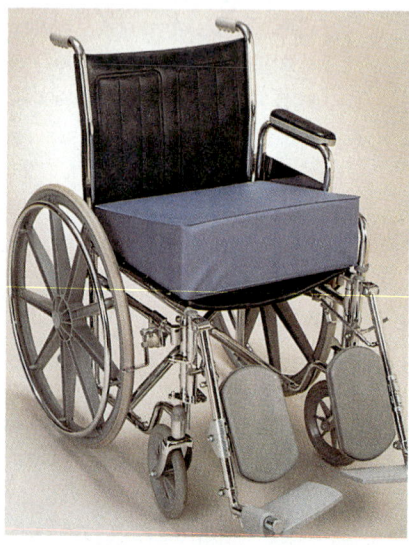

FIGURE 15-17 Some patients slide forward to the edge of the chair, and must be restrained to keep their hips back. The wedge cushion prevents sliding. A piece of gripper can be placed on top of the wedge for additional security. *(Courtesy of Skil-Care Corporation, Yonkers, NY, (800) 431-2972.)*

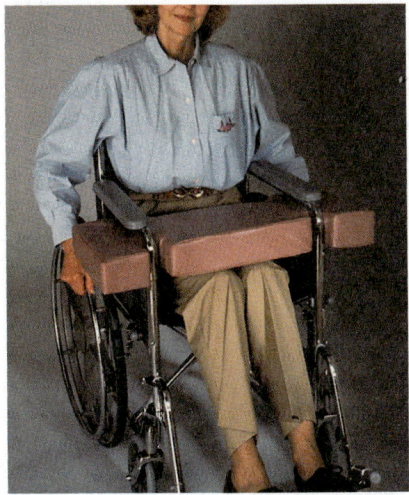

FIGURE 15-18 The lap buddy is foam covered with vinyl. It is lightweight and comfortable and may be used in place of a heavier tray. It is a restraint if the patient cannot remove it. *(Courtesy of Skil-Care Corporation, Yonkers, NY, (800) 431-2972.)*

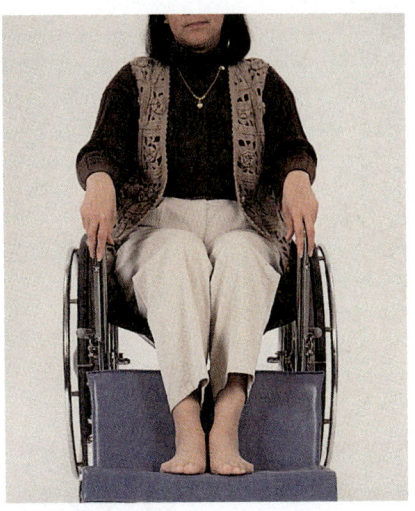

FIGURE 15-19 The patient's feet must be supported when she is sitting in a chair. The footrest elevator keeps the patient's legs from dangling and prevents her from sliding forward in the chair. *(Courtesy of Skil-Care Corporation, Yonkers, NY, (800) 431-2972.)*

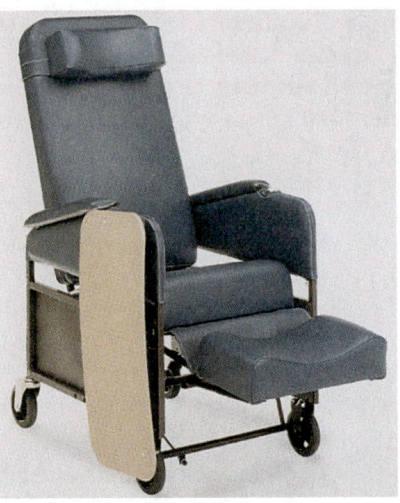

FIGURE 15-20 The geriatric chair can be used as a recliner for patient comfort. If the patient cannot stand, the chair is a restraint when in the reclining position. The tray is locked across the lap to prevent rising. It cannot be removed independently, and is considered a restraint. *(Photo courtesy of Hill-Rom® Long-Term Care Division.)*

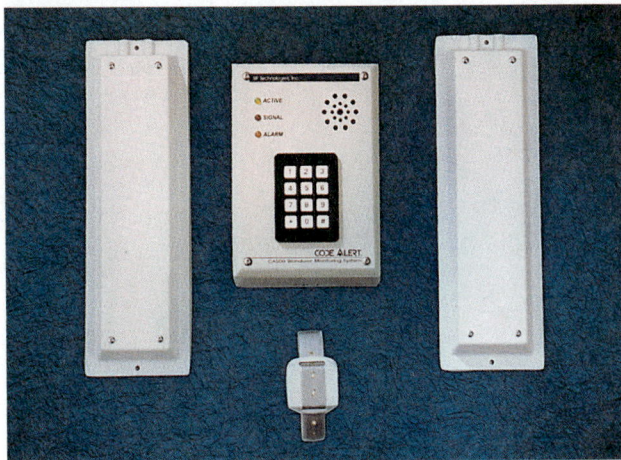

FIGURE 15-21 The magnetic sensor bracelet is used to allow cognitively impaired patients to wander within the unit. The door alarm will sound if the patient tries to exit. *(©1996, RF Technologies. Used with permission.)*

PREVENTION OF OTHER INCIDENTS

Many situations can result in an incident that may harm the patient. Incidents can be prevented when all staff members are aware of appropriate preventive measures.

Accidental Poisoning

Many common items, such as household chemicals, shaving lotion, plants, and cologne, are poisonous if ingested.

Food kept in a bedside table may spoil and also cause illness. Patients who are disoriented may eat or drink any of these items. To prevent accidental poisonings:

- Keep all chemicals and cleaning solutions in locked cupboards.
- Store patients' personal food items in the refrigerator in dated labeled containers.

Thermal Injuries

Thermal injuries are those caused by heat or cold and result in burns. To prevent thermal injuries:

- Follow procedures accurately when administering warm or cold treatments.
- Check water temperatures before helping a patient into the bathtub or shower. Turn the hot water on last and turn it off first.
- Check food temperatures before feeding patients. Using a microwave oven to reheat food can be dangerous because of the uneven temperatures the oven produces.
- Store smoking materials in a safe place and supervise patients while they smoke. (Most health care facilities do not allow smoking by anyone.)

Skin Injuries

Skin injuries include lacerations (cuts or breaks in the skin) and punctures. To prevent these injuries:

- Store knives, scissors, razors, and tools in locked cupboards.

- Store syringes and needles in locked cupboards. These should be disposed of in a sharps container immediately after use.
- Clean up broken glass immediately, as described earlier.

Choking

Aspiration is the accidental entry of food or a foreign object into the trachea (windpipe). This causes choking. Because swallowing becomes less efficient as people age, choking occurs more often in the elderly. Persons who are disoriented or who have impaired consciousness are also at risk. To prevent choking or aspiration:

1. Be aware of which patients have problems with swallowing. Follow all instructions when helping with feeding:
   - Cut food into small pieces.
   - Feed slowly.
   - Offer fluids carefully between solid foods.
   - If the patient has had a stroke, place the food in the unaffected side of the mouth.
   - Use thickeners for liquids if ordered.

2. Place patients upright in good body alignment before meals. Have them remain in this position for at least 30 minutes after eating.

3. At the end of the meal, give oral care to patients who are known to keep food in their mouths. Food may remain in the mouth for several minutes after a meal and be accidentally aspirated if the patient coughs or goes to sleep.

4. Know the procedure to clear an obstructed airway. (See Unit 51.)

INTRODUCTION TO PROCEDURES

Caring for patients safely means that you must faithfully and carefully carry out specific routines. The normal manner of carrying out a task is called a procedure.

As you progress in your studies, you will learn the procedures for many nursing assistant tasks. You have already been introduced to the procedures for washing your hands and using PPE. The procedures that follow give you step-by-step directions for carrying out tasks that involve patients.

Certain things must be done before you begin patient care procedures. These actions are called *preprocedure* or beginning procedure actions. At the end of each patient care procedure, you will carry out a standard series of procedure completion actions.

Beginning Procedure Actions

At the beginning of each procedure, do the following:
- Wash your hands thoroughly (Figure 15-22A). You may use an alcohol-based hand cleanser, if permitted by your facility.

- Assemble equipment.
- At the patient's room, knock and pause before entering (Figure 15-22B).
- Introduce yourself and identify the patient by checking his or her identification bracelet (Figure 15-22C).
- Ask visitors to leave the room and inform them where they may wait.

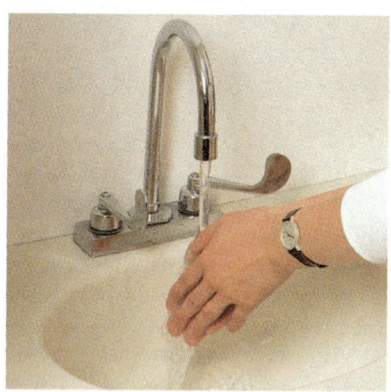

FIGURE 15-22A
Wash your hands.

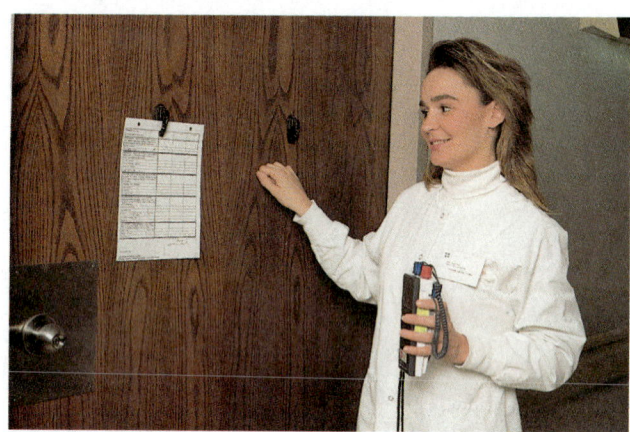

FIGURE 15-22B If the door is closed or the privacy curtains are drawn, knock or speak before entering. Allow enough time for the patient to respond.

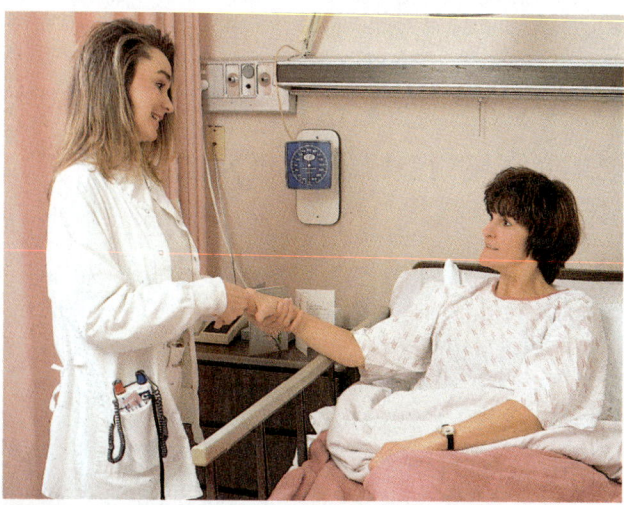

FIGURE 15-22C Identify the patient.

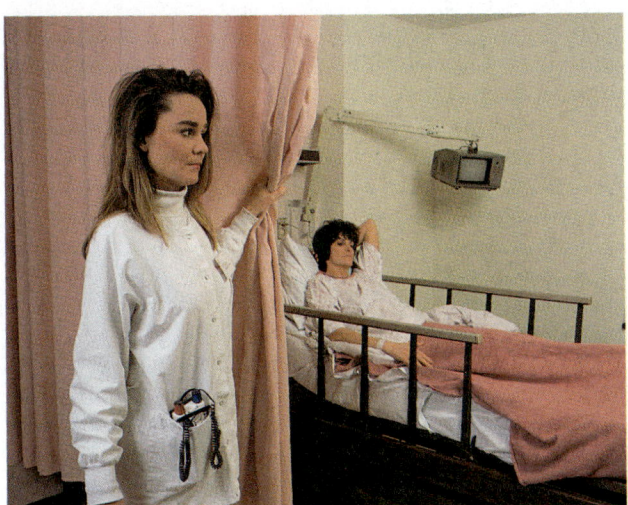

FIGURE 15-22D Draw the curtains for privacy. If the bed is near a window, also close the window curtains.

- Provide privacy (Figure 15-22D).
- Explain what will happen and answer questions.
- Allow the patient to assist as much as possible.
- Raise the bed to a comfortable working height.
- Lower the side rail on the side where you are working.
- Position the patient for the procedure. Ask an assistant to help, if necessary, or support the patient with pillows and props. Make sure the patient is comfortable and can maintain the position throughout the procedure.
- Drape the patient for modesty.
- Set up the equipment for the procedure at the bedside. Open trays and packages. Position items so that you can reach them conveniently. Avoid putting a container for soiled items in a place where you must cross over clean items to use it.
- Carry out precaution gowning and gloving.

COMMUNICATION *Highlight*

Communicate with the patient throughout the procedure. Whenever possible, use age-appropriate terms and explanations. Talk to the patient even if he or she is young, confused, may not understand, or cannot communicate verbally. Use gestures and body language to demonstrate, whenever possible. Continue to talk and smile throughout the procedure, regardless of the patient's age or level of understanding. This is important for the patient's well-being, and shows that you care. Remember that you also communicate with touch. Handle the patient gently to prevent injury and communicate caring.

- Use standard precautions when contact with blood, body fluids, mucous membranes, or nonintact skin is likely.

Procedure Completion Actions

When a procedure is completed, do the following:
- Remove gloves.
- Position the patient comfortably.
- Replace the bed covers, then remove any drapes used.
- Return the bed to the lowest horizontal position.
- Elevate the side rails, if used, before leaving the bedside.
- Leave signal cord (Figure 15-23A), telephone, and fresh water where the patient can reach them.
- Perform a general safety check of the patient and the environment.
- Open privacy curtains.
- Remove and discard personal protective equipment, if used, according to facility policy.
- Care for equipment following facility policy.
- Wash your hands (Figure 15-23B). You may use an alcohol-based hand cleanser if permitted by your facility. Do not use an alcohol product if you have protein substances on your hands.

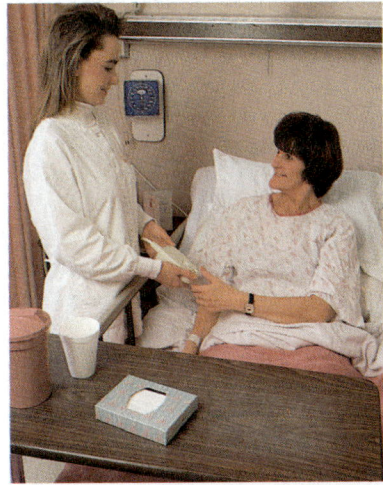

FIGURE 15-23A Lower the bed and place the signal cord within the patient's reach.

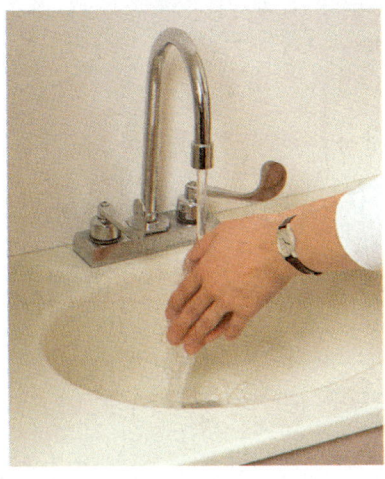

FIGURE 15-23B Wash your hands.

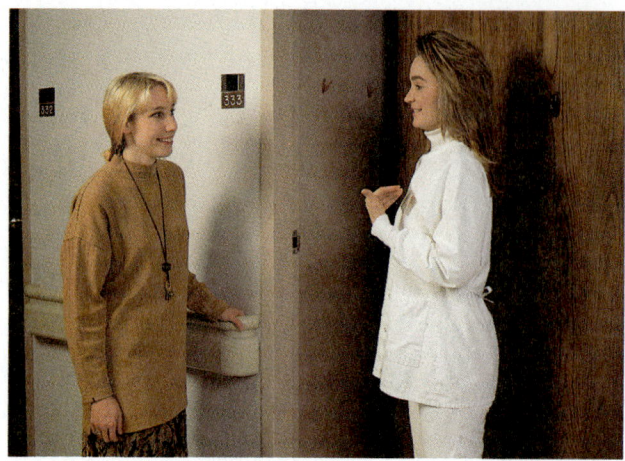

FIGURE 15-23C Let visitors know when they may reenter the room.

- Let visitors know when they may reenter (Figure 15-23C).
- Report completion of task (Figure 15-23D).
- Document action and your observations.

Note: Where there are open lesions, wet linen, or possible contact with patient body fluids, blood, secretions, excretions, mucous membranes, or nonintact skin, wear disposable gloves during the procedure. Put on gloves before contact with the patient or linen. Dispose of gloves according to facility policy after they are removed. **ALWAYS APPLY STANDARD PRECAUTIONS.**

So much handwashing may seem unnecessary, because of the short length of time that you are with the patient. Just remember that your hands can transmit germs. Patients already weakened by disease have a much lower resistance to germs.

Because the beginning procedure and procedure completion actions are the same for each patient care procedure, they are not restated in this book as individual steps with each procedure. Rather, a general reference is made to these

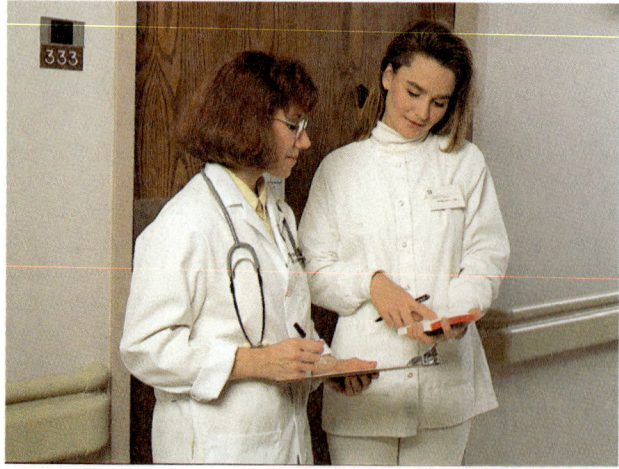

FIGURE 15-23D Report and document your actions and the patient's response.

steps at the beginning and end of each procedure. You must, however, learn and faithfully complete each of these steps for each patient care procedure you perform.

BODY MECHANICS FOR THE PATIENT

Body mechanics for the patient are very similar to those for the health care team. Although the patient probably is not doing any lifting, good posture habits should not be neglected. Good posture for the patient means that moving in bed, getting out of bed, standing, and walking are done safely.

Bed patients sometimes find it hard to stay in a position; they tend to slide toward the foot of the bed when the head of the bed is elevated (Figure 15-24). Patients who are dependent are not able to change their position. These patients need extra help to gain and maintain proper alignment. Remember to:

- Get help.
- Use turning or lifting sheets.
- Change the patient's position frequently, at least every two hours.

Body Alignment and Positioning

Body alignment means maintaining a person in a position in which the body can properly function. Patients who are weak, have impaired consciousness, are disoriented, or are

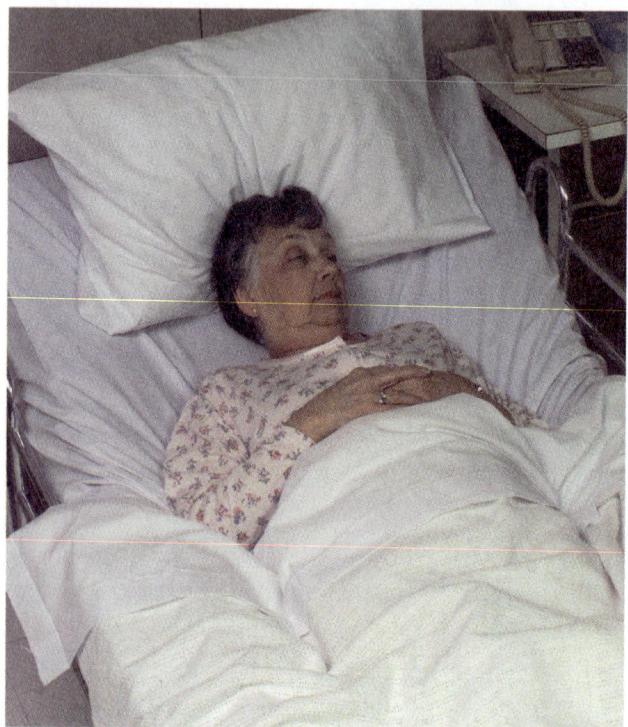

FIGURE 15-24 Patients frequently slide down in bed, causing poor body alignment.

in pain have problems keeping good alignment. Body alignment is maintained by moving, turning, and positioning the patient in a manner that:

- Helps the patient feel more comfortable
- Relieves strain
- Helps the body function more efficiently
- Prevents complications like contractures and pressure ulcers

Complications of Incorrect Positioning

Complications can occur when body alignment is not maintained or when the patient's position is not changed often enough. The two most common complications are pressure ulcers and contractures. **Pressure ulcers** (bedsores) result when unrelieved pressure on a bony prominence interferes with blood flow to the area. Pressure ulcers are dangerous and expensive to treat. (These are discussed in Unit 24.) **Contractures** occur when a joint is allowed to remain in the same position for too long (Figure 15-25). The muscles stiffen and shorten (atrophy), preventing the joint from full movement. The joint becomes fixed in a bent position (position of flexion). Contractures are permanent and can interfere with mobility.

Contractures can begin to develop within as little as four days of immobility and inactivity. After approximately 15 days, the patient loses the ability to move the joint freely. Contractures interfere with the patient's ability to move, complicate all nursing care, and interfere with proper positioning of the patient. Contractures promote the development of pressure ulcers and make treatment of existing pressure ulcers difficult. The contractures cause bony prominences to suffer reduced blood flow. Some studies have shown a relationship between the presence of contractures and the development of pressure ulcers. Contractures are a serious complication of immobility, making movement and activity painful and difficult. Voluntary movement of the contracted joint becomes impossible as the contracture worsens. Contractures can be prevented, and some can be reversed, with proper care. (Additional preventive measures for contractures are discussed in Unit 40).

Supportive Devices

Supportive devices are used to maintain proper body alignment and position in the bed or in a chair. Supportive devices include:

- Pillows and/or folded sheets, bath blankets, or mattress pads to support the trunk and extremities
- Splints and other specially designed **orthotic devices** (**orthoses**). Orthoses restore or improve function and prevent deformity.
- Special boots or shoes that are worn in bed to keep the feet in alignment (Figure 15-26A)
- Bed cradles, which prevent pressure on the feet from the bed covers (Figure 15-26B)
- Footboards to maintain foot alignment

A folded pillow placed between the soles of the feet and the foot of the bed, or a pillow resting against the footboard

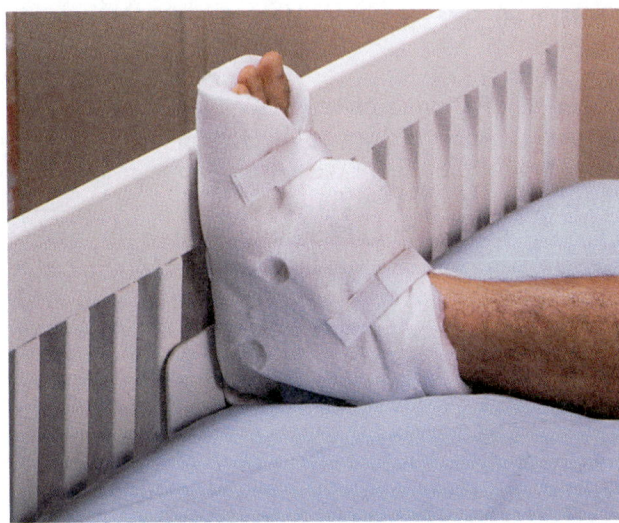

FIGURE 15-26A Special boots will maintain the ankles and feet in good alignment. *(Bunny boot support is provided by Sammons Preston, Inc., a Bissell® HealthCare Company. Reprinted with permission.)*

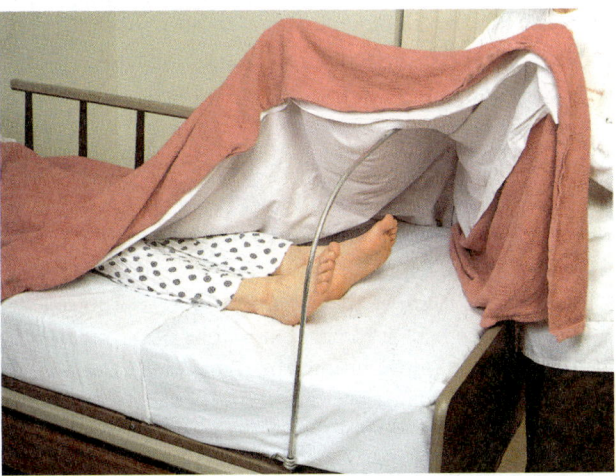

FIGURE 15-26B Bed cradles prevent pressure on the feet from the bed covers.

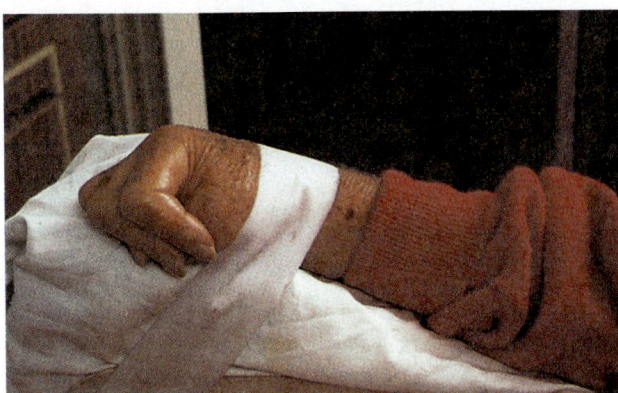

FIGURE 15-25 Contractures occur when joints are allowed to remain in the same position for too long.

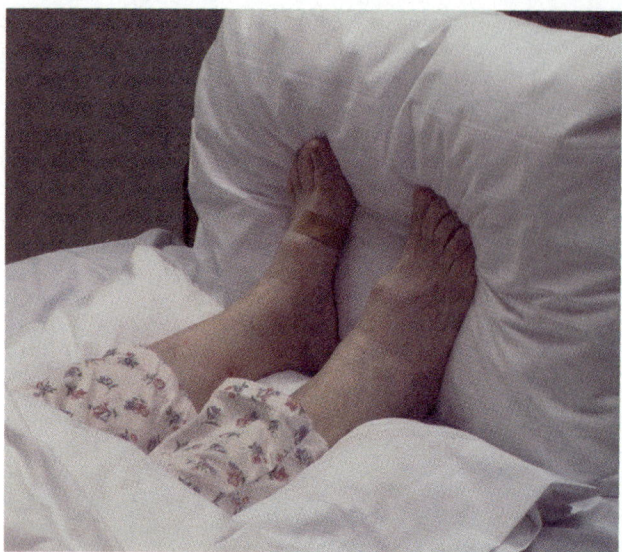

FIGURE 15-27 Footboards or a pillow resting against the footboard may be used to maintain good alignment and prevent contractures.

(Figure 15-27), can take the place of a footboard alone. In some cases, a footboard may be harmful. For example, a footboard against the soles of the feet can stimulate **spasticity** (involuntary muscle contraction) in the legs and possibly cause skin breakdown from the rubbing of the feet against the footboard. Special shoes are sometimes worn in bed to maintain the feet in correct alignment. In most cases, ankle contractures can be avoided by doing passive range-of-motion exercises consistently (Unit 40).

Many other commercial products can be used as supportive devices. Remember that a supportive device is also a restraint if it is attached or next to the patient's body, if the patient cannot easily remove it, and if it restricts freedom of movement and normal access to the patient's body.

Basic Body Positions

There are four basic positions, with variations for each one. These are:

- **Prone** (on the abdomen), with a variation of **semiprone**
- **Supine** (on the back), with a variation of **semisupine**
- **Lateral** (on either side), with a variation of **Sims' position**
- **Fowler's position**, with variations of **high Fowler's**, **semi-Fowler's**, and **orthopneic position**

Changing a patient's position involves these steps:

1. Moving the patient into proper body alignment. You may need to move the patient up in bed or to one side of the bed. If the patient will be positioned on his left side, move him to the right side of the bed. If the patient will be positioned on his right side, move him to the left side of the bed. That way he will not be too close to the edge of the bed after he is turned.

2. Turning the patient onto the back, onto the abdomen, or to the side.

3. Placing the patient's trunk and extremities in proper position and maintaining alignment with the use of supportive devices.

MOVING AND LIFTING PATIENTS

Lifting, moving, and transporting patients is a major responsibility of the nursing assistant. Using proper body mechanics and following safety rules will protect both you and your patients from injury. *Always* ask the nurse whether help is needed to lift or move a patient before pro-

OSHA *Alert*

Your spine is one of the most important parts of your body, enabling you to maintain an upright position, move freely, stand, and walk. The vertebrae protect your spinal cord, a column of nerves connecting your brain with the rest of your body. Your organs would not function without it. Keeping your spine healthy is a vital concern for nursing assistants. Unfortunately, back injuries from improper lifting and moving are common in health care workers. These are often caused by using improper lifting and moving techniques. Other contributing factors are rushing to get things done and not asking for help from others. Pay attention to your body and your position. Your back must last a lifetime.

SAFETY *Alert*

Using a lifting or turning sheet is better for the patient because it prevents injury to the skin. It prevents pain that sometimes occurs when you pull on the patient's body. It also reduces the risk of back injury in nursing assistants. When moving a patient on a sheet, make sure you have enough help. Two or three assistants may be necessary. Usually, two assistants are needed to reposition the patient's torso. A third may also be needed to prevent friction and shearing on the feet if the patient is being pulled up in bed.

ceeding with your assignment. Never be afraid to ask for help. By exercising caution, you are also preventing potentially serious injuries. Always check the care plan to see if there are special positioning instructions.

A turning sheet or draw sheet (folded large sheet or half sheet) may be placed under a heavy or helpless patient to make moving easier. The sheet must extend from above the shoulders to below the hips to be effective.

Procedures 14 to 17 should be followed when you are lifting or moving patients. As you practice these procedures, keep in mind the 10 basic rules of good body mechanics that were discussed in Unit 14.

PROCEDURE 14

TURNING THE PATIENT TOWARD YOU

1. Carry out each beginning procedure action.

2. Lower the side rail nearest to you. Cross the patient's far leg over the leg that is nearest to you.

3. Cross the far arm over the patient's chest. Bend the near arm at the elbow, bringing the hand toward the head of the bed.

4. Place your hand nearest the head of the bed on the patient's far shoulder. Place your other hand on the patient's hips on the far side. Brace your thighs against the side of the bed.

5. Roll the patient toward you (Figure 15-28A). Do it slowly, gently, and smoothly. Help the patient bring the upper leg toward you and bend it comfortably.

6. Put up the side rail. Be sure it is secure.

7. Go to the opposite side of the bed.

8. Place your hands under the patient's shoulders and then the hips. Pull toward the center of the bed (Figure 15-28B). This helps the patient maintain the side-lying position. Make sure the patient is not lying directly on the lower arm. The lower shoulder should be tipped slightly, so pressure is not centered directly over the joint.

9. Make sure the patient's body is properly aligned and safely positioned.

10. A pillow may be placed behind the patient's back. Secure it by pushing the near side under the patient to form a roll.

11. If the patient is unable to move independently, position the arms and legs. Support them with pillows between the shoulders, hands and knees, and ankles to prevent friction and contractures (Figure 15-28C). If the patient has an indwelling catheter, make sure the tubing is not between the legs, to prevent undue stress on the catheter and to prevent pressure ulcers.

12. Carry out each procedure completion action.

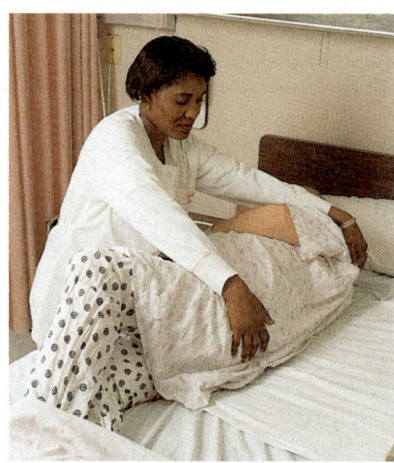

FIGURE 15-28A Place one hand on the patient's far shoulder and the other hand on the patient's hip, then turn the patient toward you.

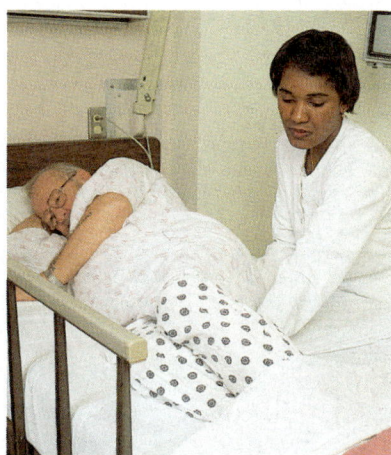

FIGURE 15-28B Move the patient to the center of the bed, keeping your back straight.

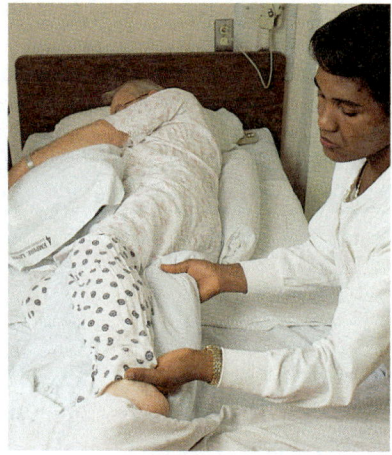

FIGURE 15-28C Place pillows to support the patient's body and maintain good alignment.

PROCEDURE 15

TURNING THE PATIENT AWAY FROM YOU

1. Carry out each beginning procedure action.

2. Lower the near side rail. Be sure the side rail on the opposite side of the bed is up and secure.

3. Have the patient bend his knees, if able. Cross the arms on the chest.

4. Place your arm nearest the head of the bed under the patient's head and shoulders. Place the other hand and forearm under the small of his back. Bend your body at the hips and knees. Keep your back straight. Pull the patient toward the edge of the bed.

5. Place your forearms under the hips and pull them toward you.

6. Move the ankles and knees toward you by placing one hand under the ankles and one under the knees.

7. Cross the near leg over the other leg at the ankles.

8. Roll the patient slowly and carefully away from you (Figure 15-29) by placing one hand under the shoulder and one hand under the hips.

9. Place your hands under the head and shoulders. Draw them back toward the center of the bed.

10. Move the hips to the center of the bed, as in step 5.

11. Place a pillow for support behind the back.

12. Make sure that the patient's body is in a good position. Support the upper leg with a pillow. Place the lower arm in a flexed position. Support the upper arm with a pillow.

13. Replace the side rail on near side of the bed. Return the bed to the lowest position.

14. Carry out each procedure completion action.

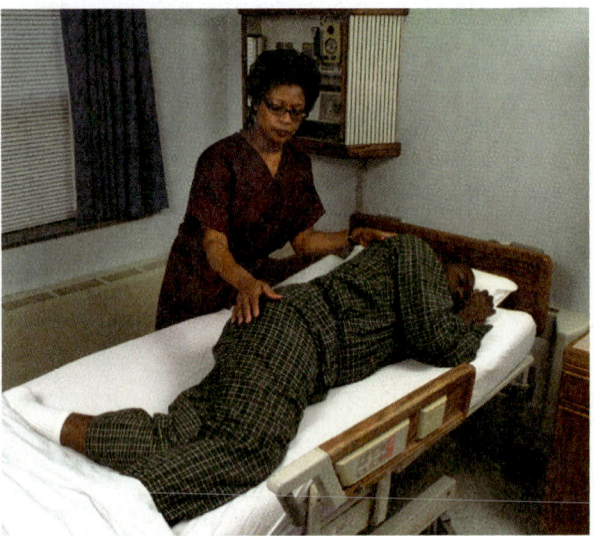

FIGURE 15-29 Roll the patient away from you.

PROCEDURE 16

MOVING A PATIENT TO THE HEAD OF THE BED

1. Carry out each beginning procedure action.

2. Ask a coworker to assist from the opposite side of the bed.

3. Lock the wheels of the bed. Raise the bed to comfortable horizontal working height. Lower side rails.

4. Lower the head of the bed if the patient can tolerate this position. Remove the pillow. Place it at the head of the bed, on its edge, for safety.

5. Lift top bedding and expose the draw sheet. Loosen both sides of the draw sheet.

continues

PROCEDURE 16

continued

6. Roll the draw sheet edges close to both sides of the patient's body (Figure 15-30).

7. Face the head of the bed. Grasp the draw sheet with the hand closest to the foot of the bed.

8. Position your feet 12 inches apart, with the foot that is farthest from the bed edge forward.

9. Place your free hand and arm under the neck and shoulders, cradling the head from both sides.

10. Bend your hips slightly.

11. Together, on a count of three, raise the patient's hips and back with the draw sheet, while supporting the head and shoulders. Move the patient smoothly toward the head of the bed.

12. Replace the pillow under the patient's head.

13. Tighten and tuck in the draw sheet. Adjust the top bedding.

14. Carry out each procedure completion action.

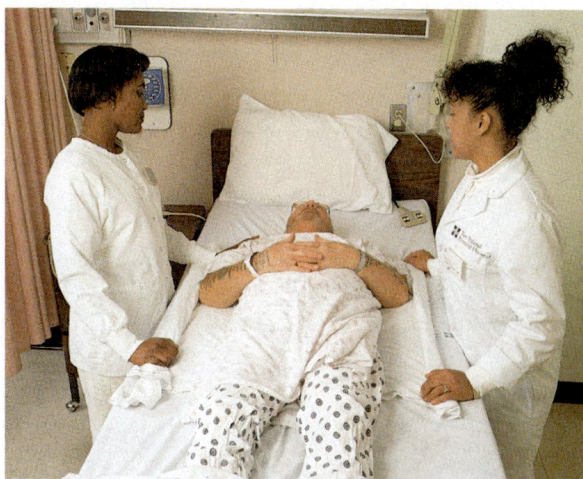

FIGURE 15-30 Using an overhand grasp, roll both edges of the turning (moving) sheet close to the patient's sides.

PROCEDURE 17

LOGROLLING THE PATIENT

📝 **Note:** *This procedure is performed when the patient's spinal column must be kept straight, such as following spinal surgery or spinal cord or vertebral column injury. It is a good procedure to use with any dependent patient.*

1. Carry out each beginning procedure action.

2. Get help from another nursing assistant.

3. Raise the bed to waist-high horizontal position. Lock the wheels.

4. Lower the side rail on the side opposite to which the patient will be turned. Both assistants should be on the same side of the bed.

5. One assistant places hands under the patient's head and shoulders. The second person places hands under the hips and legs. Then move the patient as a unit toward you.

6. Place a pillow lengthwise between the legs. Fold the patient's arm over the chest.

7. Raise the side rail. Check for security.

8. Go to the opposite side of the bed and lower the side rail.

9. Turning the patient to side may be done by:

   a. Using a turning sheet that was previously placed under the patient.

      - Reach over the patient, grasping and rolling the turning sheet toward the patient (Figure 15-31A).

      - One nursing assistant should be positioned beside the patient to keep the shoulders and hips straight.

      - A second assistant should be positioned to keep the thighs and lower legs straight.

   b. If a turning sheet is not in position, the first assistant should position hands on the patient's far shoulder and hips.

      - Second assistant positions hands on the patient's far thigh and lower leg.

continues

PROCEDURE 17

continued

10. At a specified signal, roll the patient toward both assistants in a single movement, keeping the spine, head, and legs straight. If a turning sheet is used, grasp the sheet and move the patient as a unit, onto her side (Figure 15-31B).

11. Place additional pillows behind the back to

maintain the patient's position. A small pillow or folded bath blanket may be permitted under the patient's head and neck. Leave a pillow between the legs. Position small pillows or folded towels to support the arms.

12. Carry out each procedure completion action.

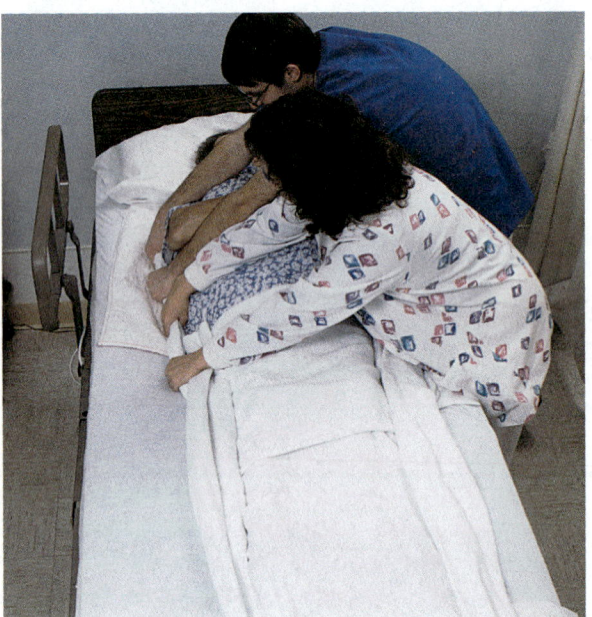

FIGURE 15-31A Roll the turning sheet against the patient.

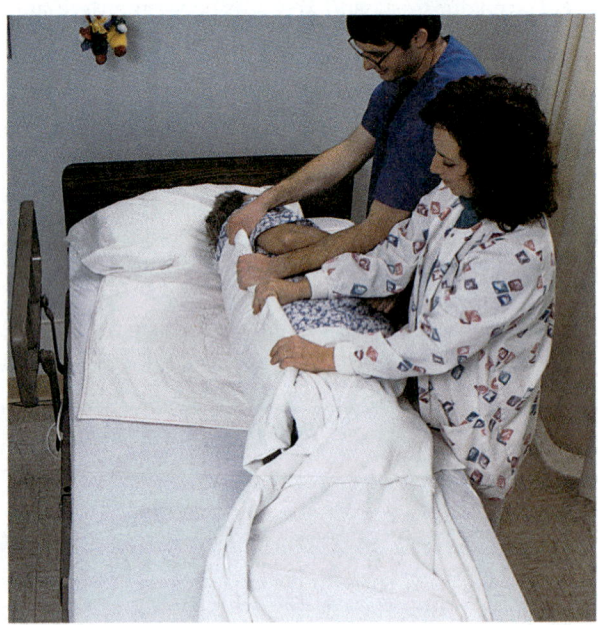

FIGURE 15-31B Pulling together, turn the patient to the side in one smooth motion.

Positioning the Patient

After you have turned and moved the patient into proper body alignment, you can place pillows and other supportive devices to help the patient maintain the position. Directions are given here for the basic four positions and their variations.

Supine Position (Figure 15-32A).

1. Start with the bed flat and the patient lying on the back. The patient's head should be about 2 to 3 inches from the head of the bed.

2. Place a pillow under the patient's head. It should extend about 2 inches below the patient's shoulders, with the head in the middle of the pillow.

3. Place a **trochanter roll** along the affected hip or along both hips if the patient has little control over the legs. A trochanter roll is devised by rolling a bath blanket into a shape about 12 inches long. The roll should be just long enough to reach from above the

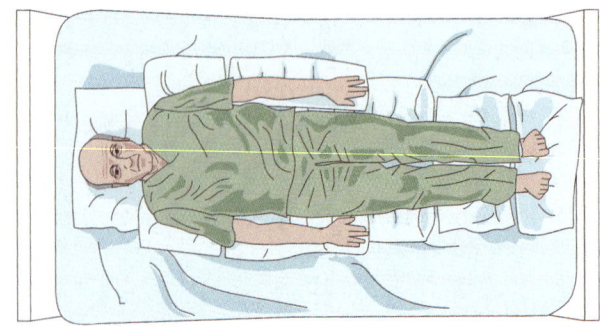

FIGURE 15-32A Supine position.

hip to above the knee (Figure 15-32B). The trochanter roll prevents external rotation (Figure 15-32C) of the hip.

4. Place pillows under the legs to reach from above the back of the knee to the ankle so that the ankles and heels do not rub on the sheets.

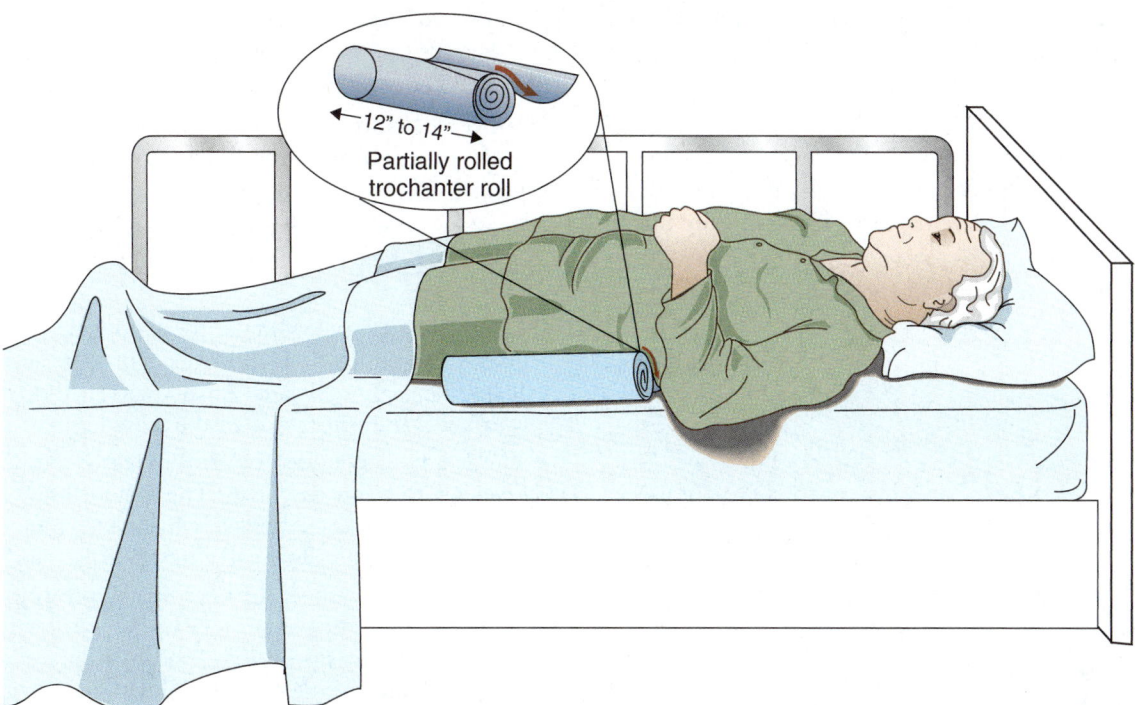

FIGURE 15-32B The trochanter roll should extend from above the hip to just above the knee.

5. If the care plan so indicates, position the footboard or place a folded pillow to support the patient's feet. The ankles should be at 90° angles.

6. Extend the patient's arms and place small pillows to reach from the elbow to below the wrist. The hand should be in alignment with the wrist and the palm should be down (Figure 15-32D).

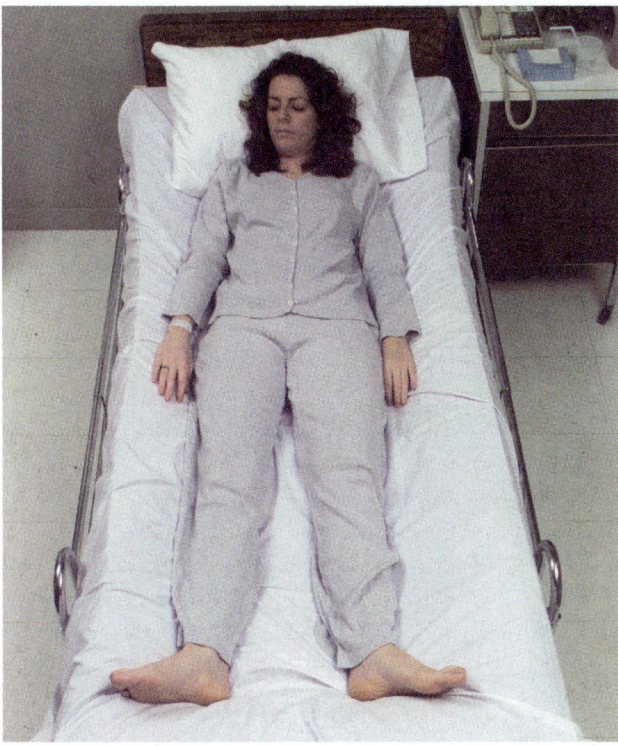

FIGURE 15-32C A correctly placed trochanter roll prevents external rotation of the hip.

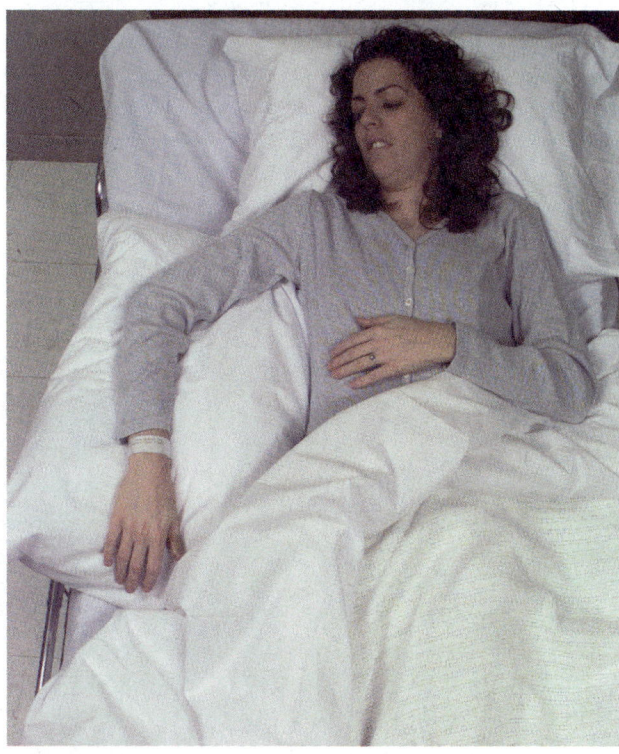

FIGURE 15-32D Pillows support the wrist and arm in good alignment and are more comfortable for the patient.

Semisupine Position (Figure 15-33). Start with the patient in supine position. Roll the trunk and shoulder away from you so that there is a 45° angle between the patient's back and the bed.

1. Place a pillow behind the back for support.
2. Bring the left shoulder forward. Flex the elbow of the left arm and place the lower left arm, palm up, on a pillow.
3. Flex the elbow of the right arm and bring the forearm across the chest with palm down.

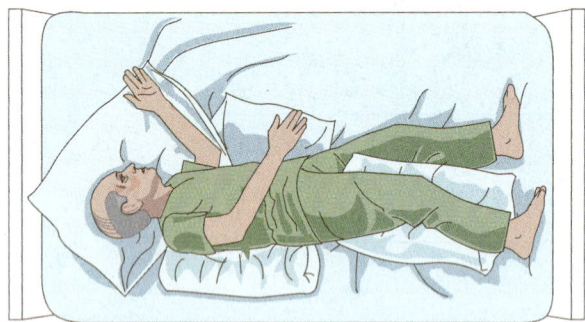

FIGURE 15-33 Semisupine position is a variation of supine that is very comfortable and prevents pressure on the major pressure points.

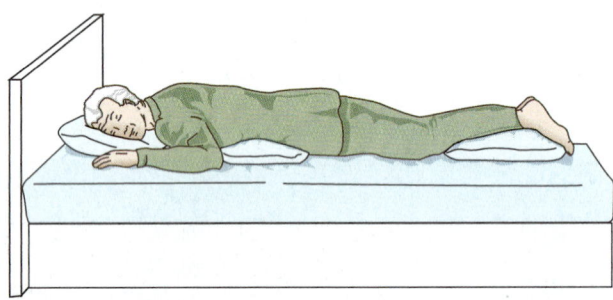

FIGURE 15-34A Prone position.

4. Extend both legs. Place the right leg a little behind the left leg. Support the right leg with two pillows folded in half that extend from groin to ankle.

Prone Position (Figure 15-34A). Start with the bed flat and the patient lying on the abdomen with the head turned to either side, spine straight and legs extended.

1. Place a small pillow under the head so that it extends to the patient's shoulders and 5 to 6 inches beyond the face.
2. Place a small pillow under the abdomen. This relieves pressure on the back and reduces pressure against a female patient's breasts. An alternate method is to roll a towel and place it under the shoulders.
3. Place a pillow under the arms to reach from the elbow to below the wrists. The shoulders and elbows may be flexed or extended, whichever is more comfortable for the patient (Figure 15-34B).
4. Place a pillow under the lower legs to prevent pressure on the toes. The patient may be moved down in bed before starting the procedure, so that the feet extend over the end of the mattress. This allows the foot to assume a normal standing position (Figure 15-34C).

Semiprone Position (Figure 15-35). This position relieves pressure on the hips. Breathing is easier in this position than in the full prone position. Directions are for the patient lying on the left side.

1. Extend the patient's left arm and tuck it slightly beneath the patient's body.
2. Place a pillow in front of and at right angles to the patient's chest.
3. Flex the patient's right knee and hip. Support with pillows that are parallel to the leg.
4. Grasp the patient's left arm from the back of the patient. Turn the patient onto the chest facing away from you. Gently pull his left arm toward you and push on the hip.

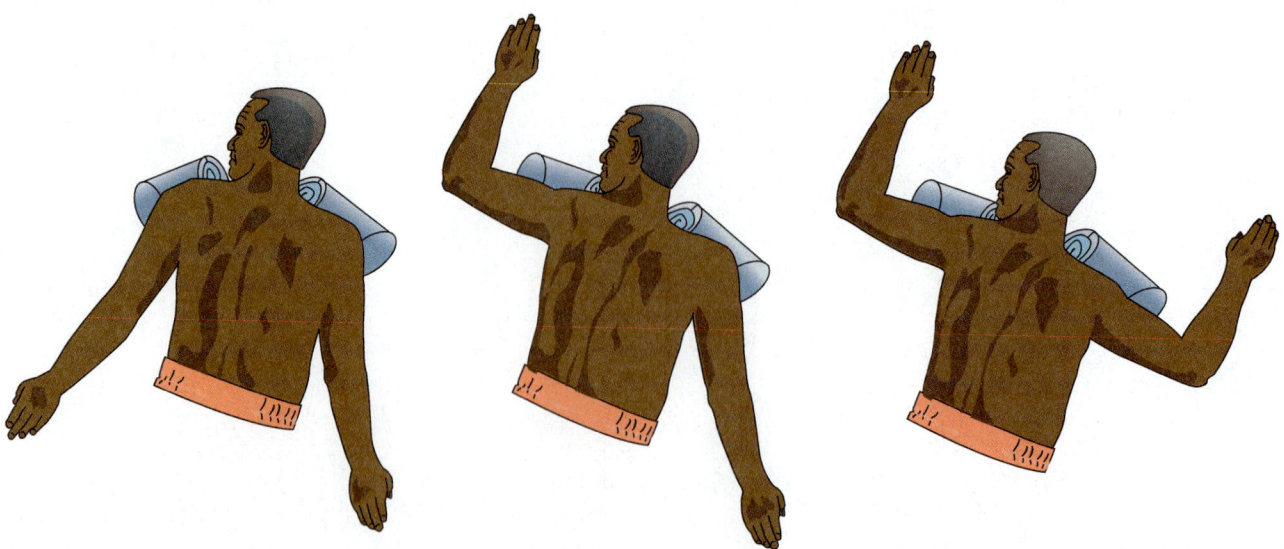

FIGURE 15-34B Position the arms in the way most comfortable for the patient.

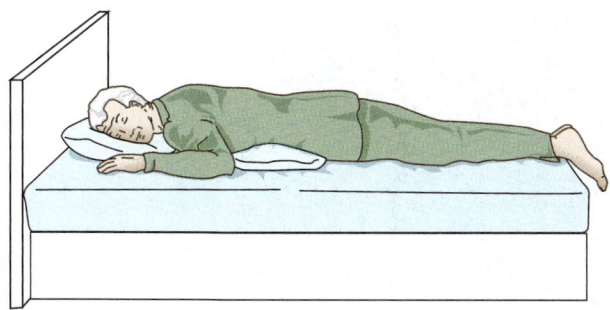

FIGURE 15-34C The patient may be moved down in bed so the feet hang over the end of the mattress.

Sheepskin

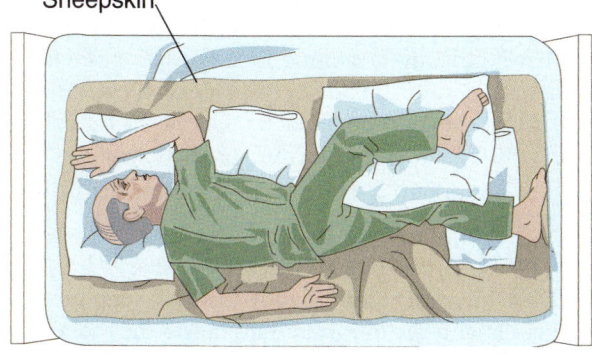

FIGURE 15-35 Semiprone position is a variation of prone.

5. Extend the right arm upward and toward the head of the bed. Place it on the head pillow with the fingers and palm against the bed.
6. Flex the upper arm on a pillow.
7. Lift up the sheepskin and place a foam block under the sheepskin above the iliac crest (hipbone).
8. Place another foam block under the sheepskin just below the iliac crest. You should be able to slide your hand between the hip and the bed.

SAFETY *Alert*

The semiprone and semisupine positions may be a source of confusion for some health care workers. These positions are not the same as the lateral positions. Patients in semiprone and semisupine positions are tilted at an angle so that pressure is not applied to the bony prominences, whereas the lateral position places pressure on many vital areas. The semiprone and semisupine positions are very comfortable and relieve pressure from all major pressure points on the patient's body.

Right Lateral Position (Figure 15-36). Reverse directions for left lateral position.

1. Start with the bed flat and the patient turned to the left side, with spine straight. Remember before turning to move the patient to the right side of the bed.
2. Place a pillow under the head so it extends 5 to 6 inches beyond the patient's face and down to the shoulders.
3. Position the right arm so the shoulder and elbow are flexed and the palm of the hand is facing up.
4. Place the left arm so it is extended or only slightly flexed and rest it on the hip or bring it forward and place it on a pillow. The patient's shoulder, elbow, and wrist should be at approximately the same height.
5. Place a pillow between the patient's legs, extending from above the knee to below the ankle. The patient's hip, knee, and ankle should be at approximately the same height.
6. A pillow may be placed behind the patient to help maintain the position.

Sims' Position (Figure 15-37). This is a variation of the lateral position with the patient on the left side, left leg extended and right leg flexed. This position is often used for rectal examinations and treatments and enemas.

1. Place a pillow under the patient's head as for lateral position.
2. Start with the bed flat and the patient moved and turned onto the left side.
3. Extend the patient's left arm and position it behind the patient's back.
4. Flex the right arm and bring it forward. Support the arm with a pillow.

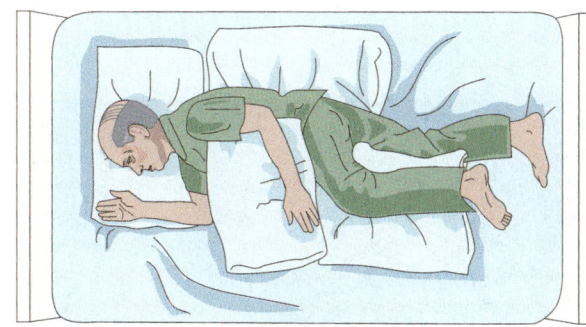

FIGURE 15-36 Right lateral position.

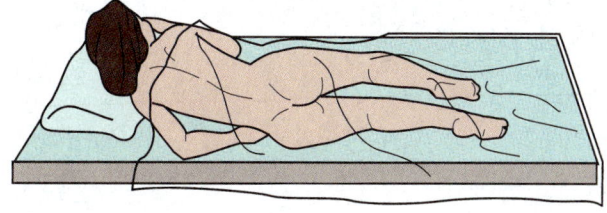

FIGURE 15-37 Sims' position.

Fowler's Position. This position, or a variation of it, is used for feeding patients in bed, for certain treatments and procedures, for the patient's comfort while visiting or watching television, and for those who have trouble breathing. This position increases pressure on the buttocks and increases the risk of skin breakdown and pressure ulcers. Because of this, patients should not be left in Fowler's position for prolonged periods. Check the care plan for instructions.

1. Start with the patient on the back, in the middle of the bed and in good alignment. The patient's hips should be at the place where the bed bends when the bed head is rolled up. Place the head of the bed at 30° for semi-Fowler's, 45° to 60° for Fowler's (Figure 15-38), and 90° for high Fowler's.

2. Place one or two pillows behind the patient's head to extend 4 to 5 inches below the patient's shoulders.

3. Flex elbows and place a pillow under each arm to prevent pull on the shoulders.

4. Place a pillow under each leg to extend from above the knee and to the ankle, to prevent pressure on heels.

5. Place a footboard or folded pillow to keep the feet in position, if necessary.

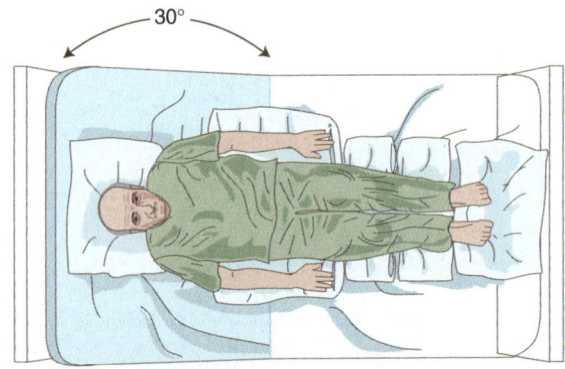

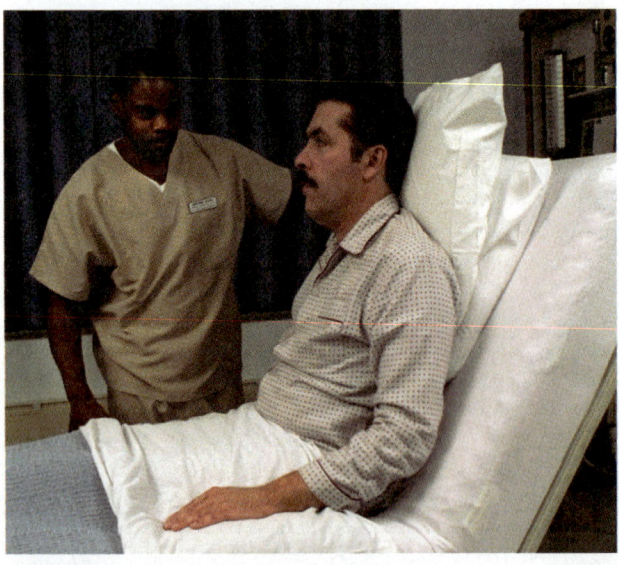

FIGURE 15-38 Fowler's position.

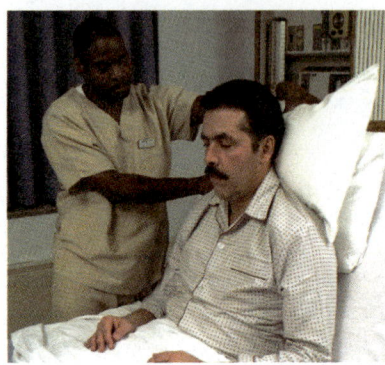

FIGURE 15-39
Orthopneic position.

Orthopneic Position (Figure 15-39). This is a variation of high Fowler's position and is used for patients who have difficulty breathing. Like Fowler's position, the orthopneic position increases the risk of pressure ulcers. Special skin care may be necessary. Check the care plan or ask the nurse manager for further instructions.

1. The position of the bed remains the same as high Fowler's.

2. Assist the patient to sit as upright as possible.

3. Have the patient lean slightly forward, supporting herself with the forearms. This makes the thorax larger, enabling the patient to inhale more air.

4. Place another pillow low behind the patient's back for support.

Sitting Position. Patients should be positioned in a comfortable, well-constructed chair, so that the head and spine are erect (Figure 15-40). The back and buttocks should be up against the chair back. The feet should be flat on the floor.

1. Pillows or postural supports may be needed to maintain the position.

2. A small pillow may be folded and placed at the small of the back to add comfort and support.

3. Do not permit the back of the patient's knees to rest against the chair.

SAFETY *Alert*

Patients can develop pressure ulcers when sitting in a chair. If the patient will be up in the chair for prolonged periods of time, make sure that the seat of the chair is padded. If the patient is able, remind him or her to push on the armrests and shift his or her weight every 15 minutes. Ambulate, stand, or reposition the patient in the chair at least every 2 hours to stimulate circulation and relieve pressure.

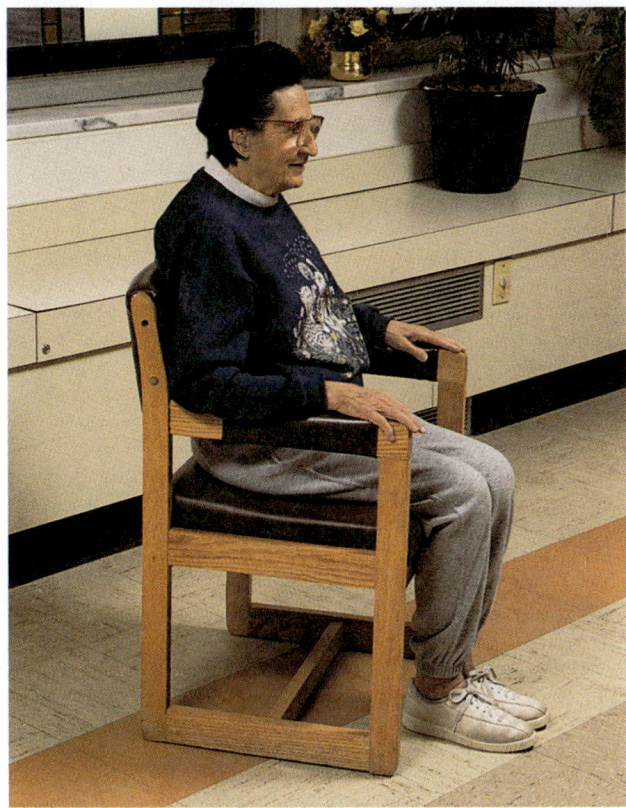

FIGURE 15-40 Maintaining good body alignment is important when patients are sitting in chairs.

Positioning Devices. Several types of devices, called orthoses, are used to maintain the position of an extremity. The correct use of these devices prevents contracture formation. Orthoses are also called splints. Figure 15-41 shows examples of orthoses for the upper extremities.

The physician may also order splints or orthoses for the lower extremities. A common type is called the *ankle foot orthosis (AFO)*. The AFO provides support for an unstable ankle and helps reduce extensor spasticity. The AFO is applied to the lower leg before the shoe is put on.

guidelines *for*

The Use of Splints

- The splint must be applied correctly. Follow the manufacturer's directions for each splint.
- Follow the care plan for the patient's wearing schedule.
- Keep the extremity under the splint clean and dry.
- Keep the splint clean. If it becomes soiled, check with the nurse to see how it should be cleaned.
- Check the skin under the splint regularly for signs of redness, irritation, and skin breakdown.

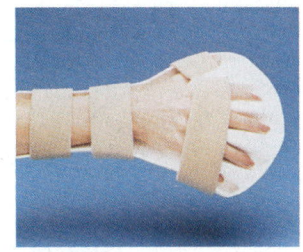
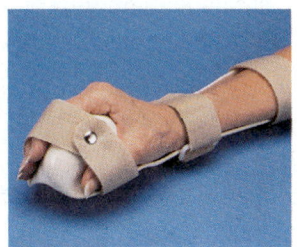
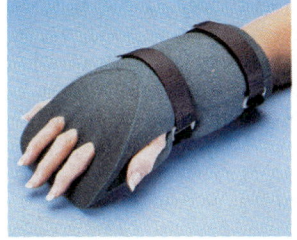
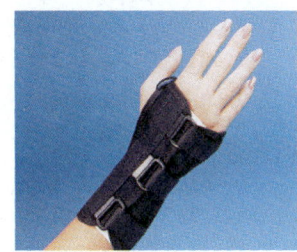

FIGURE 15-41 Several different orthoses are used to maintain good alignment of the hand, wrist, and fingers. *(Photos provided by Sammons Preston, Inc., a Bissell® HealthCare Company. Reprinted with permission.)*

REVIEW

A. Multiple Choice.

Select the one best answer for each of the following.

1. Patients may be at risk for incidents because they
   a. ambulate in the hallway.
   b. use a wheelchair for long distances.
   c. keep one side rail up for turning independently when in bed.
   d. receive certain medications affecting balance, coordination, and mental status.

2. Patient falls can be prevented by
   a. encouraging the patient to remain in bed.
   b. using restraints when the patient is up.
   c. keeping the side rails up at all times.
   d. caring for the patient's physical needs promptly.

3. Alternatives to restraints include
   a. taking patients to the bathroom regularly.
   b. giving medications to sedate the patient.

    c. playing music throughout the day to distract the patient.

    d. using side rails when in bed.

4. When restraints are used, they must be released

    a. every 2 hours.

    b. once each shift.

    c. every hour.

    d. every 4 hours.

5. When restraints are used on patients in bed,

    a. there must be full side rails on the bed, in the raised position.

    b. the bed should be elevated to the high position.

    c. the restraints should be secured to the stationary part of the bed frame.

    d. the electric bed adjustment switch should be removed to reduce the risk of injury.

6. Injuries caused by heat or cold are called

    a. lacerations.

    b. bruises.

    c. thermal injuries.

    d. aspiration.

7. Choking may be prevented by

    a. giving the patient only fluids.

    b. giving the patient finger foods.

    c. using thickeners for liquids.

    d. allowing only blended foods.

8. Beginning procedure actions include

    a. handwashing.

    b. raising side rails.

    c. placing the call signal within reach.

    d. opening the door.

9. Correct body alignment will

    a. heal disease.

    b. prevent infection.

    c. help the body function more efficiently.

    d. be harmful in certain circumstances.

10. Examples of supportive devices include

    a. belts.

    b. pillows.

    c. side rails.

    d. vests.

11. Supine position is

    a. lying on the back.

    b. lying on the abdomen.

    c. lying on the side.

    d. sitting in the chair.

12. A position used for patients who have trouble breathing is

    a. orthopneic.

    b. semiprone.

    c. lateral.

    d. supine.

13. Logrolling is a procedure performed for

    a. persons who have had both legs amputated.

    b. ambulatory patients.

    c. all conscious patients.

    d. patients who have had spinal surgery or spinal cord injury.

14. A trochanter roll is used to

    a. maintain the hip in alignment.

    b. maintain the feet in alignment.

    c. support the patient's back.

    d. prevent contractures of the hand.

15. Splints may be used to

    a. maintain position of an extremity.

    b. provide support for a fractured femur.

    c. restrain the wrists.

    d. prevent pressure ulcers.

B. True/False.

Mark the following true or false by circling T or F.

16. T F Restraints are attached to the side rails for security.

17. T F Restraints may be needed for some patients.

18. T F A physician's order is not necessary before applying restraints.

19. T F The position of bed patients should be changed at least every 2 hours.

20. T F The left Sims' position is often used for rectal treatments and enemas.

21. T F When turning a patient toward you, cross the patient's near leg over the leg that is farthest from you.

22. T F You must wash your hands before beginning and after completing every nursing assistant task.

23. T F After patient care, the bed should be left in the highest horizontal position.

24. T F Turning sheets make moving heavy patients an easier task.

25. T F You should always explain what you plan to do even if the patient seems not to hear or understand.

C. Matching.

Complete the following by matching Column I with Column II.

Column I

26. __f__ supine

27. __g__ prone

28. __e__ orthopneic

29. __a__ trochanter roll

30. __d__ splint

31. __b__ contracture

32. __c__ supportive devices

33. __h__ physical restraints

Column II

a. prevents external rotation of hip

b. joint deformity caused by shortening of the muscles

c. devices used to maintain patient's position

d. device used to maintain position of an extremity

e. position for patients with difficult breathing

f. lying on the back

g. lying on the abdomen

h. devices that inhibit movement

D. Nursing Assistant Challenge.

Sara Abrams is 76 years old, has Parkinson's disease, and is a resident in a long-term care facility. She is ambulatory, with a shuffling walk, and has tremors of her hands related to the Parkinson's. She is disoriented and frequently walks into other patients' rooms.

34. Discuss safety issues related to Ms. Abrams's condition.

35. Which of the Residents' Rights may be a special issue in this situation?

36. What steps can you take to meet Ms. Abrams's physical needs? Will doing so lower her risk of falling?

37. How can you incorporate exercise into her daily routine?

38. What types of activities might interest Ms. Abrams?

39. Are there are actions that can be taken to avoid restraints and falls?

EXPLORING THE WEB

Description	Location
Patient Safety	*http://www.patientsafety.com*
American Society for Healthcare Risk Management Hospital Connect	*http://www.hospitalconnect.com*
Before the Fall	*http://www.advancefornurses.com* (see past articles 6/24/02)
Developing Successful Strategies for Preventing Falls	*http://www.nursinghome.org*
National Center for Injury Prevention and Control	*http://www.cdc.gov/ncipc/pub-res/toolkit/toolkit.htm*
National Patient Safety Foundation	*http://www.ama-assn.org*
National Safety Council	*http://www.nsc.org*
Posey Corporation	*http://www.posey.com*
Restraint Reduction	*http://www.nursinghome.org*
The Right Steps (Orthoses)	*http://www.advancefornurses.com* (see past articles 9/25/00)
RN Plus Fall Prevention	*http://www.rnplus.com*
Skil-Care Corporation	*http://www.skil-care.com*
Untie the Elderly Newsletter	*http://www.ute.kendal.org*
Vail Beds	*http://www.vailbed.com*

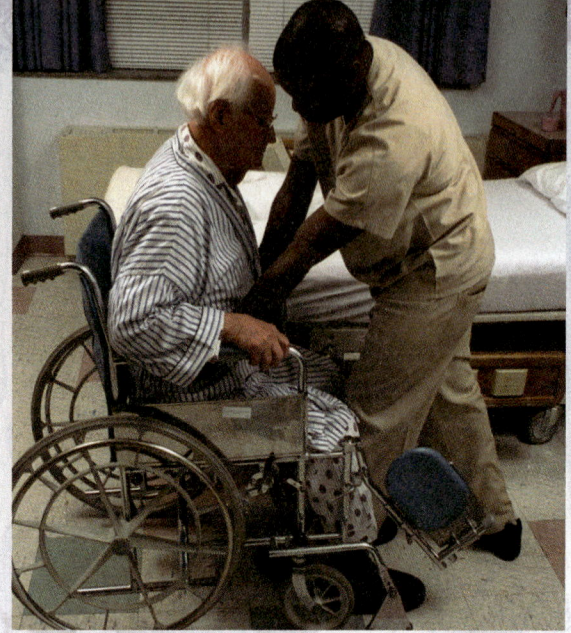

The Patient's Mobility: Transfer Skills

objectives

After completing this unit, you will be able to:

- Spell and define terms.
- List the guidelines for safe transfers.
- Describe the difference between a standing transfer and a sitting transfer.
- Demonstrate correct application of a transfer belt.
- Demonstrate the following procedures:
  - Procedure 18 Applying a Transfer Belt
  - Procedure 19 Transferring the Patient from Bed to Chair—One Assistant
  - Procedure 20 Transferring the Patient from Bed to Chair—Two Assistants
  - Procedure 21 Transferring the Patient from Chair to Bed—One Assistant
  - Procedure 22 Transferring the Patient from Chair to Bed—Two Assistants
  - Procedure 23 Independent Transfer, Standby Assist
  - Procedure 24 Transferring the Patient from Bed to Stretcher
  - Procedure 25 Transferring the Patient from Stretcher to Bed
  - Procedure 26 Transferring the Patient with a Mechanical Lift
  - Procedure 27 Transferring the Patient onto and off the Toilet
  - Procedure 28 Transferring the Patient into and out of the Bathtub
  - Procedure 29 Transferring a Patient into and out of a Car

vocabulary

Learn the meaning and the correct spelling of the following words and phrases:

contraindication	nonweight-bearing	pivot	weight-bearing
full weight-bearing	paralysis	sitting transfer	
gait belt	paresis	standing transfer	
mechanical lift	partial weight-bearing	transfer belt	

INTRODUCTION

As a nursing assistant, you will work with many patients who have impaired mobility. In the last unit you learned how to move and position patients in bed. In this unit you will learn how to transfer patients (to move them from one place to another). Patients transfer:

- Out of bed into a chair and back to bed from the chair
- Out of bed onto a stretcher and back to bed from the stretcher
- Onto and off of a toilet
- Into and out of a car
- Into and out of a bathtub or shower

Refer to Procedures 19 through 29 later in this unit.

TYPES OF TRANSFERS

There are basically two types of transfers. A **standing transfer** means the patient stands during the transfer with the help of one or two nursing assistants. A **sitting transfer** means the patient is sitting throughout the transfer, such as when a **mechanical lift** is used. A mechanical lift is a piece of equipment that is used to move dependent patients.

The nurse or the physical therapist determines which method is used to transfer a patient (Figure 16-1). It is important to follow instructions carefully to avoid injury. The method selected depends on:

1. The patient's physical condition. This takes into consideration:
   - **Paralysis** (inability to move) of any extremity
   - **Paresis**, which is weakness of an extremity
   - Absence of an extremity due to amputation
   - Recent hip surgery
2. The patient's strength, endurance, and balance. These abilities may be affected by:
   - Respiratory (lung) disease
   - Cardiac (heart) disease

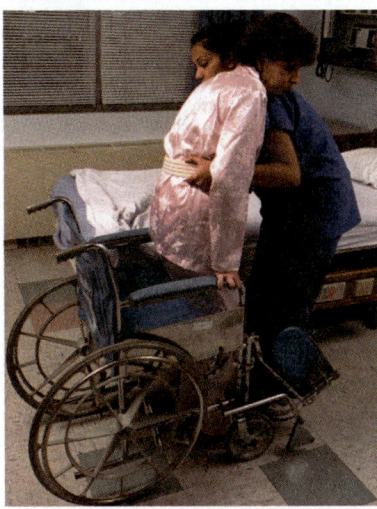

FIGURE 16-1
The nurse or physical therapist determines the method of transfer.

guidelines *for*

Safe Patient Transfers

Moving dependent patients can result in injury to you or the patient unless all safety measures are followed.

- Know the method of transfer that has been ordered by the nurse or physical therapist.
- Know the patient's capabilities.
- Use correct body mechanics.
- Place the bed in the lowest position before starting the standing transfer. Make sure the wheels on the bed and the transfer vehicle (wheelchair, stretcher) are locked before the move. It is helpful to elevate the head of the bed for bed-to-chair transfers.
- *Never allow patients to place their hands on your body during a transfer.* This is a dangerous practice. A patient who is disoriented or frightened can cause you to lose your balance. If this happens, the patient can pull you down, possibly injuring both of you.
- *Never place your hands under a patient's arms or shoulders.* This practice can cause the patient severe shoulder injury.
- Use a transfer belt for standing transfers unless it is contraindicated.
- Make sure the patient is wearing shoes with sturdy, nonslip soles and that clothing is not too loose or dragging on the floor.
- Be aware of any tubes, orthoses, or other items that must be dealt with during the transfer.
- Transfer the patient toward his strongest side if possible.
- Always explain to the patient what you are doing and how he can help.
- Test the patient's understanding and make sure she knows what you expect her to do during the transfer.
- Allow the patient to see the surface to which he is being transferred. Encourage the patient to keep his head up.
- Stand close to the patient during the transfer.
- If the patient has a weak or paralyzed leg, brace the knee of that leg with your knee or leg. If the patient has a paralyzed arm, be sure it is supported during the transfer to avoid dangling and pulling on the patient's shoulder.
- Give the patient only the assistance that she needs.
- Never have the patient use a footstool unless it is absolutely necessary.

- Neurological disease, such as multiple sclerosis or a stroke

- The ability to stand on one or both legs. This is called **weight-bearing**. For example, a patient may not be able to place full weight on a paralyzed leg. The physician may order the patient to be **non-weight-bearing** or only **partial weight-bearing** if the patient has had hip surgery. The ability to stand on both legs is called **full weight-bearing**. For a standing transfer, the patient must be able to stand and have at least partial weight-bearing on one leg.

3. The patient's mental condition. Can the patient understand and follow the instructions?

4. The patient's size. For example, transfer of a very tall or large person who cannot bear full weight would need two assistants or a mechanical lift.

In some situations you may be instructed to take the patient's pulse before and after she gets out of bed. If the patient has been inactive for a long time, the heart muscle may be deconditioned. Checking the pulse when the patient is active provides an evaluation of the heart's condition.

TRANSFER BELTS

A **transfer belt** is a webbed belt 1½ to 2 inches wide and about 54 to 60 inches long. It is an assistive and safety device used to transfer or ambulate patients who need help. (Refer to Procedure 18.) When it is used to assist a patient with ambulation, it is called a **gait belt**. Using a transfer belt avoids the need to grasp the patient around the rib cage or under the shoulders. Either of these methods can cause serious injury. It also allows you to have more control in directing the transfer. A transfer belt is not used to "lift" a patient. If the patient has no ability to bear weight, another method should be used for transferring.

OSHA *Alert*

Each year more than 12.8 million Americans consult their doctors about back problems. In fact, as many as 8 out of 10 individuals will suffer back pain during their lifetime. A transfer belt is an inexpensive item that helps protect you from injury and makes transfers safer and more secure for patients. Make the transfer belt a permanent part of your uniform. Wear it when you are on duty so it is readily available when needed to move a patient.

Contraindications (situations in which something is not indicated, inappropriate, or potentially dangerous) for use of the transfer belt include:

- Abdominal, back, or rib injuries, fractures, or recent surgery
- Abdominal pacemakers
- Advanced heart or lung disease
- Abdominal aneurysms
- Pregnancy
- Colostomy
- Gastrostomy tube or feeding tube

Medication pumps may be implanted under the skin of the abdomen in some patients. If the surgical site is well healed, it is probably safe to use the transfer belt. However, always follow the care plan or check with the nurse before using a transfer belt to move a patient with any type of implantable device.

PROCEDURE 18

APPLYING A TRANSFER BELT

1. Carry out beginning procedure actions.

2. Assemble equipment:
   - Transfer belt

3. Explain the procedure. Tell the patient that the belt is a safety device that will be removed as soon as the transfer is completed.

4. Apply the belt over the patient's clothing (Figure 16-2A). If the patient is undressed and being transferred from wheelchair to tub or shower chair, either leave the patient's shirt on, put the patient's robe on, or place a towel around the patient's waist and then apply the belt over the towel.

continues

PROCEDURE 18

continued

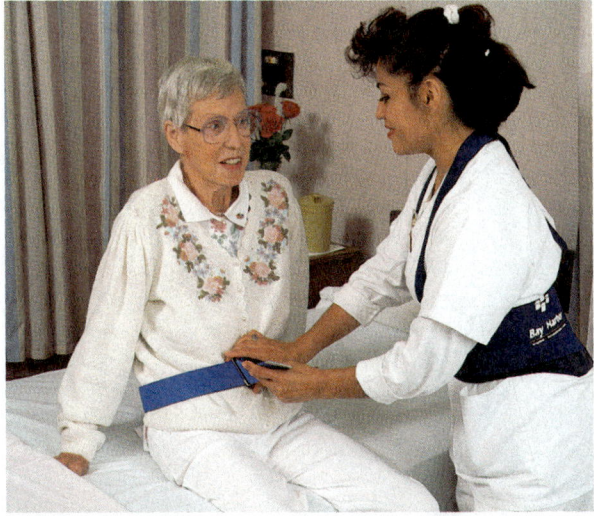

FIGURE 16-2A   Always apply the transfer belt over clothing.

5. If the patient is going to transfer from bed to chair, the belt may be applied after the patient comes to a sitting position on the edge of the bed. If the patient has inadequate balance, the belt can be applied while the patient is still lying down in bed. You may need to readjust the belt after the patient sits up.

6. Keep the belt at the patient's waist level. Avoid placing it too high. Make sure the belt is right side out and is not twisted.

7. Buckle the belt in front by threading the belt end through the teeth side of the buckle first and then through both openings (Figure 16-2B). The buckle must be in front.

8. Check female patients to be sure the breasts are not under the belt.

9. The belt should be snug, so that it does not slide up, but not tight (Figure 16-2C). Check the fit of the belt by placing three fingers under it. There should be just enough space for your fingers to fit comfortably.

10. Before attempting to move the patient, be sure her feet are flat on the floor. If they are not, use the belt to assist the patient to the edge of the bed until her feet are resting firmly on the floor.

11. If you are transferring a patient into or out of a wheelchair, keep the footrests out of the way during the transfer. After the patient is seated, her legs should not dangle. The feet are supported on the floor or on the wheelchair footrests.

12. Teach the patient to assist by pushing off the bed or arms of the chair with her hands when you count to three.

13. Use an underhand grasp when holding the belt. For transfers, one hand should be on each side of the buckle in front.

14. Do not overuse the belt by pulling the patient up with force.

15. When the patient is standing, pivot to transfer.

16. The chair should be close enough so the patient can feel it with her hands after you pivot.

17. Remove the belt after the patient is safely moved.

18. Carry out procedure completion actions.

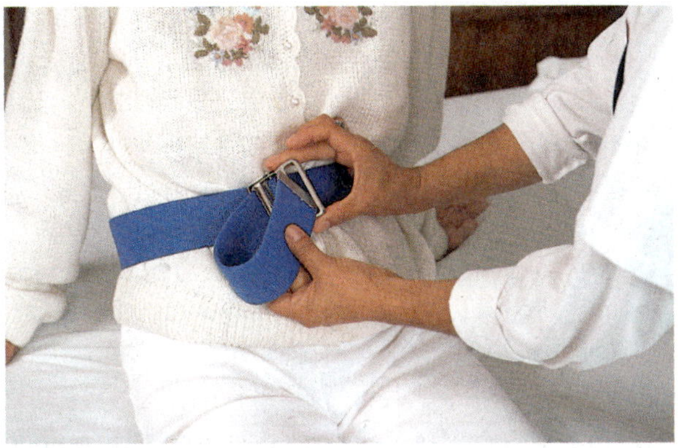

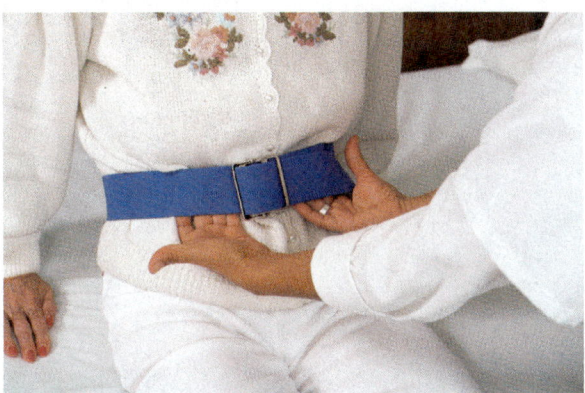

FIGURE 16-2B Thread the belt through the teeth side of the buckle first.

FIGURE 16-2C The belt should be snug but not tight.

PROCEDURE 19

TRANSFERRING THE PATIENT FROM BED TO CHAIR—ONE ASSISTANT

1. Carry out beginning procedure actions.

2. Assemble equipment:
   - Transfer belt
   - Chair for patient
   - Bath blanket
   - Robe or clothing
   - Shoes and socks

3. Place chair so the patient moves toward her strongest side. Set the chair parallel with the bed. Lock the wheelchair and raise or remove the footrests (Figure 16-3A). Cover the chair with a bath blanket, unless the patient is fully clothed.

4. Lower the bed to the lowest horizontal position and lock the bed wheels.

These instructions are for getting out of the right side (patient's right side) of the bed.

5. Stand against the right side of the bed with the side rail down. Ask the patient to slide toward the right side of the bed.

6. Have the patient roll over onto her right side, flexing the knees and bending the right arm so it can be used for propping the upper body. Bend the elbow of the left arm so this hand can be used to push off from the bed.

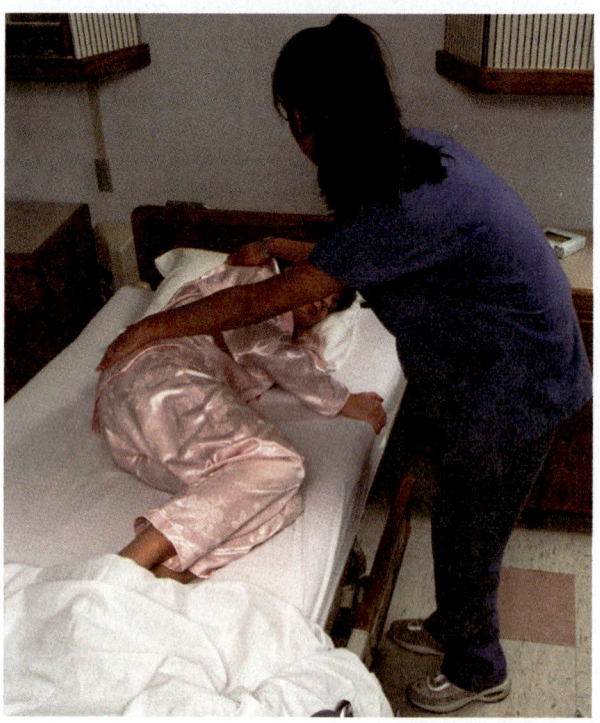

FIGURE 16-3B Instruct the patient to use her hands to push to the sitting position.

7. Instruct the patient to use the elbow of her right arm to raise the upper body and to push with the hand of the right arm so she comes to an upright position (Figure 16-3B).

8. Instruct the patient to let her legs slide off the bed at the same time.

9. If assistance is needed, place one arm under the shoulders (not the neck) and one arm over and around the knees (Figure 16-3C). Raise the patient's upper body at the same time you move the legs off the bed.

10. Give the patient time to adjust to sitting up and then apply the transfer belt. Assist to put on shoes and socks. (If the patient has problems with balance, the shoes and socks can be put on while the patient is lying down in bed.)

11. If the patient has a weak or paralyzed arm, do not let it hang or dangle during the transfer. Put it in

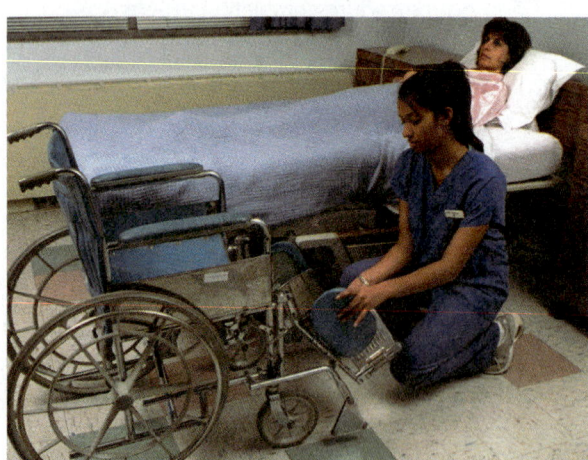

FIGURE 16-3A Lock the wheelchair and lift or remove the footrests before the patient transfers.

continues

PROCEDURE 19

continued

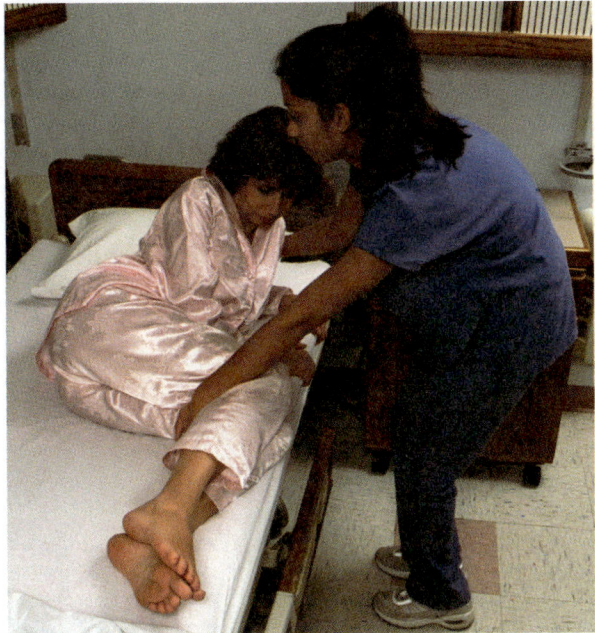

FIGURE 16-3C Place one arm under the patient's shoulders and one arm over and around the patient's knees.

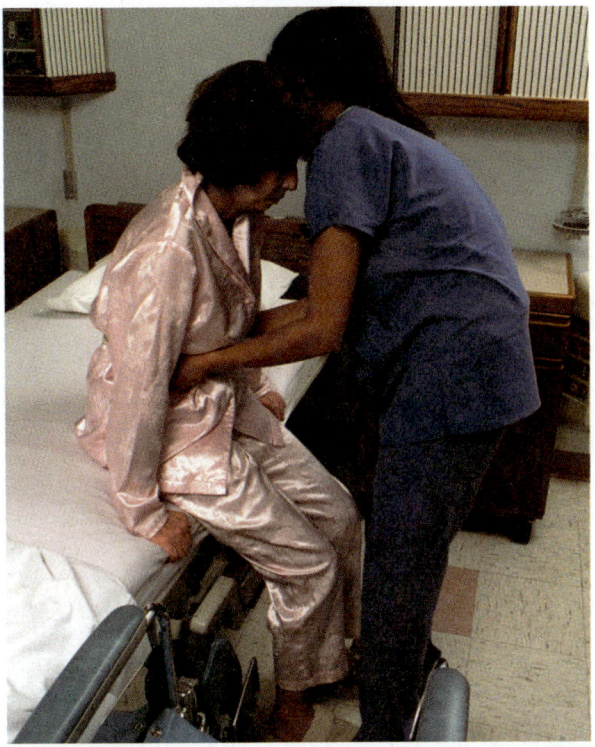

FIGURE 16-3D The stronger leg should be slightly back.

her pocket, or have her cradle it with her strong arm, or carefully tuck her weaker hand in the transfer belt or waist of the pants until she is again seated.

12. When the patient is ready to transfer:

    * Instruct her to move forward or closer to the edge of the mattress, to spread her knees, lean forward from the waist, and place her feet slightly back.

    * If one leg is weaker or should not bear weight, place this leg out in front with the strong leg slightly back (Figure 16-3D).

    * Remember to spread your feet apart and bend your knees and hips, keeping your back straight.

    * Hold the belt with an underhand grasp, one hand on each side of the front of the belt.

    * If the patient has a weaker leg, press your knee against her knee, or block the patient's foot with yours to prevent the weaker leg from sliding out from under her.

    * Tell the patient on the count of three to use her hands (if able) to press into the mattress, to straighten her elbows and knees, and to come to a standing position (Figure 16-3E).

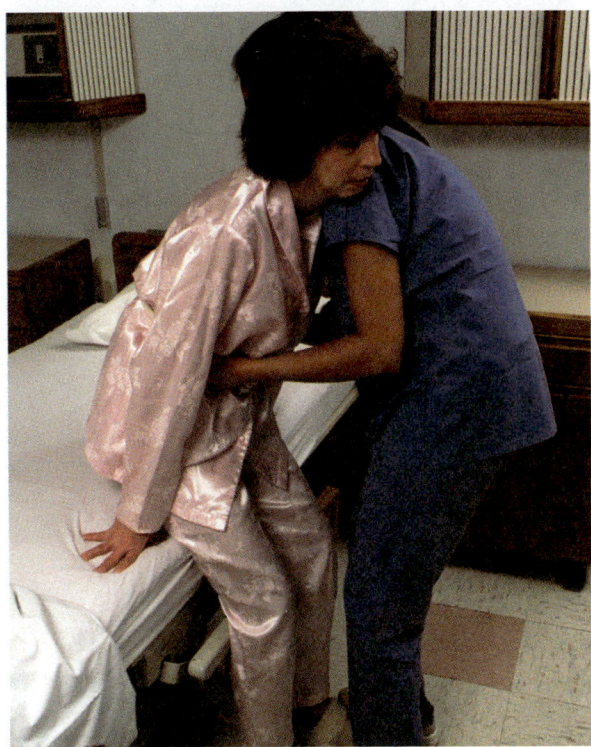

FIGURE 16-3E Tell the patient to straighten her elbows and knees to come to a standing position.

continues

PROCEDURE 19

continued

13. If patient cannot walk, have her **pivot** (turn the entire body as one unit) around to the front of the chair until the chair is touching the backs of her legs (Figure 16-3F).

14. Instruct the patient to place her hands on the arms of the chair (if able), to bend her knees, and to gently lower herself into the chair as you ease her downward (Figure 16-3G). Replace the footrests.

15. Position patient comfortably. Place the signal light within easy reach.

16. Straighten the bed and prepare it for the patient's return.

17. Carry out procedure completion actions.

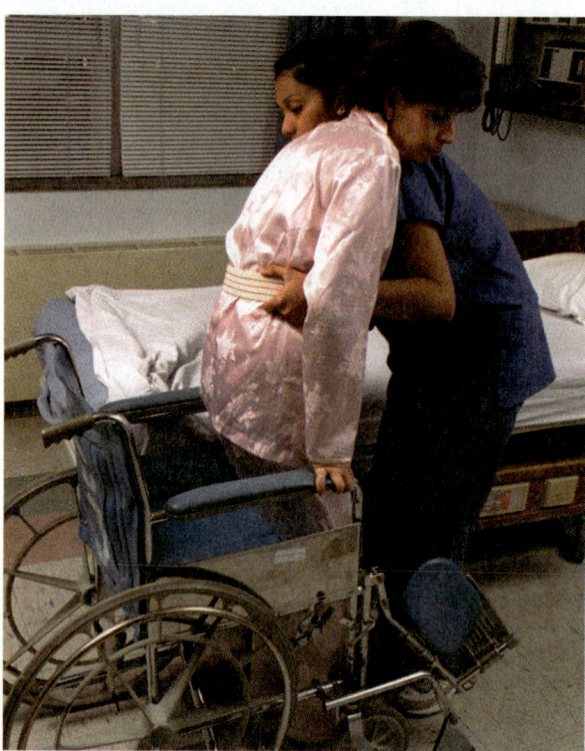

FIGURE 16-3F The patient pivots around to the wheelchair.

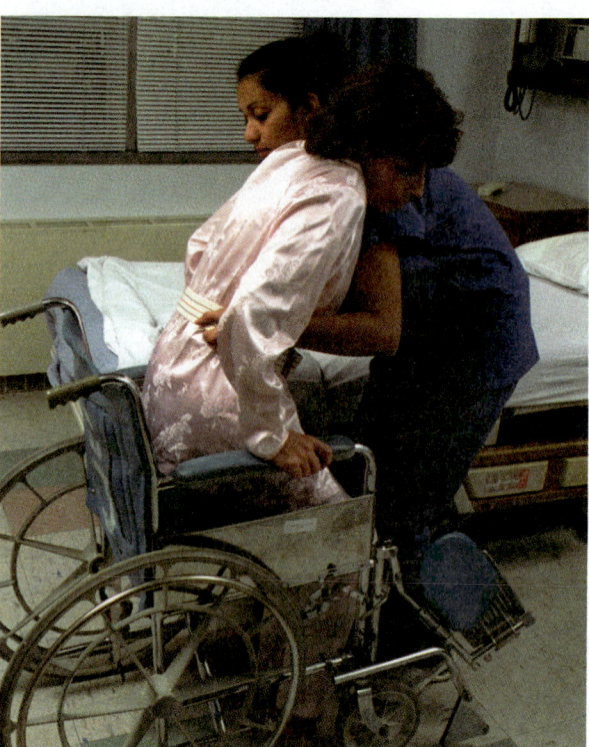

FIGURE 16-3G Tell the patient to bend her knees and lower herself into the chair.

SAFETY *Alert*

Remember to lock the brakes before transferring a patient into or out of a wheelchair. Turn the small front wheels so the large part faces forward. Lock the brakes any time the chair is parked. If you remove the wheelchair footrests during a transfer, remember to replace them.

PROCEDURE 20

TRANSFERRING THE PATIENT FROM BED TO CHAIR—TWO ASSISTANTS

Two people may be needed to transfer patients who are weak, disoriented, have limited weight-bearing ability, or are very large. Directions are given for transferring toward the patient's right side.

1. Follow steps 1 through 11 in Procedure 19.

2. The nursing assistants stand one on each side, facing the patient.

3. Each one places the hand closest to the patient through the belt, with an underhand grasp toward the front of the patient. The other hand of each assistant grasps the belt toward the back. Coordination of movement is necessary (Figure 16-4A).

4. The nursing assistant closest to the chair (on the patient's right side) stands in a position to step or pivot around smoothly to allow the patient access to the chair. This person stands with the left leg further back than the right leg.

5. The other nursing assistant uses the left knee to brace the patient's weaker left leg. This assistant's left leg is further back than the right leg.

6. Instruct the patient to bend forward and place the palms of the hands on the edge of the mattress to push off.

7. The patient's knees should be spread apart, with both feet back and the stronger foot slightly in back of the weaker foot.

8. The nursing assistants bend their knees and give a broad base of support.

9. On the count of three, the patient stands. Allow her to stand for a moment and bear weight. Tell her to keep her head up. Both nursing assistants help the patient pivot by slowly and smoothly pivoting their feet, legs, and hips to their left.

10. To sit, have the patient bend forward slightly, bend the knees, and lower onto the chair. At the same time, have her reach for the arms of the chair with both hands (Figure 16-4B).

11. Complete the procedure as instructed for a one-assistant transfer (Procedure 19).

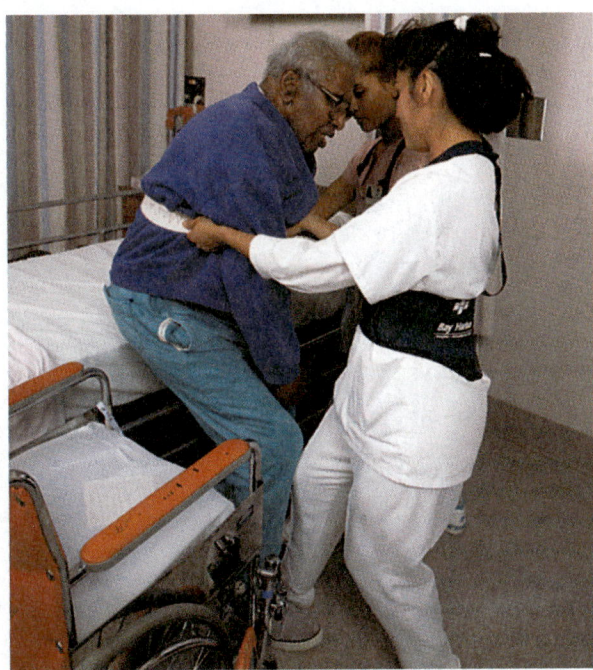

FIGURE 16-4A Coordination of movement is necessary.

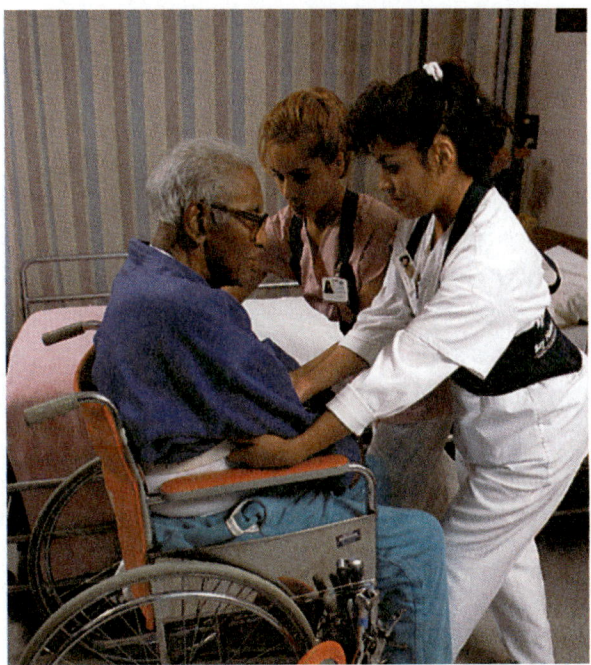

FIGURE 16-4B The patient reaches for the arms of the chair with both hands.

PROCEDURE 21

TRANSFERRING THE PATIENT FROM CHAIR TO BED—ONE ASSISTANT

1. Carry out beginning procedure actions.

2. Assemble equipment:
   - Transfer belt

3. Place chair so the patient moves toward his strongest side. Set chair parallel with bed.

4. Move the bed to the lowest horizontal position and lock the wheels. Fanfold top covers to foot of bed if necessary and raise the opposite side rail.

5. Lock the wheelchair and raise or remove the footrests.

6. Have the patient place both feet flat on the floor.

7. Place the transfer belt around the patient's waist.

8. Instruct the patient to move forward in the chair, to bend forward, and to spread his knees apart. Both feet should be back, with the stronger foot slightly in back of the weaker foot. Both of the patient's hands should be on the arms of the chair (Figure 16-5).

9. Take hold of the transfer belt with an underhand grasp. Brace the patient's weaker leg with your knee or leg, as instructed in Procedure 19. Ask the patient to push off the chair on the count of three and to stand up as you provide the necessary assistance.

10. Allow the patient to remain standing for a time to stabilize position. Keep your grasp on the transfer belt and continue to brace the weak leg if necessary.

11. To complete the transfer, instruct the patient to step or pivot around to stand in front of the bed, facing away from it. Tell the patient to sit when the edge of the mattress is touching the back of his legs. To sit, have the patient bend forward

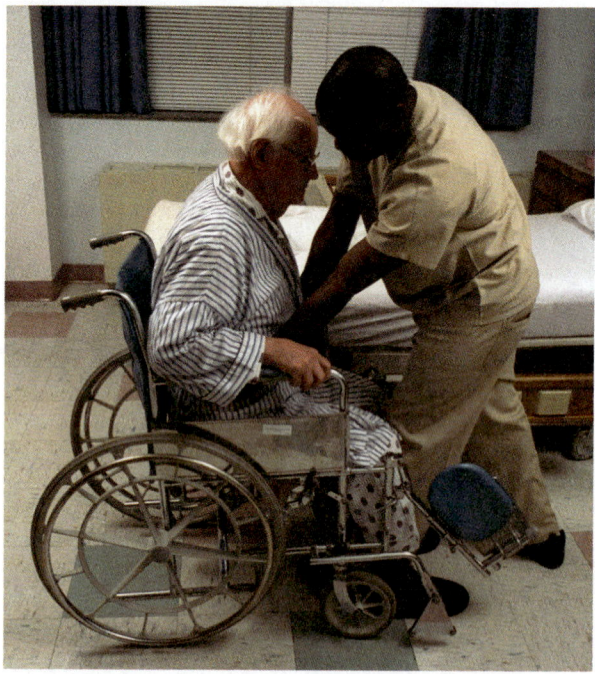

FIGURE 16-5 Instruct the patient to hold the chair arms with both hands.

slightly, bend his knees, and lower himself onto the mattress.

12. When the patient is safely in bed, remove the transfer belt.

13. Remove the patient's slippers and robe. Assist the patient to lie down. Position the patient as necessary. Draw top bedding over the patient. Fold the bath blanket (if used) from the wheelchair and return it to the bedside stand. Make sure the signal light is within reach.

14. Move the wheelchair out of the way.

15. Carry out procedure completion actions.

PROCEDURE 22

TRANSFERRING THE PATIENT FROM CHAIR TO BED—TWO ASSISTANTS

The directions given here are for moving the patient toward his left side.

1. Follow instructions 1 through 8 in Procedure 21.

2. Each nursing assistant places the hand closest to the patient through the belt with an underhand grasp in front of the patient; the other hand goes toward the back.

3. The nursing assistant closest to the bed (on the patient's left side) stands in a position to step or pivot around smoothly to allow the patient access to the bed. This person stands with the right leg further back than the left leg.

4. The other nursing assistant uses the left knee to brace the patient's weaker right leg. This person's right leg is further back than the left one (Figure 16-6A).

5. Ask the patient to push off the chair on the count of three and to stand up as you provide the necessary assistance.

6. Allow the patient to remain standing for a time to stabilize position. Keep your hands on the transfer belt and continue to brace the weak leg if necessary.

7. To complete the transfer, instruct the patient to step or pivot around to stand in front of the bed, facing away from it. Tell the patient to sit when the edge of the mattress is touching the back of his legs. To sit, have the patient bend forward slightly, bend his knees, and lower himself onto the mattress (Figure 16-6B).

8. When the patient is safely in bed, remove the transfer belt.

9. Remove the patient's slippers and robe. Assist the patient to lie down and position as necessary. Raise side rails if ordered. Draw top bedding over the patient. Fold the bath blanket (if used) from the wheelchair and return it to the bedside stand. Make sure the signal light is within reach.

10. Move the wheelchair out of the way.

11. Carry out procedure completion actions.

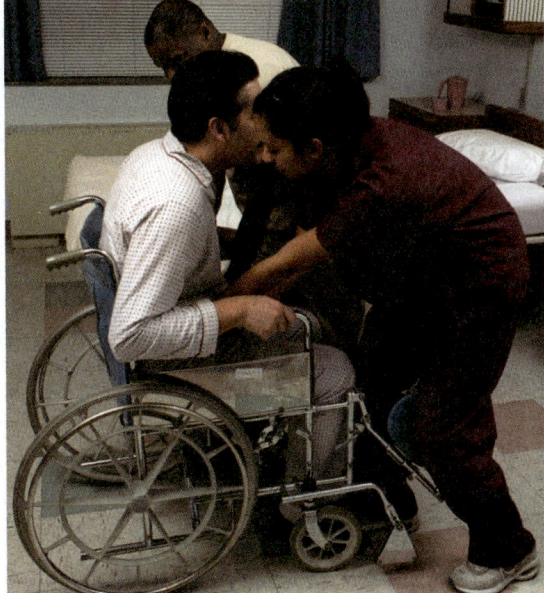

FIGURE 16-6A The nursing assistant uses the left knee to support the patient's weaker right leg.

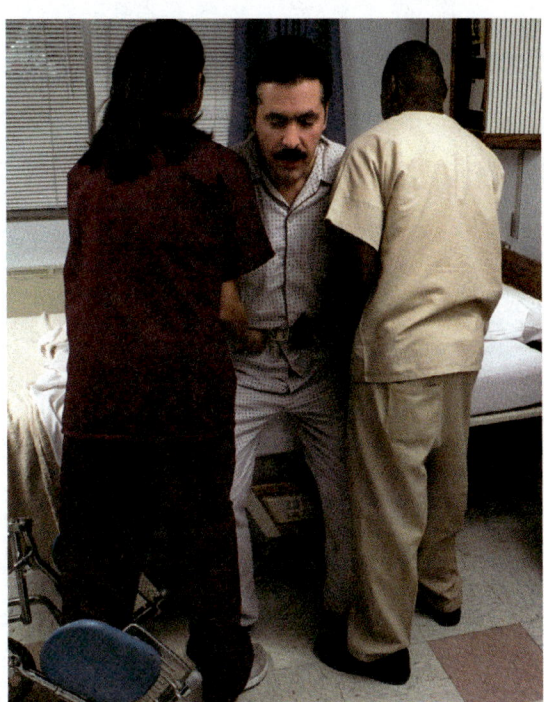

FIGURE 16-6B Tell the patient to bend forward, bend the knees, and lower himself onto the mattress.

PROCEDURE 23

INDEPENDENT TRANSFER, STANDBY ASSIST

This method is appropriate for the patient who has good balance and strength and can understand instructions. Put a transfer belt on the patient the first time this is attempted.

1. Follow the instructions for getting the patient to a sitting position on the side of the bed. (See Procedure 19.) For an independent transfer, the patient should be able to do this without help.

2. Have the patient place the strongest foot slightly in back of the other foot. The patient's knees should be spread slightly apart.

3. Instruct the patient to place the palms of the hands at the edge of the bed and to lean slightly forward.

4. Tell the patient to press the hands into the bed to push off, at the same time the legs straighten, to assume a standing position.

5. Once standing, have the patient reach for the far arm of the chair and then step or pivot to stand in front of the chair. Instruct the patient to sit when the edge of the seat is felt against the back of the legs.

6. Carry out procedure completion actions.

Reverse these directions when transferring from chair to bed.

STRETCHER TRANSFERS

This procedure is used to move a patient from her room to another room for surgery, treatments, or diagnostic tests. The procedure may be very frightening to the patient. Assure the patient that the procedure is safe.

 Note: Procedures 24 and 25 are for moving an unconscious or semiconscious patient. For alert, fully awake patients, two people may be able to perform this procedure with one person against the stretcher and the other person on the opposite side of the bed. Instruct the patient how to help you.

PROCEDURE 24

TRANSFERRING THE PATIENT FROM BED TO STRETCHER

1. Carry out beginning procedure actions.

2. Assemble equipment:
   - Stretcher
   - Bath blanket

3. You will need three to four people for transferring an unconscious or comatose patient from bed to stretcher.

4. Lock the wheels of the bed. Raise the bed to a horizontal position equal to the height of the stretcher. Lower the side rails.

5. Place a bath blanket over the patient and fanfold top covers to the foot of the bed, out of the way.

6. Roll the turning sheet up against the patient on both sides. The sheet should be long enough to support the patient's head and shoulders during the move.

7. Position the stretcher close to the bed. Lock stretcher wheels.

8. Two or three people stand along the open side of the stretcher. The other person stands on the open side of the bed. This assistant may need to get on the bed, on her knees, to avoid over-stretching her back.

Note: Use an overhand grasp on the moving sheet to avoid wrist strain.

continues

PROCEDURE 24

continued

- The assistant at the end of the bed grasps the moving sheet by placing one hand by the patient's legs and the other hand by the patient's hips.
- The middle assistant grasps the moving sheet by placing one hand by the patient's hips and the other hand by the patient's shoulders.
- The assistant at the head of the bed grasps the turning sheet by the patient's shoulder and head.
- On the count of three, all persons slide the moving sheet from bed to stretcher (Figure 16-7).

9. Center the patient on the stretcher in good body alignment. Secure the stretcher safety belt. Raise the side rails of the stretcher.

10. Transport the patient as directed.

SAFETY *Alert*

Patients on stretchers are not left alone.

11. Prepare the bed for the patient's return.

12. Carry out procedure completion actions.

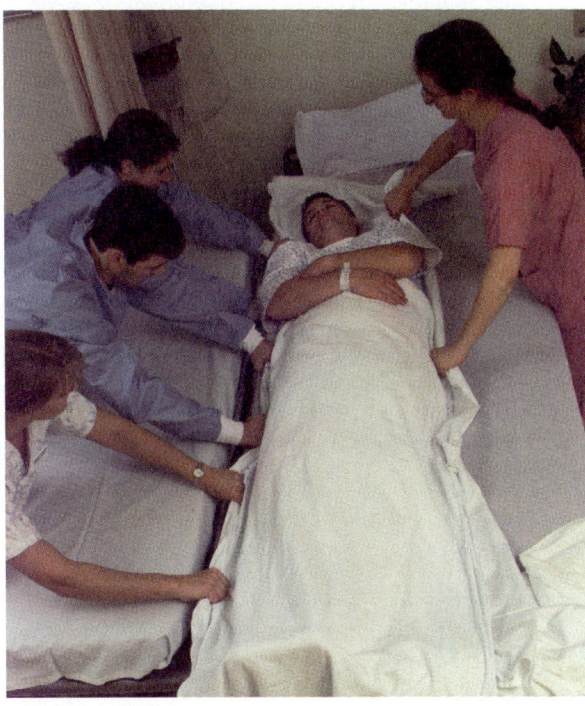

FIGURE 16-7 All persons slide the lifting sheet from bed to stretcher.

PROCEDURE **25**

TRANSFERRING THE PATIENT FROM STRETCHER TO BED

1. Carry out beginning procedure actions.

2. Assemble equipment:
   - Stretcher
   - Bath blanket (patient should already be covered with one on the stretcher)

3. You will need three to four people for transferring an unconscious or comatose patient from stretcher to bed.

4. Lock the wheels of the bed. Raise the bed to a horizontal position equal to the height of the stretcher. Lower the side rails. Fanfold top covers to the foot of the bed, out of the way.

5. Place a bath blanket over the patient if necessary.

6. Roll the turning sheet up against the patient on both sides. The sheet should be long enough to support the patient's head and shoulders during the move.

7. Position the stretcher close to the bed. Lock the wheels and lower the side rails.

continues

PROCEDURE 25

continued

8. One person stands along the open side of the stretcher. The other two or three people stand on the open side of the bed. These assistants may need to get on the bed, on their knees, to avoid overstretching their backs.

 Note: Use an overhand grasp on the moving sheet to avoid wrist strain.

- The assistant at the end of the bed grasps the moving sheet by placing one hand by the patient's legs and the other hand by the patient's hips.
- The middle assistant grasps the moving sheet by placing one hand by the patient's hips and the other hand by the patient's shoulders.
- The assistant at the head of the bed grasps the turning sheet by the patient's shoulder and head.
- On the count of three, all persons slide the moving sheet from stretcher to bed (Figure 16-8).

9. Center the patient on the bed in good body alignment. Position the patient properly. Raise the side rails of the bed if ordered.

10. Carry out procedure completion actions.

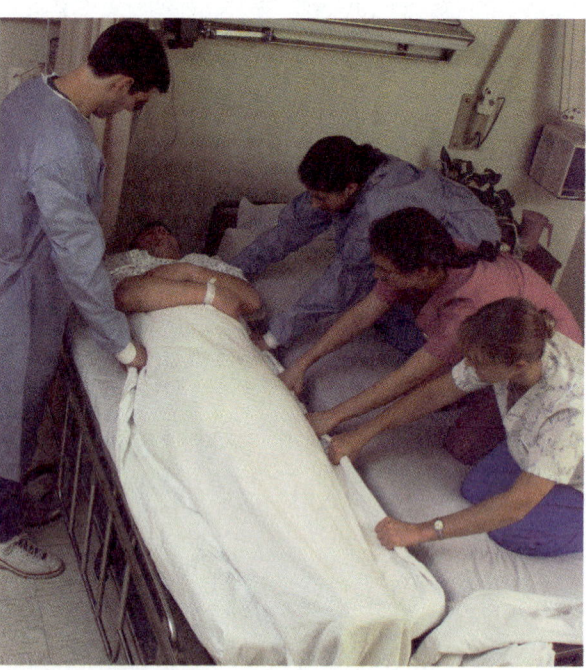

FIGURE 16-8 All persons slide the lifting sheet from stretcher to bed.

MOVING THE PATIENT WITH A MECHANICAL LIFT

The mechanical lift is used for moving heavy patients who have little or no ability to assist. Using a mechanical lift for transfers is safer for both the patient and the nursing assistant. Various types of seats are available so the patient can be moved in the sitting or supine position. Some mechanical lifts may be used to weigh bedfast patients.

Several types of mechanical lifts are available. Some are manually operated, others are electric. The most commonly used lift is the hydraulic lift. It is used when a patient is heavy, unable to assist, unbalanced, or has an amputation or other condition that makes transfer with a belt difficult or impossible. For safety reasons, the hydraulic lift should be operated by two or more nursing assistants. Never attempt to operate it alone. Some electric and battery-operated lifts can safely be used by one person. Know and follow your facility policy for use of the mechanical lift.

PROCEDURE 26

TRANSFERRING THE PATIENT WITH A MECHANICAL LIFT

This procedure is used for heavy patients who have little or no weight-bearing ability.

 Note: Check slings, chains, and straps for frayed areas or clasps that do not close properly. Check the hydraulic lift and the leg spreader to make sure they are both working. Do not use if there is oil on the floor or if equipment is defective. Report need for repair and obtain safe equipment.

continues

PROCEDURE 26

continued

1. Carry out beginning procedure actions.

2. Assemble equipment:
   - Mechanical lift
   - Sling
   - Chair

3. Place a wheelchair or other chair parallel to the foot of the bed, facing the head. Lock the wheelchair.

4. Elevate the bed to a comfortable working height. Lock the bed wheels. Lower the nearest side rail. Roll the patient toward you.

5. Position the sling beneath the patient's body behind shoulder, thighs, and buttocks. Be sure the sling is smooth (Figure 16-9A).

6. Roll the patient back onto the sling and position properly (Figure 16-9B). If the sling has inserts for metal bars, insert them now.

7. Position lift frame over bed with base legs in

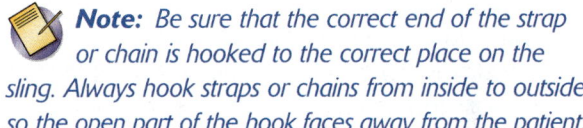

SAFETY *Alert*

Two people should carry out these procedures to ensure patient safety.

maximum open position, and lock lift legs (Figure 16-9C).

8. Attach suspension straps or chains to the sling (Figure 16-9D). Check fasteners for security.

Note: Be sure that the correct end of the strap or chain is hooked to the correct place on the sling. Always hook straps or chains from inside to outside so the open part of the hook faces away from the patient.

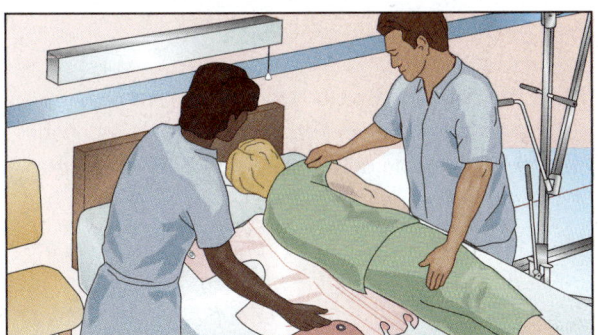

FIGURE 16-9A Position the sling under the patient.

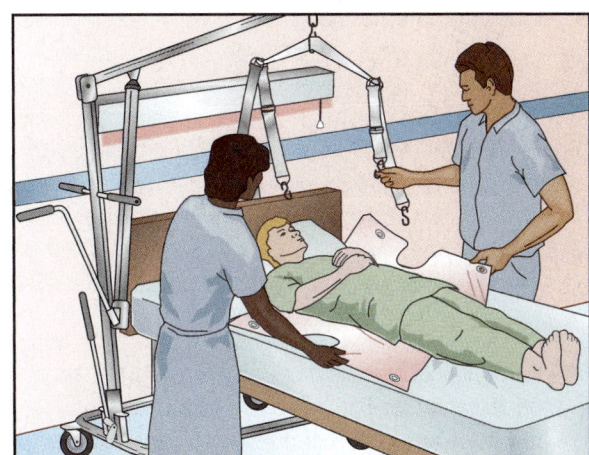

FIGURE 16-9C Position the lift frame over the bed.

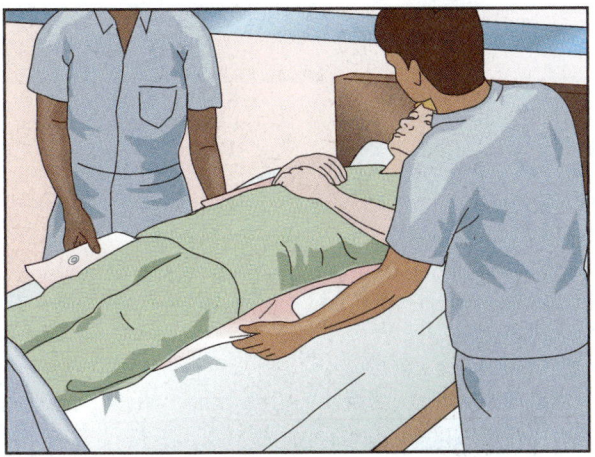

FIGURE 16-9B Roll the patient back onto the sling.

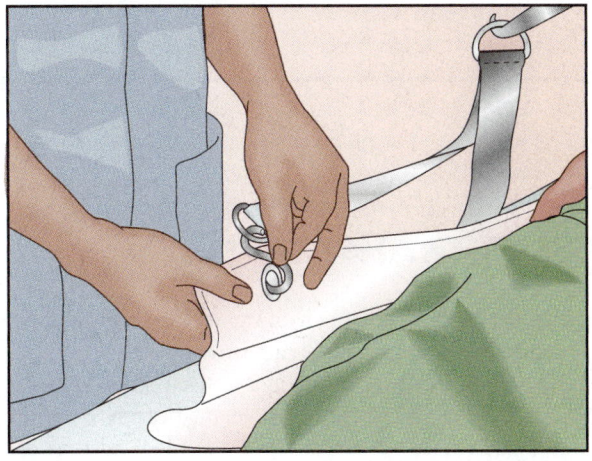

FIGURE 16-9D Attach the straps or chains to the sling.

continues

PROCEDURE 26

continued

9. Position the patient's crossed arms inside the straps.

10. Secure straps or chains if necessary.

11. One assistant operates the lift and the other assistant guides the movement of the patient. Lock the hydraulic mechanism, and slowly raise the boom of the lift until the patient is suspended over the bed. Talk to the patient while slowly lifting him free of the bed.

12. Guide the lift away from the bed.

13. Position the patient and lift over the chair or wheelchair (Figure 16-9E). Make sure that the wheels of the wheelchair are locked.

14. Slowly lower the patient into the chair or wheelchair. Pay attention to the position of the patient's feet and hands. One assistant stands behind the chair to pull and guide the patient's hips back into position.

15. Unhook the suspension straps or chains and remove the lift.

16. Position the footrests to support the feet.

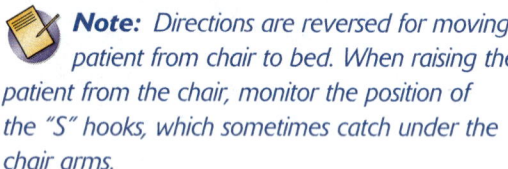 **Note:** *Directions are reversed for moving patient from chair to bed. When raising the patient from the chair, monitor the position of the "S" hooks, which sometimes catch under the chair arms.*

17. If the patient is in a chair, the sling can remain underneath the patient so it is in position for transfer back to bed. If the sling has metal bars, remove them and make sure the sling is smooth and wrinkle-free. Make sure the signal light is within reach.

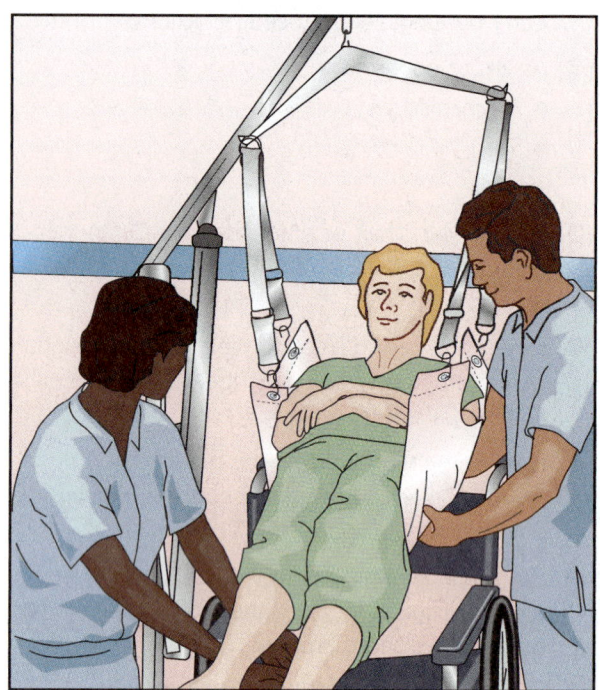

FIGURE 16-9E Position the lift frame over the chair.

18. If the patient has returned to bed, remove the sling. Pull top covers up and position the patient. Raise both side rails if necessary. Make sure the signal light is within reach.

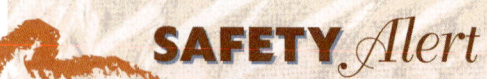 **Note:** *The method for raising and lowering the lift and for moving the base legs varies for different types of equipment. Read the manufacturer's directions and practice using equipment before using it with patients.*

19. Carry out procedure completion actions.

TOILET TRANSFERS

The bladder is emptied much more efficiently if patients can use the toilet or commode rather than a urinal or bedpan. To use the toilet, the patient must possess transfer skills. Unless the patient has full weight-bearing on both legs and good balance, a wall rail is needed for support while transferring. (Refer to Procedure 27.) Towel racks are not safe for this purpose. Male patients may find it easier and safer to sit rather than stand while urinating.

SAFETY *Alert*

Many falls occur going to and from the bathroom, as well as in the bathroom. Assist patients with toileting regularly. Respond to call signals promptly. Do not leave the patient alone if you think doing so is unsafe.

PROCEDURE 27

TRANSFERRING THE PATIENT ONTO AND OFF THE TOILET

1. Carry out beginning procedure actions.

2. Assemble equipment:
   - Toilet tissue
   - Transfer belt
   - Disposable gloves
   - Commode if toilet is not available

3. Position the wheelchair at a right angle to the toilet or commode to face the wall rail. Lock the wheels. Raise or remove footrests.

4. Place a transfer belt around the patient's waist. Use an underhand grasp with one hand toward the patient's back and the other hand toward the patient's front.

5. Tell the patient to lean forward slightly, to place the strongest foot slightly behind the other foot, to bring herself to a standing position by pushing off from the wheelchair, and to grasp the wall rail with both hands (Figure 16-10A).

6. Have the patient pivot or step around until she feels the toilet against the back of her legs.

7. Slide the pants and underwear down over the patient's knees. You may need to keep one hand in the transfer belt and use the other hand to manipulate the patient's clothing (Figure 16-10B).

8. Assist the patient to a sitting position on the toilet and allow her time to eliminate.

9. When the patient is finished, put on the disposable gloves. Instruct the patient to stand and to reach for the wall rail. Use the toilet tissue to clean the patient if she was unable to do this herself. If the patient is steady, remove and dispose of your gloves. Then pull the patient's pants or underwear up.

10. If the sink is close enough, the patient can pivot or step to the sink to wash her hands before sitting down in the wheelchair. Otherwise, unlock the wheelchair, replace the footrests, and move the wheelchair to the sink so this step can be completed while the patient is seated.

11. Wash your hands.

12. Assist the patient to leave the bathroom. Make sure she is comfortable and has a signal light within reach.

13. Carry out procedure completion actions.

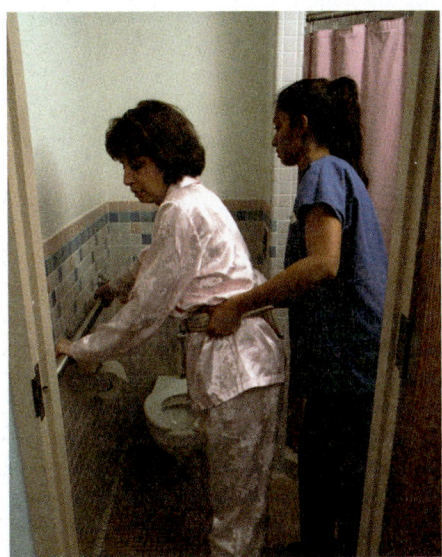

FIGURE 16-10A Tell the patient to grasp the wall rail with both hands.

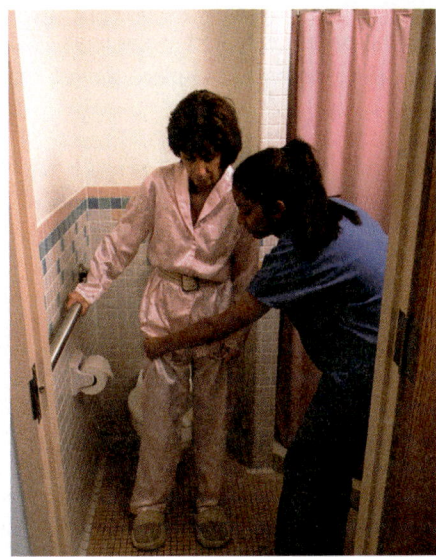

FIGURE 16-10B Keep one hand on the transfer belt and adjust the patient's clothing.

TUB TRANSFERS

In the institutional setting, a shower with chair or tub with hydraulic lift is available. If the patient is at home, a tub chair, rail on the wall beside the tub, and slip-proof mats in the tub are needed for safety. Add water to the tub after the patient has safely transferred, with cold water turned on first and off last. A hand-held shower attached to the faucet of the tub is safer and easier for self-bathing.

PROCEDURE **28**

TRANSFERRING THE PATIENT INTO AND OUT OF THE BATHTUB

1. Carry out beginning procedure actions.

2. Assemble equipment:
   - Towels and washcloths
   - Soap
   - Hand-held shower if available
   - Tub chair
   - Slip-proof bath mats for floor and tub
   - Disposable gloves if necessary
   - Sturdy straight chair if necessary

    Note: *If patient's wheelchair has a removable arm or side, remove it and place the wheelchair at the foot of the tub, facing the faucets.*

3. Place a sturdy chair beside the tub, facing the faucets, if wheelchair arm is not removable. (Use this in place of a wheelchair.)

4. Have the patient transfer from the wheelchair to the chair and then into the tub and onto the tub chair. Make sure the tub chair is even with the other chair.

5. Once the patient is seated in the chair beside the tub, instruct the patient to place the leg closest to the tub into the tub. If this is the weaker leg, the strong arm can be used to lift the leg over the side of the tub (Figure 16-11A).

6. Tell the patient to use the strongest arm to reach for the wall rail. Sliding across onto the tub chair, have the patient bring the other leg over the side of the tub (Figure 16-11B).

 Note: *For this procedure, it is safer to have the weaker side toward the tub, if possible; that way the strong arm can be brought around to the wall rail.*

7. Proceed with the bath, giving assistance as needed or allowing the patient privacy to complete the bath, if possible. Stay within hearing distance.

8. When the patient is ready to get out of the tub, the strong side will be next to the outer chair. This allows the patient to get the strong leg out of the tub and to use the strong arm to move herself onto the chair. She then uses the strong arm to move her weaker leg out of the tub.

9. Assist the patient to dry and dress if necessary.

10. Carry out procedure completion actions.

11. Disinfect tub and tub chair.

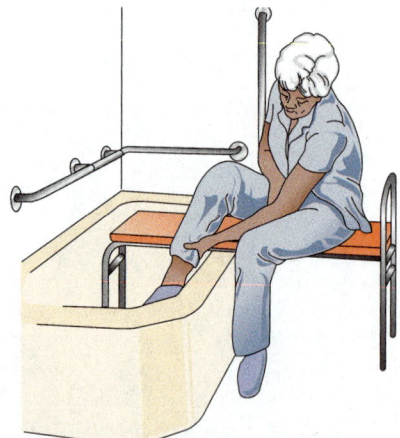

FIGURE 16-11A The patient uses the stronger arm to lift the weak leg over the edge of the tub.

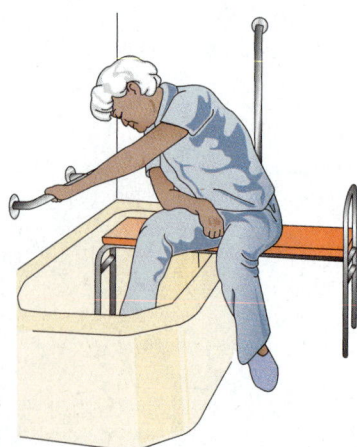

FIGURE 16-11B The patient brings the stronger leg over the side of the tub.

CAR TRANSFERS

You may need to assist a patient to transfer into a car when she is discharged from the facility. If you are working in the patient's home, you may need to be able to help the patient into and out of the car. A two-door car makes the transfer easier because the door is wider and gives more room for moving in and out of the car. With either a two-door or four-door car, the patient should always transfer onto the front seat. The front door is usually wider and opens wider.

PROCEDURE 29

TRANSFERRING A PATIENT INTO AND OUT OF A CAR

1. Carry out beginning procedure actions.

2. Assemble equipment:
   - Car
   - Wheelchair
   - Transfer belt

3. Place the wheelchair at a 45° angle to the car, with brakes set. Put transfer belt on the patient if necessary (Figure 16-12A). Have the patient come to a standing position in the usual manner.

4. If transferring to the stronger side, the dashboard and car door can be used for support (Figure 16-12B). If moving toward the weaker side, instruct the patient to use the strong arm and the door with the window open for support. Another person should hold the door for stability.

5. Tell the patient to pivot or step around so the side of the car seat is touching the back of the legs. After she sits down, have the patient raise one leg at a time into the car to face forward (Figure 16-12C). Assist with the seat belt.

6. To get the patient out of the car, reverse the procedure. Car seats are usually lower than other sitting surfaces and the patient may need help in getting to a standing position.

7. Carry out procedure completion actions.

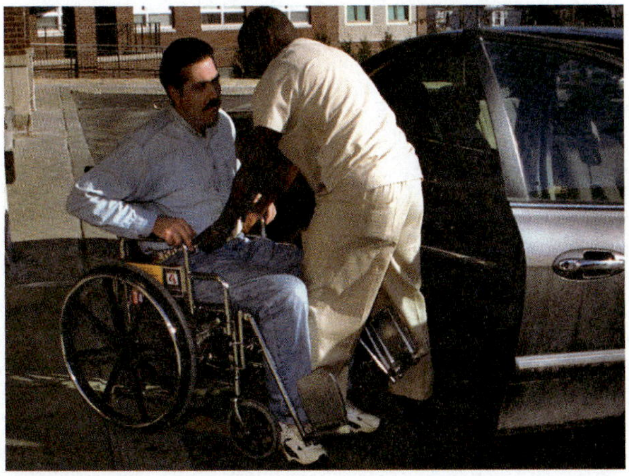

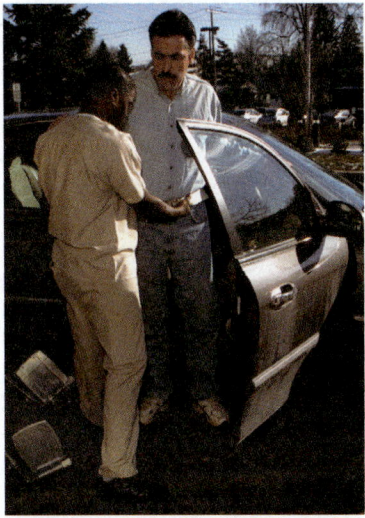

FIGURE 16-12B The dashboard and car door can be used for support.

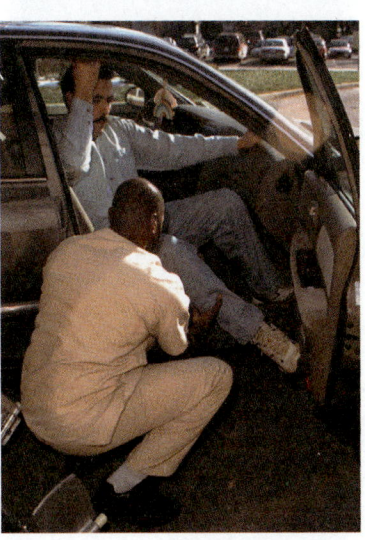

FIGURE 16-12C The patient lifts one leg at a time into the car.

FIGURE 16-12A Apply the transfer belt and prepare to assist the patient to a standing position.

REVIEW

A. Multiple Choice.

Select the one best answer for each of the following.

1. The method used for transferring a patient depends on
   a. the availability of two nursing assistants.
   b. the patient's personal preference.
   c. the patient's size, strength, endurance, and balance.
   d. where the patient is going.

2. A transfer belt should never be used on patients who
   a. have a long-term medication pump.
   b. have a colostomy.
   c. can stand on their feet.
   d. have an IV or catheter.

3. During a transfer, the patient should never
   a. be allowed to help in the move.
   b. place his hands on your body.
   c. wear shoes.
   d. be allowed to stand.

4. When transferring a patient, you should never place your hands under a patient's arms because the
   a. patient may not want you to stand so close.
   b. patient cannot see where she is going.
   c. patient's bones are fragile.
   d. patient may be ticklish.

5. Using a mechanical lift requires that
   a. there always be two persons to do the procedure.
   b. the patient be able to assist in the move.
   c. the patient be mentally alert.
   d. the patient weigh at least 300 pounds.

B. True/False.

Mark the following true or false by circling T or F.

6. T F During a transfer, the patient should place his or her hands on the nursing assistant's shoulders.

7. T F A transfer belt should always be used for standing transfers unless contraindicated.

8. T F Always transfer toward the patient's strongest side.

9. T F During a transfer, the nursing assistant should place his or her hands around the patient's trunk.

10. T F During a transfer, always explain to the patient how he or she can help.

11. T F Towel bars are not safe to use as grab bars.

12. T F Before using a mechanical lift, always check the slings and straps for frayed areas.

13. T F One person can safely transfer an unconscious patient from a stretcher to a bed.

14. T F When transferring a patient from a bed to a stretcher, raise the bed to the same horizontal height as the stretcher.

15. T F The unconscious patient should be secured with a safety belt during transport.

C. Nursing Assistant Challenge.

You are assigned to Mrs. McNeely, who is scheduled for surgery. She is alert and able to follow your directions. You know that when she returns from surgery she will be semiconscious from the medications and anesthesia. Consider the differences in procedures when she goes to surgery and when she returns to her room.

16. What instructions will you give Mrs. McNeely when she transfers from her bed to the surgical stretcher?

17. What will you need to do to transfer her back to bed after the surgery?

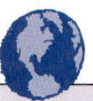 ## EXPLORING THE WEB

Description	Location
Ergonomics in Patient Transfers	http://www.osha.gov/SLTC/hospital_etool/hazards/ergo/ergoequipment/ergoequip.html
How to Use a Gait Belt	http://www.medformation.com
Lifting, Transferring, and Positioning Patients	http://911papers.virtualave.net
Policy for Gait Belt Use	http://wdhfs.state.wy.us
Transfer Procedures	calder.med.miami.edu

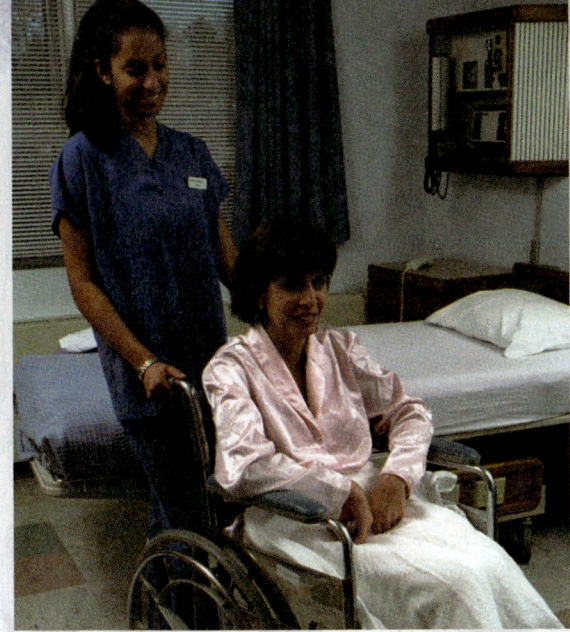

The Patient's Mobility: Ambulation

objectives

After completing this unit, you will be able to:

- Spell and define terms.
- Describe the purpose of assistive devices used in ambulation.
- List safety measures for using assistive devices.
- Describe safety measures for using a wheelchair.
- Describe nursing assistant actions for
  - Ambulating a patient using a gait belt.
  - Propelling a patient in a wheelchair.
  - Positioning a patient in a wheelchair.
  - Transporting a patient on a stretcher
- Demonstrate the following procedures:
  - Procedure 30 Assisting the Patient to Walk with a Cane and Three-Point Gait
  - Procedure 31 Assisting the Patient to Walk with a Walker and Three-Point Gait
  - Procedure 32 Assisting the Falling Patient

vocabulary

Learn the meaning and the correct spelling of the following words and phrases:

ambulate	gait	orthopedic
assistive device	gait training	prosthesis

AMBULATION

The term **ambulate** means to walk. Some patients may not be able to walk because of a disease or injury. Patients who cannot walk may be able to self-propel their wheelchairs to increase their independence.

The term **gait** refers to the way in which a person walks. Many disorders can affect a person's gait, such as:

- A stroke—one side of the body is paralyzed (hemiplegia).
- Multiple sclerosis—one or both legs are weakened and balance may be disturbed.
- Huntington's disease—the patient has involuntary movements that disturb balance.
- Parkinson's disease—the patient has stiffness and slowness of movements, causing shuffling.
- Arthritis—pain and stiffness of joints.
- Amputation—the patient has a **prosthesis** (artificial limb).
- **Orthopedic** (bones and muscles) surgery.

Evaluation for Ambulation

Before initiating an ambulation program, the nurse or physical therapist (Figure 17-1) will evaluate the patient's:

- Tolerance to movement in bed
- Ability to participate in active (as opposed to passive) exercise
- Ability to safely transfer with minimal assistance
- Ability to stand and bear weight
- Strength, endurance, and balance

- Mental state, to determine if the patient can follow directions
- Ability to walk alone (whether the assistance of a person or equipment is needed)

Normal Gait Pattern

There are two phases to a normal gait (walking). The leg is on the floor during the first phase and the leg is brought forward during the second phase. Walking begins with the ankle in *dorsiflexion* (toes pulled toward shin) and the heel striking the floor first (Figure 17-2), rolling onto the ball of the foot. The patient must be able to stand straight on this leg while bringing the other leg forward. The arms normally swing slightly during walking. Each arm moves in the same direction as the opposite leg. To walk safely, the patient must have adequate joint motion in the hips and knees and strength in the muscles of the hips, buttocks, and legs. The physical therapist may work with the patient on exercises to promote movement and strength before the patient starts walking.

Gait Training

The physical therapist may work with the patient on **gait training** (teaching the patient to walk). The therapist will teach the patient how to:

- Walk correctly
- Walk on different surfaces, such as linoleum floors, carpet, grass, gravel, etc.
- Go up and down stairs (Figure 17-3)
- Get in and out of a chair
- Use an assistive device if one is ordered

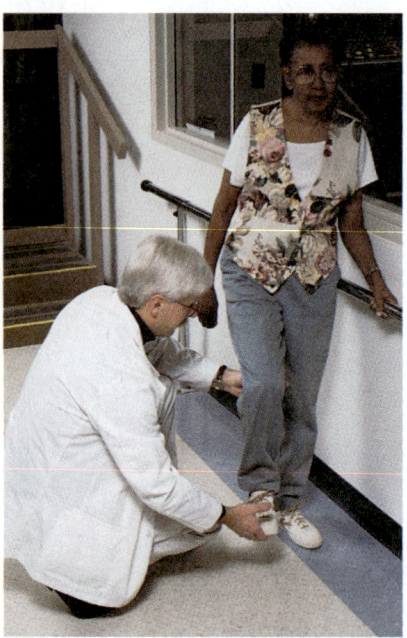

FIGURE 17-1 The physical therapist evaluates the patient's ability to ambulate and need for assistive devices.

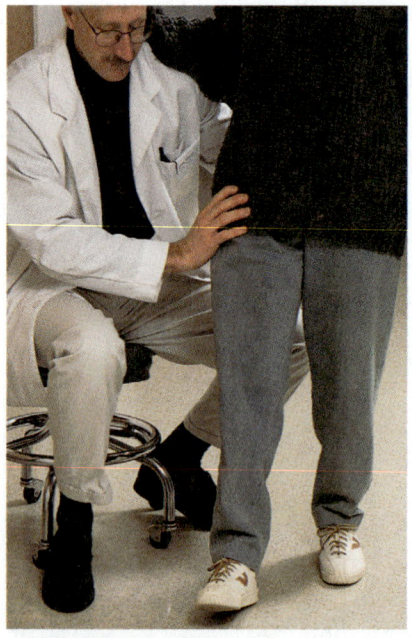

FIGURE 17-2 Walking begins with the ankle in dorsiflexion and the heel striking the floor first.

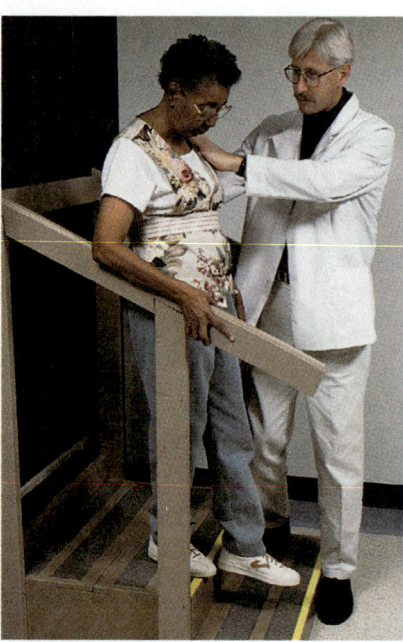

FIGURE 17-3 The physical therapist teaches the patient how to walk on stairs.

guidelines *for*

Safe Ambulation

- Encourage independent patients to use the hand rail when walking.
- Always stand on the patient's affected side when walking with her.
- Always use a gait belt (transfer belt) if the patient needs assistance with ambulation. Grasp the belt in the back with an underhand grip (Figure 17-4). Place your other hand on the patient's shoulder if balance is unsteady.
- Make sure the patient is wearing sturdy shoes with nonslip soles and that laces are tied. Clothing should not be too loose or drag on the floor.
- Check floor for clutter or puddles that could cause a fall.
- If you are unsure of the patient's endurance or balance, ask another nursing assistant to follow behind you with the wheelchair. If the patient becomes weak, dizzy, or tired, she can sit in the wheelchair.
- Check rubber tips on bottoms of canes, crutches, and walkers, and also check the rubber handgrips (Figure 17-5). These should be replaced if the ridges are cracked, loose, or worn down. If the ridges are filled with debris, use alcohol and cotton swabs to clean them. Replace the handgrip if it is loose or cracked.
- Check screws, nuts, and bolts for tightness. Do not use any device that appears unsafe. Report the problem to the appropriate person.
- Practice good body mechanics for both yourself and the patient.

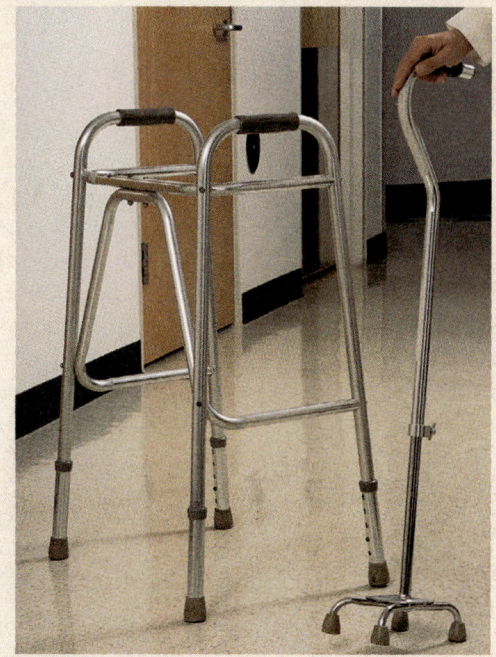

FIGURE 17-5 Check the rubber tips and handgrips.

- Teach the patient to practice safety.
- Position your body so it moves with the patient's body. You should not interfere with the patient's movement. Match the patient's stride.
- Encourage the patient to stand upright and erect when walking.
- Encourage the patient to take large, even steps. Teach him or her to maintain a wide base of support. The distance between the feet should be equal to the patient's shoulder width.
- Allow adequate time for ambulation. Avoid making the patient feel rushed.
- Allow the patient time to rest, if necessary.
- Provide only the amount of assistance needed.
- If the patient is not motivated, place a chair ahead of him or her. Tell the patient the goal is to walk to the chair.
- Stop ambulation immediately if the patient shows signs of illness, pain, extreme fatigue, shortness of breath, dizziness, sweating, or anxiety. Notify the nurse.
- Never leave the patient standing unattended. When you are through, leave the patient safely sitting in a chair.

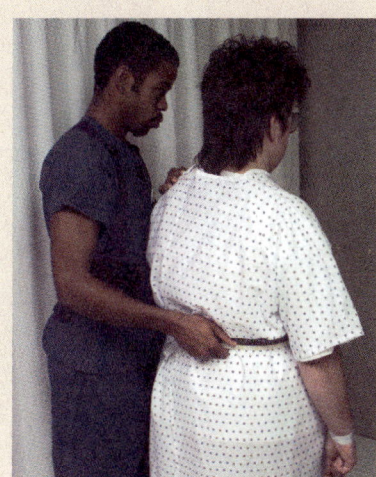

FIGURE 17-4
Hold the gait belt in back, using an underhand grip.

ASSISTIVE DEVICES

An **assistive device** is often prescribed. These devices include:

- Crutches
- Canes
- Walkers

An assistive device can help compensate for problems the patient has with walking. A walker or crutches may be ordered if the patient has only partial weight-bearing on one leg. Canes are usually ordered for persons who have problems with balance. There are several types of crutches, canes, and walkers. Each device is selected according to the needs of the patient and the cause of the problem. The nurse or physical therapist will adjust the device to fit the patient. The gait used with the device is determined by the patient's abilities, the cause of the impairment, and the type of assistive device being used. The nurse or physical therapist will select the appropriate gait. You should know the gaits that have been chosen. When you walk with the patient, you can then help make sure the patient is using the device correctly.

Use of Crutches

Standard crutches (Figure 17-6) are seldom recommended for older adults. They can be cumbersome to handle and require considerable balance and two strong arms. Metal forearm crutches may be used by patients who have weakness of both legs. These crutches are also called Lofstrand crutches or Canadian crutches. The cuff of the crutch encloses the forearm so the patient can release that hand without dropping the crutch (Figure 17-7).

Forearm crutches with platforms permit weight-bearing on the forearms, providing stability. During use, the elbows are at a constant 90° angle to the shoulder (Figure 17-8). The patient may need assistance in attaching the arm straps of

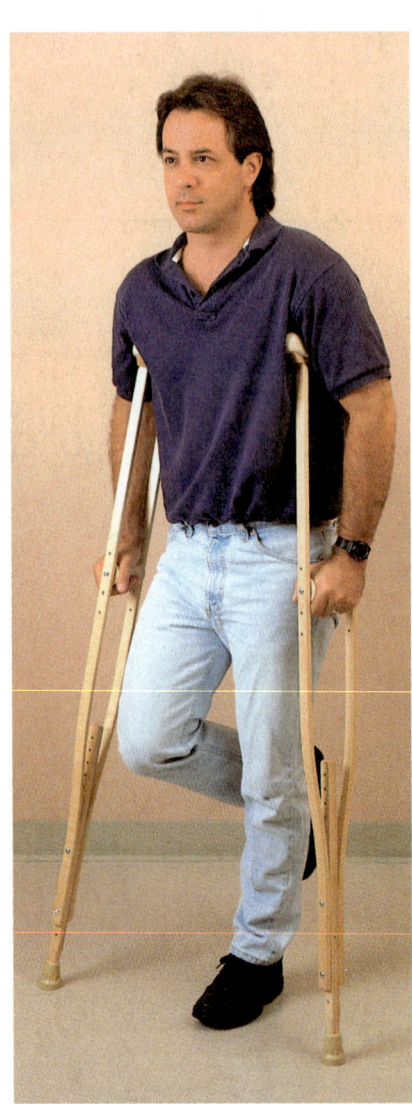

FIGURE 17-6 Standard crutches are not usually appropriate for elderly patients.

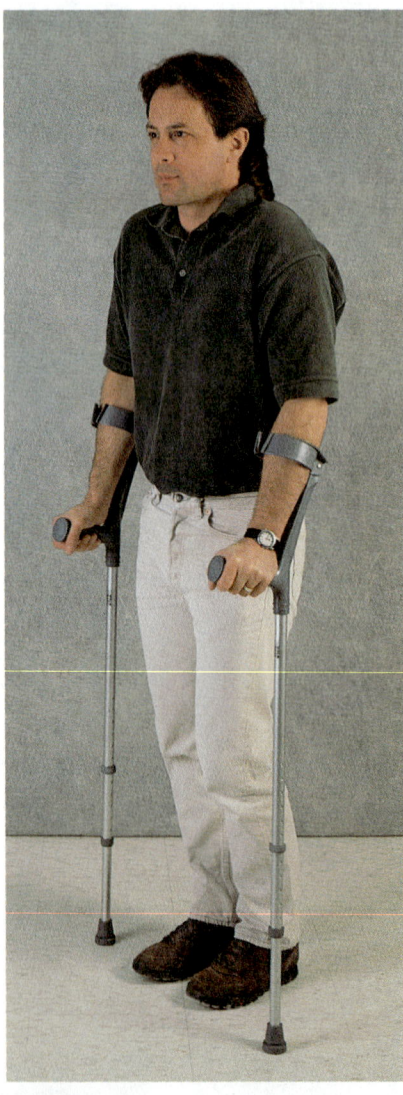

FIGURE 17-7 Forearm crutches can be released to free the hand without dropping the crutch.

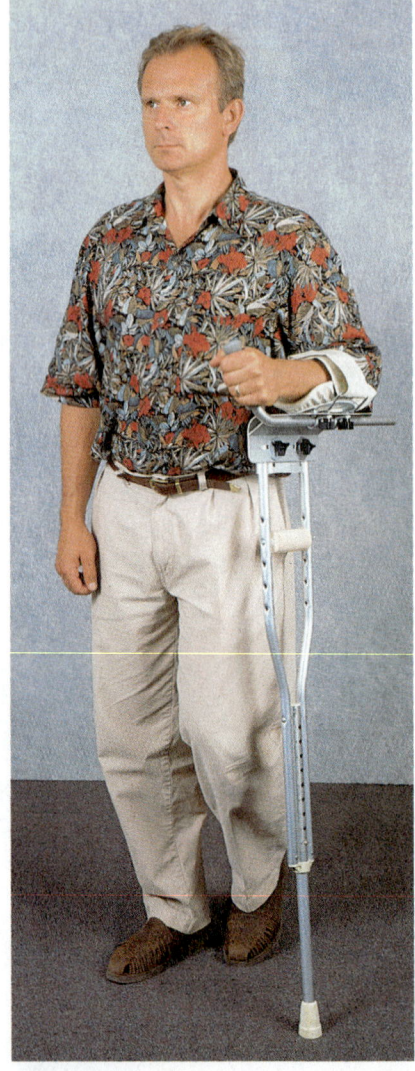

FIGURE 17-8 Forearm crutches with platforms permit weight-bearing on the forearms to provide stability.

the platforms. If you care for patients with crutches, you will be taught the gaits the patients are to use.

Use of Canes

Quad canes and tripod canes provide a wide base of support. Pyramid canes are four-pronged devices with a broad base, and are narrower at the top. Single-prong canes with T-handles or J-handles have straight handles with a handgrip and are easier to hold than half-circle handled canes. For proper fit, the elbow is flexed 30° when the hands are on the handgrip, and the patient's wrist is even with the hip joint. Canes are recommended for aiding balance rather than for providing support. (Refer to Procedure 30.) The cane is always held by the arm on the *strong* side of the body. The patient will be taught to use either a two-point gait or a three-point gait with a cane.

PROCEDURE 30

ASSISTING THE PATIENT TO WALK WITH A CANE AND THREE-POINT GAIT

1. Carry out beginning procedure actions.

2. Assemble equipment:
   - Cane as ordered
   - Gait belt

3. Make sure the patient has on sturdy shoes with nonslip soles. Check clothing to be sure it does not hang down over shoes.

4. Place the bed in the lowest horizontal position with brakes locked. Assist the patient to sit on the edge of the bed. Place a gait belt on the patient and assist the patient to a standing position. Stand on the patient's affected side. Place your closest hand in the gait belt, using an underhand grip.

5. Instruct the patient to hold the cane on her stronger side, with the tip about 4 inches to the side of the stronger foot. Her weight should be distributed evenly between her feet and the cane (Figure 17-9A).

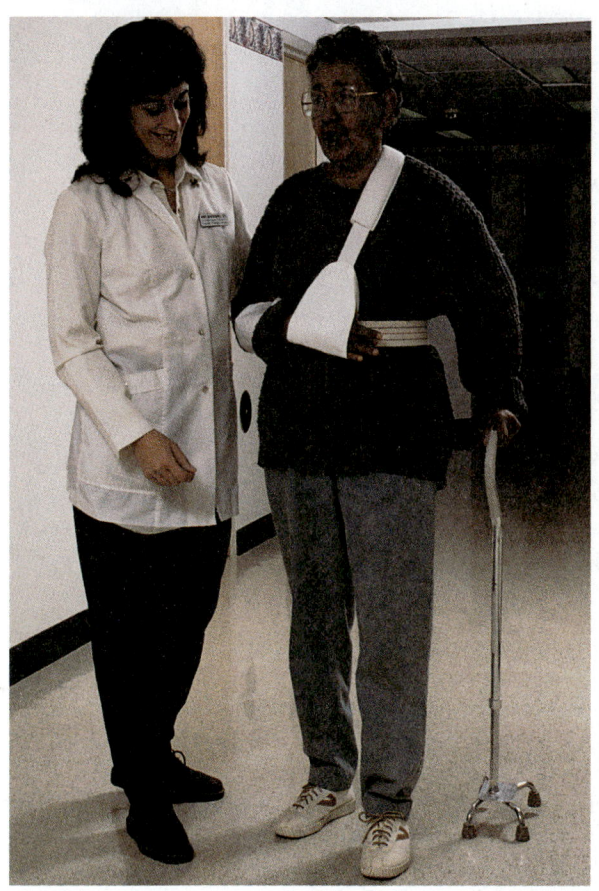

FIGURE 17-9A The patient holds the cane on the strong side of the body. The patient's weight should be distributed evenly between her feet and the cane before she starts to walk.

continues

PROCEDURE 30

continued

6. Tell the patient to shift her body weight to the strong leg and advance the cane about 4 inches so she is supporting her weight on the strong leg and the cane. Move the weak leg forward so it is even with the cane (Figure 17-9B).

7. The patient then shifts her weight to the weak leg and the cane, moving the strong leg forward, ahead of the cane. This pattern is repeated while the patient is walking.

8. Note the patient's endurance, balance, and strength while walking. Stop immediately if the patient has trouble and help her to the closest chair. Call the nurse.

9. Assist the patient to sit in the chair or to lie down in bed. Remove the gait belt. Store the cane in an appropriate area.

10. Document the distance the patient ambulated and her tolerance of the procedure.

11. Carry out procedure completion actions.

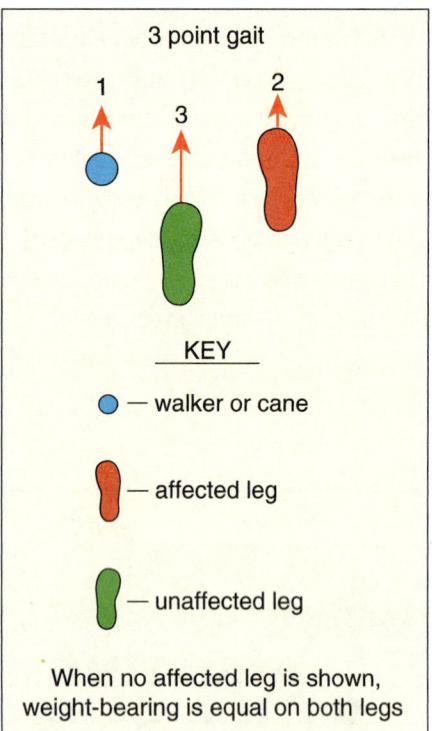

FIGURE 17-9B Three-point gait.

Two-Point Gait with Cane. The steps for this procedure are as follows:

1. Follow steps 1 through 5 in Procedure 30.
2. Tell the patient to move the cane and weaker leg forward at the same time, while his weight is on the stronger leg (Figure 17-10).
3. He then shifts his weight to the weak leg and cane, and moves the stronger leg forward.
4. This pattern is repeated while the patient is walking.
5. Repeat steps 8 through 11 in Procedure 30.

Use of Walkers

Walkers also come in a variety of styles. Walkers are recommended for individuals who have general weakness of both legs, partial weight bearing on one leg, or mild balance problems. The patient needs strength in both arms to pick up the walker. The walker should be wide enough to allow the patient to walk into it. For proper fit, the elbow is flexed 30° when the hands are on the handgrip, and the top of the walker reaches the hip joint. Most walkers are adjustable. The nurse or physical therapist will make any necessary changes. There are many additional features available from most manufacturers.

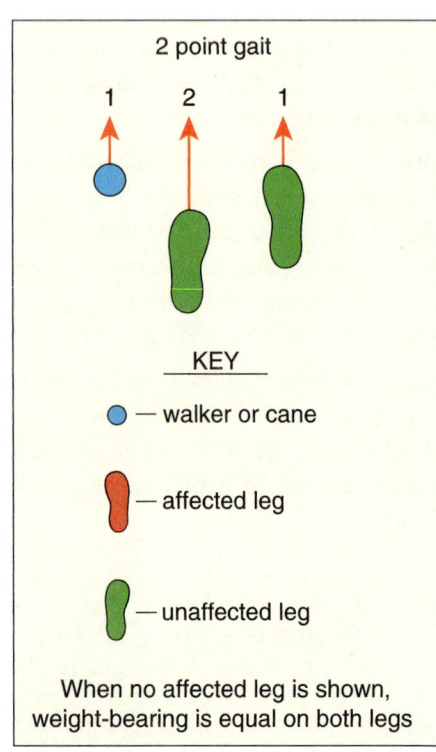

FIGURE 17-10 Two-point gait.

PROCEDURE 31

ASSISTING THE PATIENT TO WALK WITH A WALKER AND THREE-POINT GAIT

1. Carry out beginning procedure actions.

2. Assemble equipment:
   - Walker as ordered
   - Gait belt

3. Make sure the patient has on sturdy shoes with nonslip soles. Check clothing to be sure it does not hang down over shoes.

4. Place a gait belt on the patient and assist the patient to a standing position. Place the walker in front of the patient and have her grasp the walker with both hands. Stand on the patient's affected side. Place your closest hand in the gait belt, using an underhand grip (Figure 17-11).

   Note: The walker is not a transfer device and should not be used to help the patient stand up. The patient grasps the walker after she is standing. To sit, the patient releases her grip on the walker while still standing, and then places her hands on the arms of the chair before sitting.

5. Instruct the patient to stand with her weight evenly distributed between the walker and both legs, with the walker in front of her.

6. Have the patient shift her weight to the strong leg as she lifts and moves the walker 6 to 8 inches ahead. All four legs of the walker should strike the floor at the same time.

7. The patient then brings her weak foot forward into the walker.

8. Now have her bring her strong foot forward even with the weak foot.

9. This process is repeated while the patient is walking.

10. Note the patient's endurance, balance, and strength while walking. Stop immediately if the patient has trouble and help her to the closest chair. Call the nurse.

11. Assist the patient to sit in the chair or to lie down in bed. Remove the gait belt. Store the walker in an appropriate area.

12. Document the distance the patient ambulated and her tolerance of the procedure.

13. Carry out procedure completion actions.

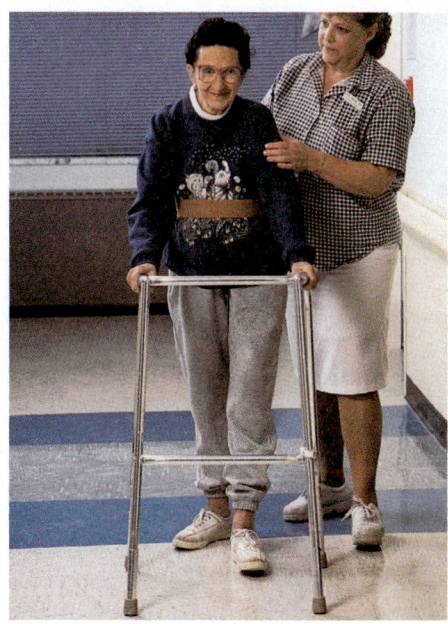

FIGURE 17-11 Stand on the patient's affected side while she grasps the walker with both hands.

Two-Point Gait with Walker. The steps for this procedure are as follows:

1. Complete steps 1 through 5 in Procedure 31.

2. Have the patient shift his weight to the strong leg as he lifts and moves the walker and the weak leg 6 to 8 inches ahead.

3. Now have him shift his weight to the weaker leg and the walker (with most of the weight on the walker).

4. He then moves his strong leg 6 to 8 inches ahead.

5. This process is repeated while the patient is walking.

6. Note the patient's endurance, balance, and strength while walking. Stop immediately if the patient has trouble and help him to the closest chair. Call the nurse.

7. Assist the patient to sit in the chair or to lie down in bed. Remove the gait belt. Store the cane in an appropriate area.

8. Document the distance the patient ambulated and his tolerance of the procedure.

9. Carry out procedure completion actions.

THE FALLING PATIENT

If a patient starts to fall, you must protect both yourself and the patient. If the patient has started to fall, do not try to hold her upright. This will strain your back and may injure the patient. *If a patient does fall, call the nurse to assess the patient for injuries before she is moved.*

SAFETY *Alert*

If you find a patient on the floor, remain in the room and call for help. Leave the patient on the floor. Provide any emergency measures that you are qualified to provide. If the nurse suspects a fracture, he or she will instruct you on how to return the patient to bed. Rolling him or her onto a sheet or blanket will make the transfer less traumatic. After proper emergency treatment and positioning on the sheet, the patient is lifted back to bed.

SAFETY *Alert*

Fall prevention is a major concern in health care facilities. Patients with a previous history of falls are always at higher risk than other patients. Other risk factors include advancing age, muscle weakness, gait and balance problems, neurological and musculoskeletal disorders, use of psychoactive medication, dementia, lower extremity disability or foot problems, and visual impairment. Environmental risk factors include slippery surfaces, uneven floors, loose rugs, poor lighting, unstable furniture, and objects on the floor.

Some elderly individuals have basic trust issues, particularly if the caregiver is young. They have their own way of doing things and believe they know best. The caregiver's way may be safest, but to gain compliance, avoid telling the individual that he or she is wrong. Rather, try to incorporate the patient's method into a safer way of accomplishing the task.

PROCEDURE 32

ASSISTING THE FALLING PATIENT

1. Keep your back straight, bend from the hips and knees, and maintain a broad base of support as you assist the falling patient. Maintain your grasp on the transfer belt.

2. Ease the patient to the floor, protecting her head.

3. As you ease the patient to the floor, bend your knees and go down with the patient (Figure 17-12).

4. Call for help.

5. Assist in returning the patient to bed or chair.

6. Carry out procedure completion actions.

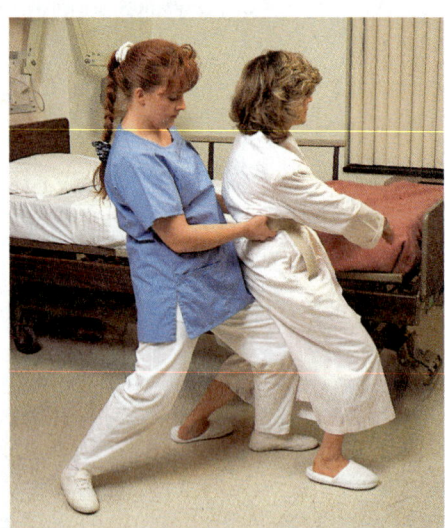

FIGURE 17-12 Ease the falling patient to the floor; bend your knees and go down with the patient.

USE OF WHEELCHAIRS

Many individuals who are unable to ambulate can gain some independence with the use of a wheelchair. A wheelchair should fit the person who is using it. Correct fit and body alignment will prevent contractures (Figure 17-13). If the chair fits correctly, there will be:

- About 4 inches between the top of the back upholstery and the patient's axillae.
- Armrests that support the arms without pushing the shoulders up or forcing them to hang.
- Two to 3 inches clearance between the front edge of the seat and the back of the patient's knee.
- Enough space between the patient's hip and the chair

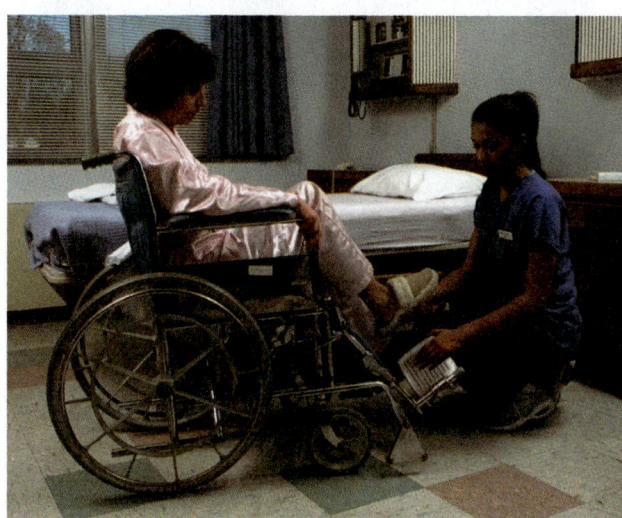

FIGURE 17-13 The wheelchair should fit the patient.

to slide your hand between the patient's hips on each side and the side of the wheelchair; the right amount of space avoids internal or external rotation of hips.

- Two inches between the bottom of the footrests and the floor.
- 90° angles between the feet and the legs, whether they are on the footrests or on the floor (when the footrests have been removed).

If the wheelchair does not fit the patient, check with the nurse or physical therapist to see how you can use pads or other devices to adapt the chair to the patient.

SAFETY *Alert*

There is no "one size fits all" wheelchair. Patients may have difficulty propelling a wheelchair that does not fit properly. A chair that does not fit correctly increases discomfort. Positioning problems are common. Patients may lean to the side, slide forward, or sit slumped in the chair. The risk of skin breakdown is increased. Positioning aids may be necessary. Sometimes unnecessary restraints are used to correct positioning problems. For many patients, a properly fit wheelchair solves the problem! If you suspect that the patient's problems are due to a wheelchair of the wrong size, inform the nurse.

guidelines *for*

Wheelchair Safety

- Check the wheelchair to see that brakes are working and wheels are securely attached. If the patient needs footrests, make sure they are in place. Replace the arm of wheelchair if it was removed during transfer.
- The small, front caster wheels of the chair provide the ability to move in all directions. The large part of the wheel faces back when the chair is moving. When the chair is parked, position the large part of the front wheel facing forward. This changes the center of gravity in the chair. Positioning the wheels to face forward prevents tipping if the patient leans forward. It helps stabilize the chair if the patient picks up an item from the floor. To reposition the wheels, back the chair up, then move it forward.

- Keep the wheelchair locked when not moving.
- Apply brakes and lift footrests out of the way when the patient is getting in or out of the wheelchair.
- Instruct the patient not to try to pick up an object off the floor. If there is satisfactory trunk stability and balance, the patient may be taught to do so, but instruct the patient to:
  - avoid shifting weight in the direction of the reach
  - not move forward in the seat
  - not reach down between the knees

The safest method is to position the chair alongside the object with casters in forward position, lock the chair, and reach only as far as the arm will extend.

continues

guidelines *continued*

- Check the patient's body alignment while in the wheelchair and reposition the patient when necessary.
- Prevent bath blankets, lap robes, or clothing from getting caught in wheels.
- Observe the patient's affected arm. A paralyzed arm may fall over the side of the wheelchair and become caught in the wheel.
- Guide the wheelchair from behind, grasping both handgrips (Figure 17-14).
- Approach corners slowly and look before you go around them.
- Take care when approaching swinging doors. Prop the door open to propel the chair through the door. If this is not possible, back through swinging doors.
- Back the wheelchair over the threshold in a doorway.
- Always back into doorways and elevators when transporting a patient by wheelchair (Figure 17-15).
- When leaving an elevator, push the stop button and ask others to step out. Turn the wheelchair around and back it out the door.
- When transporting a patient in a wheelchair down a ramp or incline, walk backward, slowly pulling the chair. Periodically look over your shoulder, as you would when backing up in a car, to make sure that the path is clear.
- When parking a wheelchair, avoid blocking a doorway. Apply the brakes.

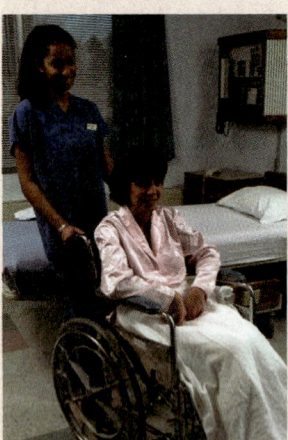 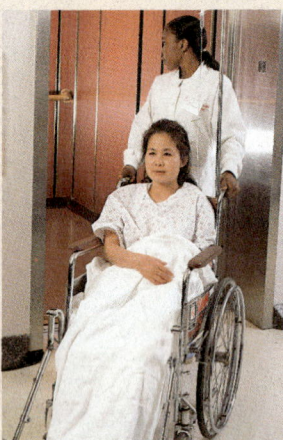

FIGURE 17-14 Guide the wheelchair from behind, grasping both handgrips.

FIGURE 17-15 Always back into doorways and elevators when transporting a patient in a wheelchair.

POSITIONING THE DEPENDENT PATIENT IN A WHEELCHAIR

The dependent person may slide down in the wheelchair, requiring assistance to regain body alignment. Several procedures can be used to correct the dependent patient's position in the wheelchair. Lock the drive wheels and position the caster wheels in the forward position before repositioning the patient.

1. Stand in front of the patient; make sure that the feet are in alignment and the arms are on the armrests. Help the patient lean forward and push with the hands and legs as you push against the patient's knees (Figure 17-16).

2. For an alternate method, place a soft towel or small sheet under the patient's buttocks and use this as a pull sheet to move the patient up in the chair. This requires two people (Figure 17-17).

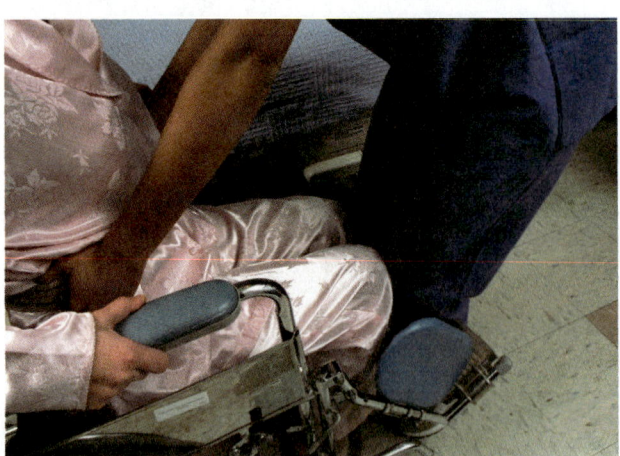

FIGURE 17-16 Push against the patient's knees as she pushes with her hands and legs.

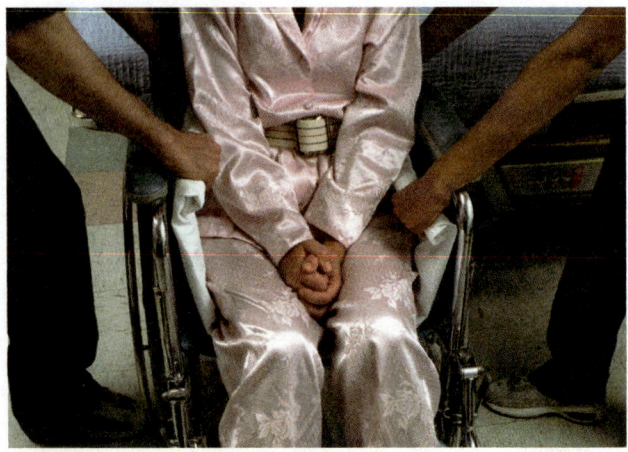

FIGURE 17-17 A draw (lift) sheet may be used to correct the patient's body alignment.

3. This method also requires two people. Place the transfer belt around the patient's waist. One assistant stands in back of the wheelchair and grasps the transfer belt with one hand on each side of the patient. The other one stands in front of the patient and places her hands and arms under the patient's knees. On the count of three, this assistant supports the lower extremities while the other one moves the patient back in the chair (Figure 17-18). This is not recommended for a heavy patient.

4. This method also requires two people. Stand in back of the wheelchair and have another assistant in front of the patient. Both assistants work with knees and hips bent and backs straight. Lean forward with your head over the patient's shoulder. Instruct the patient to fold the arms. Place your arms around the patient's trunk. Grasp the patient's right wrist with your left hand and grasp the patient's left wrist with your right hand. The other assistant encircles the patient's knees with hands and arms. On the count of three, both assistants lift and move the patient up (Figure 17-19).

5. One person can do this procedure. The patient needs to be oriented and able to follow directions. Stand in front of the patient. Flex your knees and hips and keep your back straight. Position your feet, one on each side of the patient's feet. Brace your knees against the patient's knees. Have the patient lean forward. Lean forward over the patient's right shoulder with the patient's head under your right arm. Encircle your arms around the patient's trunk. The patient's arms are folded together (Figure 17-20). Rock the patient forward and on the count of three, when the patient's weight is over the legs, push against the patient's knees to move back in the chair.

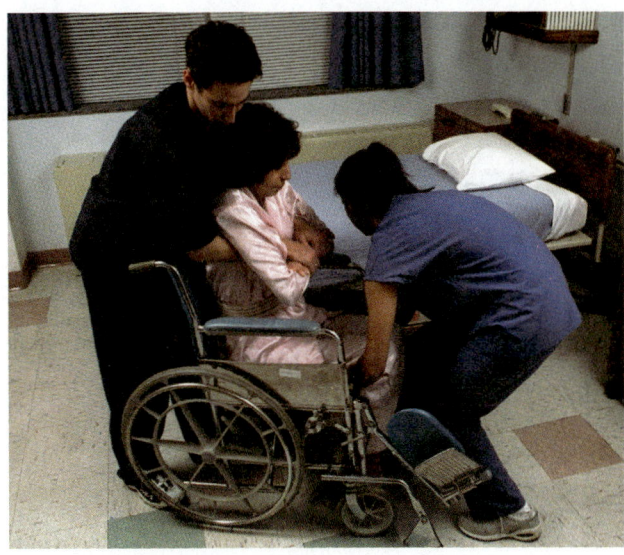

FIGURE 17-19 One assistant encircles the patient's legs with her hands and arms.

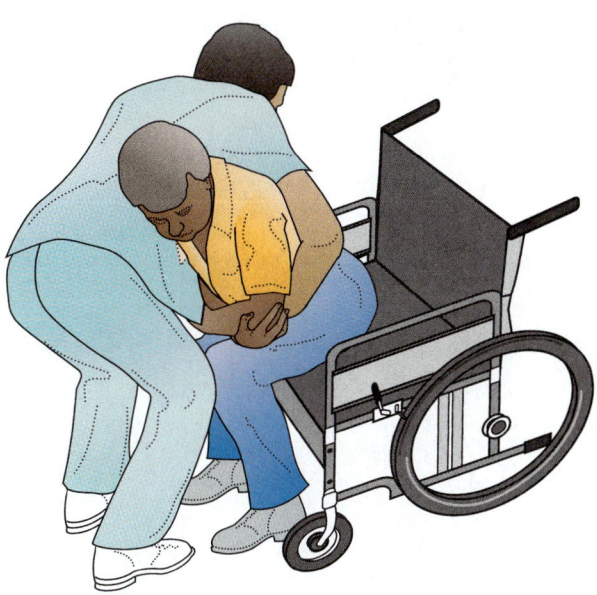

FIGURE 17-20 Put your arms around the patient's trunk.

If the patient can bear weight, it is easier and more beneficial to assist the patient to stand and then sit back down, getting the hips to the back of the chair. Wedge cushions placed in the wheelchair will prevent the patient from sliding forward.

WHEELCHAIR ACTIVITY

Pressure over the buttocks is dramatically increased when the patient is sitting. Teach the patient (and provide assistance if necessary) to periodically relieve the pressure by shifting weight every 15 minutes. *Be sure wheelchair is locked before beginning any activities involving patient movement in the chair.*

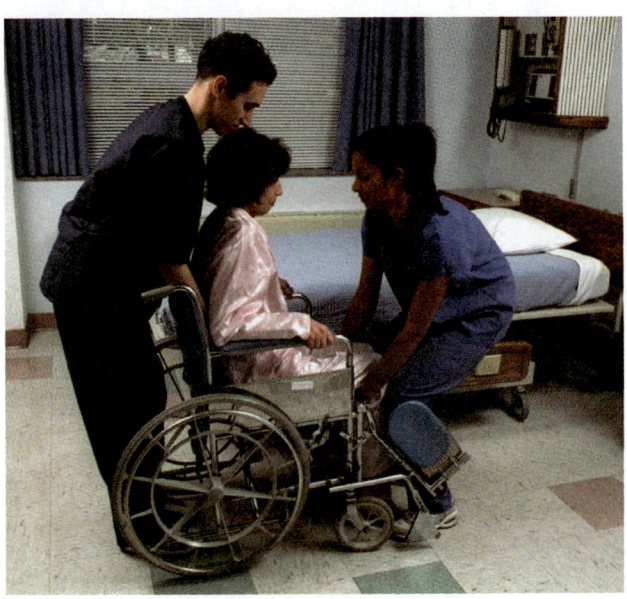

FIGURE 17-18 One assistant supports the lower extremities while the other uses the transfer belt to move the patient back in the chair.

Wheelchair Push-ups

1. Teach the patient to place one hand on each armrest, keeping both elbows bent.
2. Then have patient lean forward slightly, pushing on the armrests and straightening the elbows while lifting the buttocks off the seat of the wheelchair. Have the patient hold this position to the count of five if possible (Figure 17-21).

Leaning

If the patient cannot do push-ups, teach her to place the hands on the armrests or thighs and lean forward slightly, and then to each side to relieve pressure on the buttocks (Figure 17-22). Monitor patients who have balance problems, to avoid falling out of the chair.

Other Preventive Measures

Place a folded bath blanket in the seat of the chair if the patient is wearing a hospital gown, so the skin does not contact the vinyl chair seat. Use pressure-relieving pads in the seat of the chair if the patient will be up for a prolonged period of time. Use pillows, pads, or other props to maintain the patient in good body alignment. Patients should always sit upright, without leaning to either side.

TRANSPORTING A PATIENT BY STRETCHER

Before moving a patient on a stretcher, make sure that the side rails are up and all safety belts are fastened. Push the stretcher by standing at the patient's head. Moving the stretcher in this manner enables you to use good body mechanics and see potential hazards. Approach corners slowly and look before you go around them. Take care when approaching swinging doors. Prop the door open to propel the stretcher through the door. If this is not possible, back through swinging doors.

When entering an elevator, push the stop button to lock the doors open. Back the stretcher into the elevator by walking backward and pulling the head end of the stretcher. Stand by the patient's head while the elevator is in motion. When the elevator stops, push the stop button to lock the door open. Push the stretcher out so the feet exit the elevator first. If the threshold is uneven, go to the foot end of the stretcher and pull it out of the elevator. After the stretcher is safely out of the elevator, unlock the door mechanism.

When transporting a stretcher down a ramp or incline, walk backward, slowly guiding the stretcher from the head end. Periodically look over your shoulder to make sure that the path is clear.

When parking a stretcher, avoid blocking a doorway. Never leave a patient who is on a stretcher unattended or unsupervised.

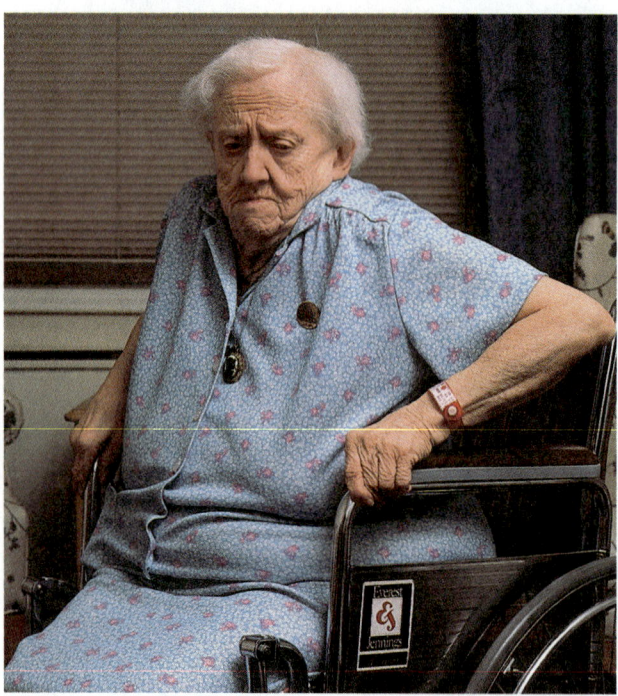

FIGURE 17-21 Wheelchair push-ups can relieve pressure on the buttocks, preventing pressure ulcers.

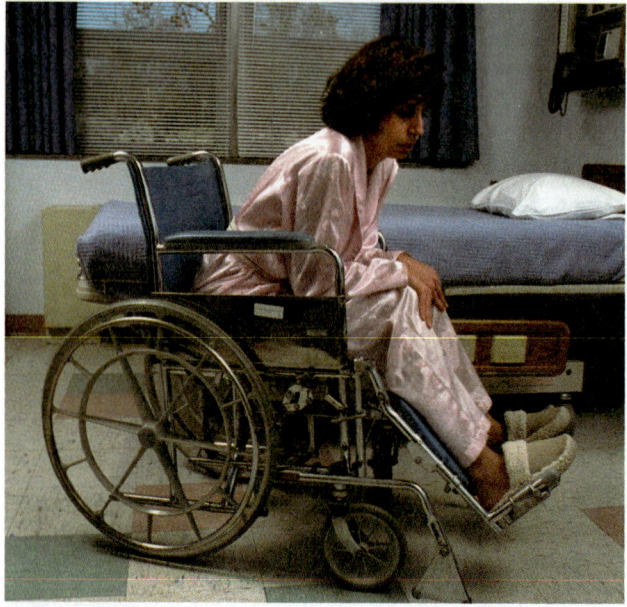

FIGURE 17-22 The patient can lean forward slightly to relieve pressure.

REVIEW

A. Multiple Choice.

Select the one best answer for each of the following.

1. When ambulating a patient with a weak right side, you should stand
   a. in back of the patient.
   b. on the patient's right side.
   c. on the patient's left side.
   d. in front of the patient.

2. When ambulating the patient, you should hold the gait belt with
   a. an overhand grasp in back of the patient.
   b. an underhand grasp in back of the patient.
   c. one hand on each side of the patient.
   d. one hand in front of the patient.

3. Before helping a patient to walk with a cane or walker, you should check the
   a. distance between the patient's feet.
   b. screws and bolts for tightness.
   c. height of the wheelchair.
   d. length of each step.

4. The cane is always held
   a. on the patient's weaker side.
   b. on the patient's stronger side.
   c. in the dominant hand.
   d. in the nondominant hand.

5. When using a two-point gait with a cane, the patient will
   a. place the strong foot forward, then the cane, then the weaker foot.
   b. place the strong foot and cane forward at the same time and then the weaker foot.
   c. place the weaker foot and cane forward at the same time and then the stronger foot.
   d. place the weaker foot forward, then the stronger foot, and then the cane.

6. If a patient starts to fall, you should
   a. try to hold the patient upright to prevent a fall.
   b. let go of the patient immediately, to avoid back strain.
   c. ease the patient to the floor.
   d. leave the patient and go for help.

7. When using a walker, the walker is set down so that
   a. the front legs strike the floor first and then the back legs.
   b. the back legs strike the floor first and then the front legs.
   c. all four legs strike the floor at the same time.
   d. how the walker is set down depends on the patient's problem.

8. When transporting a patient in a wheelchair, always
   a. stay to the right in corridors.
   b. guide the wheelchair from the front going down ramps.
   c. push the patient into an elevator frontwards.
   d. position the patient's feet at a 45° angle.

9. Conditions that can affect a patient's gait include
   a. diseases such as Parkinson's disease.
   b. having a catheter.
   c. having hand surgery.
   d. transferring independently.

10. Assistive devices are usually selected by the
    a. nursing assistant.
    b. physician.
    c. physical therapist.
    d. family.

B. True/False.

Mark the following true or false by circling T or F.

11. **T** F Always back in as you move a patient in a wheelchair into an elevator.

12. T **F** When transporting a patient in a wheelchair, always walk on the left of the corridor.

13. **T** F A wheelchair should always be locked unless the patient is being moved.

14. T **F** A cane is held in the patient's weaker hand.

15. T **F** When using a walker, the front two tips of the walker should strike the floor first and then the back two tips should strike the floor.

16. T **F** When assisting a patient to ambulate, you need to use a gait belt only if the patient is using an assistive device.

17. **T** F To relieve pressure on the buttocks, the patient should be taught how to do wheelchair push-ups or how to lean to relieve pressure.

18. **T** F To pick an article up from the floor, the patient should lean forward and reach down between the knees.

19. **T** F A cane is used for patients who are unable to bear weight on one leg.

20. **T** F The patient needs to be able to use both hands to manipulate a walker.

C. Nursing Assistant Challenge.

Mr. Santozi is 76 years old and has had right hip surgery. His physician does not want him to bear full weight on the affected leg. He uses a walker to assist his ambulation. He has been taught to use a three-point gait. When you help him out of bed, *he reaches for the walker to help pull himself up from the bed. As you watch him walk down the hall, you note that he is setting the walker down by the front legs first and then the back legs. When he walks, he pushes the walker and his strong leg ahead at the same time. What errors is Mr. Santozi making, and how can you help him?*

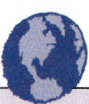

EXPLORING THE WEB

Description	Location
Ambulating with a Gait Belt	http://www.gc.maricopa.edu
Ambulation Training	http://sandiego.networkofcare.org
Articles on Falls and Risk	http://www.amda.com
Assisted Walking	http://www.ohsah.bc.ca
Preventing Falls and Fractures	http://www.crouse.org
Safety Procedures	http://www.texashste.com
Strategies for Improving Resident Mobility	http://www.nursinghome.org
Merry Walker	http://www.merrywalker.com
Making Health Care Safer	http://www.ahrq.gov/clinic/ptsafety/spotlight.htm
Procedure for Ambulation Aids	http://www-nmcp.med.navy.mil/nursing/procman/ambulationaids.doc

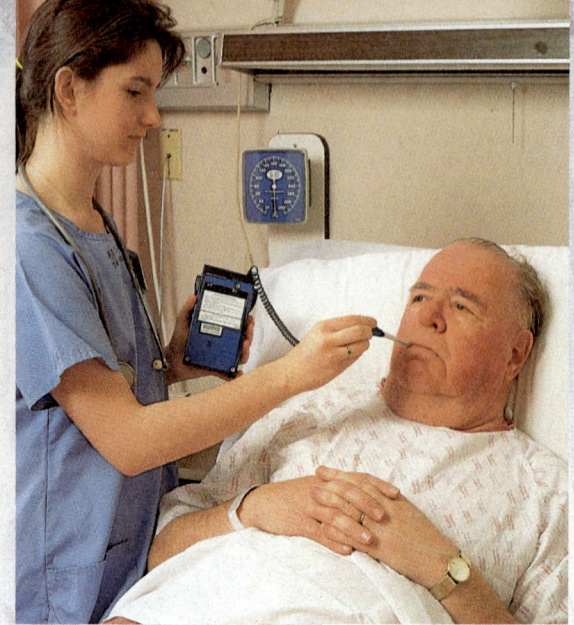

Body Temperature

objectives

After completing this unit, you will be able to:

- Spell and define terms.
- Name and identify the three types of clinical thermometers and tell their uses.
- Read a thermometer.
- Identify the range of normal values.
- Demonstrate the following procedures:
  - Procedure 33 Measuring an Oral Temperature (Glass Thermometer)
  - Procedure 34 Measuring Temperature Using a Sheath-Covered Thermometer
  - Procedure 35 Measuring a Rectal Temperature (Glass Thermometer)
  - Procedure 36 Measuring an Axillary or Groin Temperature (Glass Thermometer)
  - Procedure 37 Measuring an Oral Temperature (Electronic Thermometer)
  - Procedure 38 Measuring a Rectal Temperature (Electronic Thermometer)
  - Procedure 39 Measuring an Axillary Temperature (Electronic Thermometer)
  - Procedure 40 Measuring a Tympanic Temperature
  - Procedure 41 Cleaning Glass Thermometers

vocabulary

Learn the meaning and the correct spelling of the following words and phrases:

body core	digital thermometer	flagged	tympanic
body shell	electronic	metabolism	thermometer
Celsius scale	thermometer	probe	vital signs
clinical thermometer	Fahrenheit scale		

INTRODUCTION

Measurement of body temperature is a common nursing assistant task. Body temperature is one of the vital (living) signs. The patient's other vital signs include the pulse, respiration, and blood pressure. Although they are not part of the vital signs, the height and weight of the patient are also commonly measured.

Specific equipment is used to determine or measure these values. They must be accurately measured because they tell us a great deal about the patient's condition. Do not tell the patient the results. This is not your responsibility. Tell the patient you will ask the nurse to discuss the results with him. Although they are usually determined as a combined procedure, each vital sign is discussed in a separate unit. Measurement of height and weight is discussed in Unit 21. Many facilities use electronic equipment that automatically registers the four vital signs simultaneously.

TEMPERATURE VALUES

Temperature values may be expressed in either of two scales. They are the:

- Fahrenheit scale, which is indicated by an *F*.
- Celsius scale (centigrade scale), which is indicated by a *C*.

A small ° before either capital letter indicates degrees or levels of temperature.

A formula can be used to convert temperature readings from Celsius to Fahrenheit and from Fahrenheit to Celsius. See Table 18-1 for some important equivalents. Figure 18-1 compares the markings of the Fahrenheit and Celsius thermometers.

DEFINITION OF BODY TEMPERATURE

Temperature is the measurement of body heat. It is the balance between heat produced and heat lost.

TABLE 18-1 COMPARISON OF FAHRENHEIT AND CELSIUS TEMPERATURE SCALES

	Celsius (C)	Fahrenheit (F)
Freezing	0°	32°
Body temperature	37°	98.6°
Pasteurization	63°	145°
Boiling	100°	212°
Sterilizing (Autoclave)	121°	250°

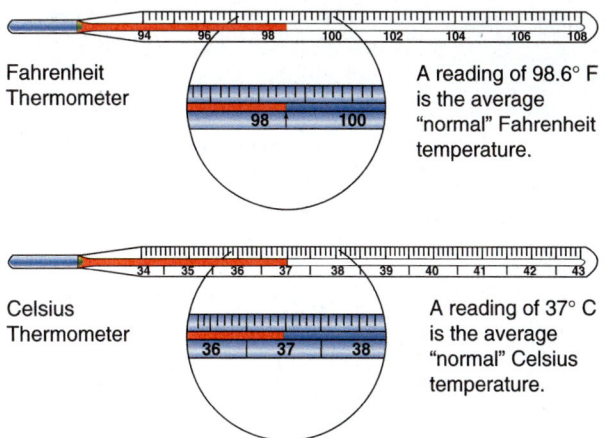

Fahrenheit Thermometer — A reading of 98.6° F is the average "normal" Fahrenheit temperature.

Celsius Thermometer — A reading of 37° C is the average "normal" Celsius temperature.

FIGURE 18-1 Fahrenheit and Celsius thermometers.

Body temperature is:

- Fairly constant. There is a daily variation of 1 to 3°F. Body temperature is lowest in the morning. It is higher in the afternoon and evening.
- Lower the closer to the body surface it is measured. The temperature at the center of the body (body core) is much higher than the temperature at the surface of the body.
- Different in the same person when determined from different body areas (Table 18-2). It is important to know the "normal" temperature for an individual, because the normal may vary from person to person.
- Less stable in children. Table 18-3 shows average temperatures in infants and children.
- Affected by
  - illness
  - external temperature/environment
  - medication
  - age
  - infection
  - time of day
  - exercise
  - emotions
  - pregnancy

TABLE 18-2 TEMPERATURE VARIATIONS IN THE SAME PERSON

	Oral	Axillary	Rectal
Average Temperature	98.6°F	97.6°F	99.6°F
Range	97.6–99.6°F (36.5–37.5°C)	96.6–98.6°F (36–37°C)	98.6–100.6°F (37–38.1°C)

TABLE 18-3	AVERAGE TEMPERATURES IN INFANTS AND CHILDREN
Age	**Temperature**
3 months	99.4°F
6 months	99.5°F
1 year	99.7°F
3 years	99.0°F
5 years	98.6°F
9 years	98.0°F

- menstrual cycle
- crying
- hydration

Excessive body temperature puts stress on vital body organs.

TEMPERATURE CONTROL

Activities to control and regulate body temperature are managed by special cells in the brain.

- Heat is produced by chemical reactions (**metabolism**) in the body core and muscular contractions. For this reason, rectal temperature is highest.
- Blood carries the heat to the skin (**body shell**). The heat is lost from the skin to the outside.
- Heat loss is largely controlled by regulating the amount of blood reaching the skin and through perspiration.
- Average oral temperature range is 96.8°F (36°C) to 100.4°F (38°C). Average temperature is 98.6°F (37°C).

MEASURING BODY TEMPERATURE

Temperature is usually measured in one of four body areas:

- mouth (oral)—most common.
- ear (aural or tympanic)—takes the least amount of time.
- rectal—most accurate of commonly used sites (mouth, rectal, axillary); rectal temperature registers 1°F higher than oral.
- axillary or groin—least accurate; measures temperature under the arm or at the groin. (This method is used only when the patient's condition does not permit the use of oral, aural, or rectal sites.) An axillary or groin temperature registers 1°F (or 0.6°C) lower than oral temperature.

The patient's condition determines which is the best site for measuring the temperature. The site used most often is the mouth. It is not, however, always the best or safest site to use. In some situations, it is wiser to use the rectal site.

For example, if the patient is a child or irrational, a glass thermometer in the mouth could result in injury. Patients with respiratory problems, those who breathe through the mouth, or those who are very weak or unconscious may not be able to keep an oral thermometer in their mouths for a long enough time to ensure an accurate recording. In these situations, the best choice is the aural site, because the care provider holds the tympanic thermometer in the ear. The reading registers within seconds, so the tympanic thermometer is a good choice for restless patients as well. If the tympanic thermometer is not available, the rectal site might be used. Use a rectal thermometer inserted in the anus for the proper time. Be sure to hold the rectal thermometer in place to avoid possible injury.

CLINICAL THERMOMETERS

A patient's temperature is determined by using a **clinical thermometer**. There are several types of clinical thermometers.

The Glass Clinical Thermometer

The glass clinical thermometer is a slender glass tube containing liquid; the liquid expands when exposed to heat and moves up or down the tube. Three types of glass clinical thermometers are in general use (Figure 18-2). They are the oral, security, and rectal thermometers. They differ mainly in the size and shape of the bulb. The bulb is the end that is inserted into the patient. When only the security or stubby type is in use, the rectal thermometers are marked with a red dot at the end of the stem.

Thermometers containing mercury have been used for many years. However, recently the trend in health care has been to avoid the use of products containing mercury, because the mercury can be very toxic to humans and wildlife, if the product is broken. This is true even if mercury exposure occurs in very small amounts.

A mercury thermometer is a small glass tube containing

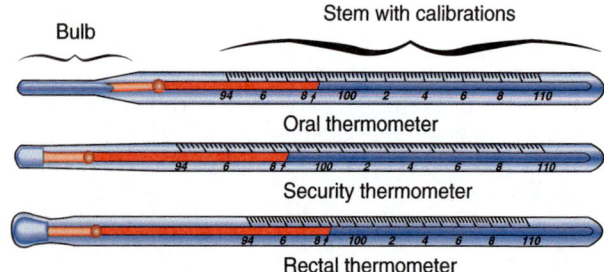

FIGURE 18-2 Clinical thermometers (from top to bottom): oral, security, rectal.

liquid mercury, a silvery-white substance that registers body heat. Alternative products are now being used in many glass thermometers because of mercury's potential for toxicity. Some thermometers contain a red or blue liquid. These are alcohol thermometers and contain no mercury. Another, less common thermometer contains galinstan, a substance similar to mercury in appearance. These thermometers are mercury-free, however, and are generally marked as such.

Mercury can be toxic in small amounts, particularly if it vaporizes and is inhaled. Even small mercury spills must be cleaned up properly to prevent contamination and illness. If you accidentally break a thermometer or other medical device containing mercury, follow your facility policies and procedures for cleaning the spill.

Electronic Thermometer

The **electronic thermometer** (Figure 18-3) is used in many hospitals. One unit can serve many patients because the nursing assistant simply changes the disposable sheath that fits over the probe.

- The electronic thermometer is battery-operated. It registers the temperature on the viewing screen in a few seconds.
- The portion called the **probe** is inserted into the patient.

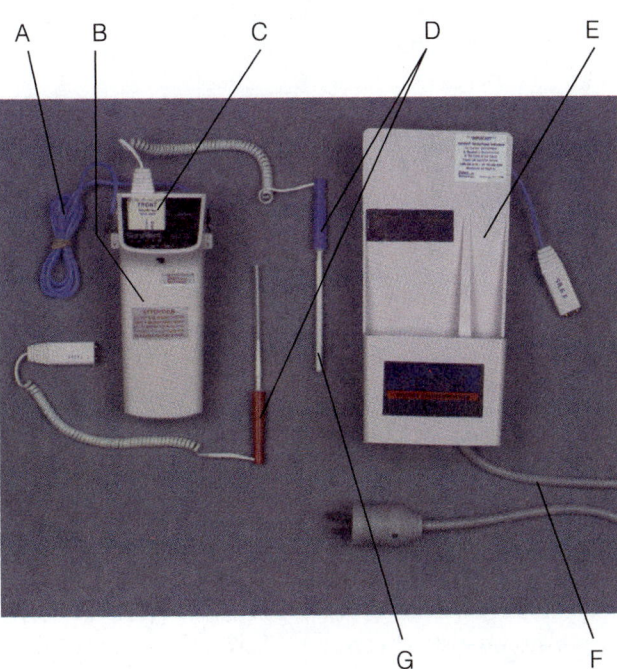

FIGURE 18-3 An electronic thermometer. The temperature is registered in large, easy-to-read numerals. The disposable protective sheath (probe cover) is placed over the probe tip. The probe is inserted in the patient's mouth in the usual manner. (A) Plastic cord goes around the nursing assistant's neck when carrying the thermometer. (B) Thermometer (C) Box of disposable probe covers (D) Probe (Blue = oral, Red = rectal) (E) Charging unit (F) Probe cord (G) Disposable probe cover.

- The probes are colored red for rectal use and blue for oral or axillary use.
- The probe is covered by a plastic sheath before use. The plastic sheath stays on during use. It is discarded after use.

Digital Thermometer

Digital thermometers are hand-held and have a probe that is inserted into the patient's mouth or rectum (Figure 18-4). Sheaths are used to cover the oral or rectal probe before use and are discarded after use. The unit is battery-operated. After the sheath-covered probe is inserted, the temperature can be read within 20 to 60 seconds. The temperature is shown as a digital (number) display.

Disposable Oral Thermometers

Plastic or paper thermometers are used for oral temperatures in some facilities. They are used once and discarded. They have dots on them. The dots change color from brown to blue, according to the patient's temperature.

SAFETY *Alert*

The disposable thermometer is made of rigid plastic. Remove the thermometer from the patient's mouth slowly. Pulling the thermometer out rapidly from between closed lips can cause tears of the lips and mucous membranes in the mouth.

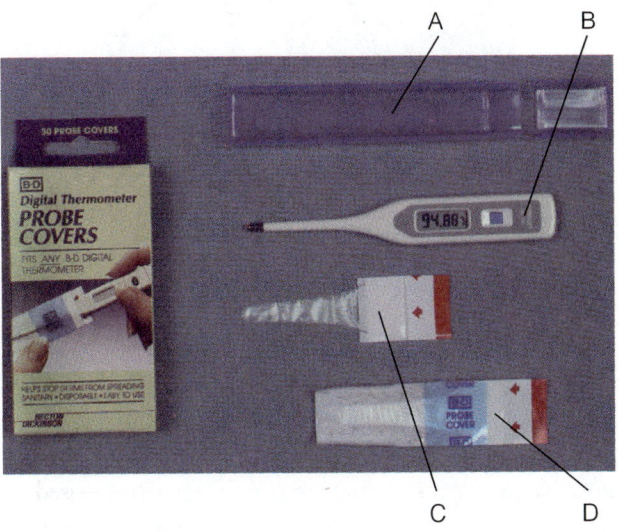

FIGURE 18-4 Digital thermometer (A) Carrying case (B) Digital thermometer (C) Probe cover less backing (D) Probe cover with backing.

Tympanic Thermometer

The **tympanic thermometer** is an instrument that measures the temperature from blood vessels in the tympanic membrane (ear drum) in the ear (Figure 18-5). The temperature reading obtained is close to the core body temperature. To obtain an accurate reading, the probe must be placed solidly into the ear canal. The instrument has a built-in converter that provides the equivalent temperature in rectal or oral values (in both the Fahrenheit and Celsius systems). The type of temperature reading (mode) is selected by the user. The disposable speculum is inserted into the ear canal, gently sealing the canal. The instrument is activated, usually by pressing a button, and within a few seconds it registers the temperature of the blood flowing through the vessels in the eardrum.

Using the Glass Thermometer

The glass thermometer is a long, cylindrical, calibrated tube that contains a column of heat-sensitive liquid (Figure 18-6).
- Starting with 94°F (34°C), each long line indicates a one-degree elevation in temperature.
- Only every other degree is marked with a number.
- In between each long line are four shorter lines.
- Each shorter line equals two-tenths (2/10 or 0.2) of 1 degree.

The liquid (the solid color line shown in Figure 18-6) in the bulb of the thermometer rises in the hollow center of the stem as heat is registered. To read the thermometer:
- Hold it at eye level.
- Find the solid column in the center.
- Look along the sharper edge between the numbers and lines.

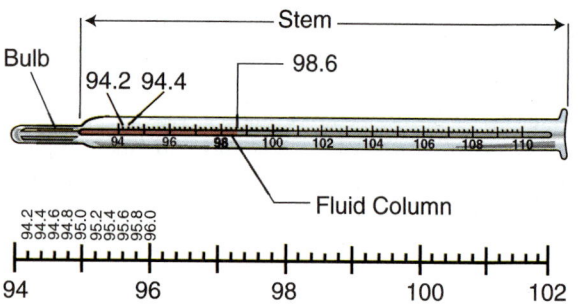

FIGURE 18-6 Reading a thermometer. This thermometer reads 98.6°F. Most Fahrenheit thermometers have an arrow indicating 98.6°F.

- Read at the point at which the liquid ends.
- If it falls between two lines, read it to the closest line.

Some glass thermometers come individually prepackaged for patient use. The patient receives it as part of the admission package.

Using the Electronic Thermometer

Battery-operated electronic thermometers are commonly used. The temperature registers in large numbers on the screen. The probe is placed into the patient. The probe stem is colored blue for oral or axillary use and red for rectal use. A new, disposable probe cover is used for each patient. Following use, the cover is discarded. The temperature registers in about 30 seconds.

Using the Tympanic Thermometer

Many facilities use tympanic thermometers. The temperature is taken by measuring the heat given off by the tympanic membrane (in the ear). This method has several advantages:
- Tympanic thermometers are accurate and easy to use.

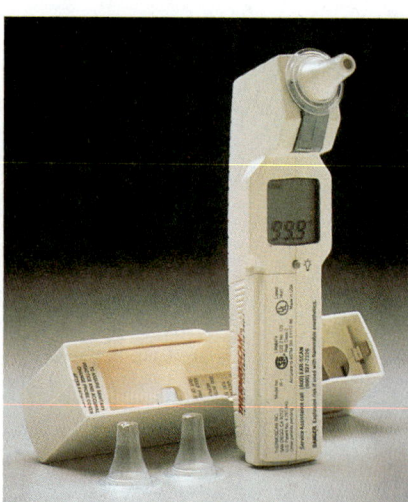

FIGURE 18-5 Cordless, hand-held tympanic thermometer that measures the temperature of the tympanic membrane in the ear. The window on the handset indicates the digital temperature reading. *(Courtesy of Thermoscan® Inc., San Diego, CA.)*

SAFETY *Alert*

If you accidentally break a mercury thermometer, apply gloves and eye protection. Your facility may also require use of a mask to prevent inhalation. Pick up broken glass and other debris and place in a puncture-resistant container. Follow facility policies for picking up mercury. Use an index card to consolidate the droplets, then seal them in a plastic bag or covered container. Small droplets can be picked up with adhesive tape or wet paper towels. Seal the container and affix a label identifying the material as "mercury spill debris."

guidelines *for*

Using an Oral or Rectal Thermometer

Oral Thermometer

1. Do not use if the patient is:
   - uncooperative
   - restless
   - unconscious
   - chilled
   - confused or disoriented
   - coughing
   - an infant or child under the age of 6
   - unable to breathe through the nose
   - recovering from oral surgery
   - irrational
   - very weak
   - receiving oxygen (except nasal prongs)
   - on seizure precautions
2. An oral temperature reading could be false on denture wearers.
3. To measure an oral temperature accurately, wait 15 minutes if patients have been smoking, eating, or drinking, then take the temperature.

Rectal Thermometer

1. Do not use if the patient has:
   - diarrhea
   - fecal impaction
   - combative behavior
   - rectal bleeding
   - hemorrhoids
   - had rectal surgery or rectal or colonic disease
   - recently had a heart attack
   - recently had prostate surgery
   - a colostomy
2. Always hold a rectal thermometer in place the entire time.

- The temperature registers in a few seconds. Because of this, taking the temperature of an agitated patient is safer and faster.
- Temperatures that cannot be taken orally can be taken by the tympanic method, eliminating the need to take rectal or axillary temperatures.

guidelines *for*

The Safe Use of a Glass Thermometer

- Make sure the thermometer is clean.
- Wear disposable gloves when measuring oral and rectal temperatures.
- Check glass thermometers for chips.
- Shake the thermometer down before use. Shake away from the patient and hard objects.
- Cover the thermometer with a disposable plastic sheath.
- Do not leave the patient alone with a thermometer in place.
- Allow a glass thermometer to register for at least 3 minutes for oral temperature, 3 minutes for rectal temperature, and 10 minutes for axillary temperature. Each facility may have it's own guidelines. Be sure to follow your facilities guidelines.
- Hold rectal and axillary thermometers in place.
- When using a rectal thermometer, lubricate the bulb end of the thermometer before inserting it into the rectum.
- After removing the thermometer and before reading it, wipe the thermometer from end to tip with an alcohol wipe or cotton ball.
- Do not touch a bulb end or disposable sheath that has been in patient's mouth (oral thermometer) or anus (rectal thermometer).
- Discard the sheath according to facility policy after use.
- Clean and disinfect the thermometer after use.

- The tympanic thermometer allows you to select a core, oral, or rectal mode. This means the reading will correlate with the mode selected. Choose the mode according to your facility's policy.
- Wait for 15 minutes to take the temperature if the patient has been outdoors or if the patient has been lying on the ear you will use.

The tympanic temperature is the fastest and most convenient method, but it can also give inaccurate readings if the user's technique is not precise. To ensure an accurate reading, insert the probe tip into the ear as far as it will go. Next, rotate the probe handle until it is aligned with the jaw, like speaking on the telephone. Quickly press the "scan" button. Using this method will help ensure accurate temperature readings.

PROCEDURE 33

MEASURING AN ORAL TEMPERATURE (GLASS THERMOMETER)

1. Carry out beginning procedure actions.

2. Assemble the following equipment on a tray:
   - Gloves (standard precautions)
   - Container with clean thermometers
   - Container for used thermometers
   - Cotton balls
   - Container for soiled tissues
   - Container with tissues
   - Pad and pencil
   - Watch with second hand

3. Have the patient rest in a comfortable position in a bed or chair. Put on gloves.

4. Remove the thermometer from the container by holding the stem end. Rinse the thermometer with cold water and wipe with tissue from stem to bulb end if the thermometer has been in disinfectant. Check to be sure the thermometer is intact. Read the center column. It should register below 96°F. If necessary, shake it down. (To shake down (Figure 18-7A), move away from tables and other hard objects. Grasp the stem tightly between your thumb and fingers. Shake down with a downward motion.) If used in your facility, place the thermometer in a disposable plastic cover sheath.

5. Ask the patient if he or she has had anything to eat or drink or has smoked within the last 15 minutes. Wait 15 minutes before taking an oral temperature if the answer is yes.

6. Insert the bulb end of the thermometer under the patient's tongue, toward the side of the mouth (Figure 18-7B). Tell the patient to hold the thermometer gently with lips closed for 3 minutes.

7. Remove the thermometer, holding it by the stem. Wipe from stem end toward bulb end (Figure 18-7C).

8. Discard tissue in the proper container.

9. Read the thermometer and record the temperature on a pad (Figure 18-7D).

10. Place the thermometer in the container for used thermometers. If the thermometer is to be reused for this patient:
    - Wash it twice in cold water and soap with two separate cotton balls, wiping from stem to bulb.
    - Rinse and dry it.
    - Return it to the individual disinfectant-filled holder.

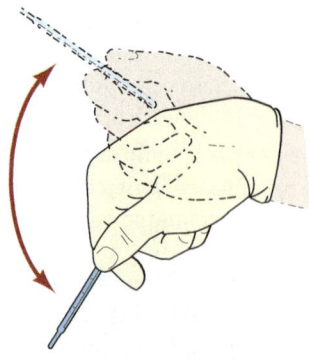

FIGURE 18-7A Shake the liquid down in the column by holding the thermometer by the stem and snapping the wrist. Check the reading. Repeat until the reading is below 96°F.

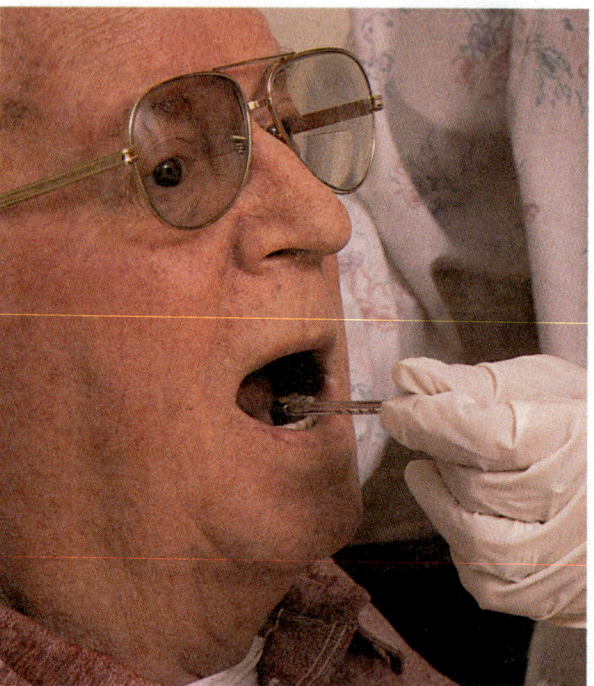

FIGURE 18-7B The bulb end of the thermometer is inserted under the tongue, left 3 minutes, then removed.

continues

PROCEDURE 33

continued

- Remove gloves and discard according to facility policy.

11. Carry out procedure completion actions.

12. Report any unusual variations to the nurse at once.

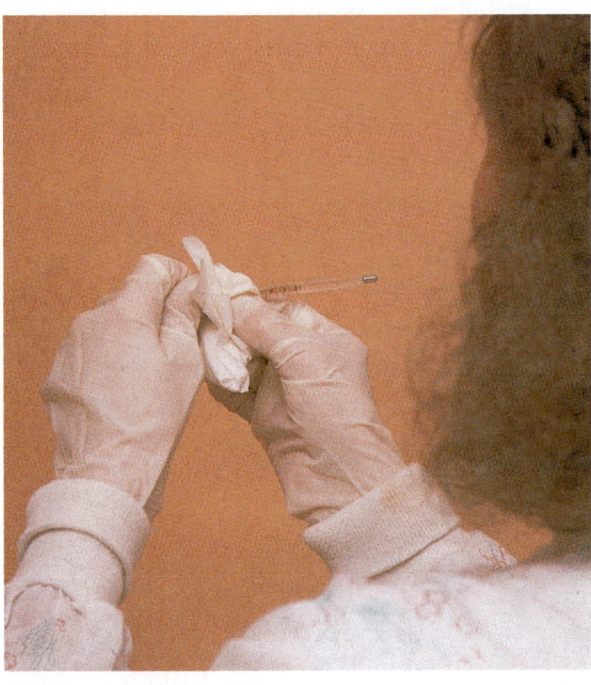

FIGURE 18-7C Wipe the thermometer after removing it from the patient's mouth or discard the disposable sheath. Always wipe from the stem to the bulb. Do not touch the bulb.

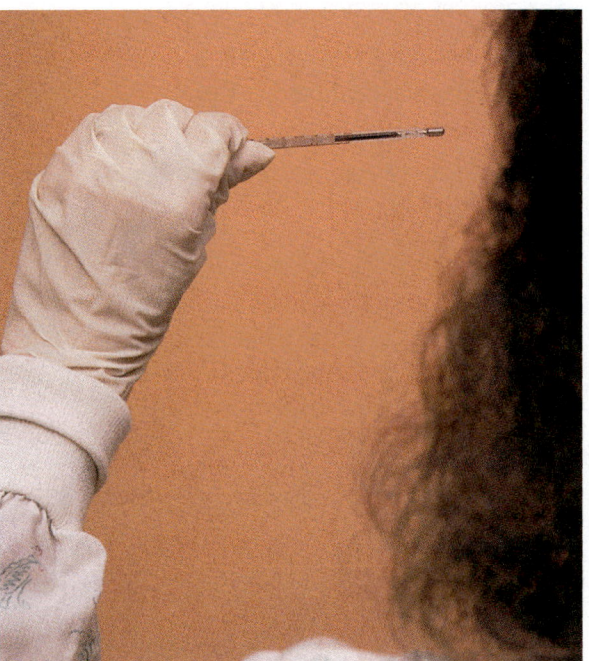

FIGURE 18-7D Hold the thermometer at eye level. Locate the column of liquid in the center and read to the next closest line.

guidelines *for*

Using a Tympanic (Ear) Thermometer

- Make sure the thermometer lens is clean and that there is no dirt or debris on the lens at the end of the probe tip.
- Use each probe cover only once. Make sure the cover is on snugly, without ripples.
- Store the thermometer out of the path of any cold air flow. If the thermometer is in a cold area, allow it to warm up before use, or it may read low.
- Make sure the patient is not directly in the path of cold air or being fanned. This action cools the ears, which can cause a low temperature reading.
- If the patient is lying on one ear, use the opposite ear.

- If the patient has a hearing aid, use the opposite ear or remove the aid and wait 15 minutes.
- The tympanic thermometer can be set to oral, core, or rectal mode. In most cases, oral is appropriate. The mode will be shown in the LCD readout screen. If the screen says "CAL," the thermometer is in the unadjusted mode, which is used only for calibration and other bench work.
- Insert the probe tip into the ear as far as possible, then rotate the handle to the correct position in alignment with the jaw.

PROCEDURE 34

MEASURING TEMPERATURE USING A SHEATH-COVERED THERMOMETER

1. Carry out beginning procedure actions.

2. Assemble needed equipment:
   - Gloves (standard precautions)
   - Clinical thermometer
   - Protective sheath (unopened package)
   - Pad and pencil

3. Have the patient rest in a comfortable position.

4. Ask the patient if he or she has had anything to eat or drink or has smoked within the last 15 minutes. Wait 15 minutes before taking an oral temperature if the answer is yes.

5. Apply gloves.

6. Shake the thermometer down to below 96°F.

7. Holding the thermometer in one hand, insert it into the marked end of a protective sheath wrapper (Figure 18-8A).

8. Holding onto the sheath tab on the stem end of the thermometer, peel back the paper cover to expose the plastic sheath (Figure 18-8B).

9. Hold the paper wrapper in one hand (Figure 18-8C). Twist on the paper wrapper to break the seal with the tab and remove the paper wrapper, leaving the plastic sheath on the thermometer (Figure 18-8D).

10. Keeping the protective sheath over the thermometer, insert the bulb end of the thermometer under the patient's tongue, toward the side of the mouth.

11. Tell the patient to hold the thermometer gently, with lips closed, for 3 minutes.

12. Remove the thermometer and discard the used sheath (Figure 18-8E). Read and shake down. Record on notepad.

13. The thermometer can be stored in the patient's bedside stand for reuse with a new sheath.

14. Remove gloves and discard according to facility policy.

15. Carry out procedure completion actions.

16. Report any unusual variations to the nurse at once.

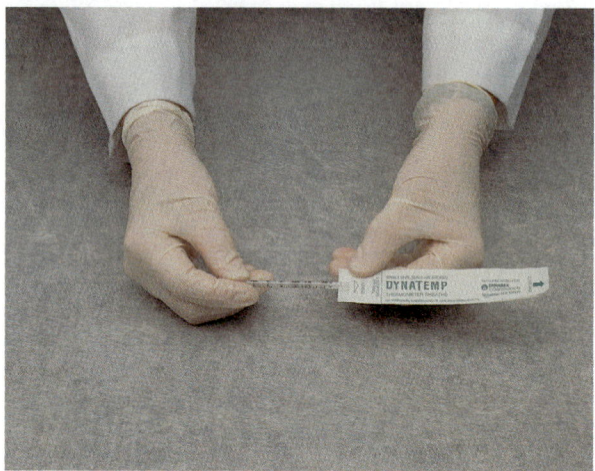

FIGURE 18-8A Inserting a thermometer into a disposable thermometer sheath.

continues

Cleaning Glass Thermometers

Glass thermometers are reusable. Therefore, they must be cleaned and disinfected between uses. If each patient has an individual thermometer kept in solution at the bedside, you must clean and disinfect it after each use. If a general supply of thermometers is used to determine routine temperature, they too must be disinfected before reuse.

Each used thermometer must be carefully washed with soapy, cold, running water to remove saliva or other body secretions. It must be rinsed to remove the soap and then carefully dried before disinfecting.

PROCEDURE 34

continued

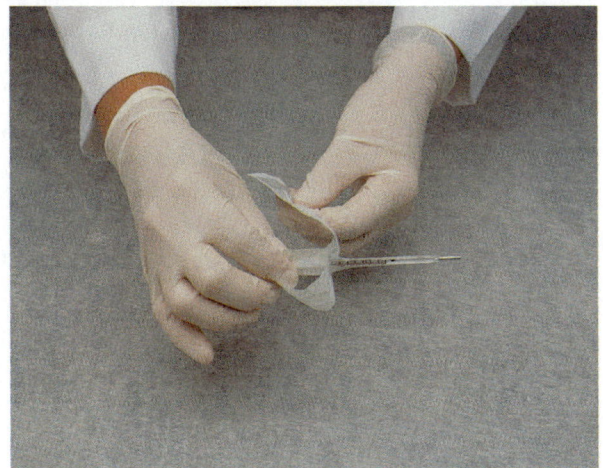

FIGURE 18-8B To remove the sheath, peel back the outer paper wrapper to expose the inner plastic sheath.

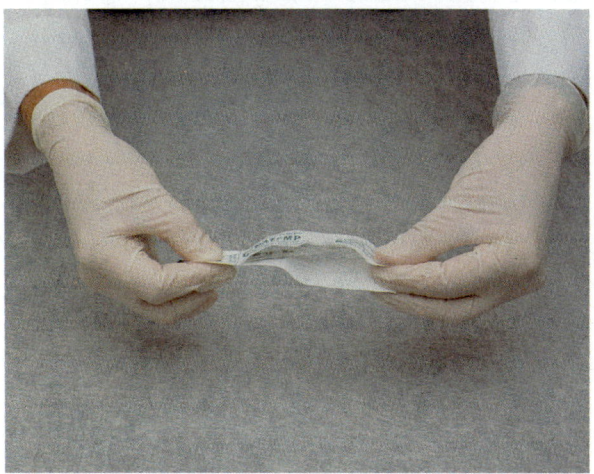

FIGURE 18-8C Grasp the outer paper wrapper.

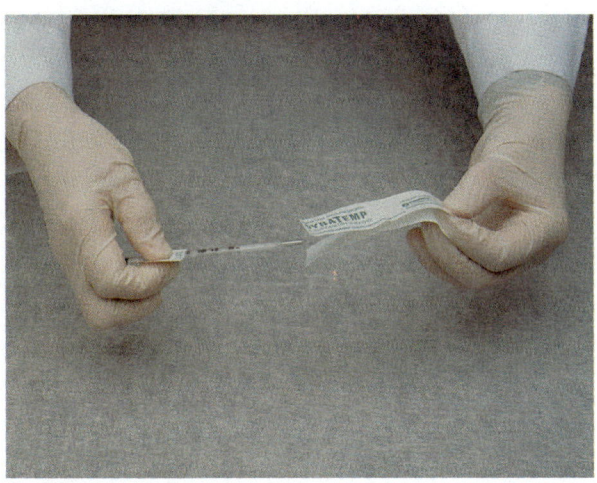

FIGURE 18-8D Holding onto the paper tab with one hand, twist and remove the outer paper wrapper.

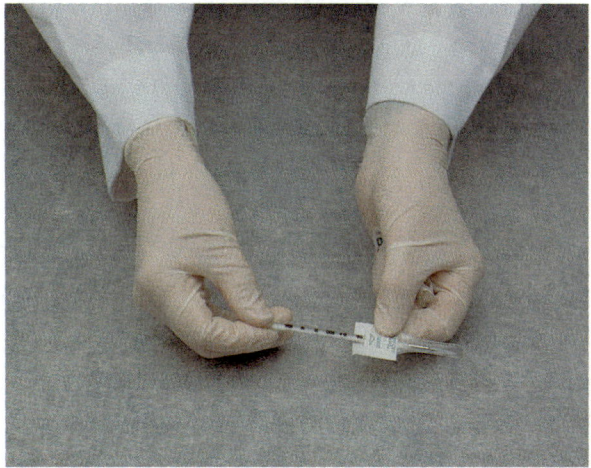

FIGURE 18-8E The sheath-covered thermometer is inserted into the patient's mouth. After the temperature is taken, the sheath is removed and discarded in the biohazard trash container.

Remember that glass breaks very easily, so be careful when washing and drying thermometers. Check each one for chips before putting it into disinfectant and before using a thermometer with a patient.

Documentation

In many facilities, temperatures are recorded on a temperature clipboard. They are then transferred to the individual patient charts. Changes in readings may be **flagged** (specially noted) by placing a circle around the reading or a star beside it. Make sure to report any changes from previous temperature readings directly to the nurse. Your accurate observations, reporting, and documentation contribute to the nurses' evaluation and assessment of the patient.

PROCEDURE 35

MEASURING A RECTAL TEMPERATURE (GLASS THERMOMETER)

1. Carry out beginning procedure actions.

2. Assemble equipment on a tray:
   - Container with clean rectal thermometer
   - Container for used thermometers
   - Container for soiled tissues
   - Lubricant
   - Container with tissues
   - Pad and pencil
   - Watch with second hand
   - Gloves (standard precautions)

3. Put up opposite side rail. Lower backrest of bed. Ask the patient to turn to the left side, if possible. Assist the patient if necessary.

4. Place a small amount of lubricant on a tissue.

5. Put gloves on. Remove the thermometer from the container by holding the stem end. Read the liquid column. Be sure it registers below 96°F. Check the condition of the thermometer.

6. Apply a small amount of lubricant to the bulb with a tissue.

7. Fold the top bedclothes back to expose the patient's anal area.

8. (Refer to Figure 18-9.) Separate the buttocks with one hand. Insert the thermometer gently into the rectum 1 inch. Hold in place. Adjust the bedclothes for privacy as soon as the thermometer is inserted.

9. The thermometer should remain inserted for 3 minutes, or according to facility policy. Hold the thermometer in place for the full time.

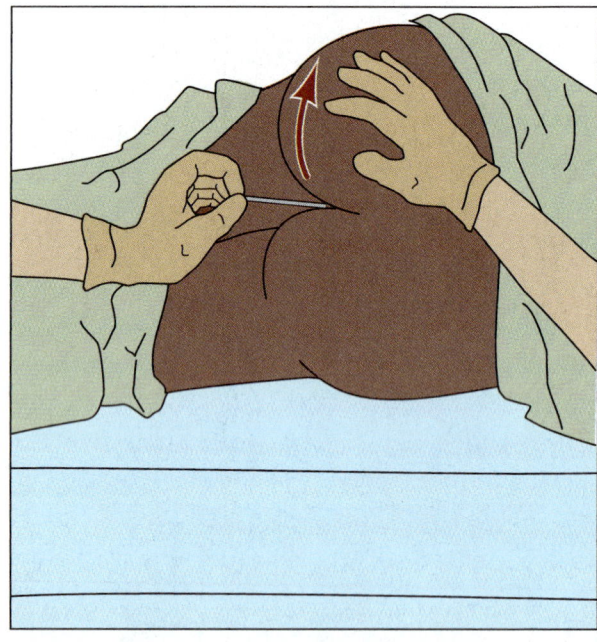

FIGURE 18-9 The rectal thermometer is lubricated and then inserted 1 inch into the rectum.

10. Remove the thermometer, holding it by the stem. Wipe from stem toward bulb end.

11. Discard tissue in the proper container.

12. Read the thermometer. Record the reading on a pad.

13. Wipe the lubricant from the patient. Discard tissue.

14. Place the thermometer in the container for used thermometers. If the thermometer is to be reused for this patient:
    a. Wash it in cold water and soap.
    b. Rinse and dry it.
    c. Return it to the individual disinfectant-filled holder.

15. Remove gloves and discard according to facility policy.

16. Lower the opposite side rail.

17. Carry out procedure completion actions.

 Note: *Remember, when a rectal temperature is recorded, you must add (R) after the reading.*

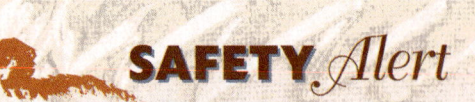

SAFETY *Alert*

Always hold the rectal thermometer in place. Never leave the patient unattended during the rectal temperature procedure.

PROCEDURE 36

MEASURING AN AXILLARY OR GROIN TEMPERATURE (GLASS THERMOMETER)

1. Carry out beginning procedure actions.

 Note: Use disposable gloves if there may be contact with open lesions, wet linens, or body fluids.

2. Assemble equipment on a tray:

- Gloves
- Container with clean oral thermometers
- Container for used thermometers
- Container for soiled tissues
- Container with tissues
- Disposable sheath, if used
- Pad and pencil
- Watch with a second hand

3. Shake the thermometer down to below 96°F. Cover the thermometer with a disposable sheath, if used.

4. Wipe the area dry and place the thermometer. Put on gloves if the groin area is used for temperature measurement.

   a. The patient's arm is held close to the body if an axillary site is used (Figure 18-10).

   b. The thermometer must be in the fold against the body if the groin site is used.

   c. Hold the thermometer in place for 10 minutes.

   d. Remove, wipe (or discard sheath, if used), and read the thermometer. Note the reading on a pad.

   e. Shake the thermometer down.

   f. Clean and replace as with an oral thermometer if the thermometer is to be reused.

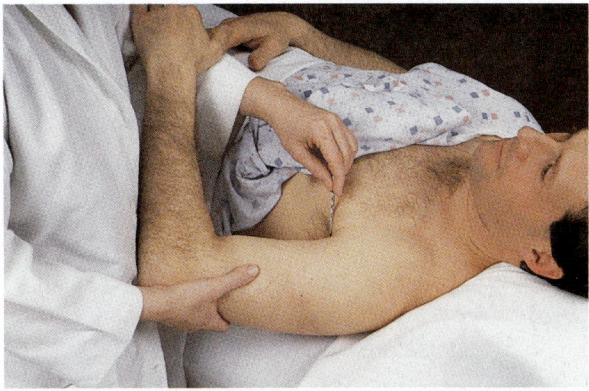

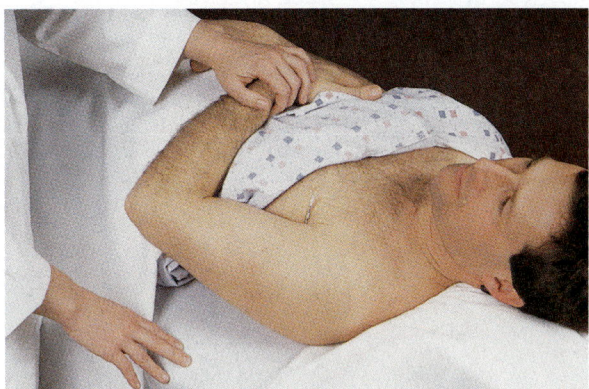

FIGURE 18-10 Hold the thermometer in place.

5. If the groin area was used, remove gloves and discard according to facility policy.

6. Carry out procedure completion actions.

 Note: Remember, when an axillary temperature is recorded, you must add (AX) after the reading.

SAFETY *Alert*

Remember that the axillary method of taking a temperature is the least accurate method. Use it only when other methods are impractical or unavailable.

Hold the glass thermometer in place for a full 10 minutes. Do not leave the bedside during this procedure.

PROCEDURE 37

MEASURING AN ORAL TEMPERATURE (ELECTRONIC THERMOMETER)

1. Carry out beginning procedure actions.

2. Obtain an electronic thermometer, disposable probe covers, and gloves, if this is your facility policy. (Gloves are not necessary with an *oral temperature* using this type of thermometer. Know and follow your facility policy.)

3. Ask the patient if he or she has had anything to eat or drink or has smoked within the last 15 minutes. Wait 15 minutes before taking an oral temperature if the answer is yes.

4. Cover the probe (blue) with a protective sheath.

5. Insert the covered probe under the patient's tongue toward the side of the mouth (Figure 18-11).

6. Hold the probe in position. Ask the patient to close the mouth and breathe through the nose.

7. When a buzzer signals that the temperature has been determined, remove the probe from the patient's mouth.

8. Discard the sheath in the appropriate container (Figure 18-12). Do not touch the sheath. Remove gloves, if used, and discard according to facility policy.

9. Return the probe to its proper position.

10. Record the temperature on your pad.

11. Return the thermometer unit to the charger.

12. Carry out procedure completion actions.

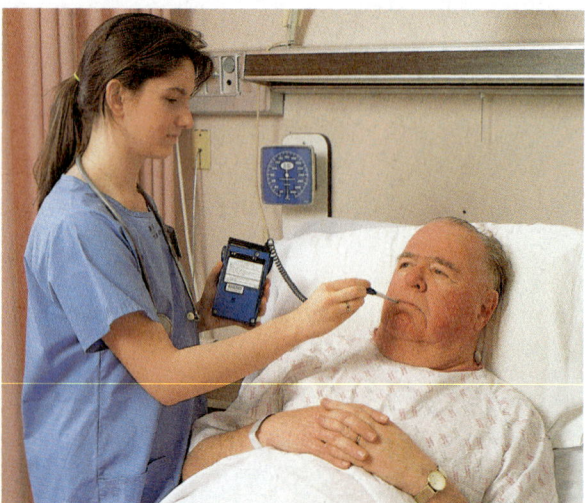

FIGURE 18-11 The thermometer probe is placed to one side of the patient's mouth and positioned under the tongue.

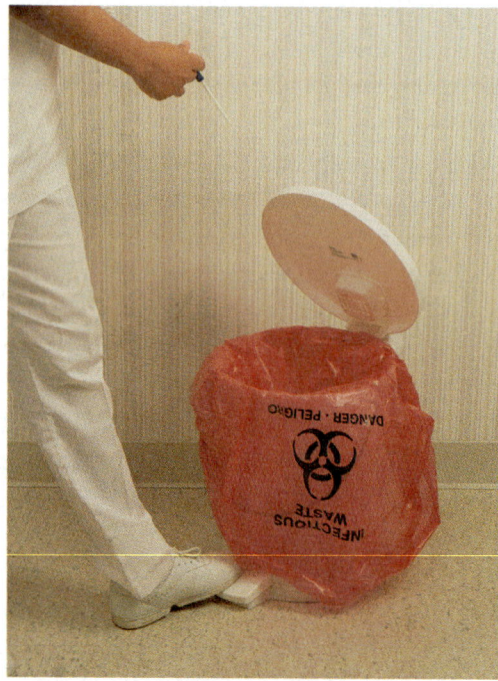

FIGURE 18-12 Once the temperature has been taken, the sheath is discarded.

PROCEDURE 38

MEASURING A RECTAL TEMPERATURE (ELECTRONIC THERMOMETER)

1. Carry out beginning procedure actions.
2. Assemble equipment on a tray:
   - Gloves
   - Electronic thermometer with rectal (red) probe
   - Probe cover
   - Lubricant
3. Lower the backrest of the bed. Ask the patient to turn on his side. Assist the patient if necessary.
4. Put on gloves. Place a small amount of lubricant on the tip of the sheath (Figure 18-13).
5. Fold the top bedclothes back to expose the patient's anal area.
6. Separate the buttocks with one hand. Insert the sheath-covered probe about 1 inch into the rectum, or as recommended by thermometer manufacturer. Hold in place. Replace the bedclothes for privacy as soon as the thermometer is inserted.
7. Read the temperature when registered on the digital display.

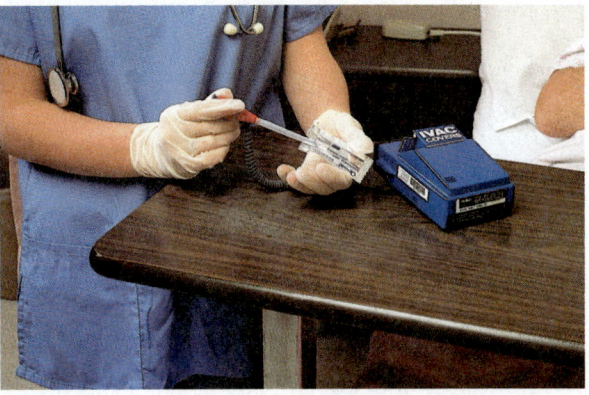

FIGURE 18-13 Remove the thermometer and apply a small amount of lubricant on the tip of the sheath.

8. Remove the probe and discard the sheath. Wipe lubricant from the patient. Discard tissue. Return probe to its proper position.
9. Remove gloves and dispose of according to facility policy.
10. Record the temperature on your pad.
11. Return the thermometer unit to the charger.
12. Carry out procedure completion actions.

PROCEDURE 39

MEASURING AN AXILLARY TEMPERATURE (ELECTRONIC THERMOMETER)

1. Carry out beginning procedure actions.

 Note: Use disposable gloves if there may be contact with open lesions, wet linens, or body fluids.

2. Equipment needed: same as for oral temperature measurement using an electronic thermometer. (See Procedure 37.)
3. Wipe the axillary area dry and put the covered probe in place. Keep the patient's arm close to the body. Hold the probe in place until the temperature shows on the digital display and the buzzer signals that it has been recorded.
4. Remove the thermometer probe. Dispose of the sheath. Return the probe to its proper position.
5. Record the temperature on your pad.
6. Return the thermometer unit to the charger.
7. Carry out procedure completion actions.

PROCEDURE 40

MEASURING A TYMPANIC TEMPERATURE

1. Carry out beginning procedure actions.
2. Assemble equipment:
   - Disposable gloves if there may be contact with blood or body fluids, open lesions, or wet linens
   - Tympanic thermometer
   - Probe covers
3. Place a clean probe cover on the probe.
4. Select the appropriate mode on the thermometer.
5. Check the lens to make sure it is clean and intact (Figure 18-14A).
6. Put on disposable gloves if you may have contact with blood or body fluids, open lesions, or wet linens.
7. Position the patient so you have access to the ear you will be using.
8. Gently pull the ear pinna back and up (Figure 18-14B). This straightens the ear canal so the thermometer can be placed for an accurate reading. Note: When this thermometer is used for children under age 3, pull the pinna down and back. In children over age 3, pull the pinna up and back. This straightens the ear canal, enabling the sensor to detect heat in the eardrum. When the probe is positioned correctly, the probe tip will point at the midpoint between the eyebrow and sideburn on the opposite side of the face.
9. Place the probe in the patient's ear, aiming it toward the tympanic membrane. Insert the probe until it seals the ear canal (Figure 18-14C). Do not apply pressure.
10. Rotate the probe handle slightly until it is aligned with the jaw, as though the patient were speaking on the telephone.

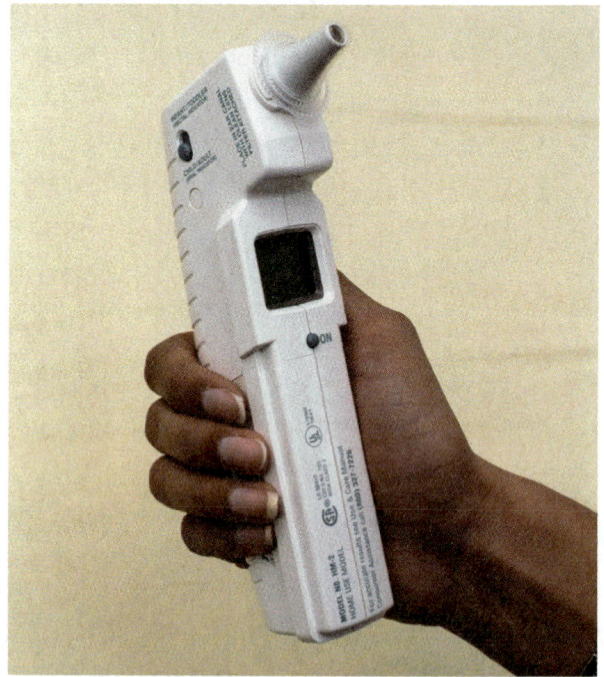

FIGURE 18-14A Check the lens of the tympanic thermometer to make sure it is clean and intact.

11. Quickly press the activation button (Figure 18-14D). Leave the thermometer in the ear for the time recommended by the manufacturer.
12. When you have a reading, remove the probe from the patient's ear and dispose of the cover. See Table 18-4 for normal ranges of tympanic temperatures by age group.
13. Record the temperature on your pad.
14. Return the thermometer unit to the charger.
15. Carry out procedure completion actions.

TABLE 18-4 NORMAL RANGES FOR TYMPANIC TEMPERATURES

Years of Age	Fahrenheit	Celsius
0–2	97.5–100.4°F	36.4–38.0°C
3–10	97.0–100.0°F	36.1–37.8°C
11–65	96.6–99.7°F	35.9–37.6°C
>65	96.4–99.5°F	35.8–37.5°C

continues

PROCEDURE 40

continued

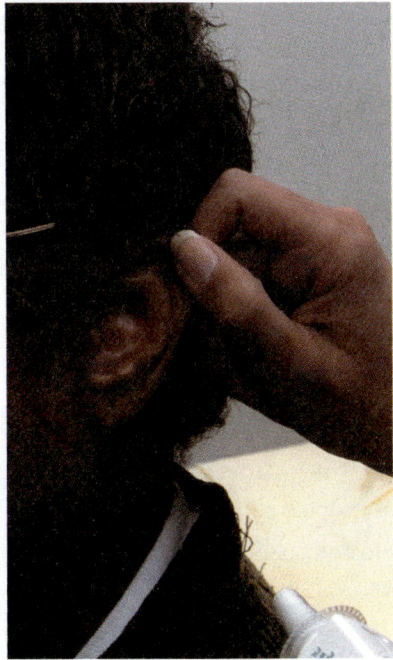

FIGURE 18-14B Gently pull the ear pinna back and up.

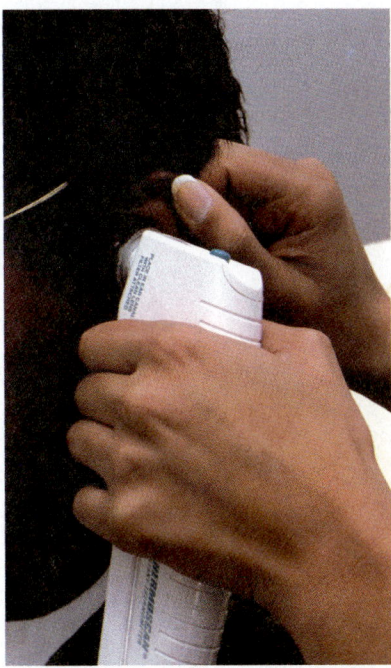

FIGURE 18-14C Place the covered probe in the patient's ear, aiming it toward the tympanic membrane. Insert the probe until it seals the ear canal.

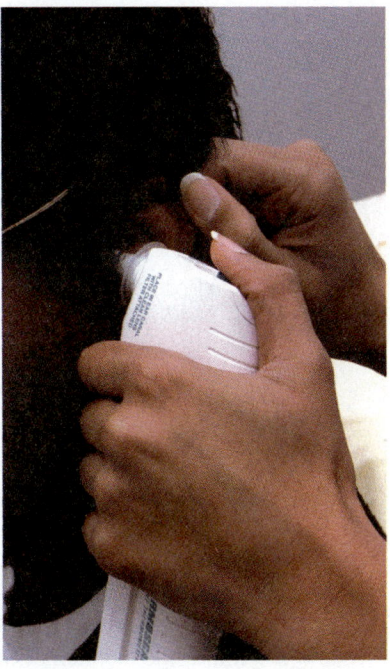

FIGURE 18-14D Press the activation button and leave the thermometer in the ear for the time recommended by the manufacturer.

PROCEDURE 41

CLEANING GLASS THERMOMETERS

1. Wash your hands.
2. Assemble equipment on a tray:
   - Towel
   - Label
   - Washcloth
   - Soiled thermometers in container of soapy water
   - Wash basin
   - Container for clean thermometers
   - Liquid soap
   - Container of cotton balls
   - Facility-approved disinfectant
   - Disposable gloves
3. Take tray of equipment to soiled utility room.
4. Place a towel on the sink side.
5. Wash and dry the container and cover for clean thermometers. Place on the towel with the cover top up.
6. Place gauze in the bottom of the container.
7. Place a clean wash basin in the sink. Line the bottom of the basin with a washcloth. (This is done to reduce the risk of breakage if you accidentally drop a thermometer.) Fill the basin one-third full with cool water. Apply gloves.
8. Slowly turn on the cold water faucet.

continues

PROCEDURE 41

continued

9. Moisten a sponge/cotton ball and apply soap.

10. Pick up one thermometer at a time, holding it by the stem.

    a. Using a circular motion, cleanse the thermometer from stem to bulb.

    b. Discard cotton ball.

    c. Carefully rinse the thermometer.

    d. Using a circular motion and a new, dry cotton ball for each, dry each thermometer.

    e. Check thermometers for chips and shake down to 96°F (21°C) or below before placing them in the clean container (Figure 18-15A).

    f. Fill the clean container half full with disinfectant (Figure 18-15B).

    g. Empty the water from the dirty container.

11. Shut off the faucet. Squeeze out the washcloth and put it into the laundry. Shut the basin drain and add hot water and soap.

12. Wash, rinse, and dry the dirty thermometer container and wash basin.

13. Remove gloves and discard according to facility policy.

14. Add disinfectant, if necessary, so that each thermometer is completely covered by it.

15. Place a cover on the container. Place a label with the date, time, and your initials on the container. Remember that disinfectants take time to be effective.

16. Place towel in laundry. Dispose of used sponges or cotton balls in trash.

17. Leave area neat and tidy.

18. After disinfecting:

    a. Remove label. Remove thermometers.

    b. Empty disinfectant.

    c. Wash and dry container.

    d. Place 4 × 4 folded sponge on the bottom of the container.

19. Rinse and dry thermometers.

20. Place dry, clean thermometers on a sponge in the container and cover (Figure 18-15C).

21. Store according to facility policy in clean area.

22. Wash your hands and report completion of task to the nurse.

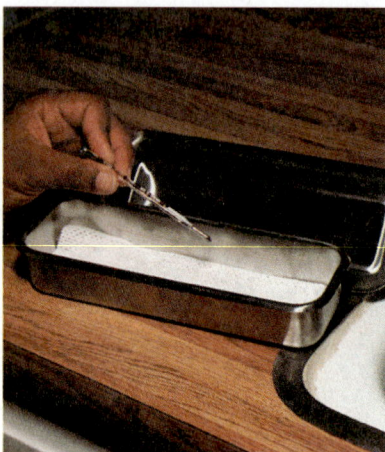

FIGURE 18-15A Place in a clean container that has folded gauze on the bottom to prevent breakage of thermometers.

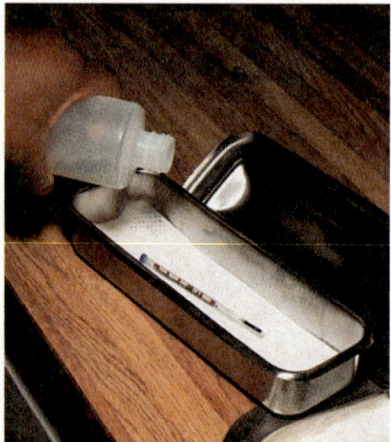

FIGURE 18-15B Add disinfectant solution, being sure to cover the entire thermometer.

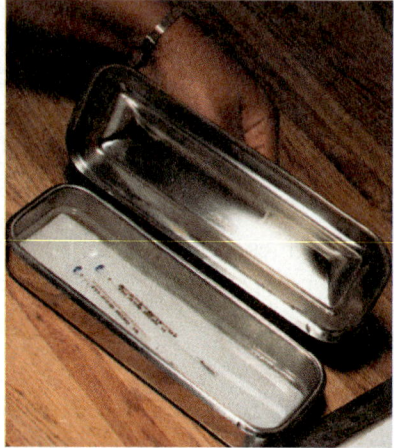

FIGURE 18-15C Allow thermometers to soak for the required time, then remove and rinse well before storing in a clean, dry container.

REVIEW

A. True/False.

Mark the following true or false by circling T or F.

1. (T) F When charting an axillary temperature, always print AX after the reading.

2. (T) F Readings taken with a plastic thermometer may not be entirely accurate.

3. (T) F Temperature is the measurement of body heat.

4. (T) F The most common method of measuring the temperature of a cooperative adult is by mouth.

5. T (F) To measure a rectal temperature, the patient is best positioned on her back.

6. T (F) 96.8°F is an average oral temperature.

7. T (F) Only temperature variations of more than 5°F should be reported to the nurse.

8. (T) F Clinical thermometers can be identified by the shapes of their bulbs.

9. T (F) The probe of an electronic thermometer is covered with a red sheath for rectal use.

10. T (F) The axillary temperature of a patient will register approximately one degree higher than his oral temperature.

11. T (F) The tympanic temperature reading is the most accurate.

12. T (F) A freezing temperature registered in Celsius readings would be 32°.

13. (T) F It would be unsafe to use glass oral thermometers with children.

14. T (F) If safely placed, rectal thermometers need not be held.

15. T (F) Wait 5 minutes after the patient has taken hot liquids to measure an oral temperature.

16. T (F) When washing used glass thermometers, always wash them in hot, soapy water.

17. (T) F Always wipe the axillary area before placing a thermometer.

18. (T) F When using an electronic thermometer, you should not allow your fingers to touch the probe sheath.

19. (T) F All rectal thermometers should be lubricated before insertion.

20. T (F) The oral thermometer should remain in place for one minute.

21. (T) F The liquid column in a glass oral thermometer should register below 96°F at the beginning of the procedure.

22. (T) F There may be times when a temperature has to be measured in the groin area.

23. T (F) Each long line on the stem of a clinical thermometer indicates an increase of 2 degrees of temperature.

24. (T) F Each short line on the stem of the clinical thermometer indicates a 0.2-degree increase in temperature.

25. T (F) Measuring the temperature in the groin area gives the most accurate indication of body temperature.

B. Completion.

Complete the statements by choosing the correct words from the following list.

~~Fahrenheit~~	~~less~~
~~higher~~	~~temperature~~
~~pulse~~	~~tympanic~~

26. Vital signs include _temp_ , _pulse_ , respiration, and blood pressure.

27. A normal temperature reading of 98.6° would be in the _F_ scale.

28. A _tympanic_ thermometer is used to measure the temperature in the ear.

29. A 3-month-old child might be expected to have a slightly _higher_ temperature normally than a child who is 9 years old.

30. Temperature is _less_ stable in children than in adults.

C. Nursing Assistant Challenge.

31. Mrs. LeJune is having difficulty breathing and is very restless. The nurse instructs you to measure her temperature. What type of thermometer would you choose if all were available?

   a. Glass oral thermometer

   b. Glass rectal thermometer

   c. Electronic oral thermometer

   d. Tympanic thermometer

32. You are about to measure a rectal temperature with a glass thermometer. You find a small chip in the glass. What should you do?

a. Use the thermometer, because it is just a small chip.

b. Throw the thermometer in the wastepaper basket.

c. Break the thermometer in half so no one else will use it.

d. Replace it with another thermometer.

33. You are assigned to measure your patient's rectal temperature using a glass thermometer. How long should you hold the thermometer in place?

a. 3 minutes

b. 10 minutes

c. 15 minutes

d. 20 minutes

 # EXPLORING THE WEB

Description	Location
Assessment	*http://www.delmarhealthcare.com/olcs/white/pnotes.asp* (see Chapter 25)
Measuring vital signs	*http://www.delmarhealthcare.com/olcs/delaune/ppt/ DeLaunechapter%2027.ppt*
Temperature regulation	*http://phy025.lubb.ttuhsc.edu*
Accuracy of Core Temperature Measurement with the IVAC® CORE·CHECK™ Tympanic Thermometer System	*http://www.alarismed.com*
Accuracy of the CORE·CHECK® Tympanic Thermometer for Pediatric Core Temperature Measurement	*http://www.alarismed.com*
The Facts About Tympanic Thermometers and Cross Contamination	*http://www.alarismed.com*
Going Green (resource kit for eliminating mercury in health care)	*http://www.noharm.org*
Mercury Free at NIH	*http://www.nih.gov/od/ors/ds/nomercury*
Mercury Thermometers and Your Family's Health	*http://www.noharm.org*
Planning and Holding a Mercury Thermometer Exchange	*http://www.noharm.org*
Sustainable Hospitals	*http://www.sustainablehospitals.org*
Taking a Tympanic Temperature	*http://www.alarismed.com*
Techniques of Vital Signs	*http://hsc.virginia.edu*
Wong on Web Sites of Temperature Measurement in Children	*http://www.us.elsevierhealth.com*

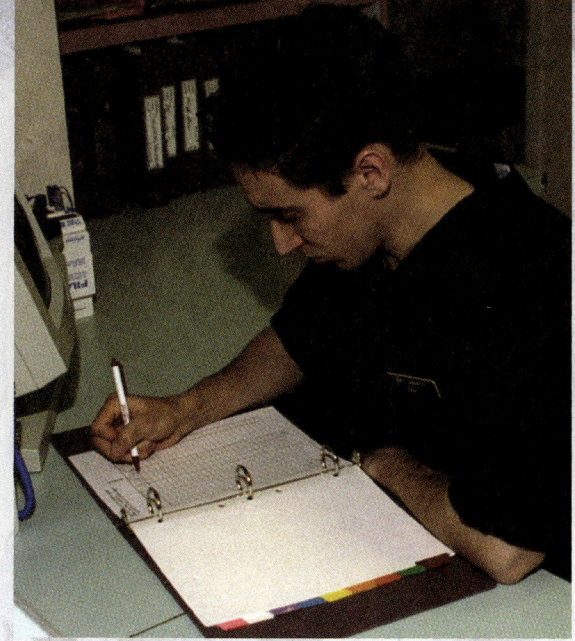

Pulse and Respiration

objectives

After completing this unit, you will be able to:

- Spell and define terms.
- Define pulse.
- Explain the importance of monitoring a pulse rate.
- Locate the pulse sites.
- Identify the range of normal pulse and respiratory rates.

- Measure the pulse at different locations.
- List the characteristics of the pulse and respiration.
- Demonstrate the following procedures:
  - Procedure 42 Counting the Radial Pulse
  - Procedure 43 Counting the Apical-Radial Pulse
  - Procedure 44 Counting Respirations

vocabulary

Learn the meaning and the correct spelling of the following words and phrases:

accelerated	cyanosis	radial pulse	symmetry
apical pulse	dyspnea	rales	tachycardia
apnea	expiration	rate	tachypnea
bradycardia	inspiration	respiration	volume
Cheyne-Stokes	pulse	rhythm	
respirations	pulse deficit	stertorous	

INTRODUCTION

The pulse and respiration of the patient are usually counted during the same procedure. Because breathing is partly under voluntary control, a person is able to stop or alter breathing temporarily for a short period. For example, when a patient realizes that her breathing is being watched and counted, she alters her breathing pattern without meaning to do so. To avoid this, the respirations are counted immediately following the pulse count without telling the patient. The patient's hand is kept in the same position, and your fingers remain on the pulse point so that you seem to still be taking the pulse.

THE PULSE

The **pulse** is:

- The pressure of the blood felt against the wall of an artery as the heart alternately contracts (beats) and relaxes (rests).
- More easily felt in arteries that come fairly close to the skin and can be gently pressed against a bone.
- The same in all arteries throughout the body.
- An indication of how the cardiovascular system is meeting the body's needs.

Radial Pulse

The **radial pulse** is the most commonly measured pulse. It is measured at the radial artery in the wrist. Figure 19-1 shows areas of the body where other large blood vessels come close enough to the surface to be used as sites for counting the pulse. Conscious patients can be checked at the radial artery. (See Procedure 42.) Unconscious patients should be checked at the carotid artery or apically (over the heart).

Pulse measurement includes determining the:

1. Rate or speed
   a. **Bradycardia**—an unusually slow pulse (below 60 beats per minute)
   b. **Tachycardia**—an unusually fast pulse (more than 100 beats per minute)
2. Character
   a. **Rhythm**—regularity
   b. Volume or fullness

Report:

- Pulse rates over 100 beats per minute (bpm) (tachycardia)
- Pulse rates under 60 bpm (bradycardia)
- Irregularities in character (rhythm and volume)

Pulse rates can be affected by:

- Illness
- Emotions

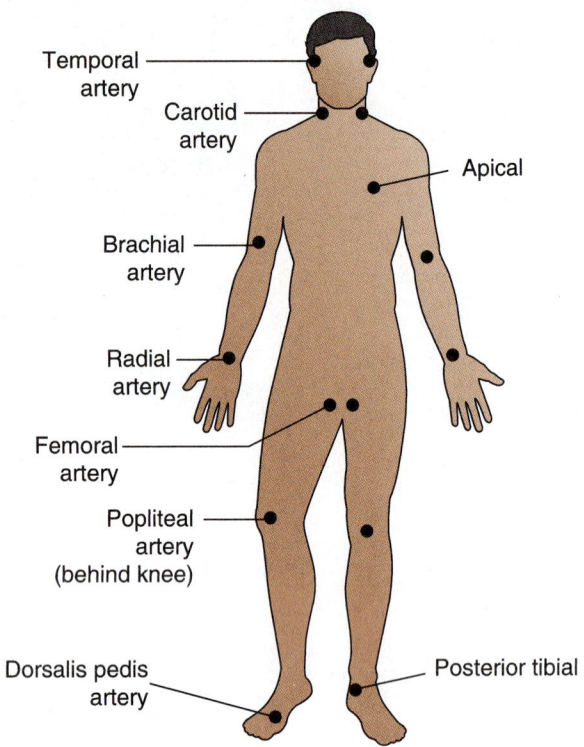

FIGURE 19-1 Common pulse sites of the body.

- Age
- Exercise
- Elevated temperature
- Sex
- Position
- Physical training
- Lowered temperature
- Drugs

Table 19-1 shows average pulse rates.

TABLE 19-1 AVERAGE PULSE RATES	
Patient	**Beats per Minute**
Adult men	60–70
Adult women	65–80
Children over 7 years	75–100
Preschoolers	80–110
Infants	120–160

PROCEDURE 42

COUNTING THE RADIAL PULSE

1. Carry out beginning procedure actions.

2. Place the patient in a comfortable position. The palm of the hand should be down and the arm should rest on a flat surface.

3. Locate the pulse on the thumb side of the wrist with the tips of your first three fingers (Figure 19-2). Do not use your thumb—it contains a pulse that may be confused with the patient's pulse.

4. When the pulse is felt, exert slight pressure. Using the second hand of your watch, count for one minute. It is the practice in some hospitals to count for one-half minute and multiply by two and to record the rate for one minute. A one-minute count is preferred and must be done if the pulse is irregular.

5. Remember the reading when counting

respirations. Record the reading on your pad as soon as possible.

6. Carry out procedure completion actions.

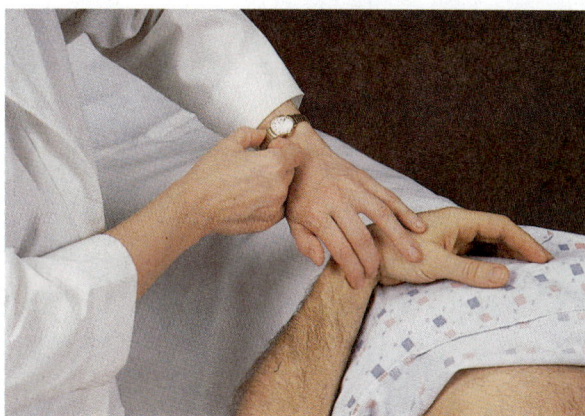

FIGURE 19-2 Locate the pulse on the thumb side of the wrist with the tips of your first three fingers.

The Apical Pulse

An **apical pulse** is measured by counting the heart contractions. The stethoscope is placed over the apex (tip) of the heart. Listen for the heart sounds that indicate closing of the valves. These sounds occur as the heart pumps blood into the arteries. The sounds should occur at the same rate as the pulse that is felt as an expansion of the radial artery. The apex of the heart is found:

- On the left side of the front of the chest
- Between the fifth and sixth ribs
- Just below the left nipple
- In women, under the left breast

Listen carefully for two sounds: lub dub. The louder sound (lub) corresponds to the contraction of the ventricles pushing the blood forward through the arteries, and the closing of the valves to prevent the backflow of blood. This is the sound to be counted. The softer sound (dub) corresponds to the relaxation of the ventricles as they fill with blood before the next contraction and the closing of the semilunar valves to prevent backflow from the arteries.

When documenting an apical pulse reading, write "AP" after the value.

Apical-Radial Pulse Rate

The apical and radial pulse rate is a comparison of the apical rate and the radial rate. Usually they are the same.

Sometimes the contraction of the heart is so weak that it fails to send enough blood to the arteries to expand them. When this happens, no pulse is felt. In this case, the number of loud sounds do not correspond with the number of pulses felt in the radial artery.

The difference between the apical pulse (the loud sounds heard over the heart) and the radial pulse (the expansion felt over the radial pulse) is called a **pulse deficit**. Two people measure the heart rate and the radial pulse at the same time. (See Procedure 43.) The nurse measures the apical pulse while the second person counts the radial pulse for 1 minute. The rates are then compared.

Apical pulse rates are checked:

- Whenever a pulse deficit exists or is suspected.

- Before the registered nurse administers drugs that alter the heart rate or rhythm.

- In children whose rapid rates might be difficult to count at the radial artery.

PROCEDURE 43

COUNTING THE APICAL-RADIAL PULSE

1. Carry out beginning procedure actions.

2. Clean the stethoscope earpieces and bell with disinfectant.

3. Place the stethoscope earpieces in your ears with tips facing slightly forward for better fit.

4. Place the stethoscope diaphragm or bell over the apex of the patient's heart. If it is cold, warm the diaphragm with your hands before placing it on the patient's chest.

5. Listen carefully for the heartbeat.

6. Count the louder sounding beats for one minute.

7. Check the radial pulse for one minute. The best way to obtain these numbers is to have the nurse count the apical pulse while you take the radial pulse (Figure 19-3).

8. Note results on a pad for comparison.

9. Clean earpieces and bell of stethoscope with disinfectant.

10. Carry out procedure completion actions.
    Example: Apical pulse = 108
    Radial pulse = 82
    Pulse deficit = 26 (108 − 82 = 26)

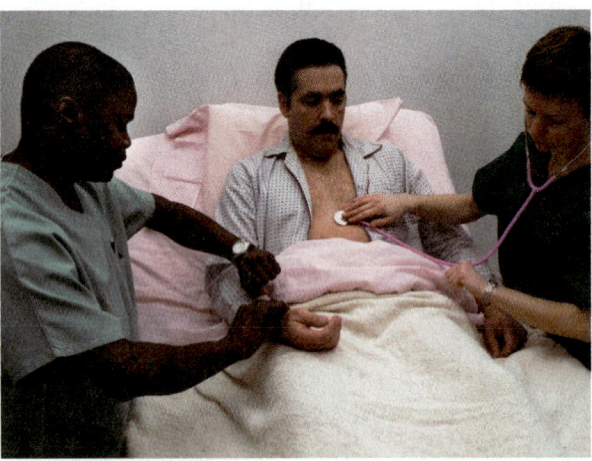

FIGURE 19-3 The nurse takes the apical pulse while the nursing assistant takes the radial pulse.

- For one full minute.
- On any child 12 months of age or younger.
- Whenever you are uncertain of the accuracy of the radial pulse or it is irregular.

Pulse deficits are found in some forms of heart disease.

RESPIRATION

The main function of **respiration** is to supply the cells in the body with oxygen and to rid the body of excess carbon dioxide. When respirations are inefficient, there is less oxygen in the blood available for body needs. In addition, carbon dioxide is released less efficiently. The skin takes on a bluish or dusky color and the patient develops a condition known as **cyanosis**.

There are two parts to each respiration: one **inspiration** (inhalation) followed by one **expiration** (exhalation). Special terms describe different breathing patterns:

- Normal—regular, 16 to 20 breaths per minute
- **Tachypnea**—rapid, shallow breathing
- **Dyspnea**—difficult or labored breathing
- Shallow—breaths that only partially fill the lungs
- **Apnea**—a period of no respirations

- **Cheyne-Stokes respirations**—a period of dyspnea followed by periods of apnea
- **Stertorous**—Snoring-like respirations
- **Rales** (crackles)—moist respirations. At times, fluid (mucus) will collect in the air passages. This causes a bubbling type of respiration. Rales are common in the dying patient.
- Wheezing—difficult breathing accompanied by a whistling or sighing sound due to narrowing of bronchioles (as in asthma) or an increase of mucus in the bronchi.

Respirations should be checked for:

- **Rate**—number of respirations per minute
- Rhythm—regularity
- **Symmetry**—ability of the chest to expand equally as air enters each lung
- **Volume**—depth of respiration
- Character—terms used to describe the character of respirations include:
  - Regular
  - Irregular
  - Shallow
  - Deep
  - Labored (difficult)

PROCEDURE 44

COUNTING RESPIRATIONS

1. When the pulse rate has been counted, you may leave your fingers on the radial pulse and start counting the number of times the chest rises and falls during one minute (Figure 19-4). Count one inhalation and one exhalation as one respiration.

2. Note the depth and regularity of respirations.

3. Record the time, rate, depth, and regularity of respirations.

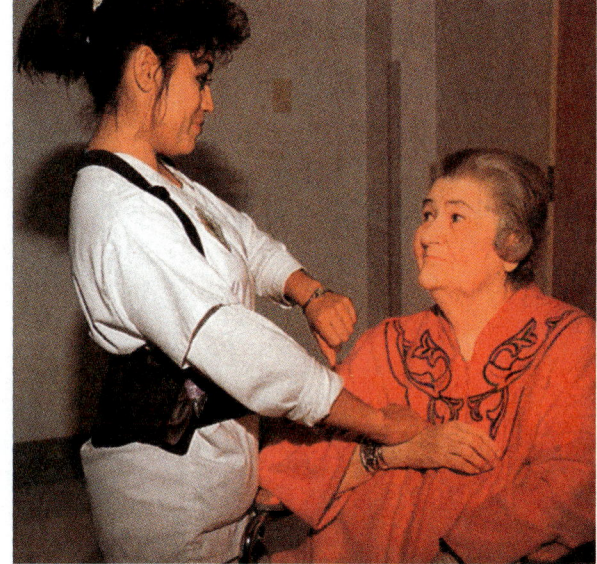

FIGURE 19-4 Continue to rest the back of the hand against the chest wall while counting respirations.

The rate of respiration is determined by counting the rise or fall of the chest for one minute, using a watch equipped with a second hand. (See Procedure 44.)

- The average rate for adults is 16 to 20 respirations per minute.
- If the rate is more than 25 per minute, it is said to be **accelerated**. Accelerated respiration should be reported.
- If the rate is less than 12 per minute, it is too slow. It should be reported.

Remember that, if possible, respirations should be counted without the patient's knowing that you are doing so; the rate and volume may change if the patient knows they are being counted. You might count respirations before or after counting the radial pulse. Continue pressing on the pulse area while counting.

The factors affecting respiratory rates include:

- Illness
- Emotions
- Elevated temperature
- Sex
- Age
- Exercise
- Position
- Drugs

Temperature, pulse, and respiration (TPR) rates and character are recorded in a notebook and then transferred to the patient's chart (Figure 19-5).

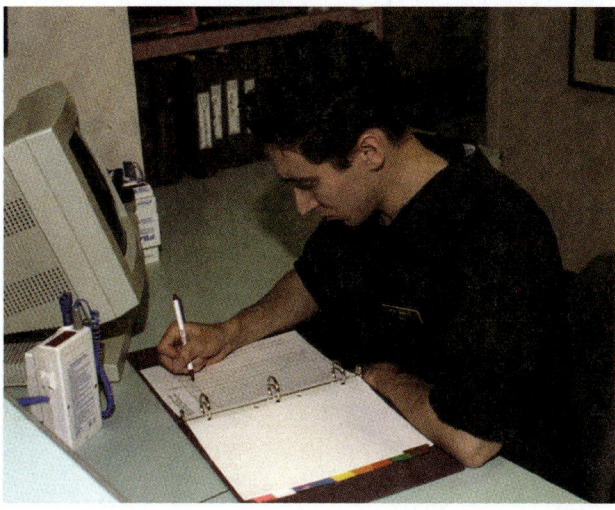

FIGURE 19-5 TPR readings are recorded in the patient's medical record.

REVIEW

A. True/False.

Mark the following true or false by circling T or F.

1. (T) F   A pulse deficit results when there is a difference between the apical and radial pulses.
2. (T) F   The pulse is the pressure of blood against the arterial wall.
3. T (F)   Cheyne-Stokes respirations are deep and regular.
4. T (F)   Pulses differ when counted at different pulse sites.
5. (T) (F)   The pulse rate of an infant is 110 to 130 bpm.   *120-160 bpm*
6. (T) F   An apical pulse should be counted in children.
7. T (F)   The most often used pulse site is the carotid artery.
8. (T) F   The respiratory system rids the body of excess carbon dioxide.
9. (T) F   Mucus in the air passages causes rales.
10. T (F)   A pulse is best counted using the thumb placed over the artery.

B. Matching.

Choose the correct word from Column II to match the words and phrases in Column I.

Column I		Column II
11.	h Snoring types of respiration	a. accelerated
12.	d Bluish discoloration to the skin	b. apnea
13.	g Regularity	c. bradycardia
14.	b Periods of no respiration	d. cyanosis
15.	e Difficult breathing	e. dyspnea
16.	i Rapid respirations	f. rate
17.	a Increased or speeded up	g. rhythm
18.	k Expiration	h. stertorous
19.	f Speed	i. tachypnea
20.	c Slow pulse	j. inspiration
		k. exhalation

C. Nursing Assistant Challenge.

21. Mrs. Morgan has a heart condition that makes her heart rate irregular and faster than normal. Her respirations are difficult or rapid, labored, and moist. She receives a medication that profoundly alters her heart action. Your orders are to assist in determining the pulse deficit. Answer the statements using the terms in the following list.

    apical   rales
    dyspnea   tachycardia
    radial   tachypnea

    a. The faster heart rate is described as _____.
    b. The difficult respirations can be charted as _____.
    c. Moist respirations are best described as _____.
    d. Rapid respirations are also called _____.
    e. Which pulse rate will you count? _____.
    f. Which pulse rate will a second person count? _____.

22. List two reasons why a radial-apical pulse rate would be ordered.

    a. _____
    b. _____

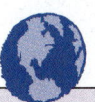 # EXPLORING THE WEB

Description	Location
Assessment	*http://www.delmarhealthcare.com/olcs/white/pnotes.asp* (see Chapter 25)
Measuring vital signs	*http://www.delmarhealthcare.com/olcs/delaune/ppt/ DeLaunechapter%2027.ppt*
Techniques of Vital Signs	*http://hsc.virginia.edu*

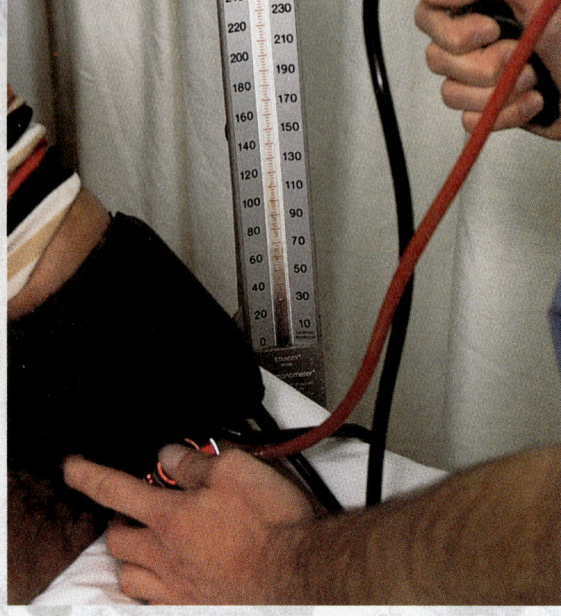

Blood Pressure

objectives

After completing this unit, you will be able to:

- Spell and define terms.
- Describe the factors that influence blood pressure.
- Identify the range of normal blood pressure values.
- Identify the causes of inaccurate blood pressure readings.
- Select the proper size blood pressure cuff.
- List precautions associated with use of the sphygmomanometer.
- Demonstrate the following procedure:
  - Procedure 45 Taking Blood Pressure
  - Procedure 46 Taking Blood Pressure with an Electronic Blood Pressure Apparatus

vocabulary

Learn the meaning and the correct spelling of the following words and phrases:

aneroid gauge	diastole	hypotension	systole
auscultatory gap	diastolic pressure	pulse pressure	systolic pressure
blood pressure	elasticity	sphygmomanometer	
brachial artery	fasting	stethoscope	
depressant	hypertension	stimulant	

INTRODUCTION

Blood pressure is the fourth vital sign. It is the measure of the force of the blood against the walls of the arteries. Blood pressure depends on the:

- Volume (amount of blood in the circulatory system).
- Force of the heartbeat.
- Condition of the arteries. Arteries that have lost their elasticity (stretch) give more resistance. The pressure is greater in these arteries.
- Distance from the heart. Blood pressure in the legs is lower than in the arms.

Pressure varies with contraction (systole) and relaxation (diastole) of the ventricles of the heart.

- Systolic blood pressure reading indicates the period when the pressure within the arteries is the greatest, during contraction of the ventricles. The systolic blood pressure is the working pressure.
- Diastolic reading indicates the lowest point of pressure between ventricular contractions. The diastolic blood pressure is the resting pressure.

Blood pressure is elevated by:

- Sex of the patient (males slightly higher than females before menopause)
- Exercise
- Eating
- Stimulants (substances that speed up body functions)
- Emotional stress, such as anger, fear, or sexual activity
- Disease conditions, such as arteriosclerosis (hardening of the arteries), elevated cholesterol, or diabetes mellitus
- Hereditary factors
- Pain
- Obesity
- Age
- Condition of blood vessels
- Some drugs

Blood pressure is lowered by:

- Fasting (not eating)
- Rest
- Depressants (drugs that slow down body functions)
- Weight loss
- Emotions (such as grief)
- Abnormal conditions such as hemorrhage (loss of blood) or shock
- Dehydration and fluid loss
- Some drugs, such as antihypertensives (drugs that lower blood pressure in persons who have hypertension)
- Diuretics (drugs that lower the volume of body fluids)

The factors affecting blood pressure are:

- Age
- Sleep
- Weight
- Emotion
- Heredity
- Gender
- Viscosity of blood
- Condition of blood vessels

EQUIPMENT

The sphygmomanometer (blood pressure measuring apparatus) consists of:

- A cuff (different sizes are available) that fits around the patient's arm. There is a rubber bladder inside the cuff. A pressure control button is attached to the cuff. It is important to use the proper size cuff when measuring blood pressure. Cuffs that are too wide or too narrow will give inaccurate readings (Figure 20-1). To check the size of the cuff, compare the length of the rubber bladder inside the cuff (Figure 20-2) with the patient's arm circumference. The bladder should be at least 80% of the circumference of the arm. If it is larger or smaller, obtain a different size cuff.
- Two tubes. One tube is connected to the pressure control bulb and to the bladder inside the cuff. The other tube is connected to the pressure gauge.
- A pressure gauge, which may be a column of mercury (Figure 20-3A) or a round aneroid gauge (Figure 20-3B) dial. Both are marked with numbers.

The stethoscope (Figure 20-4) magnifies sounds. It consists of:

- A bell or diaphragm.
- Tubing that carries sounds to the listener.
- Earpieces that direct the sounds into the listener's ears. The earpieces and diaphragm must be cleaned with antiseptic before and after each use to prevent transmission of disease.

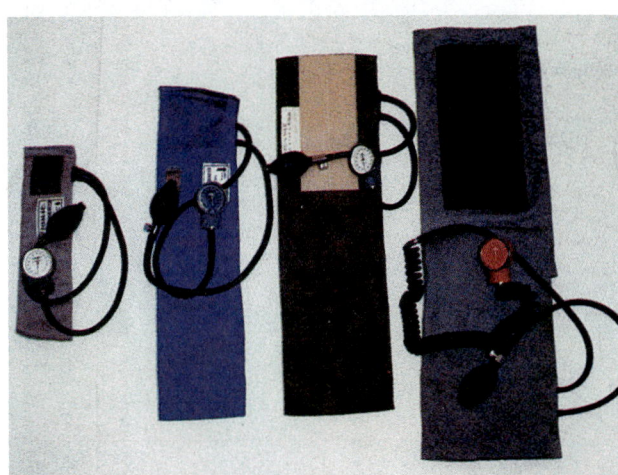

FIGURE 20-1 A variety of cuff sizes are available. The cuff must fit properly for accurate readings.

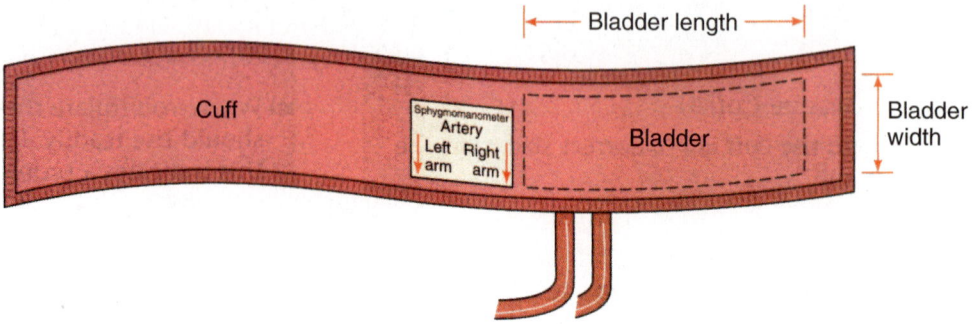

FIGURE 20-2 The bladder inside the cuff should be 80% the circumference of the patient's arm.

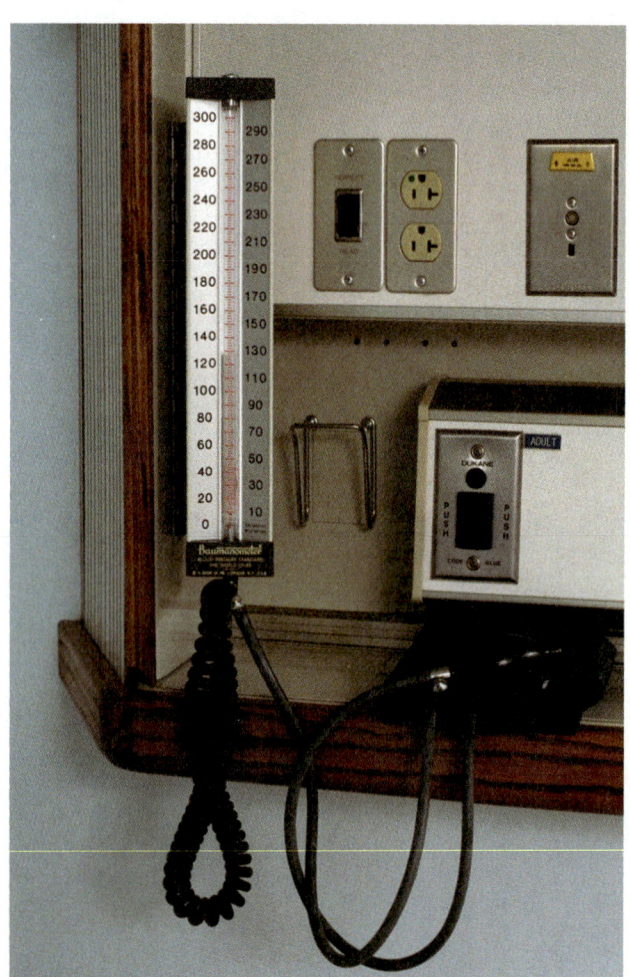

FIGURE 20-3A A mercury gravity sphygmomanometer.

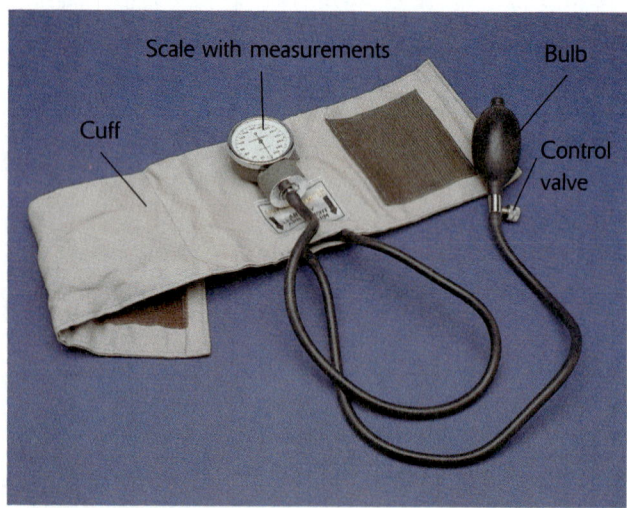

FIGURE 20-3B A dial (aneroid) sphygmomanometer.

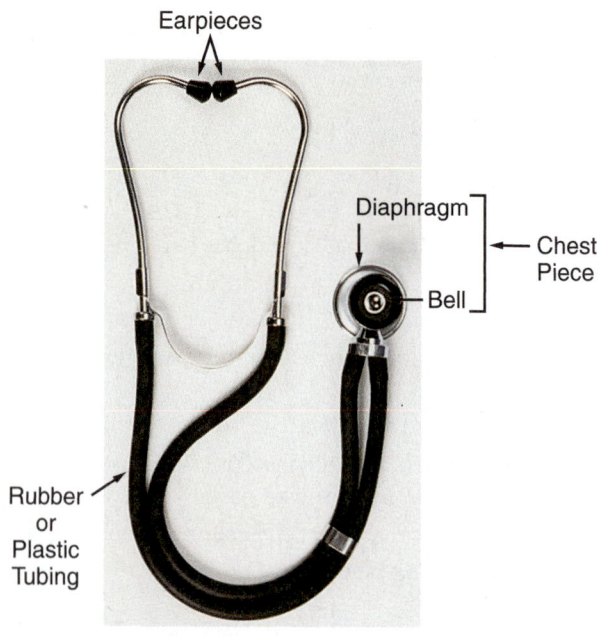

FIGURE 20-4 Stethoscope.

Electronic sphygmomanometers with attached cuffs are used in some facilities. You do not have to use a stethoscope with these units, because they automatically register the readings on a digital display. Follow the manufacturer's directions for the type of unit you are using.

Some facilities use an instrument that measures pulse rate, temperature, and blood pressure (Figure 20-5).

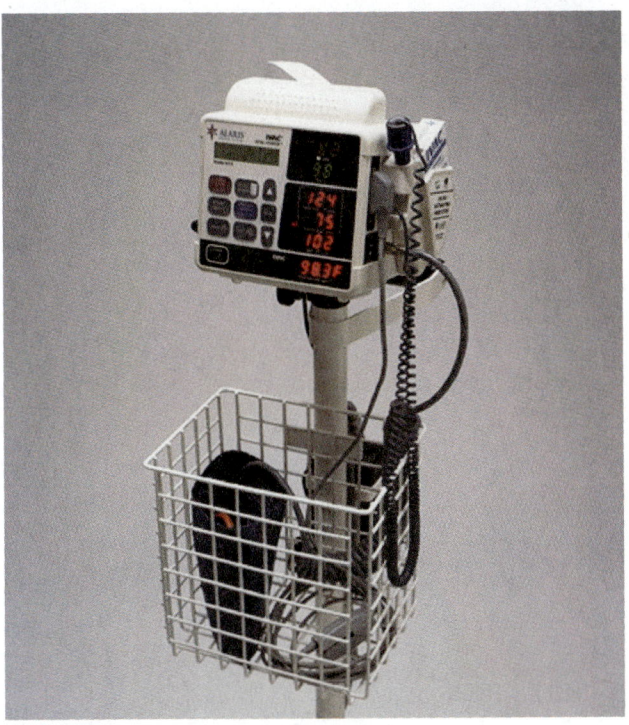

FIGURE 20-5 All vital signs may be checked with a single instrument. *(Vital•Check® patient monitor; photo courtesy of Alaris Medical Systems Inc., San Diego, CA)*

MEASURING THE BLOOD PRESSURE

Blood pressure is usually measured in the upper arm over the brachial artery. Blood pressure readings taken anywhere else must be ordered by a doctor. The values are recorded in millimeters of mercury (mm Hg).

1. The cuff is smoothly applied directly over the brachial artery (1 inch above the antecubital area).

2. The stethoscope bell is placed over the brachial artery.

3. Pressure is then increased by inflating the rubber bladder in the cuff to stop the flow of blood through the artery.

4. The pressure is slowly released and the sounds of heart valves closing can be heard. The sounds correspond to pressure changes in the blood. *at least 170*

5. The blood pressure is measured:

   a. At its highest point as the systolic pressure. This will be the first regular sound you will hear. This is the sound of the bicuspid and tricuspid valves shutting.

   b. At its lowest point as the diastolic pressure. This will be the change or last sound you will hear. This is the sound of the semilunar valves shutting.

guidelines *for*

Preparing to Measure Blood Pressure

Before using the stethoscope:

1. Clean the earpieces with an alcohol wipe (Figure 20-6) and clean the bell with a different alcohol wipe.

2. Point the earpieces forward when inserting them in your ears.

3. Use the bell portion of the stethoscope (Figure 20-7).

4. Be sure the bell portion is open so you will hear the beats.

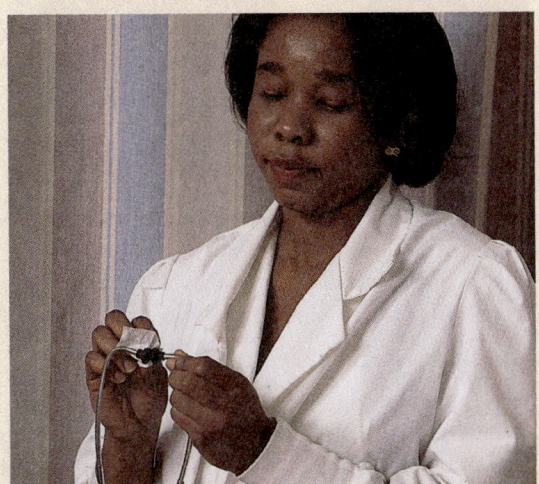

FIGURE 20-6 Clean the earpieces with an alcohol sponge before and after use.

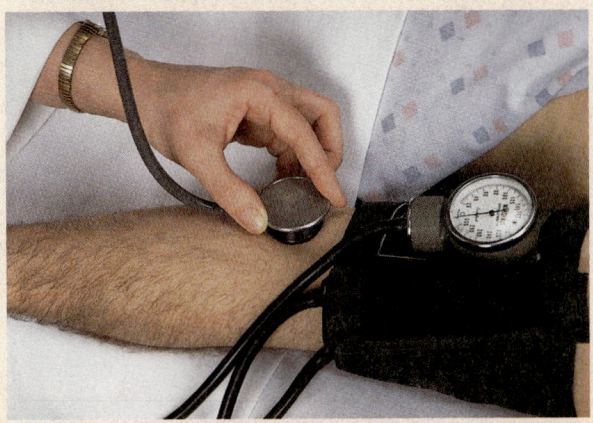

FIGURE 20-7 When taking a blood pressure, use the bell portion of the stethoscope.

continues

guidelines *continued*

Before using a sphygmomanometer:

1. If using a mercury manometer—if the mercury moves up the column very slowly (Figure 20-8), it may have oxidized. Report this to the nurse and use another sphygmomanometer.

2. If using an aneroid manometer—make sure the needle is on zero before you inflate the cuff (Figure 20-9). If it is not, report this to the nurse and use another sphygmomanometer.

Generally:

Turn off radio and television when taking blood pressure. Ask the patient not to talk. Do not take blood pressure on an arm that:

- Has an intravenous feeding or other device inserted
- Is being treated for burns, fractures, or other injuries
- Has a dialysis access device

SAFETY *Alert*

For accurate blood pressure values, check the stethoscope tubing. Do not use if it has cracks or holes in it. The bell or diaphragm of the stethoscope should not come in contact with the patient's clothing, blood pressure cuff, or other device. Place the bell or diaphragm of the stethoscope flat against the patient's skin and hold it in place. If it is at an angle, you will not be able to hear the sounds. Apply firm but gentle pressure when holding the diaphragm in place. If you press too hard, you will be unable to hear the sound.

- Is on the same side as the patient's recent mastectomy (breast removal) or other surgical procedure

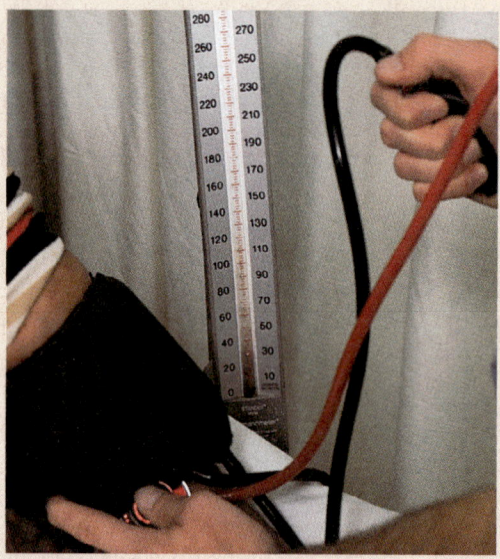

FIGURE 20-8 Do not use the sphygmomanometer if the mercury moves up the column slowly.

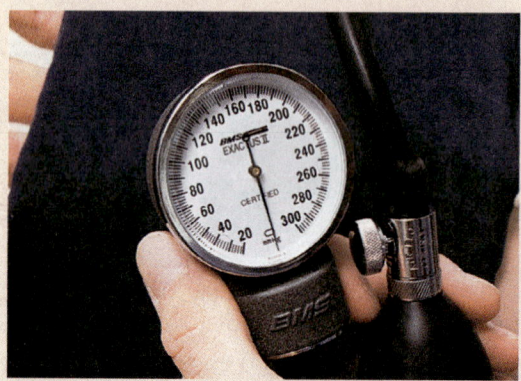

FIGURE 20-9 Make sure the needle is on zero before inflating the cuff on an aneroid sphygmomanometer.

---

c. The difference between systolic and diastolic pressure is called **pulse pressure**. The pulse pressure gives important information about the health of the arteries. The average pulse pressure in a healthy adult is about 40 millimeters (mm) of mercury (Hg) (range 30–50 mm Hg). However, factors in both health and disease can alter the pulse pressure. An increase in blood volume or heart rate or a decrease in the ability of the arteries to expand may result in an increased pulse pressure.

6. Blood pressure readings are recorded as an improper fraction; for example, systolic/diastolic or 130/92. This means the systolic pressure is 130 and the diastolic pressure is 92. Both numbers in the blood pressure are important, but for people who are 50 or older, systolic pressure gives the most accurate diagnosis of high blood pressure.

7. Blood pressure values:

a. Average resting adult brachial artery pressure is less than 120 millimeters of mercury (mm Hg) systolic and less than 80 millimeters of mercury (mm Hg) diastolic.

b. *Prehypertension* is a condition that means you are likely to develop high blood pressure in the future. In this condition, blood pressure is between 120/80 mm NG and 139/89 mm Hg. People with prehypertension can take steps to decrease their risk.

c. **Hypertension** (high blood pressure) is when values are greater than 140 mm Hg systolic and 90 mm Hg diastolic.

d. **Hypotension** (low blood pressure) is when values are less than 100 mm Hg systolic and 60 mm Hg diastolic. Excessive hypotension can lead to shock.

e. For either hypertension or hypotension, unusual or changed readings must be recorded and reported. (See Procedure 45.)

f. High blood pressure is a dangerous condition. There are no signs and symptoms. It increases the risk of several serious diseases (Unit 39). It can also cause complications of conditions such as diabetes. People with prehypertension and hypertension require regular blood pressure monitoring.

g. Blood pressure classifications are listed in Table 20-1. When systolic and diastolic blood pressures fall into different categories, the higher category is used to classify blood pressure level. For example, 172/78 mm Hg would be stage 2 hypertension (high blood pressure).

Inaccurate Blood Pressure Readings

Causes of inaccurate blood pressure readings include:

- Use of a wrong-size cuff
- An improperly wrapped cuff
- Incorrect positioning of arm
- Not using the same arm for all readings
- Not having the gauge at eye level
- Deflating the cuff too slowly
- Mistaking an **auscultatory gap** (sound fadeout for 10 to 15 mm Hg which then begins again) as the diastolic pressure

TABLE 20-1 BLOOD PRESSURE CLASSIFICATIONS				
	Blood Pressure Level (mm Hg)			
Category	**Systolic**		**Diastolic**	
Normal	<120	and	<80	
Prehypertension	120–139	or	80–89	
High Blood Pressure				
Stage I Hypertension	140–159	or	90–99	
Stage II Hypertension	≥160	or	≥100	

Legend: < means less than; ≥ means greater than or equal to

HOW TO READ THE GAUGE

The gauges on sphygmomanometers are marked with a series of lines. The large lines are at increments of 10 millimeters of mercury pressure. The shorter lines are at 2-mm intervals. For example, the first small line above 80 mm is 82 mm. The first small line below 80 mm is 78 mm (Figure 20-10).

To properly read the mercury gauge:

- It should be at eye level.
- It should not be tilted.
- The reading should be taken at the top of the column of mercury. It should not be taken at the "hump" in the middle of the mercury when you hear the first sound.

To properly read the aneroid gauge, observe the gauge at eye level. Do not read it at an angle.

Following completion of the blood pressure measurement, you will record and report the following:

- If you were unable to hear the reading.
- If blood pressure is higher than in a previous reading.
- If blood pressure is lower than in a previous reading.
- If the site where you took the reading was other than brachial artery.

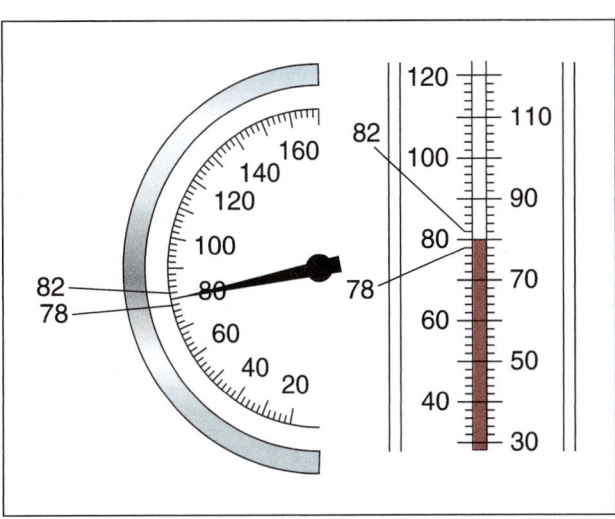

FIGURE 20-10 The aneroid gauge (left) and the mercury gauge (right). Take the reading at the closest line.

PROCEDURE 45

TAKING BLOOD PRESSURE

1. Carry out beginning procedure actions.

2. Assemble equipment:
   - sphygmomanometer with appropriate size cuff
   - stethoscope
   - alcohol wipes

3. Remove the patient's arm from sleeve or roll sleeve 5 inches above the elbow; it should not be tight or binding.

4. Locate the brachial artery with your fingertips (Figure 20-11).

5. Place the patient's arm palm upward, supported on bed or table, at heart level.

6. Wrap the cuff smoothly and snugly around the arm. Center the bladder over the brachial artery. The bottom of the cuff should be 1 inch above the antecubital space (inner elbow) (Figure 20-12).

7. Place the bulb in your dominant hand and feel for the radial pulse with the fingers of your other hand (Figure 20-13). To find out how high to pump the cuff:
   - Rapidly inflate the cuff until you no longer feel the radial pulse.
   - Add 30 mm to that reading. (If you no longer feel the pulse when the mercury or needle reaches 130, add 30 mm for a reading of 160.) Note that point.

8. Quickly and steadily deflate the cuff. Wait 15 to 30 seconds.

9. Place the stethoscope over the brachial artery (Figure 20-14).

10. Reinflate the cuff quickly and steadily to the level you calculated (in the example in step 7, to 160).

11. Release the air at an even pace, about 2 to 3 mm per second. Keep your eyes on the needle or the mercury.

12. Listen for the onset of at least two consecutive beats. Note where the needle is on the

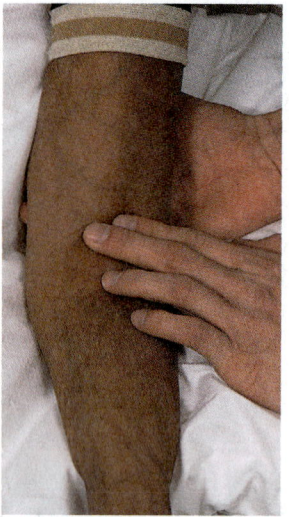
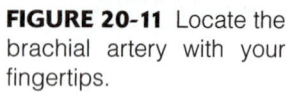
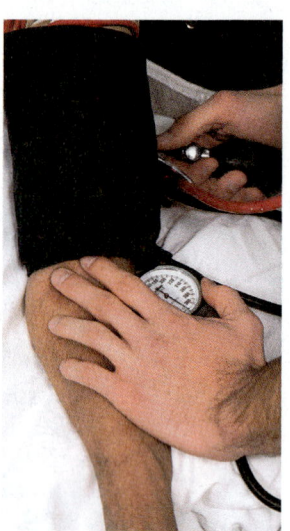

FIGURE 20-11 Locate the brachial artery with your fingertips.

FIGURE 20-12 The bottom of the cuff should be at least 1 inch above the antecubital space (inner elbow).

sphygmomanometer when you first hear the sound. (Do not stop deflating the cuff.) This is your systolic reading.

13. Continue deflating the cuff. The last sound you hear is the diastolic reading. Continue to deflate and to listen for 10 to 20 mm more to make sure you have the correct diastolic reading.

14. Record the reading (blood pressure is always recorded in even numbers, with the systolic on top and the diastolic on the bottom, e.g., 128/82). Indicate the arm used and the position of the patient (sitting, lying down, or standing).

15. If you are not sure of the reading and need to retake the blood pressure, wait 1 to 2 minutes before repeating the procedure.

16. Clean the earpieces of the stethoscope with alcohol wipes. If the tubing has contacted the patient or linen, wipe it as well.

17. Return equipment to the appropriate area.

18. Carry out procedure completion actions.

continues

PROCEDURE 45

continued

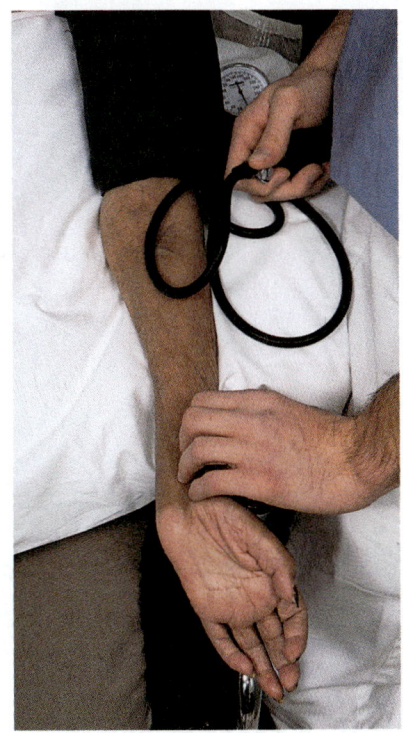

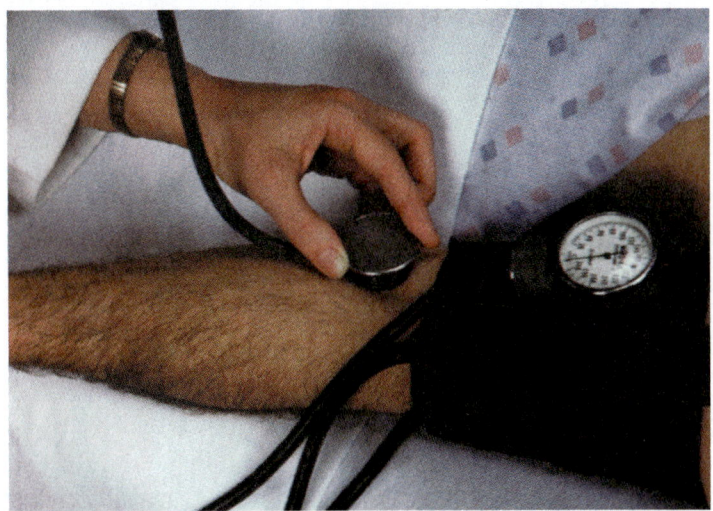

FIGURE 20-14 Position the bell of the stethoscope over the brachial artery.

FIGURE 20-13 Hold the bulb in your dominant hand and feel for the radial pulse with the fingers of the other hand.

guidelines *for*

Electronic Blood Pressure Monitoring

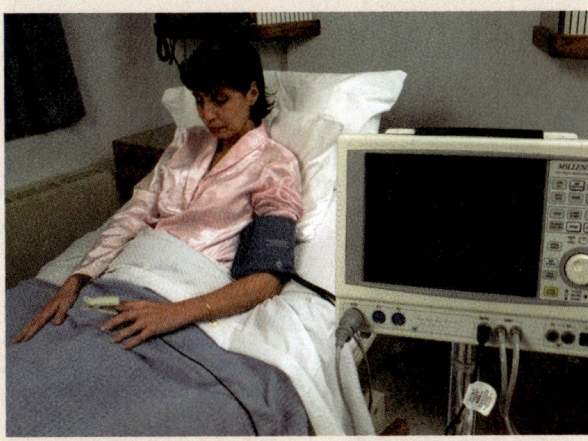

FIGURE 20-15 An electronic blood pressure monitoring unit takes the blood pressure automatically.

Patient Selection (Refer to Figure 20-15)

- This procedure can be done on patients of all ages and sizes, but appropriately sized cuffs must be used.
- At least one blood pressure reading should be taken using the auscultation method before an electronic blood pressure device is used. The auscultation reading is needed as a baseline with which to compare the values from the electronic device.

The procedure is contraindicated in patients with:

- Extreme hypertension or hypotension
- Very rapid heart rates
- Excessive body movement or tremors
- Irregular heart rhythms or atrial dysrhythmias

continues

guidelines *continued*

Patients for whom electronic blood pressure monitoring is not acceptable should be known to all caregivers and identified on the care plan or Kardex. If in doubt, check with the nurse for instructions for patients with very high blood pressure or rapid or irregular heart (pulse) rates.

Do not place the cuff on an arm that:

- Is paralyzed
- Is the site of an intravenous infusion (IV)
- Has a pulse oximeter on it
- Has impaired circulation
- Is the site of a dialysis access device

- Is fractured
- Is burned
- Is on the same side as a recent mastectomy or other surgical procedure site

Application of the Cuff

- Select the proper cuff size. The width should be equal to 40% of the arm circumference.
- The upper arm is the preferred location for the monitoring cuff, but the forearm and ankle may also be used.

PROCEDURE 46

TAKING BLOOD PRESSURE WITH AN ELECTRONIC BLOOD PRESSURE APPARATUS

1. Carry out beginning procedure actions.

2. Assemble equipment:
   - electronic blood pressure device
   - assortment of cuffs and tubes

3. Bring the electronic blood pressure unit to the bedside. Place it near the patient and plug it into a source of electricity.

4. Locate the on/off switch and turn the machine on.

5. Select the appropriate cuff for the machine and size for the patient's extremity.

6. Remove restrictive clothing.

7. Squeeze excess air out of the cuff.

8. Connect the cuff to the connector hose.

9. Wrap the cuff snugly around the patient's extremity, verifying that only one finger can fit between the cuff and the patient's skin. Make

sure the "artery" arrow marked on the outside of the cuff is correctly placed over the brachial artery.

10. Verify that the connector hose between the cuff and the machine is not kinked.

11. Set the frequency control for automatic or manual.

12. Press the start button.

13. If the cuff will take periodic, automatic measurements, set the designated frequency of blood pressure measurements.

14. Set upper and lower alarm limits for systolic, diastolic, and mean blood pressure readings.

15. Remove the cuff at least every 2 hours and alternate sites, if possible. Evaluate the skin for redness and irritation. Report abnormalities to the nurse.

16. Carry out procedure completion actions.

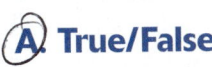

REVIEW

A. True/False.

Mark the following true or false by circling T or F.

1. **Ⓣ** F The volume of blood in the circulatory system is a factor in the blood pressure.

2. T **Ⓕ** Exercise decreases blood pressure.

3. **Ⓣ** F To accurately measure blood pressure, you will need both a sphygmomanometer and a stethoscope.

4. T **Ⓕ** Blood pressures taken over arteries closer to the heart will be lower than those taken over arteries farther from the heart.

5. **Ⓣ** F A blood pressure below 100/70 would signal hypotension.

6. T **Ⓕ** The large lines on the blood pressure gauge are in increments of 20 mm of Hg pressure.

7. T **Ⓕ** Depressant drugs elevate the blood pressure.

8. **Ⓣ** F Using a blood pressure cuff of the wrong size will give an inaccurate reading.

9. **Ⓣ** F When measuring a blood pressure, always keep the gauge at eye level.

10. **Ⓣ** F Stethoscope earpieces should be cleaned both before and after use.

B. Matching.

Choose the correct word from Column II to match each phrase in Column I.

Column I

11. __g__ high blood pressure

12. __b__ lowest blood pressure reading

13. __h__ stretch

14. __a__ most common artery used to determine blood pressure

15. __c/e__ blood pressure apparatus

Column II

a. brachial

b. diastolic

c. stethoscope

d. femoral

e. sphygmomanometer

f. hypotension

g. hypertension

h. elasticity

i. systolic

C. Completion.

Complete the statements by choosing the correct word.

16. The closing of the heart valves is heard as the __systolic__ sounds.
    (diastolic) (systolic)

17. High blood pressure is known as __hypertension__
    (hypotension) (hypertension)

18. Blood pressure is lowered when weight is __lost__.
    (gained) (lost)

19. Blood pressure is raised by __exercise__.
    (rest) (exercise)

20. The earpieces of the stethoscope should be pointed __~~backward~~ forward__ as they are placed in the ears.
    (forward) (backward)

D. Nursing Assistant Challenge.

You are assigned to take Mr. King's blood pressure at 12 noon. He is a very heavy man and has an IV inserted in his left arm. His blood pressure was 180/140 at 8 A.M. Answer the following questions:

21. What effect will his size have on your selection of cuff? __enlarged cuff__

22. On which arm will you apply the cuff? __R__

23. Will you report your findings? __yes__

24. Why? __cause its elevated__

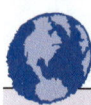 **EXPLORING THE WEB**

Description	Location
Assessment	http://www.delmarhealthcare.com/olcs/white/pnotes.asp (see Chapter 25)
Measuring vital signs	http://www.delmarhealthcare.com/olcs/delaune/ppt/ DeLaunechapter%2027.ppt
National Institutes of Health Guide to Lowering High Blood Pressure	http://www.nhlbi.nih.gov/hbp
Systolic blood pressure treatment	http://www.advancefornurses.com (see past articles October 27, 2000)
Does Accurate Blood Pressure Depend on Mercury?	http://www.noharm.org
The Elimination of Mercury Sphygmomanometers	http://www.noharm.org
Mercury Free at NIH	http://www.nih.gov/od/ors/ds/nomercury
Sustainable Hospitals	http://www.sustainablehospitals.org
Techniques of Vital Signs	http://hsc.virginia.edu/med-ed

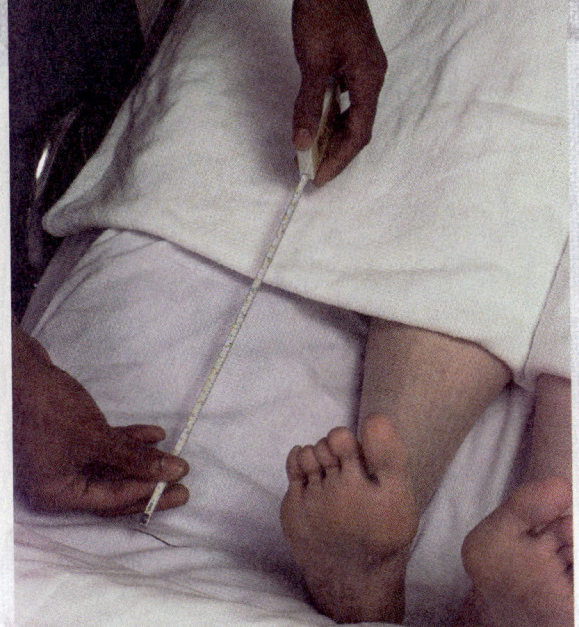

Measuring Height and Weight

objectives

After completing this unit, you will be able to:

- Spell and define terms.
- Describe the proper use of an overbed scale.
- Demonstrate the following procedures:
  - Procedure 47 Weighing and Measuring the Patient Using an Upright Scale
  - Procedure 48 Weighing the Patient on a Chair Scale
  - Procedure 49 Measuring Weight with an Electronic Wheelchair Scale
  - Procedure 50 Measuring and Weighing the Patient in Bed

vocabulary

Learn the meaning and the correct spelling of the following words and phrases:

balance bar	centimeter (cm)	kilogram (kg)
baseline	increment	pound (lb)

WEIGHT AND HEIGHT MEASUREMENTS

Changes in weight are frequently used as an indicator of the patient's condition.

- A baseline (original) measurement of height and weight is usually obtained on admission. These are usually noted on the Kardex.
- Weights are frequently measured when patients are given drugs (diuretics) to increase their urine output.
- Weight is an indicator of the patient's nutritional status.
- Measurements of weight and height must be accurately made and recorded according to facility policy because medications may be ordered according to the patient's size.
- Height measurements may be recorded in feet (') and inches (") or in centimeters (cm).
- Weight measurements may be recorded in pounds (lb) or kilograms (kg).

Note: Some facilities use the metric system, so you may be recording weight in kilograms. If your facility uses this measurement system, the scales will be calibrated for the metric system. You will not be required to convert measurements from the inch and pound system to the metric system.

- The upright scale is used for ambulatory patients who can stand unattended on the platform (Figure 21-1).
- A mechanical lift with scale can be used to weigh patients who cannot stand or sit in a wheelchair (Figure 21-2).

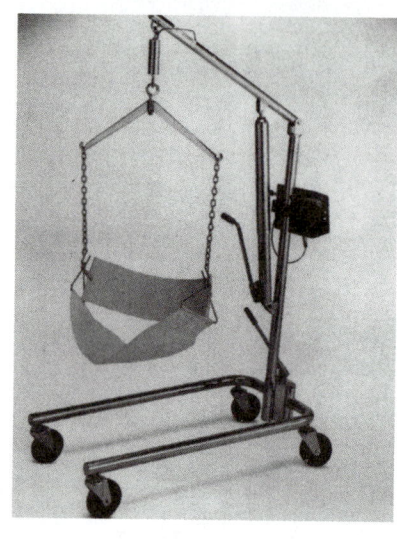

FIGURE 21-2 The scale on the mechanical lift is used when patients are not ambulatory or are too heavy or difficult to move. *(Photo courtesy Health O Meter®)*

- Sling scales can be used to weigh patients whose conditions do not permit the use of a mechanical lift/scale (Figure 21-3).
- Chair scales are used to weigh patients in wheelchairs (Figure 21-4).

(See Procedures 47 to 50.)

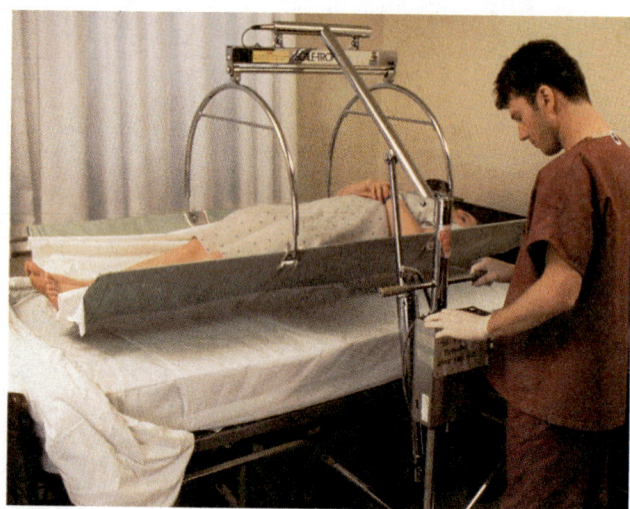

FIGURE 21-3 The sling scale is used for bedfast patients who cannot sit or stand.

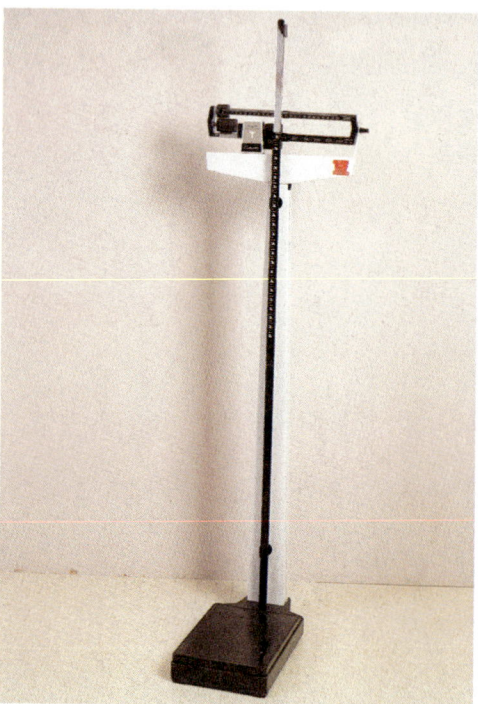

FIGURE 21-1 An upright scale is used only for patients who can stand unaided on the platform.

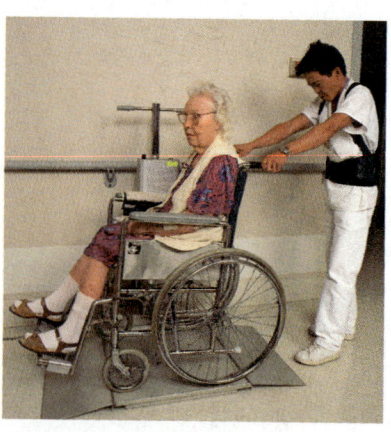

FIGURE 21-4 Electronic chair scales are used for patients who cannot stand on an upright scale.

guidelines *for*

Obtaining Accurate Weight and Height Measurements

To obtain an accurate weight measurement, you must:

- Always balance the scale before using.
- Have the patient empty his or her bladder.
- Weigh the patient at the same time of day each time.
- Have the patient wear the same type of garments each time.
- Use the same method and the same scale each time, if possible.

You must learn to read the scale correctly. There are two bars on the upright scale (see Figure 21-1). The **balance bar** should hang free to start.

- The lower bar indicates weights in 50-pound **increments** (amounts).
- The upper bar indicates one-quarter-pound increments (Figure 21-5).

- The even-numbered pounds are marked with numbers.
- The long line between each number indicates the odd-numbered pounds.
- Each small line indicates one-quarter pound, or 4 ounces.

The two figures are added and recorded as the person's total weight. The sum is recorded according to facility policy in either pounds or kilograms. For example:

Large bar = 100 pounds

Small bar = +22 pounds

Total = 122 pounds

- Height is measured with the ruler attached to an upright scale or with a tape measure when the patient is in bed.

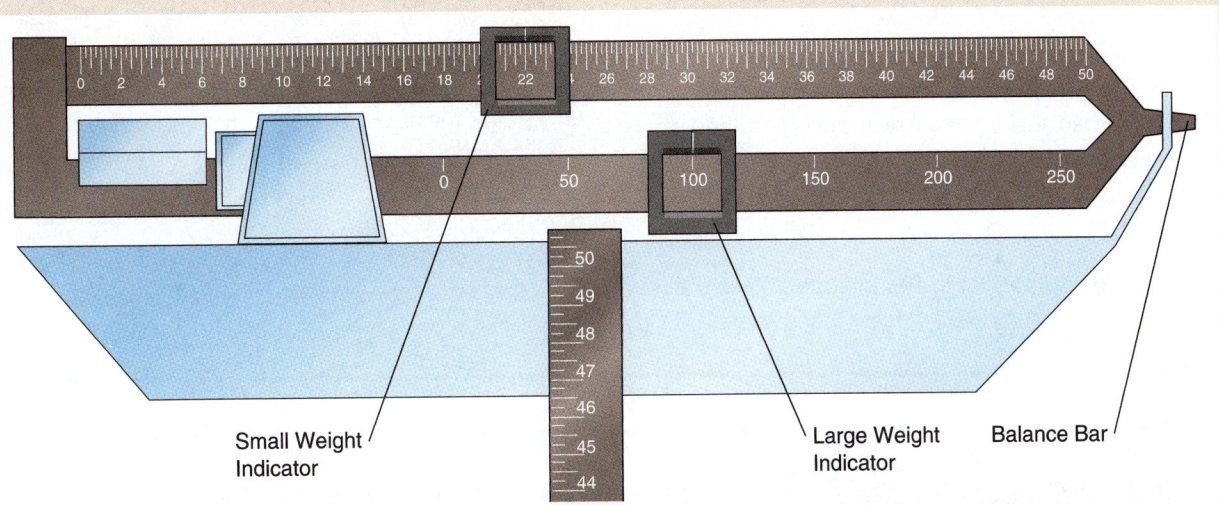

FIGURE 21-5 The upper bar indicates smaller pound weights. The weight shown on the lower bar is measured in 50-pound increments. This figure is added to the amount shown on the upper bar.

PROCEDURE 47

WEIGHING AND MEASURING THE PATIENT USING AN UPRIGHT SCALE

1. Carry out beginning procedure actions.

 Note: Use disposable gloves if there may be contact with open lesions, wet linens, or body fluids.

2. Check notes or chart for previous weight as documented. Then escort the patient to the scales.

continues

PROCEDURE 47

continued

3. Place a paper towel on the platform of the scale.

4. Be sure the weights are to the extreme left and the balance bar (bar with weight markings) is hanging free.

5. Assist the patient to remove shoes and step up onto the scale platform, facing the balance bar. The balance bar will rise to the top of the bar guide. The patient should not hold the bar or other parts of the scale.

6. Move the large weight to the right to the closest estimated patient weight.

7. Move the small weight to the right until the balance bar hangs freely halfway between the upper and lower bar guides.

8. Add the two figures and record the total as the patient's weight in pounds or kilograms, according to the type of scale used.

9. Assist the patient to turn on the platform until facing away from the balance bar. Raise the height bar until it is level with the top of the patient's head.

10. The reading is made at the movable point of the ruler (Figure 21-6).

11. Note the number of inches indicated. Record this information in inches ("), feet (') and inches ("),

or centimeters (cm), according to the type of scale. The height shown in Figure 21-6 is 62 inches. This may be recorded as 62 inches or 5 feet 2 inches (62 ÷ 12 = 5 feet 2 inches). Record the value on your notepad.

12. Assist the patient off the platform. Help the patient to put on shoes, if necessary, and return to the room.

13. Carry out procedure completion actions.

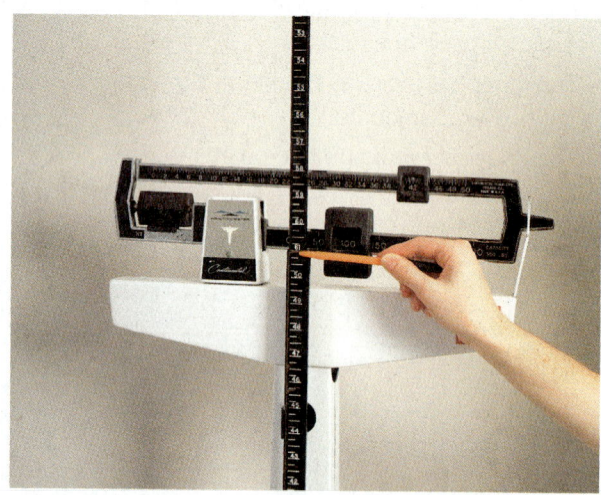

FIGURE 21-6 The height is read at the movable point of the ruler.

PROCEDURE 48

WEIGHING THE PATIENT ON A CHAIR SCALE

1. Carry out beginning procedure actions.

2. Assemble equipment:
   • chair scale

3. Take the patient in a wheelchair to the chair scale. Lock the brakes to the wheelchair. Check the brakes of the chair scale to make sure they are locked in place.

4. Apply a transfer belt to the patient and assist

in a pivot transfer to the chair on the scale. Instruct the patient to sit down when the chair is felt against the back of the legs. Be sure the patient's feet are on the footrest of the scale.

5. Walk behind the scale to obtain the reading.

6. Transfer the patient back to the wheelchair.

7. Carry out procedure completion actions.

PROCEDURE 49

MEASURING WEIGHT WITH AN ELECTRONIC WHEELCHAIR SCALE

1. Carry out beginning procedure actions.

2. Assemble equipment:
   - wheelchair scale

3. Determine empty weight of a wheelchair by weighing it on the scale.

4. Take the wheelchair to the patient's room. Help the patient into the wheelchair and take the patient to the electronic wheelchair scale.

5. Open the metal ramp sides the on scale so that they rest on the floor. This allows wheelchair access to the scale.

6. Press the "on" button; the scale zeroes automatically (Figure 21-7).

7. Roll the wheelchair with the patient in it, onto the platform of the scale. Lock wheelchair wheels.

8. The digital readout will show weight.

9. Record weight of the patient and wheelchair. Subtract the wheelchair weight to obtain the patient's weight.

10. Unlock wheelchair wheels. Roll the wheelchair with patient off the scale.

11. Fold the scale ramps back into place.

12. Carry out procedure completion actions.

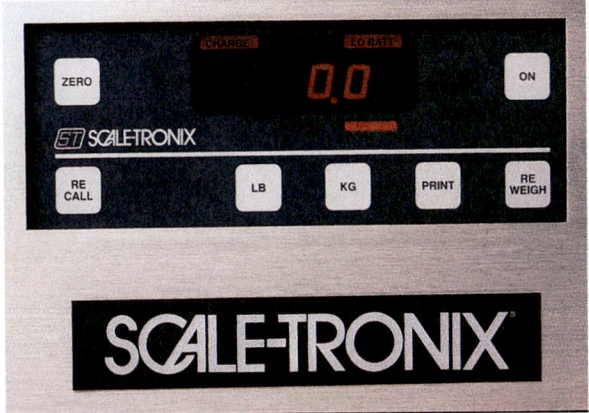

FIGURE 21-7 Press the "on" button to calibrate the scale. This will cause the reading to return to zero. *(Courtesy of Scale-Tronix, White Plains, NY)*

PROCEDURE 50

MEASURING AND WEIGHING THE PATIENT IN BED

1. Carry out beginning procedure actions.

2. Obtain assistance from a coworker.

3. Assemble equipment:
   - overbed scale
   - sheet
   - tape measure
   - pencil

4. Check scale sling and straps for frayed areas or straps that do not close properly.

5. Lower the side rail on your side. Make sure the side rail is up on the other side.

6. Fanfold top linen to foot of bed.

7. Position the patient flat on back with arms and legs straight and body in good alignment. Make sure the sheet is straight and wrinkle-free.

8. Make a small pencil mark at the top of the patient's head on the sheet.

continues

PROCEDURE 50

continued

9. Make a second pencil mark even with the heels (Figure 21-8).

10. Roll the patient on the side. Using the tape measure, measure the distance between the two pencil marks.

11. Note the patient's height in feet and inches on a pad.

12. Cover the canvas sling with a sheet. Balance the scale according to the manufacturer's directions. The scale should be balanced with the sheet, canvas sling, chains, or straps attached.

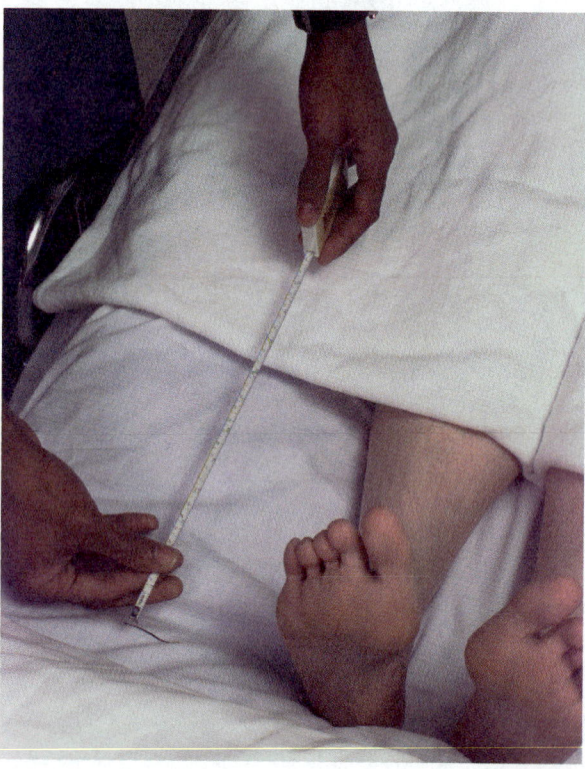

FIGURE 21-8 Measuring the height of the patient in bed. Measure from the pencil line at the heels to the pencil line at the top of the head.

13. Remove the scale sling from the suspension straps and position half of the sheet-covered sling under the patient.
   - Turn the patient away from you.
   - Place the sling, folded lengthwise, under the patient.
   - Return the patient to recumbent position and place the sling so that the patient rests securely within it.
   - Attach the sling to the suspension straps. Check to be sure attachments are secure.

14. Position the lift frame over the bed with base legs in maximum open position, and lock the frame.

15. Elevate the head of the bed and bring the patient to a sitting position.

16. Attach the suspension straps to the frame. Position the patient's arms inside the straps.

17. Slowly raise the sling so the patient's body is off the bed. Be reassuring.

18. Guide the lift away from the bed so that no part of the patient touches the bed.

19. Take and note the reading.

20. Reposition the sling over the center of the bed.

21. Release the knob slowly, lowering the patient to the bed.

22. Remove the sling by reversing the process in step 13.

23. Assist the patient to a comfortable position.

24. Move the overbed scale out of the way.

25. Replace the top bed linen over the patient. Raise the side rail and lower the bed to the lowest horizontal height.

26. Carry out procedure completion actions.

REVIEW

A. True/False.

Mark the following true or false by circling T or F.

1. T (F) The lower bar on the scale indicates pounds in increments of 25.

2. (T) F Always check the overbed scale for needed repairs before use.

3. (T) F To obtain a proper reading, the scale balance bar must hang freely.

4. (T) F The scale used most often to weigh ambulatory patients in care facilities is the upright scale.

5. T (F) A patient who cannot get out of bed cannot be measured.

6. (T) F When using an overbed scale, the patient's body must be free of the bed.

7. T (F) To measure a patient confined to bed, first help her assume the left Sims' position.

B. Short Answer.

Choose the correct word from the following list to complete each statement in questions 8–12.

1 ambulatory   4 inches
2 centimeters   5 kilograms
3 forward   6 pounds

8. Weights may be measured in __6__ or __5__.

9. Height measurements may be recorded in feet and __4__ or in __2__.

10. The upright scale is used to weigh __1__ patients.

11. A scale that is calibrated for the metric system will express weights in __5__.

12. When a patient is measured on an upright scale, he should face __3__.

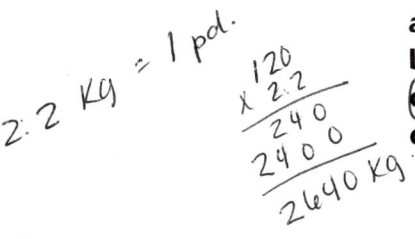

2.2 Kg = 1 pd.

2.2 Kg = 1 pd.
    120
  × 2.2
    240
  2400
  2640 Kg.

C. Nursing Assistant Challenge.

Mrs. Haughn is in bed recovering from a stroke. She is unable to walk or stand. She is receiving diuretics. Her doctor wants to order some new medication that is given according to the patient's size. You are assigned to weigh and measure the height of this patient. Answer each of the following by selecting the correct answer.

13. The best way to weigh this patient is with
  a. an upright scale.
  b. an overbed scale.
  c. a wheelchair scale.
  d. a chair scale

14. The best way to measure this patient is
  a. with a height bar.
  b. with a tape measure.
  c. to ask the patient.
  d. to estimate the height.

15. One reason the physician might have asked for the patient's weight is because the patient
  a. is receiving diuretics.
  b. has had a stroke.
  c. cannot stand.
  d. cannot walk.

16. The patient measures 63 inches. This may be expressed as
  a. 5 feet 6 inches.
  b. 5 feet 8 inches.
  c. 5 feet 3 inches.
  d. 6 feet 3 inches.

12
24
36
48
60

5
12)63

3

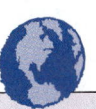

EXPLORING THE WEB

Description	Location
Assessment	http://www.delmarhealthcare.com/olcs/white/pnotes.asp (see Chapter 25)
Average height and weight charts (adult)	http://www.halls.md
Average height and weight charts (child)	http://www.halls.md
Children's growth charts	http://www.sickkid.net
Determining body mass index	http://www.state.ma.us
Height and weight converter (to metric)	http://www.mdt.state.mt.us
Height and weight tables	http://insurancepage.com
Notes on the Use of Height and Weight Charts	http://www.bradfordvts.co.uk

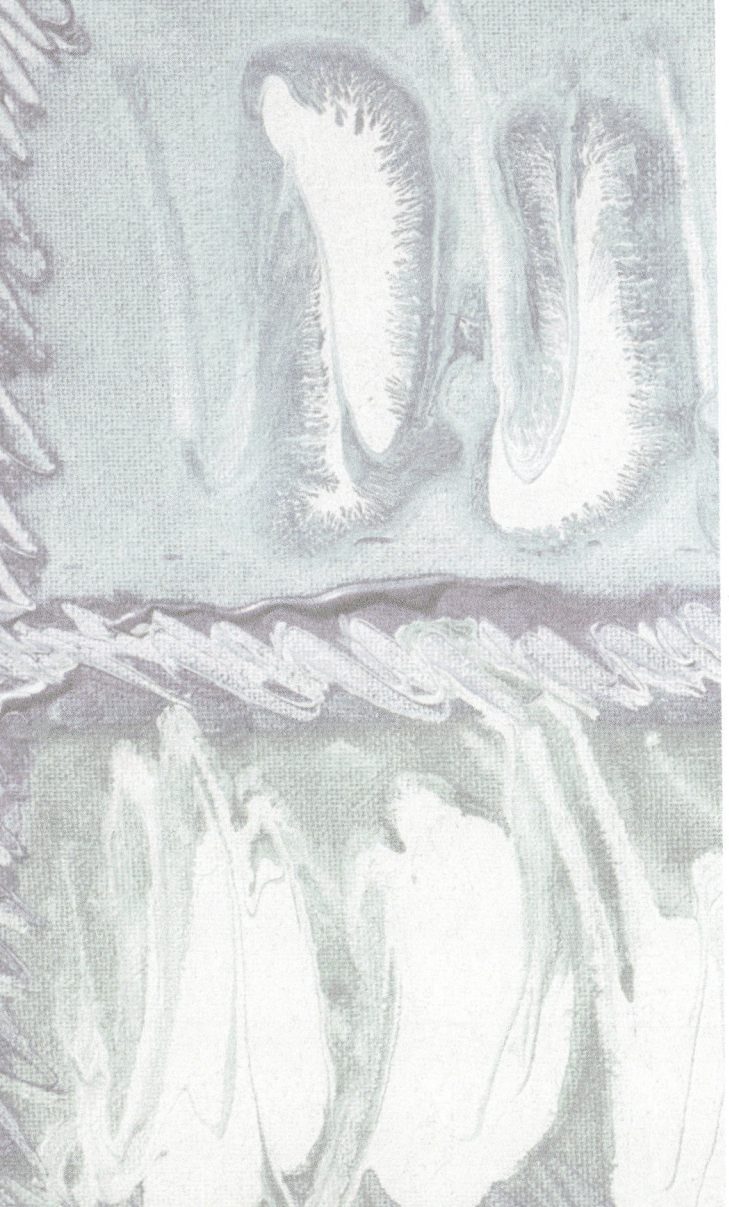

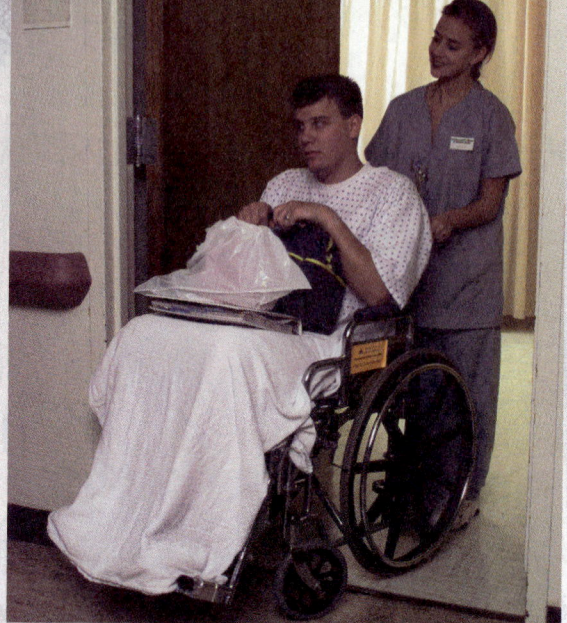

Admission, Transfer, and Discharge

objectives

After completing this unit, you will be able to:
- Spell and define terms.
- List the ways the nursing assistant can help in the processes of admission, transfer, and discharge.

- Demonstrate the following procedures:
  - Procedure 51 Admitting the Patient
  - Procedure 52 Transferring the Patient
  - Procedure 53 Discharging the Patient

vocabulary

Learn the meaning and the correct spelling of the following words and phrases:

admission
baseline assessment

discharge
transfer

INTRODUCTION

The nurse is responsible for overseeing and carrying out hospital procedures and physician's orders regarding all admissions, transfers, and discharges. You will usually help the nurse by carrying out the routine procedures associated with these activities.

A nursing assistant, a volunteer, or someone from the admissions office accompanies the new patient to the unit. Someone must always escort the patient to the unit for admission. Also, someone must always escort the patient from the unit during transfer or discharge.

You can do much to make these activities easier for the patient, family, and the other staff members by:

- Having equipment and materials prepared for the activity.
- Being very observant during each activity.
- Documenting observations carefully and accurately. These make a valuable contribution to the nurse's initial **baseline assessment** of the patient's condition.
- Reporting observations directly to the nurse.
- Giving attention to the details of each procedure.
- Being aware of the emotional stress these activities cause patients and their families.
- Being courteous to everyone (Figure 22-1).

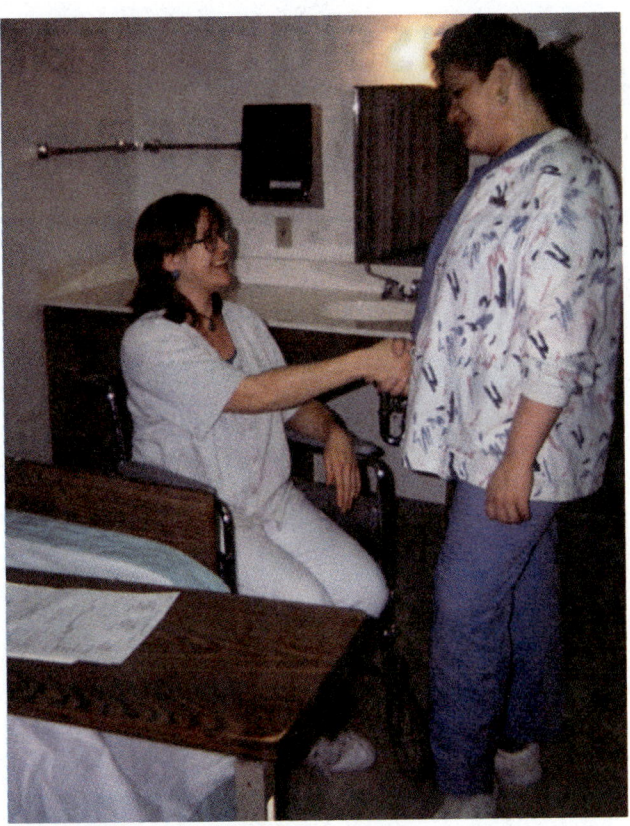

FIGURE 22-1 Treat patients and families with courtesy and respect. First impressions are lasting ones, and you represent your facility to the patient.

ADMISSION

When a person enters a health care facility for treatment of an illness or injury, the **admission** process often causes concern or stress to the patient, family, and friends. The first impression created is very important. You will be one of the first staff members the patient sees, so it is important that you be courteous, confident, and efficient. (See Procedure 51.)

When a patient is ready for admission, ask the nurse if:

- The patient requires a stretcher or wheelchair to reach the unit.
- Any special equipment such as oxygen or a fracture bed is needed.
- There are any special instructions, such as withholding fluids or foods.

Introduce yourself and observe the patient carefully. Listen for complaints as you escort and assist the patient to the room and to bed. Initial observations are very important. They become the basis of comparison for future observations.

Pay particular attention to the patient's skin condition. If you observe rashes, bruises, pressure ulcers, or other abnormalities, inform the nurse and document your findings on the admission record, or according to facility policy.

If it is necessary to ask visitors to leave, do so in a kindly and polite manner. They will be most anxious to remain and see the patient settled and comfortable, so

- Show them where they may wait.
- Let them know about how long they will have to wait.
- Tell them where they can get refreshments.
- Answer questions they may have about where to find a chapel and telephones, and visiting hours.
- After you have completed your part of the admission procedure, locate visitors and let them know they may return to the patient's room.

AGE-APPROPRIATE CARE *Alert*

Pediatric patients may fear separation from the parents. Explain the unit policies for visiting or rooming in. Orient the child and family to the playroom, bathroom, and other areas as appropriate. Speak directly to the child. Show the child how to use the signal or call for help. Ask him or her questions about normal routines. Allow the child to respond before questioning the parents. A primary goal on admission is to make the child and parents as comfortable as possible, relieving anxiety about separation.

TRANSFER

It may be necessary for the patient to be moved to another unit (Figure 22-5, see page 333). Preparations for the transfer will be handled by the nurse, but you may be asked to assist. (See Procedure 52.)

The transfer may be the patient's own preference, or may be done because a change in the patient's condition requires a different type of care. The transfer may be temporary or permanent. If it is permanent, the patient is discharged from one unit, then admitted to another. The patient may or may not fully understand the reasons for the transfer. Be positive and supportive in your attitude. Recognize that the patient may be feeling very anxious. It would be helpful to know what the patient has been told about the reasons for the transfer. You may learn this from the nurse and by carefully listening to what your patient says.

PROCEDURE 51

ADMITTING THE PATIENT

1. Wash hands.
2. Assemble equipment:
   - equipment for urine specimen collection
   - equipment for taking temperature
   - pad and pencil
   - patient's chart or worksheet
   - stethoscope
   - admission kit
     - water pitcher
     - glass
     - liquid soap
     - washcloth
     - towel
     - basin
     - lotion
     - mouthwash
   - scale
   - blood pressure cuff and manometer
   - watch with second hand
   - disposable gloves (if urine specimen is required)
3. Prepare the unit for the patient by:
   a. Making sure that all necessary equipment and furniture are in their proper places and in good working order.
   b. Checking the unit for adequate lighting.
   c. Loosening the top linen at the foot of the bed. This is called a *toe pleat*.
   d. Opening the bed (Figure 22-2).
4. Identify the patient both by asking the name and checking the identification bracelet.
   a. Introduce yourself.
   b. Take the patient and the patient's family to the unit.
   c. Do not appear to rush the patient.
   d. Be courteous and helpful to the patient and the family.

continues

PROCEDURE 51

continued

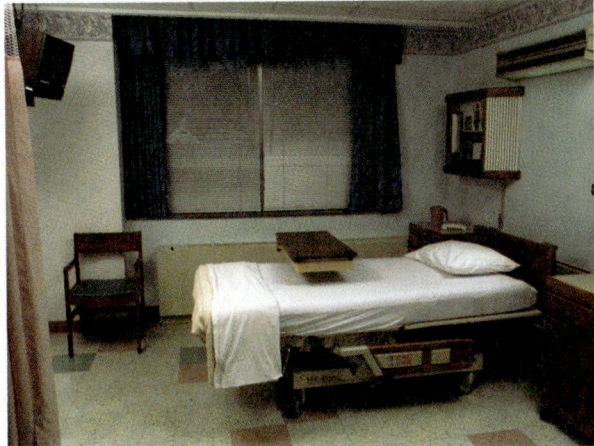

FIGURE 22-2 An open bed notifies everyone that a patient is expected.

5. Ask the patient to be seated, if ambulatory.

   a. Ask the family to go to the lounge or lobby while the patient is being admitted.

   b. Introduce the patient to the other patients in the room, unless it is a private room.

   c. As permitted, explain what will happen in the next hour.

6. Screen the unit to provide privacy (Figure 22-3).

7. Help the patient to undress and put on a hospital gown or night clothes from home. Care for clothing according to facility policy.

8. Check the patient's vital signs, weight, and height.

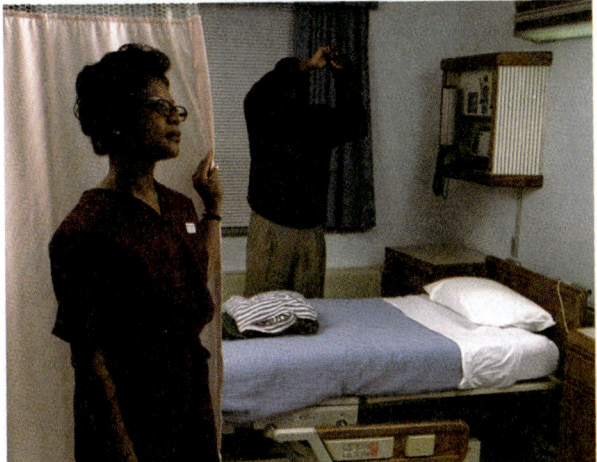

FIGURE 22-3 Provide privacy so the patient can undress.

9. Help the patient get into bed. Adjust the side rails as needed.

10. If the patient is wearing any jewelry or has valuables:

   a. Make a list of them and ask the patient to sign it. This protects the facility and the patient.

   b. Ask the relatives also to sign the list and take the valuables home, or

   c. After checking and signing, give them to the nurse to put in the hospital safe.

11. Tell the patient if a urine specimen is necessary.

   a. Put on gloves and assist the patient as necessary.

   b. Allow the patient to use the bathroom, if ambulatory, or offer the bedpan or urinal.

12. Pour the patient's specimen from the bedpan into the specimen bottle. Put on the cap. Remove gloves and dispose of them according to facility policy. Be sure to label the specimen correctly (see Unit 44).

13. An admission form is usually completed at this time (Figure 22-4). Vital information includes:

   ● observations

   ● vital signs (TPR, BP, height, weight)

   ● known allergies

   ● medications being taken

   ● food preferences and dislikes

14. If admission is to a long-term care facility, label clothing and complete the personal belongings inventory form according to facility policy.

15. Orient the patient to the unit by explaining:

   ● visiting hours

   ● how to use the telephone and/or television

   ● how to use the call light system for assistance

   ● how to operate the bed and light switches, as appropriate

   ● standard hospital regulations

   ● television rental procedures, if available

   ● any questions about facility routines

   ● when meals and refreshments are provided

16. Carry out procedure completion actions.

continues

PROCEDURE 51

continued

PATIENT PREFERS TO BE ADDRESSED AS:

_____

FROM: ☐ E.R. ☐ E.C.F. ☐ HOME ☐ M.D.'S OFFICE

COMMUNICATES IN ENGLISH: ☐ WELL ☐ MINIMAL

☐ INTERPRETER (NAME PERSON) ☐ NONE

MODE OF TRANSPORTATION:

☐ AMBULATORY ☐ OTHER **SMOKER:** ☐ Y ☐ N

☐ WHEELCHAIR _____

☐ STRETCHER _____

☐ NOT AT ALL ☐ OTHER LANGUAGE (SPECIFY) _____

HOME TELEPHONE NO. ( ) _____

WORK TELEPHONE NO. ( ) _____

ORIENTATION TO ENVIRONMENT:

☐ ARMBAND CHECKED ☐ CALL LIGHT

☐ BED CONTROL ☐ PHONE

☐ TV CONTROL ☐ SIDE RAIL POLICY

☐ BATH ROOM ☐ VISITATION POLICY

☐ PERSONAL PROPERTY POLICY ☐ SMOKING POLICY

PERSONAL BELONGINGS: (CHECK AND DESCRIBE)

☐ CLOTHING _____

☐ JEWELRY _____

☐ MONEY _____

☐ WALKER _____

☐ WHEELCHAIR _____

☐ CANE _____

☐ OTHER _____

DENTURES: CONTACT LENSES:

☐ UPPER ☐ PARTIAL ☐ HARD ☐ LT ☐ RT

☐ LOWER ☐ NONE ☐ SOFT

GLASSES: ☐ Y ☐ N **HEARING AID:** ☐ Y ☐ N

PROSTHESIS: ☐ Y ☐ N

(DESCRIBE) _____

DISPOSITION OF VALUABLES:

☐ PATIENT

☐ HOME GIVEN TO: _____

RELATIONSHIP: _____

☐ PLACED
  IN SAFE _____

(CLAIM NO.)

IN CASE OF EMERGENCY NOTIFY:

NAME: _____

RELATIONSHIP: _____

HOME TELEPHONE NO. ( ) _____

WORK TELEPHONE NO. ( ) _____

VITAL SIGNS

TEMP: _____ ☐ ORAL ☐ RECTAL ☐ AXILLARY

PULSE: _____ ☐ RADIAL ☐ APICAL RESPIRATORY
RATE _____

☐ RT

B/P: ☐ LT ☐ STANDING ☐ SITTING ☐ LYING

HEIGHT: _____ WEIGHT: _____ ☐ BEDSIDE

☐ STANDING

ALLERGIES:

MEDICATIONS: ☐ NONE KNOWN FOOD: ☐ NONE KNOWN

☐ PENICILLIN ☐ TAPE (SHELLFISH, EGGS, MILK, ETC.)

☐ SULFA ☐ OTHER (LIST) _____

☐ IODINE _____ _____

☐ ASPIRIN _____ _____

☐ MORPHINE _____ _____

☐ DEMEROL _____ _____

(PRESCRIPTIVE & NON PRESCRIPTIVE)

MEDICATIONS:	DOSE/FREQUENCY	(DATE/TIME) LAST DOSE
1.		
2.		
3.		
4.		
5.		
6.		

DISPOSITION OF MEDICATIONS:

☐ NONE BROUGHT TO HOSPITAL

☐ SENT HOME _____

WITH _____

☐ TO PHARMACY: (LIST)

_____

ADMITTING DIAGNOSIS: _____

NURSE'S SIGNATURE: _____ RN/LVN DATE _____ TIME _____

CHARTER SUBURBAN HOSPITAL
16453 SOUTH COLORADO AVENUE
PARAMOUNT, CALIFORNIA 90723
NURSING ADMISSION ASSESSMENT PAGE 1 of 6

FIGURE 22-4 Accurate admission information is an important part of the nursing assessment.

PROCEDURE 52

TRANSFERRING THE PATIENT

1. Find out which unit the patient will be transferred to. Check to see that it is ready.

2. Learn from the nurse in charge the method of transfer. Get the necessary vehicle (wheelchair, stretcher, or patient's own bed).

3. Check to see if any equipment is to be transferred with the patient.

4. Carry out beginning procedure actions.

5. Explain to the patient what you are doing.

6. Gather all the patient's belongings together.

   a. Place disposables in a paper bag to transport with you.

   b. Check against clothes list.

7. Assist the patient to put on robe and slippers, if permitted. Assist the patient into wheelchair or stretcher, as directed. The entire bed is often used. Make sure the side rails are up during transport.

8. Obtain from the nurse:
   - patient's chart
   - nursing care plan
   - medications
   - paper bag

9. Transport the patient and his belongings to the new unit (Figure 22-5). Use all precautions related to safe transport.

10. Give any transferred medications, the nursing care plan, and the chart to the nurse in charge.

11. Introduce the patient to staff. Proceed to the patient's room.

12. Assist staff in helping the patient into bed. Assist in putting away the patient's belongings and helping the patient to get settled.

13. Before leaving the unit, carry out procedure completion actions.

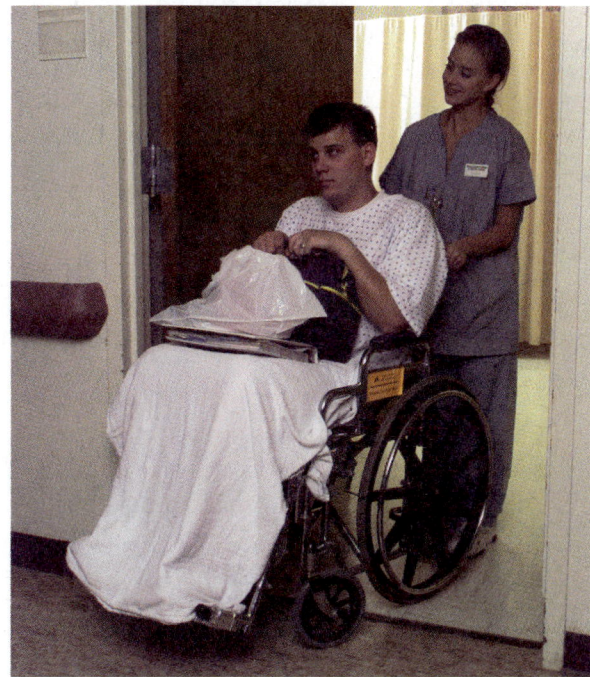

FIGURE 22-5 Transfer the patient calmly and efficiently. Never leave the patient unattended.

All details must be taken care of according to facility policy. Following facility policy ensures that there is no interruption of health care services. Some facilities have transportation services for transferring patients.

After the new unit has been notified and prepared for the move, you will:

- Tell the patient what you are doing.
- Gather all the patient's belongings together. Explain to the patient what you are doing.
- If the patient is expected to return to the unit, you may be asked to gather only a few belongings, such as glasses, dentures, and toiletries.
- Get the patient's medicines, chart, and other personal data from the nurse.
- Assist in the physical transfer.
- Give the records and medication directly to the nurse on the new unit.
- Make sure the patient is safe and comfortable in the new environment before you return to your own unit.

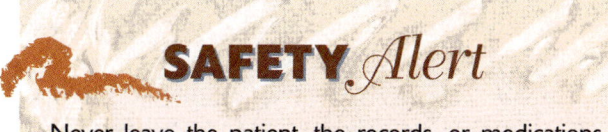

SAFETY *Alert*

Never leave the patient, the records, or medications unattended.

DISCHARGE

In recent years, the cost of health care has increased steadily. A government program known as *diagnosis-related groups* (*DRGs*) was introduced to control hospital costs. Hospitals are paid a specific amount of money for the care of an individual who has a particular condition or disease that is covered by a DRG.

If the hospital can provide the needed care and discharge the patient early, the hospital saves money and may keep the difference between the actual expenses and the DRG allotted payment. If the patient requires a longer hospital stay than is stated by the DRGs and the costs are higher, the hospital absorbs the additional cost. These standards do not apply to private patients. They apply to patients whose care is being paid for by the federal government, such as Medicare patients.

DRGs were developed for Medicare patients, but they are used today by all insurance companies to determine how many hospital days they will pay for. This has resulted in sicker patients being discharged from acute care facilities sooner.

Following hospitalization, many patients are discharged to subacute units or to long-term care facilities for further care, or to home to finish recuperation.

The discharge procedure is usually simple if the patient is going to another facility. The social worker and nurse relay information to the receiving facility. The patient and the patient's belongings are sent to the new facility. Discharge to the patient's home is more complicated and requires a number of actions called *discharge planning* (covered in Unit 34).

The Discharge Process

The **discharge**, or authorized release, of a patient requires a written order from the physician. If a patient indicates an intention to leave without an order, report it to your supervisor immediately. The nurse will make the necessary arrangements. Health care facilities have special policies that must be followed in these cases.

The patient should be spared any fatigue or unnecessary delay when being routinely discharged. (See Procedure 53.) You can help if you:

PROCEDURE 53

DISCHARGING THE PATIENT

1. Check to be sure the physician has ordered the patient to be discharged. If a discharge order has not been written, check with the supervisor before proceeding.

2. Carry out beginning procedure actions.

3. Assemble equipment
   - wheelchair
   - cart to transport items

4. Help the patient to dress, if necessary.

5. Collect the patient's personal belongings. Help the patient check them against the admission list.
   a. Pack, if necessary.
   b. Check valuables against the admission list according to facility policy.
   c. Make sure that all of the patient's belongings have been removed from the closet and bedside stand.
   d. Check to see if medications or other equipment are to be sent home with the patient.
   e. Verify that the patient has received discharge instructions from the nurse, physician, or discharge coordinator.

6. Tell the patient or a member of the family how to

collect valuables from the facility safe, if valuables were put there.

7. Help the patient into a wheelchair.

8. Take the patient to the discharge entrance of the facility.
   a. Help the patient to transfer safely into the vehicle.
   b. Be gracious as you say goodbye.

9. Return the wheelchair.

10. Return to the patient unit.
    a. Strip the bed. Dispose of linen according to facility policy.
    b. Clean and replace equipment used in patient care, according to facility policy.

11. Wash your hands.

12. Record the discharge in accordance with facility policy. Include:
    - time
    - method of transport
    - patient's reaction
    - signature

13. Report completion of task to nurse.

- Check with the nurse to make sure that the physician has written an order for discharge before preparing the patient.
- Gather all the patient's belongings and assist in packing, if necessary. Patients who are well enough usually prefer to assemble their own things. You will need to do this activity completely for other patients.
- Carefully check the closet and bedside table. Disposable equipment is often sent home with the patient. If this is the policy in your facility, be sure that the equipment is clean.

- Check with the nurse for any medications or other treatment-related equipment that should be sent home with the patient.
- Verify that the patient has received discharge instructions from the nurse, physician, or discharge coordinator.
- Never allow a patient to leave the health care facility unassisted. The patient is the staff's responsibility until she has left the building.

REVIEW

A. True/False.

Mark the following true or false by circling T or F.

1. T **F** When transferring a patient, it is all right to leave the patient unattended and return immediately to your own unit.
2. **T** F Use all precautions related to safe transport when admitting or discharging a patient.
3. T **F** You do not need to waste time introducing a new patient to others, because facility stays are very short anyway.
4. T **F** It is all right to allow patients to leave a health care facility at any time.
5. **T** F After discharge, the patient's unit is stripped, cleaned, and restocked.
6. **T** F The patient's unit should be prepared as soon as you are notified that there will be an admission.
7. T **F** During a transfer, the patient's medications remain on the original unit.
8. **T** F Measuring the patient's height and weight is part of the admission procedure.
9. **T** F The discharge order is written by the physician.
10. **T** F You should observe the patient carefully during the admission procedure.

B. Multiple Choice.

Select the one best answer for each of the following.

11. The assistant can do much to help facilitate the admission procedure by
    a. preparing equipment after the patient arrives on the unit.
    b. letting the nurse make all the observations.
    c. giving attention to the details of the procedure.
    d. recognizing that admission to the facility causes more anxiety to the staff than to the patient.

12. When dealing with the newly admitted patient's family, you should
    a. treat them with courtesy and consideration.
    b. send them home.
    c. let the nurse deal with them.
    d. allow them to stay at the patient's bedside at all times.
13. Part of the admission procedure includes
    a. securing a stool specimen.
    b. obtaining a sputum specimen.
    c. working in a hurried manner so the patient knows you are efficient.
    d. measuring vital signs.
14. Valuables that accompany the patient to her unit should be
    a. taken away.
    b. listed and signed for.
    c. left in the bedside stand.
    d. tucked under the pillow for safety.
15. When a patient is transferred, you should always include his
    a. personal belongings.
    b. bed.
    c. pillow.
    d. blood pressure cuffs.

C. Nursing Assistant Challenge.

Mrs. Leon is being admitted because her emphysema is making it very difficult for her to breathe. She is accompanied by her husband and both are obviously nervous. The next morning, her condition worsens. She is moved to the intensive respiratory care unit. Answer the following questions yes or no.

_____ 16. The anxiety of the patient and family is not natural.

_____ 17. You should answer questions about facility routines during admission.

_____ **18.** When taking vital signs, you should use an oral thermometer.

_____ **19.** When Mrs. Leon is transferred, take all of her personal articles with her.

_____ **20.** One way to prepare the unit for admission might include checking for the need for oxygen.

_____ **21.** You should turn Mrs. Leon's oxygen up to at least 6 liters to assist with her breathing.

 # EXPLORING THE WEB

Description	Location
Emory University MedWeb	http://www.medweb.emory.edu
Health Care Professionals Network Policies, Procedures, Guidelines	http://www.wlm-web.com
National Institutes of Health Nursing Policy Manual	http://www.cc.nih.gov/nursingnew/nursingresources/ nursingpolicies.shtml
Nursing Managers Policies	http://www.4nursingmanagers.com
UAMS Clinical Programs Nursing Manual	http://www.uams.edu
UTMB Nursing Practice Standards	http://www.wahoo.utmb.edu

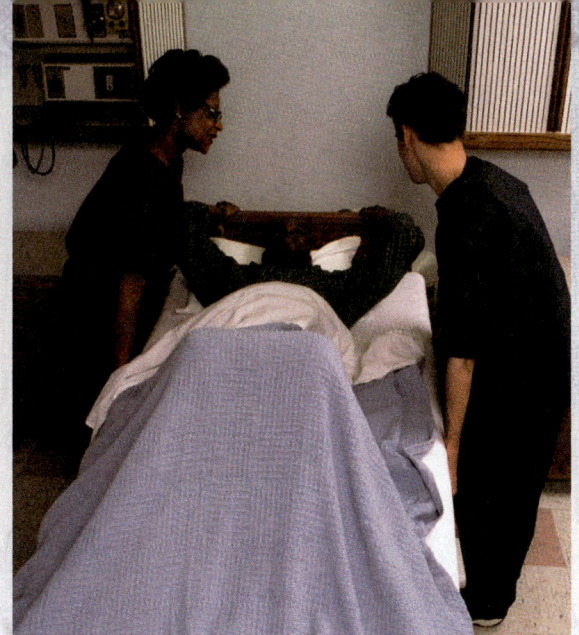

Bedmaking

objectives

After completing this unit, you will be able to:

- Spell and define terms.
- List the different types of beds and their uses.
- Operate each type of bed.
- Properly handle clean and soiled linens.

- Demonstrate the following procedures:
  - Procedure 54 Making a Closed Bed
  - Procedure 55 Opening the Closed Bed
  - Procedure 56 Making an Occupied Bed
  - Procedure 57 Making the Surgical Bed

vocabulary

Learn the meaning and the correct spelling of the following words and phrases:

box (square) corner	closed bed	gatch bed	open bed
CircOlectric® bed	electric bed	mitered corner	Stryker frame

INTRODUCTION

The room, especially the bed, is the patient's home while he or she is in the hospital or health care facility. A well-made bed offers both comfort and safety. It is an extremely important contribution to the well-being of the patient.

OPERATION AND USES OF BEDS IN HEALTH CARE FACILITIES

The types of beds and the methods used to operate them may vary in different health care facilities, but the basic principles of bedmaking are the same. The most common beds are the:

- gatch bed—a stationary bed about 26 inches high. Modern facilities are equipped with beds that can be raised to the desired height for bedside nursing or lowered to 13 inches to accommodate the out-of-bed patient. The position of the head and knee areas of the bed can be adjusted for comfort. This operation may be done manually by turning the cranks.

- electric bed—a bed similar to the gatch bed, in that it can be raised or lowered and the knee and head areas can be adjusted. It is operated electrically (Figure 23-1). You will be using this bed most often in a large facility.

- low bed—low beds are commonly used in health care facilities for patients who are at risk of falls, for whom use of side rails is not desirable. The bed frame is 4 to 6 inches from the floor to the top of the frame deck. These beds reduce the risk of injury if the patient falls from the bed. Some facilities place pads on the floor next to the bed to further reduce the risk of injury. Nursing assistants must use good body mechanics and mechanical lifts when assisting patients into and out of these beds, to prevent back injuries.

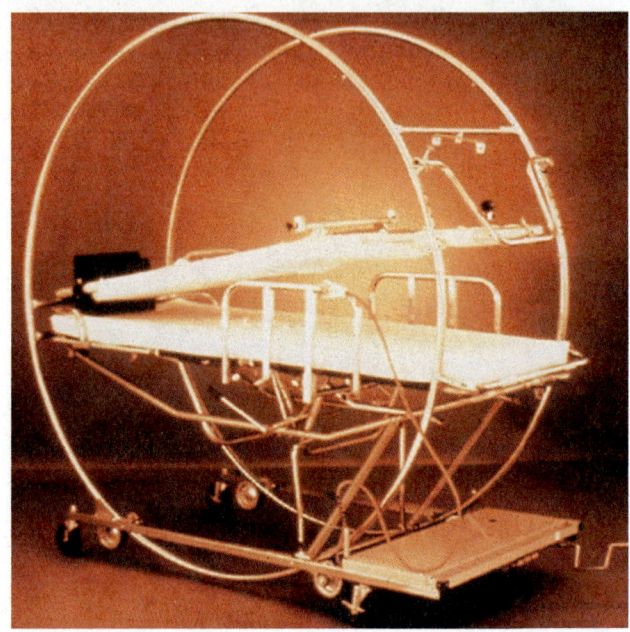

FIGURE 23-2 Turning may be frightening for patients who are in a CircOlectric® bed. Provide calm reassurance. *(Courtesy of Stryker Corporation, Kalamazoo, MI)*

- CircOlectric® bed—a special bed frame placed within a circular frame (Figure 23-2). This bed is operated electrically. The circular frame can be rotated. The patient is secured on the inner frame before the bed is moved. The entire inner frame is rotated forward. This allows for position change without any stress on the patient. After rotating, the patient is on the abdomen.

- Stryker frame, spinal bed, or wedge bed—a turning frame that serves the same purpose as the CircOlectric® but is operated manually. Once the patient is secured by placement of the upper frame, a crank is used to turn the entire frame and the patient. After turning, the patient is on the abdomen. The patient lies on the frame until turned once more (Figure 23-3).

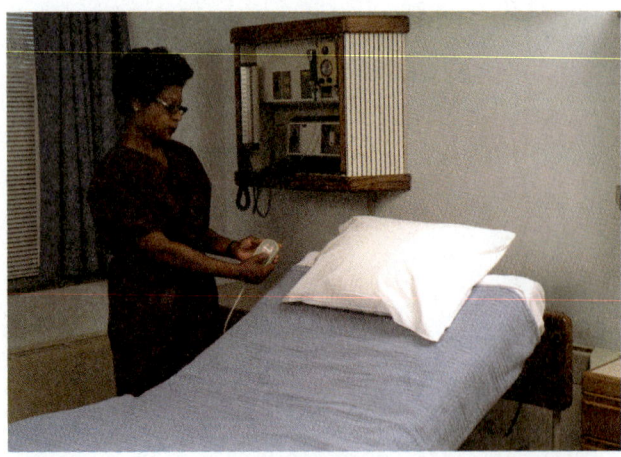

FIGURE 23-1 The typical hospital bed is electronically operated. The head and foot can be adjusted for patient comfort. The height of the bed can be raised, making it easier to give care.

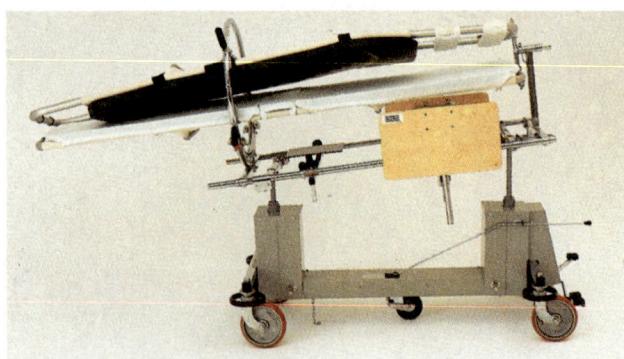

FIGURE 23-3 The Stryker® frame is similar to the CircOlectric® bed, but is manually operated. It is used for patients with pressure ulcers, paralysis, and spinal cord injuries. The patient is sandwiched between two boards when being turned, and may become very frightened. Reassure the patient when turning the frame. *(Courtesy of Stryker Corporation, Kalamazoo, MI)*

SAFETY *Alert*

Use the special turning beds only if you have been trained and are permitted to use them. In most facilities, two or more staff must be present when a patient is turned on a special bed. Make sure to follow the manufacturer's directions for use of the bed, and be certain that all safety straps are fastened properly before you move the patient. When using the Stryker frame, always turn the patient in the direction of the narrow wedge, to reduce the risk of falls. Turn the frame quickly and smoothly. Close the locks and replace the pins after the patient has been turned. If the perineal section of the frame must be removed for patient elimination, remember to replace it promptly.

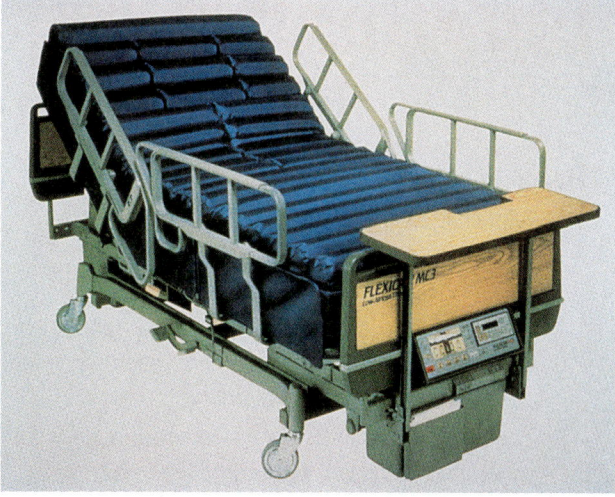

FIGURE 23-4 The low air loss bed is used for pressure ulcer prevention and treatment. Although these beds exert less pressure on the skin than a regular mattress, patients must still be turned and repositioned frequently to prevent skin breakdown. *(Courtesy of Hill-Rom, Charleston, SC)*

Patients with severe burns or spinal injuries are often placed on special beds like the CircOlectric® or Stryker frame, for safety. These beds allow patients to be repositioned with minimal handling of their bodies.

The turning procedure is frightening for many patients. Reassure the patient that he is secure and that turning will proceed without incident. In most facilities, a licensed nurse must be present during turning.

Other types of beds are available for the treatment of patients with multiple or advanced pressure ulcers, flaps, grafts, burns, and intractable pain. For example, one special unit that supports the patient's body evenly is filled with a sand-like material. Warm, dry air circulates through the material to maintain an even temperature and support the body evenly.

A low air loss bed (Figure 23-4) provides pressure relief for patients who have pressure ulcers, those who are at risk of pressure ulcers, and some patients with burns. This mattress is designed to keep the patient cooler and drier than other types of beds. Low air loss beds reduce pressure to the patient's skin, and reduce friction and shearing, which contribute to skin breakdown. These beds use a system of air-filled pillows in which inflation pressure can be adjusted so the characteristics of the support surface are matched to those of the body being supported. The pillows can be inflated and deflated to adjust the level of pressure relief. The design of the bed allows slight air escape upon movement, which reduces pressure.

Patients using a low air loss bed must still be turned and positioned regularly to prevent skin breakdown, which can occur despite the pressure-reducing mattress. Avoid tucking the bottom sheet in tightly, as this increases pressure within the bed. Some facilities use these beds with nylon covers only, without sheets. The nylon cover reduces friction and shearing. Follow the care plan and facility policies. Special underpads are used with the low air loss bed.

Correct operation of any bed or equipment is important for patient safety. Always seek help and instruction from the nurse or another health care professional when using any specialized beds. Never try to operate any bed or equipment with a patient in it without first practicing and gaining security and skill in the procedures. Although different types of hospital beds may be similar in design, the operating instructions vary. For safety, always follow the manufacturers' directions in operating the various therapeutic beds.

SAFETY *Alert*

Become familiar with the features of the low air loss bed used by your facility. Some have bed scales built in, making it possible to weigh the patient without moving her from the bed. CPR is not effective in a low air loss bed, even with a back board. The beds have a switch that rapidly deflates the air pillows in an emergency. Become familiar with the location and operation of the features of the bed.

BEDMAKING

Bed linen is always changed when soiled. It is routinely changed:

- daily in the acute care facility.
- two or three times a week in long-term care facilities.

Residents in long-term care may prefer to use their own pillows, blankets, and spreads.

guidelines *for*

Handling Linens and Making the Bed

Handling Linens

1. Wash hands and use gloves if necessary; other personal protective equipment may also be required.

2. Laundry hampers placed in the hallway should be at least one room away from clean linen carts, or placed according to facility policy.

3. The clean linen cart is always covered; replace the cover after removing required linen.

4. Take only the linens you need into the patient's room.

5. Linens that touch the floor are considered dirty and are placed in the laundry hamper; they are not used.

6. Avoid contact between the linens and your uniform (for both clean and soiled linens).

7. Unused linen is never returned to the clean linen cart; it is placed in the laundry hamper.

8. As soiled linen is removed from the bed, keep the soiled areas on the inside and fold or roll the linen toward the center.

9. Never shake bed linens, because microbes will be released into the air.

10. Soiled linen is never placed on environmental surfaces in the room, such as the overbed table, chair, or floor; soiled linens are placed in the appropriate laundry hamper (follow facility policy).

11. Fill laundry hampers no more than two-thirds full. Keep the lid of the hamper on tightly at all times.

12. Many facilities do not permit laundry hampers or barrels to be taken into the patient's room. Soiled linen may be placed in a plastic bag or a pillowcase in the room. Make a cuff at the top of the bag or open end of the pillowcase and place the cuff over the back of the chair. When the bag or case is two-thirds full, secure the top and place it in the hamper in the hallway.

13. Laundry hampers or barrels are returned to the utility room after use, or as directed by facility policy.

Making the Bed

1. Use proper body mechanics at all times to prevent back injury.

2. Work on one side of the bed at a time to complete removal of soiled linen and placement of clean linen.

3. Make sure the bottom sheet and draw sheet (if used) are smooth and unwrinkled (wrinkles in bed linens can lead to skin breakdown, especially for patients who must remain in bed).

4. Follow the care plan for positioning the head and foot of the bed, the number of pillows to be used, and the use of pillows for positioning.

OSHA *Alert*

Elevating the bed to a working height that is comfortable for you takes a minute, but it is one of the most important things you will do to protect your back. Stay on one side of the bed until it is completely made before moving to the other side. This helps organize your time and conserves energy.

SAFETY *Alert*

Be alert when removing bed linen. Look carefully for items that are a potential source of injury to yourself or the patient, such as lancets and needles. Make sure the patient's personal items are not accidentally sent to the laundry with the bed linen.

Closed Bed

The **closed bed** is made following discharge of a patient and after the unit is cleaned (terminal cleaning). It remains closed until a new patient is to be admitted. Details are important. The same procedure is followed when making an unoccupied bed, but the bed is opened as a final step when a patient is to occupy it shortly. (Refer to Procedure 54.)

PROCEDURE 54

MAKING A CLOSED BED

1. Wash your hands and assemble equipment:
   - 2 pillowcases
   - pillow
   - spread
   - blankets, as needed
   - 2 large sheets (90" × 108") (substitute one fitted sheet, if used)
   - cotton draw sheet or half sheet (if used)
   - plastic or rubber draw sheet (if used in your facility)
   - Mattress pad and cover, if mattress is not plastic-treated

   Note: Mattresses that are treated with plastic do not require a moisture-proof sheet or cotton half sheet (draw sheet). In selected cases, the half sheet is used as a lifter to assist in moving the patient. It is sometimes used simply to keep the bottom sheet clean. Some facilities use fitted bottom sheets. If this is so, use a fitted sheet in place of one of the large sheets.

2. Elevate the bed to a comfortable working height in the horizontal position. Lock bed wheels so the bed will not roll. Place a chair at the side of the bed.

3. Arrange the linen on the chair in the order in which it is to be used.

4. Position the mattress to the head of the bed by grasping the mattress handles (or the edge of the mattress, if no handles are present).

5. If used, place a mattress cover on the mattress. Adjust it smoothly for corners. You will work entirely from one side of the bed until that side is completed. Then go to the other side of the bed. This conserves time and energy.

6. Place the mattress pad even with the top of the mattress and unfold it.

7. Place the bottom sheet on the bed and unfold it, seam side down and wide hem at the top. The small hem should be brought to the foot of the mattress (Figure 23-5). The center fold should be at the center of the bed. If a fitted bottom sheet is used, fit it smoothly around one corner (Figures 23-6A and B).

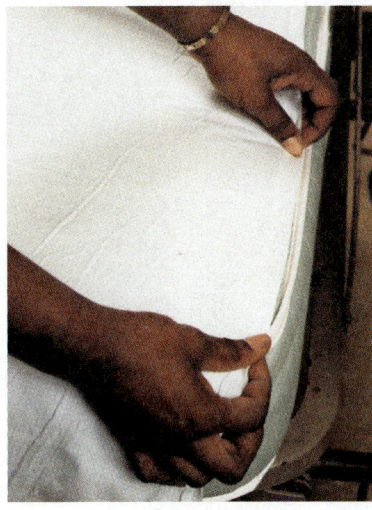

FIGURE 23-5 Place the flat bottom sheet even with the end of the mattress at the foot of the bed.

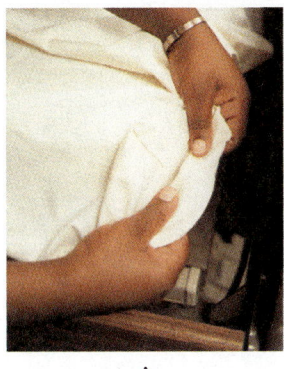
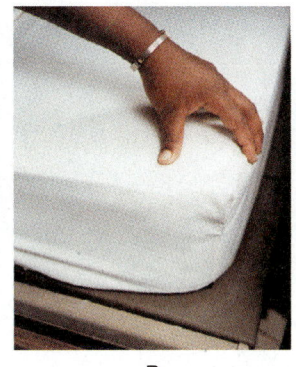

A   B

FIGURE 23-6A and **B** If a fitted bottom sheet is used, pull and smooth it around the corner.

8. Tuck 12 to 18 inches of sheet smoothly over the top of the mattress (Figures 23-7A to C).

9. Make a **mitered corner** (Figure 23-8). The square corner, preferred by some facilities, is made in a way similar to the mitered corner.

10. Tuck in the sheet on one side, keeping the sheet straight. Work from the head to the foot of the bed. If using a fitted sheet, adjust it over the head and bottom ends of the mattress.

11. If used, place the plastic draw sheet and half sheet with upper edge about 14 inches from the head of the mattress and tuck under one side. Be sure that the half sheet covers the plastic sheet.

continues

PROCEDURE 54

continued

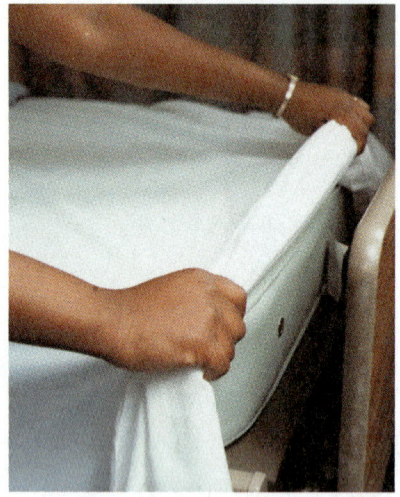

FIGURE 23-7A Gather about 12 to 18 inches of the top sheet at the bottom of the bed.

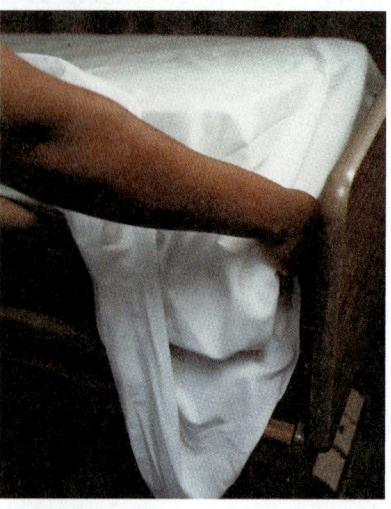

FIGURE 23-7B Face the foot of the bed and lift the mattress with your near hand.

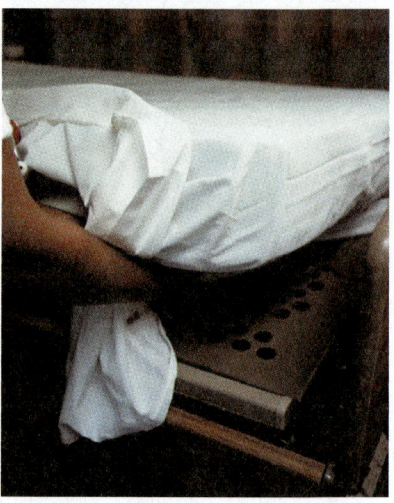

FIGURE 23-7C Bring the sheet smoothly over the end of the mattress with your opposite hand.

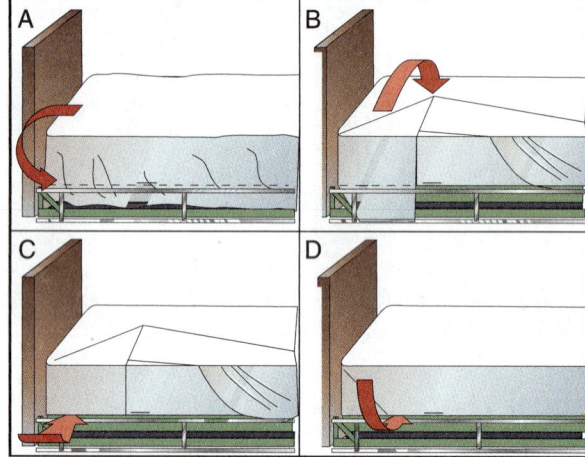

FIGURE 23-8 Making a mitered corner. A. The sheet is hanging loose at the side of the bed. B. Pick up the sheet about 12 inches from the head of the bed to form a triangle. C. Tuck in the sheet at the head of the bed. Pick up the triangle and place your other hand at the edge of the bed near the head to hold the edge of the sheet in place. Bring the triangle over the edge of the mattress and tuck it smoothly under the mattress. Tuck in the rest of the sheet along the side of the mattress. Make sure the sheet is wrinkle-free.

It should cover the area from above the patient's shoulders to below the hips.

12. Unfold and place the top sheet on the bed, seam up, top hem even with the upper edge of the mattress and the center fold in the center of the bed.

13. Spread the blanket over the top sheet and foot of mattress. Keep the blanket centered.

14. Tuck the top sheet and blanket under the mattress at the foot of the bed as far as the center only. Make a **box (square) corner** (Figures 23-9A to C).

15. Place the spread with its top hem even with the head of the mattress. Unfold the spread to the foot of the bed.

16. Tuck the spread under the mattress at the foot of the bed and miter the corner. Sometimes the spread may be placed directly on top of the sheet. Rather than tucking the sheet, blanket, and/or spread under the end of the mattress separately and forming separate corners, all of the covers may be tucked under at the same time and one corner formed (Figures 23-10A to E).

17. Go to the other side of the bed. Fanfold the top covers to the center of the bed so you can work with the lower sheets and pad.

18. Tuck the bottom sheet under the head of the mattress and miter the corner. Working from top to bottom, smooth out all wrinkles and tighten these sheets as much as possible to provide comfort. (Adjust a fitted bottom sheet smoothly and securely around the mattress corners.)

continues

PROCEDURE 54

continued

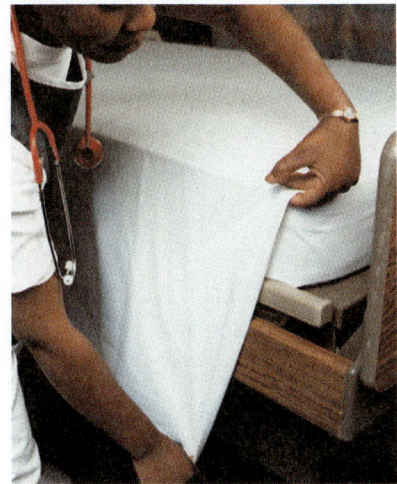

FIGURE 23-9A Make the square (box) corner following the steps shown in Figures 23-8A–C. Then, holding the corner with your left hand, grasp the bottom of the sheet and pull it straight down until the fold is even with the edge of the mattress.

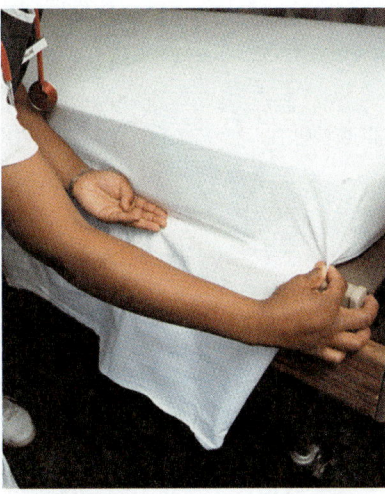

FIGURE 23-9B Holding the square corner in place, tuck the remaining sheet under the mattress.

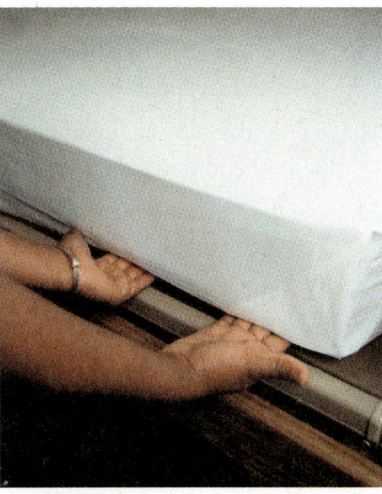

FIGURE 23-9C The finished square corner should look like this.

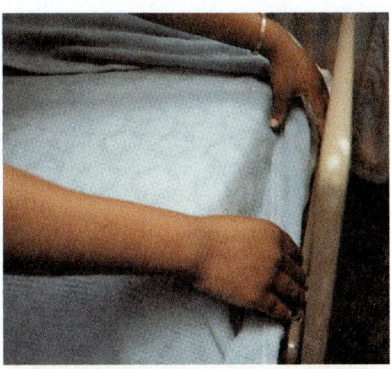

FIGURE 23-10A Gather the top sheet and bedspread together. Smooth evenly over the end of the mattress.

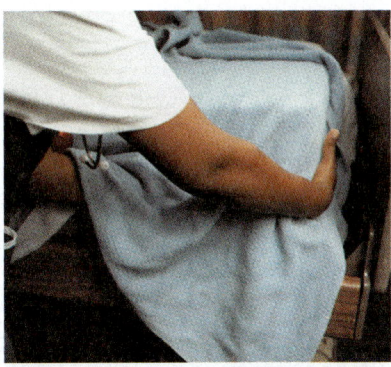

FIGURE 23-10B Tuck the sheet and spread under the mattress together.

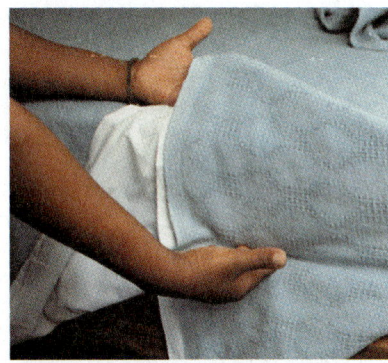

FIGURE 23-10C Continue as with the procedure for a mitered corner.

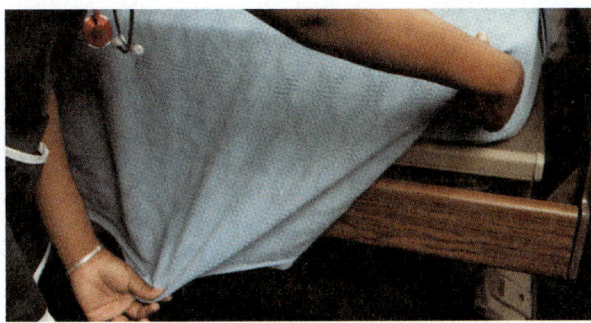

FIGURE 23-10D Slide your finger to the end to make a smooth edge.

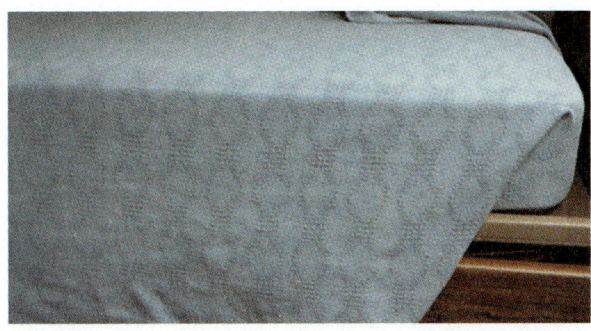

FIGURE 23-10E The completed top bedding. Repeat the procedure on the other side of the bed.

continues

PROCEDURE 54

continued

19. Grasp the protective draw sheet (if used) and cotton draw sheet in the center. Tuck these sheets under the mattress.

20. Tuck in the top sheet and blanket at the foot of the bed and miter the corner.

21. Fold the top sheet back over the blanket, making an 8-inch cuff.

22. Tuck in the spread at the foot of the bed and miter the corner. Bring the top of the spread to the head of the mattress.

23. Insert the pillow into a pillowcase:
    a. Place your hands in the clean case, freeing the corners.
    b. Grasp the center of the end seam with hand outside the case and turn the case back over your hand (Figure 23-11A).
    c. Grasp the pillow through the case at the center of one end. Pull the case over the pillow with your free hand (Figures 23-11B and 23-11C). (Do not allow the pillow to touch your uniform.)

    d. Adjust the corners of the pillow to fit in the corners of the case.

24. Place the pillow at the head of the bed with the open end away from the door.

25. Lower the bed to the lowest horizontal position.

26. Arrange the room as follows:
    a. Replace the bedside table parallel to the bed. Place the chair in its assigned location.
    b. Place the overbed table over the foot of the bed opposite the chair.
    c. Place the signal cord within easy reach of the patient.
    d. Leave the side rails down.
    e. Check for possible hazards, such as gatch handles that are out of place.

27. Leave the unit neat and tidy.

28. Wash your hands.

29. Report completion of the task to your supervisor.

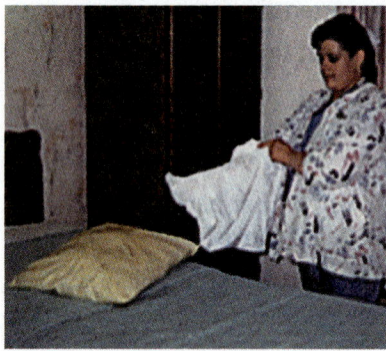

FIGURE 23-11A Grasp the pillowcase at the seam and fold it back and over your wrist, inside out.

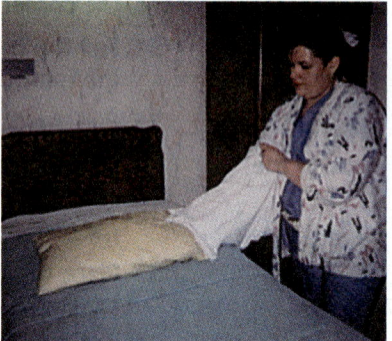

FIGURE 23-11B Grasp the end of the pillow in the center with your pillowcase-covered hand.

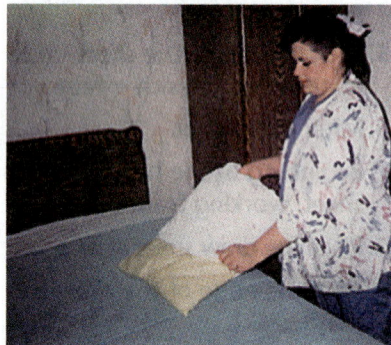

FIGURE 23-11C Unfold and smooth the pillowcase over the pillow.

INFECTION CONTROL *Alert*

Wear gloves when removing bed linen that is wet or soiled. Place the soiled linen in a plastic bag or linen hamper. Avoid contaminating environmental surfaces with gloves that have handled soiled linen. Remove one glove, if necessary. Follow facility policy for disinfecting the mattress. Allow it to dry. Discard your gloves and wash your hands. It is not necessary to wear gloves when you are handling clean linen. Cracks in the mattress are a potential source of odors and contamination. Report cracks in the mattress to the proper person in your facility.

The Unoccupied Bed

Beds are often made while patients are up in a shower or chair. Follow the procedure for making a closed bed but then fanfold the top bedding halfway down. This "opens" the bed and makes it easier for the person to get into it.

The Open Bed

The open bed is like a sign saying "welcome" to the new patient (Figure 23-12). It indicates that the patient's arrival has been made known to the assistant. It also shows that the unit has been prepared. In long-term care facilities, the bed is not opened unless the resident is going to bed soon. (See Procedure 55.)

The Occupied Bed

Unless the patient is permitted out of bed by physician's order, the bed is made with the patient in it. (See Procedure 56.) Bedmaking usually follows the bed bath, while the patient is covered with a bath blanket. It may, however, be done any time it would add to the comfort of the patient.

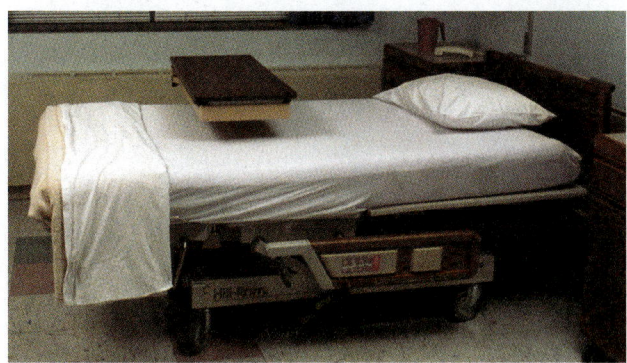

FIGURE 23-12 Open the closed bed by drawing the bedding to the foot of the bed and fanfolding it.

SAFETY Alert

Never turn your back on the patient or leave the bedside when the bed is in the high position and the side rail is down.

Surgical Bed

The surgical bed provides a safe, warm environment to receive the postsurgical patient. It must be made in such a way that movement from stretcher to bed is made with maximum safety and minimum effort. For this reason, the bed should be left open and at stretcher height. (See Procedure 57.)

All equipment needed to monitor vital signs and to supervise recovery should be in place and ready for use. You should also keep alert for the patient's return so you can help make a safe transfer from stretcher to bed.

Modern surgical techniques have shortened the time many patients stay in an acute care facility after surgery. Patients are often admitted on the morning of surgery to special units, have the surgery performed, return to these same units immediately after surgery, and are discharged the same day to recuperate at home. These units are called ambulatory, short-term, or day-care units. To prepare a postsurgical bed in one of these units:

- Tighten the bottom linen.
- Fanfold the top linen to the side or foot of bed.
- Raise the bed to stretcher height and lock the wheels.
- Place the equipment to check vital signs, emesis basin, and tissues by the recovery bed.

PROCEDURE 55

OPENING THE CLOSED BED

1. Wash your hands.
2. Check assignment for bed location.
3. Raise the bed to a comfortable working height in the horizontal position. Move the overbed table to one side.
4. Lock the bed wheels.
5. Loosen the top bedding.
6. Facing the head of the bed, grasp the top sheet and spread and fanfold it to the foot of the bed.

7. Return the bed to the lowest horizontal position. Place the overbed table over the foot of the bed.
8. Place the call bell near the pillow or within easy reach. It should be visible and within reach of the patient at all times.
9. Leave the unit neat and tidy.
10. Wash your hands.
11. Report completion of the task to the nurse.

PROCEDURE 56

MAKING AN OCCUPIED BED

1. Carry out beginning procedure actions.

2. Assemble the equipment needed:
   - disposable gloves (if linens are soiled with blood, body fluids, secretions, or excretions)
   - cotton draw sheet or turning sheet for selected patients
   - 2 large flat sheets (or one large flat sheet and one fitted bottom sheet)
   - 2 pillowcases
   - laundry hamper

3. Place the bedside chair at the foot of the bed.

4. Arrange the clean linen on the chair in the order in which it is to be used.

5. The bed should be flat, with wheels locked, unless otherwise indicated. Raise the bed to working horizontal height. Lower the side rail on your side of the bed.

6. If the bed linens are soiled with blood or other body fluids, wash your hands and put on disposable gloves.

7. Loosen the bedclothes on your side by lifting the edge of the mattress with one hand and drawing the bedclothes out with the other. Never shake the linen. This spreads germs.

8. Put the side rail up and go to the opposite side of the bed.

9. Adjust the mattress to the head of the bed (Figure 23-13). Get help, if necessary.

10. Remove the top covers except for the top sheet, one at a time. Fold to bottom. Pick up in the center. Place them over the back of chair if they are to be reused.

📝 *Note: Carefully check each piece of linen for foreign articles (such as patient care equipment, eyeglasses, dentures, items of food, or eating utensils). Remove any such items.*

11. Place the clean sheet or bath blanket over the top sheet. Have the patient hold the top edge of the clean sheet if able. If the patient is unable to help, tuck the sheet beneath the patient's shoulder.

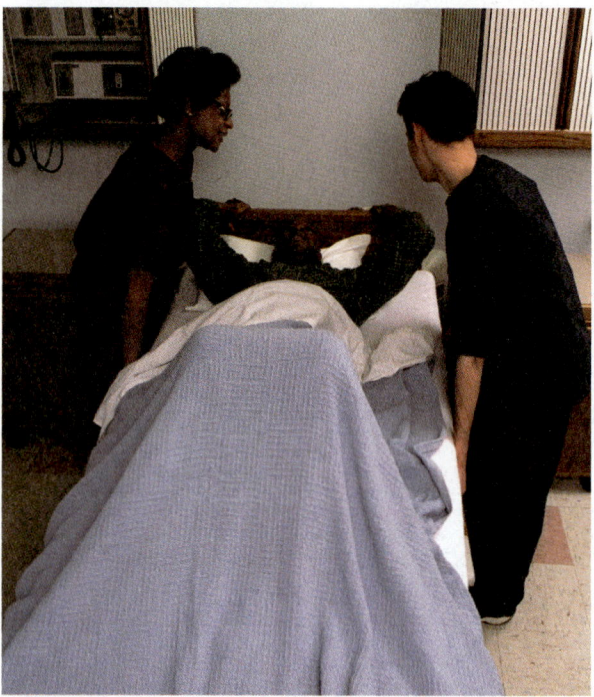

FIGURE 23-13 The patient grasps the head of the bed and pushes in with the heels while two nursing assistants pull the mattress to the head of the bed.

12. Slide the soiled sheet out, from top to bottom. Put it in a hamper or plastic bag.

13. Ask the patient to move to the side of the bed toward you. Assist if necessary. Move one pillow with the patient and remove the other pillow. Pull up the side rail. (Alternatively, you may ask the patient to turn toward the opposite side of the bed, holding onto the raised side rail. You would then fanfold the sheet, as in step 15, but there would be no need to go to the other side of the bed.)

14. Go to the other side of the bed. Fanfold the soiled cotton draw sheet, if used, and bottom sheet close to the patient (Figure 23-14).

15. Straighten the mattress pad. If the bottom sheet is to be changed, place a clean sheet on the bed so that the narrow hem comes to the edge of the mattress at the foot. The seamed side of the hem is toward the bed. The lengthwise center fold of

continues

PROCEDURE 56

continued

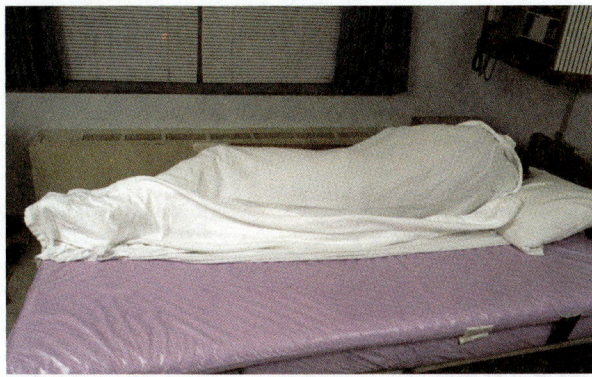

FIGURE 23-14 Fanfold the soiled bottom sheet to the center of the bed as close to the patient as possible. Note that the bottom linen is flat and the patient is positioned to the far side of the bed.

the sheet is at the center of the bed. Fanfold the opposite side of sheet close to patient.

16. Tuck the top of the sheet under the head of the mattress.

17. Make a mitered corner.

18. Tuck the side of the sheet under the mattress, working toward the foot of the bed.

19. Position a fresh draw sheet, if used. Tuck it under the mattress.

20. Ask or assist the patient to roll toward you, over the fanfolded linen. Move the pillow with the patient.

21. Raise the side rails. Test for security.

22. Go to the other side of the bed. Lower the side rail. Remove the soiled linen by rolling the edges inward. *Keep soiled linen away from your uniform.* Placed soiled linen in the hamper or plastic bag. (Raise the side rail if leaving the bedside.)

23. Remove gloves, if worn, and discard according to facility policy.

24. Wash your hands.

25. Pull the clean bottom sheet into place. Tuck it under the mattress at the head of the bed. Make a mitered corner.

26. Pull gently to eliminate wrinkles. Then tuck the side of the sheet under the mattress, working from top to bottom.

27. Pull the draw sheet smoothly into place. Tuck it firmly under the mattress.

28. Place the top sheet over the patient. Remove the bath blanket.

29. Complete the bed as an unoccupied bed. To reduce pressure on toes, grasp the top bedding over the toes and pull straight up. Some patients prefer not to have the blanket and top sheet or spread tucked in.

30. Assist the patient to turn on his or her back. Place a clean pillowcase on the pillow that is not being used. Replace that pillow. Change the other pillowcase.

31. Carry out procedure completion actions.

PROCEDURE 57

MAKING THE SURGICAL BED

1. Wash your hands.

2. Check assignment for unit location.

3. Assemble the following equipment:
   - disposable gloves (if linens are soiled with blood or body fluids)
   - articles for basic bed
   - one extra draw sheet
   - bath blanket for warmth
   - one protective (rubber or plastic) draw sheet (if used in facility)
   - roll of one-inch gauze bandage

4. Lock the bed.

5. Apply gloves if linen is wet or soiled with blood or body fluids.

continues

PROCEDURE 57

continued

6. Strip and discard used linen.

7. Remove gloves and discard according to facility policy.

8. Wash your hands.

9. Make the bottom foundation bed (steps 1–11 in Procedure 54). Repeat on the opposite side of the bed.

10. Place a protective draw sheet over the head of the mattress sheet. Cover with a cotton draw sheet. Miter the corners and tuck them in on the sides.

11. Place the top sheet, blanket, and spread in the usual manner. Do not tuck them in.

12. Fold the linen back at the foot of the bed even with the edge of the mattress.

13. Fanfold the upper covers and top sheet to the far side of the bed (Figure 23-15).

14. Tie a waterproof pillow to the head of the bed with gauze bandaging or place according to facility policy.

15. Arrange the bed so there is adequate room to position a stretcher next to it. Leave the bed locked and at the same height as a stretcher.

16. Check the unit for obvious hazards.

17. Leave the room neat and tidy.

18. Wash your hands.

19. Report completion of the task to nurse.

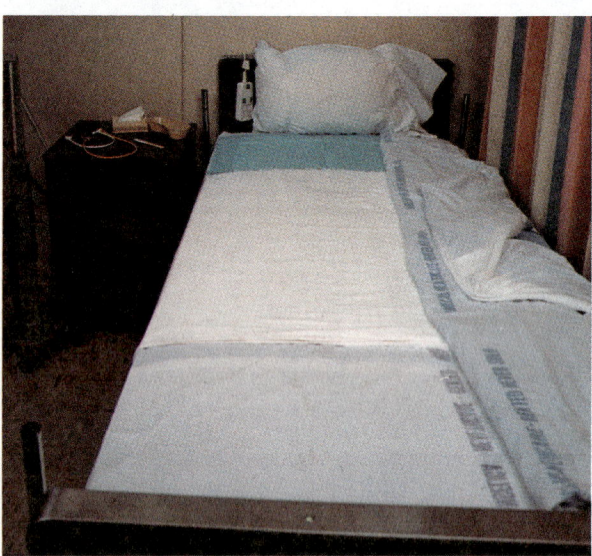

FIGURE 23-15 Prepare the surgical bed by fanfolding the covers to the far side of the bed. Raise the bed to stretcher height.

REVIEW

A. True/False.

Mark the following true or false by circling T or F.

1. T (F) The patient is most comfortable in a closed bed.

2. (T) F The Stryker frame is used to turn patients easily.

3. (T) F You should not attempt to operate a bed until you have been thoroughly supervised.

4. (T) F The closed bed is made after terminal cleaning is finished.

5. T (F) Bottom bed linen can be loosely tucked as long as there are no wrinkles when you have finished.

6. (T) F A mitered corner is tucked in, forming a triangle.

7. (T) F Shaking linen as you change the bed spreads germs.

8. (T) F The open bed is like a sign saying "welcome."

9. (T) F Before making an occupied bed, adjust the mattress to the head of the bed.

10. (T) F The side rail opposite you must be up as you make an occupied bed.

B. Multiple Choice.

Select the one best answer for each of the following.

11. Loosening the top bedding at the foot of the bed is done
    a. to improve the appearance of the bed.
    b. in unoccupied beds.
    c. as folds in the bottom sheet.
    d. to reduce pressure on the toes.

12. When making an unoccupied bed, make the
   a. entire bottom first.
   b. far side of the bottom and top first.
   c. near side of the entire bed first.
   d. far side of the bottom first.

13. Before making an unoccupied bed,
   a. elevate it to a comfortable working height.
   b. keep the bed at the lowest horizontal height.
   c. raise the head portion.
   d. raise the side rails on the opposite side.

14. Before making any bed, always
   a. raise the side rails.
   b. lower the bed to the lowest horizontal height.
   c. lock the bed wheels.
   d. raise the head of the bed.

15. Sheets should be smoothly tucked in over the head of the mattress
   a. 5 to 7 inches.
   b. 12 to 18 inches.
   c. 20 to 24 inches.
   d. 26 to 30 inches.

16. If a draw sheet or lift sheet is used, it should be placed so that it covers the area under the patient's
   a. head and shoulders.
   b. heels and lower legs.
   c. buttocks only.
   d. shoulders to buttocks.

17. When placing the case on the pillow,
   a. tuck it under your chin.
   b. lay the pillow on the chair.
   c. pull the case over while grasping the pillow with the opposite hand.
   d. lay the pillow on the bedside stand.

18. When opening a closed bed,
   a. fanfold top bedding to the foot.
   b. loosen all top bedding.
   c. leave the bed at its highest horizontal height.
   d. raise the head of the bed.

19. The top bedding in a surgical bed is
   a. untucked and draped.
   b. tucked in on two sides.
   c. untucked and fanfolded.
   d. made with toe pleats.

20. A common element to all bedmaking is
   a. fanfolding the linen.
   b. leaving the unit neat and tidy.
   c. leaving the bed in the high position.
   d. using the same linen and equipment.

C. Nursing Assistant Challenge.

21. You are assigned to make a closed bed. You have washed your hands and assembled the following equipment: pillow, blanket, spread, mattress pad, and mattress cover. What else will you need?

 # EXPLORING THE WEB

Description	Location
Hospital bed and bedrail safety advice	http://www.ecri.org
Hospital bed safety	http://www.fda.gov/cdrh/beds
Safe linen handling information	http://www.nailm.com
A Guide to Bed Safety	http://www.patientsafety.com
Hill-Rom Beds	http://www.hill-rom.com
Stryker Corporation	http://www.strykercorp.com
Stryker Medical	http://www.med.strykercorp.com

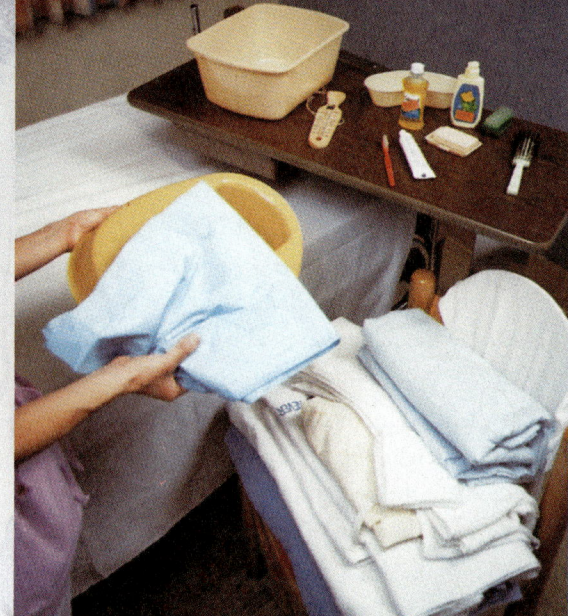

Patient Bathing

objectives

After completing this unit, you will be able to:

- Spell and define terms.
- Describe the safety precautions for patient bathing.
- List the purposes of bathing patients.
- State the value of whirlpool baths.
- Demonstrate the following procedures:
  - Procedure 58 Assisting with the Tub Bath or Shower
  - Procedure 59 Bed Bath
  - Procedure 60 Changing the Patient's Gown
  - Procedure 61 Waterless Bed Bath
  - Procedure 62 Partial Bath
  - Procedure 63 Female Perineal Care
  - Procedure 64 Male Perineal Care
  - Procedure 65 Hand and Fingernail Care
  - Procedure 66 Bed Shampoo
  - Procedure 67 Dressing and Undressing the Patient

vocabulary

Learn the meaning and the correct spelling of the following words and phrases:

axilla	genitalia	perineum
cuticle	perineal care	pubic

INTRODUCTION

A daily bath is as important for the patient as it is for you. Following the bath, the patient feels relaxed, clean, and refreshed. A bath with warm water and mild soap:

- Removes dirt and perspiration
- Increases circulation
- Provides the patient with mild exercise
- Provides an opportunity for close observation

You as the caregiver are able to see firsthand how the patient's condition is improving, declining, or changing in any way. Your observations are valuable aids to accurate nursing assessments.

With the physician's permission, the patient may be allowed to take regular tub baths or showers. Other patients will be bathed in bed.

Bathing may be performed as:

- Tub bath
- Shower bath
- Complete bed bath
- Partial bed bath
- Self-sponge bath or waterless bath
- Whirlpool bath
- Perineal care

During bathing, special attention should be given to skin areas that touch, including:

- Between the legs
- Under the arms
- Under the breasts
- Under the scrotum
- Between the buttocks
- Around the anus
- For obese people, under folds of skin or fat

Gently sponge and pat these areas dry. Follow facility policy for the use of talcum or corn starch.

A partial bath cleans the hands, face, back, axillae, buttocks, and genitals. It is very refreshing. Many patients will be able to help with bathing. Whenever possible, encourage patients to do so.

Waterless Bath

Some facilities are taking a new approach to bathing called *waterless bathing*. It may also be called *basinless bathing* or *bag bath*. The only equipment needed is a package of premoistened disposable washcloths (Figure 24-1). Each package contains washcloths moistened with a special cleansing solution that evaporates quickly after being applied so that drying is not necessary. Eight washcloths are supplied so that separate parts of the body (face, arms, legs, torso, and genitalia) can be washed. The washcloths can be warmed in the microwave for comfort. This equipment can be used by the nursing assistant to administer a bath or by the patient to self-bathe.

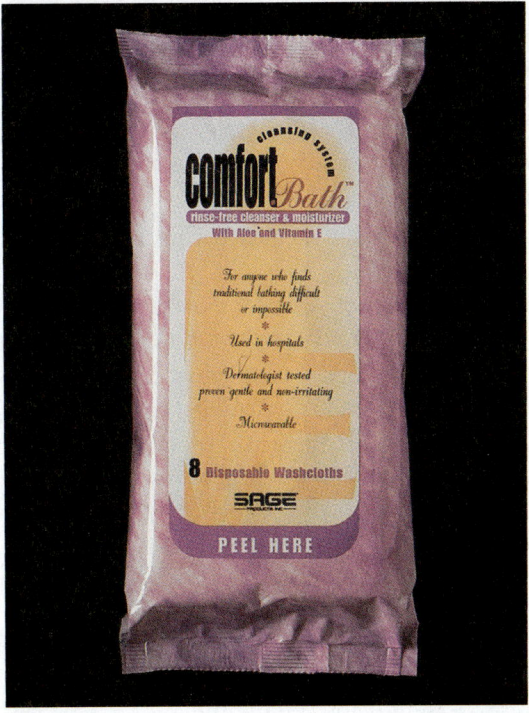

FIGURE 24-1 The waterless bathing system may be used at room temperature, or warmed for comfort. Although the product is more expensive than more conventional methods of bathing, the time savings make it worthwhile. It is gentle on the patient's skin. *(Courtesy of Sage Products, Inc.)*

The procedure is similar to a bed bath, with cleansing done in the same order:

- Face and neck
- Chest and abdomen
- Far arm and hand
- Near arm and hand
- Far leg and foot
- Near leg and foot

INFECTION CONTROL *Alert*

Waterless bathing products are designed to be used for one bath. Smaller kits containing four cloths are also available for partial baths and perineal care. The package may be resealed if not all of the cloths are used. However, the open package should be dated and discarded in 48 to 72 hours, or according to facility infection control guidelines. Follow facility policy for discarding unused cloths after the bath is completed. Discard used cloths properly, according to facility policy. Avoid flushing them down the toilet. A plastic bag at the bedside works well for cloth disposal.

- Back and buttocks
- Perineum

The waterless bathing system has several advantages:

- It is faster and more economical for the facility; each bath takes approximately 8 to 10 minutes.
- It is less fatiguing for the patient.
- It conserves moisture, reduces drying, and is gentler to skin than soaps.
- It creates less friction, because the cloths are softer than regular washcloths and towels, and drying is eliminated.

The following precautions are used when bathing patients with the waterless bathing system:

- The washcloths may be used at room temperature, but many facilities microwave them for comfort. Monitor the temperature carefully to prevent overheating and intermittent hot spots that could injure the patient.
- Peel the label back or open the package before heating to avoid bursting in the microwave.
- Follow manufacturers' directions for heating the package. One minute is usually sufficient to warm the contents to a comfortable temperature.
- The cloths in the package are for single use only.
- Discard unused cloths within 72 hours of opening the package, or immediately if they are dry.

Whirlpool Bath

The most stimulating form of bathing for patients is a therapeutic bath that is given in a whirlpool tub (Figure 24-2). The whirlpool bath benefits patients because:

- The temperature of the water can be regulated to a constant 97°F.

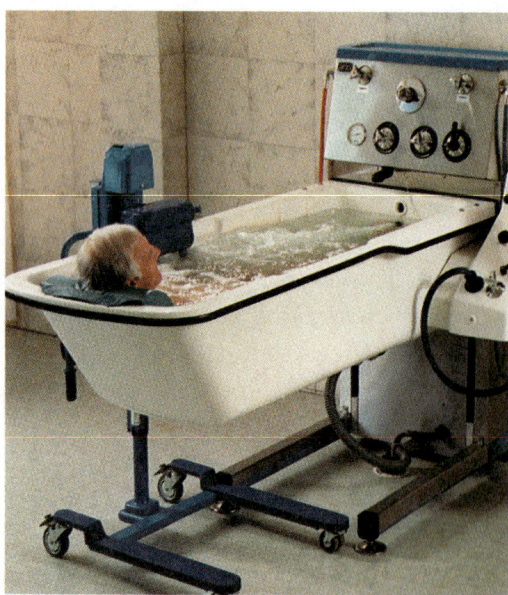

FIGURE 24-2 The water in the whirlpool circulates, maintaining a constant temperature and stimulating circulation. *(Courtesy of Arjo-Century, Inc.)*

> **INFECTION CONTROL** *Alert*
>
> The jets in some whirlpool tubs have the potential to harbor dangerous pathogens. Follow facility policies for carefully cleaning the tub with the proper disinfectant solution. Make sure that you follow directions correctly and run the disinfectant through the tub for the correct length of time.

> **INFECTION CONTROL** *Alert*
>
> Check with the nurse before giving a whirlpool bath to a patient with a surgical incision or pressure ulcer.

- The movement of the water stimulates circulation.
- Warm, circulating water is relaxing and invigorating.
- It provides the value of whirlpool activity with cleansing.

Tips: Never pour liquid soap or shampoo into a whirlpool tub. A tiny bit of liquid soap will result in an abundance of suds. If the patient accidentally creates a suds problem, rub a bar of soap against the walls of the tub to reduce the bubbles.

Care of the hair, teeth, and nails usually follows the bath procedure, but may be carried out as independent procedures. Range-of-motion exercises frequently follow bathing.

PATIENT BATHING

Nursing assistants are frequently assigned to bathe patients. It is important to follow the guidelines and the procedures for bathing carefully to ensure patient comfort and safety. (Refer to Procedures 58, 59, and 61 to 64.)

> **SAFETY** *Alert*
>
> Make sure a chair is available next to the tub or shower in case the patient needs to sit quickly. Turn the hot water on last and off first to prevent injury.

Safety Measures for Special Treatments

Patients receiving special treatments can be bathed. They include, for example, the patient who is receiving an IV, has drainage tubes, or is receiving oxygen. These patients, however, need special care.

Be careful, as you bathe and move the patient, that you:

- Do not put stress on the tubes.
- Never lower the IV container below the level of the infusion site.
- Never raise the drainage tube above the drainage site.

INFECTION CONTROL *Alert*

Think about what precautions are necessary as you perform the procedures in this chapter. Apply the principles of standard precautions. However, avoid overkill. Patients need to be touched. Do not wear gloves for the entire bathing procedure unless there is a reason to do so. When bathing patients, remove the gloves and put on a clean pair immediately prior to contact with mucous membranes and nonintact skin. Do not cross-contaminate body sites by wearing the same pair of gloves for the entire procedure. Avoid contaminating the environment with your used gloves. Discard gloves properly. Wash your hands after removing gloves.

AGE-APPROPRIATE CARE *Alert*

Most patients, young and old, have some independence with activities of daily living when they are in the home. Sometimes they are able to continue to do all or part of these skills. If so, encourage them to continue, unless contraindicated. Provide the supplies needed and arrange them conveniently so the patient can use them. Supervise the patient and assist if needed. This may take longer, but you will reinforce the patient's feelings of self-worth by allowing her to do these things. Organize your work so that you can do something else while the patient is performing self-care skills, as appropriate. This makes good use of your time. If the patient is unable to complete the task, finish it promptly without complaint.

guidelines *for*

Patient Bathing

- Wear disposable gloves if there may be contact with open lesions, blood, body fluids, secretions, or excretions.
- Make sure the shower or tub is cleaned before and after each use (Figure 24-3).
- Check that all safety aids, such as hand rails, shower chairs, tub seats/benches, and hydraulic lifts are in good repair and proper working order.
- Always fasten the safety belt when moving a patient into or out of a whirlpool tub with a hydraulic lift seat.
- Protect patients from fatigue by transporting patients to and from the tub room and carrying out the bathing procedure as efficiently as possible.
- Make sure the patient's body is covered during transport.
- If a patient falls in the tub or shower room or feels faint during bathing, do not leave him alone.

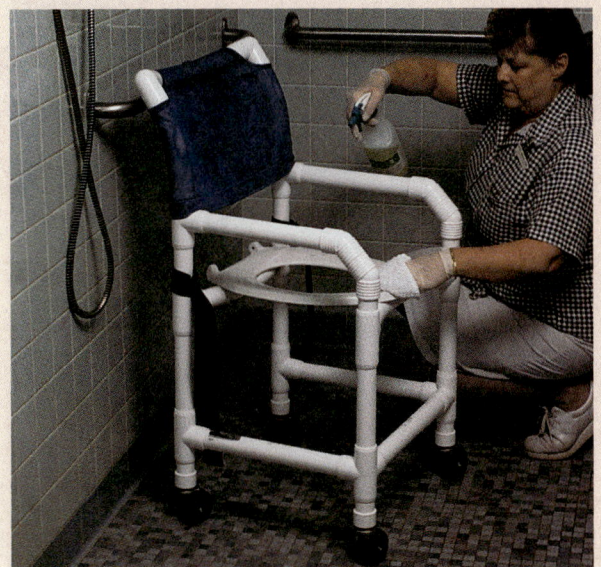

FIGURE 24-3 Clean the tub or shower chair before and after use. Wipe all areas, including the hand rails.

continues

guidelines *continued*

- Signal for help, using the emergency call button in the bathroom. Do not lock the bathroom door.
- Use good body mechanics to protect yourself and the patient.
- Nonskid strips placed in the tub and on the floor of the shower prevent slipping.
- Hand rails secured to the walls help prevent falls as the patient transfers into and out of the tub.
- The patient should be assisted in all transfer activity related to the bath. Be sure to have enough help.
- The use of a shower chair will prevent patient stress and fatigue, but it must be secured so that it does not move as the patient transfers into and out of it.

SAFETY *Alert*

Never leave the patient alone in the tub or shower. A call signal in the bathing area is used to call for emergency help.

- Wipe up all water spilled or dripped on the floor immediately, to prevent falls.
- The room should be comfortably warm (about 70°F) and free from drafts, to prevent chilling the patient.
- Cotton bath blankets should be used to cover the patient during a bed bath. They may also be used for added warmth following the tub bath or shower.
- Drape the patient's genital area with a bath towel for modesty during a tub bath or shower.
- Wrap the patient with a bath blanket for warmth and modesty immediately at the end of the tub bath or shower.
- The temperature of the water for a shower, tub bath, or bed bath should be maintained at about 105°F. The temperature of the whirlpool is set at 97°F because the whirlpool maintains a constant temperature. Use a bath thermometer to check the temperature of the water.
- Observe the patient's skin for any changes or irregularities. Note any reddened areas. Do not disturb or injure warts or moles. Report anything unusual.

Tips: It is important to use a bath blanket and towels to drape the patient during all bathing and personal care procedures, even if the room is completely private. Being exposed is uncomfortable for most people. Draping the patient properly provides a sense of dignity, reduces feelings of vulnerability, and protects the patient's modesty and self-esteem. Do not omit this important step for any patients, regardless of their age.

PROCEDURE 58

ASSISTING WITH THE TUB BATH OR SHOWER

1. Carry out beginning procedure actions.
2. Assemble equipment needed:
   - disposable gloves
   - liquid soap
   - washcloth
   - 2–3 bath towels
   - bath blanket
   - bath lotion
   - deodorant
   - chair or stool beside shower or tub
   - bath or shower chair, as needed
   - patient's gown, robe, and slippers
   - bath mat

3. Take the supplies to the bathroom. Prepare the bathroom for the patient. Make sure the tub is clean.

4. Fill the tub half full of water at 105°F or adjust the shower flow. If a bath thermometer is available, check the water temperature. If a bath thermometer is not available, test the water with

continues

PROCEDURE 58

continued

your wrist or elbow. The water should feel comfortably warm.

5. Help the patient put on a robe and slippers. Escort the patient to the bathroom. Cover the nonambulatory patient with a bath blanket when going to or from the bath or shower.

6. Help the patient to undress. Give the patient a towel to wrap around the waist.

7. Position a shower chair in tub or shower, if needed (Figure 24-4).

8. Assist the patient into the tub or shower. For the patient's safety, the bottom of the tub and the shower floor are covered with a nonskid surface.

9. Put on disposable gloves if the patient has open skin lesions.

10. Encourage the patient to wash the rest of his or her body. Assist in washing, as needed.

11. Wash the patient's back.
   - Observe the skin for signs of redness or breaks. See Unit 37 for information on caring for pressure sores or other skin lesions.

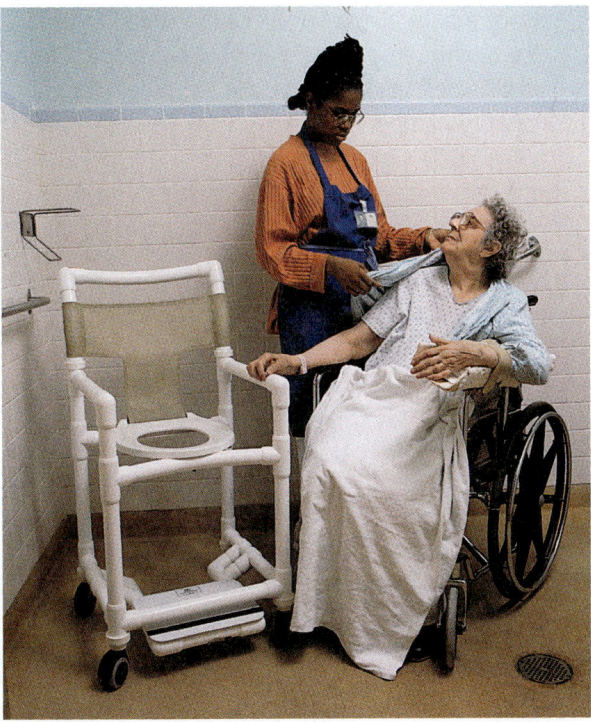

FIGURE 24-4 The shower chair is used to enable the patient to bathe safely.

12. The patient may wash the **genitalia** (external reproductive organs), if able.
   - If the patient is not able to wash the genitalia, then you will also perform this part of the bath. Apply disposable gloves before bathing the genital area.
   - After washing the genitalia, remove gloves, if worn, and discard according to facility policy.
   - Wash your hands.

13. If the patient shows any signs of weakness:
   - Get help. Use the call button.
   - Remove the plug and let the water drain.
   - Turn off the shower.
   - Allow the patient to rest until feeling better before making any attempt to assist the patient out of the tub or shower.
   - Keep the patient covered with a bath blanket to avoid chilling.

14. If the patient wants a shampoo and you have permission to do so:
   - Ask the patient to hold a washcloth over eyes.
   - Pour a small amount of water on hair (enough to wet hair thoroughly).
   - Use a small amount of shampoo to lather hair.
   - Massage scalp gently.
   - Rinse hair with warm water.
   - Repeat lathering, massaging, and rinsing, if necessary.
   - Towel hair dry.

15. Hold the bath blanket around the patient as he or she steps out of the tub. The patient may choose to remove the wet towel from under the bath blanket.

16. Assist the patient to dry, apply deodorant, dress, and return to the unit.

17. Escort the patient back to his or her unit. Return supplies to the patient's unit.

18. Carry out procedure completion actions.

19. Return to the bath or shower room. Put on gloves and clean and disinfect the tub, shower chair, and hand rails.

20. Discard soiled linen.

21. Wash your hands.

PROCEDURE 59

BED BATH

Note: *Disposable gloves should be worn if the patient has draining wounds, nonintact skin, or if contact with blood, body fluids, mucous membranes, secretions, or excretions is likely.*

1. Carry out beginning procedure actions.

2. Assemble equipment needed:
   - disposable gloves
   - bed linen
   - bath blanket
   - laundry bag or hamper
   - bath basin
   - bath thermometer
   - soap and soap dish, or liquid soap
   - washcloths
   - face towel
   - 2 bath towels
   - hospital gown/patient's night clothes
   - lotion
   - equipment for oral hygiene
   - nail brush, emery board, and orangewood stick (if needed)
   - deodorant
   - brush and comb
   - bedpan and cover or urinal
   - paper towel or protector

3. Close the windows and door to prevent chilling the patient.

4. Close the privacy curtain.

5. Put clean towels and linen on a chair in the order of use (Figure 24-5). Place a laundry hamper nearby.

6. Offer the bedpan or urinal. If the patient wants to use the bedpan or urinal, put on gloves. Empty and clean the bedpan or urinal before proceeding with the bath. Remove gloves and discard according to facility policy. Wash your hands.

7. Lower the head of the bed and the side rail on the side where you are working.

8. Loosen the top bedclothes. Remove and fold the blanket and spread and place them over the back of the chair.

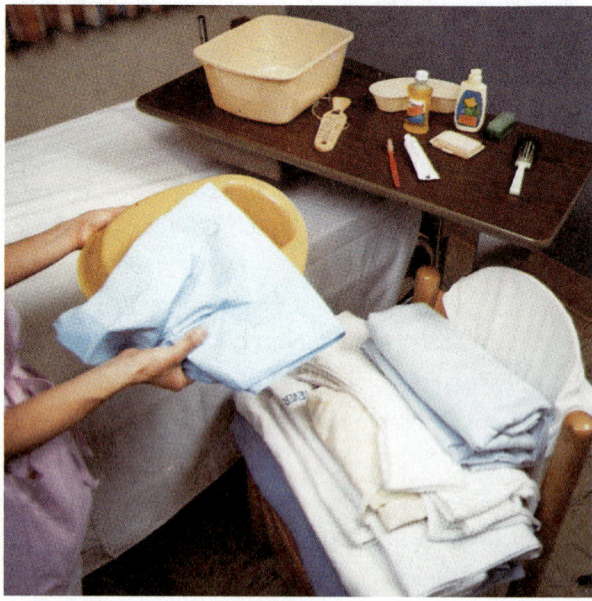

FIGURE 24-5 Assemble equipment. Place bed linens on the chair and remaining items (except bedpan) on the overbed table. If used, the bedpan or urinal should be cleaned immediately, then returned to the bedside stand.

9. Place a bath blanket over the top sheet (Figure 24-6) and remove the sheet by sliding it out from under the bath blanket. Place the sheet in a laundry hamper.

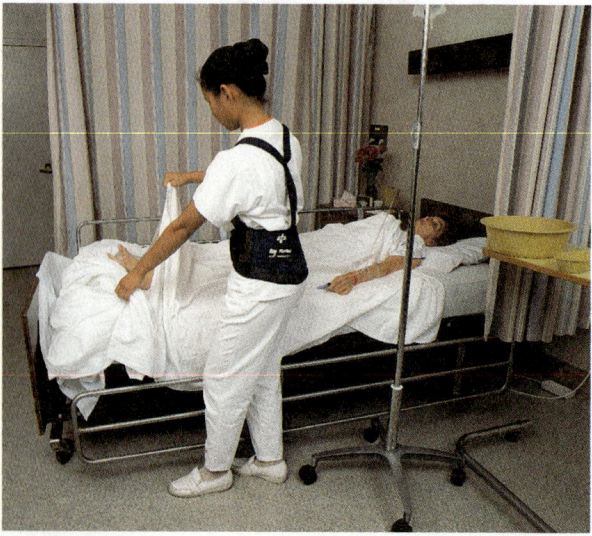

FIGURE 24-6 Replace the top bedding with a bath blanket.

continues

PROCEDURE 59

continued

10. Leave one pillow under the patient's head. Place the other pillow on a chair.

11. Remove the patient's night wear and place it in a laundry hamper (assuming the patient has no IV).

12. Fill a bath basin two-thirds full with water at 105°F. Use a bath thermometer, if available, to be sure of the proper temperature.

13. Assist the patient to move to the side of the bed nearest you.

14. Fold a face towel over the upper edge of the bath blanket to keep the blanket dry. Put on gloves.

15. Form a mitt by folding a washcloth around your hand (Figure 24-7 shows a mitt being made on a gloved hand).
    a. Wet the washcloth.
    b. Wash eyes, using separate corners of the cloth for each eye.
    c. Wipe from inside to outside corner.
    d. Do not use soap near eyes.
    e. After you have washed the eyes, remove gloves and discard according to facility policy.
    f. Do not use soap on the face unless the patient requests it.

16. Rinse the washcloth and apply soap if the patient desires. Squeeze out excess water. Do not leave soap in water.

17. Wash and rinse the patient's face (Figure 24-8), ears, and neck well. Use a towel to dry.

18. Remove gloves and discard according to facility policy.

19. Expose the patient's far arm. Protect the bed with a bath towel placed underneath the arm (Figure 24-9).
    a. Wash, rinse, and pat dry arm and hand.
    b. Be sure **axilla** (armpit) is clean and dry.
    c. Repeat for other arm.
    d. Apply deodorant if the patient requests it.

20. Care for hands and nails as necessary. Check with the nurse first to see if there are any special instructions.
    a. Place the patient's hands in a basin of water. Wash each hand carefully. Rinse and dry. Push **cuticle** (base of fingernails) down gently with a towel while wiping the fingers. Be sure to dry between fingers.
    b. Clean under the nails with orangewood stick. Shape the nails with emery board. Be careful not to file nails too close. Do not cut nails if the patient is diabetic. Inform the nurse if attention is needed.

21. Discard used bath water and refill the basin two-thirds full with water at 105°F.

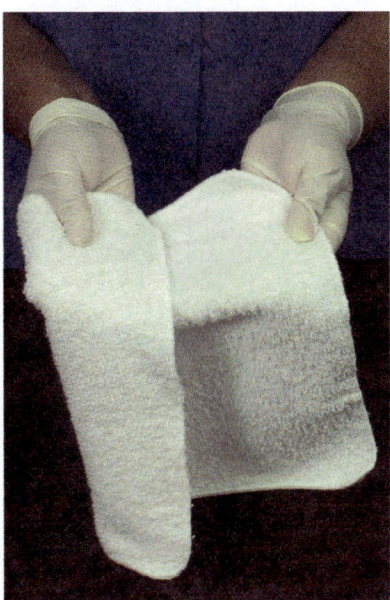
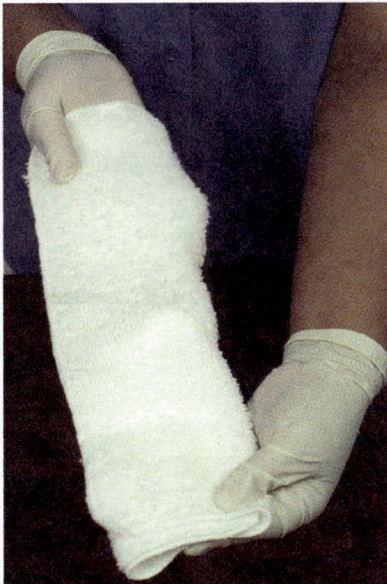
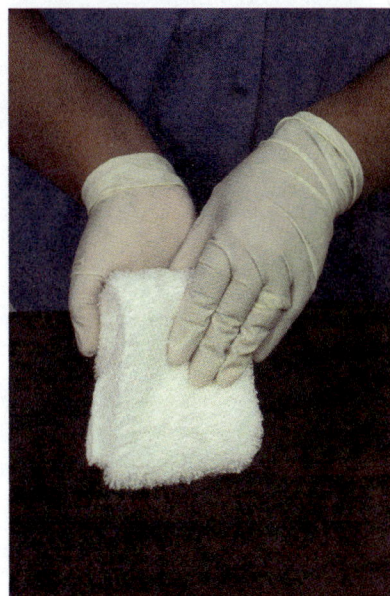

FIGURE 24-7 To make a mitt over a gloved hand, wrap the washcloth in thirds around one hand. Then bring the free end over the palm and tuck in the end. The thumb is free to hold the washcloth in place.

continues

PROCEDURE 59

continued

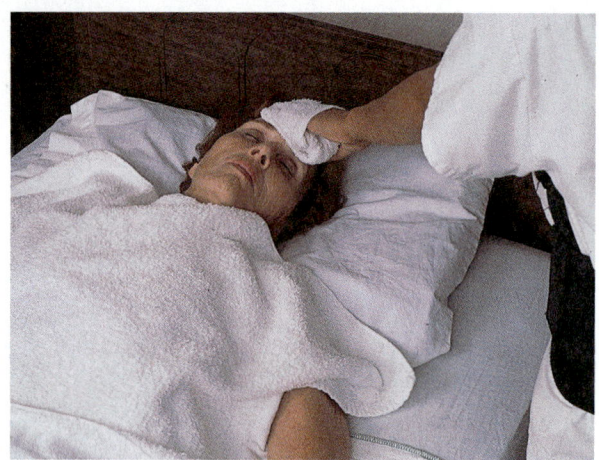

FIGURE 24-8 Wash the face carefully, doing each eye separately. Avoid soap in the eye area. Some patients do not use soap on the face.

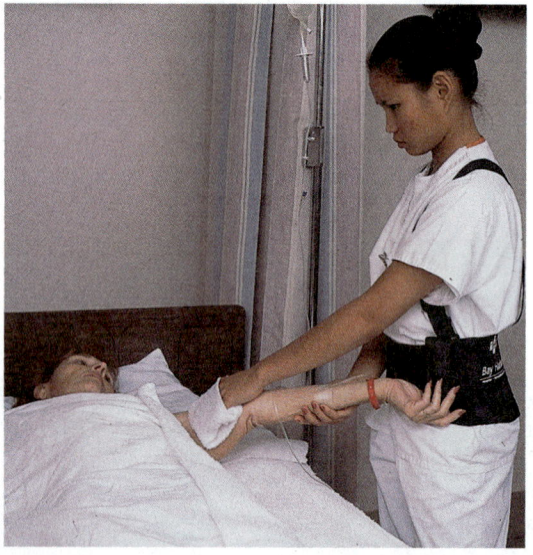

FIGURE 24-9 Place the towel under the patient's arm. Support the arm as you wash it.

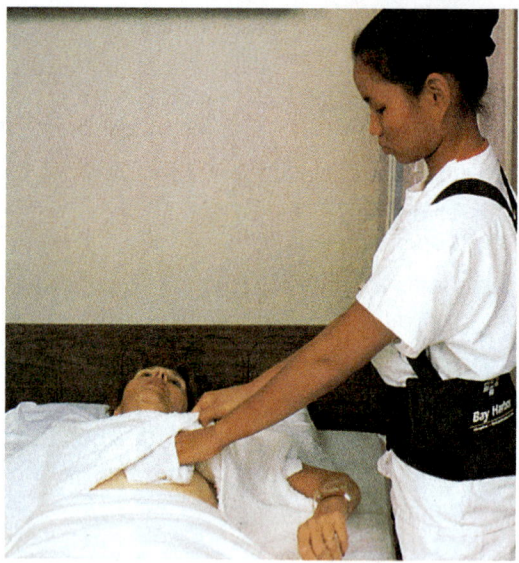

FIGURE 24-10 Lift the towel with one hand. Wash underneath with the other hand.

22. Put a bath towel over the patient's chest. Then fold the blanket to waist. Under the towel:

   a. Wash, rinse, and pat dry chest (Figure 24-10).

   b. Rinse and dry folds under the breasts of a female patient carefully to avoid irritating the skin.

23. Fold the bath blanket down to the **pubic** area (location of external genitalia). Wash, rinse, and pat dry abdomen. Fold the bath blanket up to cover the abdomen and chest. Slide the towel out from under the bath blanket.

24. Ask the patient to flex the far knee, if possible. Fold the bath blanket up to expose the thigh, leg, and foot. Protect the bed with a bath towel.

   a. Put the bath basin on the towel.

   b. Place the patient's foot in the basin (Figure 24-11).

   c. Wash and rinse the leg and foot.

   d. When moving the patient's leg, support it properly.

25. Lift the leg and move the basin to the other side of the bed. Dry the leg and foot. Dry well between toes.

26. Repeat for the other leg and foot. Take the basin off the bed before drying the leg and foot.

27. Care for toenails as necessary. Check with the nurse for any special instructions. Apply lotion to the feet of a patient with dry skin. Do not apply lotion between the toes, as this keeps the area moist and promotes fungal growth.

- Do not attempt to cut thickened nails.
- File nails straight across.
- Do not round edges.
- Do not push back the cuticle, because it is easily injured and infected.
- If the patient is diabetic, inform the nurse if toenail care is required.

continues

PROCEDURE 59

continued

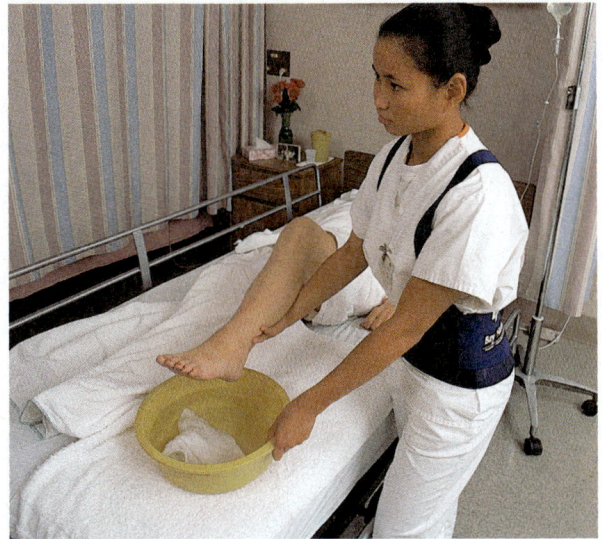

FIGURE 24-11 Support the leg and place the patient's foot in the basin.

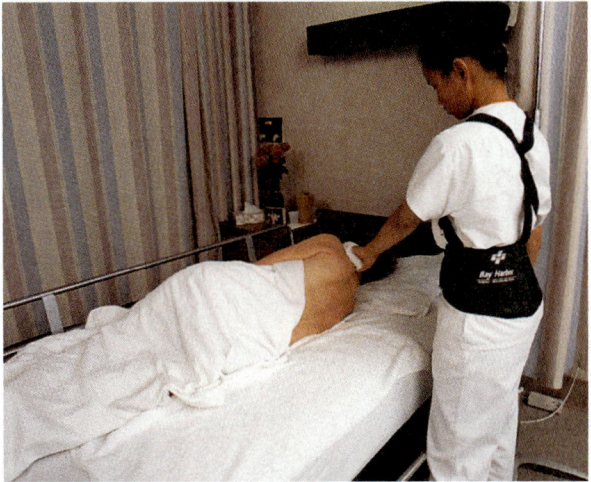

FIGURE 24-12 Change the water and wash the patient's back.

28. Change water and check for the correct temperature with a bath thermometer. It may be necessary to change the water before this point in the patient's bath if it becomes cold or too soapy.

29. Help the patient to turn on the side away from you. Help her to move toward the center of the bed. Place a bath towel lengthwise next to the patient's back.
   - Wash, rinse, and dry neck, back, and buttocks (Figure 24-12).
   - Use long, firm strokes when washing the back.

30. A back rub is usually given at this time (see Unit 25).

31. Help the patient to turn on the back.

32. Place a towel under the buttocks and upper legs. Change the water in the basin and check for the correct temperature. Place a washcloth, soap, basin, and bath towel within convenient reach of the patient. Have the patient complete the bath by washing the genitalia. Assist the patient if necessary. You must take responsibility for the procedure if the patient has difficulty. Many times patients are reluctant to acknowledge the need for help. If assisting a patient with genital washing, always put on disposable gloves.
   - For a female patient, wash from front to back, drying carefully.
   - For a male patient, carefully wash and dry the penis, scrotum, and groin area. If the patient is not circumcised, gently push the foreskin back and carefully wash and dry the penis. Then gently pull the foreskin down to its original position.

33. Remove gloves and discard according to facility policy.

34. Carry out range-of-motion exercises as ordered (see Unit 40 for procedures).

35. Cover the pillow with a towel. Comb or brush the patient's hair. Oral hygiene is usually given at this time (see Unit 25).

36. Discard towels and washcloth in a laundry hamper.

37. Provide a clean gown.

38. Clean and replace equipment according to facility policy.

39. Put clean washcloth and towels in the bedside stand, or hang according to facility policy.

40. Change the bed linen, following the procedure for making an occupied bed. Replace and discard soiled linen in a laundry hamper.

41. Remove and discard disposable gloves according to facility policy. Wash your hands.

42. Raise the side rails, if required.

43. Carry out procedure completion actions.

PROCEDURE 60

CHANGING THE PATIENT'S GOWN

Note: *Wear disposable gloves if the patient has draining wounds, nonintact skin, or if contact with mucous membranes, blood, body fluids, secretions, or excretions is likely.*

1. Carry out beginning procedure actions.

2. Assemble equipment needed:
   - disposable gloves
   - bath blanket
   - clean gown
   - laundry bag or hamper

3. Place a bath blanket over the top sheet. Pull the sheet down by sliding it out from under the bath blanket.

4. Loosen gown from the patient's neck.

5. Slip the gown down the arms.

6. Make sure the patient is covered by a bath blanket (Figure 24-13).

Note: *This procedure is to be used only when the patient has an IV that is NOT run through an electric pump. When a pump is used, the patient may wear a gown that snaps at the shoulder. In this case, the gown can be removed without touching the IV bag or tubing. If the patient is wearing a nonsnap gown, call the nurse if the gown is to be changed. Never disconnect the tubing from the pump.*

7. For a patient wearing a regular gown (nonsnap):

   a. Remove the gown from the arm without the IV and bring the gown across the patient's chest to the other arm.

   b. Place a clean gown over the patient's chest to avoid exposure.

   c. On the arm with the IV, gather the gown material in one hand so there is no pull or pressure on the IV line (Figure 24-14A), and slowly draw the gown over the tips of the patient's fingers.

   d. With your free hand, lift the IV free of the standard and slip the gown over the bag of fluid (Figure 24-14B), removing the gown from the patient's body. **Never allow the bag of fluid to be lower than the patient's arm.**

   e. Take the sleeve of a clean gown and slip it over the bag of fluid, over the tubing, and up the patient's arm.

   f. Replace the bag of fluid on the IV standard.

   g. Remove the soiled gown and place it at the end of the bed. Finish putting the clean gown on the patient's other arm. Secure the neck ties.

   h. Place the soiled gown in a laundry hamper.

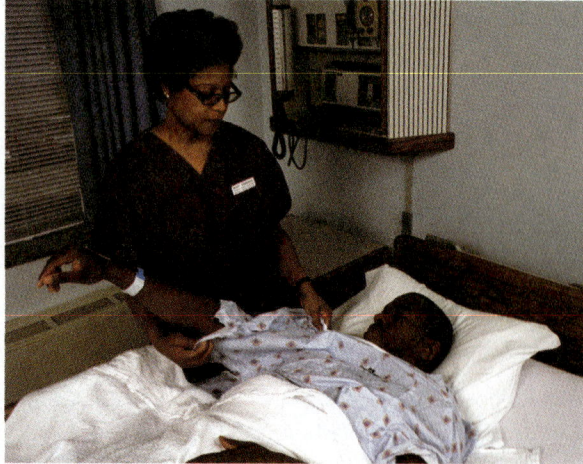

FIGURE 24-13 Keeping the patient covered with the bath blanket, remove the patient's gown.

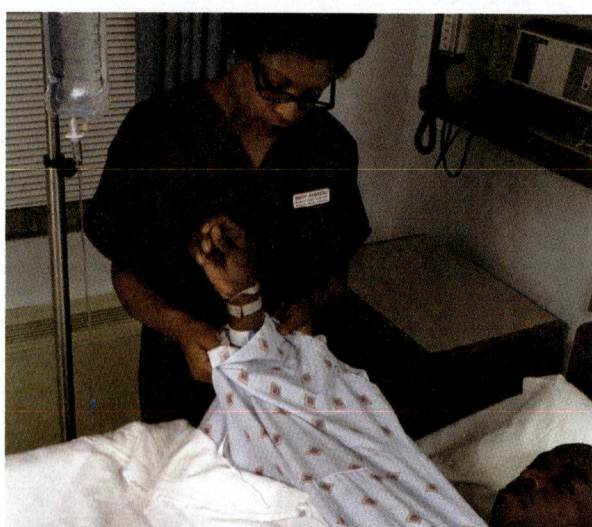

FIGURE 24-14A Gather the material of the gown in one hand so there is no traction on the IV line. Slowly draw the gown over the tips of the patient's fingers.

continues

PROCEDURE 60

continued

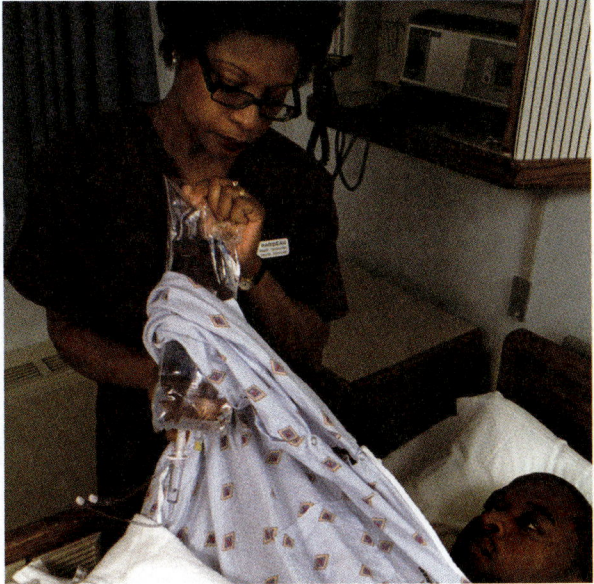

FIGURE 24-14B With your free hand, lift the IV off the standard and slip the gown over the bag of fluid.

    i. Make sure the IV is dripping at the required rate and that the tubing is not kinked or twisted.

8. If the patient has a weak or paralyzed arm, always undress the patient in the following manner:

    a. Untie the gown and remove the back sides of the gown from underneath the patient.

    b. Remove the gown from the stronger arm first.

    c. Bring the gown across the patient's chest and slide the gown down over the weak arm.

    d. Gently lift the patient's weak arm to finish removing the gown over the patient's hand.

    e. Reverse the procedure to put a clean gown on the patient, by putting the gown over the weaker arm first.

9. Pull the sheet up over the bath blanket. Remove the bath blanket.

10. Carry out procedure completion actions.

PROCEDURE 61

WATERLESS BED BATH

1. Carry out beginning procedure actions.

2. Assemble equipment:
- disposable gloves
- bed linen
- bath blanket
- laundry bag or hamper
- hospital gown/patient's night clothes
- bath towel
- lotion for back rub
- waterless bathing product, heated according to facility policy or patient wishes
- basin of warm water for soaking hands (optional)
- comb, brush
- bedpan or urinal with cover, as needed
- supplies for oral hygiene, as needed
- supplies for nail care, as needed
- small plastic bag to discard used bathing cloths
- large plastic bag or hamper for soiled linen

3. Close the windows and door to the room.

4. Pull the privacy curtain. Place clean supplies on the overbed table.

5. Offer the bedpan or urinal. Put on gloves if you will be assisting with this procedure.

6. Lower the head of the bed and the side rail on the side where you will be working.

7. Loosen the top bedclothes. Remove and fold the blanket and spread and place them over the back of the chair.

continues

PROCEDURE 61

continued

8. Place a bath blanket over the top sheet and remove the sheet by sliding it out from under the bath blanket. Place the sheet in the laundry hamper.

9. Leave one pillow under the patient's head. Place the other pillow on the chair.

10. Remove the gown (see Procedure 60) and place it in the laundry hamper.

11. Assist the patient to move to the side of the bed near you.

12. Warm the package according to facility policy and manufacturer's directions. Open the package. (If you used a microwave to heat the package, check the cloths for hot spots.) Remove one cloth and cleanse the patient's face and neck. (The solution on these cloths can safely be used around the eyes.)

13. Place a towel over the patient's chest. Fold the bath blanket down to the waist and cleanse the chest. Be sure the area under a female patient's breasts is carefully cleaned.

14. Fold the bath blanket down to the pubic area and wash the abdomen. Replace the bath blanket over the abdomen and chest. Remove the towel by sliding it out from under the bath blanket. Discard the used cloth in the plastic bag.

15. Uncover the far arm. Remove another cloth from the package and wash the arm and hand. It is nice to soak each of the patient's hands separately in a basin of warm water while you wash the opposite arm. This is refreshing for the patient who cannot be out of bed to bathe. Wash each axilla. Apply deodorant if the patient desires. Discard the used cloth in the plastic bag. Cover the arm with the bath blanket.

16. Uncover the near arm. Remove a new cloth from the package. Wash the arm, hand, and axilla. Apply deodorant. Discard the used cloth in the plastic bag. Cover the patient with the bath blanket.

17. Provide nail care as needed.

18. Ask the patient to flex the far leg, if possible. Fold the bath blanket up to expose the thigh, leg, and foot. Remove a new cloth from the package. Cleanse the thigh, leg, and foot. Be sure the area between the toes is left dry. Discard the used cloth in the plastic bag. Cover the leg and foot with the bath blanket.

19. Repeat step 18 with the near thigh, leg, and foot.

20. Make sure the side rail on the opposite side of the bed is up. Help the patient turn onto the side away from you. Place a bath towel lengthwise next to the patient's back.

21. Remove a new cloth from the package. Draw the bath blanket back to expose the back. Wash the back and buttocks. Discard the used cloth in the plastic bag. A backrub may be given at this time. Cover the patient with the bath blanket.

22. Assist the patient to turn onto the back. Position a towel under the buttocks by asking the patient to lift the hips, if possible. Remove a new cloth from the package. Hand the patient the cloth and instruct the patient to wash the perineum. Assist if necessary. (Wear gloves if you will be assisting.) Discard gloves and the used cloth in the plastic bag. Remove the towel.

23. Wash your hands.

24. Assist the patient to put on a clean gown.

25. Cover the pillow with a towel. Comb or brush the patient's hair. Assist with oral hygiene, if needed.

26. Change the bed linen, following the procedure for making an occupied bed (see Procedure 56). Put soiled linen in a plastic bag or linen hamper.

27. Carry out procedure completion actions.

PROCEDURE 62

PARTIAL BATH

1. Carry out beginning procedure actions.

2. Assemble equipment needed:
   - disposable gloves
   - bed linen
   - bath blanket
   - bath thermometer
   - soap and soap dish or liquid soap
   - washcloth
   - face towel
   - bath towel
   - gown and robe
   - laundry bag or hamper
   - bath basin
   - lotion
   - equipment for oral hygiene
   - nail brush, emery board, and orangewood stick
   - brush, comb, and deodorant
   - bedpan or urinal and cover
   - paper towels or protector

   Note: A package of premoistened washcloths can be substituted for the basin of water, soap, washcloth, and towel if the facility has approved the use of the waterless bath. The nursing assistant or the patient (condition permitting) can use the premoistened washcloths for the partial bath.

3. Close windows and door and turn off fans to prevent chilling the patient.

4. Put the towels and linen on the chair in the order of use. Make sure a laundry hamper is available.

5. Put on disposable gloves.

6. Offer the bedpan or urinal (see Unit 25). Empty and clean it before proceeding with the bath. Remove gloves and discard according to facility policy. Wash your hands.

7. Elevate the head of the bed, if permitted, to a comfortable position.

8. Loosen the top bedclothes. Remove and fold the blanket and spread and place them over the back of the chair. Place a bath blanket over the top sheet. Remove the top sheet by sliding it out from under the bath blanket.

9. Leave one pillow under the patient's head. Place the other pillow on the chair.

10. Assist the patient to remove the gown. Place the gown in the laundry hamper. Make sure the patient is covered with a bath blanket.

11. Place paper towels or a bed protector on the overbed table.

12. Fill a bath basin two-thirds full with water at 105°F. Place the basin on the overbed table.

13. Push the overbed table comfortably close to the patient.

14. Place towels, washcloth, and soap on the overbed table within easy reach.

15. Instruct the patient to wash as much as she is able and tell her that you will return to complete the bath.

16. Place the call bell within easy reach. Ask the patient to signal when ready.

17. Wash hands and leave unit.

18. Wash hands and return to unit when the patient signals. Put on a new pair of gloves.

19. Change the bath water. Complete bathing those areas the patient could not reach. Make sure the face, hands, axillae, buttocks, back, and genitals are washed and dried.

20. Remove gloves and discard according to facility policy.

21. Wash your hands.

22. Give a backrub with lotion.

23. Assist the patient in applying deodorant and a fresh gown.

24. Cover the pillow with a towel. Comb or brush the patient's hair. Assist with oral hygiene, if needed (see Unit 25).

25. Clean and replace equipment according to facility policy.

26. Put a clean washcloth and towels in the bedside stand, or hang according to facility policy.

27. Change the bed linen, following the procedure for making an occupied bed. Put soiled linen in the laundry hamper.

28. Carry out procedure completion actions.

Perineal Care

The **perineum** is the area between the legs. In females, it is the area between the vagina and the anus. In males, it is the area between the scrotum and the anus.

Perineal care may be performed as part of general bathing or as a separate procedure, as needed. **Perineal care** means to wash the area including the genitals and anus (see Procedures 63 and 64). Always wear gloves and use standard precautions when caring for the perineal area.

Tips: If the patient has been incontinent, remove the wet pad or linen and replace with a dry pad before beginning perineal care. Clean excess stool off with toilet tissue before beginning.

COMMUNICATION *Highlight*

Patients who need assistance with perineal care and those who become incontinent may feel guilty and embarrassed. Avoid showing disgust. Be sensitive to the patient's feelings. Communicate with the patient tactfully. Use proper terms when referring to body parts and excretions.

INFECTION CONTROL *Alert*

Providing perineal care is one of the most important procedures you will perform as a nursing assistant. Always apply the principles of standard precautions. Remember that there are mucous membranes in the genital area. If you are wearing gloves, change them before beginning care. Using proper technique is critical because of the high risk of contamination and infection. Avoid scrubbing back and forth. Always wipe from clean to dirty with a single wipe, then turn or discard the cloth, according to facility policy. Guidelines for female perineal care vary with the institution. In some facilities, you will be instructed to clean the center first, then each side. In others, you will clean the sides of the genitalia first, then the center. Know and follow your facility policies. Discard your gloves properly and avoid contaminating environmental surfaces with your used gloves.

PROCEDURE 63

FEMALE PERINEAL CARE

1. Carry out beginning procedure actions.

2. Assemble equipment:
   - disposable gloves
   - bath blanket or top sheet
   - bedpan and cover
   - liquid soap
   - basin
   - bath thermometer
   - bed protector
   - washcloth and towel
   - plastic bag(s), if needed to discard linen or trash
   - laundry barrel or hamper

3. Lower the side rail on the side where you will be working. Be sure the opposite side rail is up and secure.

4. Remove the bedspread and blanket. Fold and place them on the back of the chair.

5. The patient is to be on her back. Cover the patient with a bath blanket and fanfold the sheet to the foot of the bed.

6. Put on disposable gloves. Fill a basin with water at 105°F.

7. Ask the patient to raise her hips while you place a bed protector underneath the patient.

8. Offer the bedpan to the patient.
   a. If used and the patient is on intake and output, record the amount.
   b. Empty and clean the bedpan before continuing with the procedure.

continues

PROCEDURE 63

continued

c. Remove gloves and discard according to facility policy.

d. Wash your hands and put on a new pair of gloves.

9. Position the bath blanket so that only the area between the legs is exposed.

10. Ask the patient to separate her legs and flex her knees.

    Note: If the patient is unable to spread her legs and flex her knees, turn the patient on her side with the legs flexed. This position provides easy access to the perineal area.

11. Wet the washcloth, make a mitt, and apply a small amount of liquid soap.

    Note: Heavy soap application may be difficult to rinse off completely. Soap residue is irritating.

12. Use one gloved hand to stabilize and separate the vulva (Figure 24-15). With the other gloved hand, proceed as follows.

   a. Bring the soaped washcloth in one downward stroke along the far side of the outer labia to the perineum.

   b. Rinse the washcloth, remake the mitt, and rinse the area just cleaned.

   c. Repeat steps a and b, washing and rinsing the inner far labia.

   d. Repeat steps a and b, washing and rinsing the inner near labia.

   e. With gloved hands, separate the labia. Clean and rinse the inner part of the vulva to the perineum.

f. Dry the washed area with a towel.

13. Turn the patient away from you. Flex the upper leg slightly if permitted.

14. Make a mitt, wet it, and apply soap lightly.

15. Expose the anal area. Wash the area, stroking from perineum to coccyx (front to back) (Figure 24-16).

16. Rinse well in the same manner.

17. Dry carefully.

18. Return the patient to her back.

19. Remove and dispose of the bed protector according to facility policy.

20. Cover the patient with a sheet or bath blanket.

21. Remove and dispose of gloves according to facility policy. Wash your hands.

22. Remove, fold, and store the bath blanket according to facility policy.

23. Replace the top covers, tuck them under the mattress, and make mitered corners. (Some patients prefer that the top covers not be tucked in.)

24. Put up the side rail.

25. Put on gloves. Empty the water. Clean equipment and dispose of or store it, according to facility policy.

26. Remove gloves and discard according to facility policy. Wash your hands.

27. Carry out procedure completion actions.

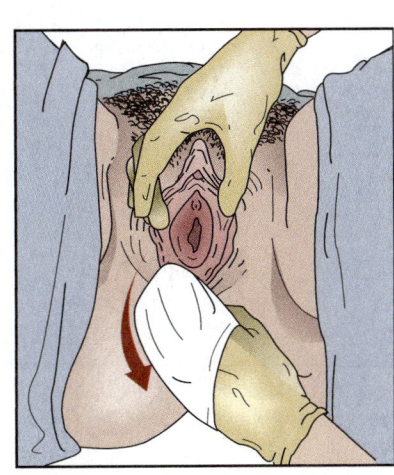

FIGURE 24-15
Spread the vulva with one hand. With the washcloth in the other hand, start in the front and stroke downward along the outer labia.

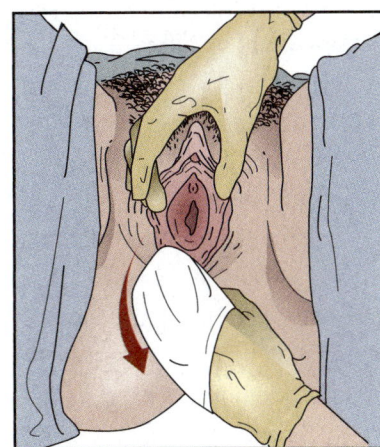

FIGURE 24-16
With one hand, lift up on the buttocks to expose the anal area. Wipe from the perineum back toward the anus.

PROCEDURE 64

MALE PERINEAL CARE

1. Carry out beginning procedure actions.

2. Assemble equipment:
   - disposable gloves
   - bath blanket
   - bath thermometer
   - urinal and cover or bedpan and cover
   - soap, washcloth, and towel
   - plastic bag
   - bed protector or bath towel
   - ordered solution (if other than water)
   - basin
   - laundry hamper

3. Fill a basin with warm water at approximately 105°F.

4. Lower the side rail on the side where you will be working.

5. Fanfold the blanket and spread to the foot of the bed. Remove, fold, and place them on the back of the chair.

6. Cover the patient with a bath blanket and fanfold the sheet to the foot of the bed.

7. Put on disposable gloves.

8. Place a bed protector under the patient's buttocks.

9. Offer the bedpan or urinal.
   a. If used and the patient is on intake and output, record the amount.
   b. Empty and clean the bedpan or urinal before continuing with the procedure.
   c. Remove gloves and discard according to facility policy.
   d. Wash your hands and put on a new pair of gloves.

10. Have the patient flex and separate his knees.

 Note: If the patient is unable to spread his legs and flex the knees, the perineal area can be washed with the patient on his side with the legs flexed. This position provides easy access to the perineal area.

11. Draw the bath blanket upward to expose the perineal area only.

12. Make a mitt with a washcloth and apply a small amount of soap.

 Note: Heavy soap application may be difficult to rinse off completely. Soap residue is irritating.

13. Grasp the penis gently with one hand and wash. Begin at the meatus and wash in a circular motion (Figure 24-17).

14. If the patient is not circumcised, draw the foreskin back (Figure 24-18). Be sure the entire penis is washed. Rinse thoroughly.

15. Continue to wash down the penis and the rest of the perineal area, including the scrotum, using downward strokes and working outward to the thighs. Lift the scrotum and wash the perineum.

16. Rinse the washcloth and remake a mitt. Rinse the urethral and perineal areas well, working in the same direction until the entire area is clean and soap-free.

17. Dry the washed area with a towel. Reposition the foreskin if necessary.

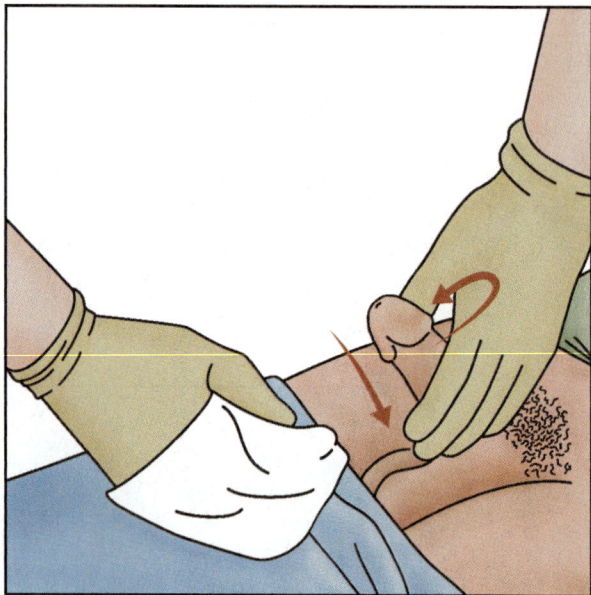

FIGURE 24-17 Grasp the penis gently with one hand. With the other, wipe in a circular motion, beginning with the urinary meatus, working outward over the glans (head of the penis). Continue to wash down the penis and the rest of the perineal area, including the scrotum, using downward strokes and working outward to the thighs.

continues

PROCEDURE 64

continued

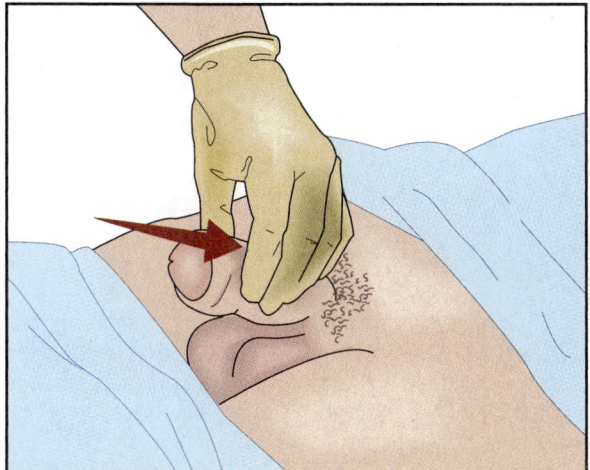

FIGURE 24-18 If the patient is not circumcised, gently push the foreskin back so the glans can be washed. Once the penis is washed and dried, return the foreskin to its normal position.

18. Turn the patient away from you. Flex his upper leg slightly if permitted.

19. Make a mitt, wet it, and apply soap lightly.

20. Expose the anal area. Wash the area, stroking from perineum to coccyx.

21. Rinse well in the same manner.

22. Dry carefully.

23. Return the patient to his back.

24. Remove and dispose of the bed protector according to facility policy.

25. Cover the patient with a sheet.

26. Remove and dispose of gloves according to facility policy. Wash your hands.

27. Remove, fold, and store the bath blanket, according to facility policy.

28. Replace the top covers, tuck them under the mattress, and make mitered corners. (Some patients prefer that the top covers not be tucked in.)

29. Put up the side rail, if required.

30. Put on gloves. Empty the water. Clean equipment and dispose of or store it, according to facility policy.

31. Remove gloves and discard according to facility policy. Wash your hands.

32. Carry out procedure completion actions.

PROCEDURE 65

HAND AND FINGERNAIL CARE

Note: Check with the nurse and nursing care plan to learn if this procedure is permitted for the patient or if it is to be modified because of the patient's condition.

This procedure can be carried out independently or can be modified and added to the bath procedure.

1. Carry out beginning procedure actions.

2. Assemble equipment:
   - basin
   - bath thermometer
   - soap
   - bath towel and washcloth
   - lotion
   - plastic protector
   - nail clippers
   - emery board
   - orangewood stick
   - nail polish (optional)

3. Elevate the head of the bed, if permitted, and adjust the overbed table in front of the patient. If the patient is allowed out of bed, assist the patient to transfer to a chair and position the overbed table waist-high across the patient's lap.

4. Place a plastic protector on the overbed table.

continues

PROCEDURE 65

continued

5. Fill a basin with warm water at approximately 105°F, using the bath thermometer to test temperature. Place the basin on the overbed table.

6. Instruct the patient to put hands in the basin and soak for approximately 5 minutes. Place a towel over the basin to help retain heat. Add warm water if necessary. Remember to remove the patient's hands before adding water.

7. Wash the patient's hands. Push cuticles back gently with a washcloth or an orangewood stick (Figure 24-19A). (A cream may be used to soften the cuticles first.) Use a soft brush or orangewood stick to clean under nails. (Check with the nurse before using an orangewood stick for a patient with diabetes.)

8. Dry the patient's hands with a towel. Remember to dry between the fingers.

9. Use nail clippers to cut fingernails straight across, if permitted by facility policy (Figure 24-19B).
   - Do not cut below the tips of the fingers.
   - Keep nail clippings on the protector to be discarded.

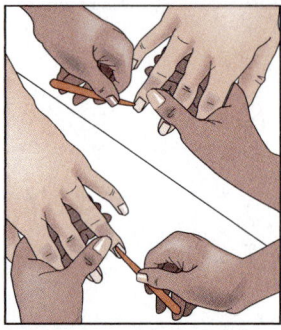 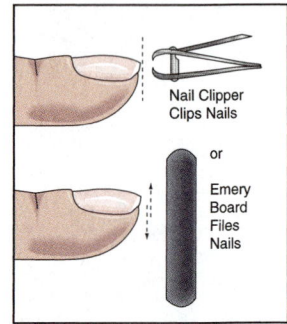

FIGURE 24-19A Gently push the cuticles back with a washcloth, or orangewood stick, if permitted.

FIGURE 24-19B Clip the nails straight across, then round the edges.

10. Shape and smooth the fingernails with an emery board. Apply polish to nails if the patient desires.

11. Pour a small amount of lotion in your palms and gently smooth it on the patient's hands.

12. Empty the basin of water. Gather equipment. Clean and store it according to the facility policy.

13. Return the overbed table to the foot of the bed. If the patient has been sitting up for the procedure, assist the patient to get into bed.

14. Carry out procedure completion actions.

PROCEDURE 66

BED SHAMPOO

1. Carry out beginning procedure actions.

2. Assemble equipment needed:
   - shampoo tray
   - shampoo
   - washcloths
   - 3 bath towels
   - bath blanket
   - pitcher of water (105°F)
   - safety pin
   - 2 bed protectors
   - waterproof covering for pillow
   - large bucket to collect used water
   - hair dryer, if available (portable)
   - hairbrush and comb
   - small empty pitcher or cup
   - larger pitcher of water (105°F)—use if additional water is needed

3. Place a large, empty basin on the floor under the spout of the shampoo tray.

4. Arrange on the bedside stand, within easy reach (Figure 24-20A).
   - large pitcher of water (105°F)

continues

PROCEDURE 66

continued

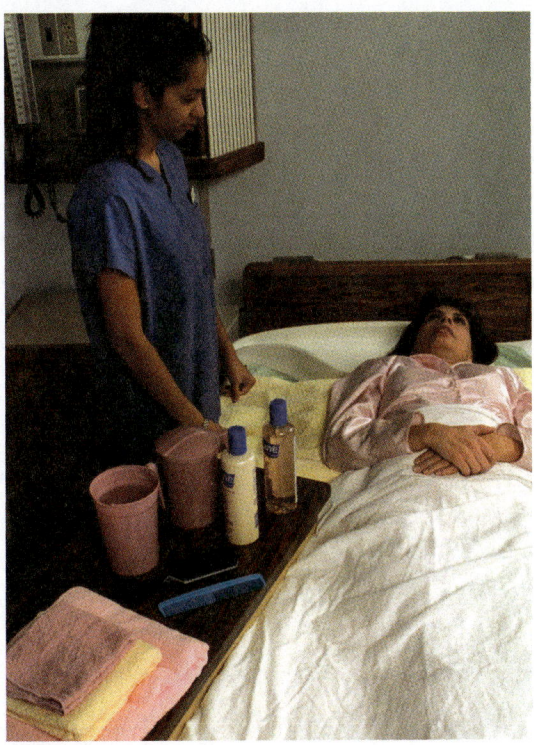

FIGURE 24-20A Assemble equipment.

- washcloth
- 2 bath towels
- shampoo
- small pitcher of water (105°F)

5. Replace the top bedding with a bath blanket.

6. Ask the patient to move to the side of the bed nearest you. Assist as needed.

7. Replace the pillowcase with a waterproof covering.

8. Cover the head of the bed with a bed protector. Be sure it goes well under the patient's shoulders.

9. Loosen neck ties of the gown.

10. Place a towel under the patient's head and shoulders. Brush hair free of tangles, working snarls out carefully.

11. Bring the towel down around the patient's neck and shoulders and pin it. Position the pillow under shoulders so that the patient's head is tilted slightly backward.

12. Raise the bed to high horizontal position.

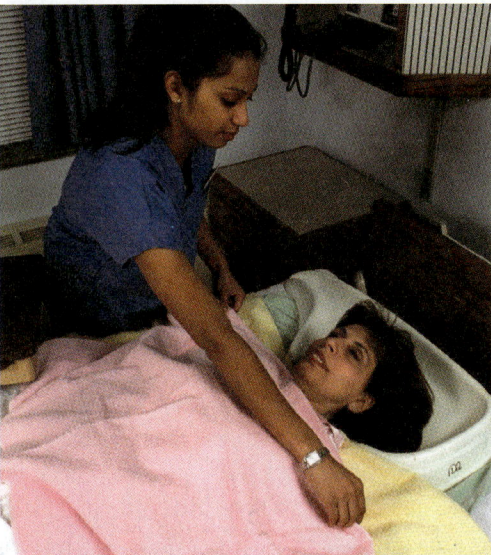

FIGURE 24-20B Position the patient's head on the shampoo tray. Protect the patient with a towel and the bed with a protector.

13. Raise the patient's head and position the shampoo tray (Figure 24-20B) so that the drain is over the edge of the bed directly above the basin.

14. Give the patient a washcloth to cover eyes (Figure 24-20C).

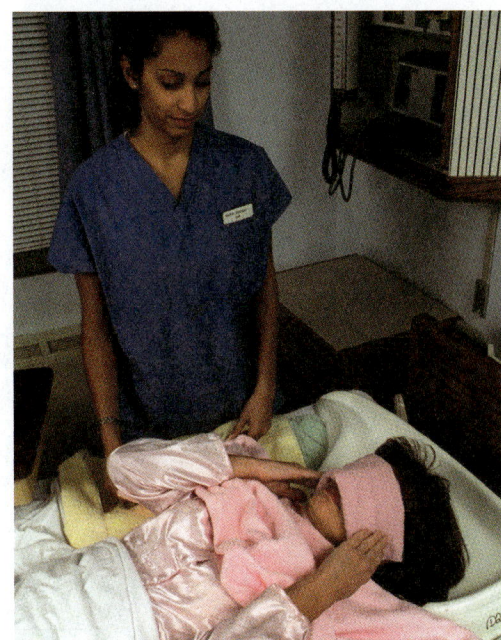

FIGURE 24-20C Give the patient a folded washcloth to protect her eyes.

continues

PROCEDURE 66

continued

15. Recheck the temperature of water in the basin.

16. Using the small pitcher (Figure 24-20D), pour a small amount of water over hair until thoroughly wet. Use one hand to help direct the flow away from the face and ears.

17. Apply a small amount of shampoo, working up a lather (Figure 24-20E). Work from scalp to hair ends.

18. Massage the scalp with your fingertips. Do not use your fingernails.

19. Rinse thoroughly, pouring from hairline to hair tips. Direct the flow into the drain. Use water from the pitcher if needed, but be sure to check the water temperature before use.

20. Repeat lathering and rinsing (steps 16–19).

21. Lift the patient's head. Remove the tray and bed protector. Adjust the pillow and slip a dry bath towel underneath the head.

22. Place the tray on the basin. Wrap hair in a towel. Be sure to dry face, neck, and ears as needed.

23. Dry hair with the towel. If available and not otherwise contraindicated, a portable hair dryer may be used to complete the drying process. Brushing the hair as you blow-dry helps the hair to dry. Be sure to keep the dryer moving and not too close to the hair.

24. Comb hair appropriately. Remove the protective pillow cover. Replace with a cloth cover.

25. Lower the bed to a comfortable working position.

26. Replace the bedding and remove the bath blanket.

27. Help the patient assume a comfortable position. Lower the bed to the lowest horizontal position. Leave the call bell within reach.

28. Allow the patient to rest undisturbed. The length of this procedure may tire the patient.

29. Empty the water from the collection basin.

30. Carry out procedure completion actions.

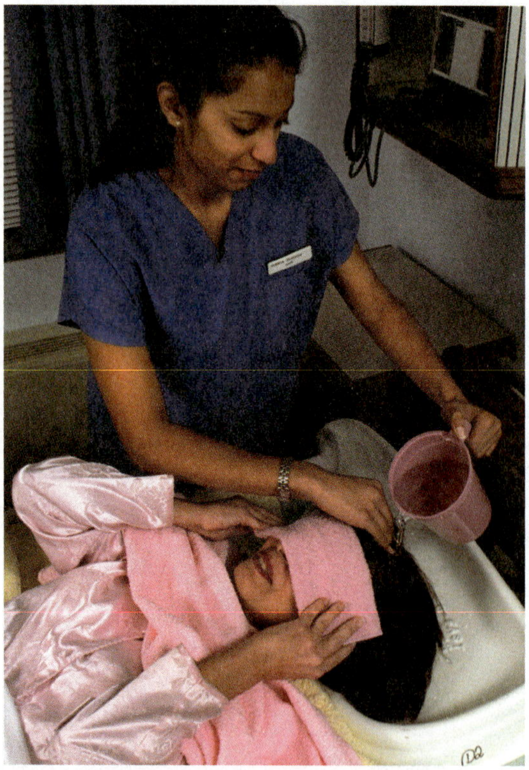

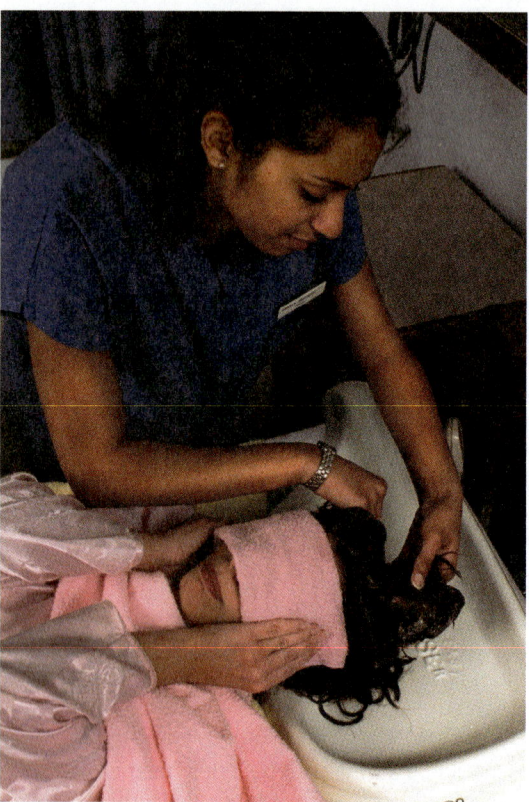

FIGURE 24-20D Wet the hair by slowly pouring warm water.

FIGURE 24-20E Apply shampoo and work into a lather, using your fingertips.

DRESSING A PATIENT

Patients in hospitals generally wear hospital gowns because they are in bed most of the time. However, some patients may prefer to wear their own nightgowns or pajamas and will need assistance in dressing. You may also need to assist patients to dress when they are discharged from the hospital. It is usually easier to help people dress while they are still in bed. (See Procedure 67.)

guidelines *for*

Dressing and Undressing Patients

The patient who requires help in dressing may wish to sit in a chair with clothing placed nearby. You can help by:

- Allowing the patient to choose the clothing to be put on.
- Encouraging the patient to participate in the dressing or undressing procedure as much as he or she is able.
- Being prepared to assist with shoes and stockings even for patients who can do much themselves. Bending over to adjust shoes and stockings can result in dizziness and loss of balance.
- Putting clothing on the affected or weakest side first if the patient has difficulty moving one side or is paralyzed.
- Removing clothing from unaffected or strongest side first if the patient has difficulty moving one side or is paralyzed.

PROCEDURE 67

DRESSING AND UNDRESSING THE PATIENT

1. Carry out beginning procedure actions.

2. Select appropriate clothing and arrange in order of application. Encourage the patient to participate in selection.

3. Cover the patient with a bath blanket and fanfold top bedclothes to the foot of the bed.

4. Elevate the head of the bed to sitting position.

5. Assist the patient to a comfortable sitting position.

6. Remove night clothing, keeping the patient covered with the bath blanket. Remove from strong side first and then from weaker side. Place night clothes in a laundry hamper or fold them to be taken home.

7. If the patient wears a bra, slip the straps over the patient's hands (weak side first), move the straps up her arms, and position them on her shoulders. Adjust the breasts in the bra cups. Then hook the bra in back (assist the patient to lean forward so the bra can be fastened).

8. For an undershirt, or any garment that slips on over the head:

   a. Gather the undershirt and place it over the patient's head (Figure 24-21A).

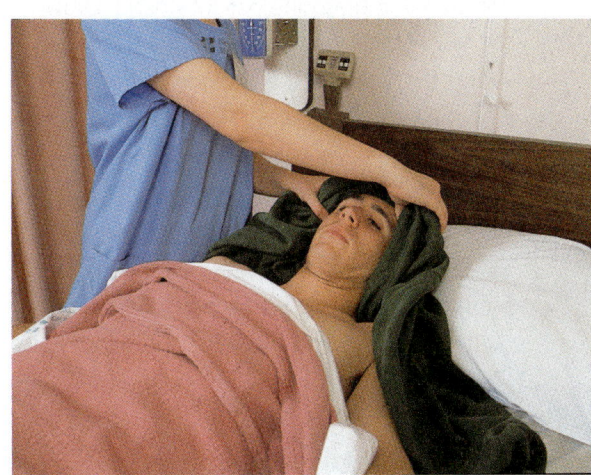

FIGURE 24-21A Gather the garment and pull it over the patient's head.

continues

PROCEDURE 67

continued

    b. Grasp the patient's hand and guide it through the armhole by reaching into the armhole from the outside.

    c. Repeat the procedure with the opposite arm.

    d. Assist the patient to lean forward, and adjust the undershirt so it is smooth over the upper body.

9. Alternate procedure for slipover garments:

  Note: *A garment must be large enough or made of stretchy fabric for this procedure.*

    a. Place the garment front side down on the patient's lap, with the bottom opening facing the patient.

    b. Put the patient's hands into the bottom of the garment and, one at a time, into the sleeve holes.

    c. Pull the sleeves up as far as possible on the patient's arms and pull the hands through at the wrist if it is a long-sleeved garment. The garment should now be high on the patient's chest.

    d. Gather up the back of the garment with your hand and slip the garment over the patient's head.

    e. Smooth the garment down and position it comfortably about the patient's body. Adjust sleeves and shoulders as needed.

10. Shirts or dresses that fasten in the front:

    a. Insert your hand through the sleeve of the garment and grasp the patient's hand. Draw the sleeve over your hand and the patient's.

    b. Adjust the sleeve at the shoulder.

    c. Assist the patient to sit forward. Arrange clothing across the patient's back.

    d. Gather the sleeve on the opposite side by slipping your hand in from the outside.

    e. Grasp the patient's wrist and pull the sleeve of the garment over your hand and the patient's hand. Draw the sleeve upward and adjust it at the shoulder.

    f. Button, zip, or snap the garment.

11. Underwear or slacks:

    a. Facing the foot of the bed, gather the patient's underwear from waist to leg hole.

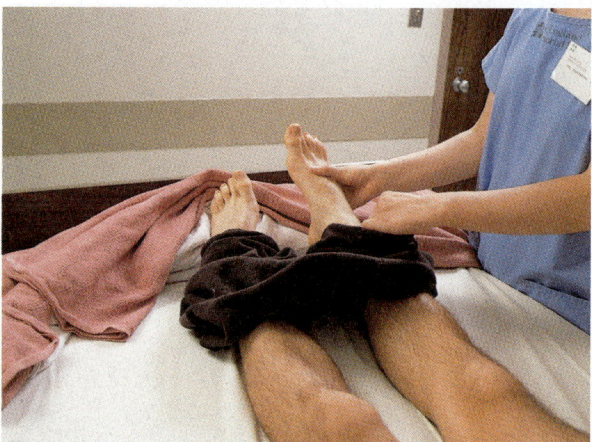

FIGURE 24-21B Slip pants over the feet and lower legs.

    b. Slip the underwear over one foot at a time (Figure 24-21B). Pull underwear up legs as high as possible.

    c. Assist the patient to raise the hips. Draw the garment over buttocks and up to waist. If patient cannot raise the buttocks, assist the patient to roll first to one side, as you pull up the garment, and then the other side (Figure 24-21C). Adjust the garment until comfortable.

    d. Fasten the garment, if required.

12. Socks or knee-high (or thigh-high) stockings:

    a. Roll a sock or stocking with heel in back and place it over the toes (Figure 24-21D).

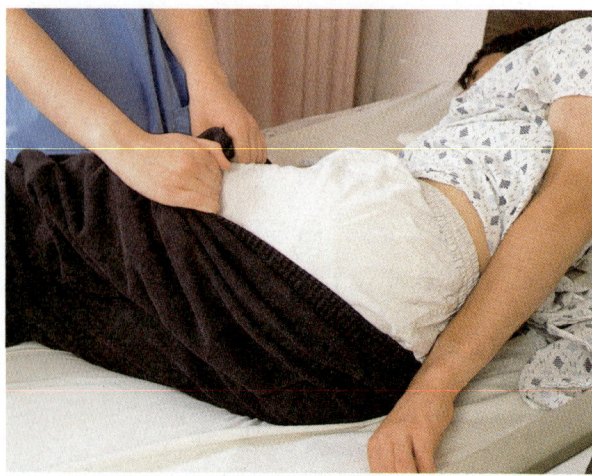

FIGURE 24-21C Have the patient roll onto the strong side first, then pull the pants over the upper hip. Then roll the patient to the other side and pull up pants. Adjust for comfort.

continues

PROCEDURE 67

continued

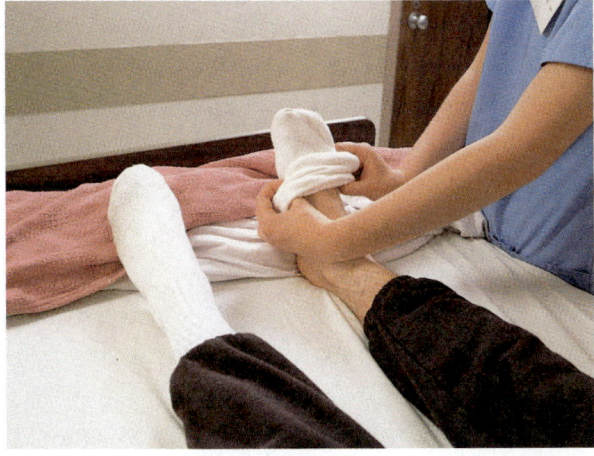

FIGURE 24-21D Adjust socks smoothly over the toes.

   b. Draw the sock up over the foot and adjust until smooth. Pull stockings smoothly up to knee or thigh.

   c. Repeat for other foot.

13. Pantyhose:

   a. Gather pantyhose and adjust over toes and feet. Draw up legs as high as possible.

   b. Draw over hips as described in step 11c. Adjust until comfortable at waist.

14. Shoes:

   a. Slip shoe on, using a shoe horn if necessary. Open laces of shoes completely so the foot can easily slip into the shoe (Figure 24-21E).

   b. Be sure the shoe is fastened securely (Velcro tabs or ties). If the shoes tie, be sure that the ends of the shoelaces do not drag on the floor. The shoes should be fastened tight enough to prevent them from slipping off the patient's feet but not so tight that circulation is impaired.

   c. Shoes should be appropriate to the floor surface.

15. To undress, reverse order of steps.

16. Carry out procedure completion actions.

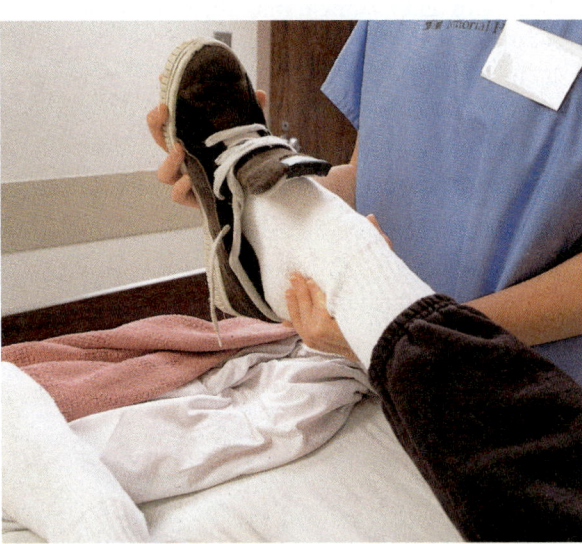

FIGURE 24-21E Open shoelaces completely so that the foot can easily slip into the shoe.

REVIEW

A. True/False.

Mark the following true or false by circling T or F.

1. T F The nursing assistant should carefully observe the patient during the bath procedure.

2. T F Perineal care is given with the patient positioned on a bedpan.

3. T F Range-of-motion exercises are often performed after the bath procedure begins.

4. T F The bath can be omitted if the patient is receiving an IV.

5. T F During the bed bath, only the part being bathed should be exposed.

6. T F Patients should be encouraged to use handrails when getting in and out of the bathtub.

7. T F Traction may be placed on drainage tubes as long as they are not disconnected.

8. T F Because soap is used during the bathing procedure, the tub need not be cleaned between patient uses.

9. T F The bathing procedure can provide the patient with mild exercise.

10. (T)F   Disposable gloves should be worn during bathing if the patient has draining wounds.

B. Matching.

Match the words in Column II with the statements in Column I.

Column I	Column II
11. _C_ External reproductive organs	**a.** axillae
12. _d_ Area at base of nails	**b.** midriff
13. _a_ Area under the arms	**c.** genitalia
	d. cuticle
	e. shampoo

C. Multiple Choice.

Select the one best answer for each of the following.

14. The room temperature during the bath procedure should be about
   a. 62°F.
   b. 68°F.
   c. 70°F.
   d. 78°F.

15. Patients needing special care during the bath period are those who
   a. have drainage tubing.
   b. are confused.
   c. are paralyzed.
   d. are independent.

16. Bath water temperature should be approximately
   a. 105°F.
   b. 90°F.
   c. 100°F.
   d. 115°F.

17. When giving hand and nail care, the hands should be soaked approximately
   a. 1 hour.
   b. ½ hour.
   c. 20 minutes.
   d. 5 minutes.

18. When a patient takes a bath, the bathroom door should
   a. not be locked.
   b. be left wide open for easier access.
   c. be locked for privacy.
   d. be left partially open.

D. Nursing Assistant Challenge.

Mr. Rodriguez is taking a shower before going home. He had bowel surgery four days ago. Answer the following about his care by selecting the correct word.

19. The person responsible for the cleanliness of the shower is the _____.
   (patient) (nursing assistant)

20. The patient _____ be assisted into and out of the shower.
   (should not) (should)

21. You can protect the patient from fatigue by _____ to the shower.
   (walking slowly) (transporting him by wheelchair)

22. If Mr. Rodriguez feels faint during his shower, you should turn the water _____.
   (to cold) (off)

23. To prevent chilling when Mr. Rodriguez felt weak, you should _____.
   (turn on the warm water) (wrap him in a bath blanket)

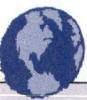

EXPLORING THE WEB

Description	Location
Bag bath	http://www.bag-bath.com
Infection control and bathing articles	http://www.infectioncontroltoday.com
Towel bath procedure	http://www.dementiasolutions.com
Ergonomics and Safety in Patient Bathing	http://www.patientsafetycenter.com
A Gentle Bathing Program Inservice	http://www.dementiasolutions.com
Procedure for Using the Arjo Bathing System	http://www-nmcp.med.navy.mil/nursing/procman/Arjo_Bath_SOP.doc
Skin Care Rituals That Do More Harm Than Good	http://www.woundheal.com
Using the Folding Bathtub for Bedfast Patients	http://www.puntukas.it

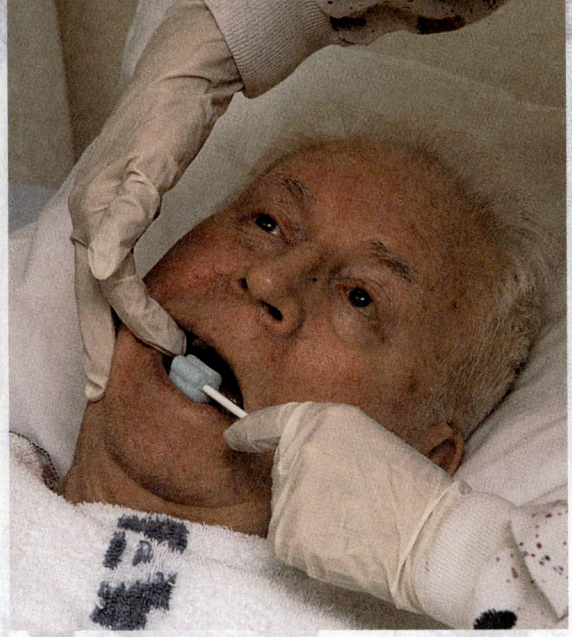

General Comfort Measures

objectives

After completing this unit, you will be able to:

- Spell and define terms.
- Discuss the reasons for early morning and bedtime care.
- Identify patients who require frequent oral hygiene.
- List the purposes of oral hygiene.
- Explain nursing assistant responsibilities for a patient's dentures.
- State the purpose of backrubs.
- Describe safety precautions when shaving a patient.
- Describe the importance of hair care.
- Explain the use of comfort devices.
- Demonstrate the following procedures:

- Procedure 68 Assisting with Routine Oral Hygiene
- Procedure 69 Assisting with Special Oral Hygiene
- Procedure 70 Assisting the Patient to Floss and Brush Teeth
- Procedure 71 Caring for Dentures
- Procedure 72 Backrub
- Procedure 73 Shaving a Male Patient
- Procedure 74 Daily Hair Care
- Procedure 75 Giving and Receiving the Bedpan
- Procedure 76 Giving and Receiving the Urinal
- Procedure 77 Assisting with Use of the Bedside Commode

vocabulary

Learn the meaning and the correct spelling of the following words and phrases:

AM care	caries	footboard	oral hygiene
anticoagulants	dentures	foot drop	PM care
bridging	feces	halitosis	trochanter roll

INTRODUCTION

You can do many things for your patients that will add to their general comfort and feeling of well-being. This includes:

- Providing AM and PM care
- Giving oral hygiene care
- Giving backrubs
- Brushing hair
- Shaving
- Using pillows and special equipment to maintain comfortable positions

AM CARE AND PM CARE

Early morning (AM) care prepares the patient for a day of activities and PM care prepares the patient for a night of rest. Each provides an opportunity for the patient to meet elimination needs and to be refreshed. The nursing assistant has an opportunity to closely observe the patient's condition and to interrelate supportively with the patient.

Early Morning (AM) Care

Early morning or AM care helps to set the tone for the entire day. If the patient is refreshed and comfortable before eating breakfast, the day is off to a good start. The nursing assistant provides AM care by:

- Awakening the patient gently—never abruptly—by saying the patient's name (Figure 25-1). If necessary, gently touch the arm.
- Awakening the patient before breakfast.
- Giving the patient the opportunity to use the bathroom, if permitted, or to use the bedpan or urinal.
- Helping the patient to wash hands and face.

The patient is not awakened early if he or she is:

- Going to surgery
- Having tests that prohibit eating

Bedtime (PM Care)

The care given to the patient just before bedtime is similar to that given in the early morning. Bedtime care is called PM care (or HS care). The nursing assistant gives PM care:

- In a quiet, unrushed manner that will help prepare the patient for sleep (Figure 25-2)
- Before medication for sleep is given by the nurse

Other routine procedures that may be carried out during AM and PM care include:

- Measuring vital signs
- Giving a backrub
- Providing mouth and hair care
- Giving the patient the opportunity to use the bathroom, if permitted, or to use the bedpan or urinal.

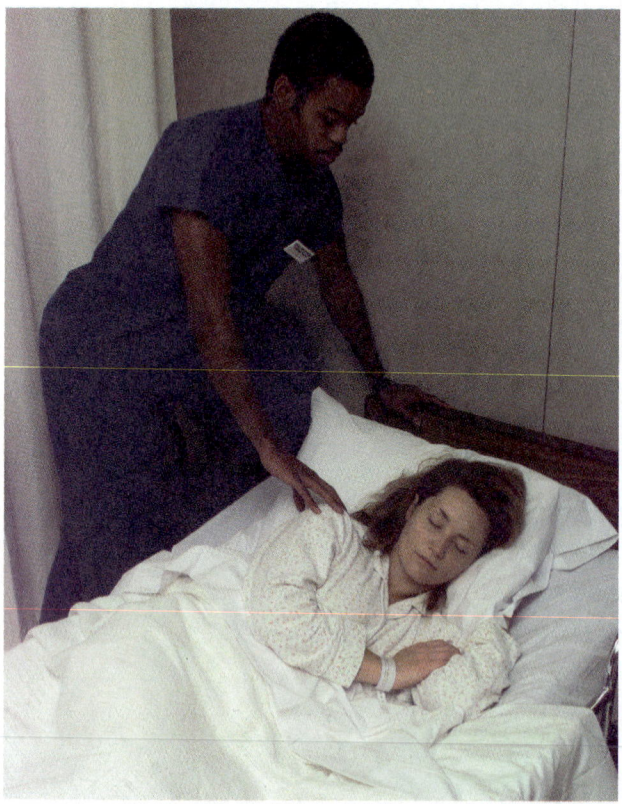

FIGURE 25-1 Early AM care. Wake the patient by saying the patient's name, then gently touching the arm, if necessary.

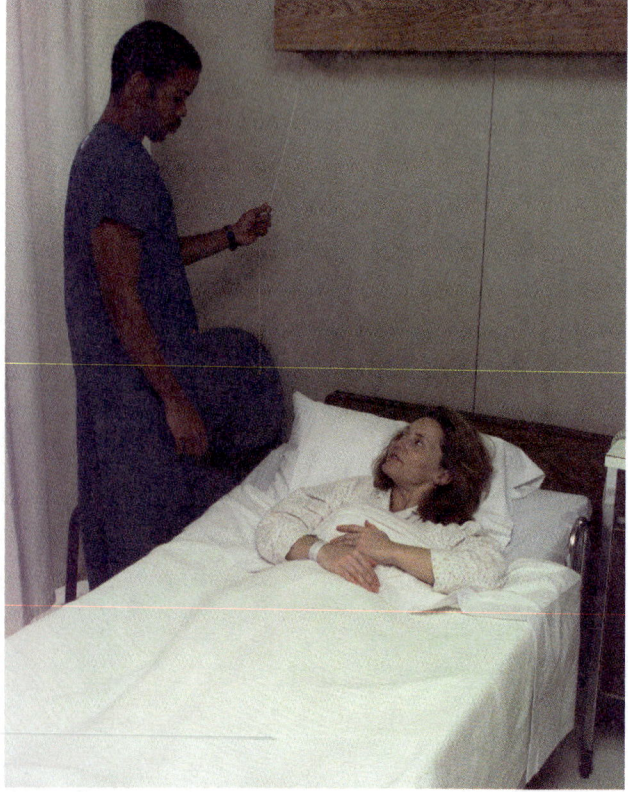

FIGURE 25-2 Turn off the light when the patient is settled and comfortable.

ORAL HYGIENE

Oral hygiene is the care of the mouth and teeth. (Refer to Procedures 68 to 70.)

- Routine oral hygiene (including brushing and flossing the teeth) should be performed at least three times a day.
- Patients should be encouraged to do as much as possible for themselves.
- *Special oral hygiene* is the cleansing of the mouth of the helpless patient using commercially prepared lemon and glycerine swabs, Toothettes®, and other preparations.

Patients requiring more frequent oral hygiene include those who are:

- unconscious
- vomiting
- experiencing a high temperature
- receiving certain medications
- dehydrated
- breathing through the mouth
- receiving oxygen
- receiving tube feeding
- dying

Proper cleansing of the teeth and mouth helps:

- prevent tooth decay (**caries**)
- eliminate bad breath (**halitosis**)
- contribute to the patient's comfort

INFECTION CONTROL *Alert*

Take care in storing the patient's toothbrush. Make sure it is covered or stored away from other items, such as the hairbrush.

INFECTION CONTROL *Alert*

Apply the principles of standard precautions when selecting protective equipment for assisting with dental procedures. Always wear gloves. If there is a chance of spraying or splashing of oral secretions, you will need a gown, gloves, mask, and face shield.

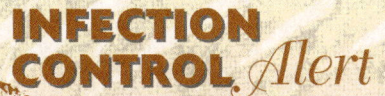

PROCEDURE 68

ASSISTING WITH ROUTINE ORAL HYGIENE

1. Carry out beginning procedure actions.
2. Assemble equipment:
   - disposable gloves and face mask
   - toothbrush
   - toothpaste
   - dental floss
   - mouthwash solution in cup
   - emesis basin
   - bath towel
   - straw
   - tissues
   - cup of fresh water
   - plastic bag
   - bed protector

3. Raise the head of the bed so that the patient may sit up, if his condition permits.
4. Lower the side rails and position the overbed table across the patient's lap.
5. Cover the table with a protector and place equipment on the table.
6. Place a bath towel over the patient's gown and bedcovers.
7. Be prepared to help as the patient brushes and flosses teeth.
8. Pour water over the toothbrush and put toothpaste on the brush.
9. Put on disposable gloves. A face mask may be used.

continues

PROCEDURE 68

continued

10. Brush teeth as follows (Figure 25-3):

    a. Insert the toothbrush into the mouth with bristles pointing downward.

    b. Turn the toothbrush with bristles toward teeth.

    c. Brush all tooth surfaces with a back-and-forth motion using short (tooth-wide) strokes.

    d. Use the "toe" end of the brush to clean the inner surfaces of the front teeth, using a gentle up-and-down motion.

    e. Brush the front of the tongue gently, if tolerated by the patient. Avoid the back of the tongue, as touching this area may cause gagging and coughing.

11. Give the patient water in a cup to rinse the mouth. Use a straw, if necessary. Turn the patient's head to one side, with the emesis basin near the chin, for return of fluid.

12. Repeat steps 10 and 11 as necessary.

13. To floss the patient's teeth:

    a. Select a piece of dental floss about 12 inches long. Wrap the end of the floss around your middle fingers, leaving the center area free (Figure 25-4).

    b. Ask the patient to open her mouth. Gently insert the floss between each tooth down to, but not into, the gum line.

    c. Ask the patient to rinse her mouth using the emesis basin.

14. Offer the patient mouthwash. Dilute the mouthwash if the patient wishes.

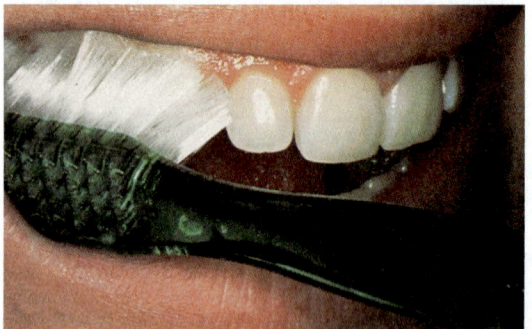

A. Place the head of the toothbrush beside the teeth, with the bristle tips at a 45-degree angle against the gum line. Move the brush back and forth in short (half-a-tooth-wide) strokes several times, using a gentle scrubbing motion. Brush the outer surfaces of each tooth, upper and lower, keeping the bristles angled against the gum line.

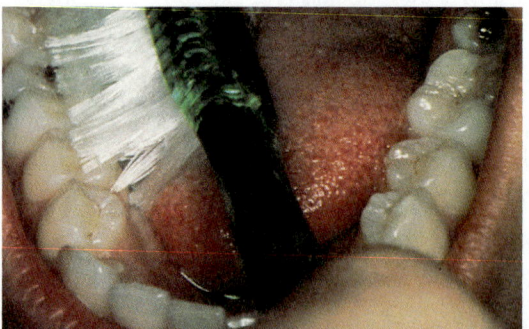

B. Use the same method on the inside surfaces of all the teeth, still using short back-and-forth strokes.

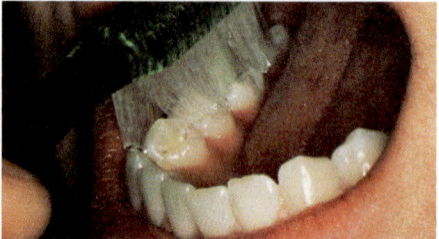

C. Scrub the chewing surfaces of the teeth.

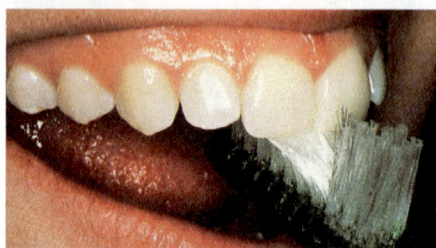

D. To clean the inside surfaces of the front teeth, tilt the brush vertically and make several gentle up-and-down strokes with the "toe" (the front part) of the brush.

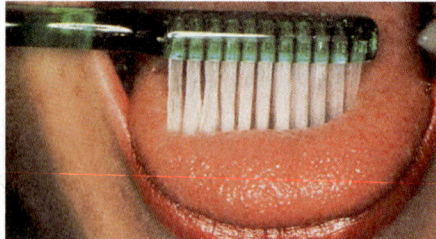

E. Brushing the patient's tongue will help freshen breath and clean the mouth by removing bacteria.

FIGURE 25-3 Brush teeth in the direction they grow and across the chewing surfaces. *(Toothbrushing photos and descriptions compliments of the American Dental Association)*

continues

PROCEDURE 68

continued

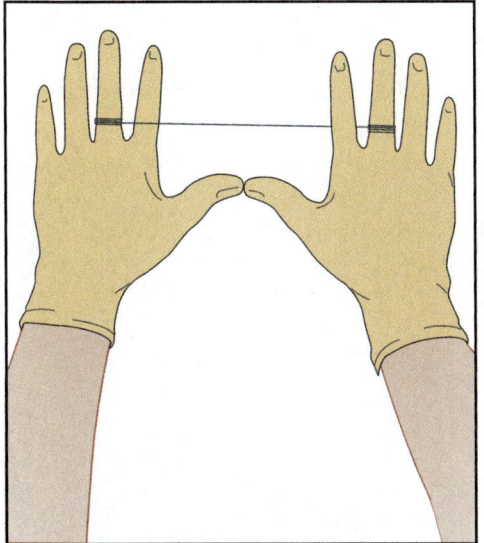 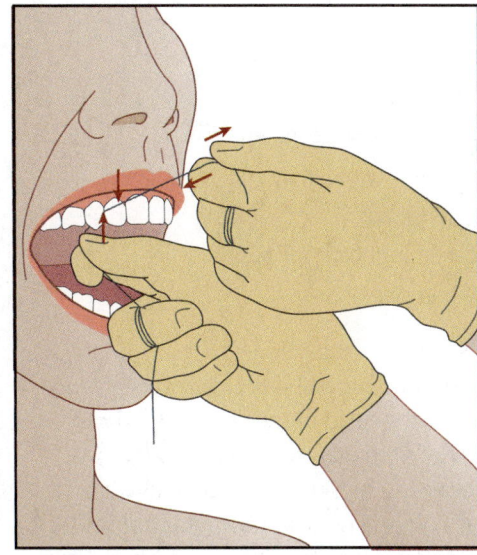

FIGURE 25-4 Floss is wrapped around the middle fingers (left). The proper method of using the floss to clean between the teeth (right).

15. Remove the basin. Wipe the patient's mouth and chin with tissue. Discard the tissue in a paper bag.

16. Remove the towel.

17. Rinse the toothbrush with water.

18. Remove and dispose of gloves and mask according to facility policy.

19. Carry out procedure completion actions.

CULTURE *Alert*

Many individuals have tongue piercings for fashion or cultural reasons. Many risks accompany this procedure. Inform the nurse promptly if a patient with a tongue piercing has pain, bleeding, increased flow of saliva, swelling, or signs of infection in the mouth. Swelling of the tongue can become severe, closing off the airway.

PROCEDURE 69

ASSISTING WITH SPECIAL ORAL HYGIENE

 Note: *Special oral hygiene is provided when the patient cannot participate actively in such care.*

1. Carry out beginning procedure actions.

2. Assemble equipment:
- disposable gloves
- Toothettes® or lemon and glycerine applicators

continues

PROCEDURE 69

continued

- emesis basin
- 2 bath towels
- plastic bag
- premoistened applicators
- tissues
- tongue depressor
- water-based lubricant for lips
- laundry hamper

3. Put on gloves.

4. Cover pillow with a towel. If the patient is able to sit up, elevate the head of the bed. If the patient is unable, or not permitted to sit up, turn the patient's head to one side and slightly forward so any excess fluid will not run down the throat. Cover the patient's upper chest with a towel. Place an emesis basin under the patient's chin.

5. Gently pull down on the chin to open the mouth, or open the mouth gently with a tongue depressor.

6. Using moistened Toothettes®, wipe gums, teeth, tongue, and inside of mouth (Figure 25-5).

7. Discard used applicators in a plastic bag.

8. Using clean applicators, apply lubricant to the patient's lips. Place used applicators in a plastic bag.

9. Remove towels. Clean and replace equipment.

10. Remove and dispose of gloves properly. Wash your hands.

11. Carry out procedure completion actions.

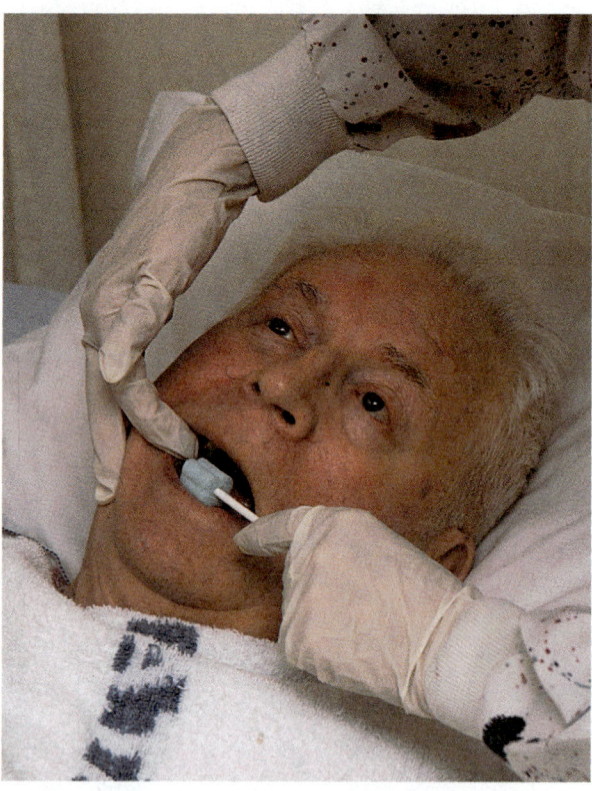

FIGURE 25-5 Using premoistened applicators, wipe gums, teeth, and tongue.

PROCEDURE 70

ASSISTING THE PATIENT TO FLOSS AND BRUSH TEETH

1. Carry out beginning procedure actions.

2. Assemble equipment:
   - disposable gloves
   - emesis basin
   - toothbrush
   - toothpaste
   - dental floss
   - glass of cool water
   - straw
   - mouthwash (if permitted)
   - hand towel
   - bed protector
   - plastic bag
   - laundry hamper

continues

PROCEDURE 70

continued

3. Elevate the head of the bed. Help the patient into a comfortable position.

4. Lower the side rails and position the overbed table across the patient's lap.

5. Cover the table with a plastic protector.

6. Place the emesis basin and a glass of water on the overbed table.

7. Place a towel across the patient's chest.

8. Be prepared to help as the patient flosses and brushes teeth. Remind the patient to clean the tongue and gums. Apply gloves and use standard precautions if you will be assisting with the procedure.

9. After the patient has flossed and brushed his teeth:
   a. Push the overbed table to the foot of the bed.
   b. Remove the emesis basin, clean it, and replace it according to facility policy.
   c. Rinse toothbrush.
   d. Remove the towels and put them with the soiled linen.
   e. Remove gloves and discard according to facility policy. Wash your hands.

10. Carry out procedure completion actions.

AGE-APPROPRIATE CARE *Alert*

Elderly patients may experience dry mouth and reduced saliva production. This commonly occurs as a side effect of medications. Related complaints are burning or sore throat, difficulty in swallowing, hoarseness, and dry nasal passages. Saliva is needed to help break down food for digestion. It also neutralizes acids in the mouth caused by plaque. Artificial saliva products are available, as are medicated oral rinses. The dentist may recommend that the patient use sugar-free gum or candy to increase saliva production. Inform the nurse if the patient experiences problems with saliva production.

DENTURES

Some patients have full sets of dentures. Other patients have partial plates that are removable, but attach by small metal clips to existing teeth. Partial plates should be given the same care as full dentures. **Dentures** are artificial teeth that are removable. They must be cleaned. The patient may feel embarrassed about wearing dentures and may dislike being seen after the dentures have been removed. Therefore, always provide privacy when dentures are to be removed and cleaned. (See Procedure 71.)

Denture Care

Denture care includes the following:
- Cleaning dentures daily under cool running water.
- Handling dentures carefully to prevent damage.
- Storing dentures in a safe place when they are out of the patient's mouth, such as in the drawer of the bedside stand in a container labeled with the patient's name (Figure 25-6).

SAFETY *Alert*

Remove dentures from a comatose patient to prevent accidental airway obstruction by the denture. Remove dentures from patients preoperatively to prevent potential damage to the dentures and accidental airway obstruction in surgery.

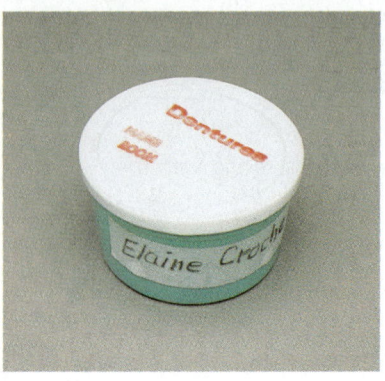

FIGURE 25-6 Dentures are stored in a cup labeled with the patient's name. The dentures are usually kept covered with water.

- Cleaning and checking the patient's mouth for signs of irritation.
- Checking the patient's lips for cracking and dryness.
- Applying cream, petroleum jelly, or glycerin to lips to avoid excessive dryness.

PROCEDURE 71

CARING FOR DENTURES

1. Carry out beginning procedure actions.
2. Assemble equipment:
   - disposable gloves
   - tissues
   - emesis basin
   - tongue depressor
   - brush
   - toothpaste or tooth powder
   - mouthwash, if permitted
   - cup of water
   - straw
   - gauze squares
   - applicators
   - denture cup
3. Apply disposable gloves.
4. Allow the patient to clean the dentures if she is able to do so. If the patient cannot, give a tissue to the patient and ask her to remove the dentures. Assist if necessary.
   a. To remove upper dentures, grasp the dentures firmly, ease them downward and then forward, and remove them from the mouth (Figure 25-7).

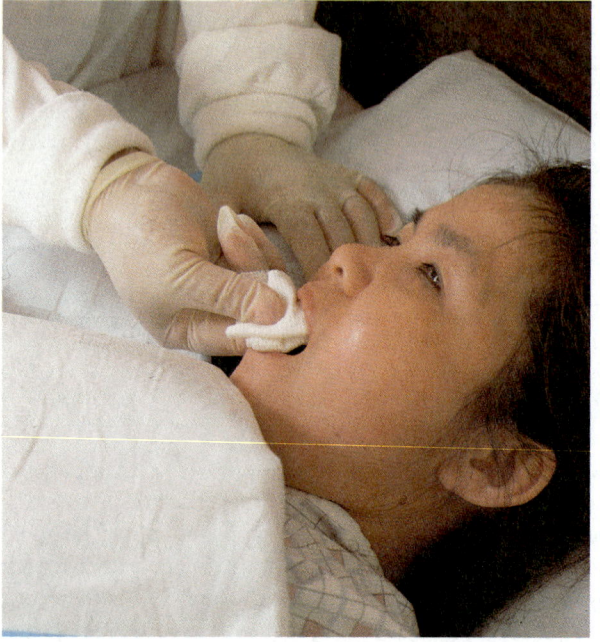

FIGURE 25-7 Grasp the upper dentures firmly with gauze-covered fingers, to prevent slipping. Ease them down and forward to remove.

   b. To remove lower dentures, grasp the dentures firmly, ease them upward and then forward, and remove them from the mouth.

continues

PROCEDURE 71

continued

5. Place the dentures in a denture cup padded with gauze squares. Take them to the bathroom or utility room.

6. Place a paper towel or washcloth in the bottom of the basin to protect the dentures (Figure 25-8). Fill the sink half full with cool water. The combination of water and towel protect the dentures from chipping or breaking if they are accidentally dropped in the sink.

7. Dentures may be soaked in a solution with a cleansing tablet before brushing, if desired.

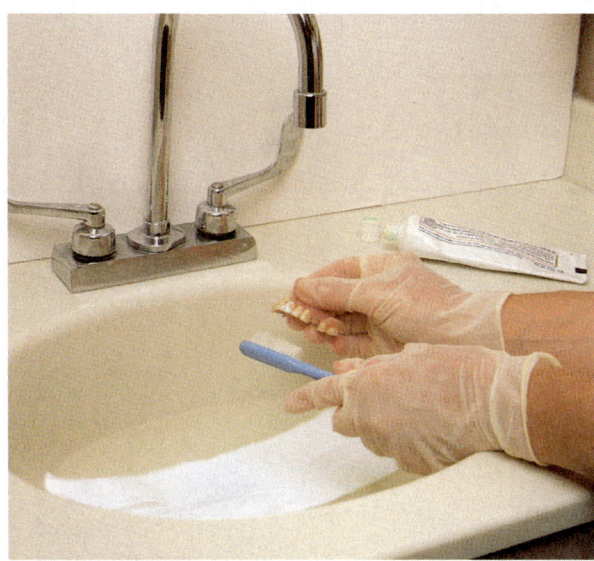

FIGURE 25-8 Brush dentures until all surfaces are clean.

8. Wet the dentures by rinsing under cool water.

9. Put toothpaste or tooth powder on a brush. Hold the dentures and brush until all surfaces are clean.

10. Rinse the dentures thoroughly under cool running water. Never use hot water. Rinse the denture cup.

11. Place fresh gauze squares in the denture cup with clean, cool water unless instructed otherwise.

12. Place the dentures in the gauze-lined cup and take them to the bedside.

13. Assist the patient to rinse her mouth with mouthwash, if permitted. Otherwise, use water. Hold the mouth open gently with a wooden tongue depressor. Clean the gums and tongue with applicators moistened with mouthwash, or use foam Toothettes.®

 Note: *Carefully observe and report the condition of the teeth, mouth, tongue, lips, and dentures.*

14. Use a paper towel or gauze to hand wet dentures to the patient. If the patient is able, she can remove the dentures from the cup. Insert if necessary, upper denture first.

15. Clean and replace equipment according to facility policy.

16. Remove and dispose of gloves according to facility policy.

17. Carry out procedure completion actions.

BACKRUBS

When properly given, backrubs can be:
- stimulating to the patient's circulation.
- a major aid in preventing skin breakdown (*decubiti*).
- soothing.
- refreshing.

Keep your nails short to prevent injuring the patient. The backrub procedure provides a good opportunity for you to observe the condition of the patient's skin. (See Procedure 72.) Report all observations to the nurse. Look for:
- Reddened areas that do not blanch (whiten) when pressed
- Raw areas of skin
- Condition of skin over bony prominences

Unless contraindicated, the backrub is given:

- routinely as part of the bed bath or partial bath.
- following use of the bedpan.
- when changing the position of the helpless patient.

OSHA *Alert*

When giving a backrub, make sure the bed is elevated to a comfortable height for you. Stand with one foot slightly ahead of the other, with knees bent slightly. Use your arm and shoulder muscles to massage the back. Rock back and forth, using the strong muscles in your legs. Avoid bending from the waist.

- at bedtime.
- when it could be a comfort to the patient.

Long, smooth strokes are relaxing. Short, circular strokes tend to be more stimulating. Avoid massaging red areas over bony prominences.

The backrub is given with warmed lotion.

DIFFICULT *Situations*

For many years, backrubs were almost a sacred, routine part of nursing care. Over time, we have become much more dependent on technology. When we are busy or staffing is short, it seems as if there is no time to give backrubs. Yet, calming the agitated patient who cannot sleep is time-consuming; the pregnant mother with a backache may use the call signal frequently; the patient with spasticity just cannot get into a comfortable position.

You may find that taking a few minutes to give a backrub will save you a great deal of time in caring for your patients. A good backrub is comforting and relaxing. Agitated patients often calm down. Uncomfortable patients become more comfortable and demand less attention. Do not omit this important part of nursing care that pays such large dividends in patient comfort and satisfaction. In the long run, it may even make your job easier.

PROCEDURE 72

BACKRUB

1. Carry out beginning procedure actions.

2. Assemble equipment:
   - disposable gloves
   - basin of water (105°F)
   - bath towel
   - soap and lotion

3. Put up the far side rail.

4. Place the lotion in a basin of water to warm (Figure 25-9).

5. Put on disposable gloves if the patient has open lesions.

6. Turn the patient on the side with the back toward you.

7. Expose and wash the back; dry carefully. This step is not necessary if the backrub is given after a bath.

8. Pour a small amount of lotion into one hand and warm it in the palm of your hand. Cold lotion may be very uncomfortable to the patient.

9. Apply the lotion to the patient's skin and rub with gentle but firm strokes. Give special attention to

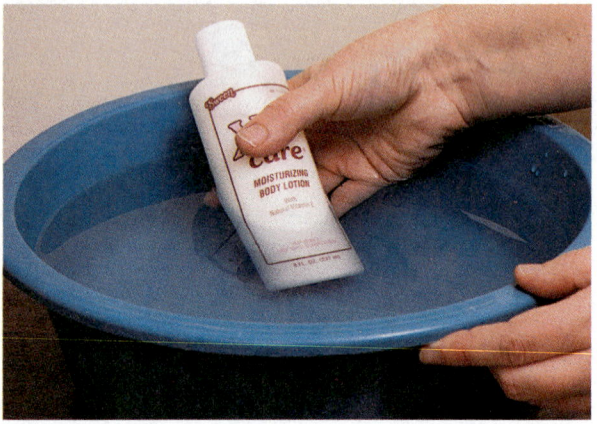

FIGURE 25-9 Warming the lotion in water for several minutes will make it more comfortable for the patient.

all bony prominences (Figure 25-10). Do not rub red areas. Report these to the nurse, if noted.

10. Begin at the base of the spine:
   - With long, soothing strokes, rub up the center of the back, around the shoulders, and down the sides of the back and buttocks (Figure 25-11, *left*).

continues

PROCEDURE 72

continued

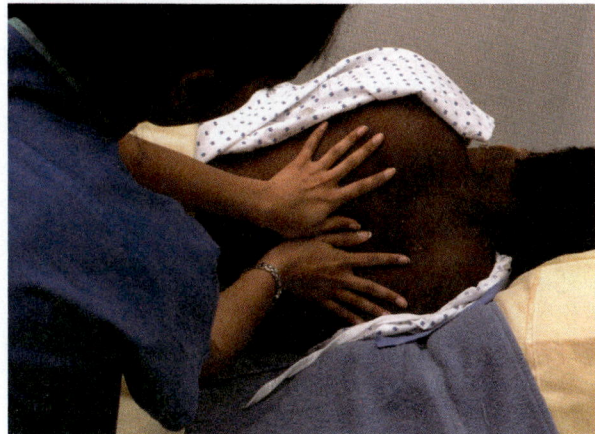

FIGURE 25-10 Use long, smooth, firm strokes to apply lotion.

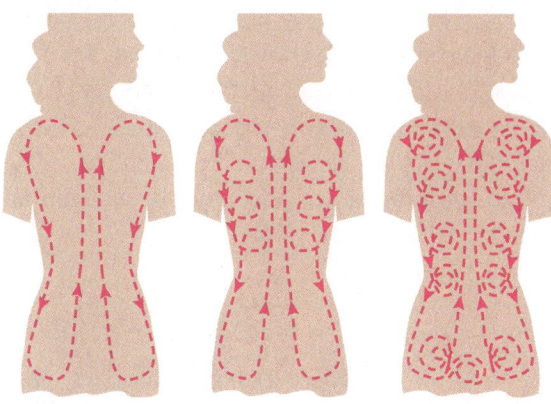

FIGURE 25-11 Strokes to be used during the backrub: soothing strokes (left), circular movement (middle), passive movement (right).

- Repeat the previous step four times, using long, soothing upward strokes and a circular motion on the downstroke (Figure 25-11, *middle*).

- Repeat, but on the downward stroke rub in small circular motions with the palm of your hand. Include areas over the coccyx (base of the spine) (Figure 25-11, *right*).

- Repeat long, soothing strokes on muscles for 3 to 5 minutes (Figure 25-11, *left*).

- Dry the area well.

- If redness on pressure areas is noted, report it to the nurse. Straighten and tighten the bottom sheet and draw sheet.

11. Change the patient's gown, if necessary.

12. Remove gloves if used. Discard according to facility policy and wash your hands.

13. Replace equipment.

14. Carry out procedure completion actions.

DAILY SHAVING

Daily shaving is part of the routine self-care of most men. It should not be neglected in a care facility. When patients are unable to shave themselves and a barber is not available, it is your responsibility. (See Procedure 73.)

Older women have an increase in the growth and coarseness of hairs on the chin and upper lip. Many women find this distressing. Tweezers can be used to remove some of the hairs, but a more permanent method is to have the hairs removed professionally with an electric needle. Some women may require a shave. In some facilities nursing assistants are not permitted to shave women patients. Be sure to check the policy of your facility.

OSHA *Alert*

Always wear gloves when shaving patients with a nonelectric razor, because of the high risk of contact with blood. Discard the razor in a puncture-resistant (sharps) container.

AGE-APPROPRIATE CARE *Alert*

Elderly women may grow facial hair as a result of hormonal changes during aging. Coarse hair is common on the chin. Most women prefer to have facial hair removed. Many women also prefer to have hair removed from their legs and underarms. Honor the patient's preferences. Know your facility policy for removing facial hair from female patients. Some facilities use depilatories. Although some facilities shave women, check with the nurse before performing this procedure because shaving may worsen the problem, causing the hair to become thicker and coarser.

guidelines *for*

Safety in Shaving

- Use the patient's own shaving equipment if possible. For safety, use an electric razor or rotary razor.

- If the patient is receiving **anticoagulants** (medications that thin the blood and increase the risk of bleeding), a special procedure may be required. For example, an electric razor provides the greatest safety. Check with the nurse for the proper procedure.

- If oxygen is being given, it may be possible to discontinue it during this procedure. Consult the nurse and follow hospital policy.

INFECTION CONTROL *Alert*

Shaving may be done with an electric razor, which is the patient's personal property. Such a razor is used for one patient only and cleaned according to manufacturer's directions after each use. This usually involves brushing the heads with a small brush designed for this purpose. All hair should be removed from the head of the razor. Some electric razors must be recharged periodically. Electric razors are expensive. Handle the razor carefully and avoid dropping it. If the electrical cord is frayed or worn, report to the nurse and remove the razor from use. If an electric razor is not available, use a disposable safety razor. Wearing gloves is usually not necessary when an electric razor is used.

PROCEDURE 73

SHAVING A MALE PATIENT

1. Carry out beginning procedure actions.

2. Assemble equipment:
   - disposable gloves
   - electric shaver or safety razor
   - shaving lather or preshave lotion for electric razor
   - basin of water (105°F)
   - face towels
   - mirror
   - washcloth
   - aftershave lotion

3. Raise the head of the bed. Place equipment on overbed table.

4. Put on gloves.

5. Place one face towel across patient's chest and one under head.

6. Moisten face and apply lather (or preshave lotion).

7. Starting in front of ear:
   a. Hold skin taut and bring razor down over cheek toward chin (Figure 25-12).
   b. Repeat until lather on cheek is removed and area has been shaved. Rinse frequently.
   c. Repeat on other cheek.
   d. Use firm, short strokes. Shave in direction of hair growth.
   e. Rinse razor frequently.

continues

PROCEDURE 73

continued

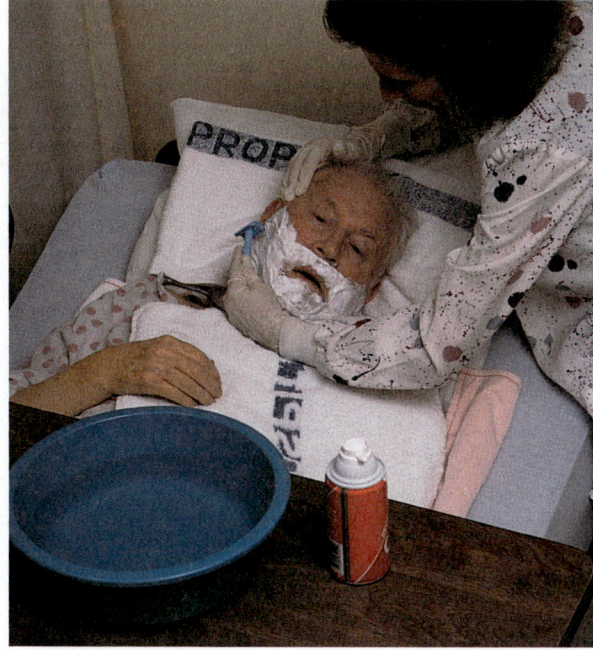

FIGURE 25-12 Shaving is part of the daily routine for most men.

8. Ask the patient to tighten his upper lip. Shave from the nose to the upper lip in short, downward strokes.

9. Ask the patient to tighten his chin. Shave the chin in downward strokes.

10. Assist the patient to tip his head back.

11. Lather the neck area and stroke up toward the chin. Rinse and repeat until all lather is removed.

12. Wash the patient's face and neck and dry thoroughly.

13. Apply aftershave lotion if desired.

14. If the skin is nicked, apply a small piece of tissue and hold pressure directly over the area. Then apply an antiseptic and bandage. Report the incident to the nurse.

15. Clean and replace equipment. Dispose of razor according to facility policy. Remove the head of an electric razor. Use a razor brush to remove clippings. Store the razor according to facility policy.

16. Remove and dispose of gloves according to facility policy.

17. Carry out procedure completion actions.

DAILY HAIR CARE

Daily care of the hair, for both male and female patients, is usually performed after the patient's bed bath. (See Procedure 74.)

The hair should be combed and brushed each morning. Tangles can be loosened by sectioning the hair with a comb or brush, working with one section at a time. Grasp the hair near the scalp to reduce pulling (Figure 25-13). Start combing or brushing tangles out starting at the ends and working toward the scalp. Braiding long hair after brushing can help reduce tangles. Tangles can be reduced in wiry, dry hair by using conditioner and keeping the hair short or in braids.

Tips: Avoid braiding a patient's hair tightly, because it can be uncomfortable. Secure the braids with hair ties. Avoid rubber bands, if possible. If the hair is very tangled, applying a small amount of alcohol or oil to the tangle will make it easier to remove.

Brushing the hair:

- stimulates circulation of the scalp.
- refreshes the patient.
- removes dust and lint.
- helps to keep the hair shiny and attractive.

If additional care is needed, a fluid dry cleaner to shampoo the hair is available. It leaves the hair soft and manageable and the hairstyle intact. This procedure is so simple that it

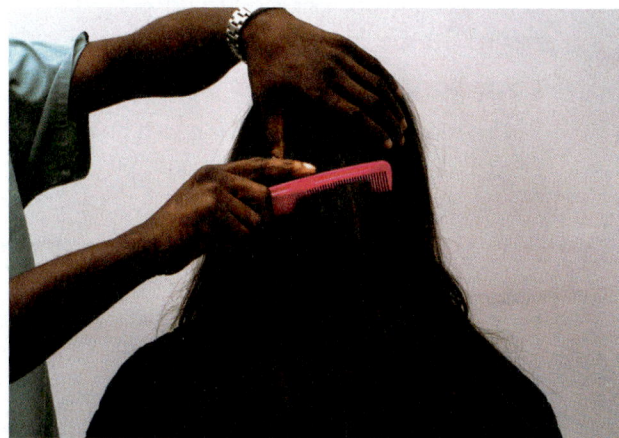

FIGURE 25-13 To remove tangles from long hair, divide the hair into sections. Work with one section at a time. Hold the hair near the scalp to reduce pulling and start combing at the end of the hair, working up toward the scalp.

is often used instead of the regular shampoo for patients who must remain in bed.

Sometimes, however, a shampoo may be advisable for the patient in bed. Approval for the procedure must be obtained from the doctor. Bed shampoos should be given every two weeks when the patient is bedbound for an extended period. (See Unit 24, Procedure 66.)

The following procedure assumes that the patient is a female. Hair care for a male is very similar, however, so the procedure can easily be adapted.

DIFFICULT *Situations*

Hair is important to everyone's self-esteem and appearance. Some diseases and medications cause hair loss. Some cause changes to the volume and texture of hair. Some medications cause hair to become dry and brittle. Patients who have problems with their hair may become anxious or angry because the appearance of the hair affects their self-esteem. If the patient is experiencing problems with hair, treat it gently. Use products such as baby shampoo and conditioner. Use tepid water. Pat the hair dry rather than rubbing it with a towel. Use a wide-toothed comb to style the hair gently. Avoid braids and rubber bands, which may worsen the problem. Assist the patient to wear a scarf or turban, if desired.

PROCEDURE 74

DAILY HAIR CARE

1. Carry out beginning procedure actions.

2. Assemble equipment:
   - towel
   - comb and brush

3. Ask the patient to move to the side of the bed nearest you; or the patient may sit in a chair if permitted. If the patient is sitting up, put a towel around her shoulders.

4. Cover the pillow with a towel.

5. Part or section the hair and comb with one hand between the scalp and the ends of the hair.

6. Brush carefully and thoroughly.

7. Have the patient turn so that you can comb and brush the hair on the back of her head. If the hair is tangled, work section by section to unsnarl it, beginning near the ends and working toward the scalp.

8. Complete brushing and arrange the hair attractively. Braid long hair to prevent repeated snarling. Allow the patient to choose the style, if able.

9. Clean and replace equipment according to facility policy.

10. Carry out procedure completion actions.

COMFORT DEVICES

The physician, nurse, or physical therapist orders comfort devices such as bed cradles, footboards, and pillows. They are designed to relieve pressure on specific areas or to help maintain body position.

Bed Cradle

A bed cradle (Figure 25-14) prevents the weight of the bed-clothes from falling on some part of the body. It can be used therapeutically or as a comfort device. It is used:

- over fractured limbs

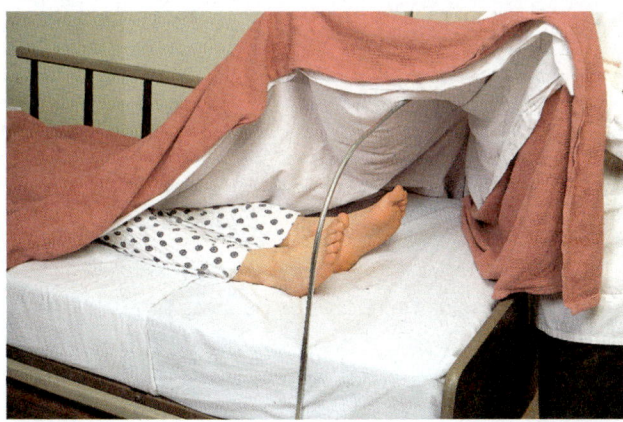

FIGURE 25-14 A bed cradle keeps the sheet and blanket from putting pressure on the feet.

- when there are burns
- to prevent skin lesions
- over widespread skin conditions, such as psoriasis or eczema
- to prevent contractures of the feet
- over a wet cast until it dries

Coverings that maintain some degree of warmth within the cradle may also be needed to keep the patient comfortable. Care must be taken to position the limb within the cradle. It may be necessary to pad the cradle edges.

Footboard or Footrest

The **footboard** or footrest is a device placed between the mattress and bed to keep the feet at right angles to the legs (natural standing position). A footboard is always padded. It is used to prevent a type of contracture called **foot drop**. In foot drop, the muscle in the calf of the leg tends to tighten, causing the toes to point downward. Foot drop may happen when the patient must remain in bed over a long period of time. Even a brief period in bed is sufficient to cause a degree of foot drop that makes walking difficult when the patient does get out of bed.

If a footboard is not available, a pillow folded lengthwise may be placed against the foot of the bed to serve the same purpose. Some facilities use special tennis shoes or soft boots to prevent foot drop in patients who are at risk because they are bedfast.

Pillows and Bath Blankets

Pillows can be used as comfort devices and to maintain alignment when properly arranged. For directions on properly altering the patient's positions, refer to Unit 15.

The **trochanter roll** is used to prevent external rotation of the hip. Trochanter rolls should be used routinely for bedfast patients, to prevent deformities. Unless a specific medical condition, such as a hip fracture, is present, no special order is necessary.

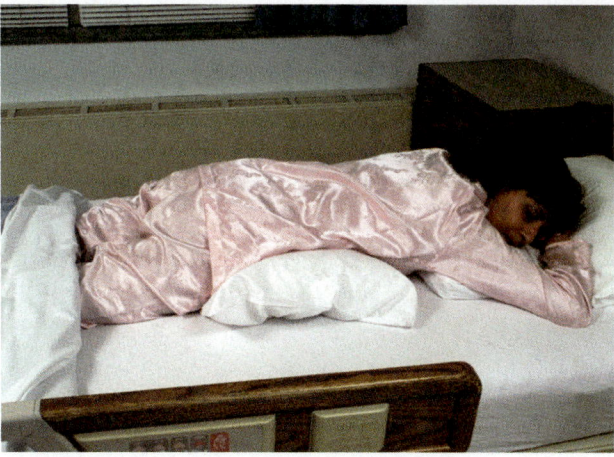

FIGURE 25-15 The patient is positioned on her abdomen and pillows are used to form a bridge, preventing pressure on her breasts.

A trochanter roll or support can be made as follows:

1. Fold a bath blanket lengthwise in thirds.
2. Position the patient in the center of the folded bath blanket. The blanket should extend from mid-thigh to above the waist.
3. Roll each side of the blanket under and toward the patient until the blanket roll is firmly against the patient. Then tuck the roll inward toward the bed and patient to maintain the patient's position.

Pillows are also used to relieve pressure in such a way that spaces are left for specific areas (Figure 25-15). This technique is called **bridging**. Bridging elevates an area of the body off the surface of the bed. It is useful for patients with healing pressure ulcers. Bridging is commonly used for the sacrum, hips, heels, and ankles. No special equipment is necessary. Facilities may use a combination of pillows, foam props, and bath blankets to support an area.

ELIMINATION NEEDS

Regular, periodic elimination of body wastes is essential for maintaining health. Patients who are confined to bed must rely on you to help them with this physical task. (See Procedures 75 to 77.) You should know that:

- The patient must regularly empty the bladder by urinating (voiding).
- A urinal (duct or bottle) is used by male patients when they need to urinate. A bedpan is used by female patients to void when they are confined to bed.
- A regular bowel movement (which is the discharge of solid waste from the body) is also important to a patient's health.
- The solid waste produced by the patient is called **feces** or *stool*.
- Both male and female patients use a bedpan for solid waste elimination when confined to bed.

- Many patients are somewhat sensitive about using a bedpan or urinal.
- Personal hygiene is exceedingly important in carrying out these procedures properly.
- Bedpans are very uncomfortable.

Four important points must be kept in mind. You must:

1. Wear disposable gloves.
2. Wash your hands immediately before and after the procedure. This will help prevent the transmission of any disease to others and to yourself.
3. Provide privacy for the patient. Obtain the proper bedpan according to patient needs.
4. As soon as possible, answer the light indicating that the patient is finished.

One-Glove Technique

Some facilities require health care providers to use the one-glove technique when removing bedpans, urinals, and other contaminated items. Gloves are worn on both hands when the contaminated item is removed. The bedpan or

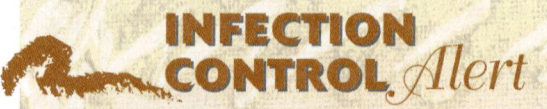

INFECTION CONTROL *Alert*

Make sure that bedpans and urinals are labeled with the patients' names for patients in rooms with two or more beds. After cleaning the bedpan or urinal, store it properly in the bedside stand or according to facility policy. Do not leave uncovered bedpans and urinals in the bathroom.

contaminated item is covered if it is to be carried to the bathroom or into the hallway. A glove is then removed from one hand. Do not put the glove on an environmental surface. The gloved hand carries the glove that you removed and the contaminated item. The ungloved hand is used to open doors and turn on faucets. By using this method, you avoid contaminating the environment with your gloves.

PROCEDURE 75

GIVING AND RECEIVING THE BEDPAN

1. Carry out beginning procedure actions.
2. Assemble equipment:
   - disposable gloves
   - bedpan and cover
   - basin
   - washcloth
   - bath blanket
   - paper towels/protector
   - toilet tissue
   - soap
   - towel
3. Lower the head of the bed, if necessary.
4. Put on gloves.
5. Take the bedpan and toilet tissue from the bedside stand.
   - Place a protector on the chair. Place the bedpan (Figure 25-16) on it.
   - Never place a bedpan on the bedside stand or overbed table.

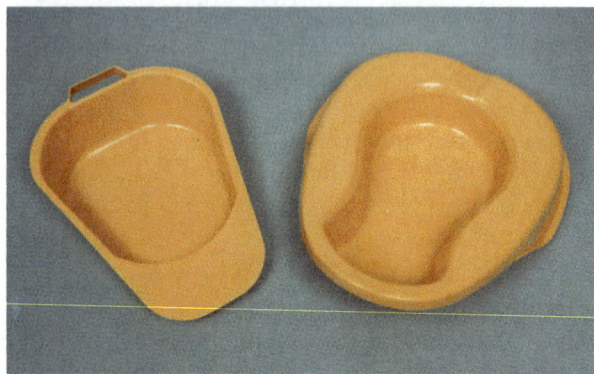

FIGURE 25-16 Orthopedic (fracture) bedpan (left) and regular bedpan (right).

   - Put the remainder of the articles on the bedside table.
6. Place the bedpan cover at the foot of the bed.
   - The bedpan may be warmed by running warm water into it and then emptying and drying it.
   - Plastic bedpans may be comfortable without warming.

continues

PROCEDURE 75

continued

> 📝 **Note:** *Never carry or allow a used bedpan to sit uncovered. If a bedpan cover is not available, cover the bedpan with a towel, bed protector, pillowcase, or paper towels.*

7. Cover the patient with a bath blanket. Fold the top bedcovers back at a right angle. Raise the patient's gown. If the patient is thin or has a pressure sore, consult the nurse for the appropriate action. The nursing care plan may have specific instructions for such cases. For example, it may be necessary to pad the bedpan with a folded towel or to take some other action.

8. Ask the patient to flex the knees and rest weight on the heels, if able.

9. Help the patient to raise the buttocks by:
   - Putting one hand under the small of the patient's back and lifting gently and slowly with that hand.
   - With the other hand, place the bedpan under the patient's hips.
   - If the patient is unable to raise the buttocks, two assistants may be needed to lift the patient.
   - The pan may also be placed by rolling the patient to one side, positioning the bedpan against the buttocks, and rolling the patient back onto the pan (Figure 25-17). Check to be sure the bedpan is positioned properly.

- Alternatively, if a trapeze is in place over the bed, place the bedpan under the patient as the patient lifts self using the trapeze (Figure 25-18).
- The patient's buttocks should rest on the rounded shelf of the regular bedpan.
- The narrow end should face the foot of the bed.

10. Replace the top bedcovers. Raise the head of the bed to a comfortable height. Remove gloves and dispose of properly.

11. Make sure the toilet paper and signal cord are within easy reach of the patient. Leave the patient alone unless contraindicated in the nursing care plan.

12. Wash your hands.

> 📝 **Note:** *If a specimen is to be taken, instruct the patient that toilet tissue is not to be placed in the bedpan. In this case, the nursing assistant will clean the patient and provide perineal care.*

13. Watch for the patient's signal.

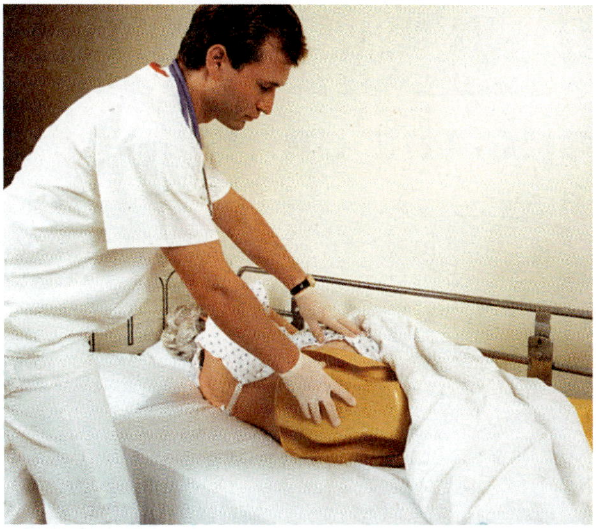

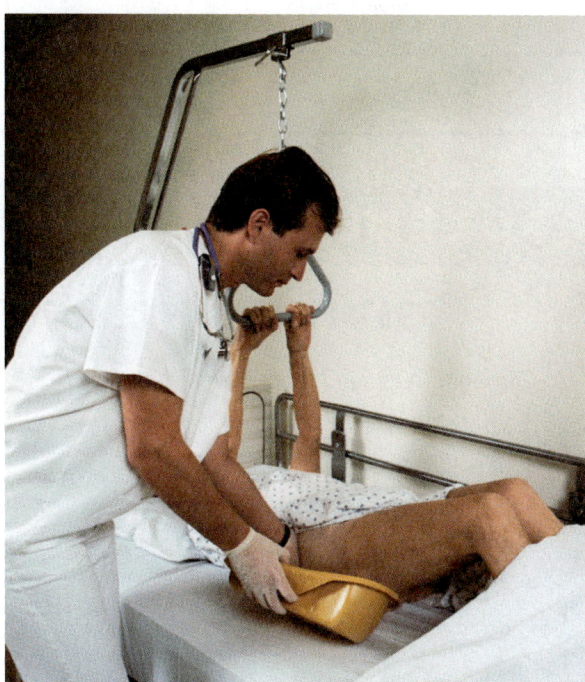

FIGURE 25-17 Roll the patient away from you while supporting the patient with one hand on the patient's hip. Place the bedpan with the other hand, then roll the patient back onto the bedpan.

FIGURE 25-18 The patient assists by lifting with the trapeze as the nursing assistant places the bedpan under the patient. Note that the nursing assistant supports the patient's back with his hand.

continues

PROCEDURE 75

continued

14. Answer the patient's call signal immediately. Wash your hands and put on disposable gloves. Fill the basin with warm water (105°F) and place it next to soap, washcloth, and towel on the overbed table.

15. Fold the top bedcovers back so that the patient remains covered only with the bath blanket.

16. Remove the bedpan from under the patient.

    - Ask the patient to flex the knees and rest weight on the heels. Place one hand under the small of the back and lift gently to help raise the buttocks off the bedpan. Take the bedpan with the other hand. Cover it and place it on the chair.

    - If the patient is unable to raise the buttocks, two assistants may be needed to lift. Otherwise, roll the patient off the pan to the side and remove the pan. Lift and move carefully. Hold the pan firmly with one hand.

    - Many patients have difficulty cleaning adequately after using the bedpan. You may need to clean and dry the patient yourself.

17. Assist the patient to a clean area of the bed, if necessary. Provide perineal care.

- Discard used toilet tissue in the bedpan unless a specimen is to be collected.
- Cover the bedpan again.
- Cleanse the patient with warm water and soap, if necessary.

18. Replace the bedclothes, changing linen or protective pads as necessary.

19. Cover the patient with top bedding and remove the bath blanket.

20. Encourage the patient to wash hands and freshen up after the procedure.

21. Take the bedpan to the bathroom or utility room and observe its contents. Measure, if required.

22. Empty the bedpan.

23. Turn on the faucet, using a paper towel. Rinse the bedpan with cold water and disinfectant. Rinse, dry, and return the bedpan to storage in the patient's bedside stand.

24. Remove gloves and dispose of them properly. Wash your hands.

25. Carry out procedure completion actions.

PROCEDURE 76

GIVING AND RECEIVING THE URINAL

1. Carry out beginning procedure actions.

2. Assemble equipment:
   - urinal (Figure 25-19)
   - basin
   - soap
   - washcloth
   - towel
   - disposable gloves

3. Put on gloves. Lift the top bedcovers and place the urinal under the covers so the patient can grasp the handle. Instruct the patient to place his penis in the urinal opening. If he cannot do this,

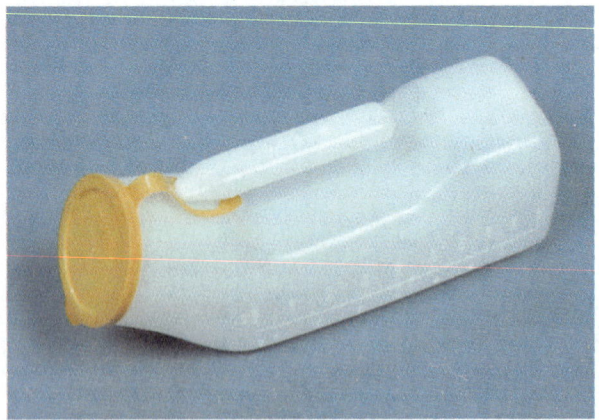

FIGURE 25-19 Male urinal with lid.

continues

PROCEDURE 76

continued

you must position the urinal and ensure that the penis is placed in the opening.

4. Remove gloves and dispose of them properly. Wash your hands. Make sure the signal cord is within easy reach of the patient. Leave the patient alone if possible. Watch for his signal.

5. Answer the patient's signal immediately. Wash your hands. Use a paper towel to turn on the faucet. Fill a basin with warm water (105°F), and place it next to soap, washcloth, and towel so the patient can wash and dry his hands.

6. Put on gloves. Ask the patient to hand the urinal to you. Cover it. Rearrange the bedclothes if necessary.

7. Take the urinal to the bathroom or utility room and observe the contents. Measure, if required. Do not empty the urinal if you observe anything unusual (such as blood). Rather, save the contents of the urinal for the nurse's inspection.

8. Empty the urinal. Use a paper towel to turn on the faucet and another towel to turn the faucet off. Rinse the urinal with cold water and clean it with warm soapy water. Rinse, dry, and cover the urinal. Remove gloves and dispose of them properly. Wash your hands.

9. Place the urinal inside the patient's bedside table. Clean and replace other articles.

10. Carry out procedure completion actions.

PROCEDURE 77

ASSISTING WITH USE OF THE BEDSIDE COMMODE

1. Carry out beginning procedure actions.

2. Assemble equipment:
   - disposable gloves
   - portable commode
   - toilet tissue
   - basin
   - washcloth
   - soap
   - towel
   - bath blanket

3. Position the commode beside the bed, facing the head. Lock the commode wheels and open the lid. Be sure a receptacle is in place under the seat.

4. If the bed and side rails are elevated, lower the side rail nearest you and lower the bed to the lowest horizontal position. Lock bed wheels.

5. Put on gloves.

6. Assist the patient to a sitting position. Swing the patient's legs over the edge of the bed.

7. Assist the patient to put on a robe. Put slippers on the patient. Assist the patient to stand. If needed, use a transfer belt.

8. Support the patient with hands on either side of the chest. Remember to use proper body mechanics. Pivot the patient to the right and lower her to the commode.

9. Cover the patient's legs with a bath blanket.

10. Leave the call bell and toilet tissue within reach.

11. Remove gloves and discard according to facility policy.

12. When the patient signals, return promptly. Wash your hands and put on gloves. Fill a basin with water at 105°F. Bring the basin to the bedside along with soap, a towel, and a washcloth.

13. Remove bath blanket. Assist the patient to stand.

continues

PROCEDURE 77

continued

14. Cleanse the anus or perineum if the patient is unable to do so.

15. Allow the patient to wash and dry her hands. Remove gloves and dispose of according to facility policy. Wash your hands.

16. Assist the patient to return to bed. Adjust bedding and pillows for comfort.

17. Leave the signal cord within easy reach.

18. Put on gloves.

19. Remove the receptacle from the commode and cover it. Close the commode lid.

20. Take the receptacle to the bathroom. Note its contents and measure if required.

21. Empty and clean the receptacle per facility policy. Replace it in the commode. Remove and dispose of gloves properly.

22. Put the commode in its proper place.

23. Carry out procedure completion actions.

REVIEW

A. True/False.

Mark the following true or false by circling T or F.

1. T (F) Dentures should be stored in an antiseptic solution.

2. (T) F Backrubs are routinely given as part of the bath procedure.

3. (T) F A padded footboard is used to prevent foot drop.

4. (T) F Routine oral hygiene should be carried out once daily. 3X

5. (T) F Proper oral hygiene helps prevent tooth decay.

6. T (F) When not in the patient's mouth, dentures should be left on the bedside stand.

7. (T) F Patients should never be awakened abruptly.

8. (T) F When giving PM care, the bottom sheet should be tightened and the top linen straightened.

9. (T) F Disposable gloves should be used by a nursing assistant who is giving oral care.

10. T (F) The unconscious patient needs no oral care because he is not eating.

B. Matching.

Choose the correct word from Column II to match the phrases in Column I.

Column I

11. _e_ bad breath
12. _a_ mouth care
13. _b_ tooth cavities
14. _d_ means of relieving pressure
15. _c_ artificial teeth

Column II

a. oral hygiene
b. caries
c. dentures
d. bridging
e. halitosis
f. foot drop

C. Completion.

Complete the statements in items 16–20 by writing in the correct word from the following list.

arm	~~name~~
~~breakfast~~	~~PM care~~
~~down~~	removed
early AM care	~~surgery~~
~~hand~~	

16. After PM care, the bed should be left with the backrest _down_.

17. _pm care_ should be completed before sleep medication is given.

18. The best way to awaken a patient is to place your _hand_ on the patient's arm and say his _name_.

19. Patients are not wakened early if they are going to have _surgery_.

20. Early morning care awakens the patient before _breakfast_

D. Multiple Choice.

Select the one best answer for each of the following.

21. Which of the following patients should be given special mouth care?

  a. One who can brush her own teeth

  b. One who is drinking water ad lib

  c. One who has a broken leg

  (d.) One who has a high fever

22. To warm lotion before giving a backrub,

  a. hold it under running water.

  (b.) soak it in a basin of warm water.

  c. let the patient hold the bottle for a few minutes.

  d. microwave the bottle for 15 seconds.

23. The best way to support a patient in a side-lying position is to

  a. use a footboard to keep the feet aligned.

  b. place a pillow doubled under the head.

  c. place two pillows lengthwise between the legs.

  (d.) double a pillow lengthwise behind the back.

24. When brushing a patient's teeth, the best technique includes

  (a.) inserting the toothbrush with the bristles down.

  b. brushing in a circular motion.

  c. inserting the toothbrush with bristles facing the teeth.

  d. brushing the teeth in a downward motion only.

25. Backrubs are given

  (a.) routinely as part of the pericare procedure.

  b. before use of the bedpan.

  c. routinely every two hours.

  d. only for patients with red areas.

E. Nursing Assistant Challenge.

Your patient, Mrs. Ubanan, has a history of heavy smoking and breathes through her mouth. She has plastic dentures and her care plan indicates that she needs assistance with denture care. Complete the following statements regarding this patient.

26. State two reasons why special oral hygiene has been ordered for Mrs. Ubanan.

  a. smoker

  b. mouth breather

27. Where are the dentures stored when not in use? denture cup

28. Should the dentures be kept dry or wet? wet

29. Should you wear gloves when removing her dentures? yes

30. Will you clean the dentures in cool or hot water? cool

EXPLORING THE WEB

Description	Location
Infection control and patient hygiene	http://www.infectioncontroltoday.com
American Dental Association	http://www.ada.org
Patient Hygiene PowerPoint Slides	http://www.sonser4.nur.uth.tmc.edu

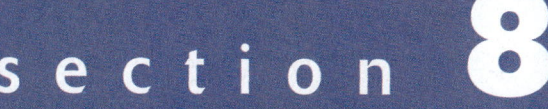

section 8

Principles of Nutrition and Fluid Balance

UNIT 26
Nutritional Needs and Diet
Modifications

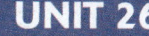

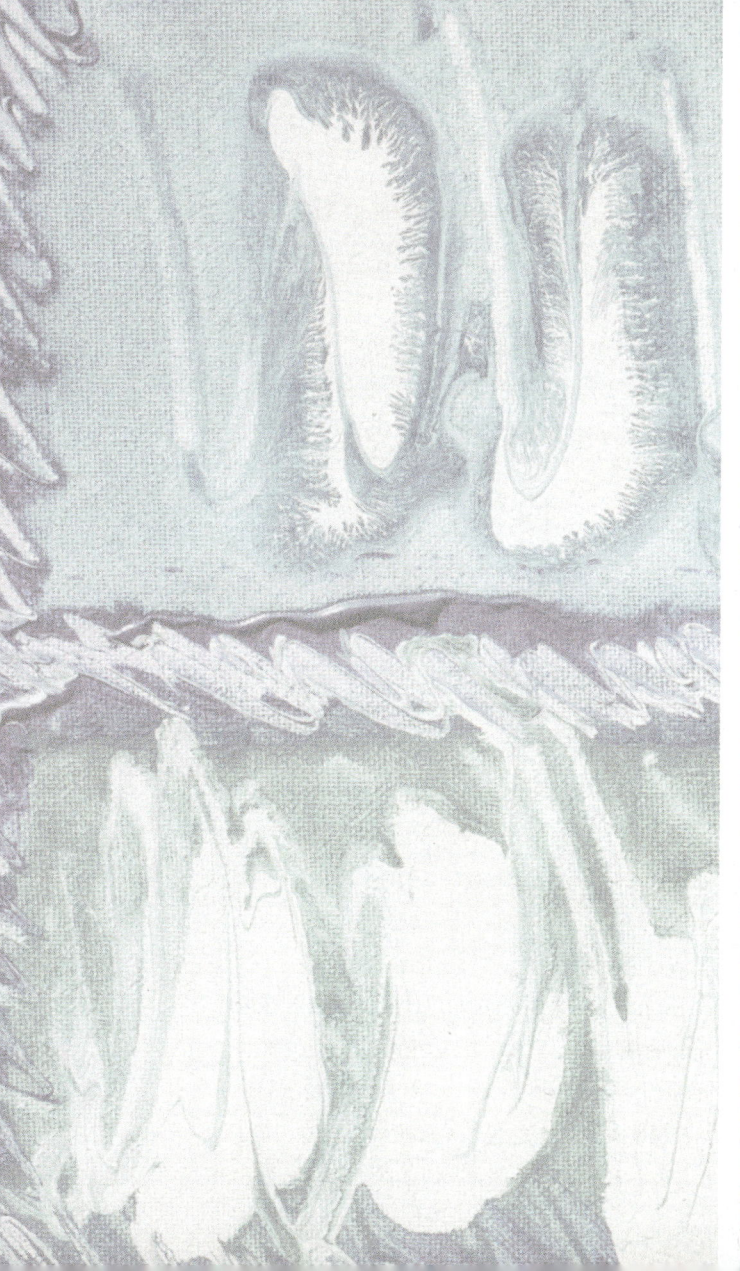

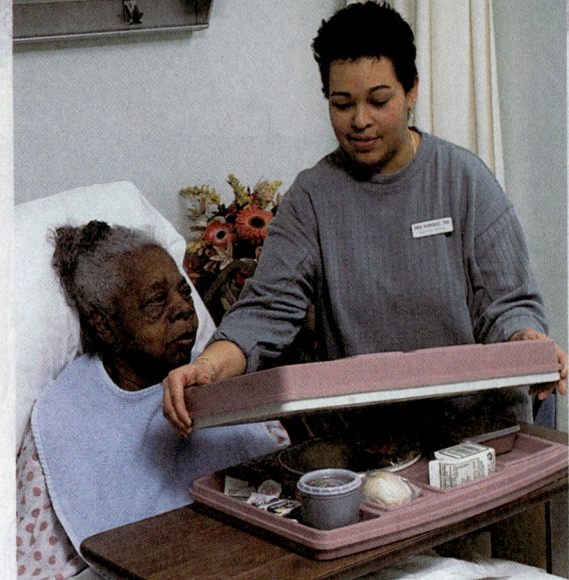

Nutritional Needs and Diet Modifications

objectives

After completing this unit, you will be able to:

- Spell and define terms.
- Define normal nutrition.
- List the essential nutrients.
- Name the five food groups and list the foods included in each group.
- State the liquids/foods allowed on the four basic facility diets.
- Describe the purposes of the following diets:
  - clear liquid
  - full liquid
  - soft
- State the purpose of calorie counts and food intake studies.

- Define dysphagia and explain the risks of this condition.
- Describe general care for the patient with dysphagia and swallowing problems.
- State the purposes of therapeutic diets.
- List types of alternative nutrition.
- Describe the nursing assistant actions when patients are unable to drink fluids independently.
- Demonstrate the following procedures:
  - Procedure 78 Assisting the Patient Who Can Feed Self
  - Procedure 79 Feeding the Dependent Patient

vocabulary

Learn the meaning and the correct spelling of the following words and phrases:

amino acids	edema	graduate	nutrients
aspiration	emesis	hyperalimentation	nutrition
carbohydrates	enteral feeding	intake and output	protein
cellulose	essential nutrients	(I&O)	pureed diet
clear liquid diet	exchange list	intravenous infusion	push fluids
defecation	excrete	(IV)	soft diet
dehydration	fats	mechanical soft	supplement
diaphoresis	fluid balance	mechanically altered	therapeutic diets
digestion	force fluids	minerals	total parenteral
diuresis	full liquid diet	nasogastric feeding	nutrition (TPN)
dysphagia	gastrostomy feeding	(NG feeding)	vitamins

INTRODUCTION

Nutrition is the entire process by which the body takes in food for growth and repair and uses it to maintain health. The signs of good nutrition include:

- Shiny hair
- Clear skin and eyes
- A well-developed body
- An alert expression
- A pleasant disposition
- Healthy sleep patterns
- Appropriate appetite
- Regular bowel habits
- Body weight appropriate to height

NORMAL NUTRITION

Food is normally taken into the body through the mouth. The mouth is the beginning of the digestive tract. **Digestion** is the process of breaking down foods into simple substances that can be used by the body cells for nourishment. These substances are called **essential nutrients**.

ESSENTIAL NUTRIENTS

To be well nourished, we must eat foods that:

- supply heat and energy.
- build and repair body tissue.
- regulate body functions.

These foods are called **nutrients**. The six nutrients essential to maintain health are:

- Proteins
- Carbohydrates
- Fats
- Minerals
- Vitamins
- Water

Protein

Protein is an essential nutrient. It is the basic material of every body cell. It is the only nutrient that can make new cells and rebuild tissue. The foods that contain the greatest amount of protein come from animals. They include:

- Meat
- Poultry
- Eggs
- Milk
- Cheese

Proteins are made of small building blocks called **amino acids**. The body can manufacture some of the amino acids, but not all of them.

- *Complete proteins* are proteins that contain all the amino acids the body cannot manufacture. Examples of complete proteins are meat, fish, eggs, and poultry.
- *Incomplete proteins*, although still important, do not contain all the essential amino acids. Essential amino acids are those that must be obtained through foods. Examples of incomplete proteins are corn, soybeans, peas, and nuts.

Carbohydrates and Fats

Carbohydrates and **fats** are called energy foods because the body uses them to produce heat and energy. When a person eats more energy foods than the body needs, the remainder is stored as fat. Foods that contain the greatest amount of carbohydrates come from plants. They include:

- Fruits
- Vegetables
- Foods that are made from grains, such as breads, cereals, and pasta products

Carbohydrate foods also supply the body with fiber or roughage (**cellulose**). Cellulose is important in maintaining bowel regularity.

Fats come from both plants and animals. Examples of foods that are rich in fat include:

- Pork
- Butter
- Nuts
- Egg yolk
- Cheese

Vitamins and Minerals

Vitamins and minerals are present in a wide variety of foods. The best way to be sure that you are getting enough vitamins and minerals is to include a variety of foods in your daily diet.

Vitamins are substances that regulate body processes. They help to:

- build strong teeth and bones.
- promote growth.
- aid normal body functioning.
- strengthen resistance to disease.

You probably know the vitamins by their letter names:

- Vitamin A
- B-complex vitamins
- Vitamin C
- Vitamin D
- Vitamin E
- Vitamin K

Fat-soluble vitamins do not dissolve easily in water. They can be stored in the body. Vitamins A, D, E, and K are fat-soluble vitamins.

Vitamins B and C are water soluble. Water-soluble vitamins dissolve in water, so they can be lost in the cooking process.

In general, these vitamins are not stored in large amounts in the body. Deficiencies in water-soluble vitamins are more common.

Minerals help to build body tissues, especially the bones and teeth. They also regulate the chemistry of body fluids such as the blood and digestive juices. Minerals needed in the daily diet include:

- Calcium
- Phosphorus
- Iodine
- Iron
- Copper
- Potassium

THE FIVE FOOD GROUPS

The U.S. Department of Agriculture revised the recommendations for a balanced food intake. The guidelines now include:

- Eat a variety of foods.
- Maintain a healthy body weight.
- Select foods low in fat, saturated fat, and cholesterol.
- Select plenty of vegetables, fruits, and grain products.
- Use sugar in moderation.
- Use salt and sodium in moderation.
- Drink alcoholic beverages in moderation, if at all.

Food Guide Pyramid

Figure 26-1 shows the five food groups. Although the pyramid has six levels, the items in the small triangle do not fit in any of the major food categories. The sixth level at the top of the food pyramid is not considered a food group. The guide to daily food choices recommends:

- 6–11 servings daily from the bread, cereal, rice, and pasta group
- 2–4 servings from the fruit group
- 3–5 servings from the vegetable group
- 2–3 servings from the milk, yogurt, and cheese group
- 2–3 servings from the meat, poultry, fish, dry beans, eggs, and nuts group
- Use fats, oils, and sweets sparingly

The food pyramid shape represents the need for the foods at the bottom (grain foods) and gives equal importance to fruit and vegetables. Persons eating the lowest number of servings from each group will take in about 1,600 calories daily if low-fat foods are chosen. This may be adequate for most older women and some older men. Younger and more active people need more calories and can obtain them by choosing the larger number of servings.

Average servings of foods include:

- One medium-size fruit or its equivalent
- ½ cup cooked fruit or vegetable
- 2–3 ounces of meat
- ½ to 1 ounce of pasta/bread

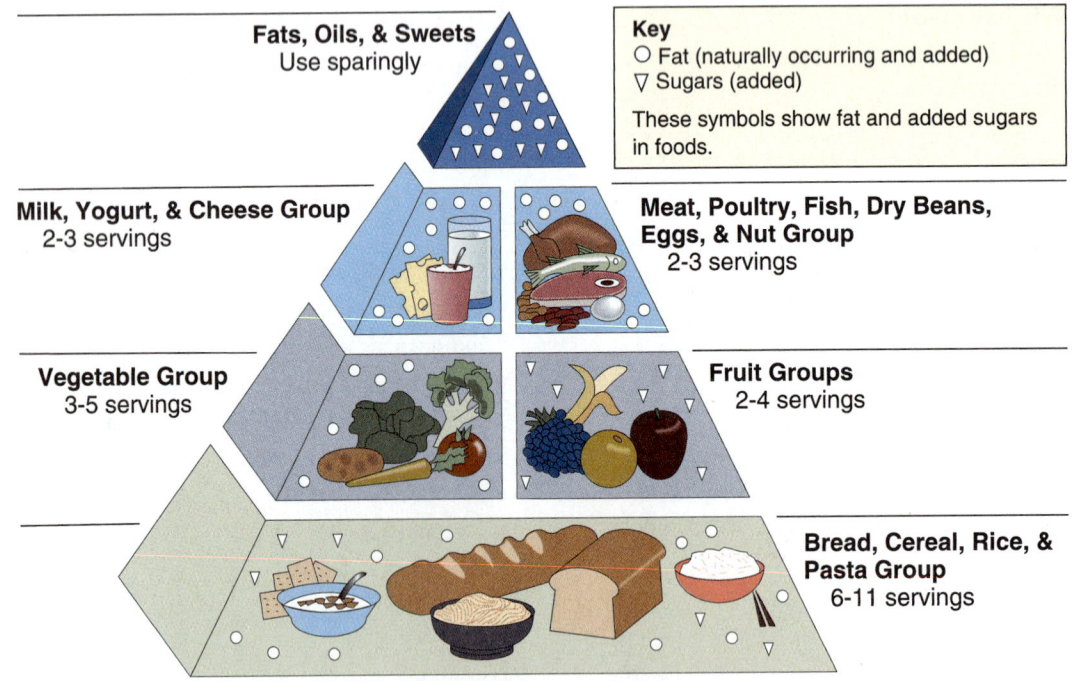

The Food Guide Pyramid
A guide to daily food choices

FIGURE 26-1 The USDA Food Guide Pyramid. *(Courtesy of US Department of Agriculture)*

Table 26-1 shows average servings for selected foods. The food guide pyramid emphasizes foods from the five major food groups shown in the three lower sections of the pyramid. Each of these food groups provides some, but not all, of the nutrients you need each day. Foods in one group cannot replace those in another. No one food group is more important than another. For good health, you need them all.

Vegetable Group

- Select three to five servings. Include:
  - Dark green or yellow vegetables
  - Tomatoes
  - Leafy, green, and yellow vegetables

TABLE 26-1 AVERAGE SERVINGS FOR SELECTED FOODS

Food	Serving Size
Fruit	
Apple	1 medium
Banana	1 medium
Peach	1 medium
Apricots	2–3
Figs	2–3
Canned—	
Grapefruit	½ can
Pineapple	2 slices
Peaches	½ cup
Juice	6 ounces
Vegetables	
Fresh	3–4 ounces
Cooked	½ cup
Milk	8 ounces
Eggs	1 medium
Meat, Fish, Poultry	2½–3 ounces, cooked
Cereal (dried)	½ cup, uncooked
Bread	1 slice
Pasta	½ cup, cooked

- Use vegetables raw, cooked, frozen, or canned.
- This group provides vitamin A, vitamin C, B-complex vitamins, calcium, and iron.
- Leafy green vegetables furnish riboflavin and niacin, which are both B vitamins.

Three to Five Servings Daily

asparagus	mustard greens
beans	okra
broccoli	onions
brussels sprouts	parsley
cabbage	parsnips
carrots	peas (green)
cauliflower	peppers
celery	potatoes
corn	pumpkin
cucumber	radishes
eggplant	rutabaga
escarole	spinach
kale	squash
leeks	sweet potatoes
lettuce	tomatoes
other greens	turnips
mushrooms	

Fruit Group

- Select two to four servings daily.
- Use foods in this group raw, cooked, frozen, canned, or dried.
- When eaten in fairly large amounts, foods in this group provide thiamine, vitamins A and C, calcium, and phosphorus.

Two to Four Servings Daily

apples	kumquats
apricots	lemons
artichokes	limes
avocados	oranges
bananas	peaches
berries	pears
cantaloupe	persimmons
cherries	pineapple
cranberries	plums
currants	prunes
dates	raisins
figs	rhubarb
fruit juice	strawberries
grapefruit	tangerines
grapes	watermelon

Milk, Yogurt, Cheese Group

- This group provides calcium, phosphorus, riboflavin, protein, vitamin A, and fat.
- People need varying amounts of the nutrients in dairy foods at different periods of their lives.
  - Children should have three or four glasses of milk daily.
  - Teenagers need four or more glasses.
  - Adults should drink two or more glasses.
  - Pregnant women should drink at least one quart of milk, or the nutritional equivalent, daily.
  - Nursing mothers should increase the amount of milk in their diet to 1½ quarts daily.
- Daily calcium requirement for postmenopausal women is 1,500 mg.
- Cheese, ice cream, and other milk-made foods can be substituted for part of the milk requirement. (This increases fat and sodium content.)

The following dairy foods contain calcium equal to that in one cup of milk and may be substituted for milk:

Milk Substitutes

1½ ounces cheddar-type cheese

2 ounces cream cheese

2 cups cottage cheese

1½ cups ice cream

1 cup plain, lowfat yogurt

½ ice cream or ice milk

½ cup frozen yogurt

Milk is available in the following forms:

whole milk

skim milk

evaporated milk

condensed milk

buttermilk

dried milk

Grain Group

- Select six to eleven servings daily.
- This group provides carbohydrates, thiamine, niacin, iron, and roughage (fiber).

Six to Eleven Servings Daily

breads: whole wheat, dark rye, enriched cornmeal, whole grain enriched, or oatmeal

rolls or biscuits made with whole wheat or enriched flour

flour: enriched, whole wheat, other whole grain

grits, enriched cereals: whole wheat, rolled oats, brown rice, converted rice, other cereals, if whole grain or restored

noodles, spaghetti, macaroni

Meat Group

- Select two to three servings daily.
- Alternate dried beans, peas, or nuts. These are incomplete protein foods.
- This group provides protein, some fat, iron, phosphorus, and B-complex vitamins.
- Choose low-fat items.
- Remove skin from poultry and trim fat from meat.

Two to Three Servings Daily

beef	lunch meats, such as bologna
eggs	
lamb	dried beans
game	dried peas
veal	lentils
pork (except bacon and fatback)	nuts
	peanuts
poultry: chicken, duck, goose, turkey	peanut butter
	soybeans
fish, shellfish	soya flour and grits

Fats, Oils, and Sweets

The small triangle at the top of the food pyramid represents food items that should be consumed in very limited quantities, such as fats, sweets, and oils. Examples of foods in this category are salad dressings, cream, butter, margarine, sugars, soft drinks, candies, and sweet desserts. These foods are usually very high in calories, but have little nutritional value. Most people should use them sparingly. Some fat or sugar symbols are shown in the food groups to remind you that some food choices in these food groups can also be high in fat or added sugars. When choosing foods, consider both the fats and sugars in your choices from the food groups, as well as the fats, oils, and sweets from the pyramid tip.

Fats. As a rule, foods that come from animals (milk and meat groups) are naturally higher in fat than foods that come from plants. Many lowfat dairy and lean meat choices are available, and foods can be prepared in ways that lower fat. Fruits, vegetables, and grain products are naturally low in fat. However, fat may be used in food preparation or at the table, such as for french-fried potatoes, buttered vegetables, or croissants, making them higher-fat choices.

Added Sugars. The triangular symbols on the chart represent sugars added to foods in processing or at the table, not natural sugars. The added sugars provide calories with few vitamins and minerals. Most of the added sugars in the typical American diet come from foods in the pyramid tip: soft drinks, candy, jams, jellies, syrups, and table sugar that we add to foods like coffee or cereal.

Fat and Sugar Tips

- Select lower-fat foods from the food groups most often.

- Limit fats and sugars added to foods in cooking or at the table, such as butter, margarine, gravy, salad dressing, sugar, and jelly.
- Select fewer high-sugar foods, such as candy, sweet desserts, and soft drinks.

BASIC FACILITY DIETS

The food you will serve to patients in the health care facility will be prepared by the dietary department (Figure 26-2). It includes the essential nutrients. The way in which it is prepared and its consistency will depend on the individual patient's condition and needs. Sometimes very strict dietary control is needed.

The trays will usually be delivered to the patient floors in large food containers. Each tray will be labeled with the patient's name and type of diet. You will:

- Prepare the patient for the meal.
- Check the tray card for the patient's name.
- Check the tray card against the patient's armband.
- Check the items on the tray to make sure they are allowed on the patient's diet.
- Serve the tray to the patient.
- Assist with feeding as necessary.

Health care facilities usually have many types of diets. Four common diets are:

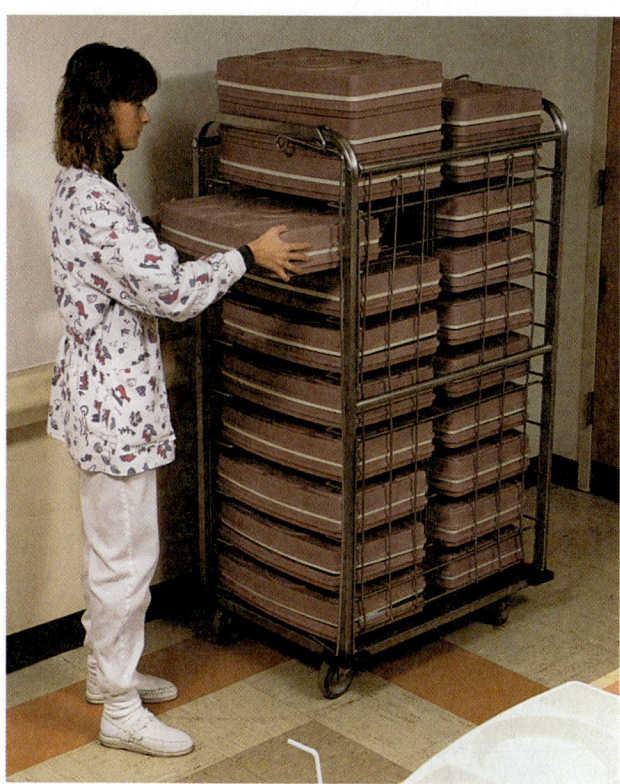

FIGURE 26-2 Patient diets are prepared in the dietary department and transported to the units in containers designed to maintain the temperature.

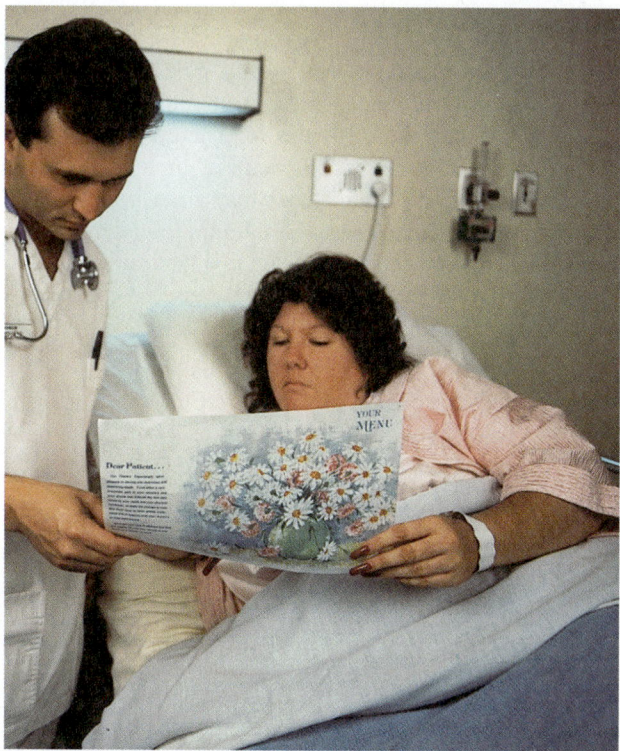

FIGURE 26-3 Patients on a house diet can select foods from a menu.

- Regular or house, sometimes called a general diet (Figure 26-3)
- Full liquid
- Clear liquid
- Soft

The progression of diets a patient is allowed following surgery is as follows:

1. Ice chips/sip of water
2. Clear liquids
3. Full liquids
4. Soft diet
5. Regular diet

In addition, the dietary department prepares special or **therapeutic** (treatment) **diets**. Therapeutic diets are discussed later in this unit.

Regular Diet

The regular-select or house diet is a normal or full diet based on the five food groups. The regular diet:

- Includes a great variety of foods.
- Excludes only very rich foods: pastries, heavy cakes, fried foods, and highly seasoned foods, which might be difficult for inactive people to digest.
- Has a lower caloric count, because an inactive person does not require as many calories as an active person.

In many health care facilities, patients may select foods from a menu.

Liquid Diets

Clear Liquid Diet. A clear liquid diet is a temporary diet because it is an inadequate diet. It is made up primarily of water and carbohydrates for energy. Feedings are given every two, three, or four hours as prescribed by the physician. It replaces fluids that may have been lost by vomiting or diarrhea. When a clear liquid food item is held up to the light, you can see through it. The clear liquid diet consists of liquids that do not irritate, cause gas formation, or encourage bowel movements (defecation).

Foods allowed on the clear liquid diet include:

- Tea, coffee with sugar but without cream
- Strained fruit or vegetable juice with gelatin (occasionally)
- Fat-free meat broths
- Ginger ale (usually), 7Up®, Coke®, strained grape or apple juice
- Gelatin (occasionally)
- Popsicles

Full Liquid Diet. The full liquid diet does supply nourishment and may be used for longer periods of time than the clear liquid diet. Six to eight ounces are usually given every two to three hours.

The full liquid diet is given to:

- Those with acute infections
- Patients who have difficulty chewing
- Those who have conditions involving the digestive tract

The diet includes all of the foods allowed on the clear liquid diet, in addition to the following:

- Strained cereal (gruel)
- Strained soups
- Sherbet
- Gelatin
- Eggnog
- Malted milk
- Milk and cream
- Plain ice cream
- Strained vegetables and fruit juices
- Junket
- Solids that liquefy at room temperature
- Yogurt

Soft Diet

The soft diet usually follows the full liquid diet. Although this diet nourishes the body, between-meal feedings are sometimes given to increase the calorie count. Foods allowed on the soft diet are:

- Low-residue, which are almost completely used by the body
- Mildly flavored, slightly seasoned, or unseasoned
- Prepared in a form that requires little digestion

The diet includes liquids and semisolid foods that have a soft texture and are easily digested. It is given to patients who:

- Have infections and fevers
- Have difficulty chewing
- Have conditions involving the digestive tract
- Are on a progressive postoperative dietary regime

The following foods are usually allowed on the soft diet:

- Soups
- Cream cheese and cottage cheese
- Crackers, toast
- Fish
- White meat of chicken or turkey (boiled or stewed)
- Fruit juices
- Cooked fruit (sieved)
- Tea, coffee
- Milk, cream, butter
- Cooked cereals
- Eggs (not fried)
- Beef and lamb (scraped or finely ground)
- Cooked vegetables (mashed or sieved)
- Angel food or sponge cake
- Small amounts of sugar
- Gelatin, custard
- Pudding
- Plain ice cream

Foods to be avoided include:

- Coarse cereals
- Spices
- Gas-forming foods (onions, cabbage, beans)
- Rich pastries and desserts
- Foods high in roughage/fiber
- Fried foods
- Raw fruits and vegetables
- Corn
- Pork (except bacon)

SPECIAL DIETS

Special diets are planned to meet specific patient needs. Patients may need special diets because of religious preferences or health needs.

Religious Restrictions

Religious practice requires changes in diet for some patients. For example, persons of the conservative Jewish faith follow strict food laws.

- There are strict prohibitions against shellfish and nonkosher meats such as pork.
- Certain fishes, such as tuna and salmon, are permitted.

- Foods may not be prepared with utensils that have been used for nonkosher food preparation.
- There are strict rules regarding the sequence in which milk products and meat may be consumed.

Some other faith restrictions are summarized in Table 26-2.

Therapeutic Diets

Standard diets can be changed to conform to special dietary requirements. For example, an order might be written for a low-sodium soft diet when a patient has ill-fitting dentures and heart disease. These therapeutic diets are planned and prepared according to a patient's individual health problems. Commonly prescribed therapeutic diets include the diabetic diet, sodium-restricted diet, and low-fat diet.

The Diabetic Diet

Diet is an integral part of the therapy of the patient with diabetes mellitus. The diet is nutritionally adequate. It provides enough energy in the form of calories for a 24-hour period. Sometimes a proper diet is all that is needed to control the disease. Usually, however, the food intake is balanced by the administration of insulin or hypoglycemic drugs.

It is important for you to accurately evaluate and report the patient's intake. Foods and liquids have a major impact on diabetes management. Illness increases the need for insulin because the liver releases more glucose in response to the stress. Dehydration is a particularly serious problem for the diabetic. This can occur when not enough foods and fluids are taken in. Insulin administration may depend on your observations. Not all physicians prescribe dietary intake in the same way.

TABLE 26-2 RELIGIOUS DIETARY PRACTICES

Faith	Coffee	Tea	Alcohol	Pork/Pork Products	Caffeine-Containing Foods	Dairy Products	All Meats
					Restricted Food		
Christian Science	•	•	•				
Roman Catholic							1 hour before communion, Ash Wednesday, Good Friday
Latter Day Saints (Mormons)	•	•	•		•		
Seventh Day Adventist	•	•	•	•	•		
Some Baptist	•	•	•				
Greek Orthodox (on fast days)						•	Fasting from meat and dairy products on Wed./Fri. during Lent and other holy days
Jewish Orthodox				• Also shellfish		Certain holy days	Forbids the serving of milk and milk products with meat; regulates food preparation; forbids cooking on the Sabbath
Moslem, Islamic		•	•				Fasting during Ramadan during day, feasting at night
Hindu							Some are vegetarians
Buddhist							Meat must be blessed and killed in special ways; some sects are vegetarians

- Some physicians prescribe a very carefully balanced diet and insulin to maintain the level of blood sugar (glucose) within normal limits. All foods must be measured and repeated injections of insulin are required.
- Other physicians are much more liberal in their approach. They permit an unmeasured diet, limiting only sugar and high-sugar foods. This diet is known as a no-concentrated-sweets diet. It may be balanced by insulin or hypoglycemic drugs.
- Many physicians treat diabetes with an approach that is midway between the preceding two methods. They prescribe the American Dietetic Association diets with specific calorie levels, such as the 1,200-calorie diet or the 1,500-calorie diet. The dietitian teaches the patient about the diet and acts as a major resource for health care providers. The diet is balanced by insulin or hypoglycemic drugs.

The Exchange List. The exchange list method of balancing the diabetic diet:

- is based on standard household measurements, to make it easier to measure.
- excludes sugar or high-sugar-content foods, to prevent rapid swings in blood sugar.
- divides foods into six groups.
- allows equivalent exchanges to be made within a group but not from group to group.

The six groups are:

- Milk exchanges
- Vegetable exchange: Group A, Group B
- Fruit exchange
- Bread exchange
- Meat exchange
- Fat exchange

Sodium-Restricted Diet

Sodium-restricted diets may be ordered for patients with chronic renal failure and cardiovascular disease. Sodium-restricted diets are some of the most difficult diets to follow. The average American consumes 2 to 6 grams of sodium in food each day. Table salt is a major source of sodium in the diet.

The physician may order several different levels of sodium restriction. These are listed in Table 26-3, in order of most to least salt content.

Processing may add significant amounts of sodium to foods. Food preservatives such as sodium citrate and sodium benzoate are added to many processed foods. This factor is considered in planning and selecting foods for the sodium-restricted diet. It is important to carefully read the labels for the contents of all commercially prepared foods.

Some foods naturally contain relatively large amounts of sodium. These foods may be restricted for this diet. They include:

TABLE 26-3 SODIUM-RESTRICTED DIETS

Type of Low-Sodium Diet	Amount of Sodium
No added salt (limited salt used in cooking, no salt added at meals)	3 to 4 grams daily
2 grams sodium	2 grams daily
1 gram sodium	1 gram daily
500-mg sodium	½ gram daily

- Meat
- Fish
- Poultry
- Milk and milk products
- Eggs

Avoid:

- Pork, ham
- Breads
- Potato chips, pretzels, and similar snacks
- Saltine crackers
- Pop (soda)
- Pickles
- Processed meats
- Canned foods, such as vegetables and soups

Some foods are naturally low in sodium. They can be used more liberally. They are:

- Some cereals, such as shredded wheat
- Vegetables
- Fruits

Calorie-Restricted Diet

As long as activity remains constant, a person must take in approximately 500 calories a day less than usual (3,500 calories deficit per week) to lose one pound.

Calorie-restricted diets are prescribed for patients who are overweight. These diets are planned to meet general nutritional needs. They take into consideration the patient's energy output, general nutritional state, and weight goal.

In planning the calorie-restricted diet, the dietitian tries to create a realistic balance between fats, proteins, and carbohydrates. This type of diet encourages the patient to develop better, more consistent eating habits. Exact amounts of the three nutrients are not uniformly prescribed, but they may be balanced as follows:

- Proteins, 20%
- Fats, 25–35%
- Carbohydrates, 45–65%

Some physicians use a factor of 10 calories multiplied by the desired weight in calculating the daily calorie requirements. For example:

- Desired weight 120 lb. × 10 = 1,200 calories per day
- Desired weight 160 lb. × 10 = 1,600 calories per day

Low-Fat/Low-Cholesterol Diet

Low-fat/low-cholesterol diets are prescribed for patients who suffer from vascular, heart, liver, or gallbladder disease, and for those who have difficulty with fat metabolism. Fats are limited and calories are balanced by increasing proteins and carbohydrates. Foods are baked, roasted, or broiled, and the skin is removed from chicken. Low-fat foods include:

- Low-fat cottage cheese (no other allowed)
- Skim milk, buttermilk, yogurt
- Lean meats, fish, chicken
- Vegetables and fruits
- Jams, jellies, ices
- Cereals, pasta, bread, potatoes, rice
- Carbonated beverages, tea, coffee

Mechanically Altered Diets

Any diet may be **mechanically altered**. This means that the consistency and texture are modified, making the food easier to chew and swallow. The **mechanical soft** diet is commonly served to patients who have no teeth, or those with serious dental problems. Meats and hard foods are ground to the consistency of hamburger. Soft items, such as bread, are not ground. The **pureed diet** (Figure 26-4) is blended with gravy or liquid until it is the consistency of pudding. This diet is used for patients who have difficulty swallowing. Pureed foods should not be watery. Properly prepared food items will support a plastic spoon in the upright position.

SUPPLEMENTS AND NOURISHMENTS

Many patients receive a nutritional **supplement** or between-meal nourishments. Supplements are ordered by the physician and have a definite therapeutic value. Patients who have wounds may receive supplements high in protein to facilitate healing. These supplements may be liquid or in any form that is easy to eat and digest. It is essential that the patient consume the entire serving. Between-meal nourishments are snacks served to patients to provide the required nutrient daily intake or to prevent between-meal hunger.

Serving between-meal snacks and supplements is an important function of the nursing assistant (Figure 26-5). Between-meal nourishments are usually served:

- Midmorning—between 9:30 and 10:00 AM
- Midafternoon—between 2:30 and 3:00 PM
- At bedtime—between 8:00 and 10:00 PM

Snacks served include:

- Milk
- Juices

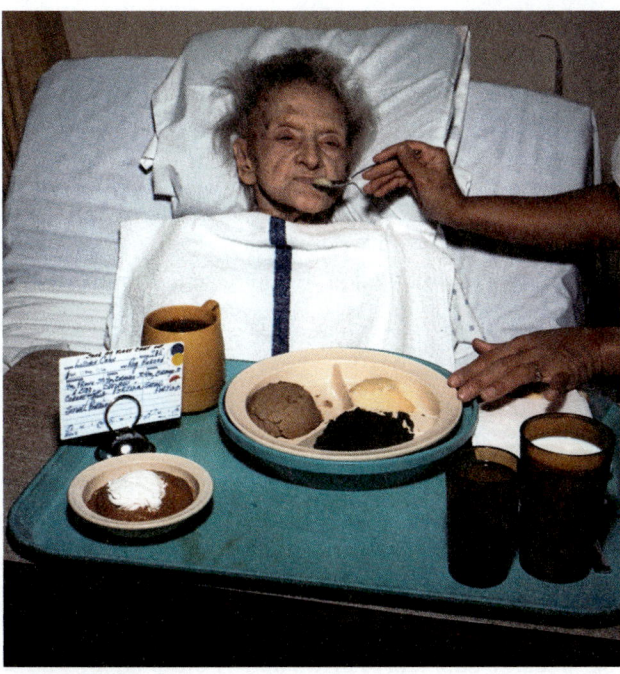

FIGURE 26-4 The pureed diet is given to patients who have difficulty swallowing.

DIFFICULT *Situations*

Liquid nutritional supplements are very filling, which is why they are usually served between meals and not with meals. Most patients prefer them cold. If the beverage is warm, the patient may not accept it. Because some of these products are milk-based, serving them warm can also be an infection control hazard. When serving supplements and nourishments, make sure the patient is able to consume the beverage independently. Do not just set it on the table and walk out. Pour the beverage into a cup, if that is what the patient prefers. Provide a straw. If the patient cannot consume the product independently, assist him or her. Document the percentage consumed on the proper form. Record the amount if the patient is on intake and output. Inform the nurse if the patient expresses a preference or dislike for a certain product or flavor.

FIGURE 26-5
Supplements and nourishments are an important, planned part of the diet. They are usually given to patients who have had undesirable weight loss, and are served between meals. *(Photo used with permission of Ross Products Division, Abbott Laboratories, Columbus, Ohio)*

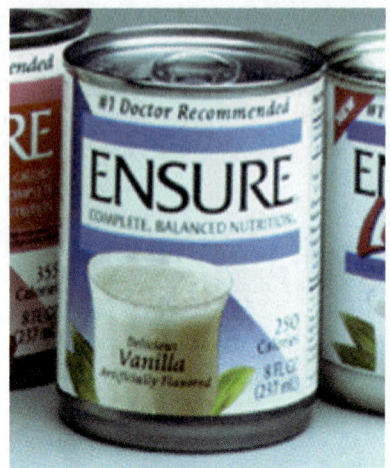

- Gelatin
- Custard
- Ice cream
- Sherbet
- High-protein drinks
- Fruits

To serve nourishments:

- Wash your hands.
- Check the nourishment list of each patient for any limitations or special dietary instructions.
- Allow patients to choose from the available nourishments whenever possible.
- Assist those who are unable to take their nourishment alone.
- Remember to pick up used glasses and dishes after the patient has finished and return them to the proper area.
- Notice what the patient was or was not able to take.
- Record on intake and output (I&O) sheet if required.

CALORIE COUNTS AND FOOD INTAKE STUDIES

The physician or dietitian may order special food intake studies for patients with special nutritional needs. The patient's food intake is carefully recorded for a period of time, usually three days. The food intake is analyzed for nutritional adequacy and number of calories consumed. The dietitian uses this information to plan a diet to meet the patient's special medical needs.

If the physician orders a food intake study, nursing personnel will notify the dietary department. A special food documentation form (Figure 26-6) is prepared and placed on the medical record or other designated location. The food intake study usually begins with the breakfast meal on the day after the physician writes the order. Some facilities post a sign in the room or on the door to remind staff and visitors

that a study is in progress. In some facilities, each food item is weighed or measured. At the end of each meal, you will accurately record the patient's food intake on the form. Facility policies vary on how food intake is documented, but this is usually done by recording an accurate percentage of each individual meal item consumed. You will also accurately document intake of all snacks, liquid nutritional beverages, and food items brought from home by visitors.

At the end of the study period, the form is returned to the dietitian or dietetic technician. He or she uses the information to calculate the amount of protein, carbohydrates, fat, and calories the patient consumed each day. In some facilities, nutrient, vitamin, and mineral intake are also calculated. The dietitian uses this information to adjust the patient's diet and nutritional plan of care. The results of the study and the dietitian's recommendations are communicated to the physician, who may order extra vitamin or mineral supplements necessary for the patient's medical condition. Completing a food intake or calorie count study requires a team effort, good communication, and accurate documentation.

DYSPHAGIA

Some patients have **dysphagia**, or difficulty swallowing food and liquids. This condition may occur in patients who have:

- had a stroke
- neurological diseases
- cancer of the head, neck, or esophagus
- undergone radiation therapy to the head or neck
- dementia

People who take medications that cause sedation or reduce saliva production are also at risk of dysphagia. Signs and symptoms of dysphagia are:

- taking a long time before beginning to swallow
- swallowing three or four times with each bite of food
- frequent throat clearing or coughing
- lack of a gag reflex or weak cough
- difficulty controlling liquids and secretions in the mouth
- wet, gurgling voice
- refusing to eat, spitting food out, or pocketing food in cheeks
- unintentional weight loss
- tightness in the throat or chest
- feeling as if food is sticking in the esophagus or sternal area

If you observe any of these signs or symptoms, inform the nurse. Patients with dysphagia are at high risk of developing malnutrition and dehydration. Consultation with a speech language pathologist and diagnostic tests for dysphagia may be necessary.

Diet _____

CALORIE/PROTEIN SUMMARY

PATIENT _____   ROOM # _____

DAY 1					DAY 2					DAY 3				
DATE ___ / ___ / ___					DATE ___ / ___ / ___					DATE ___ / ___ / ___				
	% 0–25	% 25–50	% 50–75	% 75–100		% 0–25	% 25–50	% 50–75	% 75–100		% 0–25	% 25–50	% 50–75	% 75–100
Breakfast					**Breakfast**					**Breakfast**				
Meat					Meat					Meat				
Milk					Milk					Milk				
Fruit					Fruit					Fruit				
Starch					Starch					Starch				
Fat					Fat					Fat				
Other					Other					Other				
AM Supp.					AM Supp.					AM Supp.				
Noon Meal					**Noon Meal**					**Noon Meal**				
Meat					Meat					Meat				
Milk					Milk					Milk				
Juice					Juice					Juice				
Starch					Starch					Starch				
Vegetable					Vegetable					Vegetable				
Bread					Bread					Bread				
Fat					Fat					Fat				
Dessert					Dessert					Dessert				
Other					Other					Other				
PM Supp.					PM Supp.					PM Supp.				
Evening Meal					**Evening Meal**					**Evening Meal**				
Meat					Meat					Meat				
Milk					Milk					Milk				
Juice					Juice					Juice				
Starch					Starch					Starch				
Vegetable					Vegetable					Vegetable				
Bread					Bread					Bread				
Fat					Fat					Fat				
Dessert					Dessert					Dessert				
Other					Other					Other				
PM Supp.					PM Supp.					PM Supp.				
Total Kcal					**Total Kcal**					**Total Kcal**				
Total Pro					**Total Pro**					**Total Pro**				
Avg. for 3 days Kcal:						**Avg. Protein for 3 days:**								

PLEASE RETURN COMPLETED FORM TO NUTRITION CARE MANAGER

FIGURE 26-6 The calorie count provides an accurate picture of the patient's calorie and nutrient intake over a three-day period. The information is used to adjust the patient's diet and nutritional plan of care.

Dysphagia is treated with swallowing exercises, practice of proper swallowing techniques, and alteration of the consistency of food and beverages. The dietitian works closely with the speech language pathologist to ensure that the food is the proper consistency to meet the patient's needs and reduce the risk of aspiration. The goal is to keep the look, taste, and food consistency as close to normal as possible, considering the patient's safety needs. Extra gravies or sauces may be added to some foods. Adults may be resistant to eating pureed food because it resembles baby food. Molds and special methods of preparation are used to enhance the appearance of pureed foods, making them more acceptable to the patient. You may be instructed to monitor the patient's food and fluid intake accurately. Inform the nurse if the patient has special dietary requests. The physician may order frequent weight monitoring.

Patients with dysphagia will use special approaches to eating and drinking to prevent aspiration and ensure proper intake. The speech therapist works closely with these patients. Liquids are usually the most difficult to swallow. The speech professional may recommend using food thickeners (Figure 26-7) to slow the movement of fluid through the esophagus. Thickeners are nonprescription, powdered products that are mixed into beverages and some foods to make swallowing easier and prevent aspiration. The consistency of the liquid depends on the amount of powder added. It is important to add exactly the amount that has been ordered. Thickeners do not change the taste of food or liquids, but they may change the intensity, making it taste stronger. Prethickened liquids are also available.

The care plan will specify the type and amount of thickener to use to achieve the necessary texture. For example, the therapist may recommend that liquids be mixed to the consistency of peach juice, nectar, honey, or pudding. Add the thickener immediately before serving the product. Follow the therapist's directions exactly. When adding thickeners:

- Use the correct product
- Use the correct amount
- Follow the manufacturer's directions
- Stir the thickener well
- Follow the speech therapist's instructions and plan of care for positioning and feeding

FLUID BALANCE

Fluid balance is the balance between liquid intake and liquid output. Because two-thirds of the body's weight is water, there must be a balance between the amount of fluid taken into the body and the amount lost under normal conditions. Generally, we do not need to concern ourselves about this balance. It usually takes care of itself.

The metric system is used for fluid measurements: milliliters (mL) or cubic centimeters (cc). A mL and a cc are the same amount. Table 26-4 provides a comparison of U.S. customary and metric measurements.

Intake

We take in approximately 2½ quarts (2,500 mL) of fluid daily:

- In liquids such as water, tea, and soft drinks.
- In foods such as fruits and vegetables.
- Artificially, such as by intravenous infusions or gavage.

Most adult patients need to consume an average 600 to 800 mL of fluid during each eight-hour shift. Because patients may sleep during most of the night shift, additional fluids must be provided during waking hours to keep

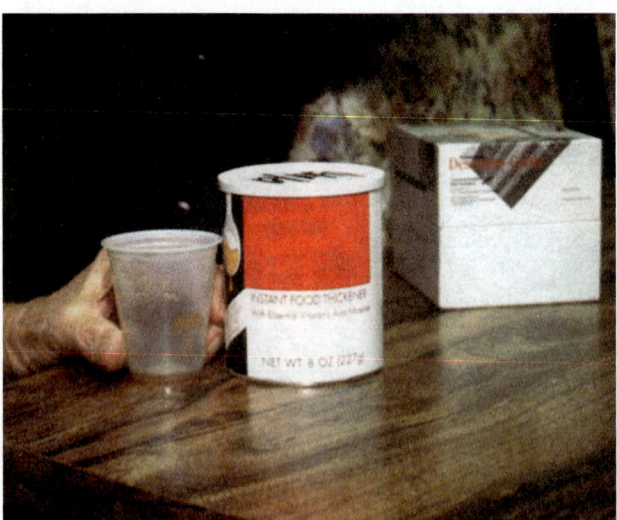

FIGURE 26-7 Food thickener is used to change the texture and consistency of liquids to prevent choking.

TABLE 26-4 COMPARISON OF U.S. CUSTOMARY AND METRIC MEASUREMENTS	
U.S. Customary Units	**Metric Units**
1 minim	0.06 milliliter (mL)
16 minims	1 mL
1 ounce	30 mL
1 pint	500 mL
1 quart	1,000 mL (1 liter)
2.2 pounds	1 kilogram (kg)
1 inch	2.5 centimeters (cm)
1 foot	30 cm

the body in balance. Excessive fluid retention is called **edema**. Inadequate fluid intake results in **dehydration**, or the lack of sufficient fluid in body tissues. Some disease conditions may change the amounts of fluid the patient is allowed to have.

Output

Typical output equals about 2½ quarts daily in the form of:

- Urine, 1½ quarts (1,500 mL)
- Perspiration
- Moisture from the lungs
- Moisture from the bowel

Excessive fluid loss results in dehydration. This can occur through:

- Diarrhea
- Vomiting
- Excessive urine output (**diuresis**)
- Excessive perspiration (**diaphoresis**)
- Wound drainage or blood loss

Recording Intake and Output

An accurate recording of **intake and output** (**I&O**), or fluid taken in and given off by the body, is basic to the care of many patients. Intake and output records are kept when specifically ordered by the physician and when patients:

- are dehydrated.
- receive intravenous infusion.
- have recently had surgery.
- have a urinary catheter.
- are perspiring profusely or vomiting.
- have specific diagnoses such as congestive heart failure or renal disease that require accurate monitoring of I&O.

Fluid intake may have to be encouraged in some patients. This is called **push fluids** or **force fluids**. In some situations (as in kidney disease), fluid intake may have to be restricted.

Fluid intake and output is calculated by measuring and recording the fluids the patient takes in and the fluids the patient **excretes** (eliminates from the body) (Table 26-5). Because the fluids taken in by the patient cannot actually be measured, an estimate is made and recorded. This is done by:

- Knowing what the liquid container holds when full.

Note: Sizes of containers vary. Learn the fluid content of the containers used at your facility. Remember that there are 30 mL per ounce (240 mL ÷ 30 mL = 8 oz).

- Coffee/tea cup, 8 oz = 240 mL
- Water carafe, 16 oz = 480 mL
- Foam cup, 8 oz = 240 mL
- Water glass, 8 oz = 240 mL

TABLE 26-5 COMPUTING INTAKE AND OUTPUT

Intake	
IV	1,500 mL
By mouth	2,000 mL
Total	3,500 mL
Output	
Urine	1,500 mL
Vomitus	500 mL
Drainage	600 mL
Total	2,600 mL

- Soup bowl, 6 oz = 180 mL
- Jello, 1 serving = 130 mL
- Ice chips, full 4 oz glass = 120 mL

- Estimating how much is gone from the container (what the patient drank), such as one-third of a glass of juice or half of a cup of coffee
- Converting this to mL. *Example:* A water glass holds 240 mL when filled. The patient drinks ¾ of the glass of water. ¾ × 240 = 180 mL. Intake for the glass of water is recorded as 180 mL. Fluids that are calculated and recorded include all liquids, such as water, juices, soda, coffee, tea, milk, and soup. Also included are foods that melt at room temperature: ice cream, sherbet, and gelatin.

Note: Containers may vary from one facility to the next. Each facility should have a chart available that tells you what each size of glass, cup, and bowl holds when full.

Fluids taken by mouth, through intravenous infusion, or through gastric feeding are all recorded separately (Figure 26-8). At the end of each 8-hour shift and the end of 24 hours, the figures are totaled.

Fluid output amount is obtained by measuring all fluids excreted from the body. This includes urine, **emesis** (vomitus), and drainage from body cavities, such as gastric drainage. A container called a **graduate** is marked in mL or cc. The substance is poured into the graduate to determine the amount of output. Urine and any other excretions are recorded separately.

Note: Standard precautions must be followed when measuring any body excretion. Gloves are required for measuring all forms of output (Figure 26-9).

Date	Time	Method of Adm.	Solution	Intake Amounts Rec'd	Time	Output Urine Amount	Others Kind	Amount
7/16	0700	PO	water	120 mL		500 mL		
	0830	PO	coffee	240 mL				
			or. ju.	120 mL				
	1030	PO	cran.ju.	120 mL				
	1100					300 mL		
	1230	PO	tea	240 mL				
	1400	PO	water	150 mL				
Shift Totals	1500			990 mL		800 mL		
	1530	PO	gelatin	120 mL				
	1700	PO	tea	120 mL				
			soup	180 mL				
	2000					512 mL		
	2045						vomitus	500 mL
	2205						vomitus	90 mL
Shift Totals	2300			420 mL		512 mL		590 mL
	2345						vomitus	80 mL
	0130	IV	D/W	500 mL				
	0315					400 mL		
Shift Totals	0700			500 mL		400 mL		80 mL
24 Hour Totals				1910 mL		1712 mL		670 mL vomitus

FIGURE 26-8 Sample intake and output record.

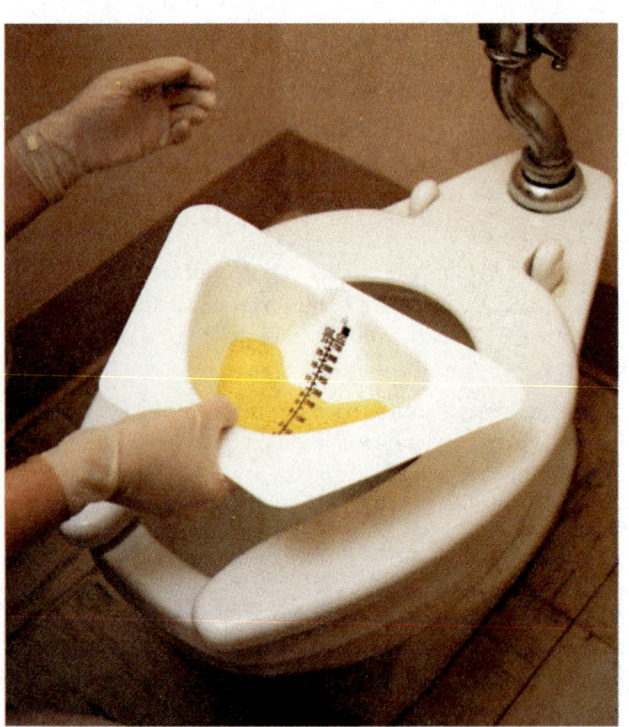

FIGURE 26-9 The specimen collection container is placed under the toilet seat when the patient eliminates. Wear gloves when measuring output, then clean and replace the collection device.

CHANGING WATER

It is important to provide fresh water for patients, because water is essential to life. In all cases, you should know whether a patient is allowed ice or tap water and if water is

INFECTION CONTROL *Alert*

Avoid contaminating the ice chest or ice scoop when filling pitchers and passing drinking water. Keep the ice scoop covered when not in use. Note that the handle is contaminated and should not touch the clean ice supply. Avoid filling the pitcher over the source of clean ice. (If ice hits the rim of the pitcher and drops back into the clean ice supply, it is contaminated.) Do not allow the scoop to touch the pitcher. Always keep water pitchers covered at the bedside. If more than one patient shares the room, make sure each pitcher and cup are labeled with a single patient's name.

to be especially encouraged. Even without an order to force fluids, you must encourage patients to take 6 to 8 glasses of fluids daily, unless the patient is NPO (nothing by mouth) or on restricted fluids. Give special attention to confused patients, patients who may not be able to reach a source of water, and the elderly. The need for adequate water intake cannot be overstressed. Because patients often do not drink enough water, sometimes the physician will leave orders that fluids are to be forced to a specific number of mL per day.

Forcing fluids is an old term that is not quite accurate. Patients should never actually be forced to consume water or other beverages. When "force fluids" is ordered, encourage the patient to drink each time you are in the room. Offer to assist, if necessary. Some patients will not drink water. Find out what beverages the patient likes, and provide these, if possible.

Providing fresh water is one way to encourage the patient to increase intake of fluids. The procedure for providing fresh water varies greatly.

- In some hospitals, the water pitcher and glass are replaced with a new disposable set each time water is provided.
- In others, the pitcher and glass are washed, refilled, and returned to the patient's bedside table.

In all cases, be sure you know whether a patient is allowed ice or tap water.

FEEDING THE PATIENT

Eating should be an enjoyable experience. (See Procedures 78 and 79.) Prepare the patient for the meal tray before it arrives by:

- Offering the bedpan or helping the patient to the bathroom.
- Assisting the patient to wash hands and face.
- Assisting with oral hygiene, if needed.
- Raising the head of the bed, if permitted, or assisting the patient out of bed and into a chair, if permitted.
- Adjusting the in-bed patient's position with pillows.
- Clearing away anything that is unpleasant, such as the emesis basin and bedpan.
- Clearing the overbed table.
- Encouraging the patient to do as much as possible.

When you have served the tray and after you have washed your hands, assist the patient as needed by:

- Being unhurried and pleasant.
- Opening prepackaged items.
- Cutting meat.
- Pouring liquids.
- Buttering bread.
- Explaining the arrangement of the tray as if items were on the face of a clock (Figure 26-10) if the patient cannot see.

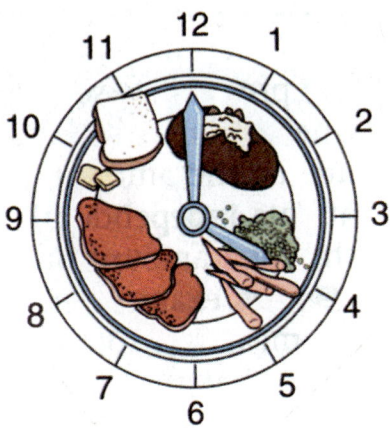

FIGURE 26-10 Describe the location of each food item compared with its position on the face of a clock.

There are times when you will be responsible for the entire feeding procedure.

 Note: Carry some extra straws with you during meal times. It can save you steps.

INFECTION CONTROL *Alert*

Keep the soiled linen hamper and housekeeping cart separated from the food cart by *at least* one room's width (approximately 12 to 16 feet). Some facilities remove the linen hampers and housekeeping carts from the hallway when food is being served. Know and follow facility policies and state requirements. When passing trays, close the door to the food cart as soon as each tray is removed. This maintains food temperature (which prevents pathogen growth), and prevents environmental contamination of food items. Serve food promptly when it arrives on the unit. Maintaining proper food temperature is key to preventing foodborne infection. If a patient must be fed, leave the tray on the cart to maintain temperature until you are ready to feed the patient. Avoid placing used meal trays back on the food cart until all fresh trays have been served. Avoid placing lab specimens in the refrigerator with food and beverages. Store these biohazardous items separately in a refrigerator or cooler marked with a biohazard label.

PROCEDURE 78

ASSISTING THE PATIENT WHO CAN FEED SELF

1. Carry out beginning procedure actions.

2. Assemble equipment:
   - bedpan/urinal
   - disposable gloves
   - basin of warm water
   - towel
   - soap
   - washcloth
   - oral hygiene items
   - tray of food

3. Offer bedpan/urinal. (If used, follow Procedure 75 in Unit 25—"Giving and Receiving the Bedpan.") Use standard precautions if you anticipate contact with blood, body fluids, mucous membranes, or nonintact skin when assisting the patient with elimination or feeding.

4. If permitted, elevate the head of the bed or assist the patient out of bed.

5. Provide a washcloth to wash the patient's hands and face.

6. Assist with oral hygiene or assist with dentures.

7. Remove and discard personal protective equipment, if used, according to facility policy.

8. Clear the overbed table and position it in front of the patient. Remove unpleasant equipment from the sight.

9. Wash your hands. Obtain the meal tray from the dietary tray conveyor.

10. Check the diet with the dietary card and with the patient's identification band (Figure 26-11A).

11. Place the tray on the overbed table and arrange food in a convenient manner.

12. Assist in food preparation as needed (Figure 26-11B). Encourage the patient to do as much as possible.

13. Remove the tray as soon as the patient is finished. Make sure to note what the patient has and has not eaten.

14. Record fluids on intake record, if necessary. Record food intake.

15. Push the overbed table out of the way.

16. Carry out procedure completion actions.

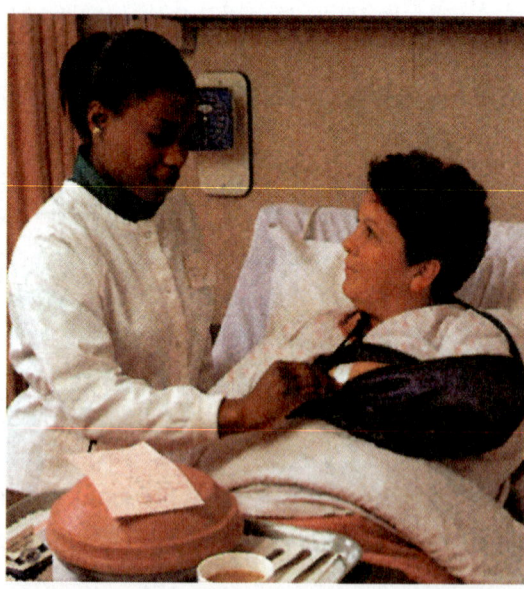

FIGURE 26-11A Check the patient's identification band against the tray card.

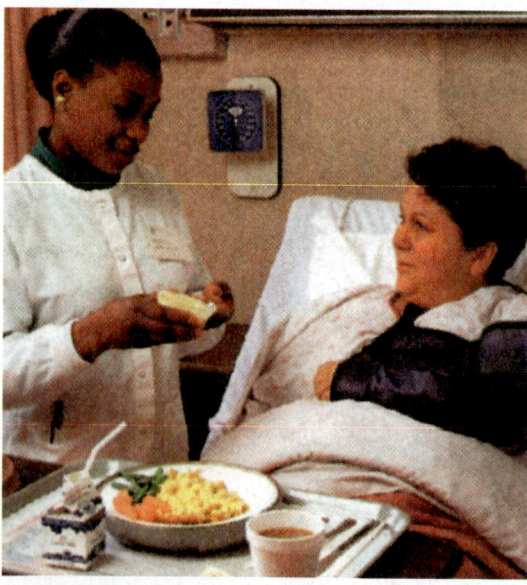

FIGURE 26-11B Assist with food preparation as needed.

PROCEDURE 79

FEEDING THE DEPENDENT PATIENT

1. Carry out beginning procedure actions.

2. Assemble equipment:
   - bedpan/urinal
   - basin
   - soap
   - towel
   - washcloth
   - clothing protector
   - oral hygiene items
   - tray of food

3. Offer the bedpan or urinal. (If used, follow Procedure 75 in Unit 25—"Giving and Receiving the Bedpan.") Follow standard precautions.

4. Provide oral hygiene, if desired.

5. Remove unnecessary articles from the overbed table.

6. Elevate the head of the bed with the patient's head bent slightly forward.

7. Place a towel or protector under the patient's chin (Figure 26-12A). Avoid calling this item a "bib," which is demeaning to adults.

8. Obtain the meal tray. Check the diet against the patient's identification band and dietary card.

9. Place the tray on the overbed table (Figure 26-12B).

10. Butter bread and cut meat. Do not pour a hot beverage until the patient is ready for it.

11. Use different drinking straws to give each fluid, or use a cup. Thick fluids are more easily controlled by using a straw. Use adaptive devices as indicated on the care plan.

12. Sit down while you are feeding the patient, so that you are at eye level.

13. Holding the spoon at a right angle:
    - Give solid foods from the point of the spoon (Figure 25-12C).
    - Alternate solids and liquids.
    - Ask the patient in what order she would like the food.
    - Describe or show the patient what kind of food you are giving.
    - If the patient has had a stroke, direct food to the unaffected side and check for food stored

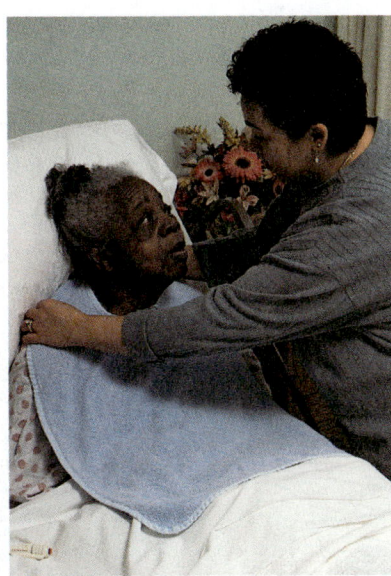

FIGURE 26-12A Place a towel or garment protector over the patient.

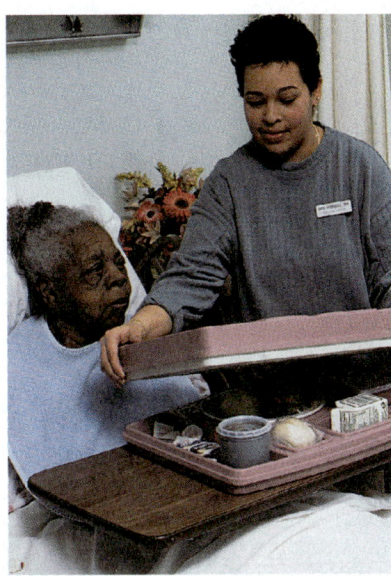

FIGURE 26-12B Uncover the food and arrange it on the overbed table.

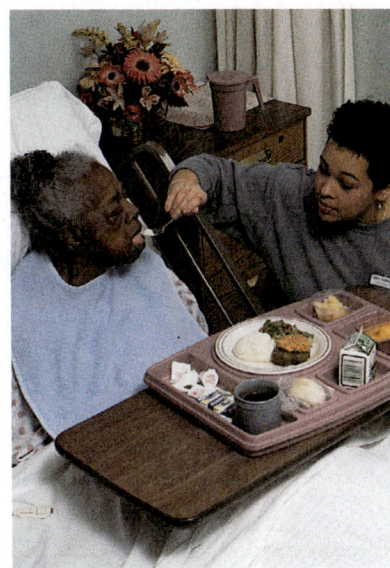

FIGURE 26-12C Give solid foods from the tip of the spoon.

continues

PROCEDURE 79

continued

in the affected side. Watch the patient's throat to check for swallowing.

- Test hot foods by dropping a small amount on the inside of your wrist before feeding them to the patient.
- Never blow on the patient's food to cool it.
- Never taste the patient's food.
- Do not hurry the meal.

14. Allow the patient to assist to the extent that he or she is able.

15. Use a napkin to wipe the patient's mouth as often as necessary.

16. Remove the tray as soon as the patient is finished. Record percentage of food eaten. Record fluid intake.

17. Carry out procedure completion actions.

Mealtime Assistance for Patients Who Have Swallowing Problems

Patients who have difficulty swallowing may require one-to-one assistance, prompting, or supervision at meals. The speech therapist will recommend special techniques and positions for improving swallowing and preventing aspiration. These will be listed on the care plan. The therapist may work closely with each staff member who may feed the patient. In general:

- Before serving food or beverages, make sure the patient is fully awake and alert.
- Position the patient as upright as possible.
- The head should face forward, with the neck flexed forward slightly.
- During the meal, reduce distractions.
- Limit conversation. The patient with dysphagia should not try to carry on a conversation while eating. Focus the patient on eating.
- Prompt or feed the patient slowly, offering small bites. Remind the patient to chew the food well.

The speech language pathologist may order other special positions and exercises, depending on the patient's medical condition and needs. The care plan will provide additional directions, such as reminding the patient to tuck the chin in when swallowing. In some types of dysphagia, this changes the position of the airway, further reducing the risk of aspiration. In other types, this technique increases the risk. Because dysphagia care is highly individualized, many staff members must work as a team to ensure that the patient's nutritional needs are safely met.

ALTERNATIVE NUTRITION

There may be situations in which the patient is unable to take in food in the usual way. This may occur if the patient:

- is unconscious.
- has a disease of the digestive tract.
- has persistent vomiting and cannot hold down food.

- is unable to swallow without **aspiration** (choking).

To maintain life, the body must meet its requirements for daily essential nutrients. This may be done by:

- administration of **total parenteral nutrition** (**TPN**) (also called **hyperalimentation**), which is a form of **intravenous infusion** (**IV**), or by
- **enteral feedings** (tubes inserted into digestive tract).

Total Parenteral Nutrition

TPN is a technique in which high-density (concentrated) nutrients are introduced into a large vein, such as the subclavian or the superior vena cava. This method of feeding is used for patients with diseases of the digestive tract. Caring for patients with TPN is discussed in Unit 35 (Subacute Care).

Enteral Feedings

Enteral feedings may be administered by a tube that is

- Inserted through the nose and into the stomach (**nasogastric** or **NG feeding**) (Figure 26-13).
- Inserted directly through the abdominal skin and into the stomach (**gastrostomy feeding**) (Figure 26-14).

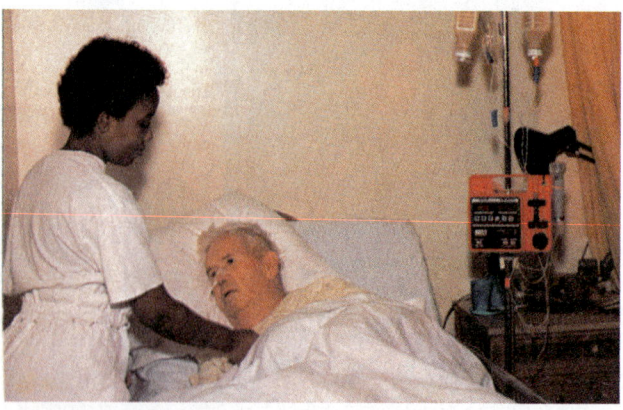

FIGURE 26-13 An NG tube is inserted through the patient's nose into the stomach.

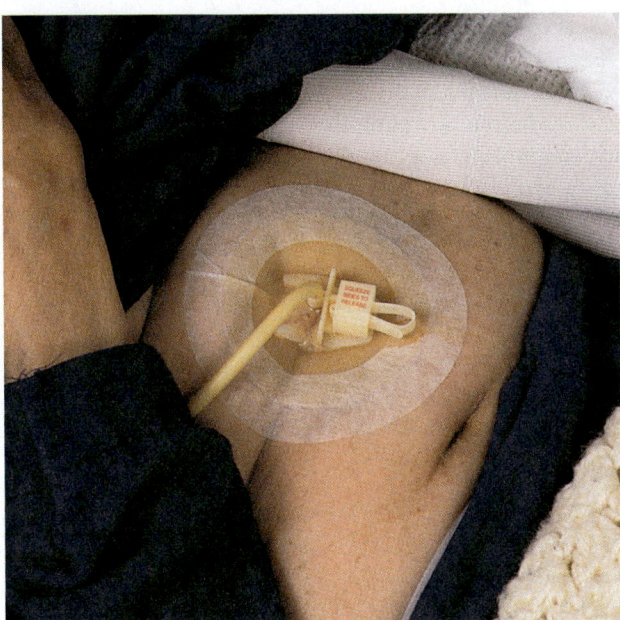

FIGURE 26-14 Gastrostomy tubes are surgically inserted through the abdominal skin into the stomach. This type of tube is used when long-term tube feeding is anticipated.

Many different types of tubes may be used for these feedings. The nurse or physician inserts the feeding tube. Specially prepared solutions contain all the nutrients required by the body. The feeding may be administered intermittently or it

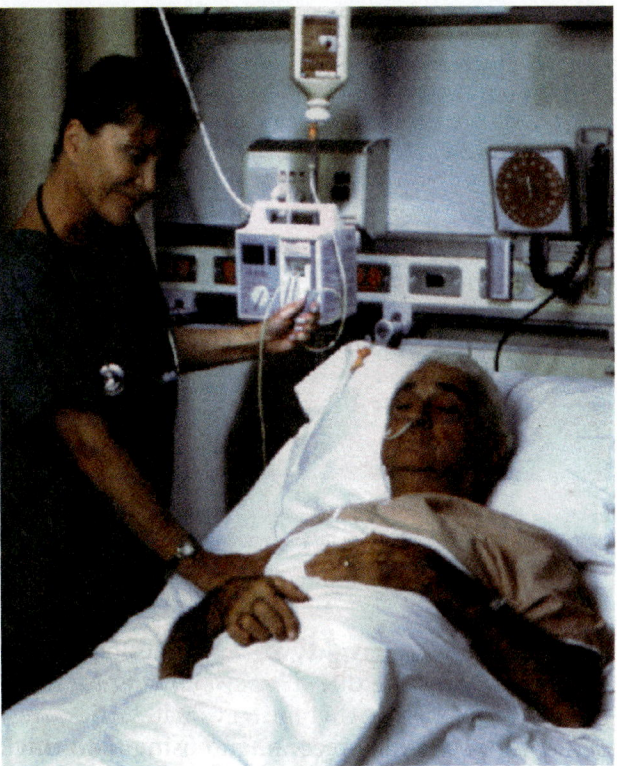

FIGURE 26-15 Enteral feedings are usually administered through a mechanical pump. *(Photo used with permission of Ross Products Division, Abbott Laboratories, Columbus, Ohio)*

may run continuously. In either case, the container of solution is hung from an IV (intravenous) pole and is usually attached to a device that automatically controls the administration (Figure 26-15).

When caring for the patient with tube feedings, you need to:

- Keep the head of the bed elevated 45° to 60° during feeding and for 30 to 60 minutes after feeding.
- Check the taping of tubes. If tape is loose, or pulls, or is causing skin irritation, inform the nurse.

SAFETY *Alert*

Most patients receiving tube feedings are NPO, but some are also permitted to have food or liquids orally. Verify the orders for that patient before giving food or fluids. When a patient receives a continuous tube feeding with a pump, the head must be elevated at all times. Keeping the head of the bed elevated when the tube feeding is infusing is critical to prevent accidental aspiration of formula into the lungs. Monitor the patient for signs of respiratory distress. If formula is aspirated into the lungs, the patient will begin coughing, choking, or gurgling, or will become cyanotic. If any of these occur, call for the nurse immediately. Monitor the skin on the hips and buttocks frequently, as this position increases pressure and the risk of skin breakdown. Move the patient in bed with an assistant. The elevation of the head of bed also increases the risk of skin damage from friction and shearing.

SAFETY *Alert*

Know the location of the tube at all times and avoid pulling on it. Avoid pulling on the tube when moving and transferring the patient. Serious complications can result if a feeding tube is dislodged. The skin around the feeding tube must be kept clean and dry. Sometimes the skin around a gastrostomy tube is covered with gauze. After the incision has healed, no dressing is necessary. If the patient has a nasogastric tube, it may be clipped to the gown or clothing to prevent pulling.

- Report any retching, nausea, or vomiting immediately.
- Check the tubing for kinks. Be sure the patient is not lying on the tubing.
- Provide frequent mouth hygiene. Patients with an NG tube will also need nasal care.
- Notify the nurse if a controlling device alarm sounds.

Adjusting to tube feeding formula can be difficult for the patient. The rate and strength of formula must be adjusted to meet the patient's needs. In some patients, the formula causes diarrhea. Inform the nurse if the patient's bowel activity increases, or if the patient experiences multiple loose or liquid stools. Keep the perineum clean and dry, and wash the patient well after each bowel activity.

REVIEW

A. True/False.

Mark the following true or false by circling T or F.

1. T F Vitamins are nutrients that help regulate body activities.
2. T F The exchange lists are used by patients on low-salt diets.
3. T F Fats are one of the six essential nutrients.
4. T F Ice cream would be served to a patient on a clear liquid diet.
5. T F Labels of canned foods must be checked when planning their use in low-sodium diets.
6. T F A gastrostomy tube introduces nutrients directly into the stomach.
7. T F Carbohydrate foods are used to make new body cells and build tissues.
8. T F Green leafy vegetables are a good source of calcium, iron, and B vitamins.
9. T F Complete protein foods like poultry contain all of the essential amino acids.

B. Matching.

Match the correct term from Column II with the words and phrases in Column I.

Column I

10. _____ difficulty swallowing
11. _____ roughage
12. _____ encourage liquid intake
13. _____ all the processes involved in taking in food and building and repairing the body
14. _____ treatment
15. _____ calcium

Column II

a. therapeutic
b. mineral
c. dysphagia
d. force fluids
e. cellulose
f. gastrostomy
g. nutrition

C. Multiple Choice.

Select the one best answer for each of the following.

16. Feeding the patient through a nasogastric tube is known as a/an
    a. intravenous infusion.
    b. gastrostomy feeding.
    c. enteral feeding.
    d. hyperalimentation.

17. Which of the following is a water-soluble vitamin?
    a. Vitamin C
    b. Vitamin E
    c. Vitamin A
    d. Vitamin D

18. An example of a fat-soluble vitamin is
    a. vitamin C.
    b. vitamin B-complex.
    c. vitamin D.
    d. vitamin N.

19. An average serving of meat is
    a. 1 ounce.
    b. 2 to 3 ounces.
    c. 8 ounces.
    d. 16 ounces.

20. Which of the following is part of the meat group?
    a. Peas
    b. Rice
    c. Poultry
    d. Cottage cheese

21. Foods naturally high in sodium include
    a. milk.
    b. cereals.
    c. vegetables.
    d. fruits.

22. Supplemental nourishments might include
   a. hot fudge sundaes.
   b. mashed potatoes.
   c. scrambled eggs.
   d. high-protein drinks.

23. A serving of cooked vegetables would be approximately
   a. ½ cup.
   b. ¾ cup.
   c. 1 cup.
   d. 1½ cups.

24. It is especially important to report to the nurse that the patient only ate two-thirds of her meal when the patient is on a
   a. low-salt diet.
   b. calorie-restricted diet.
   c. diabetic diet.
   d. house diet.

D. Nursing Assistant Challenge.

Mrs. Gole is one of your assigned patients. She is 72 years old, is on a 1,500-calorie diabetic diet, and is a member of the Seventh Day Adventist Church. She also has Parkinson's disease with tremors of her hands, and occasionally has trouble swallowing. Mrs. Gole sometimes eats food brought in by family and friends that is not on the 1,500-calorie diet. Consider Mrs. Gole's care:

25. Discuss safety issues that you need to think about when Mrs. Gole is eating.

26. Are there conflicts between the ordered diet and the dietary restrictions of her church? If so, what are the conflicts and how might they be resolved?

27. Do you anticipate that Mrs. Gole will have any problems feeding herself? If so, what are those problems, and what can you do to help her eat independently?

28. Discuss the issues of residents' or patients' rights that may arise because of the conflict between the patient's desire to eat more food than ordered and foods different from what the physician has prescribed.

 EXPLORING THE WEB

Description	Location
Basic nutrition	*http://www.delmarhealthcare.com/olcs/white/pnotes.asp* (see Chapter 18)
Carbohydrates	*http://www.delmarlearning.com/companions/content/ 0766835677/student/student4.asp*
Diet and weight control	*http://www.delmarlearning.com/companions/content/ 0766835677/student/student16.asp*
Diet during young and middle adulthood	*http://www.delmarlearning.com/companions/content/ 0766835677/student/student14.asp*
Digestion, absorption, and metabolism	*http://www.delmarlearning.com/companions/content/ 0766835677/student/student3.asp*
Food-related illness and allergies	*http://www.delmarlearning.com/companions/content/ 0766835677/student/student10.asp*
Lipids or fats	*http://www.delmarlearning.com/companions/content/ 0766835677/student/student5.asp*
Minerals	*http://www.delmarlearning.com/companions/content/ 0766835677/student/student8.asp*
Nutritional care of clients	*http://www.delmarlearning.com/companions/content/ 0766835677/student/student23.asp*
Planning a healthy diet	*http://www.delmarlearning.com/companions/content/ 0766835677/student/student2.asp*

continues

EXPLORING THE WEB *continued*

Description	Location
Proteins	*http://www.delmarlearning.com/companions/content/ 0766835677/student/student6.asp*
Relationship of food and health	*http://www.delmarlearning.com/companions/content/ 0766835677/student/student1.asp*
Vitamins	*http://www.delmarlearning.com/companions/content/ 0766835677/student/student7.asp*
Water	*http://www.delmarlearning.com/companions/content/ 0766835677/student/student9.asp*
American Diabetes Association	*http://www.diabetes.org*
American Dietetic Association	*http://www.eatright.org*
American Society on Parenteral and Enteral Nutrition	*http://www.nutritioncare.org*
Center on Nutrition	*http://navigator.tufts.edu*
Dysphagia Diet	*http://www.dysphagia-diet.com*
Dysphagia Information	*http://www.nidcd.nih.gov/health/pubs_vsl/dysph.htm*
Dysphagia Online	*http://www.dysphagiaonline.com*
Dysphagia Resource Center	*http://www.dysphagia.com*
Dysphagia Resource Society	*http://www.shs.uiuc.edu*
Education through Nutrition	*http://www.advancefornurses.com* (see past articles July 22, 2002)
Ethnic, Cultural, Special Audience Food Pyramids	*http://www.nal.usda.gov/fnic/etext/000023.html*
Food Guide Pyramid for Kids	*http://www.usda.gov/cnpp/KidsPyra*
Guide to Daily Food Choices	*http://www.nal.usda.gov:8001/py/pmap.htm*
Infusion Nurses Society	*http://www.ins1.org*
National Policy Center on Aging and Nutrition (also hydration information)	*http://www.fiu.edu*
Ross Laboratories	*http://www.ross.com*
Tufts University Nutrition Navigator	*http://navigator.tufts.edu*
United States Food and Drug Administration	*http://www.fda.gov*
Water Soluble Vitamins	*http://www.advancefornurses.com* (see past articles April 22, 2002)

section 9

Special Care Procedures

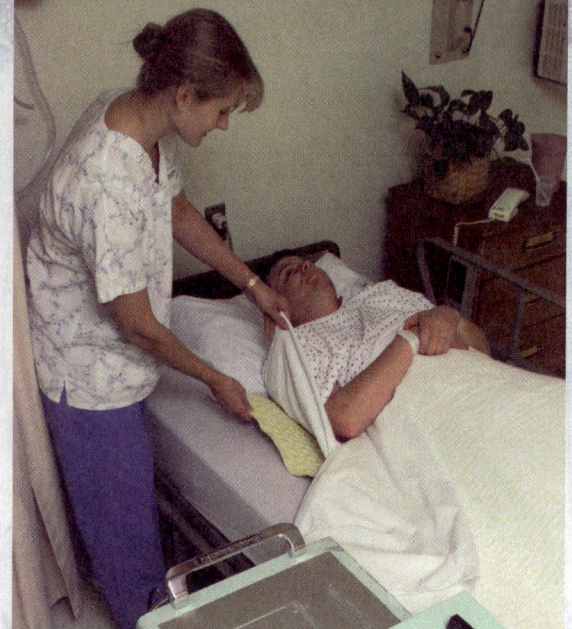

Warm and Cold Applications

objectives

After completing this unit, you will be able to:
- Spell and define terms.
- List the physical conditions requiring the use of heat and cold.
- Name types of heat and cold applications.
- Describe the effects of local cold applications.
- Describe the effects of local heat applications.
- List safety concerns related to application of heat and cold.
- Demonstrate the following procedures:

– Procedure 80 Applying an Ice Bag
– Procedure 81 Applying a Disposable Cold Pack
– Procedure 82 Applying an Aquamatic K-Pad®
– Procedure 83 Performing a Warm Soak
– Procedure 84 Applying a Warm Moist Compress
– Procedure 85 Assisting with Application of a Hypothermia Blanket

vocabulary

Learn the meaning and the correct spelling of the following words and phrases:

Aquamatic K-Pad®	hypothermia	ice bag	warm soak
cold pack	hypothermia-	thermal blanket	wet compress
diathermy	hyperthermia	vasoconstriction	
hemorrhage	blanket	vasodilation	

INTRODUCTION

Heat and cold applications are used only on written orders from the physician or nurse, and only for a specific length of time. Some facilities allow only professional personnel to apply heat and cold. **Some states have laws against nursing assistants applying heat or cold in a home health setting.** In other facilities, nursing assistants who have been specially trained are permitted to carry out these procedures under the supervision of the nurse. Be sure you know and follow the policy of your facility and are adequately prepared and *supervised*.

THERAPY WITH HEAT AND COLD

The physician orders the use of heat or cold applications to:
- relieve pain.
- combat local infection, swelling, or inflammation.
- control bleeding (**hemorrhage**).
- reduce body temperature.

Local applications of heat and cold are made with:
- Ice bags.
- Electronically operated Aquamatic K-Pads®. K-Pads® come in many shapes and sizes. They can be used to apply dry heat. By using an attachment, they can also be used for cooling.
- Prepackaged, single-use units for the application of hot and cold. A single hit on the surface activates the contents, providing a controlled temperature.
- Gel packs that can be cooled or heated as needed.

General treatments of heat and cold consist of thermal mattresses known as **hypothermia-hyperthermia blankets**. These are widely used to:
- lower body temperature when there is fever.
- elevate body temperature in cases of hypothermia.

Applications of warm and cold may be either dry or moist. Moisture makes both heat and cold more penetrating. Therefore, moist heat or moist cold is more likely to cause injury. Extra care must be taken to protect the patient when moist treatments are used. Be sure you know:
- Exact method to be used
- Correct temperature and placement
- Proper length of time the warm or cold application is to be performed
- How often the area being treated is to be checked

Table 27-1 summarizes types of warm and cold applications.

Commercial Preparations

Easy-to-use commercial warm and cold packs are available for dry applications. For one type of pack, a single hit or blow to the pack before application activates it. The pack is discarded after one use. Reusable packs are also available, but infection control issues make them less desirable.

TABLE 27-1 WARM AND COLD APPLICATIONS

Dry Warm Applications	Dry Cold Applications
Aquamatic K-Pad®	Ice cap
Disposable warm pack	Ice bag
Electric heating pads	Disposable cold pack
Aquathermia blanket	Aquamatic K-Pad®
	Hypothermia blanket

Moist Warm Applications	Moist Cold Applications
Warm soaks	Compresses
Compresses	Soaks
Tub baths	Packs
Sitz baths	

guidelines *for*

Warm and Cold Treatments

You must be very watchful when applying cold or warm treatments. When assigned to this task, keep in mind the following:
- The age and condition of the patient. Give extra care to:
  - Young children
  - The aged
  - Patients with cognitive impairment
  - Patients who are uncooperative
  - Patients who are unconscious
  - Patients who are paralyzed

continues

guidelines *continued*

  - Patients with tissue damage
  - Patients with poor circulation
- Apply the principles of standard precautions if your hands will contact blood, moist body fluids (except sweat), secretions, excretions, nonintact skin, or mucous membranes.
- If the patient has a dressing covering the area to be treated, consult the nurse for directions.
- Check the temperature of the solution with a thermometer. You may need to add more liquid during the treatment to maintain the temperature. Avoid pouring hot or cold liquid directly over the patient.
- Remove all metal jewelry, buttons, or zippers that could conduct heat or cold and thereby injure the skin.
- Avoid using heat treatments with temperatures over 110°F. Temperatures greater than this can cause burns, particularly in infants and the elderly.
- Avoid using heat in the first 48 hours after an injury.
- Follow all safety rules to prevent spills and falls.
- An electric heating pad must not be used with moist dressings unless a rubber cover is placed over the pad. If the wires become damp, a short circuit may result. The patient must not lie on the pad, because severe burns can result. Sensitivity to heat varies, so patients receiving heat treatments must be checked frequently. Although heating pads are not used in health care facilities, they are used by individuals in homes.

- Heat is not applied to the head because it could make blood vessels in the area dilate, causing headache.
- Heat should not be applied to the abdomen if there is any chance that the patient has appendicitis, because it would increase the chance of the appendix rupturing.
- Check the skin under the application every 10 minutes, or according to facility policy. If the skin under a heat application appears red, or a dark area appears, stop the treatment. Notify the nurse immediately. Stop a cold application and notify your supervisor if the patient's skin appears cyanotic, pale, white, or bright red; if the patient complains of numbness; or if the patient is shivering. Cover the patient with a blanket.
- Rubber or plastic should never touch the patient's skin. Be sure all appliances are covered with cloth.
- Heat and cold applications are usually not left in place longer than 20 minutes, according to the purpose and type of treatment. Follow the care plan and the nurse's instructions.
- After the treatment, pat the skin dry. Make the patient comfortable. Clean and store used equipment. Remove gloves, if worn, and dispose of them according to facility policy. Wash your hands. Report to your supervisor that the procedure was completed and the patient's reaction to the treatment.

USE OF COLD APPLICATIONS

Applications of cold are given only with a physician's order. The application of cold:

- Constricts or decreases the size of blood vessels (**vasoconstriction**) and reduces swelling
- Decreases sensitivity to pain
- Reduces temperature
- Slows inflammation
- Reduces itching

Cautions

Remember, moisture intensifies the effect of cold just as it does heat. Caution must be used in the application of moist cold.

- Excessive cold can damage body tissues.
- Report color changes such as *blanching* (turning white) or *cyanosis* (becoming bluish).
- Report feelings of numbness or discomfort experienced by the patient.
- Stop the cold treatment if the patient starts to shiver. Cover the patient with a blanket and report immediately to the nurse. (See Procedures 80 and 81.)

Dry Cold Applications

There are several methods for applying therapeutic cold. Careful attention to the application is needed to prevent injury.

- Disposable **cold pack**—This single-use commercial pack can be stored until needed. Reusable commercial packs are also available (for both warm and cold

Cold therapy should not be used for patients with:

- Deep vein thrombosis
- Peripheral vascular disease
- Open wound(s)
- Skin sensation impairment
- Severe cognitive impairment
- Cold intolerance, cold allergy
- Some medical conditions such as rheumatoid arthritis and Reynaud's phenomenon.

If a patient has any of these conditions, check with the nurse before applying a cold application.

applications). The pack remains effective for approximately 15 to 30 minutes. If the cold pack must be activated, follow the manufacturer's instructions exactly. When activating the pack, do not hold it in front of your face. If the pack leaks or bursts, the chemicals inside the pack may splash. Check the area being treated every 10 minutes. Discard the chemical cold pack after one use, or when the pack warms. Do not attempt to refreeze it.

- **Ice bag**—This reusable, waterproof, canvas or rubber container can be filled with ice to provide temporary local cold. An ice bag is never placed directly on the affected area because the weight of the bag will cause the patient discomfort.

- **Thermal blanket**—This is a large, fluid-filled blanket that is placed over or around the patient. The temperature of the fluid in the blanket may be raised or lowered. The blanket is used to lower or raise the patient's body temperature. However, it is most often used in care facilities to lower the body temperature. This process is called inducing **hypothermia**. A licensed professional usually monitors the use of this type of blanket.

Tips: Paper or styrofoam cups of ice are sometimes used to gently massage an injured area. To apply cold this way, hold the cup and make small, overlapping circles on the affected area for 20 minutes. An examination glove filled with ice and secured with a rubber band is also sometimes used as an alternate ice application.

Moist Cold Applications

- **Wet compresses** are moistened with a solution and placed on the affected area.
- A syringe may be used to add water to the compresses to keep them moist.
- The compresses can be kept cold by placing a covered ice bag against the affected area. Make sure the patient can tolerate the weight of the ice bag without increased pain.
- Each time the pad is removed and replaced, be careful to reposition the protective covering.

Follow facility policy for:
- method of applying the treatment.
- length of time the treatment is to be applied.
- how often the patient is to be checked for condition of the skin in the treatment area and general response to the treatment.
- signs that treatment should be discontinued.

PROCEDURE 80

APPLYING AN ICE BAG

1. Assemble equipment:
   - ice bag
   - cover (usually cotton, such as a towel, or cover specified by your facility)
   - paper towels
   - spoon or similar utensil
   - ice cubes or crushed ice

2. Prepare the ice bag as follows:
   a. Fill the ice bag with cold water and check for leaks.
   b. Empty the bag.
   c. If ice cubes are used, rinse them in water to remove sharp edges. The use of crushed ice makes the bag more flexible and is more comfortable for the patient.

continues

PROCEDURE 80

continued

d. Fill the ice bag half full, using an ice scooper, paper cup, or large spoon (Figure 27-1). Avoid making ice bags too heavy. Do not allow the scoop to touch the ice bag.

e. To remove air from the ice bag:

- Rest the ice bag flat on a paper towel on a flat surface.
- Put the top in place, but do not screw it on.
- Press the bag until the air is removed (Figure 27-2).

f. Fasten the top securely.

g. Test for leakage.

h. Wipe the ice bag dry with paper towels. Place it in a cloth cover.

Note: As an alternative, a gel pack stored in the freezer can be used for cold applications. These packs can be refrozen and reused if this is facility policy.

3. Take the equipment to the bedside on a tray. Carry out beginning procedure actions.

4. Apply the ice bag to the affected part.

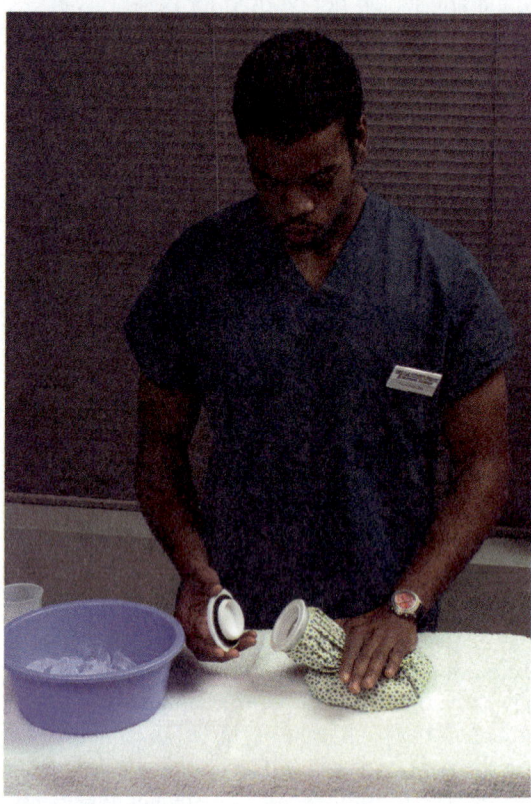

FIGURE 27-2 Place the ice bag on a flat surface, then press firmly to remove the air.

5. Refill the ice bag before all the ice has melted.

6. Check the skin area under the ice bag every 10 minutes. Report to supervising nurse immediately if skin is discolored or white or if the patient reports that the skin is numb.

7. Continue the cold application for the amount of time specified by your supervisor. If the patient feels cold, cover with a blanket, but do not cover the area being treated.

8. Carry out procedure completion actions.

9. When the treatment is complete, wash the bag with soap and water. Rinse and dry it completely, and then screw the top on. Wipe the bag with a disinfectant if this is your facility policy. Leave air in the ice bag to prevent the sides from sticking together.

10. If a reusable cold pack is used, wash it thoroughly with soap and water or wipe with a disinfectant, according to facility policy. Return the pack to the refrigerator. Discard a disposable pack.

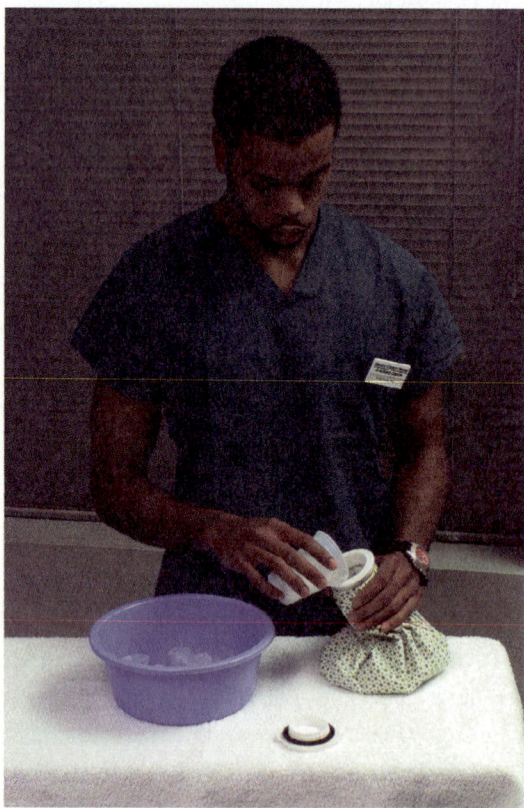

FIGURE 27-1 Fill the ice bag half full.

PROCEDURE 81

APPLYING A DISPOSABLE COLD PACK

1. Carry out beginning procedure actions.

2. Assemble equipment:
   - disposable commercial cold pack
   - cloth covering (towel, warm water bag cover, or other cover specified by the facility)
   - tape or rolls of gauze

3. Expose the area to be treated. Note the condition of the area.

4. Place the cold pack in a cloth covering (Figure 27-3).

5. Strike or squeeze the cold pack to activate chemicals. (Follow manufacturer's instructions.)

6. Place the covered cold pack on the proper area and cover it with a towel (Figure 27-4). Note time of application.

7. Secure the cover with tape or gauze, if necessary, to hold it in place.

8. Leave the patient in a comfortable position, with the signal cord within easy reach.

9. Return to the bedside every 10 minutes. Check the area being treated for discoloration or numbness. If these signs and symptoms occur, discontinue treatment and report them to your supervisor.

10. If no adverse symptoms occur, remove the pack after 30 minutes, or after the amount of time given in your instructions. Note the condition of the area. Continuous treatment requires application of a fresh pack.

11. Remove the pack from the cover and discard according to facility policy. Return unused gauze and tape.

12. Put the cover in a laundry hamper.

13. Carry out procedure completion actions.

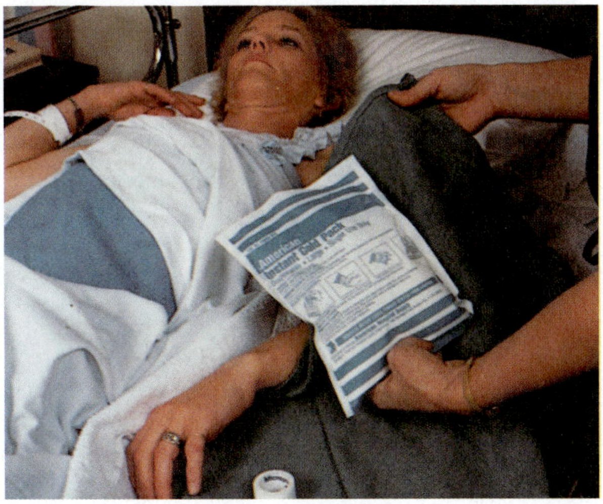

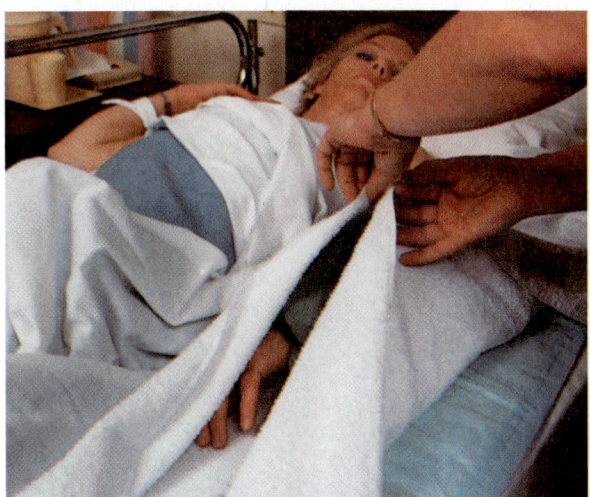

FIGURE 27-3 Cover the disposable cold pack with a cover before applying it to the patient.

FIGURE 27-4 After positioning the cold pack, cover the application with a towel.

USE OF WARM APPLICATIONS

Warm applications are ordered to:
- relieve muscle spasms.
- reduce pain.
- reduce inflammation.
- promote healing.
- combat local infection.
- increase circulation.
- improve mobility before exercise periods.
- soothe the patient.

SAFETY *Alert*

The heat application should feel comfortably warm to the patient, not uncomfortably hot. If you will be applying a pack or pad, touch the device to your forearm to check the temperature before applying it. If the patient complains of burning, remove the application and consult the nurse.

The value of heat treatments (diathermy) is that heat dilates or increases the size of blood vessels (vasodilation). This brings more blood to the area to promote healing. Warmth is very soothing when there is pain.

There must be a specific order for a warm application. Some groups of people require extra care when they receive warm applications. (See Procedures 82 to 84.)

Cautions

Follow these cautions when working with patients:

- Constant warmth must be carefully monitored.
- Moisture intensifies the effect of warmth. Use extra caution.

SAFETY *Alert*

Heat therapy should not be used for patients with:

- Acute inflammation
- Dermatitis
- Deep vein thrombosis
- Peripheral vascular disease
- Open wound(s)
- Recent soft tissue injuries in which swelling or bleeding would be increased by heat
- Skin sensation impairment
- Severe cognitive impairment

Some physicians also recommend avoiding heat use with children and women during pregnancy. If a patient has any of these conditions, check with the nurse before applying a heat application.

- Hot packs are contraindicated for paralyzed areas or areas without sensation, acute edema or inflammation, infection, and hemophilia. They must be used with caution for patients with many medical conditions, including impaired circulation, sensory impairment, cancer, rashes, and open skin conditions. Take extra care with hot packs for very young and very old patients.
- Never allow a patient to lie on a constant heat unit, because heat may be trapped and build up to dangerous levels.
- Temperature of a constant heat unit should be between 95° and 100°F.
- Always use a bath thermometer to check solution temperatures.
- Always remove the body part being soaked before adding warm solution.
- Always stay with the patient during the treatment.
- Protect areas not being treated from excessive exposure.
- Warmth is not applied to the head because it could cause blood vessels in the area to dilate, resulting in headache.
- Rubber or plastic should never touch the patient's skin. Be sure all appliances are covered with cloth.

Dry Warm Applications

The Aquamatic K-Pad® is commonly used to provide dry warmth. It consists of a plastic pad with fluid-filled coils and a control unit that maintains a constant temperature of the fluid.

The fluid in the pad is distilled water that is supplied from a reservoir in the control unit. The control unit is placed on the bedside stand and is plugged into an electrical outlet. In most facilities, the temperature is preset by the central supply department. The temperature is usually set at 95° to 100°F.

Tips: When setting up the K-Pad® for the first time, check the pad for leaks. Tip it back and forth several times to eliminate air pockets, which cause hot spots. Place the control unit on the bedside stand so it is higher than the patient, so that water will run into the pad by gravity. Make sure the tubing is free of kinks.

Moist Warm Applications

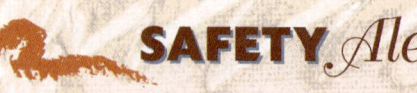

SAFETY *Alert*

Moisture intensifies heat and you must use extra care.

For each of the warm treatments, follow facility policy for:

- method of applying the treatment.
- length of time the treatment is to be applied.
- how often the patient is to be checked for condition of the skin in the treatment area and general response to the treatment.
- signs that treatment should be discontinued.

Moist warm treatments include:

- **Warm soaks**—The patient, or the part of the patient's body that is being treated, is immersed in a tub filled with water at a specific temperature, usually 105°.
- Wet compresses—The same cautions apply to warm compresses as to cold compresses. They may be kept wet with a syringe and warm by covering them with an Aquamatic K-Pad®.

PROCEDURE 82

APPLYING AN AQUAMATIC K-PAD®

1. Carry out beginning procedure actions.

2. Assemble equipment:
   - K-Pad® and control unit
   - distilled water
   - covering for pad

3. Check the cord for frayed or damaged insulation. Also check that the tubing between the control unit and the pad is intact.

4. Place the control unit on the bedside stand (Figure 27-5).

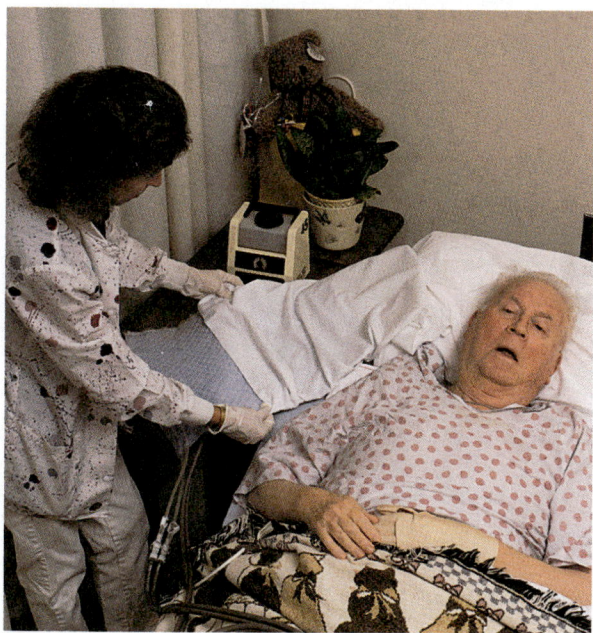

FIGURE 27-5 The control unit for the aquathermia pad maintains a constant temperature.

5. Remove the cover of the control unit and check the level of the distilled water. If it is low, fill the unit two-thirds full or to the fill line using distilled water. Tilt the unit back and forth gently to clear the tubing of air.

6. Screw the cover in place and loosen it one-quarter turn.

7. If the temperature was not preset, check with the nurse for the proper setting before turning on the unit. Remove the key after setting the temperature.

8. Plug in the unit.

9. Cover the pad with an appropriate cover, according to facility policy or as specified by the manufacturer of the unit. Do not use pins to hold the cover in place.

10. Expose the area on the patient to be treated. Place the covered pad on the patient and note the time.
    - Be sure the tubing between the control unit and the pad does not hang over the side of the bed. It should be coiled on the bed to promote the flow of liquid.

11. Following facility policy, periodically check the skin under the pad.

12. Check the level of the water in the control unit. Refill if necessary to the fill line.

13. Remove the pad after the prescribed amount of time.

14. Carry out procedure completion actions.

PROCEDURE **83**

PERFORMING A WARM SOAK

1. Carry out beginning procedure actions.

2. Assemble equipment:
   - bath thermometer
   - soak basin
   - pitcher
   - large plastic sheet
   - bath towel
   - bath blanket

3. Bring equipment to the bedside.

4. Cover the patient with a bath blanket.

5. Fanfold bedding to the foot of the bed.

6. Expose the limb to be soaked.

7. Position the patient for comfort on the far side of the bed (opposite the part to be soaked). Be sure the side rail is up and secure.

8. Cover the bed with a plastic sheet and towel.

9. Fill the soak basin half full with water at the prescribed temperature (usually 105°F). Check the temperature with a bath thermometer.

10. Take the soak basin from the overbed table and position it on the bed protector.

11. Assist the patient to gradually place the limb in the basin (Figure 27-6). Cover the basin with a towel to help maintain temperature.

12. Check the temperature every 5 minutes. Use a pitcher to get additional water and add to the soak basin to maintain temperature. Remember to remove the patient's limb before adding water to the container.

13. Discontinue the procedure at the end of the prescribed time.

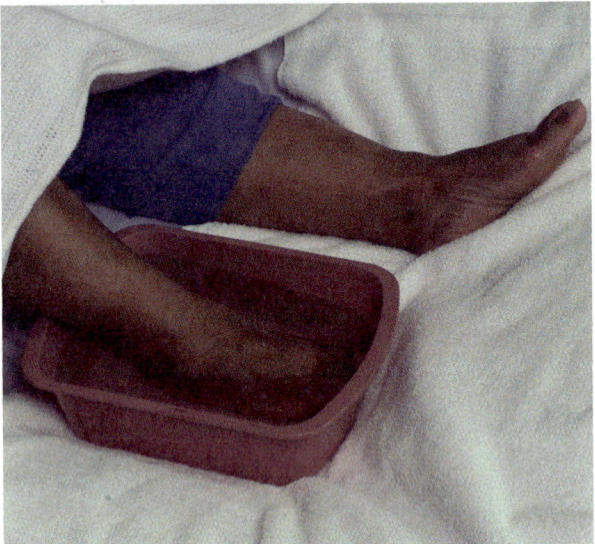

FIGURE 27-6 The patient is receiving warm soak therapy.

   a. Lift the patient's limb out of the basin.
   b. Slip the basin forward and allow the limb to rest on the bath towel.
   c. Place the basin on the overbed table. Gently pat the limb dry with a towel.

14. Remove the plastic sheet and towel.

15. Adjust bedding and remove the bath blanket. If the treatment is to be repeated, fold the bath blanket and place it in the bedside stand. Leave the unit tidy and the call bell within reach.

16. Lower the head of the bed and make the patient comfortable.

17. Take equipment to the utility room. Clean and store it according to facility policy.

18. Carry out procedure completion actions.

PROCEDURE 84

APPLYING A WARM MOIST COMPRESS

1. Carry out beginning procedure actions.

2. Assemble equipment:
   - disposable gloves
   - syringe
   - bed protector
   - compresses
   - bath thermometer
   - binder or towel
   - pins or bandage
   - basin with prescribed solution at temperature ordered

3. Bring equipment to the bedside.

4. Expose only the area to be treated.

5. Protect the bed and the patient's clothing with a bed protector (Figure 27-7A).

6. Put on disposable gloves.

7. Check the temperature of the solution. Moisten the compresses; remove excess liquid (Figure 27-7B). Apply to treatment area (Figure 27-7C).

8. Secure the compresses with a bandage or binder.

The compress must be in contact with the patient's skin.

9. Help the patient to maintain a comfortable position throughout the treatment.

10. Unscreen the unit. Leave the unit neat and tidy, with the signal cord within easy reach.

11. Maintain proper temperature and moisture.
    - If the compresses are to be kept warm, a K-Pad® may be applied.
    - If the compresses are to be kept cool, an ice bag may be applied.
    - A syringe may be used to apply more solution to keep the compresses wet.

12. Remove the compresses when ordered. Change as ordered or once in 24 hours. Check skin several times each day.

13. Discard the compresses.

14. Remove and dispose of gloves according to facility policy.

15. Carry out procedure completion actions.

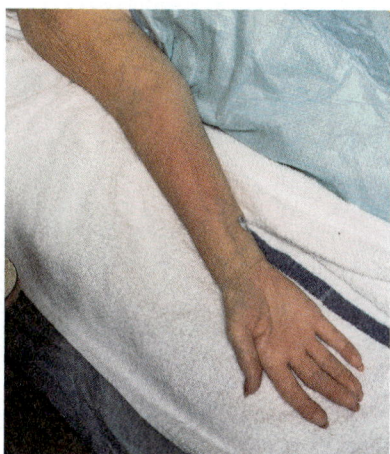

FIGURE 27-7A Protect the bed with a towel or underpad.

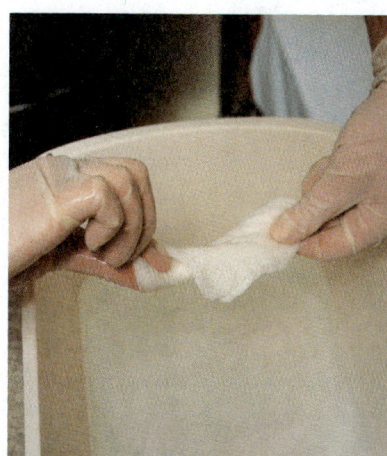

FIGURE 27-7B Dip the compress into a basin of warm (105°F) water. Grasp the edges, then squeeze out excess liquid.

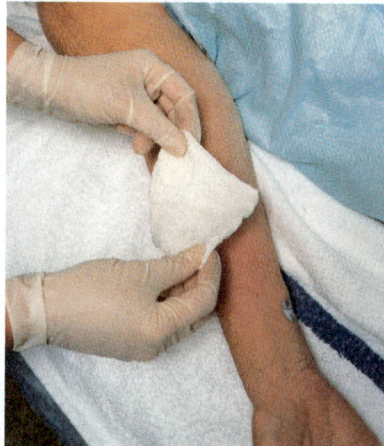

FIGURE 27-7C Open the compress and apply it to the inflamed area.

TEMPERATURE CONTROL MEASURES

Excessively high or low body temperatures are treated in acute care facilities by placing hypothermia-hyperthermia blankets (Figure 27-8) over and under the patient. These blankets are units filled with water. The blankets may be called *aquathermia blankets*. "Aqua" is the Latin term for *water*. The temperature of the water can be adjusted higher or lower depending on whether the patient's body temperature is to be raised or lowered.

Using the Aquathermia Blanket

The aquathermia blanket is operated either manually or automatically. For manual operation, the licensed nurse will set the blanket to a predetermined temperature, which is ordered by the physician. The blanket maintains this temperature regardless of changes in the patient's body temperature. When the unit is set for automatic operation, it monitors the patient's temperature through a rectal, skin, or esophageal probe. The probe is secured to the body with tape to prevent injury. The blanket temperature changes according to the patient's temperature. The goal is to main-

tain the patient's body temperature. An alarm will sound for abnormal temperature variations. Before using the blanket, check it for cracks, tears, or leaks in the system. Do not use it if there are cracks or an electrical malfunction.

The patient should wear a hospital gown when the aquathermia blanket is used. Use a gown with tie closures. Snaps, pins, or other metal may cause injury to the skin. Before beginning the procedure, check and record the patient's baseline vital signs as a basis for comparison.

One or two aquathermia blankets may be used. The nurse may instruct you to place one under the patient, and to cover him or her with the other. The blankets must be covered with a disposable cover, sheet, or bath blanket to absorb perspiration and prevent complications. Avoid using pins to cover the blanket. These can puncture the unit or injure the patient's skin by creating hot or cold spots. Use tape or Velcro® fasteners, if necessary, to cover the unit.

The blanket should be set up and preheated or precooled before it is applied to the patient. Connect the blanket to the control unit by plugging in the tubing. The nurse will set the blanket for automatic or manual operation. He or she will also set the desired body temperature or blanket temperature and instruct you as to what temperature values are being used. Turn the device on, then add distilled water to the reservoir. Position the controls at the foot of the bed. After the blanket has reached the designated temperature, apply it to the patient. If the patient will be lying on a blanket, place a pillow or folded bath blanket under the patient's head.

The patient's head should not contact the blanket directly. The combination of heat or cold and the surface of the blanket promotes skin breakdown on the back of the head. The nurse may instruct you to apply lanolin or another designated product to the skin in exposed areas that contact the blanket directly. You may wrap the patient's hands and feet to prevent chilling, if desired.

Complications. Immediately notify the nurse if you observe any of these complications:

- Changes in skin color
- Cyanosis of the lips or nail beds
- Sudden changes in body temperature
- marked changes in pulse, respirations, and blood pressure
- respiratory distress
- pain
- changes in sensation
- edema
- shivering and chills
- urinary output below 50 mL/hour

Discontinuing Blanket Use. The nurse will inform you when to discontinue use of the blanket. Follow the manufacturer's directions for the type of blanket you are

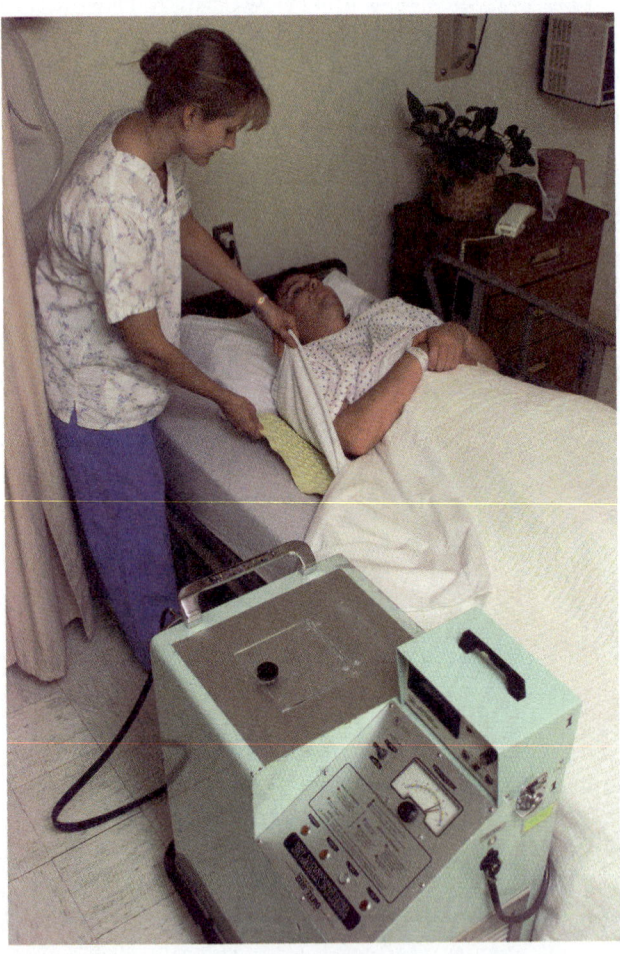

FIGURE 27-8 Hypothermia-hyperthermia blanket.

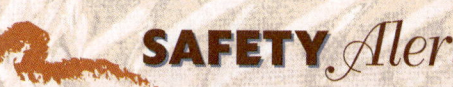

SAFETY *Alert*

The nurse will instruct you on the frequency for monitoring vital signs when an aquathermia blanket is being used. The patient's temperature and the blanket temperature are usually monitored and documented every 15 to 30 minutes. Inform the nurse immediately if the patient's temperature drops more than one degree in 15 minutes. Continued temperature monitoring is necessary after the blanket is removed because the patient's temperature can continue to drop as much as 5 degrees after the procedure ends.

AGE-APPROPRIATE CARE *Alert*

In children, temperatures tend to rise higher than in adults. This puts children at greater risk for seizures.

using. Turn the unit off. (Some types must remain plugged in for 30 to 60 minutes to dry condensation inside the unit.) Dry the patient's skin and assist him or her into a dry gown. Position the patient in a comfortable position. Remove the aquathermia blanket from the bed after the designated time. Continue checking vital signs and intake and output every 30 minutes for the first 2 hours, then hourly or as directed by the nurse. (See Procedure 85.)

Hypothermia

Hypothermia is a drop in core body temperature below 95°F (35°C) rectally. This can occur:

- when people are exposed to cold without adequate protection.
- in the elderly, when a person is exposed to external temperatures as warm as 60°F.
- when deliberately induced before surgery to slow body metabolism.

Indications of hypothermia to report include:

- Drop in body temperature
- Poor coordination and confusion
- Slurred speech
- Decreased respiratory and heart rates

Nursing Assistant Actions

- Report observations to the supervisor.
- Check the environmental temperature and adjust it.

- Provide external warmth with a sweater or blanket.
- Reduce drafts with screens or curtains.
- If permitted, give something warm to drink.
- Check vital signs.

Hyperthermia

Hyperthermia is an elevation of core body temperature to 104°F (40°C) rectally or higher. This can occur:

- when a person is exposed to high external temperature.
- with serious injuries such as burns.
- when there is damage to the temperature control center in the brain.
- with infections.

Indications of hyperthermia to report include:

- Elevated body temperature
- Hot, flushed skin
- Faintness
- Headache
- Nausea
- Convulsions

Fever or *pyrexia* occurs when core body temperature rises to at least 101°F (rectally). Fever is often associated with infections, injury, surgery, and serious trauma. Indications of fever are the same as those for general hyperthermia.

Nursing Assistant Actions

- Report observations to the supervisor.
- Check environment temperature and adjust it.
- Reduce external warmth. Cover the patient only with a gown or sheet.
- If permitted, give cooling drink.
- Carry out cooling procedures as ordered. For example, give cooling baths or enemas.
- Check vital signs frequently.

PROCEDURE 85

ASSISTING WITH APPLICATION OF A HYPOTHERMIA BLANKET

Applying a hypothermia blanket and monitoring a patient who is receiving a hypothermia treatment is a professional nursing responsibility. The nurse will supervise the procedure and monitor the patient throughout the treatment. The nurse will check the specific gravity of the patient's urine, vital signs, and nervous system response. The nursing assistant may be asked to assist in setting up equipment, positioning the patient and the thermal blanket, observing the patient during the treatment, and keeping the patient comfortable. In addition, the nursing assistant may be asked to transport equipment to and from the central supply service.

1. Wash your hands, collect equipment, and take equipment to the bedside.

2. Assemble equipment:
   - disposable gloves
   - hypothermia-hyperthermia control unit
   - fluid for control unit
   - thermometer probes (rectal or skin)
   - adhesive tape
   - sphygmomanometer
   - stethoscope
   - hypothermia-hyperthermia blanket (disposable or reusable), one or two as ordered
   - bath blanket or sheet, one or two as ordered
   - lanolin-based skin cream

3. Follow manufacturer's directions for setting up equipment. Check equipment for safety. Be sure the control unit is grounded.

4. Connect the blanket(s) to the control unit and set the control.

5. Turn on the control unit and add liquid.

6. Allow the blanket(s) to precool as you prepare the patient.

7. Carry out beginning procedure actions.

8. Place the patient in a hospital-type gown with ties.

9. Measure vital signs and record.

10. Place the hypothermia-hyperthermia blanket on the bed and cover it with a sheet. Position the patient on the sheet-covered thermal blanket in the recumbent position, with the head on a pillow that does not touch the blanket.

11. Wash your hands. Put on gloves.

12. Insert a rectal thermometer probe into the patient's rectum (unless contraindicated) and tape it in place. (Alternatively, place a skin probe into an axilla and tape it in place.)

13. Plug the end of the probe into the proper jack on the control panel.

14. Place a second sheet over the patient and place a second thermal blanket over the sheet, if ordered.

15. Apply lanolin-based cream to the patient's skin where it contacts the blanket.

16. Remove gloves. Discard according to facility policy. Wash your hands.

17. Monitor vital signs, neurologic response, and intake and output every 5 minutes until the desired body temperature is reached, and then every 15 minutes, or as ordered.

18. Report color changes in skin or excessive shivering.

19. The blanket's texture increases the risk of skin breakdown. The patient should be repositioned every 30 minutes to 1 hour. Reapply skin cream as necessary. Change the gown and top sheet as often as necessary if the patient is actively perspiring. Put on gloves each time you care for patient. At the end of care, remove gloves, discard according to facility policy, and wash your hands.

20. At completion of the treatment, follow manufacturer's instructions for turning off the unit, disconnecting the blanket(s), and returning them to storage.

21. Put on gloves. Continue to monitor the patient as you remove the equipment.

22. Replace any damp bedding or garments and cover the patient. Continue to monitor the patient every 30 minutes until he or she has been stable for 2 hours.

23. Clean the thermometer probe and store it according to facility policy.

24. Remove gloves and discard according to facility policy.

25. Carry out procedure completion actions.

REVIEW

A. True/False.

Mark the following true or false by circling T or F.

1. T F Heat and cold treatments should be supervised by the nurse.

2. T F If a patient has a possible diagnosis of appendicitis, heat should not be applied to the abdomen.

3. T F The temperature of a warm soak solution should be approximately 100°F.

4. T F Special blankets used to alter the patient's temperature are called infrared blankets.

5. T F A patient who is unconscious must receive special attention during a heat treatment.

6. T F Hyperthermia is an elevation of core body temperature to below 95°F.

7. T F Heat is frequently applied to the head.

8. T F When charting an application of cold, always include the length of time of the application.

9. T F Aquamatic K-Pads® are usually set at 115°F.

B. Multiple Choice.

Select the one best answer for each of the following.

10. Heat affects the body by
   a. causing constriction.
   b. increasing blood supply to the area.
   c. reducing oxygen in tissues.
   d. increasing white blood cells.

11. Special care with heat and cold treatments must be taken when the patient is
   a. alert and oriented.
   b. very young.
   c. cooperative.
   d. ambulatory.

12. Dry cold is provided by
   a. compresses.
   b. a hyperthermia blanket.
   c. ice caps.
   d. soaks.

13. Cold affects the body by
   a. reducing pain sensations.
   b. stimulating life processes.
   c. promoting inflammation.
   d. promoting healing.

14. Moist cold is applied with
   a. ice bags.
   b. ice caps.
   c. ice collars.
   d. soaks.

15. When applying heat and cold treatments, the nursing assistant should
   a. always remain in the room for the duration of the treatment.
   b. check the temperature of the solution with an elbow.
   c. monitor the skin under the application every 30 minutes.
   d. remove jewelry, buttons, or zippers that may conduct heat or cold.

16. When caring for a patient who is using an aquathermia blanket, the nursing assistant should
   a. regulate blanket temperature at least every 15 minutes.
   b. give the patient plenty of iced liquids to drink to reduce fever.
   c. monitor the patient for cyanosis or changes in vital signs.
   d. turn the patient at least every 2 hours.

C. Matching.

Choose the correct word from Column II to match each blank in Column I.

Column I	Column II
17. _____ excessive blood loss	**a.** diathermy
18. _____ increase in size of blood vessel	**b.** vasoconstriction
	c. vasodilation
19. _____ heat treatment	**d.** hypothermia blanket
20. _____ decrease in size of blood vessel	**e.** hemorrhage
	f. infrared
21. _____ used to lower body temperature	

D. Nursing Assistant Challenge.

Peggy, 17 years of age, was admitted to your unit from the emergency room. She fractured an ankle and will require internal repair with screws and wire. You will care for her prior to surgery. The physician has ordered an ice bag for her ankle and her leg is to be elevated. Answer the following questions.

22. What are two reasons for applying the ice bag?

23. How full should the ice bag be filled?

24. Why should ice cubes be rinsed?

25. How should the metal cap be positioned when the ice bag is placed on the patient?

26. When should the ice bag be refilled?

27. How is the ice bag held in place?

28. What important observation should be reported immediately to the nurse?

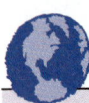 # EXPLORING THE WEB

Description	Location
Aquatic Therapy	*http://www.advancefornurses.com* (see past articles February 11, 2002)
Heat and Cold Therapy	*http://www.genufix.com*
Hot and Cold Therapies	*http://www.spineuniverse.com*
Managing Pain with Heat and Cold	*http://www.orthop.washington.edu*
	http://www.arthritis.org
Post Acute Pools	*http://www. advancefornurses.com* (see past articles September 9, 2002)
Principles of Heat and Cold: Clinical Application	*http://jan.ucc.nau.edu*
Use of Heat and Cold in Pain	*http://www.kasenterprises.com*
Using Heat and Cold	*http://www.silvercross.org*
Water World	*http://www.advancefornurses.com* (see past articles October 7, 2002)

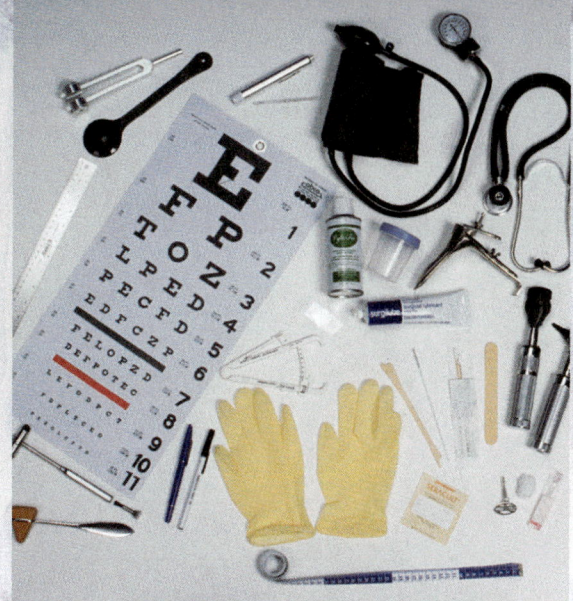

Assisting with the Physical Examination

objectives

After completing this unit, you will be able to:

- Spell and define terms.
- Describe the responsibilities of the nursing assistant during the physical examination.
- Name the positions for the various physical examinations.

- Drape patient for the various positions.
- Name the basic instruments necessary for physical examinations.
- Demonstrate the following procedure:
  – Procedure 86 Assisting with a Physical Examination

vocabulary

Learn the meaning and the correct spelling of the following words and phrases:

dorsal lithotomy position	dorsal recumbent position	ophthalmoscope	speculum
	knee-chest position	otoscope	Trendelenburg
		percussion hammer	position

INTRODUCTION

Physical examinations are done in the physician's office, in clinics, after the patient's admission to the facility, and in the patient's home. Remember to carry out each beginning procedure action and procedure completion action as you assist. The physical examination helps the physician:

- evaluate the patient's current status.
- establish a diagnosis.
- determine the patient's progress and response to therapy.

Nursing physical assessments will be performed by the nurse in the facility after the patient is admitted. This information is used by the nurse to establish a nursing diagnosis.

Both of these procedures are carried out in a similar manner. The responsibilities of the nursing assistant include:

- providing for the comfort and privacy of the patient.
- trying to anticipate the examiner's needs.
- draping and positioning patients.
- using proper body mechanics and exposing only the part of the patient being examined.
- preparing equipment that might be needed.
- reassuring the patient.
- caring for and labeling specimens.
- handing equipment as needed.
- cleaning equipment after use.
- adjusting lighting.
- remaining available during the examination.
- assisting the patient after the examination.

Tips: Adjust the room temperature for comfort and make sure the room is free of drafts. Cover the examination table with a clean sheet or disposable paper. Instruct the patient to empty the bladder before beginning.

POSITIONING THE PATIENT

When the physical examination takes place on an examination table, extra attention must be given to safety. The examination table may be raised or lowered in sections and stirrups and shoulder braces applied to assist in positioning. Be sure you know how to properly operate the examination table before positioning a patient on it. In Figures 28-2 to 28-9, an examination table is shown.

Modifications

Some of the positions discussed here may be modified and used for other purposes. For example, they might be used to change the position of a patient who is confined to bed, or to perform specific procedures. Pillows must be used to support a patient who is to be kept in position for a period of time. Remember, the patient who "feels" covered and comfortable will be able to cooperate more fully. Providing privacy for the patient is one of your tasks (Figure 28-1).

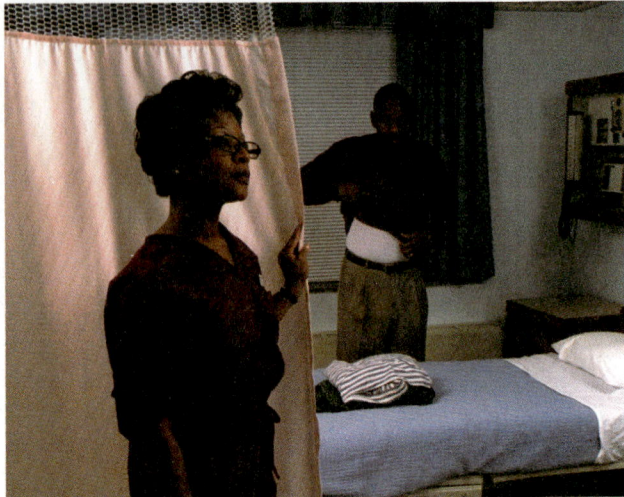

FIGURE 28-1 Provide privacy before the examination begins.

Dorsal Recumbent Position

The **dorsal recumbent position** is the basic examination position.

- Assist the patient to be flat on the back, with knees flexed and slightly separated. The feet should be flat on the bed or table (Figure 28-2).
- Place a small pillow under the patient's head.
- Loosen the gown at the neck.
- Cover the patient with a sheet.

Supine or Horizontal Recumbent Position

- Assist the patient to lie flat on the back. The legs are extended and slightly separated (Figure 28-3).
- Place a pillow under the patient's head.
- Cover the patient with a sheet.
- Loosen the gown at the neck.

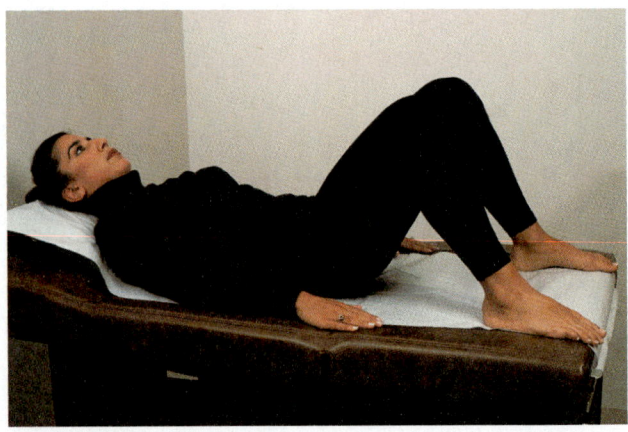

FIGURE 28-2 Dorsal recumbent position. (Draping has been omitted for clarity.)

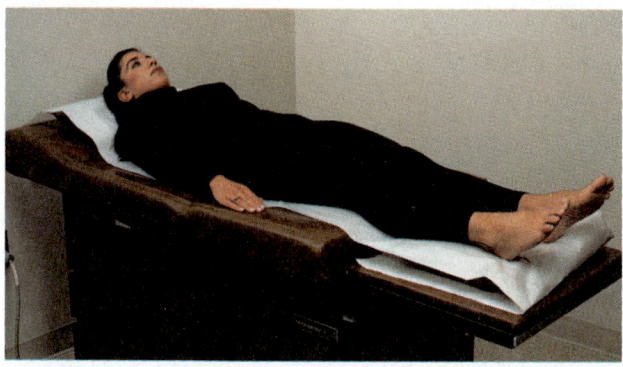

FIGURE 28-3 Supine or horizontal recumbent position.

Knee-Chest Position

The knee-chest position may be used to examine the rectal or vaginal areas and to relieve pain following childbirth. This is a difficult position to maintain, so never leave the patient alone. Position the patient in a prone position until the examiner is ready.

- Draping may be done with one or two sheets.
- Place a small pillow under the patient's head.
- Assist the patient to turn and lie on the abdomen with head turned to one side.
- Have the patient flex the arms and bring them up on either side of the head.
- Assist the patient to flex the knees and draw them up as far as possible toward the chest (Figure 28-4).

Prone Position

This position is used to examine the patient's back.

- Assist the patient to lie on the abdomen with head turned to one side.
- Place a small pillow under the patient's head.
- Arms may be extended at the patient's side or flexed and brought up on either side of the head (Figure 28-5).
- One sheet is used for draping.

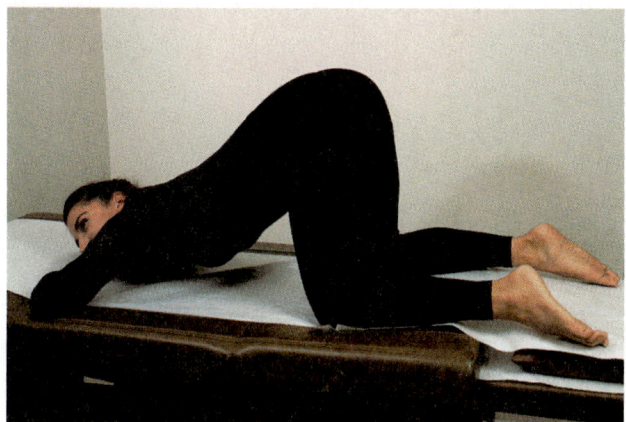

FIGURE 28-4 Knee-chest position.

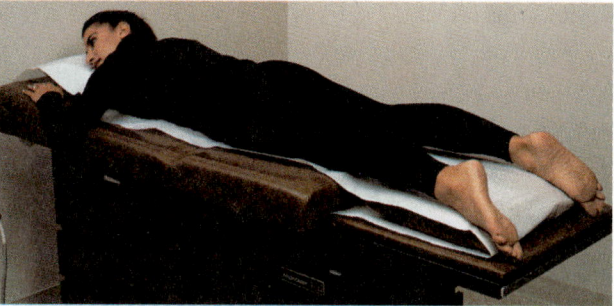

FIGURE 28-5 Prone position.

Sims' Position

This position is used for vaginal and rectal procedures, including enema administration.

- Assist the patient to turn on the left side, with the head turned to the same side and resting on a small pillow.
- Position the left arm extended behind the body.
- Flex the right arm and position it in front of the patient.
- The left leg is slightly bent, while the right leg is sharply flexed (Figure 28-6).
- One drape is usually adequate.

Semi-Fowler's Position

This is a common position for head and neck examinations of the in-bed patient.

- Assist patient to a semi-sitting position with backrest elevated at a 45-degree angle to the bed.
- The knees are supported in a slightly flexed position (Figure 28-7).

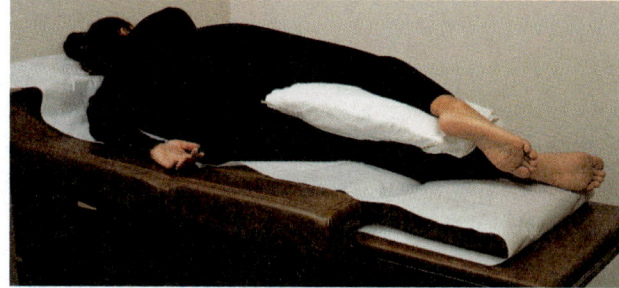

FIGURE 28-6 Sims' position.

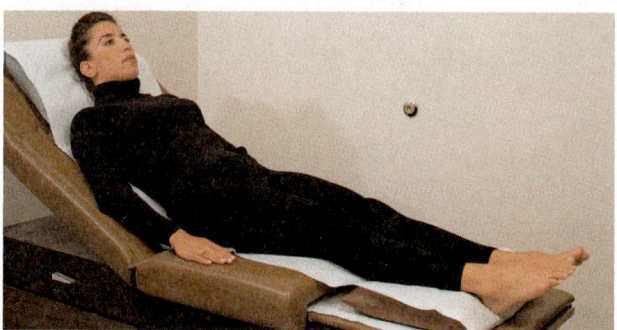

FIGURE 28-7 Semi-Fowler's position.

- The arms rest at the sides.
- One drape is usually enough.

Trendelenburg Position

The Trendelenburg position encourages circulation to the patient's heart and brain. It is used when the patient is in shock.

- Assist the patient to lie flat on the back with the head lower than the rest of the body.
- If possible, the lower half of the bed or table is tilted so the legs are slightly flexed (Figure 28-8). In an emergency, the entire bed frame may be supported on blocks, tilting the bed to a 45-degree angle. Some hospital beds, stretchers, and examination tables have a switch that enables the user to position the device in the Trendelenburg position quickly in emergencies.
- Beds that are electrically powered may be adjusted to this position.
- Shoulder braces may be needed to prevent the patient from slipping.
- One drape is usually sufficient.

Dorsal Lithotomy Position

The dorsal lithotomy position is frequently used for the pelvic examination of female patients. This is a difficult examination for most women, so make sure your draping makes the patient feel covered.

- Make sure the patient voids her bladder before the examination.
- The patient is positioned on her back.
- The knees are well separated and flexed.
- Usually this position is achieved by placing the feet in stirrups (Figure 28-9).
- One or two drapes may be used to cover the patient. The draping may be similar to draping for the knee-chest position.
- This position can be difficult and uncomfortable for the patient to maintain. Do not place the patient's legs in the stirrups until the physician is in the room and ready to begin the examination.

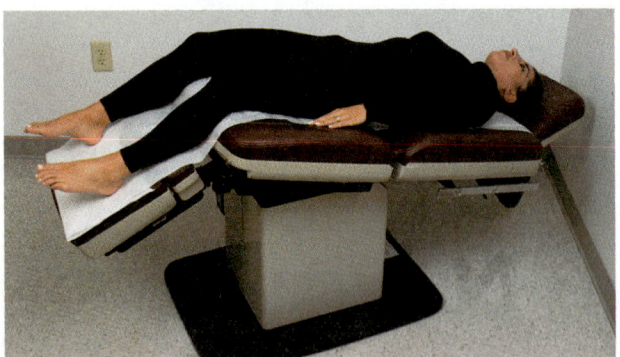

FIGURE 28-8 Trendelenburg position.

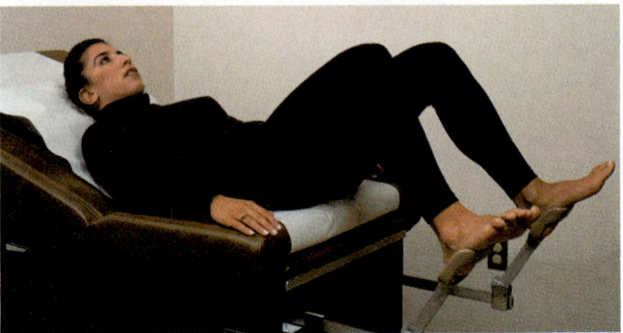

FIGURE 28-9 The patient's feet are placed in stirrups for the dorsal lithotomy position, with the knees flexed and separated.

PHYSICAL EXAMINATION

Some health care facilities have examining instruments and equipment collected on trays. At other facilities, you will gather the necessary equipment and assemble it (Figure 28-10).

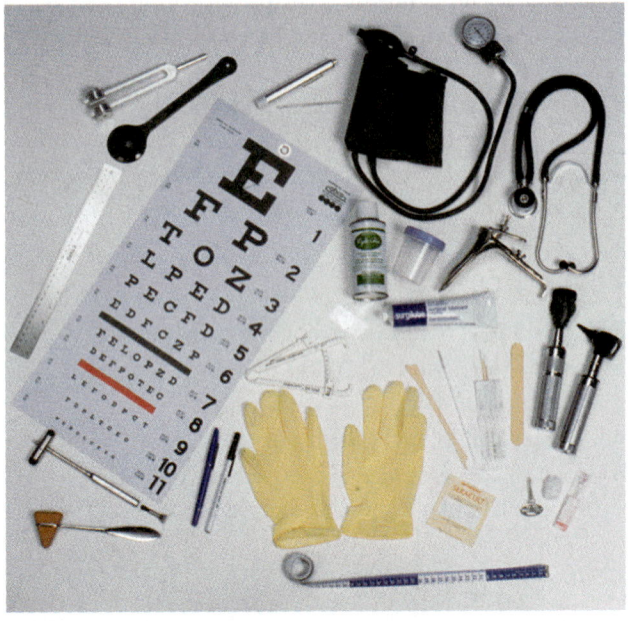

FIGURE 28-10 Equipment and supplies for the physical examination.

OSHA *Alert*

Apply the principles of standard precautions when assisting with a physical examination. Anticipate the equipment that will be needed and make sure it is available to you and to the physician or nurse who is doing the examination.

PROCEDURE 86

ASSISTING WITH A PHYSICAL EXAMINATION

1. Carry out beginning procedure actions.

2. Assemble equipment:
   - gloves
   - flashlight or penlight
   - **percussion hammer** (tests nerve reflex)
   - tongue depressors
   - thermometer
   - cotton balls
   - emesis basin (lined with paper towel)
   - specimen cup
   - vaginal speculum
   - cervical brush
   - cotton-tip applicator
   - cervical spatula
   - slide and fixative
   - lubricant
   - tape measure
   - nasal speculum
   - sterile needle
   - **otoscope** (used to examine ears)
   - **ophthalmoscope** (used to examine eyes)
   - blood pressure cuff (sphygmomanometer)
   - stethoscope
   - visual acuity chart
   - tuning fork
   - pen and paper
   - marking pen
   - guaiac material
   - goniometer
   - scale

   Note: *A* **speculum** *is an instrument used to spread a body opening. If only a female pelvic examination is to be performed, the following equipment will be needed (Figure 28-11).*

   - gloves
   - linens for draping
   - microscope slides and cover slips
   - fixative spray
   - reagents

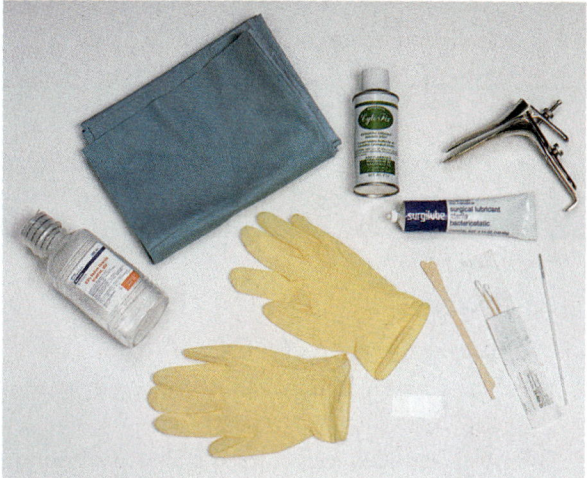

FIGURE 28-11 Equipment and supplies for the pelvic examination.

   - cotton-tipped applicators
   - vaginal speculum
   - spatulas
   - cytobrushes
   - lubricant

3. Ask the patient to void, if ambulatory. If the patient is in bed, follow the procedure for giving the bedpan or urinal.

4. Help the patient onto the examination table.

   Note: *If the examination is done with the patient in bed, cover the patient with a bath blanket and fanfold the top bedding to the foot of the bed.*

5. Cover the patient with a drape.

6. Assist as the examination is performed.
   a. Provide privacy.
   b. Position the patient and equipment as necessary.
   c. Hand equipment as required to the examiner.
   d. Adjust lighting as necessary.

7. After the examination is complete, help the patient to:
   a. Sit up slowly.
   b. Get off the table and stand.
   c. Dress.
   d. Return to the unit or office.

continues

PROCEDURE 86

continued

8. Wash your hands and return to the examination room.

9. Put on gloves.

10. Clean equipment according to facility policy.

11. Care for specimens according to facility policy.

12. Remove gloves and dispose of properly.

13. Wash your hands.

REVIEW

A. True/False.

Mark the following true or false by circling T or F.

1. T F The physical examination helps the physician establish a nursing assessment.

2. T F A patient who feels covered is able to cooperate more fully.

3. T F Positions used for the physical examination can only be used for that purpose.

4. T F The nursing assistant performs the actual physical exam.

5. T F When a patient is placed in the Trendelenburg position, the feet must be at the same level as the knees.

6. T F When positioning a patient for a physical examination, you must maintain proper body mechanics.

7. T F Once you have the patient positioned for a physical examination, you should leave the room.

8. T F The nursing assistant assists in the physical assessment by draping and positioning the patient.

9. T F Lighting may have to be adjusted during the examination.

10. T F The semi-Fowler's position encourages blood flow to the head and heart.

B. Multiple Choice.

Select the one best answer for each of the following.

11. The basic examination position is
    a. Sims'.
    b. dorsal recumbent.
    c. dorsal lithotomy.
    d. Trendelenburg.

12. The patient is to have a pelvic examination. In what position should she be positioned?
    a. Sims'

    b. Lithotomy
    c. Trendelenburg
    d. Semi-Fowler's

13. Your female patient is to have a pelvic examination. Which instrument would you be sure to have ready?
    a. Otoscope
    b. Vaginal speculum
    c. Nasal speculum
    d. Ophthalmoscope

14. The patient has vaginal bleeding and the physician orders you to place her in a position that will increase blood flow to the head. Which position would you prepare for?
    a. Sims'
    b. Semi-Fowler's
    c. Trendelenburg
    d. Lithotomy

15. Stirrups are used in which position?
    a. Dorsal lithotomy
    b. Semi-Fowler's
    c. Sims'
    d. Trendelenburg

C. Matching.

Choose the correct word from Column II to match the word or phrases in Column I.

Column I	Column II
16. _____ instrument to examine the ear	a. apprehensive
17. _____ instrument to examine the eye	b. drape
18. _____ instrument to spread (dilate) a body opening	c. ophthalmoscope
19. _____ fearful	d. otoscope
20. _____ covering	e. speculum
	f. percussion hammer

D. Nursing Assistant Challenge.

Robert Ubek is to have a physical examination in the doctor's office. He is 88 years of age and appears very nervous. He tells you that he is afraid he has prostate cancer. You are to assist the doctor. Complete the following statements using words from the following list.

anticipate	off
dorsal recumbent	on
drape	reassure

21. One of your responsibilities will be to _____ the patient.

22. Because of Mr. Ubek's age, you will be especially careful in assisting him to get _____ and _____ the table.

23. You can help him feel more comfortable if you _____ him properly.

24. You can help the examination go more smoothly if you _____ the examiner's needs.

25. You will position Mr. Ubek in the _____ position to begin the examination.

EXPLORING THE WEB

Description	Location
The Complete Physical Exam	*http://www.mtmonthly.com*
Physical Exam Encyclopedia	*http://www.nlm.nih.gov/medlineplus/ency/article/002274.htm*
Physical Exam Terms and Phrases	*http://mtdesk.com*
Physical Examination by ADAM	*http://health.yahoo.com*
Screening Physical Examination	*http://www.meddean.luc.edu*
What to Expect from a Physical Exam	*http://webmd.lycos.com*

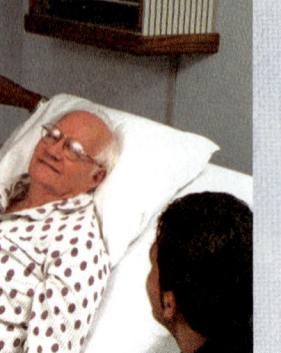

unit**29**

The Surgical Patient

objectives

After completing this unit, you will be able to:

- Spell and define terms.
- Describe the concerns of patients who are about to have surgery.
- List the various types of anesthesia.
- Shave the area to be operated on.
- Prepare the patient's unit for the patient's return from the operating room.
- Give routine postoperative care when the patient returns to the room.
- Assist the patient with deep breathing and coughing.
- Apply elasticized stockings or bandages and pneumatic hosiery.

- Demonstrate the following procedures:
  - Procedure 87 Shaving the Operative Area
  - Procedure 88 Assisting the Patient to Deep Breathe and Cough
  - Procedure 89 Performing Postoperative Leg Exercises
  - Procedure 90 Applying Elasticized Stockings
  - Procedure 91 Applying Elastic Bandage
  - Procedure 92 Applying Pneumatic Compression Hosiery
  - Procedure 93 Assisting the Patient to Dangle

vocabulary

Learn the meaning and the correct spelling of the following words and phrases:

ambulation	disruption	NPO	sequential
anesthesia	distention	operative	compression
anti-embolism hose	drainage	orifice	therapy
aspirate	dressings	perioperative	singultus
atelectasis	embolus	postanesthesia care	spinal anesthesia
bandages	general anesthetic	unit (PACU)	stable
binders	hypoallergenic tape	postoperative	surgical bed
dangling	hypoxia	preoperative	TED hose
deep vein	local anesthetic	prosthesis	thrombophlebitis
thrombosis (DVT)	Montgomery straps	pulmonary embolism	umbilicus
depilatory	nosocomial	recovery room	vertigo

INTRODUCTION

Patients facing any surgical procedure tend to be fearful. Remember that these patients require great emotional as well as physical support (Figure 29-1). Such support should be given from the time the patient is admitted through the discharge.

Patients are concerned with:

- Disfigurement
- Pain
- Loss of control as they undergo anesthesia
- What serious conditions might be found
- Length and cost of recovery
- Possibility of death

Surgery is often associated with anxiety, pain, and discomfort. For this reason, medications are given before, during, and after surgery.

PAIN PERCEPTION

When a person feels pain sensations, the:

- pain receptors record the sensation.
- sensation is sent by the spinal nerves to the spinal cord and then to the brain.
- sensation is received and interpreted in the brain.

Before surgery, the patient is given medication to promote relaxation. During surgery, anesthetics are given to prevent pain (Figure 29-2). After surgery, medications are given to reduce discomfort.

ANESTHESIA

Anesthesia is given to prevent pain, to relax muscles, and to induce forgetfulness. The anesthetic agent (drug) and method of administration used are determined by the loca-

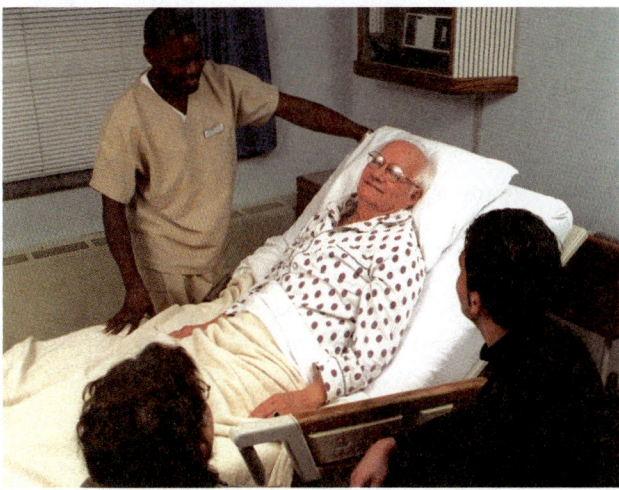

FIGURE 29-1 Patients and family members need support during the preoperative period.

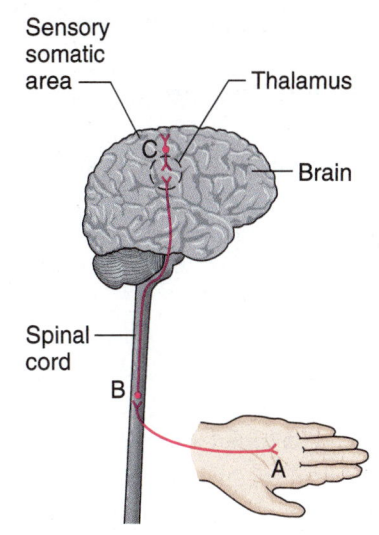

A **Pain messages are picked up by free nerve endings in the skin. Local anesthetic blocks this.**

B **Message is carried into the spinal cord. Spinal anesthetic blocks this.**

C **Message is then carried to the cortex of the brain. General anesthetic blocks this.**

FIGURE 29-2 Anesthetics will block pain impulses at points A, B, or C.

tion and type of surgery to be performed, the length of time needed for surgery, and the patient's physical condition. There are two main types of anesthetics:

1. General anesthetics—These induce the patient to become unconscious.
2. Local anesthetics—These induce loss of feeling in a specific area.

General Anesthetics

General anesthetics block reception of pain in the brain. They are usually given in one of two ways:

1. Inhalation—Some gases that are used as anesthetics include nitrous oxide and cyclopropane.
   - Inhaled anesthetics are apt to make the patient secrete more mucus and to experience nausea.
   - Special attention must be given after surgery to keep the respiratory tract clear.
   - There is a real danger that the patient may aspirate (inhale) vomitus into the respiratory tract.
2. Intravenous—Drugs are introduced directly into the veins.
   - These drugs, such as sodium pentathol, act rapidly.
   - The patient quickly loses consciousness.
   - IV anesthetics are often used with other types of anesthesia for short operations.

Local Anesthetics

Local anesthetics act by:

1. Blocking pain receptors in the operative area.
   - Drugs such as procaine hydrochloride may be injected into the patient around the operative area.

– These drugs stop the sensation of pain only in that area.

– The patient remains awake but free from pain during the operation.

2. Blocking transmission of the pain sensation at the level of the spinal cord.

– A drug injected into the spinal canal prevents feeling in any point below the level of the injection.

– The patient remains awake.

– This type of anesthesia is commonly used for abdominal surgery because it produces good relaxation of the muscles.

– This technique is called spinal anesthesia.

After getting this type of anesthetic, the patient is unable to feel or move the legs for a period of time. If not prepared ahead of time, the patient may be frightened by this experience.

SURGICAL CARE

The care of the surgical patient (perioperative) can be divided into three parts:

- Preoperative (before surgery)
- Operative (in the operating room)
- Postoperative (after surgery)

PREOPERATIVE CARE

Preoperative care begins when surgery is planned by the physician with the patient. Your responsibilities begin when the patient is admitted to the hospital. Remember that you may answer general questions that the patient asks, but you must refer specific questions about the surgery, its possible outcome, and anesthesia to your team leader.

Although it is the responsibility of the physician and nurse to answer questions and give explanations, it is helpful if you are aware of the information that has been given. Refer any questions the patient has to the nurse.

Teaching

Time spent with the patient in the preoperative period is very helpful. Patients who are prepared are able to cooperate more successfully in their recovery. Ideally, this time is spent shortly after the patient's admission. Sometimes much of the information is given in the doctor's office or clinic.

During the preoperative period, the nurse will determine the patient's specific needs. The nurse also does preoperative teaching. The other staff members support this effort.

- Tests, medications, and preoperative procedures are explained.
- Questions regarding the postoperative period are answered.

- The patient is taught and given an opportunity to practice postoperative exercises, such as leg exercises and respiratory exercises.
- The patient and staff discuss the events of the preoperative period, and what the patient may experience while being taken to the operating room and being given anesthesia.
- The recovery period is outlined and the purpose of special procedures or equipment, such as tubes or intravenous fluid lines, that may be used after surgery is explained.
- Play therapy may be used to explain to children.
- Every effort is made to teach ways of decreasing discomfort and to assure the patient that means for pain relief will be available.
- Planning for the discharge period begins now.

Psychological Preparation

The nursing staff spends as much time as possible helping patients deal with their emotional stress.

All members of the health team need to be sensitive and responsive to the psychological needs of the patient. Because you will be in frequent contact with the patient, you may be the first person to recognize signs of fear or concern. Listen to what the patient says and observe the patient's body language carefully. Report your observations to the nurse so that appropriate nursing intervention may be carried out.

Build patient confidence by:

- Performing your work in an efficient, calm manner.
- Being available to listen.
- Explaining what you plan to do before carrying out any procedure.
- Encouraging the patient to participate in his own care as much as possible. This helps the patient feel he still has a measure of control over his life.
- Immediately transmitting requests for clergy visits.

Physical Preparation

The Evening Before Surgery. If the patient is in the hospital the evening before surgery, part of the surgical preparation may be done then. It usually includes:

- Bath or shower with surgical soap
- Enema
- Surgical prep (shaving of the operative site)
- Special tests
- Medication to ensure a good night's rest, when indicated
- Insertion of special tubes for draining body cavities
- Being placed on NPO (nothing by mouth) orders after midnight
- Removal of the water pitcher from the bedside table and having the NPO notice posted over the bed,

bedside stand, on the door, on the patient's chart, and on the Kardex.

Nosocomial infections are those acquired during the hospital stay. It is known that such infections:

- are more likely to occur the longer the patient is in the hospital.
- add days to the hospital stay.
- increase the cost of hospitalization.
- can be life-threatening.

To decrease costs and the potential for nosocomial infections, patients are often admitted on the morning of surgery and are sometimes discharged on the day of surgery or the day after. In this circumstance, much of the preoperative care must be done at home or immediately upon admission. This is called outpatient or "short-term" surgery.

The Surgical Prep Area. Skin preparation before surgery may or may not include hair removal. There is a trend away from removing the hair unless its thickness will interfere with the surgery. In fact, some studies have shown more infections among shaved patients compared with unshaved patients.

If shaving is ordered, it must be done according to the procedure provided. (See Procedure 87.) It must be performed skillfully in a well-lighted area. Also, the area to be washed and shaved will be larger than the surgical incision area (Figure 29-3A and Figure 29-3B). In some cases, a depilatory (hair-removing) cream will be ordered for use the night before surgery. If a depilatory is to be used, check the skin for sensitivity. Apply a small amount to the skin of the forearm and wait 10 minutes. If redness occurs, do not continue, but report to the nurse.

Skin preparation may be performed by:

- Special surgical prep team
- Operating room (OR) staff in the OR
- Nursing staff in the patient's unit just prior to surgery

SAFETY *Alert*

All personnel involved in perioperative care of the patient must be alert to make sure that the correct surgical procedure is done on the correct patient, and that the surgery is done on the correct site. This often involves marking the site of the surgery. Various forms and checklists are used to verify the patient and surgical site. Take your responsibilities for identifying the patient and operative site seriously. There is no room for error in this area of nursing practice.

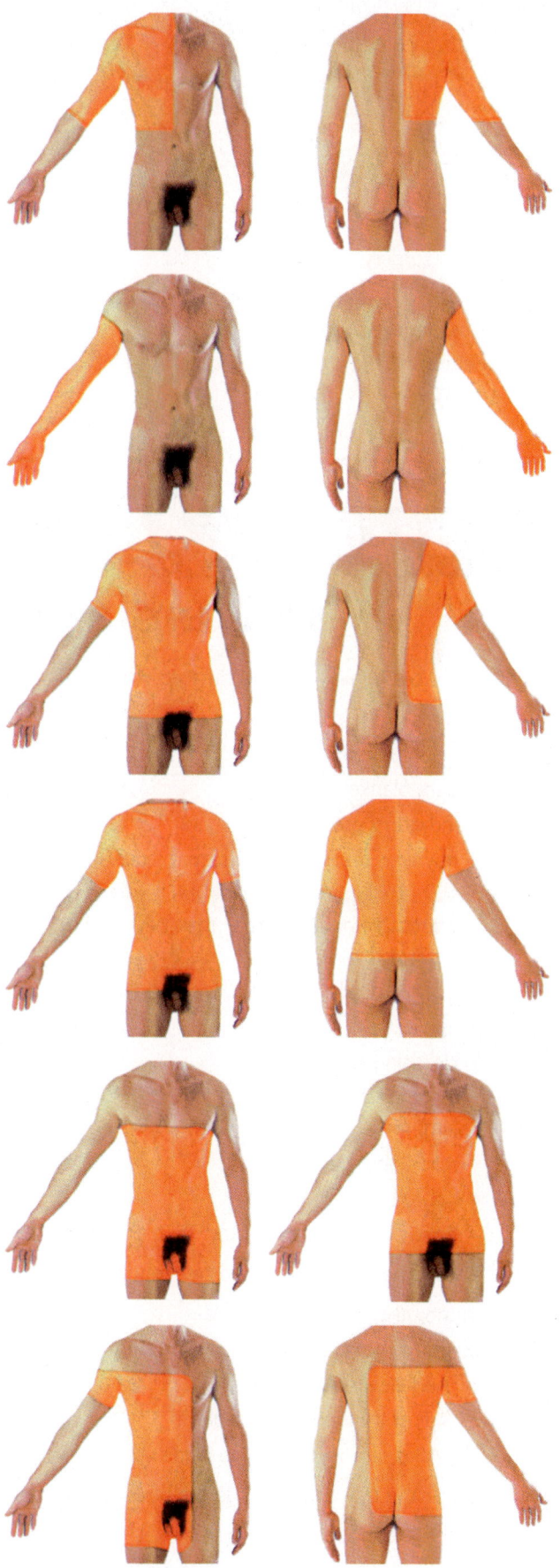

FIGURE 29-3A Surgical preparation sites for the upper extremities and torso.

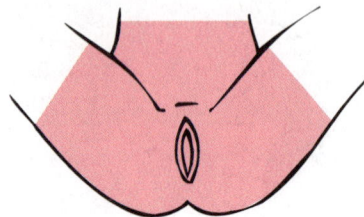

FIGURE 29-3B Surgical preparation sites for vaginal, rectal, and perineal surgery.

To prepare the surgical area by shaving:
- Make sure you know exactly what area is to be shaved. Most hospitals have routine prep areas.

- Do not shave the neck or face of a female patient. If in doubt, check with the nurse.
- Never shave the eyebrows.
- Be aware that the preparations for cranial surgery are usually performed after the patient has been medicated and taken to the operating suite. Doctors have special preferences in this regard.
- Remember that if a spinal anesthesia is to be given, the back may also be shaved.

Calm the patient's fears by explaining that the area prepared is much larger than the actual incision area. This is to prevent contamination of the surgical site, which may lead to possible complications after surgery.

PROCEDURE 87

SHAVING THE OPERATIVE AREA

1. Carry out beginning procedure actions.

2. Assemble equipment:
   - disposable gloves
   - bath blanket
   - individual prep pack, *or*
   - tray with razor and new razor blades, *or*
   - electric clipper—make sure the heads are disposable or, if reusable, that they have been sterilized
   - 2 small bowls
   - applicators
   - cleansing soap
   - lighting—for example, a spotlight or gooseneck lamp
   - 4 × 4 sponges
   - paper towels
   - towels or disposable Chux® (bed protector)

3. Determine the exact area to be prepped.

4. In the utility room:
   a. Fill the small bowls with warm water.
   b. Add cleansing soap to one.
   c. Adjust the razor and blade.
   d. Make sure the razor and blade are tight.

5. Cover the tray and take it to the bedside.

6. Drape the patient with a bath blanket. Place a towel or bed protector under the area to be shaved.

7. Put on disposable gloves.

8. If a safety razor and blade are used, soften hairs with soapy solution and wait 1 minute. This makes hair removal easier and helps avoid skin injury.

9. Holding the skin taut with one hand, lather the area to be shaved. If hair is very long, such as on the pubis and axilla, it may be clipped with scissors before shaving. Take care when clipping—do not nick the skin. If an electric clipper is used, attach the heads and check for security.

10. Shave the area with strokes in the same direction as the hair grows. Be careful not to cut the skin or to remove any warts or moles. Work carefully around such areas.

11. Using the applicators, clean the **umbilicus** (navel) and shave it if it is in the operative area.

SAFETY *Alert*

Hold the razor at a 45-degree angle. Maintain contact with the skin. Try to avoid lifting the razor and then putting it down again. Doing this increases the risk of nicks and cuts.

continues

PROCEDURE 87

continued

12. Check carefully for hairs after shaving is complete.
- Unattached hairs are easily removed by gently pressing a piece of tape against the area.
- Discard hair in a paper towel.

13. Cleanse the skin with warm, soapy water. Rinse and dry thoroughly.

14. Dispose of equipment according to facility policy.

15. Remove the towel from under the patient.
- Make sure the side rails are up.
- Make sure linen is dry.
- Change, if necessary.

16. Remove and dispose of gloves according to facility policy.

17. Carry out procedure completion actions.

Immediate Preoperative Care. Approximately one hour before surgery, the patient will be given additional medication by the nurse. Your responsibilities regarding the patient must be completed before this time. You may be asked to do the following:

- Take and record vital signs (Figure 29-4) (see Section 6).
- Take care of valuables according to hospital policy. Remove dentures and any other **prosthesis** (artificial part), such as a hearing aid or glasses. See that they are safely marked with the patient's name and stored appropriately.
- Remove nail polish, makeup, hairpins, and jewelry. Long hair should be neatly braided or capped. Plain wedding bands may be taped in place.
- Dress the patient in a gown and cover the hair with a surgical cap.
- See that the patient voids and measure the urine. Drain the catheter, if present, and record.
- Make sure that the room is quiet and comfortable.

As soon as the nurse gives the preoperative medication:

- Be sure the side rails are in place for safety.

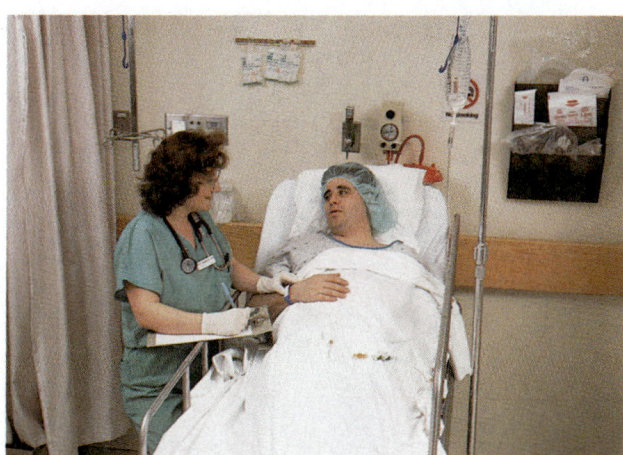

FIGURE 29-4 Taking vital signs is an important part of preoperative care.

- Remove all unnecessary equipment.
- Push the bedside table, overbed table, and chair out of the way to make room for the stretcher when it arrives from surgery.
- Complete the surgical checklist:
  1. Admission sheet
  2. Surgical consent
  3. Sterilization consent (if necessary)
  4. Consultation sheet (if necessary)
  5. History and physical
  6. Lab reports (pregnancy test also if necessary)
  7. Surgery prep done and charted, if required
  8. Latest TPR and blood pressure charted
  9. Preoperative medication given and charted (if required)
  10. Identification band on patient
  11. Fingernail polish and makeup removed
  12. Metallic objects removed (wedding ring may be taped)
  13. Dentures removed
  14. Other prostheses removed (such as artificial limb or eye, wigs and hairpieces)
  15. Glasses or contact lenses removed
  16. Bath blanket and head cap in place
  17. Bed in high position and side rails up after preop medication is given
  18. Patient has voided
  - Check off those duties to which you were assigned.
  - Note the time your patient leaves for surgery.
- Follow facility policy regarding visitors. Sometimes they are allowed to wait quietly with the patient. Sometimes they should be directed to the visitors' waiting room.
- Elevate the bed to stretcher height when the transporter arrives to take the patient to surgery.

The nurse and surgical attendant will check the patient's identification and surgical checklist before the patient is moved.

A staff member, and sometimes a family member, accompanies the patient to the doors of the operating room. You will probably be asked to assist in transferring the patient from the bed to the stretcher and, after surgery, from the stretcher to the bed. Review Procedures 24 and 25 in Unit 16.

DURING THE OPERATIVE PERIOD

While the patient is in the operating room, you will prepare the room for the patient's return.

- A special surgical bed will be prepared. This was described in Unit 23. The surgical bed is also called a postop bed or recovery bed.
- Everything should be removed from the top of the bedside stand except an emesis basin, tissue wipes, tongue depressors, and equipment to check vital signs.
- A pencil and small pad to record the signs should also be available.
- Check with your team leader for any special equipment, such as oxygen, IV poles, suction, or drainage bags, that might be necessary for your patient.
- Be watchful while carrying out your other assignments for the return of your patient from surgery.
- Follow facility policy regarding the location of visitors and family during surgery. They are sometimes permitted to wait in the patient's room. In most cases they are directed to a special waiting area.

POSTOPERATIVE CARE

During the immediate postoperative period, the patient recovers from anesthesia. For this period, the patient is placed in a special area called the recovery room (Figure 29-5). The recovery room is located next to the operating room and is sometimes called the postanesthesia care unit (PACU).

SAFETY *Alert*

Remember that most patients receive many drugs when they are in surgery. Many of these drugs can alter the patient's mental status. The drugs are excreted from the body slowly. The patient may sleep soundly upon return to the unit. Keep the side rails up and follow all safety precautions until the patient is fully awake and the nurse instructs you that side rails are no longer necessary. Do not leave liquids at the bedside until the nurse instructs you that it is safe to do so. Check on the patient regularly.

When the patient's condition is stabilized, the patient is returned to the unit. Upon the patient's return from the recovery room, you should:

- Identify the patient.
- Assist in the transfer from stretcher to bed (see Unit 16).
- Never leave the unconscious patient alone at any time.
- Check with the nurse for any special instructions.
- Realize that the patient may be drowsy for several hours after return.
- Have an extra blanket available—many patients complain of feeling cold upon return (Figure 29-6).

The following are routine instructions to be followed unless otherwise ordered.

- Always wear gloves and follow standard precautions when contact with blood, body fluids, mucous membranes, or nonintact skin is likely.

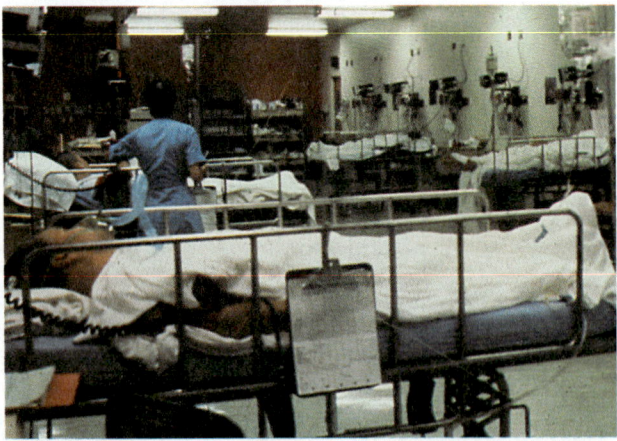

FIGURE 29-5 Postanesthesia Care Unit (PACU)—the unit where the patient wakes up from anesthesia after surgery. *(Courtesy of Memorial Medical Center of Long Beach, CA)*

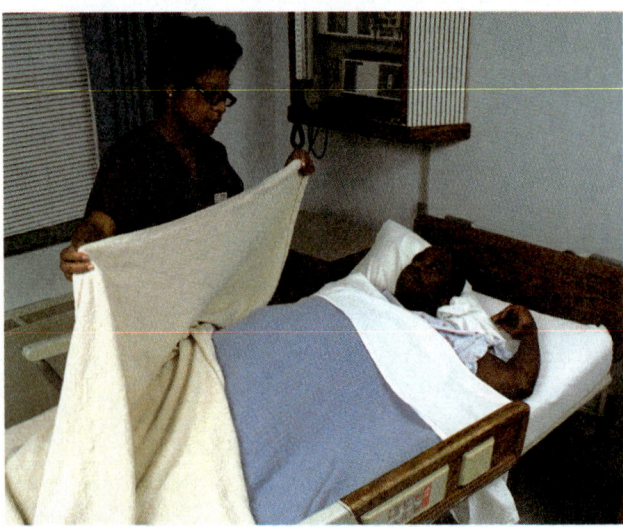

FIGURE 29-6 Patients may be cold after surgery. Cover them to prevent chilling.

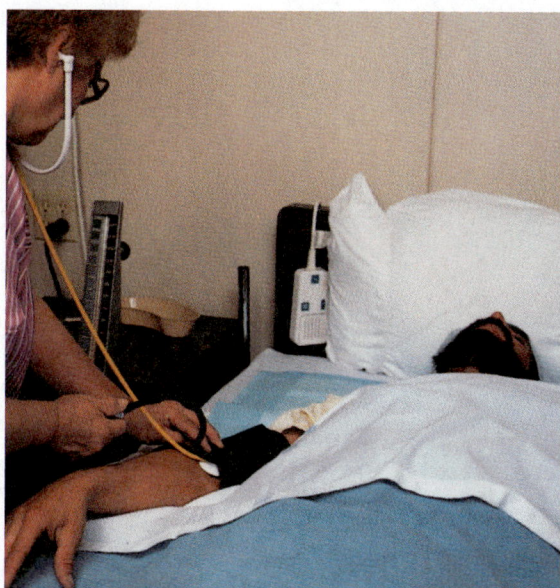

FIGURE 29-7 Check the vital signs regularly until they are stable.

- Take vital signs of the patient upon arrival on the unit (Figure 29-7) and every 15 minutes for four readings (see Section 6). The patient's temperature may not always be taken at this time.

When taking postoperative vital signs, count pulse and respiration for one full minute. Most facilities have policies for postoperative vital signs at specified frequencies that decrease if the vital signs are **stable** (approximately the same), such as:

- every 15 minutes for 1 hour
- if stable, every 30 minutes for 1 hour
- if stable, every hour for 2 hours
- if stable, every 4 hours for 24 hours

Always follow the protocol for vital signs used by your facility. The vital sign schedule may be altered by the RN if the patient's condition warrants. The physician may also order vital signs at a specifically designated frequency. Monitor the patient's level of consciousness (drowsy, unresponsive, alert) each time you check the vital signs.

Many facilities consider pain to be the fifth vital sign, so you should ask the patient if he or she is having pain each time you check the vital signs. Inform the nurse if pain is present.

SAFETY *Alert*

Anesthesia reduces body temperature. Keep the patient warm. If the patient's temperature is below 97°F, inform the nurse promptly.

- Check dressings for amount and type of any drainage. The nurse may reinforce them as necessary.
- Check IV solution for flow rate. Restrain the infusion site whenever ordered by the physician and report to the nurse. Remember that the flow rate is ordered by the physician.
- Encourage the patient to breathe deeply, cough, and move in bed. Position should be changed every 2 hours.
- Turn the patient's head to one side and support if he is vomiting. Have an emesis basin ready, as well as tissues and wet cloth. If the patient is conscious, allow the patient to rinse the mouth with water after vomiting. Note the type and amount of vomitus and record on the output worksheet.
- Check the pulses distal to the operative site. Inform the nurse if the pulse is weak or cannot be felt.
- If the patient was given a spinal anesthetic:
  - Give extra care in turning frequently and maintaining proper alignment.
  - Remember that the patient will be unable to move independently until sensation and motor functions return. Make sure to calm the patient's fear about this.
  - Some physicians require that the patient remain flat on the back and without a pillow for 8 to 12 hours following spinal anesthesia, to avoid headaches.
  - Any complaints of a headache following spinal anesthesia should be reported promptly.
  - Provide extra blankets if the patient is cold.
- Be sure all drainage tubes have been connected (the nurse will usually attend to this). If you notice a tube clamped shut, check with the nurse.
- Measure and record the first postoperative voiding. Inform the nurse.
- Report any patient complaints of discomfort or pain to the nurse (Figure 29-8).

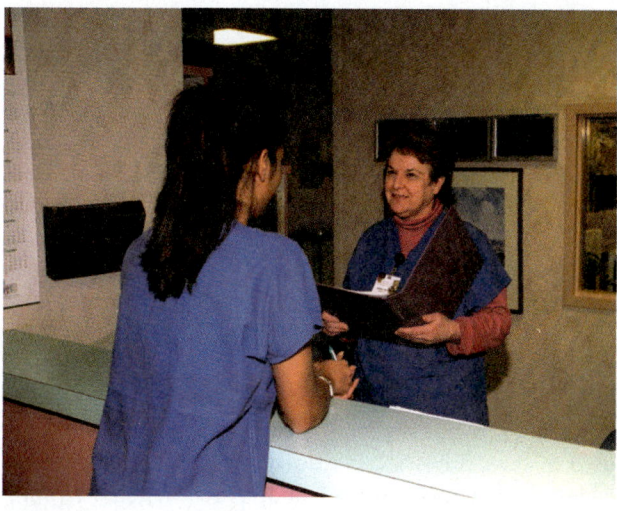

FIGURE 29-8 Report complaints of pain or discomfort to the nurse.

Tubes

Patients often return from surgery with a variety of tubes and drains in place.

- Some tubes may deliver materials into the patient. Examples are oxygen tubes or intravenous tubes.
- Other tubes may have been placed in the patient to provide drainage from wounds or body cavities. Examples are drains in the incision or urinary catheters.

The following are some special precautions to be taken:

- Always wear gloves if contact with drainage from the tube is likely.
- Learn the type, purpose, and location of each tube.
- Check drainage for character and amount.
- Check for obstructions to the tube system.
- Check flow rate of infusions from intravenous lines.
- Keep orifices (body openings) clear of secretions and discharge.
- Never disconnect tubes or raise drainage bottles above the level of the drainage site.
- Never lower infusion bottles below the level of the infusion site.
- Never put stress on the tubes when moving the patient or giving care.
- Restrain infusion sites as necessary to prevent dislocation.

 Note: A physician's order is needed.

- Monitor levels of infusions and report to the nurse before they run out.
- Report any signs of leakage or disconnected tubes immediately.
- Report pain, discoloration, or swelling at sites or drainage and infusion.

Dressings and Bandages

Caring for surgical wounds, injuries, and ulcers is very important. Dressings are gauze, film, or other synthetic substances that cover a wound, ulcer, or injury. Some dressings have an adhesive backing. Some are affixed with tape. Many different types of tape are available in the health care facility. Some patients need special hypoallergenic tape, which reduces the incidence of a skin reaction in patients who are allergic to the adhesive backing. Bandages are sometimes used to hold dressings in place. These are fabric, gauze, net, or elasticized materials used to cover the dressing and keep it securely in place. Bandages are available in different sizes and shapes. Gauze bandages are commonly used to cover dressings. Elastic bandages are used to reduce edema and support injured body parts. When wrapping bandages, avoid wrapping them so tightly that they restrict circulation.

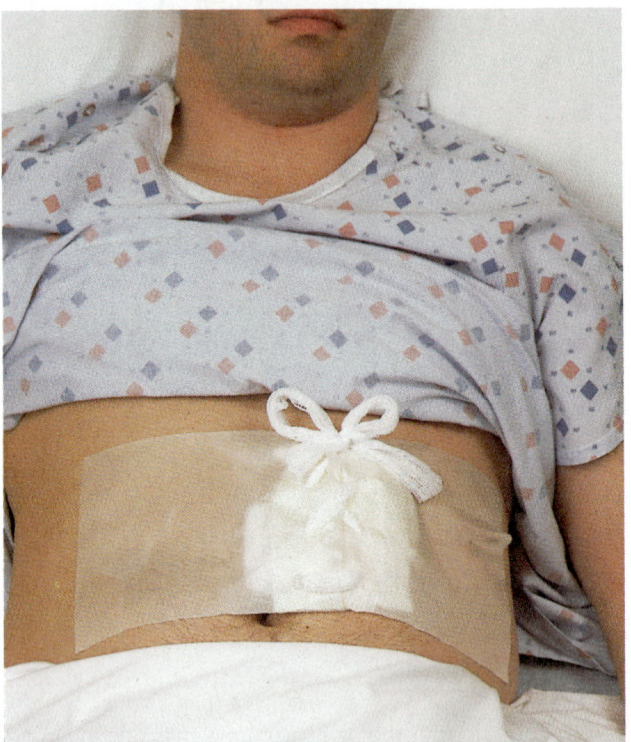

FIGURE 29-9 Montgomery straps hold dressings securely in place so they can be observed, changed, and reinforced without tape. This is much less traumatic for the patient.

Occasionally, Montgomery straps (Figure 29-9) are used to hold dressings in place. These are long strips of adhesive attached to the skin on either side of the wound. They are less traumatic to the skin because the adhesive is not removed with each dressing change unless the straps are soiled. After the dressing is in place, the straps are tied to hold the dressing securely. Binders (Figure 29-10) may also be used to hold dressings in place.

Drainage

When a body cavity is the operative site, it may be necessary to drain fluid such as blood, pus, serous drainage caused by tissue trauma, or gastric contents from it before or after surgery. Always wear gloves if contact with drainage is likely. The drainage outlet may be a:

- Catheter

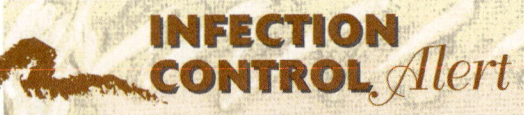

INFECTION CONTROL *Alert*

Body sites with tubes, drains, and surgical dressings are managed using sterile technique. Never open a tube or drain or remove a dressing. The nurse will use sterile technique to manage these areas.

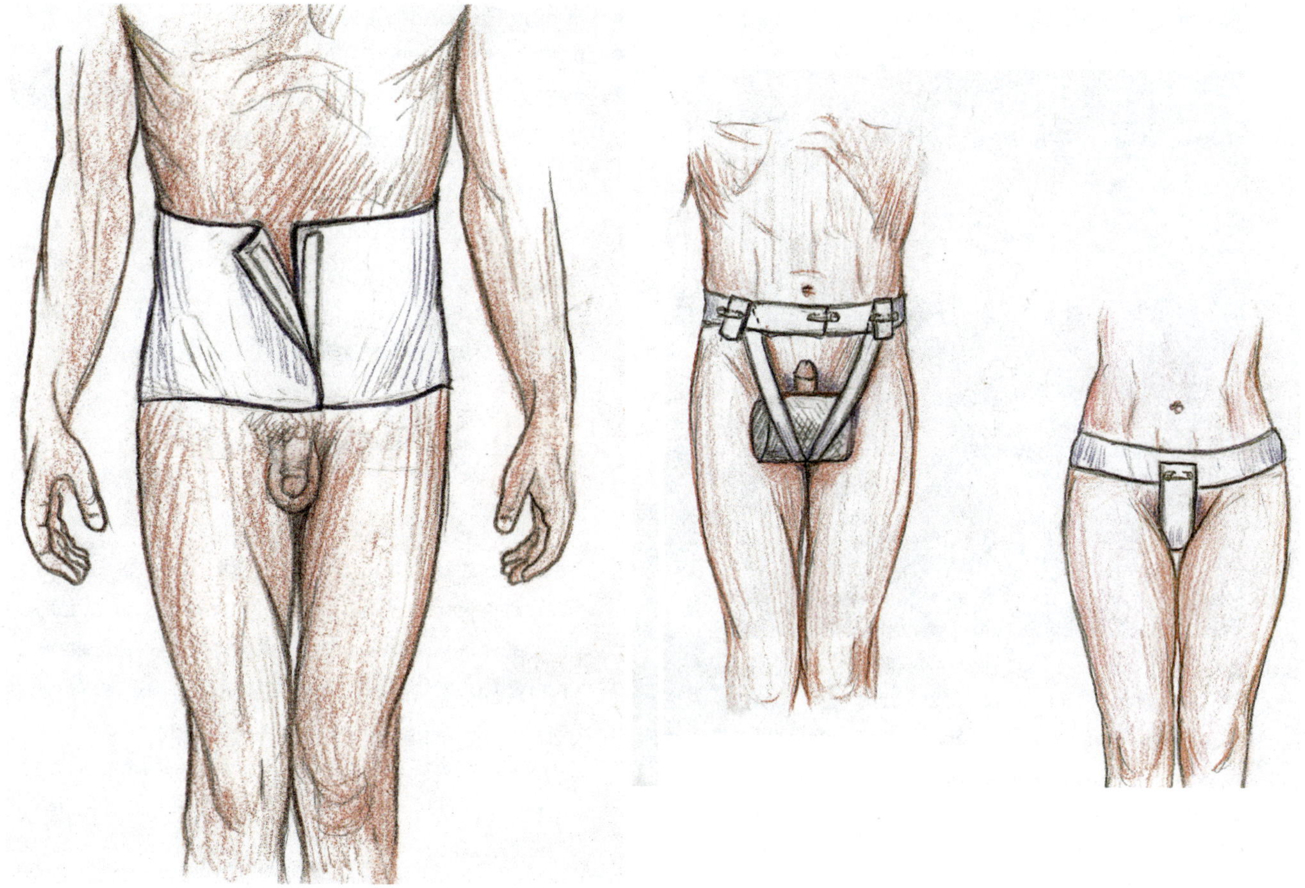

FIGURE 29-10 Various surgical binders support the body part and hold dressings in place.

- T-tube
- Jackson-Pratt (J–P)® or Hemovac® drain
- Penrose drain
- Cigarette drain

When such a drain is in place, the drainage accumulates on the dressing (Figure 29-11). You should:

- note the amount and character of the drainage.

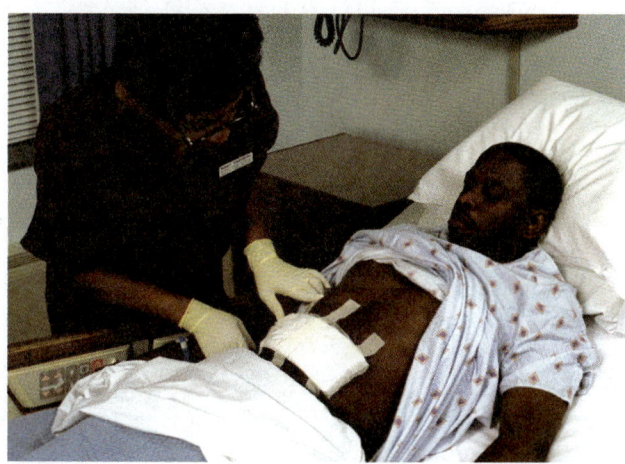

FIGURE 29-11 Check the dressings regularly for drainage or bleeding.

- inform the nurse when the dressing needs to be changed or reinforced.

At times, the withdrawal of fluids is controlled by attaching the drainage tube to a connecting tube and then a suction apparatus. The drainage accumulates in a container. The container is emptied and the contents measured at the end of each shift. The Jackson-Pratt or Hemovac drains are closed drainage systems. The drains are placed directly in the wound, and drainage goes directly into an expandable container. A record of the amount and character of the drainage is entered in both the output chart and the nurses' notes.

It is your responsibility to:

- Report either heavy or light drainage.
- Report a change in the character or amount of the drainage.
- Make sure that the flow of drainage is not blocked by kinking of the tube (Figure 29-12).

Never assume responsibility for chest drainage or attempt to empty chest bottles. Chest bottles and irrigations require the nurse's or physician's attention.

Careful preoperative preparation and postoperative care can help limit the extent of postoperative discomfort and complication.

The patient must be carefully observed, especially during the first 24 hours, for possible complications. Possible

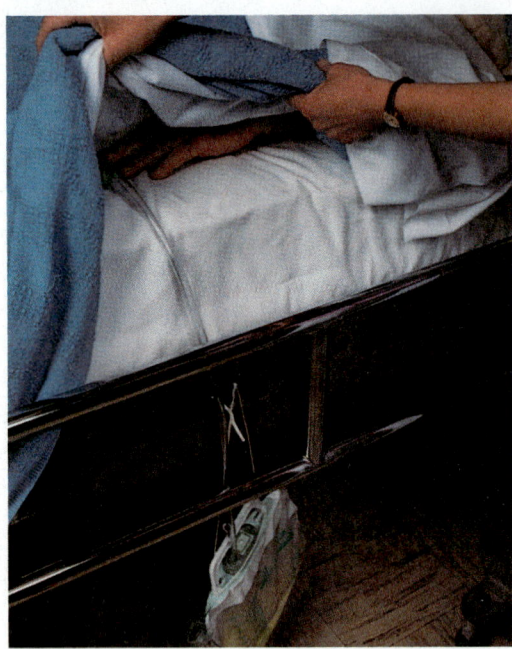

FIGURE 29-12 Monitor the drainage tubes to make sure they are not twisted, kinked, or obstructed.

postoperative discomfort and complications and appropriate nursing assistant actions are summarized in Table 29-1. When the patient has responded sufficiently and vital signs are stable, the patient may be refreshed by:

- washing the hands and face.
- changing the linen.
- being given a light backrub.

The patient is now ready to participate more actively in recovery. Exercises taught in the preoperative period are practiced, including:

- Deep breathing and coughing
- Leg exercises.

Deep Breathing and Coughing

SAFETY *Alert*

Although we routinely encourage postoperative patients to cough and deep breathe, there are a few exceptions you must be aware of. Avoid this procedure with patients who have had eye, nose, or neurologic surgery. Coughing and deep breathing will increase pressure, causing complications in these patients. Check with the nurse if you are unsure of what action to take.

TABLE 29-1 POSTOPERATIVE COMPLICATIONS AND NURSING ASSISTANT ACTIONS

Possible Discomfort	Report	What You Can Do*
Thirst	Patient complaints of dryness of lips, mouth, and skin	Carefully check I&O. Give ice chips or increase fluid intake by mouth with permission. Monitor IV if ordered. Give mouth care. Check BP and pulse. Watch for signs of shock and hemorrhage.
Singultus (hiccups)—intermittent spasms of the diaphragm	Incidence of hiccups	Allow the patient to rest; hiccups can be tiring. Support the incisional area. Assist the patient to breathe into a paper bag.
Pain	Location, intensity, type	Change position. Apply warmth if instructed. Monitor carefully for and report effects of medication given by nurse.
Distention (accumulation of gas in bowel)	Distention of abdomen, complaints of pain	Increase mobility. Insert a rectal tube if instructed and permitted.
Nausea, vomiting	Nausea, character of vomitus	Keep an emesis basin at the bedside. Monitor IV fluids, which are substituted for oral fluids. Give mouth care. Limit fluids by mouth. Encourage the patient to breathe deeply.

continues

TABLE 29-1 *continued*

Possible Discomfort	Report	What You Can Do*
Urinary retention	Amount and time of first voiding. Distention, restlessness, imbalance between I&O	Monitor I&O carefully. Check for distention.
Hemorrhage (excessive blood loss)	Fall in blood pressure; cold, moist skin; weak, rapid pulse; restlessness; pallor/cyanosis; condition of dressing; thirst	Report immediately to nurse. Keep the patient quiet. Check vital signs.
Shock	Fall in blood pressure; weak, rapid pulse; cold, moist skin; pallor	Report immediately to nurse. Keep the patient quiet. Monitor ordered oxygen. Be prepared to follow additional instructions.
Hypoxia (lack of oxygen)	Restlessness, dyspnea, crowing sounds to respirations, pounding pulse, perspiring	Report immediately to nurse. Monitor oxygen, if ordered.
Atelectasis (failure of lungs to expand)	Dyspnea; cyanosis/pallor	Report immediately to nurse.
Wound infection	Increased pain in incisional area; fever; chills, anorexia, increased drainage on dressing	Be observant. Report findings promptly to nurse. Check dressing.
Wound disruption (separation of wound edges)	Pinkish drainage. Complaints by the patient that he "feels open," "broken," "given away"	Report immediately to nurse. Keep the patient quiet. Support incisional area.
Pulmonary emboli	Anxiety, difficulty breathing; feelings of "heaviness in chest," cyanosis, chest pain	Keep the patient quiet. Report immediately to nurse. Elevate head of bed.

*In all cases, be prepared to follow the nurse's additional instructions.

Deep breathing and coughing clear the air passages. This helps to prevent postoperative respiratory complications such as pneumonia and atelectasis, which is the collapse of the alveolar air sacs. This may be an uncomfortable task when the patient has a new incision and feels fatigued. (See Procedure 88.) You can best assist the patient by:

- Explaining the value of the exercise and carrying out the following procedure.
- Checking with the nurse to see if medication for pain is to be administered before the exercise. If so, wait for 45 minutes after the medication has been given before carrying out the exercise.
- Learning from the nurse how many deep breaths and coughs should be attempted. The usual number is 5 to 10 breaths and 2 to 3 coughs.
- Using a pillow or binder to support the incision during the procedure.

OSHA *Alert*

Apply the principles of standard precautions when assisting with coughing and deep breathing procedures. If the patient is expelling loose secretions, select and wear appropriate protective equipment, including gloves, gown, mask, and face shield. Show the patient how to contain secretions in a tissue. Assist him or her with handwashing after the activity.

PROCEDURE 88

ASSISTING THE PATIENT TO DEEP BREATHE AND COUGH

1. Carry out beginning procedure actions.
2. Assemble equipment:
   - disposable gloves
   - a pillowcase-covered pillow or binder, if ordered
   - tissues
   - emesis basin
3. Elevate the head of the bed and assist the patient to assume a comfortable semi-Fowler's position.
4. Have the patient place his hands on either side of his rib cage or over the operative site (Figure 29-13). A pillow over the operative site can be used to support an incision during respiratory exercises.
5. Ask the patient to take as deep a breath as possible and hold it for 3 to 5 seconds; then exhale slowly through pursed lips.
6. Repeat this exercise about five times unless the patient seems too tired. If so, stop the procedure and report to nurse.
7. Place the pillow across the incision line as a brace. Have the patient hold the pillow on either side or have the patient interlace fingers across the incision to act as a brace.

8. Pass tissues to the patient and instruct the patient to take a deep breath and cough forcefully twice with the mouth open, collecting any secretions that are brought up in tissues (Figure 29-14).
9. Put on disposable gloves to handle the tissues.
10. Dispose of tissues in an emesis basin.
11. Assist the patient to assume a new, comfortable position.
12. Clean the emesis basin.
13. Remove and dispose of gloves according to facility policy.
14. Carry out procedure completion actions.
15. Report to nurse on the number of times the patient performed each exercise, how the patient tolerated the exercise, and the type and amount of any sputum coughed up.
    - Be sure the patient does not become overly fatigued.
    - Encourage the patient to cough and clear the respiratory passages.
    - Report to your team leader if the patient seems overly fatigued during the procedure.
    - Carefully observe and report any unusual responses such as pain, dizziness, or throat and airway irritation.

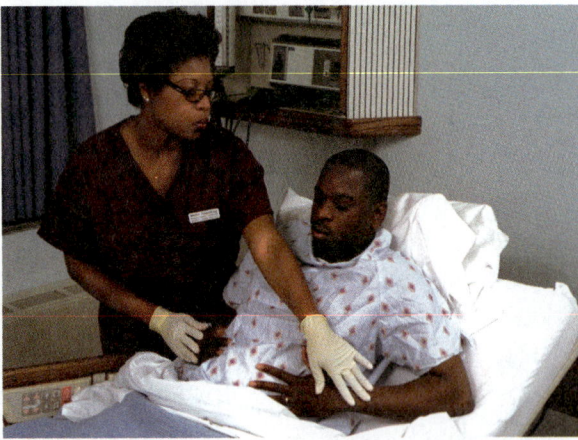

FIGURE 29-13 Encourage the patient to perform deep breathing exercises.

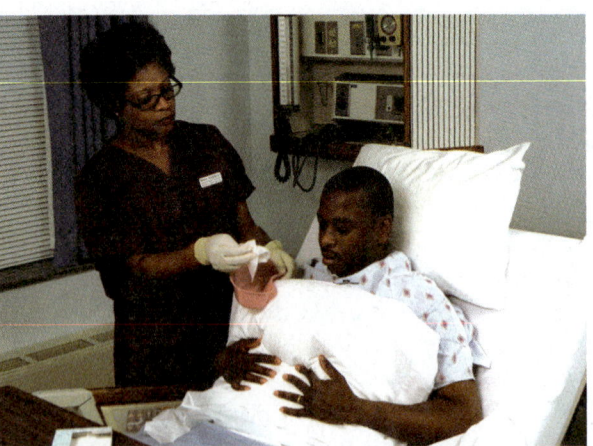

FIGURE 29-14 A pillow helps support the abdomen and splint the incision during coughing and deep breathing.

Leg Exercises

Leg exercises following surgery encourage steady circulation. This helps to prevent another serious complication of the postoperative period—the development of blood clots. (See Procedure 89.)

A blood clot or **deep vein thrombosis** (**DVT**) could develop in the venous system and block the essential blood flow. A small piece of thrombus broken off (**embolus**) could travel throughout the vascular system and block a vessel in the lungs.

A specific order must be written for leg exercises when there has been surgery on the legs themselves. Otherwise, leg exercises are routinely performed by the patient. If the patient is very weak, you may need to assist.

- Encourage leg exercises and be sure they have been performed.
- Each exercise should be performed 3 to 5 times at least every 1 or 2 hours, and at other times as well.
- Carry out leg exercises as you assist with position changes.
- Apply or reapply support hose (TED) after exercises if ordered.

PROCEDURE 89

PERFORMING POSTOPERATIVE LEG EXERCISES

1. Carry out beginning procedure actions.

2. Explain how the exercise is to be performed. Have the patient:
   a. Brace the incisional area with laced hands.
   b. Rotate each ankle by drawing imaginary circles with the toes.
   c. Dorsiflex (bring toes toward knee) and plantar flex (point toes and foot down) each ankle (Figure 29-15).
   d. Flex and extend each knee.
   e. Flex and extend each hip.
   f. Repeat each exercise 3 to 5 times. Assist as needed.

3. Lower the side rail.

4. Cover the patient with a bath blanket and draw the top bedding to the foot of the bed.

5. Supervise exercises or assist. Apply or reapply support hose (TED hose) as ordered after exercises.

6. Draw bedding up and remove the bath blanket.

7. Fold the bath blanket and place in the bedside stand for reuse.

8. Carry out procedure completion actions. Report to nurse on the number of exercises done and how they were tolerated by the patient.

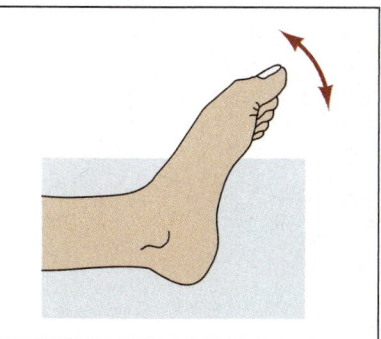

A. Curl the toes down and up. Repeat 5 times.

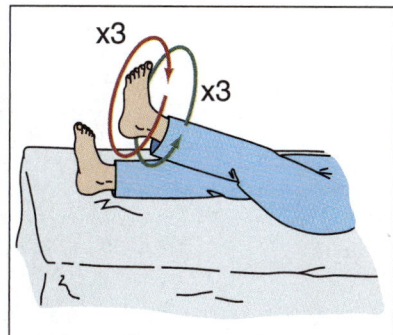

B. Make circles with the feet clockwise 3 times and counterclockwise 3 times. Repeat 5 times.

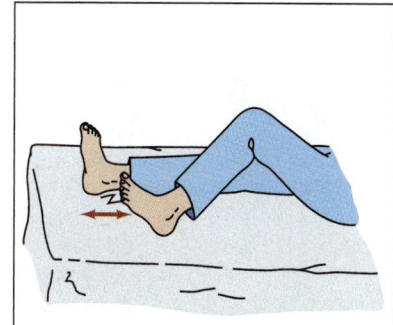

C. Slide one leg up and down in bed. Do the same with the other leg. Repeat 5 times.

FIGURE 29-15 Help the patient perform leg exercises to encourage circulation.

Elasticized Stockings

Elasticized stockings, called **TED hose** or **anti-embolism hose**, or Ace bandages that extend from the ankle or foot to calf or mid-thigh, are often applied during the preoperative and postoperative periods to support the veins of the legs. This reduces the incidence of **thrombophlebitis**, which is inflammation of the veins that can lead to blood clots. The stockings must be applied smoothly and evenly before the patient gets out of bed. They should be removed and reapplied at least every eight hours—more often if necessary or as ordered.

Several different types of anti-embolism hose are used.

Some have closed toes, but most have an opening near the toe end. The hole is positioned on the top or the bottom of the foot, just proximal to the toes. Check the heel placement on the stocking. By using the heel as a landmark, you will see where to position the hole in the stocking. (Refer to Procedure 90.)

Make sure the legs are dry before attempting to apply the hose. Elastic hosiery fit tightly. An apparatus is used in some facilities to make them easier to apply. If this is not available, the nurse may permit you to dust the legs lightly with baby powder, making the hose easier to apply. Avoid using powders if the patient has respiratory difficulty, a rash, or dressings on the legs.

PROCEDURE 90

APPLYING ELASTICIZED STOCKINGS

1. Carry out beginning procedure actions.

2. Assemble equipment:
   - elasticized stockings of proper length and size

3. Always apply stockings with the patient lying down. Expose one leg at a time.

4. Grasp the stocking with both hands at the top and roll it toward the toe end (Figure 29-16A).

5. Adjust over the patient's toes, positioning the opening at the base of the toes (unless the toes

are to be covered) (Figure 29-16B). Remember that the raised seams should be on the outside.

6. Apply the stocking to the leg by rolling it upward toward the body (Figure 29-16C).

7. Check to be sure the stocking is applied evenly and smoothly and that there are no wrinkles (Figure 29-16D).

8. Repeat the procedure on the opposite leg.

9. Carry out procedure completion actions.

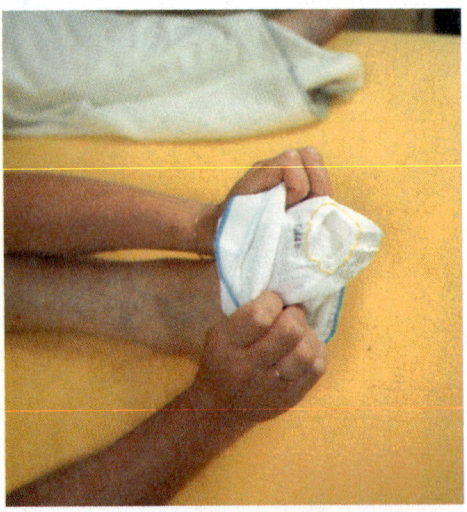

FIGURE 29-16A Gather the stocking and slip it over the patient's toes.

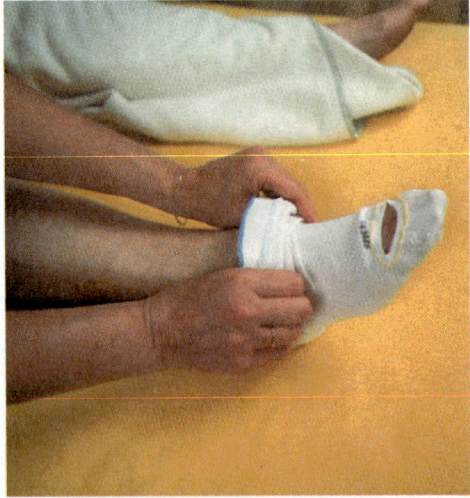

FIGURE 29-16B Position the opening on the top of the foot, at the base of the toes.

continues

PROCEDURE 90

continued

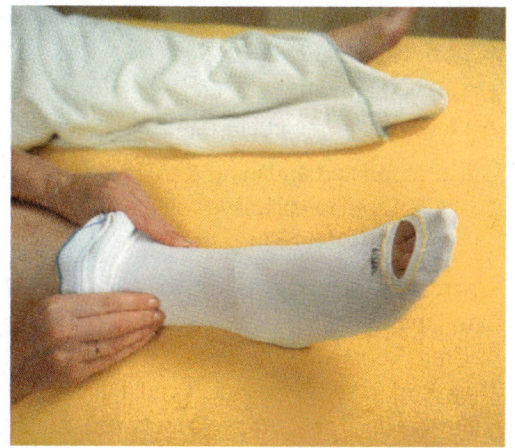

FIGURE 29-16C Draw the stocking smoothly up to the knee.

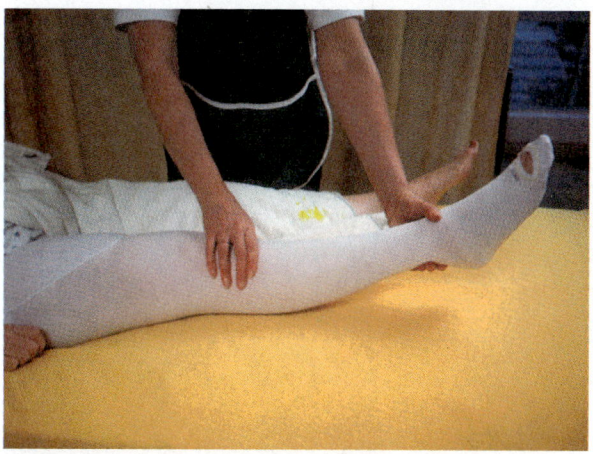

FIGURE 29-16D Check to make sure the stocking is free of wrinkles.

Elastic Bandage

An elasticized bandage (Ace bandage) may be used to keep dressings in place, especially on an extremity or on the head. You may need to remove and reapply the bandage once or twice on your shift. Elastic bandages are also used on nonsurgical patients, to promote venous blood flow in the legs, and for injuries of the musculoskeletal system, to reduce swelling. Elastic bandages come in 2-inch to 6-inch widths and in 4-foot and 6-foot lengths (Figure 29-17). Check with the nurse for the appropriate size bandage. (Refer to Procedure 91.)

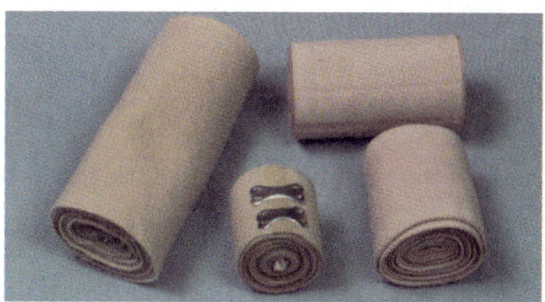

FIGURE 29-17 Elastic bandages are available in a variety of widths.

PROCEDURE 91

APPLYING ELASTIC BANDAGE

1. Carry out beginning procedure actions.

2. Assemble equipment:
   - appropriate size bandage (check for cleanliness)
   - tape, pins, or self-closures that come with bandage

3. Check the area to be bandaged.
   a. If there are lesions or signs of skin breakdown, report to the nurse before bandaging.
   b. If there are dressings underneath the bandage, the nurse may want to check them before you reapply the bandage.
   c. If an arm or leg is to be bandaged, elevate it for 15 to 30 minutes before application to promote venous blood flow.
   d. Apply the bandage so that two skin surfaces do not rub together (toes, fingers, under breasts and arms). Place gauze or cotton to prevent friction (Figure 29-18A).

continues

PROCEDURE 91

continued

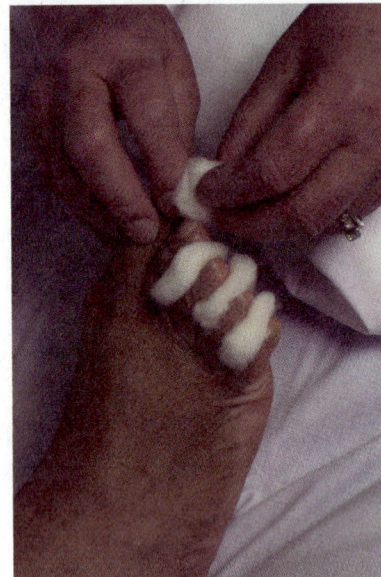

FIGURE 29-18A
Pad the toes with cotton to keep them from rubbing together.

4. Hold the bandage with the roll facing upward in one hand and the free end of the bandage in your other hand (Figure 29-18B).

   a. Hold the roll close to the part being bandaged so that pressure is even.

   b. When bandaging an extremity, always wrap from the distal (far) area to the proximal (near) area (Figure 29-18C).

   c. Unroll the bandage as you wrap the body part. Never unroll the entire bandage at once.

5. Use appropriate bandaging technique (Figure 29-18D). Overlap each layer of bandage by one-half the width of the strip.

6. When finished rolling, secure the bandage with pins, tape, or self-closures. Avoid using the clips that may come with the bandage, if possible. They tend to come loose and could injure the patient's skin. The bandage should be smooth and wrinkle-free.

7. Check distal circulation just after the bandage has been applied and once or twice every 8 hours thereafter (check the skin under the bandage for color and temperature; note patient complaints of burning, tingling, or other discomfort).

8. Remove and reapply the bandage every shift, or more often if needed. The patient should have two bandages so that they can be laundered daily. Ask the nurse whether the bandage is to be worn continuously or only at specified times.

9. Carry out procedure completion actions.

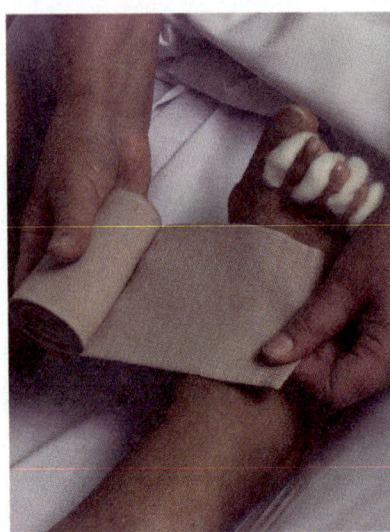

FIGURE 29-18B Hold the bandage with the roll facing upward in one hand and the free end of the bandage in your other hand.

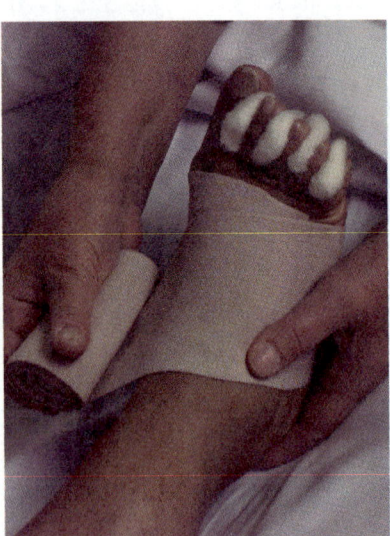

FIGURE 29-18C Always wrap from distal to proximal.

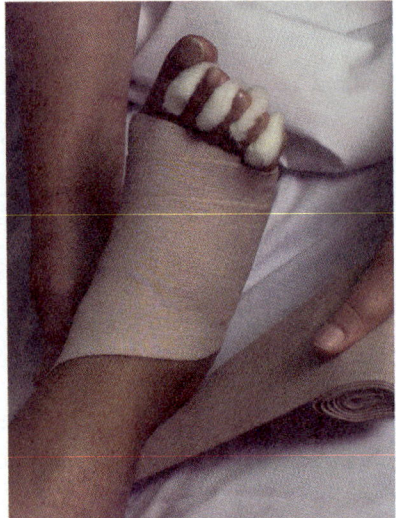

FIGURE 29-18D Use the correct bandaging technique. Overlap each layer of bandage by one-half the width of the strip. The finished bandage should be smooth and wrinkle-free.

Sequential Compression Therapy

Deep vein thrombosis and **pulmonary embolism** (blood clot in the lungs) are serious postoperative complications. Approximately 10% of all patients with DVT die from pulmonary embolism. Most have no symptoms until they develop the pulmonary embolus. The femoral vein, the large blood vessel in the groin, is particularly susceptible to clot formation. Because of the high risk and serious consequences associated with blood clots, the physician may order **sequential compression therapy** to reduce the risk. Sequential compression therapy massages the legs using a milking, wavelike motion.

Pneumatic hosiery (Figure 29-19) are also called *sequential compression hosiery*. This device prevents blood clots by massaging the legs mechanically. Pneumatic hosiery inflate and deflate rhythmically to produce the milking, wavelike massaging motion. The device should not be used on patients with lower leg ulcers, blood clots, massive edema, deformities, infected or broken skin, or arterial disease. Shiny, hairless skin is an indication of arterial problems. If you observe any hard nodules, red areas, or warm areas on the patient's lower legs, inform the nurse before applying the hosiery.

Measuring and Connecting the Hosiery. Before beginning this procedure, you must determine the proper size hosiery for the patient. Do this by measuring the circumference of the patient's upper thigh with a tape measure when she is in bed. Hold the measure snugly against the leg and note the circumference. Compare the measurement with the sizing chart, and select the proper size hosiery.

Familiarize yourself with the hosiery and compression controller if you have not used them before. Open the package and lay the hose on a flat surface. Open them completely, with the cotton lining facing up. Inside you will notice markings for the ankle and knee. When you apply the garment to the patient's leg, line it up exactly with these landmarks. Next, familiarize yourself with the compression controller. The device may have a cooling adjustment. This is used to cool the patient. It is turned off during routine use. Follow your facility policy and the nurse's instructions

for activating this feature. The controller also has arrows to adjust the pressure inside the hose. It should be set at 35 mm Hg to 55 mm Hg. The unit may automatically set at 45 mm Hg, the midway point. The nurse will set the unit or instruct you on the setting to use.

Both hosiery must be connected to the controller for the unit to operate. Position the arrows on the hose opposite the arrows on the tubing. Push the ends together firmly until you hear a clicking sound. If the patient will be using only one sleeve, such as when she has a cast on one leg, leave the unused sleeve in the sealed plastic bag. Cut a small hole in the bag and connect the tubing.

Applying Pneumatic Hosiery. Before applying the hosiery, palpate the pedal (Figure 29-20A) and posterior tibial pulses (Figure 29-20B). In most facilities, staff mark the location of these pulses with a marker, making a small

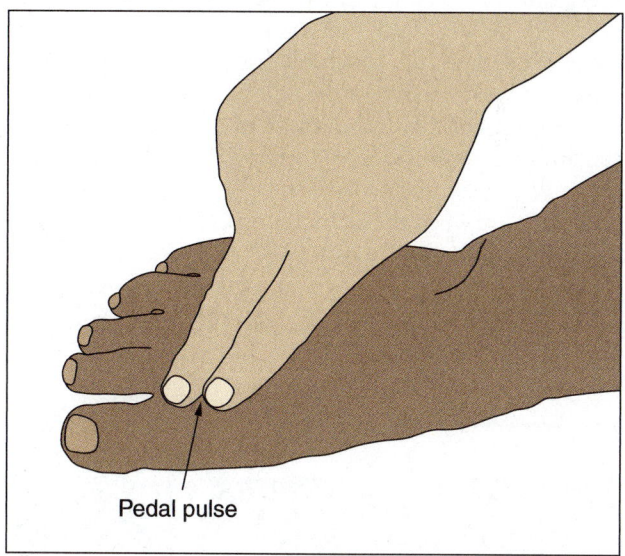

FIGURE 29-20A The pedal (dorsalis pedis) pulse.

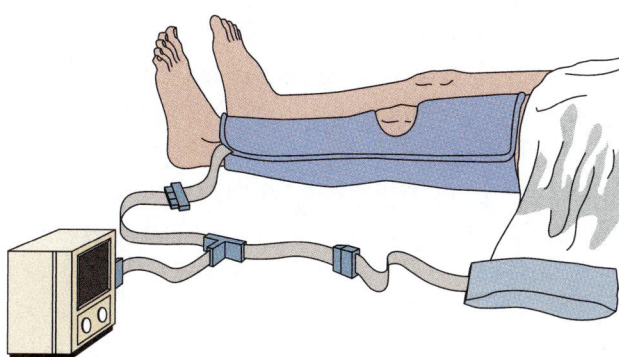

FIGURE 29-19 Pneumatic compression hosiery is used to prevent blood clots.

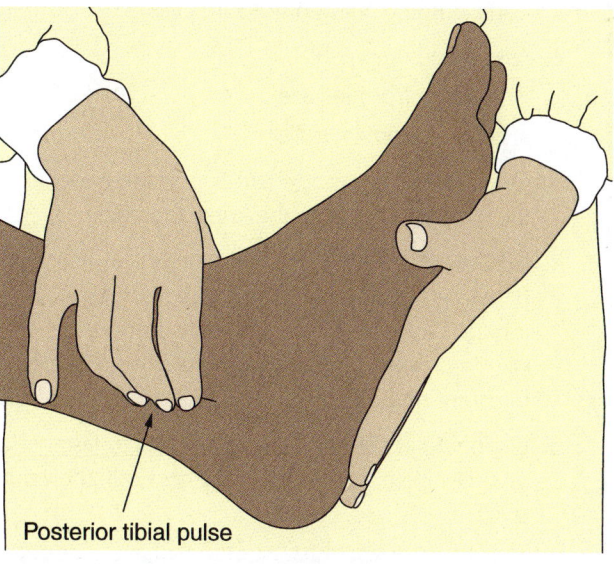

FIGURE 29-20B The posterior tibial pulse.

"X" on the patient's skin. Compare the movement, sensation, and color in both feet. If abnormalities are noted, consult the nurse before continuing. The nurse will assess the patient's legs and check for contraindications. Follow the nurse's instructions.

Pneumatic hosiery may be applied over anti-embolism hose, but both the sleeves and the anti-embolism hose must be smooth and wrinkle-free to reduce the risk of skin breakdown. The device is used 24 hours a day, when the patient is lying down, until the patient is completely ambulatory. It may be removed for bathing and ambulation, then reapplied immediately. The nurse may instruct the patient to perform certain leg exercises while the device is being used. (Refer to Procedure 92.)

Caring for the Patient with Pneumatic Hosiery.

The compression controller has a visual display that notes which chamber is inflated. When the chambers decompress, the unit will say "vent." Make sure the audible alarm is turned on, and check that the key has been removed. If the alarm sounds, the panel will display a message code. A card in a slot in the top of the unit will display the numerical message code with the nature of the problem. Follow the directions on the card to correct the problem, or notify the nurse, according to facility policy. The hose deflates automatically when the alarm sounds.

Turn the power off and remove the hose every 4 hours. Disconnect the sleeves from the tubing by releasing the latches on each side of the connectors, then pulling the connectors apart. Observe the skin under the device, and provide skin care as ordered. Avoid massaging the legs. Massage may dislodge a blood clot, which will quickly migrate to the lungs. Inform the nurse when you will be removing the device so that he or she can assess the patient's legs.

Use of the hose will be discontinued when the patient is fully ambulatory. The unit is not disposable. Clean and store the device according to facility policy after use, or return it to central supply.

Documentation. Follow your facility policy for documenting use of the pneumatic compression device. You may be asked to document the procedure, pulse checks in the feet, skin color, the patient's response, and the settings, including use of the alarm and cooling settings.

Initial Ambulation

Some time after surgery, a patient is permitted to sit up with the legs over the edge of the bed. This position is called **dangling**.

- Watch carefully for signs of fatigue or dizziness (**vertigo**).
- Assist the patient to assume the position slowly.

The first **ambulation** (walk) is usually short. The patient usually dangles for a short time before ambulating. Dangling is an important part of postoperative care because it stimulates circulation and helps prevent the formation of blood clots (thrombi). (Refer to Procedure 93.)

PROCEDURE 92

APPLYING PNEUMATIC COMPRESSION HOSIERY

1. Carry out beginning procedure actions.

2. Assemble equipment:
   - hosiery of proper size
   - compression controller

3. Open the hose, laying them flat on the bed with the markings opposite the knee and ankle.

4. Lift the patient's leg, and slide the hose under it. Begin on the side of the leg opposite the plastic tubing. Wrap the sleeve smoothly around the leg with the opening in front, over the knee. Make sure there are no dents, folds, or creases in the garment.

5. Beginning at the ankle, fasten the Velcro fasteners securely. Next, secure the ankle and calf, then the thigh.

6. Check the fit by inserting two fingers between the sleeve and the patient's leg. The fit should feel snug and secure, but not tight.

7. Wrap the other leg in the same manner, beginning on the side opposite the plastic tubing. After wrapping the leg, check the fit.

8. Attach the plastic tubing on each leg to the compression controller by lining up the arrows on the tubing.

9. Plug the controller in and turn on the power.

10. Remain with the patient for one complete cycle (usually 60 to 90 seconds) to ensure that she tolerates the procedure.

11. Carry out procedure completion actions.

PROCEDURE 93

ASSISTING THE PATIENT TO DANGLE

1. Carry out beginning procedure actions.

2. Assemble equipment:
   - bath blanket
   - pillow

3. Check the pulse (see Unit 19).

4. Lower the side rail nearest to you. Lock the bed at the lowest position.

5. Drape the patient with a bath blanket and fanfold the top bedcovers to the foot of the bed.

6. Gradually elevate the head of the bed.

7. Help the patient to put on a bathrobe.

8. Place one arm around the patient's shoulders and the other arm under the knees.

9. Gently and slowly turn the patient toward you. Allow the patient's legs to hang over the side of the bed.

10. Roll a pillow and tuck it firmly against the patient's back for support.

11. After putting slippers on the patient, ask the patient to swing the legs.

12. Have the patient dangle as long as ordered.
    - If the patient becomes dizzy or faint, help him lie down.
    - Report to the supervising nurse immediately.

13. Check the patient's pulse.

14. Rearrange the pillow at the head of the bed. Remove the patient's bathrobe and slippers.

15. Place one arm around the patient's shoulders and the other arm under the knees. Gently and slowly swing the patient's legs onto the bed.

16. Check the patient's pulse. Lower the head of the bed and raise the side rails.

17. Carry out procedure completion actions. Remember to wash your hands, report completion of your task, and document the time dangled (duration), pulse, and the patient's reaction.

SAFETY Alert

Remain next to the patient during the first dangling and ambulation. For patient safety, do not turn your back or leave the bedside. These precautions will probably not be necessary as the patient recovers and gains strength. Use common sense and follow the care plan and the nurse's instructions.

The patient may need assistance the first few times he stands up to ambulate. The anesthesia and medications administered before, during, and after surgery may affect the patient's balance, endurance, and strength. There may be drainage tubes or an intravenous feeding that must be moved with the patient (Figure 29-21).

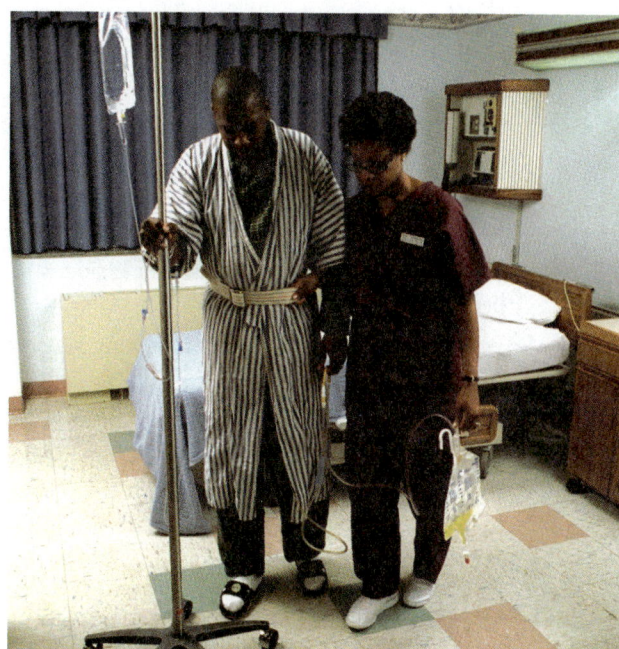

FIGURE 29-21 Drainage tubes and intravenous lines may be in place after surgery. Carefully move these with the patient.

guidelines *for*

Assisting the Patient in Initial Ambulation

- Check with the nurse to see if a transfer belt can be used.
- Assist the patient to sit on the edge of the bed with the bed in low position.
- Assist the patient to put on footwear appropriate to the floor surface. Never allow a patient to ambulate with bare feet or socks.

- Take the patient's pulse before and after standing. If there is more than 10 points difference, return the patient to bed and inform the nurse.
- If the patient becomes dizzy or faint, return the patient to bed and inform the nurse.
- Walk with the patient as instructed in Unit 17.

REVIEW

A. True/False.

Mark the following true or false by circling T or F.

1. T F Patients receiving local anesthetics lose consciousness during the surgery.
2. T F When spinal anesthetics are used, patients may lose feeling and movement in their legs.
3. T F Preoperative teaching has little effect on the patient's postoperative recovery.
4. T F You help build patient confidence when you explain what you plan to do when carrying out procedures.
5. T F Skin preparation involves shaving an area larger than the size of the incision.
6. T F The nursing assistant has no responsibilities related to the patient while the patient is in surgery.
7. T F Patients should be dangled without incident before initial ambulation.
8. T F Patients who are unconscious following surgery should not be left alone.
9. T F Nosocomial infections do not affect the cost or length of hospital stay.
10. T F Patients who are faced with surgery are often filled with apprehension and fears.

B. Matching.

Choose the correct word or phrase from Column II to match each item in Column I.

Column I

11. _____ inflammation of a vein leading to clot formation
12. _____ period before surgery
13. _____ medicine given to prevent pain
14. _____ hospital-acquired
15. _____ opening
16. _____ walking
17. _____ dizziness
18. _____ lung collapse
19. _____ blood clot
20. _____ area where immediate postoperative care is given

Column II

a. ambulation
b. orifice
c. nosocomial
d. PACU
e. umbilicus
f. vertigo
g. anesthesia
h. preoperative
i. aspiration
j. embolism
k. atelectasis
l. thrombophlebitis

C. Multiple Choice

Select the one best answer for each of the following.

21. When assisting a patient with coughing and deep breathing exercises, teach him or her to
    a. inhale through the nose.
    b. inhale through the mouth.
    c. exhale through the nose.
    d. keep the hands behind the neck to expand the lungs fully.

22. The main purpose of coughing and deep breathing exercises is to prevent

    a. pneumonia.

    b. dizziness.

    c. pain.

    d. anxiety.

23. The main purpose of pneumatic compression hosiery is to prevent

    a. edema.

    b. pneumonia.

    c. blood clots.

    d. pain.

24. Pneumatic compression hosiery are contraindicated

    a. in patients who have had abdominal surgery.

    b. if the patient is using oxygen.

    c. if a rash or open areas are present.

    d. for patients with a cast on one leg.

25. Check the postoperative patient's vital signs every

    a. 5 minutes for the first hour, then every 15 minutes for 4 hours.

    b. 15 minutes for an hour, then every 30 minutes for an hour.

    c. 30 minutes for 4 hours, then every 8 hours for 72 hours.

    d. 60 minutes for 4 hours, then every 4 hours for 16 hours.

D. Nursing Assistant Challenge.

Mr. Dovetski is a 47-year-old patient on the surgical unit. He has had abdominal surgery. When he is returned to his room from surgery, you note that he has a Foley catheter, an intravenous feeding running, dressings on the abdominal incision, and elastic stockings. Think about what procedures you will include in your care of Mr. Dovetski.

26. How often will you take his vital signs? Which procedures are included in vital signs? What are the "normal" ranges for each vital sign for a person of this age? If there are changes in the vital signs, these changes may be indications of what complications?

27. What observations will you make regarding the Foley catheter? Why do you think he has the catheter in place?

28. What observations will you make regarding the intravenous feeding? Why do you think the physician ordered an IV?

29. You know you will need to have Mr. Dovetski perform deep breathing exercises and deep coughing. Why is this important? How can you help him do the exercises with the least discomfort?

30. Why do you think he has elastic stockings on? How often should you take the stockings off and reapply them? What do you need to remember when putting the stockings back on?

31. How will you report any complaints of pain?

32. How will you check for bleeding from the incision?

EXPLORING THE WEB

Description	Location
Articles on preoperative and postoperative infection control	*http://www.infectioncontroltoday.com*
Nutrition and the surgical patient	*http://www.facs.org*
Perioperative client needs	*http://www.delmarhealthcare.com/pdf/0766824527.pdf*
Perioperative nursing slides	*http://www.indstate.edu*
Postoperative care of children	*http://www.musckids.com*
Preoperative and postoperative care procedures	*http://www.delmarhealthcare.com/olcs/acello/11checklists.pdf*
Procedure for transferring a patient to the OR	*http://www.cc.nih.gov/nursingnew*
Association of PeriOperative Registered Nurses	*http://www.aorn.org*
Guidelines for Preventing Surgical Site Infection	*http://www.nailm.com*
Nursing Specialties Perioperative Nursing	*http://allnurses.com/Nursing_Specialties*
PowerPoint Slides: Perioperative Care	*http://nursing.uaa.alaska.edu*

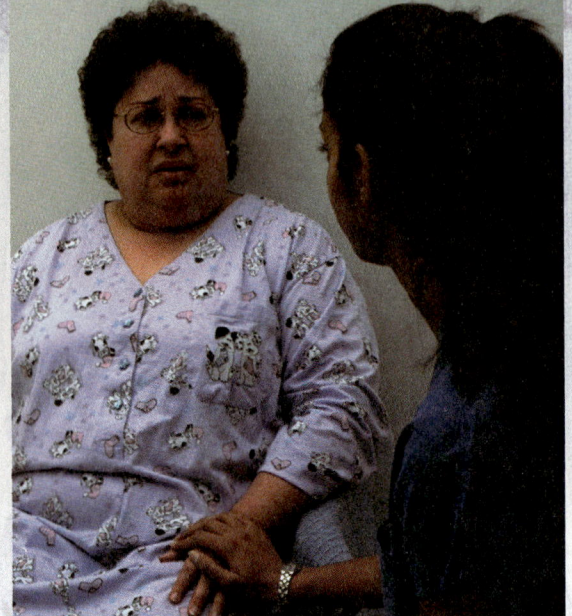

Caring for the Emotionally Stressed Patient

objectives

After completing this unit, you will be able to:

- Spell and define terms.
- Define mental health.
- Explain the interrelatedness of physical and mental health.
- Understand mental health as a process of adaptations.
- Identify commonly used defense mechanisms.

- Describe ways to help patients cope with stressful situations.
- Identify the signs and symptoms of maladaptive behaviors that should be documented and reported.
- List nursing assistant measures in providing care for patients with adaptive and maladaptive reactions.
- Identify professional boundaries in relationships with patients and families.

vocabulary

Learn the meaning and the correct spelling of the following words and phrases:

adaptation	denial	mental illness	reality orientation
agitation	depression	paranoia	repression
alcoholism	disorientation	professional	stressors
coping	enabling	boundaries	suicide
defense mechanisms	hypochondriasis	projection	suppression
delusions	maladaptive behavior	reaction formation	

INTRODUCTION

There are varying degrees and differing aspects of health. A person who is in poor physical health may be mentally healthy. Because of good mental health, the person may be self-reliant and able to make decisions and to live an effective, productive life (Figure 30-1).

In contrast, a person with good physical health may not be able to cope with and adapt to changes. This inability limits the person's chances to participate successfully in society.

MENTAL HEALTH

Mental health means exhibiting behaviors that reflect a person's **adaptation** or adjustment to the multiple stresses of life, such as:

- Illness
- Hospitalization
- Loss of a loved one
- Loss of a job
- Loss of status

Stresses or **stressors** are situations, feelings, or conditions that cause a person to be anxious about his or her physical or emotional well-being. Good mental health leads to positive adaptations. Poor mental health is demonstrated by maladaptive behaviors (behaviors that harm the person or her adjustment).

Physical and mental health are interrelated. Physical illness is often preceded by stressful life situations. Ill health causes emotional stress. It is easy to understand that each of these factors contributes to the total health pattern of each person.

Ways of **coping** with (handling) stressful situations (Figure 30-2) are learned early in life. As people grow, they find the behaviors that work best for them. They learn to use those behaviors to reduce stress and protect self-esteem. These coping patterns become part of the individual's habitual responses, becoming more and more obvious as the person ages.

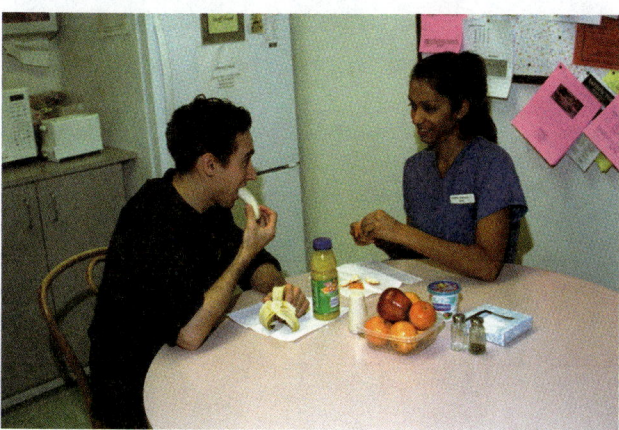

FIGURE 30-1 A mentally healthy person leads a productive life.

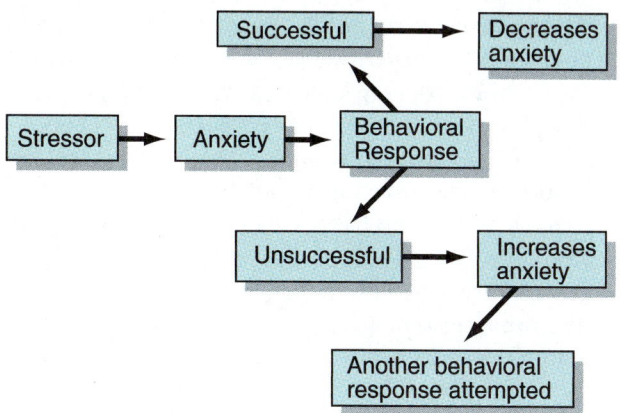

FIGURE 30-2 Each individual has different ways of coping with stress.

DEFENSE MECHANISMS

When any person feels unable to cope with stress and the situation threatens self-esteem, the person tends to act in protective ways. These ways are called **defense mechanisms**. A diagnosis of cancer, for instance, may be so overwhelming that a person must temporarily defend himself against acknowledging the truth. Everyone uses these defense-oriented behaviors from time to time to protect themselves. You use them. Patients use them. Your coworkers use them.

You must recognize and understand the need to use defense mechanisms. Do not be critical of their occasional use. Most people do not use one mechanism all the time. They usually rely on a combination of defenses. They may not even be aware that they are behaving in a defensive way.

Defensive behavior becomes harmful only when it is the major means of coping with stress. In such cases, the person continuously avoids recognizing and responding to reality with problem-solving methods. The person's stress is temporarily reduced, but the stressor (feeling or situation) is not resolved. Such a person needs counseling from a trained mental health provider.

Some of the commonly used defense mechanisms include:

- **Repression**—The involuntary exclusion from awareness of a painful or conflict-creating thought, memory, feeling, or impulse. For example, a woman has a lump in her breast, but refuses to go to a physician for examination and diagnosis. She has recently lost her husband, her house, and her job. She feels that she cannot "acknowledge" any other illness or crisis, so she unconsciously represses the knowledge of the lump in her breast. She is not going to take the chance that the lump may be cancer. She cannot face the possibility of a terminal disease.

- **Suppression**—This mechanism differs from repression because the person is aware of the unacceptable feelings and thoughts but deliberately refuses to acknowledge them. For example, a man becomes immobilized with the fear of rejection by his wife if he tells her he has a diagnosis of AIDS. Therefore, he consciously suppresses the knowledge of the AIDS diagnosis because he cannot handle the anxiety associated with telling his wife.

- **Projection**—A person's own unacceptable feelings and thoughts are attributed to others. The person blames others for his own shortcomings. For example, a person blames his wife or family for his alcoholism and loss of jobs. He projects his failings onto his wife and children.

- **Denial**—Blocking out painful or anxiety-producing events or feelings. This is one of the most common defenses against the stress of diagnosis and illness. For example, a patient with very high blood pressure refuses to stop smoking. She continues to eat a diet high in fats. She cannot deal with her fear of disability and unemployment, so she refuses to accept the seriousness of her condition.

- **Reaction formation**—A person using this defense mechanism represses the reality of a situation and then behaves in a manner that is the exact opposite of the real feelings. For example, a woman dislikes one nursing assistant but is fearful that if she expresses that feeling, the assistant will be less caring. This patient may be overly friendly and cooperative with that assistant.

Other adaptive behaviors are as follows:

- **Displacement**—Substituting an object or person for another and behaving as if it were the original object or person. *Example:* Being angry with the nursing assistant because another patient is annoying.

- **Identification**—Behaving like another person whom one holds as an ideal. *Example:* Speaking to coworkers with the same tone the supervisor uses with you.

- **Compensation**—Excelling in one area to make up for feelings of failure in another. *Example:* The nursing assistant who overachieves in the skill area because her ability to read written directions is poor.

- **Conversion**—Offering a socially acceptable reason to avoid an unpleasant situation. *Example:* The nursing assistant who calls saying she cannot report for duty because she has the flu, when she is just tired from staying up too late.

- **Fantasy**—The use of imagination to solve problems. *Example:* The supervisor criticizes the nursing assistant, who then daydreams of a time when she is the head of nursing and can fire the supervisor.

- **Undoing**—A method of reversing something wrong that was done. *Example:* The person who used his hands to hurt another may wash his hands repeatedly to try to undo the deed.

ASSISTING PATIENTS TO COPE

Here are some ways to help patients become better able to cope and adapt:

- Be a good listener.
- Try to determine the source of stress so it can be removed and the stress reduced.

DIFFICULT *Situations*

Patients with coping and behavior problems usually have a behavior management care plan that lists steps to follow when certain problems are exhibited. Become familiar with the care plan. Implement the approaches in the order listed. Modify your behavior in response to the patient's behavior by monitoring how the patient responds to you, then adjusting your approach to achieve results. Vary routines and equipment, if necessary. Put yourself in the patient's shoes and try to understand what is happening.

- Be sensitive to nonverbal messages (body language) that may give clues to the source of stress.
- Treat the person with respect, recognizing him as a unique individual.
- Understand the behavior in the same way the patient is viewing it, without labeling the behavior and passing judgment.
- Let the patient know that you are reliable and that you respect her privacy and feelings.
- Never argue, enter into a power struggle, or debate with a patient, even when you know the patient is wrong.
- Be supportive of the person's own attempts to overcome the stress (Figure 30-3).

Remember that illness, age, and separation from family and home are major stress factors.

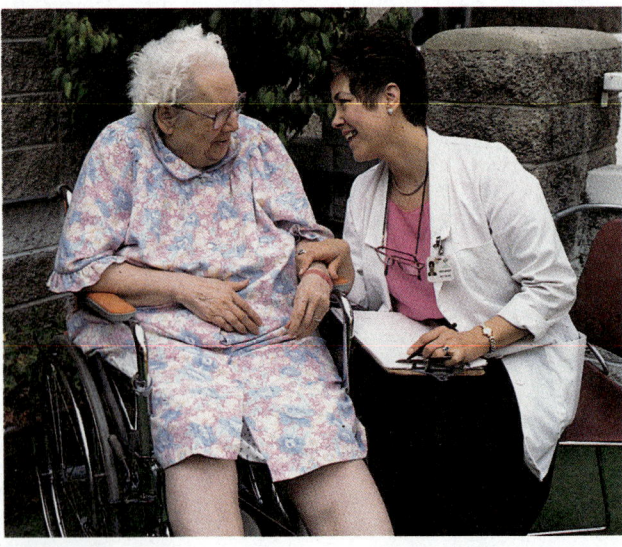

FIGURE 30-3 Staff can help patients find acceptable ways of coping with stress.

THE DEMANDING PATIENT

In every nursing care situation, you will meet patients who are very demanding. This can be a difficult experience for everyone if it is not handled correctly.

Being demanding is another way in which patients show their frustration. It is a coping behavior. Patients who are very demanding are usually frustrated by their loss of control. To be successful in caring for these patients, the nursing assistant must:

- Try to learn and understand the factors that are causing the demanding behavior.
- Show that you care about the patient's situation, but keep control of your emotions.
- Maintain open communications by listening to the patient's words and by being sensitive to the patient's body language.
- Provide opportunities that allow the patient to regain some control by making choices.
- Be consistent in the manner of care. This builds the patient's sense of security (Figure 30-4).
- Do not take the patient's demands personally.
- Report observations to the supervisor with suggestions for changes in the care plan.

ALCOHOLISM

Some people use alcohol as a means of coping with stress. The National Institute for Alcohol Abuse reports that two-thirds of the senior population uses alcohol. Fifteen percent of them become alcoholics. **Alcoholism** is regarded as a disease. Factors that contribute to the excessive use of alcohol include:

- Retirement
- Lowered income

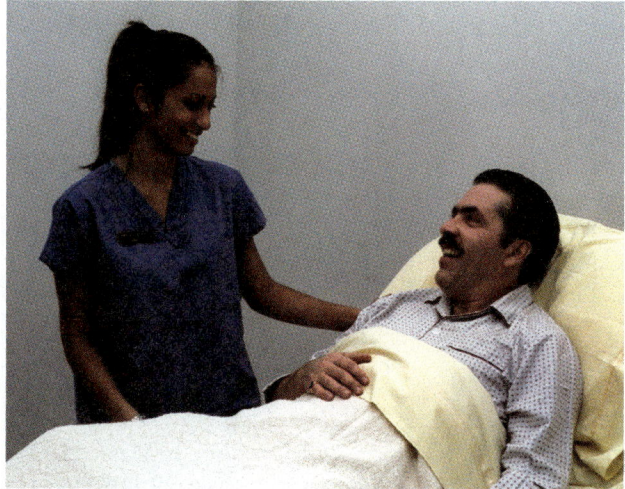

FIGURE 30-4 Being attentive and consistent builds the patient's security.

- Grief
- Loss of spouse and/or friends
- Loneliness
- Stress in the family
- Decline in health
- Pain

Alcohol toxicity may be associated with an acute onset of:

- Altered levels of awareness
- Mild confusion
- Progressive stupor
- Acute delirium
- Disorientation similar to that seen in irreversible brain syndrome

Alcohol slows down brain activity. It impairs mental alertness, judgment, physical coordination, and reaction time—increasing the risk of falls and accidents.

Alcohol can affect the body in unusual ways. It can make it difficult to diagnose diseases and conditions of the cardiovascular system. It can mask pain that might otherwise serve as a warning sign of heart attack. Alcohol can also produce:

- Symptoms similar to dementia
- Forgetfulness
- Reduced attention
- Restlessness
- Impatience
- Agitation
- Confusion

Alcohol is a drug. It mixes unfavorably with many other drugs (Table 30-1). The use of alcohol can cause some drugs to metabolize more rapidly, producing exaggerated responses. Such drugs include:

- Anticonvulsants
- Anticoagulants
- Antidiabetic drugs
- Diuretics

The alcoholic in withdrawal feels depressed and defensive. He needs to identify the stressors that bring on his need for alcohol and to find new ways of coping. This process takes professional skill, but you can:

- not allow the alcoholic to manipulate you.
- listen with empathy (Figure 30-5).
- reflect the person's ideas and thoughts.
- be sure alcohol is not available.
- be consistent in the limits that have been set.

Care of the intoxicated patient includes:

- caution during feeding to prevent choking or strangling.
- supervision of activities to prevent injury and falls.
- safety checks during bathing to prevent burns.
- close supervision if there is confusion or delirium.

TABLE 30-1	COMMON ALCOHOL-DRUG INTERACTIONS
Drug Taken by Patient	**Effects to Report**
Narcotics	Increased central nervous system (CNS) depression with acute intoxication
Salicylates	Gastrointestinal bleeding
Sedatives and psychotropic drugs	Increased CNS depression with acute intoxication
Barbiturates	Decreased sedative effect after chronic alcohol abuse
Chloral hydrate	Prolonged hypnotic effects
Chlordiazepoxide (Librium, Librax)	Increased CNS depression
Chlorpromazine (Thorazine)	Increased CNS depression
Diazepam (Valium)	Increased CNS depression
Oxazepam (Serax)	Increased CNS depression
Antihistamines	Increased CNS depression
Antabuse	Flushing, vomiting, excessive sweating, hyperventilation, confusion, and drowsiness

Problem drinkers and alcoholics have a good chance for recovery. Getting help should start with the family physician, a member of the clergy, the local mental health association, or the local chapter of Alcoholics Anonymous.

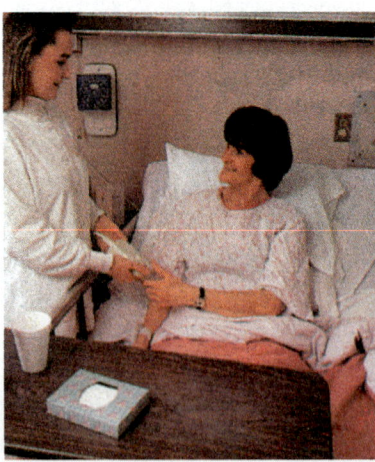

FIGURE 30-5
Listen with empathy.

MALADAPTIVE BEHAVIORS

Mental illness or maladaptive behavior occurs when behaviors and responses disrupt the person's ability to function smoothly within the family, environment, or community.

You must be careful about labeling anyone as mentally ill. Even when an official diagnosis of mental illness has been made, take care not to stereotype the patient.

Remember that stereotypes are often associated with *myths* (false beliefs). It is far better to view the person as an individual who is demonstrating poor behavioral responses.

As a nursing assistant, you need to be aware that sometimes signs and symptoms such as fatigue, loss of appetite, insomnia, and pain may reflect either physical or emotional stress. Note and report any unusual behavior or symptoms. Be careful, however, to be objective. Do not make judgments about your findings.

Remember also that confusion, disorientation, and aggressive behavior may only be temporary responses to a fever, drug interaction, or a full bladder. Continuation of such behavior may be the result of organic brain changes. Blaming and judging a patient is inappropriate and unhelpful.

Assessing the Patient's Behavior

An initial assessment of the patient's mental and emotional state will be made by the licensed care provider. Because you make frequent contact with the patient, you can make a valuable contribution to the nursing assessment process by making careful and sensitive objective observations.

Report observations regarding:

- Physical responses related to eating, personal hygiene, sleeping, participation in activities, or any strange or unusual behaviors
- Emotional responses related to interactions between the patient and yourself or between the patient and other patients, emotional outbursts, or inappropriate responses
- Patient behavior as it relates to judgment and affects memory, comprehension, and orientation

When working in long-term care, you will find many people whose coping ability has failed and so are demonstrating maladaptive behaviors. The many losses these people have suffered add to their inability to cope. Physical problems make dealing with reality more difficult.

Common maladaptive responses result in:

- Depression
- Disorientation or delirium
- Agitation
- Paranoia

Tips: Reward patients for positive behavior. Behavior that is rewarded is usually repeated. The goal is to show the patient a healthy way of directing energy. Verbal praise, positive feedback, and other signs of approval are rewards. Nonverbal rewards such as a hug, smile, or pat on the back may also be used, when appropriate. Snacks and privileges are sometimes used as rewards.

Depression

Depression is the most common functional disorder in older people (Figure 30-6), but younger people also may experience depression. Depression may be shown in a variety of ways:

- Preoccupation with constipation
- Flatulence
- Bad taste in the mouth
- Burning tongue
- Vague oral discomforts associated with dentures
- Burning on urination
- Pain in lower abdomen
- Crying spells
- Trouble sleeping (insomnia)
- Excessive sleep
- Loss of appetite or increased appetite
- Significant weight loss or weight gain
- Fatigue
- Headaches
- Backaches
- Stiff joints
- Apathy
- Impaired concentration
- Lethargy
- Agitation
- Poor personal hygiene
- Feeling of dejection
- Less interest in sex
- Depressed mood most of the day, nearly every day (irritability in children)

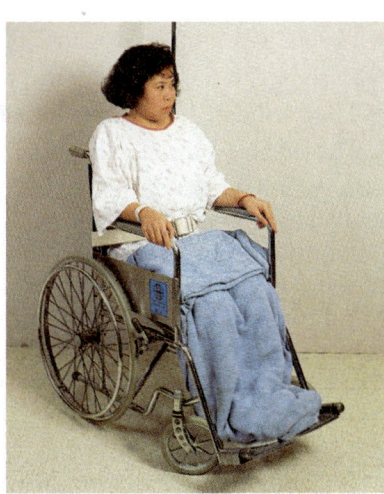

FIGURE 30-6 Withdrawal is common when a person is depressed.

- Markedly diminished interest or pleasure in almost all activities, most of the day and nearly every day
- Psychomotor agitation or retardation
- Feelings of worthlessness or guilt
- Recurrent thoughts of death or suicide

Depression is often masked by symptoms that make it seem as though the patient is physically ill. Your observations are doubly important because a patient who is depressed may actually have minor or major illnesses. These infirmities may in turn cause depression. Remember, physical and mental health are interrelated.

Some drugs that are used to treat actual physical illness in the elderly may cause depression. They are:

- Digitalis
- Reserpine
- Inderal
- Diuretics
- Most of the antihypertensive drugs

If your patient is receiving any of these drugs, be alert for signs of depression. If the depression is drug-induced, it will be relieved when the drug is withdrawn.

Severely depressed patients may be treated with:

- Antidepressants
- Electroshock therapy (in severe cases)
- Talk therapy

A mental health clinical nurse specialist, psychologist, or psychiatrist will direct and support the staff efforts.

When depression is severe, suicidal thoughts and attempts are a real possibility. You must be sensitive to the possibility of such a situation and report and document your observations. The suicidal patient must be carefully protected. Watch for and report:

- Change in response such as deepening depression or sudden elevation of mood
- Evidence of withdrawal or secretiveness
- Sudden loss of a support system (such as the death of a family member)
- Repeated, prolonged, or sporadic refusal of food (oral or through nasal tubes), care, medications, or fluids
- Hoarding of medication (stockpiling of pills)
- Sudden decision to donate body parts to a medical school
- Changes in behavior, especially episodes of depression, screaming, hitting, throwing things, or a sudden failure to get along with family, friends, or peers
- Sudden interest or disinterest in religion
- Purchase of a gun
- Purchase of razor blades and hiding them
- Statements such as: "I just want out," "I want to end it all," "I'll never get well," "I'm going to kill myself," or "You would be better off without me."

guidelines *for*

Assisting the Patient Who Is Depressed

- Reinforce the person's self-concept by emphasizing her continued value to society and helping the patient to use the support systems that are available (Figure 30-7).
- Do not act in a pitying way. This only validates the person's depressed feelings.
- Make sure physical supports, such as eyeglasses and hearing aids, are in place. These help the person to focus on reality.
- Report all complaints so that actual physical problems may be identified and corrected rather than being attributed to the depression.
- Provide the person with activities within her limitations to help her think beyond herself. For example, engage the person in some meaningful activity such as reading, making puzzles, or conversing with others (Figure 30-8).
- Avoid tiring activities.
- Use simple language and speak slowly when giving instructions.
- Monitor elimination carefully; constipation is common.
- Provide fluids frequently, because the depressed patient may be too preoccupied to drink.
- Be alert to the potential for **suicide** (the taking of one's own life).

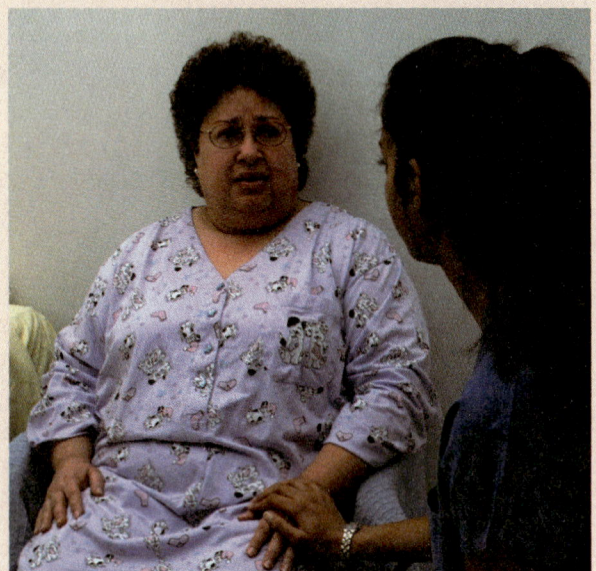

FIGURE 30-7 Try to reinforce the depressed person's sense of self-worth.

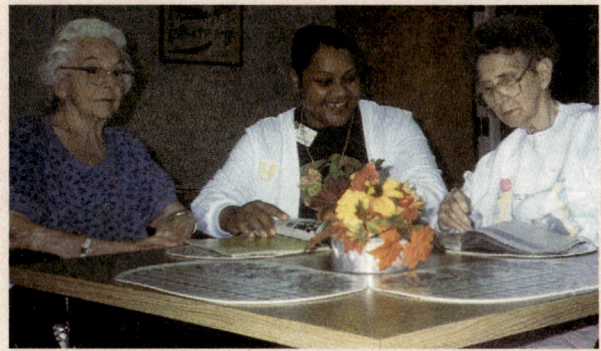

FIGURE 30-8 Socializing with others may help a person who is depressed.

- Increased use of alcohol and drugs
- Behavioral manifestations of anger, hostility, belligerence, loss of interest, or inability to concentrate
- Inability to do simple tasks, confusion, slurred speech, or retarded motor skills
- Deep preoccupation with something that cannot be explained

Nursing Care of a Patient with the Potential for Suicide. Never assume that a suicide attempt is a means of getting the attention of the staff or family. At least 15% of people who try to commit suicide do it again. Keep in mind the at-risk individuals. These include:

- White males over the age of 65 who live alone
- The very old (75 years and above)

- Persons with a recent diagnosis of a terminal illness
- Persons with unrelieved chronic pain
- Those suffering the sudden loss of a spouse
- The elderly with recent multiple losses

Be aware that the suicide rate is higher in acute medical units than it is on psychiatric units. Most of the suicides occur while the patient is under the supervision of a health provider, who frequently either misses or ignores the clues of suicide. Suicide attempts may occur either when the patient is successfully recovering or is getting worse. It is the responsibility of all staff members to observe their patients carefully and immediately report any signs of depression and/or suicide. You should:

- Be observant for clues to suicide attempts, and report them to the appropriate person.

- Be consistent in approaches and care.
- Encourage the patient to review his life, emphasizing the positive aspects.
- Give the patient hope while being realistic (Figure 30-9).
- Work to restore the person's self-esteem, self-worth, and self-respect, to preserve positive self-concept.
- Help the patient find a support network within the family, religious groups, and self-help groups.
- Make the person feel accepted as a unique, valued person.
- Never ignore the person's statements or threats about suicide.

Disorientation (Disordered Consciousness)

Disorientation is a condition in which a person shows a lack of reality awareness with regard to time, person, or place (Figure 30-10). In some cases, the disorientation is mild, sometimes severe; sometimes temporary but at times prolonged. It is important to report patient behavior, actions, and responses. The disoriented person has impaired:

- Judgment
- Memory
- Comprehension
- Orientation

Physical ailments and stresses that can bring about a disoriented state include:

- Recovery from surgery
- Pneumonia
- Myocardial infarction
- Renal infection
- Head trauma
- Organic brain disease
- Fevers

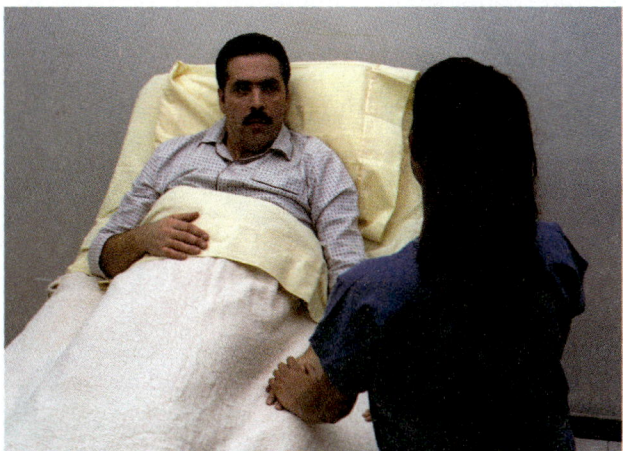

FIGURE 30-9 Be hopeful but realistic with a depressed person who is at risk of suicide.

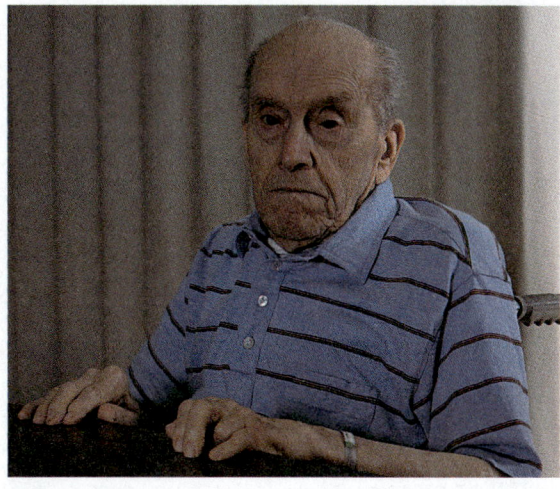

FIGURE 30-10 The person who is disoriented lacks awareness of reality.

- Dehydration
- Malnutrition
- Drug interaction

The signs and symptoms that identify the disoriented person are:

- Inability to think clearly
- Bewilderment
- Faulty memory
- Inability to follow directions
- Misinterpretation of stimuli
- Confusion about time
- Confusion about place
- Confusion about who he or she is

Nursing Assistant Responsibilities. The nursing assistant must realize that disoriented people cannot be responsible for their actions or for protecting themselves adequately. The patient's sensory misinterpretations (delusions or hallucinations) may put others at risk. The disorientation does not allow the patient to take action for self-protection. *Protection of the patient is the most important nursing responsibility.* In addition, you should:

- Be calm and gentle when approaching the patient. Disoriented patients are startled by even minor stimuli.
- Give instructions slowly, clearly, and in simple words.
- Give only one instruction at a time.
- Provide activities of short length that do not require much concentration.
- Build the patient's self-esteem with the reward of positive comments.
- Assist patients to participate in reality orientation activities (Figure 30-11). **Reality orientation** is making the disoriented patient aware of person, place, and time by visual reminders, activities, and verbal cues. See the guidelines for reality orientation activities.
- Maintain a constant, limited routine.

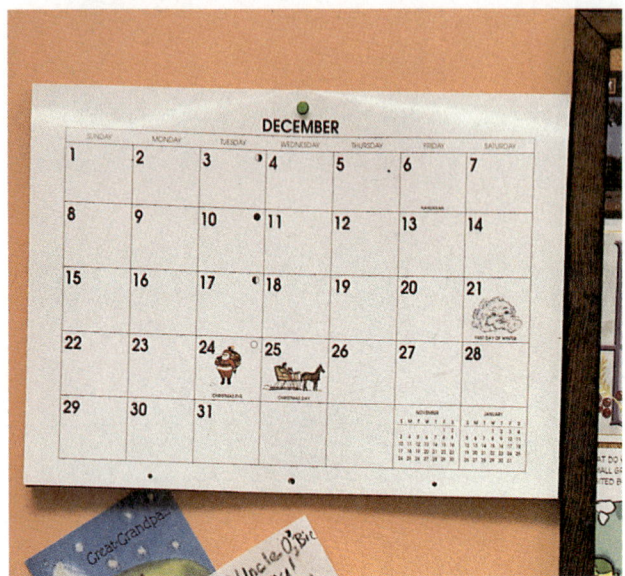

FIGURE 30-11 Calendars and clocks may help maintain orientation.

- Address the patient by name with each contact.
- Identify yourself to the patient each time there is contact.
- Avoid reinforcing illusions, delusions, or hallucinations.
- Keep glasses, dentures, and hearing aids in place.
- Speak often with the patient.
- Be patient and repeat instructions.
- Keep clock and calendar in view.
- Encourage the presence of and refer to familiar objects.
- Post an activity board and draw attention to it.
- Call attention to color-coding of facility areas.
- Introduce day, date, time, season, and weather into conversation.

- Use restraints only when absolutely necessary and with a physician's order, making sure all safety practices are followed. Medications that chemically restrain patient responses and the presence of a friend or family member may make physical restraints unnecessary.
- Reduce disorientation by keeping rooms well lighted, cool, and quiet. Also, provide reality orientation according to the nursing care plan.
- Make sure patients wear glasses and hearing aids, if used.

To maintain a safe environment for disoriented patients:

- Keep all sharps, such as knives, out of reach.
- Remove and store valuable or breakable items. If patient is at home, make sure the family knows where you put these items.
- Use sturdy chairs and couches.
- Put rails on windows that are close to the floor.
- Provide adequate lighting.
- Protect stairways with gates.
- Do not permit poisonous plants.
- Control matches and smoking materials.
- Supervise use of stoves and appliances.
- Keep all medications out of reach.

Agitation

Agitation is defined as inappropriate verbal, vocal, or motor activity due to causes other than disorientation or real need. It includes behavior such as:

- Aimless wandering
- Pacing
- Cursing
- Screaming
- Repeatedly asking the same question
- Spitting
- Biting
- Fighting or arguing constantly
- Demanding attention
- Restlessness
- Constant activity

Agitation is a significant problem for the elderly, their families, and the nursing staff. It is probably one of the foremost management problems in acute care hospitals, in home care, and in long-term care facilities.

The major factors contributing to agitation are:

- Noise
- Frustration at loss of control
- Feelings that the patient's space has been invaded
- Loneliness and need for attention
- Unresolved personal difficulties in the patient's past
- Drug interactions
- Organic brain disease
- Boredom
- Behavior of others around the patient
- Depression
- Constipation
- Restraints
- Too much sensory stimulation

Study this list carefully, because your awareness can lead to early intervention. Early intervention can often prevent serious problems.

guidelines *for*

Managing the Patient Who Is Agitated

- Do not argue with or confront the person.
- Make the environment safe (secure the windows and lock the doors).
- Make sure each patient wears an identification bracelet or patch, and that it is fastened securely.
- Keep a recent photo of the patient in case the patient wanders off.
- Notify the physician, the administrator, the family, or the police department if the patient wanders away from his unit, facility, or home.
- Assign the patient brief tasks.
- Engage the patient in games, walks, swimming, and other activities if not contraindicated. These should be activities that enhance the patient's self-esteem.
- Use bean-bag seats and rocking chairs in the parlors of the nursing home or the patient's home.
- Care for the patient—watch for injuries.
- Engage the patient in conversations and in reality therapy or remotivation groups.
- Engage the patient in short-term activities. Realize that the patient's attention span is short. Thus, the patient needs rewards for short-term activities.
- Prevent the patient from becoming exhausted.
- Carefully monitor the patient's activities, because the agitated patient is at risk for falls and injuries.

Hypochondriasis

The patient suffering from **hypochondriasis** imagines or magnifies each physical ailment. Some authorities feel that hypochondriasis is an expression of depression and is one way these individuals reduce stress. These patients need reassurance and understanding but should not be encouraged to focus or believe in their supposed illnesses. However, the staff must be careful not to overlook real illness when it occurs, just because they have become used to hearing the patient complain. Nursing assistants should report all complaints and never make a judgment that a patient is a hypochondriac.

Paranoia

Paranoia is another extreme maladaptive response to stress. It is characterized by a heightened, false sense of self-importance and delusions of being persecuted. **Delusions** are false beliefs about oneself, other people, and events. People with paranoia believe that everyone is against them. When treating the paranoid patient, you should:

- Find ways to reduce the patient's feelings of insecurity and misunderstanding.
- Keep the person as involved as possible in reality activities.
- Report and document observed responses to medication and psychotherapy.
- Monitor nutrition and fluid balance—these patients often refuse to eat or drink for fear of poisoning.
- Observe sleep patterns—the person may be fearful of being harmed while sleeping.
- Be direct and honest in all interactions.
- Not support any misconceptions or delusions that the person exhibits.
- Never argue with anyone who has delusions. It can trigger a serious confrontation.

PROFESSIONAL BOUNDARIES

As a nursing assistant, you must stay within certain **professional boundaries** in the care of each patient. Boundaries are unspoken limits on the physical and emotional relationship with patients. They limit and define how a health care worker acts with patients. They involve using your best behavior, ethical practices, and good judgment when caring for patients. Respecting boundaries is one way that you will act appropriately when on the job.

It takes good judgment and experience to identify boundaries and keep from crossing them. When driving down the road, you do not see the boundary lines when you cross from one city to the next. Professional boundaries are the same way. They exist, but you cannot see them. You must be aware of boundaries and take active steps to avoid crossing them. You may cross them inadvertently or deliberately, thinking you are meeting a patient's need.

Being aware of boundaries is particularly important when caring for patients with emotional stress. Patients who are at risk of inappropriate relationships with health care workers usually have one or more of these risk factors:

- mental or emotional problems
- poor impulse control
- marital problems
- low self-esteem

- loneliness and/or need for caring

Health care workers who are at greatest risk for inappropriate relationships and boundary problems usually have one or more of these risk factors:

- family or marital problems
- näivete
- low self-esteem
- loneliness, feelings of isolation
- addiction (chemical or sexual)
- financial problems
- stress, burnout

To avoid crossing professional boundaries, strive to act professionally, as you were taught in class. Avoid putting yourself in a position in which you think and act as a family member or friend. You must use good judgment and determine the amount of contact and assistance that are right for the patient. Too much or too little contact can be unhealthy for both the assistant and the patient. Treat all patients professionally. Consult your charge nurse if you are uncertain.

Ethical Behavior with Patients and Families

As a nursing assistant, patients expect you to act in their best interests and treat them with dignity. You do this by not taking advantage of a patient's situation and by avoiding inappropriate involvement in the patient's personal and family relationships. Some relationships with patients and families are not healthy for the patient or the nursing assistant. It is not always easy to recognize unhealthy relationships until it is too late. Once you have crossed over a boundary line, it is difficult to turn back. Be aware of boundaries at all times, and strive to keep your relationships professional.

Actively work to find a balance in your relationships with patients and families. If any of the following occur, you are probably crossing professional boundaries and may be in a relationship danger zone:

- Discussing your personal problems with the patient or family members
- Being flirtatious with a patient, including making sexual innuendos, telling jokes that are sexual in nature, or using offensive language
- Discussing your feelings of sexual attraction with a patient
- Feeling that you may become involved in a sexual relationship with the patient
- Keeping secrets with a patient and becoming defensive when someone questions your relationship or involvement in the patient's personal life
- Thinking you are immune from having an unhealthy relationship with a patient
- Believing that you are the only nursing assistant who can meet the patient's needs

- Spending an inappropriate amount of time with the patient, including off-duty visits or trading assignments with others to be with the patient
- Reporting only partial information about the patient to your charge nurse, because you fear disclosing unfavorable information or secrets the patient has told you
- Feeling that you must protect the patient from other health care workers and always siding with the patient's position

Questions to ask yourself that will help you decide whether you are crossing a professional boundary line are listed in Table 30-2. If you have trouble staying objective, or think you may cross a boundary, seek help from your charge nurse, pastor, or another professional person whom you trust.

Consequences of Boundary Violations

Boundary violations lead to inappropriate relationships with patients or families. These cloud your clinical judgment, and may lead to serious consequences, such as inappropriate sexual relationships. They often carry over into your personal life. The improper relationship may cloud your judgment, causing you to do things that you would not ordinarily do (such as stealing from your employer). There are many serious personal, legal, and professional consequences to inappropriate relationships. For your own well-being, be aware that professional boundaries exist, and actively take steps to keep from crossing them.

TABLE 30-2 QUESTIONS TO ASK

- Is this in the patient's best interest?
- Whose needs are being served?
- Does this action benefit me rather than the patient?
- Will this affect the care I am delivering?
- Should I be concerned or consult with a colleague?
- How would the patient's family view this?
- How would I feel telling a colleague about this?
- Am I treating this patient differently from other patients?
- Does this patient mean something special to me?
- Am I taking advantage of the patient?
- Am I comfortable about documenting this in the medical record?
- Is this a violation of nursing assistant ethics?

Enabling

Enabling behavior is reacting to a patient in a manner that shields the person from experiencing the full impact or consequences of his or her actions or behavior. Enabling behavior differs from helping behavior in that it allows the person to be irresponsible. As a paraprofessional health care worker, the nursing assistant should be aware of enabling behavior and avoid it when caring for patients, particularly those with mental and emotional problems. By learning and respecting professional boundaries, you will avoid helping others inappropriately. Likewise, you must learn to set limits for yourself and prevent patients from crossing into your own personal territory. Enabling behavior with patients creates dependency rather than moving the patient toward independence and good mental health. Methods of enabling patients that you should avoid include:

- Protecting the patient from the natural consequences of his or her behavior
- Keeping secrets about a patient's behavior from others
- Making excuses for a patient's behavior
- Taking steps to get a patient out of personal trouble
- Blaming others for the patient's behavior
- Seeing the patient's problems as a result of something else
- Giving money to patients
- Attempting to control patients' lives and activities
- Doing things for the patient that she should do herself

Strive to keep your behavior in the zone of helpfulness (Figure 30-12) to avoid crossing professional boundaries and enabling patients.

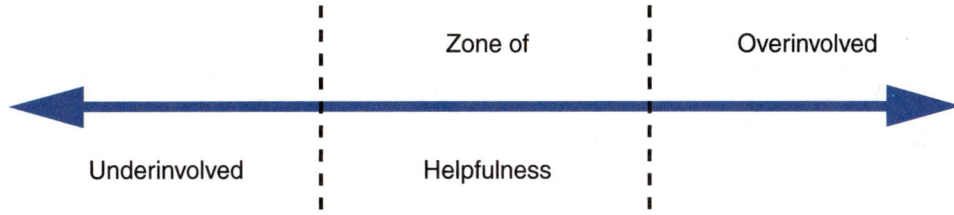

FIGURE 30-12 Keep your relationship with patients and families in the zone of helpfulness.

guidelines *for*

Assisting Patients with Behavior Problems

- Follow the care plan.
- Control your own responses and reactions.
- Be a good communicator.
- Avoid lying to the patient.
- Avoid making promises you cannot keep.
- Avoid discussing facility or staff problems with the patient. If the patient complains, inform the nurse or other appropriate person.
- Protect the safety of the patient and others.
- If the care plan tells you to respond to a specific behavior, apply the approaches when the behavior starts. Do not wait until the patient loses control.
- Use good communication and listening skills.
- Practice empathy.
- Attempt to learn the cause of the behavior. Communicate with other team members.
- Remove the cause (or trigger) of the behavior, if known.

- Let others know if you discover an approach that works.
- Modify your own behavior in response to the patient's behavior.
- Watch the patient's response to your approaches. Adjust your approach, equipment, routine, and other care, if necessary.
- Discuss family, friends, or other pleasant information with patients. This provides a source of strength, comfort, and support.
- Meet the patient's physical needs.
- Give patients as much control as possible. Offer choices in care and routines. Encourage them to direct their own care.
- Be patient. Control your reaction to the patient. Make sure your body language does not send the wrong message.
- Be happy. Smile. Make sure your body language sends a positive message. Positive behavior is contagious.

REVIEW

A. True/False.

Mark the following true or false by circling T or F.

1. T F Mental health refers to the adaptations a person makes to the multiple stressors of life.

2. T F Stressors are the physical and emotional problems that a person encounters throughout life.

3. T F Defense mechanisms are used only by mentally unhealthy persons.

4. T F If you know that the patient is wrong about something she is saying, it is proper to debate the issue with the patient.

5. T F The best way to handle the demanding patient is by trying to determine the underlying factors causing the patient's distress.

6. T F Very few senior adults use alcohol and even fewer become alcoholics.

7. T F The use of alcohol impairs mental alertness, judgment, reaction time, and physical coordination.

8. T F It is dangerous for a person to drink alcohol when taking other medications.

9. T F Alcohol is a drug.

10. T F When intoxicated, a person could choke on food.

11. T F Alcoholics have a poor chance for recovery.

12. T F Maladaptive behaviors reflect the failure of usual defense mechanisms.

13. T F Depression is the least common of the functional disorders in older people.

14. T F The depressed patient needs to be encouraged not to be overactive.

15. T F Dehydration can lead the patient into a state of disorientation.

16. T F The disoriented patient needs a stimulating environment.

17. T F It is best to give a disoriented patient one instruction at a time.

18. T F If a patient threatens suicide, you need not be concerned.

19. T F The white male who is over age 65 and living alone is at high risk for suicide.

20. T F It is the responsibility of only the licensed staff to guard against suicide attempts.

21. T F Suicides are attempted only by patients in psychiatric institutions.

22. T F The patient who is agitated may ask the same question repeatedly.

23. T F Agitation is a significant problem for the elderly, their families, and facility staff.

24. T F Paranoia is a maladaptive response that usually requires medication and psychotherapy.

25. T F Paranoid individuals believe that others are out to get them.

B. Matching.

Choose the correct word from Column II to match each phrase or statement in Column I.

Column I	Column II
26. ____ conscious refusal to recognize the reality of a situation	**a.** repression
27. ____ shielding a patient from the consequences of behavior	**b.** suppression
28. ____ blocking out painful or anxiety-producing events or feelings	**c.** projection
29. ____ involuntary exclusion of the awareness of reality	**d.** denial
30. ____ lack of awareness of reality	**e.** professional boundaries
31. ____ handling stressful situations	**f.** enabling
32. ____ attributing one's own failing to another	**g.** coping
33. ____ invisible lines that define relationships with patients	**h.** disorientation

C. Multiple Choice.

Select the one best answer for each of the following.

34. The patient tells you that her doctor says she has AIDS, but she knows that isn't possible. She most likely is using the defense mechanism of
a. repression.
b. displacement.
c. projection.
d. denial.

35. The best way to enhance the patient's capability to cope with an unpleasant situation that has developed with another patient is to
a. tell him to ignore it.
b. let him know he can talk to you safely.

c. tell him everyone has problems, his aren't so important.

d. suggest he discuss it with his clergyperson.

36. The patient who refuses to eat or drink because she is convinced that she is being poisoned is suffering from

a. paranoia.

b. depression.

c. agitation.

d. disorientation.

37. The patient is depressed. You can best help him by

a. pitying him.

b. keeping him from interacting with others.

c. agreeing that he probably deserves the way he feels.

d. stressing his continued value to society.

38. The best way to help the patient remain oriented to reality is to

a. keep glasses in the bedside stand so they will not be broken.

b. isolate the patient.

c. place a clock and calendar nearby.

d. explain things in detail.

39. The person holding a doll and acting as if it were a baby probably is experiencing

a. repression.

b. denial.

c. projection.

d. displacement.

40. Agitation may be demonstrated by

a. talking a lot.

b. boredom.

c. smiling for no reason.

d. repetitive questions.

41. Professional boundaries

a. apply only to licensed nursing personnel.

b. involve assisting patients with activities of daily living.

c. are set out in the job description.

d. are unspoken limits on relationships with patients.

42. Health care workers who are at risk of having inappropriate relationships with patients

a. are usually friendly and happy.

b. may have financial or marital problems.

c. exercise regularly to relieve stress.

d. occasionally drink alcoholic beverages.

43. Enabling behavior

a. is used when caring for patients who require total care.

b. involves orienting patients to person, place, and time.

c. is used to help patients relieve stress.

d. shields an individual from the consequences of his or her actions.

D. Nursing Assistant Challenge.

You are assigned to care for Mr. Simonson, who was recently diagnosed with diabetes. He is a top executive in a large corporation and has a wife and three adult children. He is learning how to administer his insulin, how to plan his diet, and how to test his blood sugar. He has been very quiet and keeps his eyes closed most of the time, although he is not sleeping. One day as you enter the room, he screams at you to get out and then picks up his water pitcher and throws it. Think about what you learned in this unit about human behavior as you consider these questions.

44. What examples of nonverbal communication is Mr. Simonson displaying?

45. Do you think he is using defense mechanisms to cope with his diagnosis? If so, which ones?

46. If Mr. Simonson displays this kind of behavior again, what would be an appropriate response from the nursing staff?

47. How would you document this episode?

48. How can the nursing staff show respect and concern for this patient?

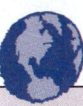

EXPLORING THE WEB

Description	Location
About Alcoholism	*http://www.alcoholism.about.com*
American Council on Alcoholism	*http://www.aca-usa.org*
American Psychiatric Nurses' Association	*http://www.apna.org*
Enabling Behavior	*http://www.cita1.com*
—Early Warning Signs of Enabling	*http://shalomplace.com*
National Council on Alcoholism and Drug Dependence	*http://www.ncadd.org*
National Institute on Alcohol Abuse	*http://www.niaaa.nih.gov*
Nursing Specialties Psychiatric Nursing	*http://allnurses.com*
Online Dictionary of Mental Health	*http://human-nature.com/odmh*
Professional boundaries	*http://www.ncsbn.org*
—Maintaining Healthy Boundaries in Professional Relationships	*http://www.mnnurses.org*
—Professional Boundaries for Therapeutic Relationships	*http://www.crnm.mb.ca*
—Professional Boundaries—Guidelines	*http://www.nbv.org.au*
—Professional Boundaries in Health Care Relationships	*http://www.cpo.on.ca*
—Pushing the Limits of Professional Boundaries	*http://www.nurseweek.com*
Tools for Coping with Life's Stressors	*http://www.coping.org*

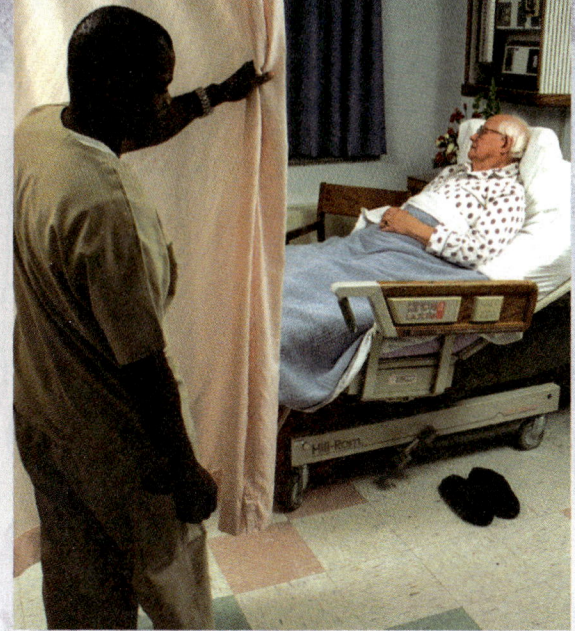

Death and Dying

objectives

After completing this unit, you will be able to:

- Spell and define terms.
- Describe how different people handle the process of death and dying.
- Describe the nursing assistant's responsibilities for providing supportive care.
- Describe the spiritual preparations for

death practiced by various religious denominations.

- Describe the hospice philosophy and method of care.
- List the signs of approaching death.
- Demonstrate the following procedure:
  - Procedure 94 Giving Postmortem Care

vocabulary

Learn the meaning and the correct spelling of the following words and phrases:

acceptance	critical list	hospice care	rigor mortis
advance directive	denial	life-sustaining	Sacrament of the
anger	depression	treatment	Sick
autopsy	DNR	living will	supportive care
bargaining	durable power of	moribund	terminal
cardiac arrest	attorney for health	no-code order	
cardiopulmonary	care	postmortem	
resuscitation (CPR)	harvested	postmortem care	

INTRODUCTION

Death is the final stage of life. It may come suddenly, without warning, or it may follow a long period of illness. It sometimes strikes the young but it always awaits the old. As a nursing assistant, you will be providing care throughout the period of dying and into the after-death (**postmortem**) period. Accepting the idea that death is the natural result of the life process may help you respond to your patient's needs more generously.

The concept of death and dying is handled differently by different people (Figure 31-1). There are many reactions to the diagnosis of a **terminal** (life-ending) illness:

- Some patients may have had time to prepare psychologically for their deaths. They may accept or be resigned to the inevitable.

- Some may actually look forward to relief from the pain and emotional burden of a long illness and await death calmly.

- Some may be fearful or angry and demonstrate moods that swing from outright denial to depression.

- Others may reach out, trying to verbalize feelings and thoughts of an uncertain future.

- In others, despair and anxiety may give way to moments of active hostility or periods of searching, groping questions.

None of the reaction states are predictable and no patient falls into one rigid pattern or another. You must accept the patient's behavior with understanding, interpret the patient's very real need for family support, and support the family in meeting their own needs during this adjustment period.

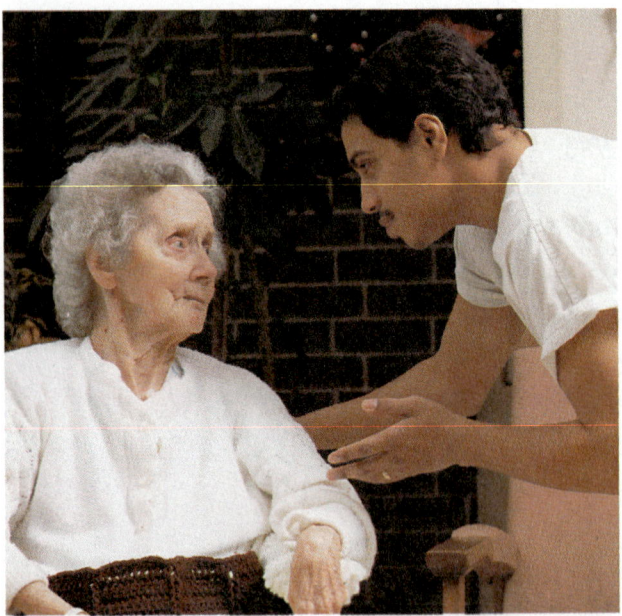

FIGURE 31-1 Each person handles death differently.

COMMUNICATION *Highlight*

Health care workers may feel helpless when caring for a dying patient. Remember that active listening is a means of therapeutic communication. Listening to a patient's concerns shows honest and caring concern for the patient. Using touch can also communicate caring and acceptance. When you are at a loss for words, consider these other means of showing the patient that you care.

FIVE STAGES OF GRIEF

Dr. Elisabeth Kübler-Ross identified five stages of grief that can occur in the dying patient. They are denial, anger, bargaining, depression, and acceptance (Table 31-1). If there is adequate time and support, some patients may be able to move psychologically through each stage to a point of acceptance of their illness and death.

- **Denial** begins when the person is made aware that he is going to die. He may not accept this information as truth, and may instead deny it. Making long-range plans that are not likely to be fulfilled may indicate that the patient is in the denial stage. Most people with a terminal illness must go through denial before they are able to eventually reach acceptance. This is a necessary and therapeutic stage. Other people should not try to convince the patient of his diagnosis or argue with the person. If denial begins to interfere with the person's adjustment, then professional counseling may be required.

- **Anger** comes when the patient is no longer able to deny the fact that she is going to die. The patient may blame those around her, including those who are giving care, for her illness. Added stresses, however small, are likely to upset the patient who is in the anger stage (Figure 31-2). Statements such as, "It's all your fault. I should never have come to this hospital," are typical of a patient in the anger stage. Remember, if the patient expresses anger, that she is angry about her diagnosis, not with you personally. Remain calm and avoid saying anything that may make her angrier. If you think the patient is angry about something other than the diagnosis, report this to the nurse so the situation can be remedied.

- **Bargaining** is the stage in the grief process in which the patient attempts to bargain for more time to live. He may ask to be allowed to go home to finish a task before he dies, or he may make private "deals" with

TABLE 31-1 EMOTIONAL RESPONSES TO DYING

Stages of Grief	Response of the Nursing Assistant
Denial	Reflect patient's statements, but try not to confirm or deny the fact that the patient is dying. **Example:** *"The lab tests can't be right—I don't have cancer."* *"It must have been difficult for you to learn the results of your tests."*
Anger	Understand the source of the patient's anger. Provide understanding and support. Listen. Try to meet reasonable needs and demands quickly. **Example:** *"This food is terrible—not fit to eat."* *"Let me see if I can find something that would appeal to you more."*
Bargaining	If it is possible to meet the patient's requests, do so. Listen attentively. **Example:** *"If only God will spare me this, I'll go to church every week."* *"Would you like a visit from your clergyperson?"*
Depression	Avoid clichés that dismiss the patient's depression ("It could be worse—you could be in more pain"). Be caring and supporting. Let the patient know that it is all right to be depressed. **Example:** *"There just isn't any sense in going on."* *"I understand you are feeling very depressed."*
Acceptance	Do not assume that, because the patient has accepted death, she or he is unafraid, or that she or he does not need emotional support. Listen attentively and be supportive and caring. **Example:** *"I feel so alone."* *"I am here with you. Would you like to talk?"*

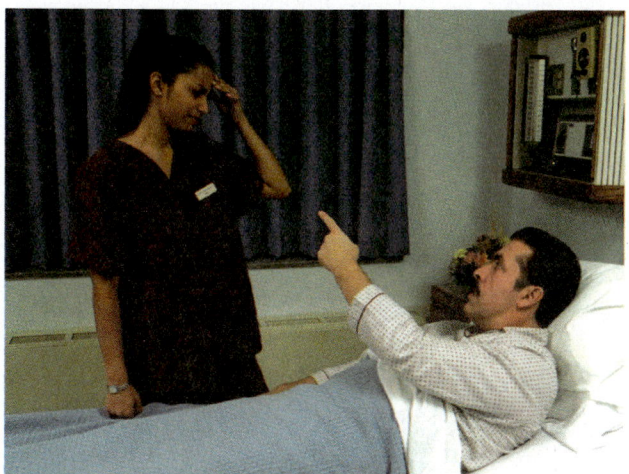

FIGURE 31-2 Patients may demonstrate feelings of frustration and anger.

God: "If you will let me live another two months, I promise I will try to be a better person." Bargaining frequently involves an important event that the patient has been looking forward to, such as a child's wedding or the birth of a grandchild. The patient in this stage is basically saying, "I know I'm going to die and I'm ready to die, but not just yet." This may be done in private and not stated verbally.

- **Depression** is the fourth stage identified in the grief process. During this stage, the patient comes to a full realization that he will die soon (Figure 31-3). He is saddened by the thought that he will no longer be with family and friends, and by the fact that he may not have accomplished some goals that he had set for himself. He may also express regrets about not having gone somewhere or done something: "I always promised my wife that we would go to Europe and now we'll never go."

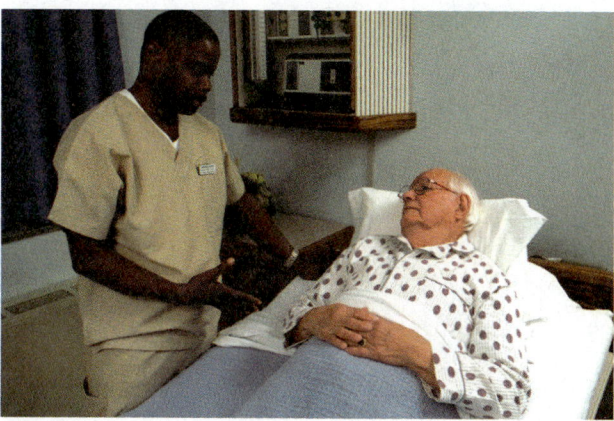

FIGURE 31-3 Depression is a normal part of the grieving process.

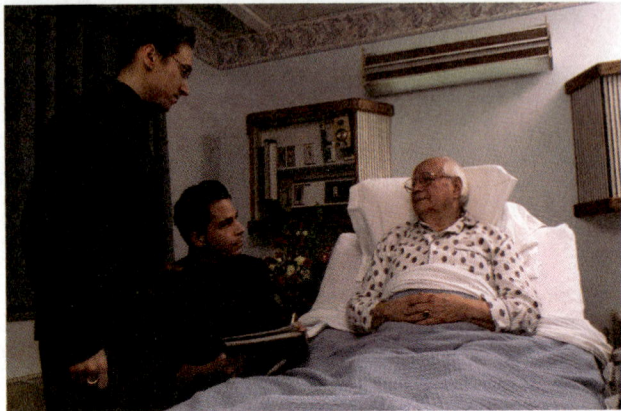

FIGURE 31-4 The patient may strive to complete unfinished business during the acceptance phase of the grieving process.

- **Acceptance** is the stage during which a patient understands and accepts the fact that he is going to die (Figure 31-4). During this stage, he may try to complete unfinished business. Having accepted his eventual death, he may also try to help those around him to deal with it, especially family members.

Not all patients progress through these stages in sequential order. Nor does movement from one level to the next mean that the previous level will be completely left behind. The staff must be aware of the possible psychological positions and be able to identify the patient's current reactions. For example, a patient who displays anger one day may be full of optimism and denial the next.

Denial frequently comes first, followed by anger and despair. Frustrated by feelings of helplessness, the person lashes out at those who are nearby. If each of these stages is expressed with some degree of success, the person is then able to move on to a level of grieving, for himself and for loved ones. When all five stages have been passed, it is believed that the patient is better able to accept the termination of life. If there is adequate time and support (Figure 31-5),

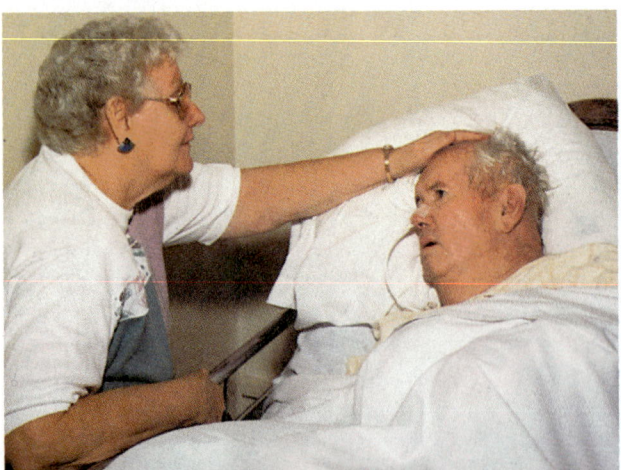

FIGURE 31-5 The support of family and friends is very important to the dying patient.

many patients can be helped to reach a more accepting frame of mind.

The family and staff move through these same stages, but not necessarily at the same time. It is particularly difficult when the patient is in one stage and the family is at another stage.

PREPARATION FOR DEATH

The knowledge of impending death comes to the patient directly from the physician or indirectly from the staff. A diagnosis of terminal illness is very difficult to conceal from the patient. The staff may, without realizing it, reveal the information by:

- Exhibiting false cheerfulness
- Being evasive
- Making fewer visits to the patient's room
- Spending less time with the patient

You must realize that most terminally ill patients do eventually come to accept that death is part of their near future. Keep the following in mind:

- Each patient reacts to this understanding in a unique way.
- How many feelings the patient wishes to share and with whom are very personal decisions.
- You should be available to listen, but do not force the issue.

Upon being told of the terminal diagnosis, the patient may proceed through several stages of emotional adjustment. Initially, the

- patient may react to the situation by denying the truth.
- patient may refuse all opportunities to discuss his illness with the staff or with family.
- patient's interpersonal relationships with family and staff may become greatly strained.
- patient may become defeated and full of despair, actively expressing a loss of hope.

THE PATIENT SELF-DETERMINATION ACT

The Patient Self-Determination Act of 1990 requires health care providers to supply written information about state laws regarding **advance directives**. An advance directive is a document that is put into effect if the patient later becomes unable to make decisions. All health care providers, including hospitals, long-term care facilities, and home health care agencies, must have policies and procedures covering these issues. The patient must be informed of the right to execute an advance directive before or at the time of admission. The patient may choose to execute an advance directive at the time of admission or at any time during his or her stay. Likewise, the patient may choose not to execute an advance directive.

Decisions often must be made when a patient is terminally or critically ill. These decisions involve provision of supportive care or life-sustaining treatment. The Patient Self-Determination Act was passed to assure patients and their families that their wishes will be followed. **Supportive care** means that the patient's life will not be artificially prolonged but that the patient will be kept comfortable physically, mentally, and emotionally. Supportive care includes:

- Oxygen to ease breathing if the patient needs it
- Food and fluids that the patient can consume by mouth
- Medications for pain, nausea, anxiety, or other physical or emotional discomforts
- The continuation of physical care such as grooming and hygiene, cleanliness, positioning, and range-of-motion exercises
- Caring and emotional support of staff

All patients deserve supportive care, but for terminally or critically ill patients, supportive care means the absence of life-sustaining treatment. **Life-sustaining treatment** means giving medications and treatments for the purpose of maintaining life. Life-sustaining treatments include all of the items listed under supportive care and may also include:

- Being placed on a ventilator to maintain breathing
- Receiving **cardiopulmonary resuscitation** (**CPR**) if **cardiac arrest** occurs (the heart and lungs stop functioning)
- Artificial nutrition through a feeding tube or hyperalimentation device
- Blood transfusions
- Surgery
- Radiation therapy
- Chemotherapy
- Other treatments that will maintain life

 Note: Radiation therapy and chemotherapy may also be given to relieve pain, not to extend life.

There are basically two types of advance directives: the living will and the durable power of attorney for health care. The **living will** is a request that death not be artificially postponed if the patient has an incurable, irreversible injury, disease, or illness that the physician judges to be a terminal condition. A living will must be witnessed by two other individuals who do not stand to benefit because of the person's death.

The **durable power of attorney for health care** is a directive that assigns someone else the responsibility for making medical decisions for the patient if the patient becomes unable to do so himself. It must be signed by the *agent* (the person given the durable power of attorney) and by the *principal* (the person appointing the agent). It also must be signed by an adult witness. The durable power of attorney may indicate whether the person:

- Does not want his life to be prolonged and does not want life-sustaining treatment

LEGAL *Alert*

Health care workers sometimes become confused about the meaning of a living will in which the patient specifies that no heroic procedures are to be undertaken if the patient is in terminal, irreversible condition. If the patient is not known to be in terminal condition, resuscitation will be done (unless otherwise ordered). For example, a 32-year-old patient in good health enters the hospital for a diagnostic procedure that involves the injection of contrast material into the veins. The patient has an allergic reaction to the contrast material and suffers a cardiac arrest. In this case, *CPR would be done*, because the patient is not known to be in terminal condition.

In another instance, an elderly patient enters the hospital for insertion of a central intravenous catheter to be used for pain management as part of terminal care for cancer. The patient is known to have inoperable cancer, as documented by two or more physicians. The patient experiences a complication during the procedure and has a cardiac arrest. In this case, the provisions of the living will would be observed, and *CPR would not be done*.

- Wants his life prolonged and wants life-sustaining treatment to be provided unless the physician believes he is in an irreversible coma
- Wants his life to be prolonged to the greatest extent possible without regard to his condition

The durable power of attorney is one way to ensure that the wishes and rights of an individual will be followed and protected when the person is no longer able to make personal decisions. As a nursing assistant, you must be aware of the patient's status for supportive care or life-sustaining treatment. The person on supportive care will have a **no-code order** or **DNR** (do not resuscitate) order. This means that no extraordinary means, such as CPR to resuscitate the person, will be used to prevent death. This allows a person to die peacefully with maximum dignity. A no-code decision is reached after discussion by the patient with her family and physician. Once made, the no-code decision is entered in the patient's chart. All staff members are made aware of the decision, but it is kept confidential. If the patient changes her mind, the order in the chart is changed.

LEGAL *Alert*

The person designated as the agent in a durable power of attorney for health care should be familiar with the patient's wishes. The authority for making decisions takes effect only if the patient becomes physically or mentally unable to speak for herself. If the patient subsequently regains the ability to make decisions, the power of attorney and the agent's power are inactivated. Your facility will have a procedure for securing another person, usually a relative, to make decisions on the patient's behalf if she has not designated a durable power of attorney for health care. The durable power of attorney for health care covers only health care decisions, and only for the period of time during which the patient is unable to make decisions. It does not cover management of finances or other areas of the patient's life.

Witnessing Advance Directives

The nursing assistant must become familiar with facility policies and state laws for witnessing advance directives. In many states, persons who care for the patient are not permitted to witness advance directives. In most states, caregivers cannot legally be appointed to be the agent (medical decision maker) for a patient unless they are related by blood or marriage.

Withdrawing or Modifying Advance Directives

Patients may withdraw or modify their advance directives at any time. For example, a patient's advance directive states

LEGAL *Alert*

Your facility may have designations for different levels of emergency care, ranging from comfort care to full advanced life support. Become familiar with the criteria for these levels. Many facilities have ethics committees made up of professionals from many disciplines. The committee meets to review some difficult care situations.

that he wants full life support if his heart and breathing stop. The patient later finds out that he has cancer, and wants only supportive care at the end of life. If a patient informs you of changes that affect the advance directive, notify the nurse promptly.

THE ROLE OF THE NURSING ASSISTANT

As a nursing assistant, you spend much time with the patient. You have a unique opportunity to be a source of strength and comfort. You must behave in a way that instills confidence in both the patient and the patient's family. Developing the proper attitude and approach for this type of situation is not easy. It will come with experience. There are some things to keep in mind:

- Your response should be consistent. It should be guided by the patient's attitude and the care plan.
- You must be open and receptive, because the terminal patient's attitude may change from day to day.
- Make sure you inform the nurse of incidents related to the patient that reflect moods and needs.
- Remember that each person's idea of death and the hereafter differs. You must be open to patients' ideas and not force your own upon them.
- Your own feelings about death and dying influence your ability to care for the dying patient. Honestly explore your feelings by talking about them with others until you can resolve any conflicts you may have. Your acceptance of death as a natural occurrence will enable you to meet patient needs in a realistic manner.
- Give your best and most careful nursing care, with special attention to comfort measures such as mouth care and fluid intake.
- You should be quietly empathetic and carry out your duties in a calm, efficient way.

When a patient's condition is critical, the physician will place his name officially on the **critical list**. Then the family and the chaplain will be notified.

Providing for Spiritual Needs

Many people find spiritual faith to be a source of great comfort during difficult times.

- Some religions have specific rituals that are carried out when a person is very ill or dying (Table 31-2). Your role is to cooperate with the patient, family, and clergyperson so that these rituals may be performed in a dignified, caring manner.
- Other religions do not have specific practices, but patients of those religions may spend time in prayer. Allow the patient and family privacy, but let them know you are close by if you are needed.
- Some patients may have no formal religious affiliation. This does not mean they do not have spiritual needs.

TABLE 31-2 BELIEFS AND PRACTICES RELATED TO DYING AND DEATH FOR MAJOR RELIGIONS

Religion	Autopsy	Organ Donation	Beliefs and Practices
Judaism (Orthodox)	Only in special circumstances	With consultation of rabbi	Visits to the dying are a religious duty.
			Witness must be present if death occurs, to protect family and commit soul to God.
			Torah and Psalms may be read and prayers recited.
			Conversation is kept to a minimum.
			Someone should be with the body after death until burial, usually within 24 hours.
			Body must not be touched 8 to 30 minutes after death.
			Medical personnel should not touch or wash body unless death occurs on Jewish Sabbath; then care may be given by nurse wearing gloves.
			Water is removed from the room.
			Mirrors may be covered at family's request.
Hinduism	Permitted	Permitted	Priest ties thread around neck or wrist of deceased and pours water in the mouth.
			Only family and friends touch body.
Buddhism	Personal preference	Permitted	Buddhist priest is present at death.
			Last rites are chanted at the bedside.
Islam (Muslim)	Only for medical or legal reasons	Not permitted	Before death, read Koran and pray.
			Patient confesses sins and asks forgiveness of family.
			Only family touches or washes body.
			After death, body is turned toward Mecca.
Roman Catholic	Permitted	Permitted	Sacrament of the Sick administered to ill patients, to patients in imminent danger, or shortly after death.
Christian Scientist	Unlikely	Not permitted	No ritual is performed before or after death.
Church of Christ	Permitted	Permitted	No ritual is performed before or after death.
Jehovah's Witness	Only if required by law	Not permitted	No ritual is performed before or after death.
Baptist	Permitted	Permitted	Clergy ministers through counseling and prayers.
Episcopalian	Permitted	Permitted	Last rites are optional.
Lutheran	Permitted	Permitted	Last rites are optional.
Eastern Orthodox Christian	Not encouraged	Not encouraged	Last rites are mandatory and are given by ordained priest.

They may request the services of a clergyperson and may not know who to call on. Relay this request to the nurse, because most health care facilities have chaplains to provide the services.

- Some patients do not believe in any higher spiritual being. This is their right and no one should try to change their feelings.

- Always respect the beliefs or nonbeliefs of any patient. Treat all religious items, such as holy books, medals, and rosaries, with respect.
- When a Catholic patient is ill, a priest may be called for the Sacrament of the Sick (Figure 31-6). It is preferable that the family be present and leave the room only while the confession is heard. The practicing Catholic and his family consider it a privilege to have the opportunity for confession. Many patients recover completely, but this hope should not prevent the reception of this sacrament if this is the patient's wish.
- A Bible or spiritual reading of the patient's faith, if requested, may be of some spiritual help through this crisis. Be courteous and provide privacy when the patient's clergyperson visits.

Be aware that dying is a lonely business, a journey each person must finish alone. Until the final moment comes, privacy, but not total solitude, should be the guiding rule (Figure 31-7).

It is important to remember the family and other loved ones when a patient is dying. Check the policies of your health care facility and assist in the following actions:

- Allow the family to be with the patient as they desire.
- Allow the family to assist with some of the care, if they wish to do so; for example, moistening the patient's lips or giving a backrub.
- Inform the family where they can get a cup of coffee or a meal.

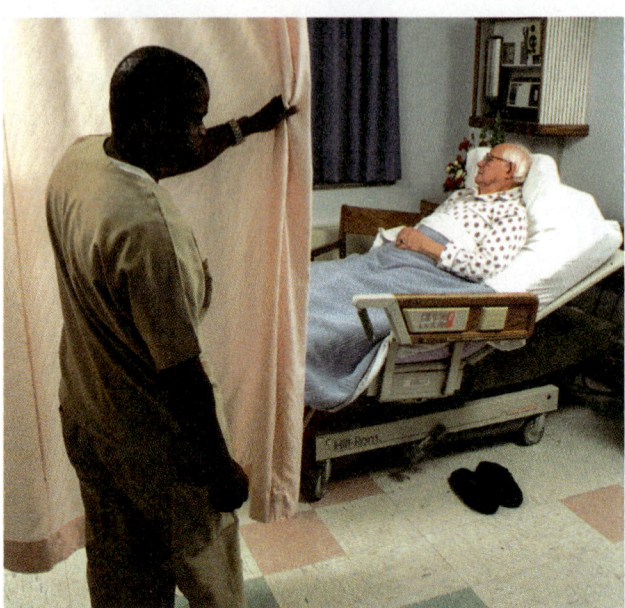

FIGURE 31-7 The dying patient needs privacy, but not total solitude.

- Show the family where they can use a telephone in private.
- If a family member stays during the night, offer a pillow and blanket. Some facilities provide recliners or cots for family members.
- Avoid being judgmental of family members. Remember that each person grieves in his or her own way. The emotions that others see are not necessarily an accurate indication of what the individual is feeling.

HOSPICE CARE

Hospice care has evolved around the philosophy that death is a natural process that should neither be hastened nor delayed and that the dying person should be kept comfortable. Hospice care is:

- Provided to terminally ill people with a life expectancy of six months or less
- Involved with direct physical care when needed
- Supportive to both the family and the patient
- Provided in special hospice facilities, in other care facilities, and at home
- Largely carried out by a home health assistant or a nursing assistant under the direction of professional health care providers
- Follow-up bereavement counseling to help survivors accept the death of a loved one
- A program in which volunteers play an important role, making regular personal visits to the patient and family

Hospice care is provided by teams who work in conjunction with the terminally ill person and his family. The team usually consists of a physician, professional nurse, nursing

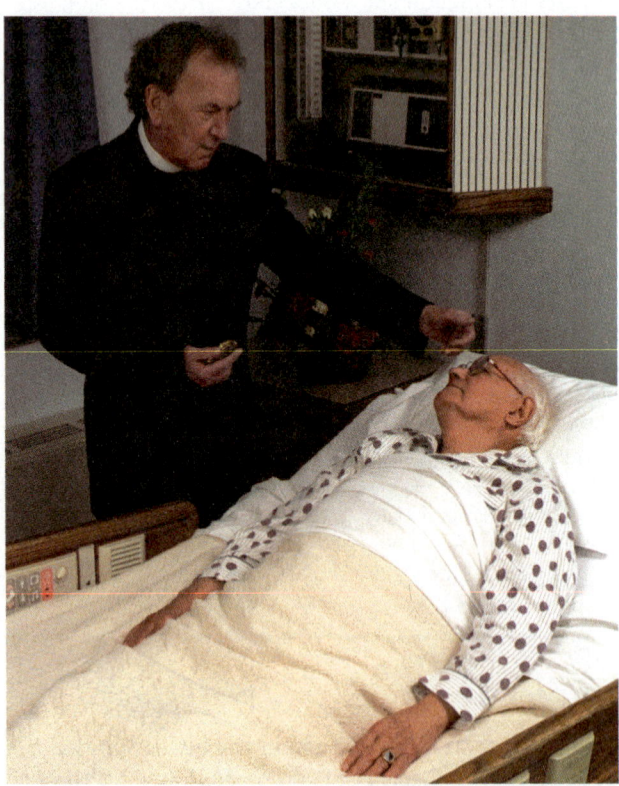

FIGURE 31-6 The Sacrament of the Sick may be administered to Roman Catholics who are gravely ill.

assistant, and other professionals (such as social workers and clergy) as needed and desired.

The goals of hospice care include:

- Control of pain so the individual can remain an active participant in life until death
- Coordinating psychological, spiritual, and social support services for the patient and the family
- Making legal and financial counseling available to the patient and family

Because hospice care is a philosophy, it becomes part of the guide for your actions when caring for the terminally ill. Hospice care is provided as you give your usual care. Some things to keep in mind, however, are:

- Report pain immediately and give close attention to comfort measures.
- Encourage the person to carry out as much self-care as possible.
- Be readily available to listen. Spend as much time with the patient as possible and desired by the patient.
- Get to know the family and be supportive to them.
- Give the same care you would if a terminal diagnosis had not been made.
- Carry out all activities with dignity and respect.

PHYSICAL CHANGES AS DEATH APPROACHES

As death approaches, there are notable physical changes. As these changes occur, report them immediately to the charge nurse.

- The patient becomes less responsive (Figure 31-8).
- Body functions slow down.
- The patient loses general voluntary and involuntary muscle control.
- The patient may involuntarily void and defecate.
- The jaw tends to drop.

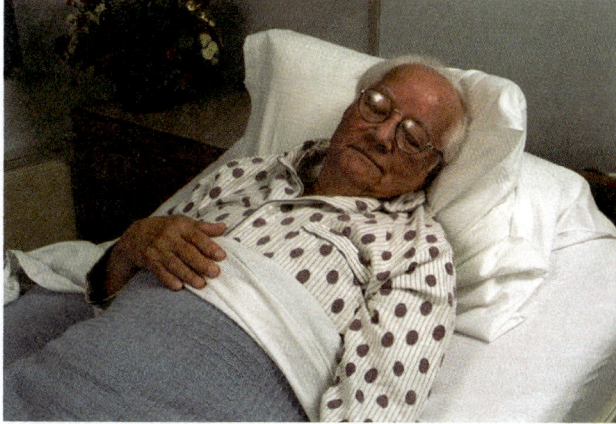

FIGURE 31-8 The patient becomes less responsive and body functions slow down as death approaches.

- Breathing becomes irregular and shallow.
- Circulation slows and the extremities become cold. The pulse becomes rapid and progressively weaker.
- Skin pales.
- The eyes stare and do not respond to light.
- Hearing seems to be the last sense to be lost. Do not assume that because death is approaching, the patient can no longer hear. You must be careful what you say.

In the period before death, the patient with a terminal diagnosis needs and receives the same care as the patient who is expected to recover. Attention is paid to physical as well as emotional needs.

As it becomes clear that death will occur very soon, you should call the nurse, who will supervise the care during the final moments of life.

Signs of Death

After death, changes continue to take place in the body. These changes are called **moribund** (dying) changes.

- Pupils become permanently dilated.
- There is no pulse or respiration.
- Heat is gradually lost from the body.
- The patient may urinate, defecate, or release flatus.
- Blood pools in the lowest areas of the body, giving a purplish discoloration to those areas.
- Within 2 to 4 hours, body rigidity, called **rigor mortis**, develops.
- Unless embalmed within 24 hours, there is indication of progressive protein breakdown.

POSTMORTEM CARE

The patient's body should be treated with respect at all times. Before death occurs, the limbs should be straightened and the head elevated on a pillow. The body should be cleaned by gently washing it with warm water. Discharges must be washed off and wiped away.

Care of the body after death is called **postmortem care** (Figure 31-9). This may be your responsibility. You may find it easier if you ask a coworker to assist.

- Use gloves when giving postmortem care. The body may continue to be infectious following death.
- Treat the body with the same dignity you would a living person.
- Some facilities prefer to have the patient left alone until the mortuary staff arrive. Your responsibility will be only to prepare the body for viewing by the family.
- Check the hospital procedure manual before proceeding with postmortem care.

The contents of morgue kits vary (Figure 31-10), but they usually include:

- A shroud of some kind (paper or cloth)

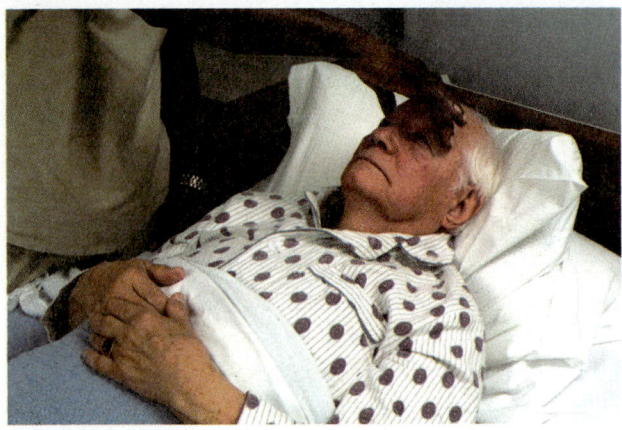

FIGURE 31-9 Postmortem care is given after death occurs.

- A clean gown
- Tags used to identify the body
- Gauze squares for padding
- Safety pins

One procedure for postmortem care is described here (refer to Procedure 94). See also Figure 31-11 for instructions on using a shroud.

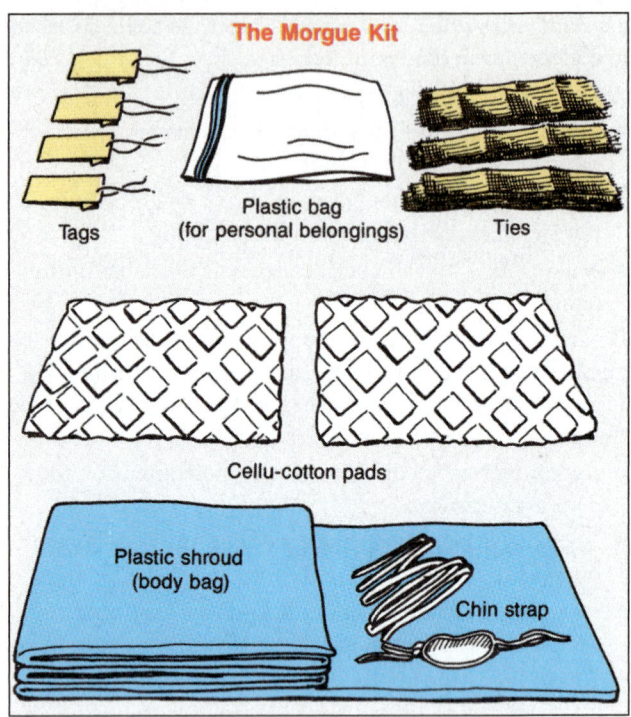

FIGURE 31-10 Supplies needed for postmortem care.

PROCEDURE 94

GIVING POSTMORTEM CARE

1. Carry out beginning procedure actions.

2. Assemble equipment:
   - shroud or clean sheet
   - basin with warm water
   - washcloth
   - towels
   - disposable gloves
   - identification tags
   - cotton
   - bandages
   - pads as needed

3. Put on disposable gloves.

4. Remove all appliances, tubing, and used articles, if instructed to do so.

5. Work quickly and quietly; maintain an attitude of respect.

6. With the bed flat, place the body on the back, with head and shoulders elevated on a pillow.

   a. Close the eyes by grasping the eyelashes, gently pulling the eyelids down, and holding shut for a few seconds.

   b. Replace dentures in the patient's mouth, if used. Replace an artificial eye, if used.

   c. The jaw may have to be secured with light bandaging.

   d. Pad beneath the bandage. Handle the body gently, as tight bandaging or undue pressure from your hands may leave marks.

   e. Straighten the arms and legs and place the arms at the sides.

7. Bathe as necessary. Remove any soiled dressings and replace with clean ones. Groom hair.

8. Place a disposable pad underneath the buttocks. If the family is to view the body:

   a. Put a clean hospital gown on the patient.

   b. Cover the body to the shoulders with a sheet.

   c. Remove disposable gloves and wash your hands.

continues

PROCEDURE 94

continued

   d. Make sure the room is neat.

   e. Adjust the lights to a subdued level.

   f. Provide chairs for the family.

   g. Allow the family to visit in private.

9. Return to the patient's room after the family leaves. Wash your hands and put on disposable gloves.

10. Collect all belongings and make a list. Wrap properly and label. Valuables remain in the hospital safe until they are signed for by a relative.

11. Fill out the identification cards or tags in the morgue kit and attach them as follows:

   a. Place one card on the right ankle or right great toe.

   b. Attach one card to the bag with the patient's valuables.

12. Put the shroud on the patient and attach an identification card or tag to the outside.

13. Transport the body to the morgue.

   a. Call an elevator to the floor and keep it empty.

   b. Close patient corridor doors.

   c. Empty the corridor.

   d. With an assistant, place the body on a gurney.

   e. Keep the patient supine, with a rubber head elevator under the neck.

   f. Cover the body with a sheet.

   g. Remove disposable gloves and discard according to facility policy. Wash your hands.

   h. Take the body to the morgue.

   i. Attach one identification card or tag to the morgue compartment.

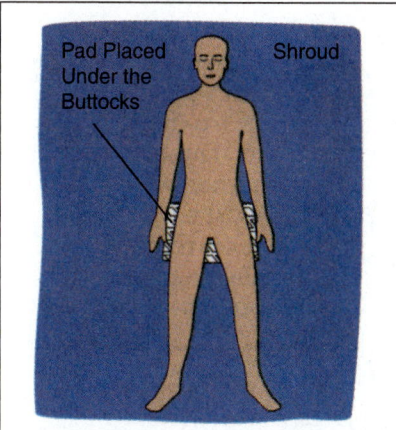

FIGURE 31-11A Position the shroud under the deceased with the pad under the buttocks.

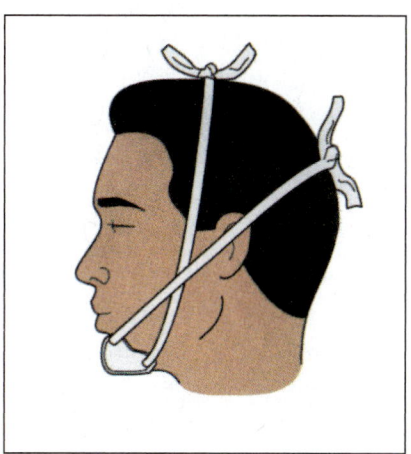

FIGURE 31-11B Apply the chin strap as shown to keep the mouth closed.

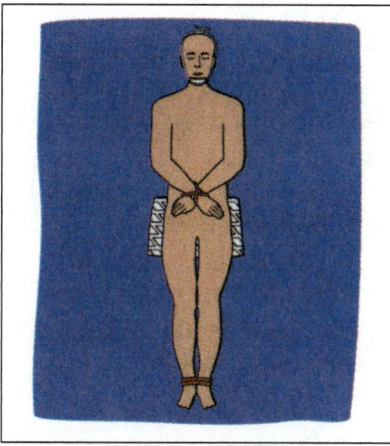

FIGURE 31-11C Fasten the wrists and ankles together with the ties. Use gauze sponges under the ties so they do not make marks on the skin.

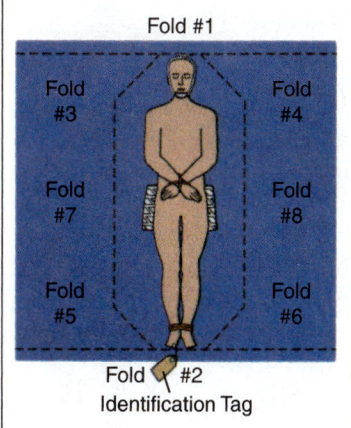

FIGURE 31-11D Fill out and attach four identification tags. Place one tag on the:
- right big toe or right ankle
- outside of the shroud
- patient's personal belongings (securely wrapped)
- compartment in the morgue

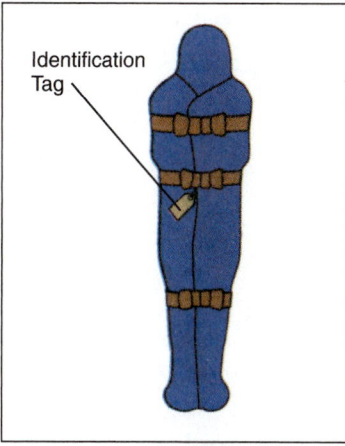

FIGURE 31-11E Fold the shroud around the body as shown. Use the long ties or tape to hold the shroud closed. Fasten a tag to the outside of the shroud.

ORGAN DONATIONS

Some people desire to share their organs with others after death. They use an organ donor card that is part of the driver's license. The card specifies if particular organs or the whole body is being donated. At times, because of a special need, the patient's family is asked for permission so that certain body organs may be removed and saved or removed and harvested (reused). Such a request is made by the physician or the nurse, never by the nursing assistant.

If the patient or family make their wishes known to you without your asking, it is important to report this to the nurse.

POSTMORTEM EXAMINATION (AUTOPSY)

In certain situations, the law requires a medical postmortem examination or autopsy of the body. At other times, the family and physician may desire such an examination to understand the reasons for the patient's death. It is possible that information learned from the examination can be used to protect other family members. As in the case of organ donations, however, requesting family permission for an autopsy is not part of the nursing assistant's responsibilities. The nursing assistant is responsible for being supportive of the family and the decision that has been made.

REVIEW

A. True/False.

Mark the following true or false by circling T or F.

1. T **F** All people respond to a terminal diagnosis in the same way.
2. T **F** Hearing is the first sense to be lost in the dying patient.
3. **T** F Death is the final stage of life.
4. T **F** The nursing assistant should call the physician when the patient dies.
5. **T** F Sometimes the staff, without realizing it, allow the patient to learn of a terminal diagnosis through their behavior.
6. **T** F The dying patient receives the same complete care that would be given to someone expected to recover.
7. **T** F The hospice philosophy has pain relief as one of its goals.
8. **T** F Permanent dilation of the pupils is a moribund sign.
9. T **F** Hospice-type care is only possible in the acute care facility.
10. **T** F The dying person needs a great deal of understanding and realistic support.

B. Matching.

Choose the correct word from Column II to match each phrase or statement in Column I.

Column I

11. _c_ refusal to accept reality
12. _e_ after death
13. _f_ covering for the body after death
14. _b_ stiffening of the body after death
15. _a_ dying

Column II

a. moribund
b. rigor mortis
c. denial
d. hospice
e. postmortem
f. shroud
g. anger

C. Multiple Choice.

Select the one best answer for each of the following.

16. Organs from a dead person may be
    a. harvested without permission.
    b. obtained on an as-needed basis.
    c. donated with permission of the family at the time of death.
    d. donated only if listed in the patient's will.

17. Postmortem examinations
    a. are never performed.
    b. may provide valuable information.
    c. are arranged by the nursing assistant.
    d. are forbidden by law.

18. As death approaches, changes include
    a. constriction of the pupils.
    b. muscle spasm.
    c. slowing of circulation.
    d. skin develops a yellow hue.

19. Moribund changes include
   a. permanent pupil constriction.
   b. increased body heat.
   c. pulse and respiration increase.
   d. blood pools in the lower body.

20. A "no-code" order on a patient's chart means
   a. to start CPR immediately.
   b. do not resuscitate.
   c. begin postmortem care at once.
   d. to call the family if the patient seems in danger of dying.

D. Nursing Assistant Challenge.

Mrs. Goldstein is a patient in the hospital where you work. She was diagnosed with cancer of the ovaries two years ago. She has been at home but is admitted periodically for chemotherapy. You have taken care of her each time she has been in the hospital. The first time was right after Mrs. Goldstein was diagnosed. She seemed happy and made frequent comments like, "I'm glad I don't have cancer." The last time she was a patient, she refused to follow the suggestions of the nursing staff, but did allow her chemotherapy to be administered. When her family visited, she was irritated and hostile toward them. This time, she is agreeable with the staff on all matters and seems genuinely happy to see her family. She has told you that if she can live to see her granddaughter get married in two months, she will become a volunteer at the hospital so she can help other patients. She is not receiving chemotherapy anymore because the cancer is in an advanced stage. She is hospitalized for pain management now but plans to go home for hospice care. Consider these questions about Mrs. Goldstein:

21. Do you think she is preparing for her death?

22. How would you describe the stages of dying she has been experiencing?

23. What response is appropriate to her comments about the wedding?

24. Do you think hospice care will benefit Mrs. Goldstein? Give reasons for your answer.

25. Mrs. Goldstein is Jewish. What considerations must you give to her postmortem care?

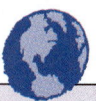

EXPLORING THE WEB

5 pts.

★ tell how you would care for a patient who has died when you come on duty/shift? postmortem care

Description	Location
Care of the dying patient	http://ccm-l.med.edu
Hospice and home care resources	http://www.growthhouse.org
Hospice Patient's Bill of Rights	http://www.hospice-america.org
Loss, grief, and death	http://www.delmarhealthcare.com/olcs/white/pnotes.asp (see Chapter 17)
	http://www.delmarhealthcare.com/olcs/whiteduncan/pnotes.asp (see Chapter 9)
Principles for end-of-life care	http://www.milbank.org
Resources for end-of-life care	http://www.public-health.uiowa.edu
Compassion in Dying	http://www.compassionindying.org
Hospice and Palliative Care Nurses Association	http://www.hpna.org
Last Acts	http://www.lastacts.org
National Hospice and Palliative Care Organization	http://www.nhpco.org
Nursing Specialties Hospice Nursing	http://allnurses.com
Oncology Nursing Society	http://www.ons.org
Partnership for Caring	http://www.partnershipforcaring.org
Project Grace	http://www.p-grace.org

Other Health Care Settings

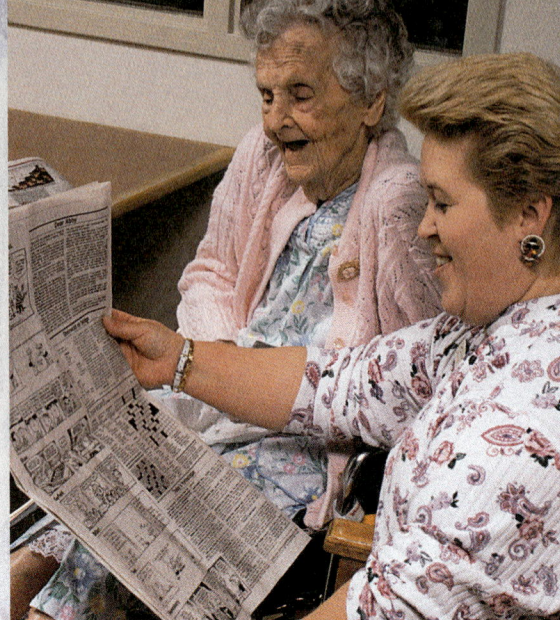

Care of the Elderly and Chronically Ill

objectives

After completing this unit, you will be able to:

- Spell and define terms.
- List the federal requirements for nursing assistants working in long-term care facilities.
- Identify the expected changes of aging.
- Identify residents who are at risk of malnutrition and list measures to promote adequate food intake.
- Explain why elderly individuals are at risk of dehydration and list nursing assistant actions to prevent dehydration.

- List the actions a nursing assistant can take to prevent infections in the long-term care facility.
- Define delirium. List potential causes and signs and symptoms of delirium to report.
- Recognize unsafe conditions in the long-term care facility.
- Describe actions to use when working with residents who have dementia.
- Describe the management of wandering residents.

vocabulary

Learn the meaning and the correct spelling of the following words and phrases:

Alzheimer's disease	dementia	intermediate care	skilled care
animal-assisted therapy	diverticula	long-term care	subacute care
assisted living	diverticulitis	music therapy	sundowning
catastrophic reaction	diverticulosis	pigmentation	superimpose
chronologic	eloping	reality orientation	validation therapy
debilitating	flatulence	reminiscing	vitality
delirium	hand-over-hand technique	residents	
		sepsis	

INTRODUCTION

Many individuals require continuing health care (Figure 32-1). These individuals are frequently elderly. This is because as people age, their risk of acquiring a chronic disease increases. A young person may also require continuing care for a chronic illness or severe injury. Persons of any age who are chronically ill or severely injured may require **long-term care**. This care is provided either in the patient's home or in a long-term care facility. This unit provides information about caring for the elderly and working in a long-term care facility. Units 33 and 34 will teach you about home care.

Nursing assistants are valuable members of the health care team in these facilities (Figure 32-2). The skills you use in acute care facilities, such as hospitals, are also used in long-term care facilities. There are some changes in the application of these skills because of the differences between long-term and acute care.

TYPES OF LONG-TERM CARE FACILITIES

Many types of facilities provide health care for persons with ongoing medical problems:

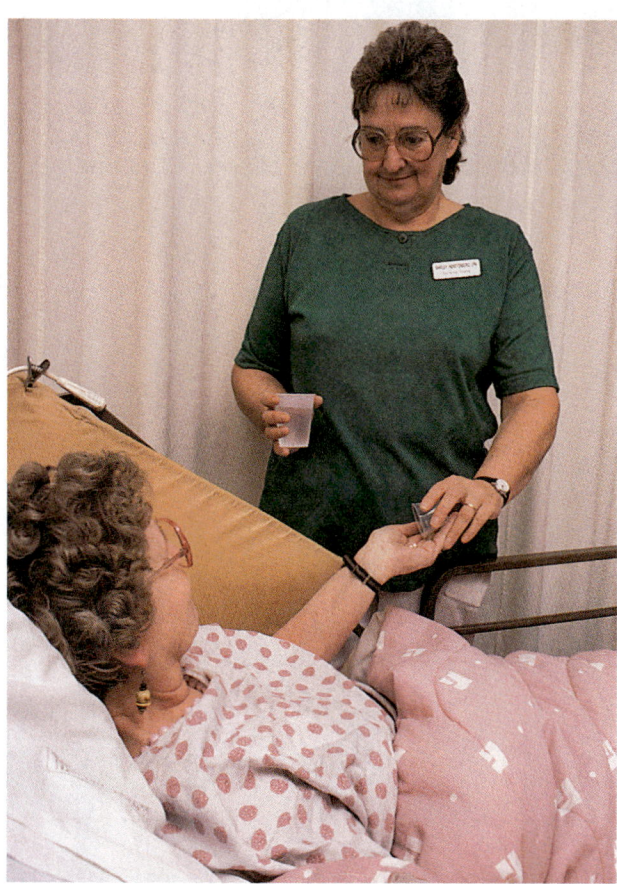

FIGURE 32-1 People of all ages need continuing health care.

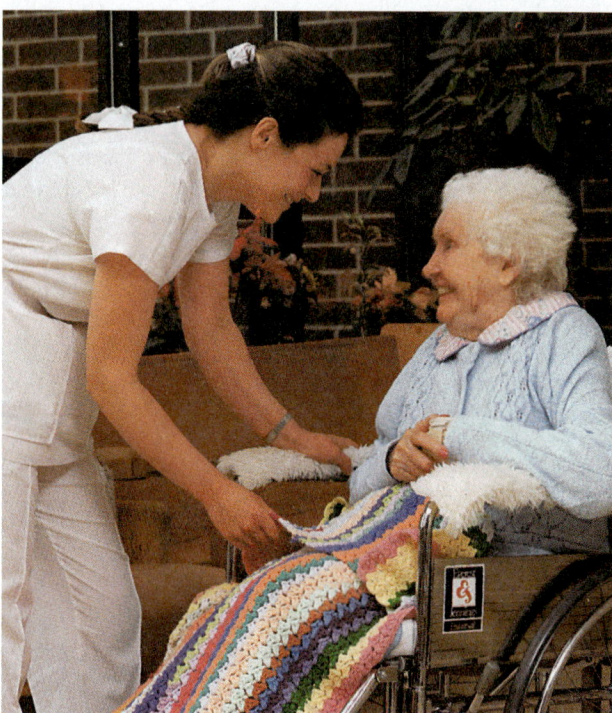

FIGURE 32-2 Nursing assistants are valuable caregivers in long-term care facilities.

- **Assisted living** is designed for persons who need minimal assistance. The assisted living residence does not provide medical or nursing care. Residents receive daily supervision or assistance with activities of daily living and instrumental activities of daily living. The facility also coordinates services by outside agencies, and monitors the activities of the residents to ensure their health, safety, and well-being.

- **Intermediate care** is available for people who have health problems that are stable and who need assistance with activities of daily living. These facilities are designed for individuals with chronic conditions who are unable to live independently, but do not need constant care. Such a facility provides supportive care and nursing supervision under medical direction 24 hours per day, but not continuous nursing care.

- **Skilled care** facilities are licensed to provide care to persons with chronic health problems or who require specialized nursing care. Skilled facilities provide the most intensive level of care on the residential care continuum. Residents of these facilities have 24-hour nursing needs or complex medical care demands. Some are chronically ill and can no longer live independently.

Some skilled care facilities have units called **subacute care**. The subacute care unit may provide services to persons who need rehabilitation, special cancer treatments, wound care, or pain management. Subacute care is discussed in Unit 35. Subacute care units may also be located in some hospitals.

Long-term care facilities used to be called *nursing homes*. The long-term care facilities of today bear little resemblance to those of the past. Employees must participate in staff development to maintain and update the knowledge and skills that are required to meet the needs of the consumers.

Some long-term care facilities specialize in the care of people with a specific diagnosis or unusual care needs. Some are licensed to care only for children. The majority care for adults with various diagnoses and problems.

One important issue facing our country today is the financing of long-term health care. Few hospital insurance policies cover expenses of a resident in a long-term care facility. Insurance specifically for long-term care is now available. People who pay for care from private funds may find that their money is soon used up.

Medicaid is a government reimbursement system through which the federal government issues money to the states. The states determine how to distribute the money to health care facilities. These funds are used for the care of people who have no money of their own.

Medicare is another government program that partially pays for health care for persons over the age of 65 or who are permanently disabled. However, Medicare covers only limited long-term care expenses.

These funds are available only to facilities that participate in the Medicaid and Medicare programs.

LONG-TERM CARE POPULATION

People living in long-term care facilities are usually called residents. This is because the facility is considered their home as well as a place to receive health care. Many admissions are permanent, but some residents are able to go home or to a less restrictive environment.

Residents are admitted to skilled-care facilities because they have problems that require ongoing monitoring and health care. They are not admitted just because they are old. The problems of residents are a result of a disease process and are not a natural part of aging. Most facilities also have younger residents who are mentally or physically disabled due to chronic disease or injuries (Figure 32-3).

The number of people requiring long-term care is growing rapidly, for several reasons:

● There are more people alive today.
● More people are living longer (Figure 32-4).
● Modern science has enabled people to recover from illnesses or injuries that would have been fatal in the past.

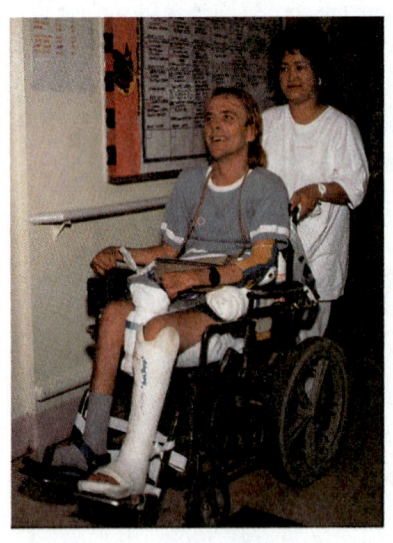

FIGURE 32-3 Most facilities also have young residents.

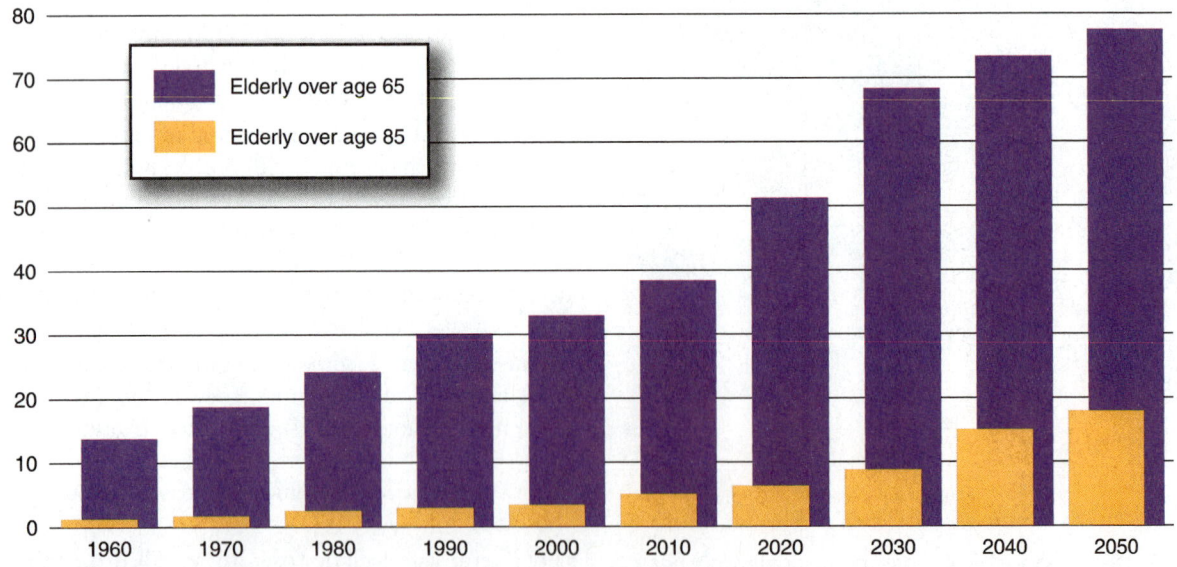

Elderly Population (in Millions) 1960 to 2050

Legend:
- Elderly over age 65
- Elderly over age 85

FIGURE 32-4 The number of elderly is increasing rapidly. *(Source: U.S. Bureau of the Census)*

- The longer a person lives, the greater the risk of acquiring a chronic, degenerative disease.
- Families are unable to provide care because of geographic distances or because everyone in the family is employed.

Here are some examples of residents in a long-term care facility:

- Rose Johnson is 78 years old and had surgery in the hospital to repair a fractured hip. She is receiving rehabilitation to learn how to walk correctly on her affected leg. She will go back to her own home after the rehabilitation is completed.
- Antony Donali is 86 years old and has Alzheimer's disease. He wanders and paces constantly, and has poor safety judgment and awareness. He is incontinent of urine, and needs supervision to ensure that he eats his meals. His family can no longer provide the 24-hour attention that he needs. He will remain in the facility for the rest of his life.
- Ted McMurry is 47 years old and has cancer of the lung. He is receiving chemotherapy. He may be able to go home after finishing the therapy unless his condition worsens.
- Jill Green is 18 years old and suffered severe, permanent head injuries in a motorcycle accident. She will never be able to care for herself and will need 24-hour-a-day care for the rest of her life. She will probably remain in the facility for this care.

- Tom Hernandez is 35 years old and has had multiple sclerosis for 10 years. The disease has progressed to the point where Tom can no longer care for himself. He will probably remain in the facility.
- Sara Pembkoski is 64 years old and has had a stroke. She is receiving intensive rehabilitation and hopes to return home. If she is not able to do so, she will be transferred to an assisted living facility.

The percentage of persons living in long-term care facilities is only 1 percent for those 65 to 74 years of age. However, this increases to 22 percent for people 85 years and older. As people grow older, the consequences of chronic disease increase. Varying degrees of functional deficits (disabilities) result. Therefore, the person requires assistance in performing the activities of daily living (Figure 32-5).

LEGISLATION AFFECTING LONG-TERM CARE

Federal legislation has mandated improvements in the quality of long-term care. This legislation is called the Nursing Home Reform Act. It is the result of the Omnibus Budget Reconciliation Act of 1987 (OBRA). Each state is responsible for implementing this legislation.

The OBRA regulations require facilities to assist residents to attain and maintain the highest level of mental, physical, and psychosocial well-being possible in their individual

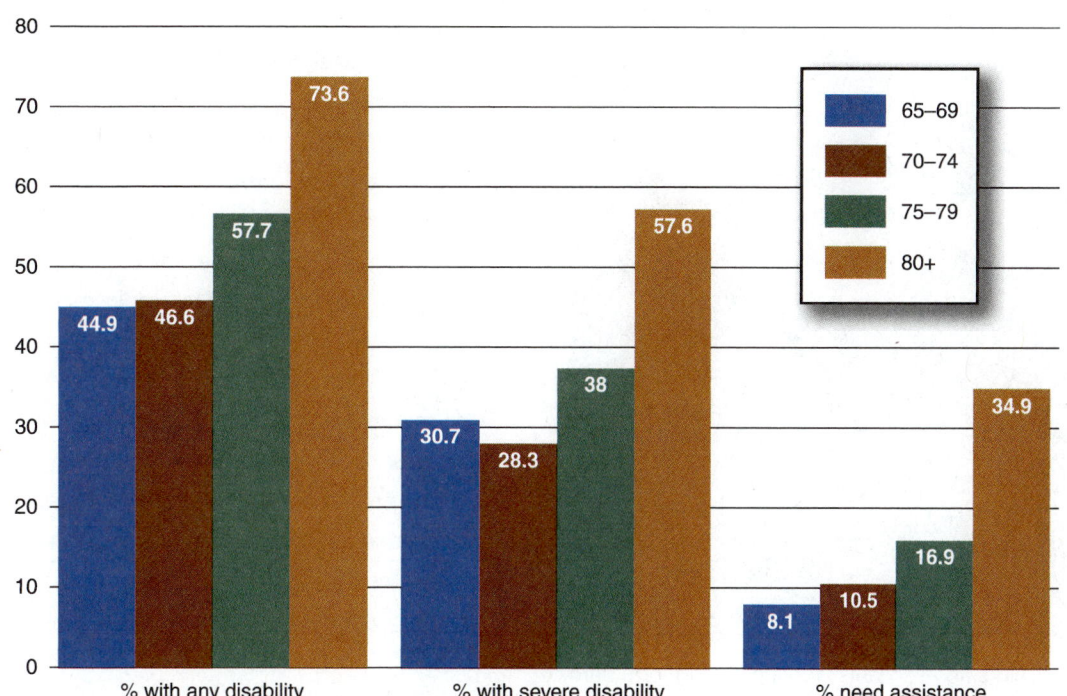

Percent with Disabilities, by Age

FIGURE 32-5 A profile of older Americans in 2001. *(Source: Administration on Aging; http://www.aoa.dhhs.gov/aoa/stats/profile/2001/12.html)*

circumstances. Care must be provided in a home-like environment.

Much of the OBRA content affects nursing assistants directly or indirectly:

- OBRA requires all nursing assistants working in long-term care to complete a course of at least 75 clock hours. The course must be approved by the state agency appointed to oversee OBRA regulations. Many states require more than the minimum of 75 hours.

- After completing the course, written and manual (skills) competency tests must be passed. The tests may be taken three times.

- Nursing assistants must complete specific hours of in-service education (12 hours) per year (Figure 32-6). (Some states may require more.)

- Nursing assistants who are not employed as such for 24 months must repeat the course or competency tests.

Federal regulations specify the content that must be included in a nursing assistant course:

- Residents' rights
- Communication and interpersonal skills
- Infection control
- Safety and emergency procedures

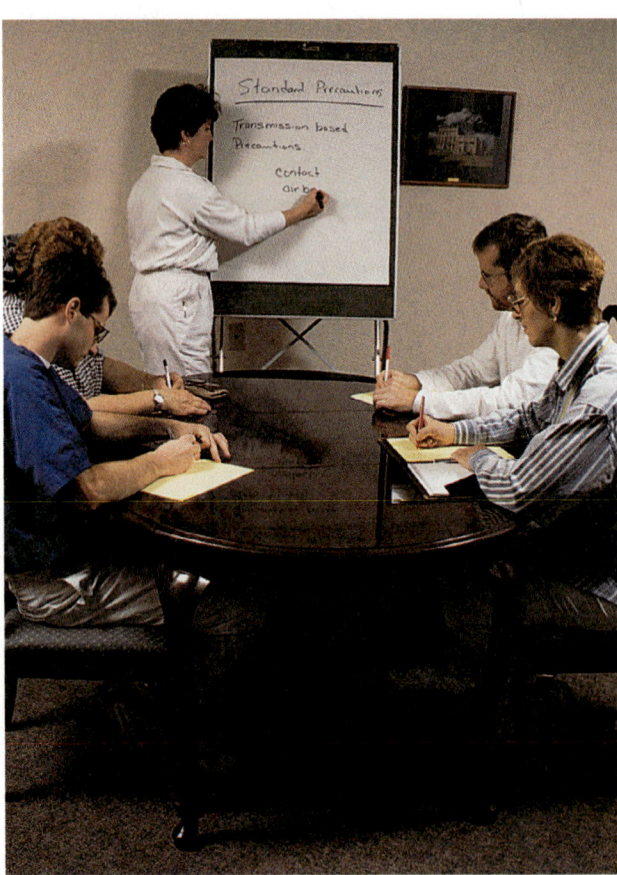

FIGURE 32-6 Nursing assistants working in long-term care facilities must complete at least 12 hours of in-service education each year.

LEGAL *Alert*

OBRA nursing assistant requirements apply only to long-term care facilities, including those in a hospital, such as the skilled nursing unit. The federal requirements do not apply to acute care hospitals, although many have voluntarily adopted the nursing assistant education as the minimum entry standard for employment.

- Basic nursing skills
- Personal care skills
- Mental health and social service needs
- Care of residents with Alzheimer's disease or other dementias
- Basic restorative services

These topics are covered in other units of this textbook. This chapter provides specific information about long-term care and OBRA requirements.

LEGAL *Alert*

All states have developed nursing assistant rules based on the federal requirements. Some states exceed the federal requirements and have additional rules for nursing assistants. Become familiar with the rules and agency regulating nursing assistant practice in your state. Many of these maintain Web sites, and information is readily available online. If a nursing assistant has completed a training and competency evaluation program prior to employment, the facility must check with the nursing assistant registry in all states in which the assistant has worked to verify that the registration is active and that there are no reports of abuse or neglect. The facility must conduct an annual performance review of each nursing assistant. In-service education programs will be developed based on the results of this review. Programs will address areas of weakness and special needs of residents in the facility.

ROLE OF THE NURSING ASSISTANT IN A SKILLED CARE FACILITY

As in the acute care facility, the nursing assistant carries out the procedures as taught, assisting in the health care of residents under the direct supervision of a nurse. Basic physical care, as well as special procedures, is done to help these residents reach their maximum degree of well-being.

To be successful in this setting, you must:

- be patient and caring.
- understand the character of the older age group.
- be able to care for persons who may be your own age and have chronic illnesses.
- be comfortable with the thought of your own aging.
- have the stamina to provide the assistance needed by the residents.
- be able to derive satisfaction from being part of slow progress and small, if any, gains.
- have a sense of humor.
- be able to communicate effectively (Figure 32-7).

These attributes are important in any health setting, but in the long-term care facility they are essential.

Many of the residents will remain under your care for long periods of time, even for years. You will develop relationships that become important to both caregiver and care receiver. In those circumstances, communications take on greater importance. Greater significance may be attached to the attention to care or even the way thoughts are expressed in words. Thus, the long-term caregiver is a *very special person* who works in an important area of health care.

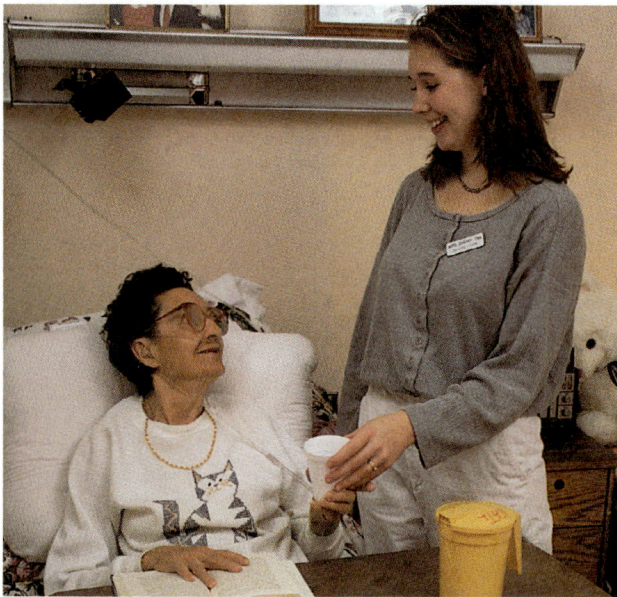

FIGURE 32-7 Persons working in long-term care must have excellent communication skills.

EFFECTS OF AGING

Many residents in the long-term facility are advanced in age and have one or more chronic, somewhat **debilitating** (weakening) conditions. Some are mentally alert. Others are confused and disoriented.

There are, however, some features of aging that are characteristic of most elderly residents. Do not expect every resident to exhibit the same characteristics at the same **chronologic** (year) age. Remember that aging is a natural, progressive process that begins at birth and extends to death. Remember also that every resident is unique and must be treated with dignity and respect.

Physical Changes in Aging

Some investigators believe we are born with a biological time clock. This clock is programmed for a specific life span, barring accidents and disease. As we move toward old age, changes that have been taking place gradually become more evident. For example, the elderly person:

- May lose vitality.
- May sleep less at night.
- May benefit from rest periods during the day.
- Stores less fluid in body tissue and is apt to become dehydrated. This results in a loss of elasticity and resiliency in tissues.
- Has fibrous tissue changes. These decrease the tone, mass, and strength of skeletal and smooth muscle.
- Has secretory and endocrine cells that become less functional and reduced nerve sensitivity.

Certain changes occur in every body system. These are listed in Table 32-1. They do not necessarily occur at the same rate in each system.

AGE-APPROPRIATE CARE *Alert*

You may find that caring for elderly individuals is time-consuming. Aging changes may cause the person to move more slowly than he or she did previously. Do not complete tasks that residents can do themselves, just for the sake of saving time. Avoid assuming that the resident cannot do something because of physical or mental problems related to aging. Test his or her ability, without making assumptions. Be patient and encourage independence, according to the care plan.

TABLE 32-1 PHYSICAL CHANGES OF AGING

Body System	Physical Changes
Integumentary	• Hair loses color and becomes thinner • Skin dries, becomes less elastic; wrinkles develop • Skin is fragile and tears easily • Bruises easily (senile purpura common) • Reduced blood flow in vessels that nourish the skin results in delayed healing • Fingernails and toenails thicken • Sweat glands do not excrete perspiration as readily • Oil glands do not secrete as much oil • There is increased sensitivity to cold • Skin discolorations (age spots) become more common • Blood supply to the feet and legs is reduced, increasing the risk of injury and ulcers, and sensations of cold
Nervous	• Tasks involving speed, balance, coordination, and fine motor activities take longer because of slowed transmission of nerve impulses • Balance and coordination problems result from deterioration in the nerve terminals that provide information to the brain about body movement and position • Temperature regulation is less effective • Deep sleep is shortened; the person awakens more during the night • Brain cells are lost, but intelligence remains intact unless disease is present • Decreased sensitivity of nerve receptors in skin (heat, cold, pain, pressure) • Risk of injury increases because of decreased ability to feel pressure and temperature changes • There is decreased blood flow to the brain, which may result in mental confusion and memory loss
Sensory	• More difficult to see close objects • Night vision may decrease • Cataracts (clouding of the lens of the eye) are more common • Dryness and itching of the eyes may result from decreased secretion of fluids • Side vision and depth perception diminish • Hearing diminishes in most elderly persons • Smell receptors and taste buds become less sensitive, so foods have less taste
Musculoskeletal	• Loss of elasticity of muscles and decrease in size of muscle mass result in reduced strength, flexibility, endurance, muscle tone, and delayed reaction time • Slower movements • Bones lose minerals, become brittle, and break more easily; arthritis and osteoporosis are common • Spine becomes less stable and flexible, increasing the risk of injury • Posture may become slumped because of weakness in back muscles • Degenerative changes in the joints result in limited movement, stiffness, and pain
Respiratory	• Lung capacity decreases as a result of muscular rigidity in the lungs • Coughing is less effective; this results in pooling of secretions and fluid in the lungs, increasing the risk of infection and choking • Shortness of breath on exertion, as a result of aging changes in the lungs • Gas exchange in the lungs is less effective, resulting in decreased oxygenation

continues

TABLE 32-1 *continued*

Body System	Physical Changes
Urinary	• Kidneys decrease in size • Urine production is less efficient • Bladder capacity decreases, increasing the frequency of urination • Kidney function increases at rest, causing increased urination at night • Bladder muscles weaken, causing leaking of urine or inability to empty the bladder completely; complete emptying of bladder becomes more difficult • Enlargement of the prostate gland in the male, causing frequency of urination, dribbling, urinary obstruction, and urinary retention
Digestive	• Saliva production in the mouth decreases, causing difficulty with swallowing and digestion of starches, and increasing risk of tooth decay • Tastebuds on the tongue decrease, beginning with sweet and salt; changes in tastebuds may result in appetite changes and increase in condiment use • Gag reflex is less effective, increasing the risk of choking • Movement of food into the stomach through the esophagus is slower • Food in the stomach is digested slower, so food remains there longer before moving to the small intestine • Flatulence increases • Indigestion and slower absorption of fat result from a decrease in digestive enzymes • Food movement through the large intestine is slower, resulting in constipation
Cardiovascular	• Heart rate slows, causing a slower pulse and less efficient circulation. This results in decreased energy and a slower response, causing the individual to tire easily • Blood vessels lose elasticity and develop calcium deposits, causing vessels to narrow • Blood pressure increases because of changes to the blood vessel walls • Heart rate takes longer to return to normal after exercise • Veins enlarge, causing blood vessels close to the skin surface to become more prominent • Heart may not pump as efficiently, leading to decreased cardiac output and circulation
Endocrine	• Decrease in levels of estrogen, progesterone • Hot flashes, nervous feelings • Higher levels of parathormone and thyroid-stimulating hormone • Delayed release of insulin, increasing blood sugar level; incidence of diabetes increases greatly with age • Metabolism rate and body functions slow, reducing the amount of calories needed for the body to function normally. This increases the risk of overweight and obesity
Reproductive	*Females:* • Fewer female hormones are produced • Ovulation and menstrual cycle cease • Vaginal walls are thinner and drier • Vagina becomes shorter and narrower • Breast tissue decreases and the muscles supporting the breasts weaken *Males:* • Scrotum less firm • Prostate gland may enlarge • Hormone production decreases, decreasing size of testes and lowering sperm count • More time required for an erection

Emotional Adjustments to Aging

Emotional adjustments to aging are basically extensions of the adjustments the individual has made throughout life to the many changes in circumstances. Personality characteristics and ways of reacting to stress are developed fairly early in life and tend to become a constant in an individual's personality. In fact, as a person ages, personality traits become even more pronounced. The stress produced by the circumstances and illnesses that accompany old age do not drastically alter the individual's personality, but they do tend to magnify, and in some cases distort, the basic traits.

Old people have the same emotional needs and require the same supports for good mental health as young people (Figure 32-8). They need:

- to be loved.
- to have a sense of self-worth.
- to feel a sense of achievement and recognition.
- to have a degree of economic security.

Although these needs are common to all human beings, regardless of age, the means of achieving satisfaction and gratification of these needs are greatly reduced for older people. The opportunities for social exchange and sexual expression, the two major means of gratification, are lessened as the years advance. The need for them does not change, however.

The attitude of the Western world toward old people tends to relegate (place) them to positions of lesser and lesser significance. The older people become, the more their self-image is depreciated (devalued), both in their own eyes and in the eyes of others.

Physical ailments, far more common in the elderly because of slowed body processes, are **superimposed** (layered on top of) upon the changes brought about by the natural aging process. Change of body image and loss of the vigor

and **vitality** (lively character) of former years are major losses that older persons must accept—losses that further alter their self-image and self-esteem. The caregiver can make an important contribution by promoting the self-esteem of those being cared for.

In old age, some accommodations must be made in the attitudes or psychological outlooks of all persons. The most healthy emotional responses are based:

- on philosophies that accept aging as a natural progressive stage.
- in life attitudes that recognize the strengths as well as the limitations of the body.
- on a form of behavior that demonstrates interest in living here and now.

Healthy psychological adjustments mean both a realistic appraisal of the present circumstance and building on the positive values while coming to terms with the negative aspects.

Some of your long-term care residents will have already made these adjustments. Some will be in the process. Your supportive caring will be important and helpful to each.

Specific Emotional Responses. The elderly or infirm resident is apt to experience some common emotional responses. Frustration is an emotion frequently felt by the elderly—frustration at physical limitations and at having less control over their own lives. That is why it is important to allow the elderly the opportunity to make as many decisions as possible. Signs of frustration are often demonstrated by:

- Aggressive behavior
- Anger
- Hostility
- Demanding behavior
- Complaining
- Crying

Some residents even resort to manipulating families, staff, or other residents in an attempt to relieve their feelings of helplessness (Figure 32-9).

Anxiety and fear may be expressed in periods of depression and withdrawal. The depression experienced by the elderly is easily understood. In many instances, they:

- are cut off from their social support systems.
- have had to make major adjustments in their lifestyles.
- may have lost loved ones and friends.
- may have very limited finances.
- may truly feel that they no longer have any control over their destinies or even of their day-to-day activities.
- may have stretched their coping ability to the breaking point because of physical weakness and disease processes.

Withdrawal, a common frustration response, is shown by:

- Lack of communication
- Temporary confusion

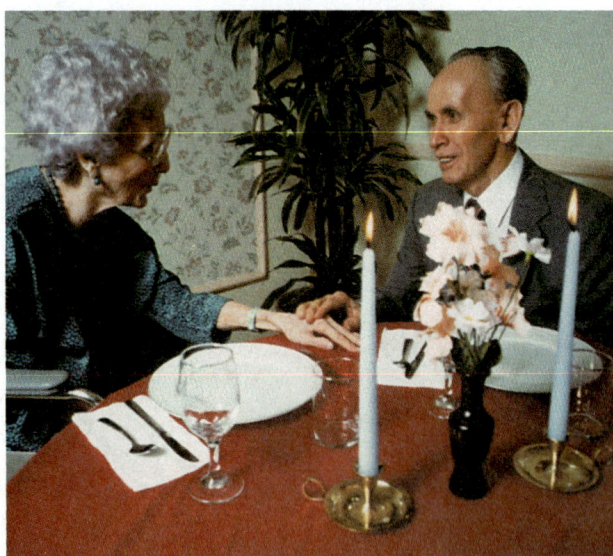

FIGURE 32-8 Older people have the same emotional needs as younger people.

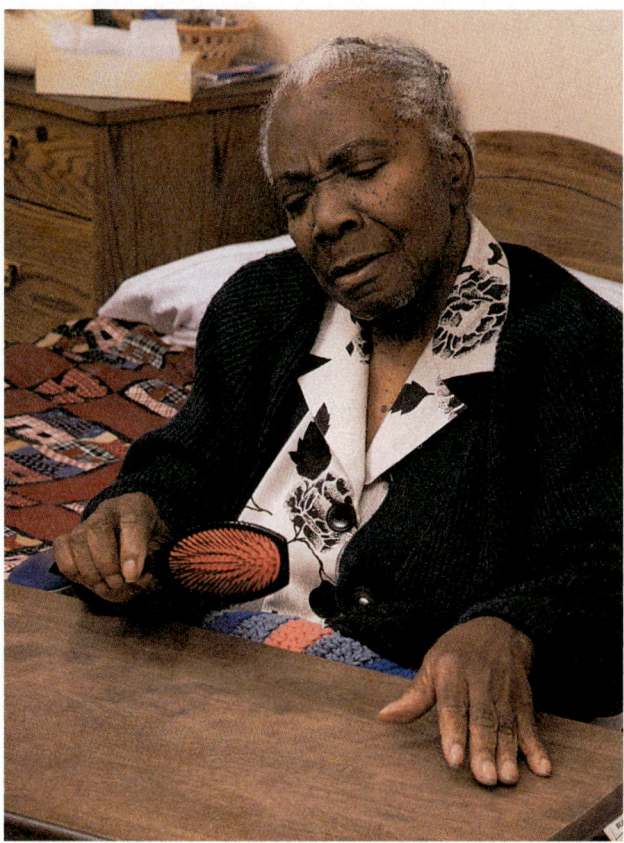

FIGURE 32-9 Residents may exhibit feelings of frustration and anger.

- General disorientation as to time and place

You can play a major role in helping residents move successfully through these periods by:

- reassuring them that they will not be abandoned now that they are no longer able to care for themselves.
- treating each person with respect, to reinforce self-esteem.
- calmly helping your residents keep in touch with reality while conveying your own feelings of compassion and caring.
- reporting changes in behavior, mood swings, and emotional responses to your supervisor so that the entire staff can form a supporting network.
- responding to the residents' negative attitudes by being willing to listen and interact with them and emphasizing the positive.

NUTRITIONAL NEEDS

Malnutrition is a problem for the aged because the older person may develop an apathy toward food that becomes progressive. Malnutrition can and does occur in long-term care facility residents, despite the fact that a balanced diet is served and nutritional supplements are available. Factors that contribute to lack of appetite are:

- Decreased activity
- Inadequate teeth
- Bad dentures
- Decreased saliva
- Diminished smell and taste
- Poor oral hygiene
- Eating alone

The diet for the elderly person should:

- Be easy to chew and digest.
- Contain decreased amounts of refined sugars, fats, and cholesterol.
- Have adequate proteins and vitamins to provide for best bodily function and repair.
- Have many complex carbohydrates, found in fruits, vegetables, and grains (Figure 32-10). These foods are also good sources of vitamins and minerals, which tend to be deficient in the elderly diet.
- Be monitored for weight control. Obesity is a major nutritional problem among the elderly and those who are inactive. The excess weight increases the stress of existing conditions. Calories are generally limited to about 2,000 calories for the average woman and 2,400 to 2,500 calories for the average man.

Because of loss of muscle tone, three intestinal problems are commonly seen. They are:

- Constipation—difficulty in eliminating solid waste
- Flatulence—gas production
- Diverticulosis—small pockets (diverticula) of weakened intestinal wall

Dietary adjustments can help reduce these problems.

- Soft bulk foods, such as whole-grain cereals and fruits and vegetables, are helpful in overcoming constipation.
- Skins and seeds should be avoided to prevent diverticulitis, which is an inflammation of the diverticula.

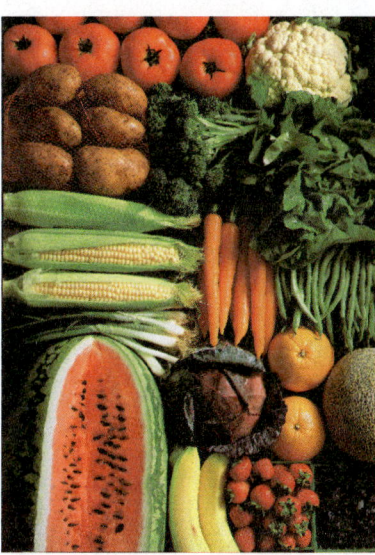

FIGURE 32-10 Elderly people require complex carbohydrates for a healthy diet. *(From: How to Eat for Good Health, Courtesy of National Dairy Council)*

The presentation and service of food are important in stimulating appetites. Keep in mind the following:

- Several smaller meals seem to be more easily tolerated than three large meals.
- Residents should be allowed to feed themselves as much as possible. You may assist by cutting up the food into bite-sized pieces. Even if you must do most of the feeding, allow the resident to participate as much as possible.
- Fruit and vegetable juices, eggnogs, and soups can serve the dual purpose of providing both nourishment and fluids.

Nursing Assistant Actions

Meal time is a very busy time in the long-term care facility, especially on the day shift, when two meals are served. Do not get so busy that you overlook residents who are having difficulty or who are not eating. Residents who are at greatest risk of malnutrition and unintentional weight loss are those who:

- need help eating and drinking (Figure 32-11).
- eat less than half their meals and/or planned snacks.
- have mouth pain.
- have no dentures, or have dentures that do not fit correctly.
- have difficulty chewing or swallowing.
- have difficulty getting utensils or glasses to the mouth.
- cough or choke while eating.
- are sad, have crying spells, or are withdrawn from others.
- are confused, wander, or pace.
- have diabetes, lung disease, cancer, HIV, or other chronic diseases.

To increase food intake and prevent weight loss and malnutrition, create a pleasant, positive dining atmosphere for the residents. Be aware of each resident's self-feeding ability

and changes in eating patterns. Report your observations and changes in residents' conditions and appetite to the nurse. You should also:

- provide oral care before meals.
- position residents correctly for feeding.
- honor food preferences, likes, and dislikes.
- offer substitutes according to facility policy.
- serve meals promptly so foods are at the proper temperature; check foods by dropping a small amount on your wrist (Figure 32-12).
- offer a variety of foods and beverages.
- help residents who are having trouble feeding themselves.
- provide adaptive utensils and dishes, as ordered (Figure 32-13).
- notify nursing staff if a resident has difficulty feeding himself, eating, or using utensils.
- prompt and encourage residents to eat.
- allow enough time for residents to finish eating; avoid rushing.
- reheat cold food items, if necessary.

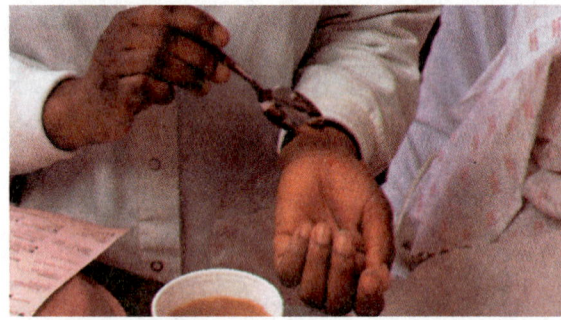

FIGURE 32-12 Serve foods promptly to maintain temperature. Check hot food temperature by dropping a small amount on your wrist.

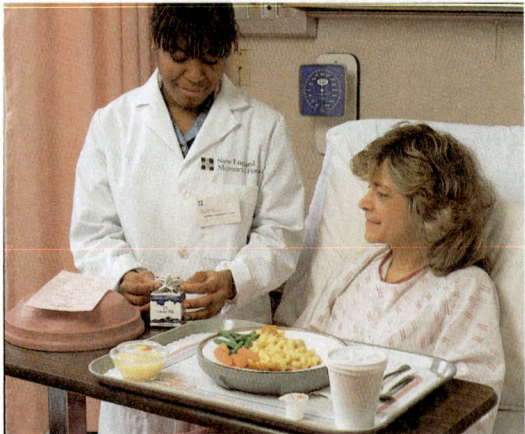

FIGURE 32-11 Assisting residents with meals helps prevent weight loss and malnutrition.

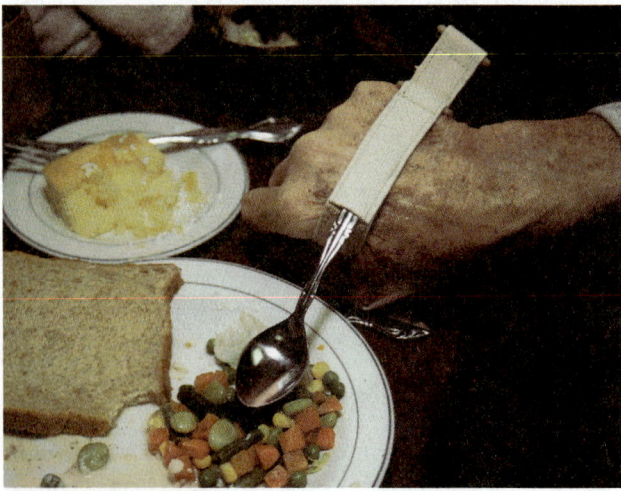

FIGURE 32-13 Adaptive utensils enable residents with physical problems to feed themselves.

- if a resident's appetite decreases, or she seems sad, ask what's wrong.
- accurately record the resident's intake at each meal.
- assist and prompt residents to consume planned, ordered snacks and supplements.

Residents Receiving Tube Feedings

Tube feedings are common treatments in the long-term care facility. Residents receiving tube feedings are also at nutritional risk. Their medical needs sometimes change, and tube-feeding formula and fluid orders must be adjusted to keep up with their bodies' demands. Signs and symptoms that a resident is at risk for or experiencing tube-feeding complications are:

- Nausea
- Vomiting
- Diarrhea
- Swollen stomach
- Constipation
- Excessive flatus, cramping
- Pain, redness, heat, swelling, crusting, or fluid oozing from the site where the feeding tube enters the body
- Cough
- Wet breathing
- Feeling that something is caught in the throat
- Complaints of dryness or discomfort in the mouth or throat
- Pulling at or removing the feeding tube

Nursing assistant actions to take when residents are at risk of tube-feeding complications are:

- Keep the head of the bed elevated 30° to 45° any time the tube feeding is running (Figure 32-14), and for one hour after feeding is completed.
- Provide frequent oral care.
- Follow the nurse's instructions and care plan for care of the skin around the feeding tube.

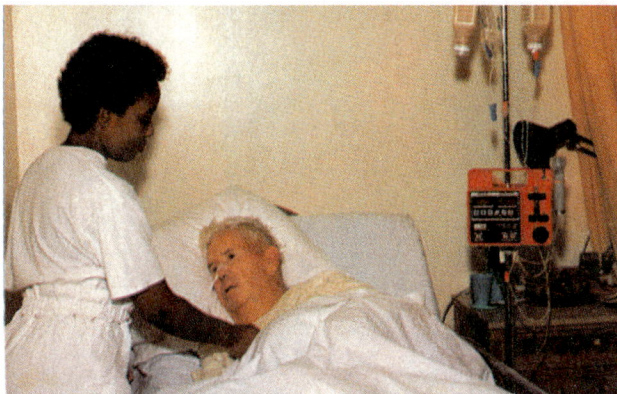

FIGURE 32-14 Keep the head of the bed elevated at least 30° to 45° when the tube feeding is running, and for at least an hour after to prevent reflux and choking.

- Move the resident carefully and position him to avoid tension or traction on the tube.
- Make sure that the tube is not kinked or obstructed.
- Give the resident something to hold if she is pulling on the feeding tube; notify the nurse promptly.
- Turn the resident on the side if coughing or choking.
- Report observations and warning signs to the nurse promptly.

HYDRATION NEEDS

Like malnutrition, dehydration can and does occur in long-term care facility residents. This is partially due to decreased thirst in the elderly. Some residents deliberately avoid fluids because they fear incontinence. Some residents do not like to drink water, but willingly accept other liquids when provided. The majority of residents who become dehydrated do so because of medical illness and the physical or mental inability to ask for liquids; many cannot reach for or hold the cup, pour from the pitcher, or drink from a straw without assistance. Extra fluid is needed by all residents in very hot weather. Dehydration can be a very serious condition in the elderly, causing delirium and other complications. Residents who are becoming dehydrated or are at high risk for dehydration are those who:

- Drink less than 6 cups of liquid a day.
- Have dry mouth.
- Have cracked lips.
- Have sunken eyes.
- Have dark urine.
- Need help drinking from a glass.
- Have trouble swallowing liquids.
- Have diarrhea, vomiting, or fever.
- Are mentally confused.
- Are weak or tired.
- Are lethargic and have difficulty staying awake.

Nursing Assistant Actions

Nursing assistant actions to prevent dehydration are:

- Offer the resident a drink each time you enter the room; set a goal, such as 2 to 4 ounces of liquid each time.
- Drink with the resident, if permitted.
- Provide fluids the resident likes, as permitted on the diet.
- Make sure that fresh water is available (Figure 32-15), that the resident can reach it, and that the pitcher and cup are light enough to hold.
- Provide physical assistance to pour and consume fluids, as needed.
- Offer ice chips, if permitted.
- Follow all swallowing precautions listed on the care plan.

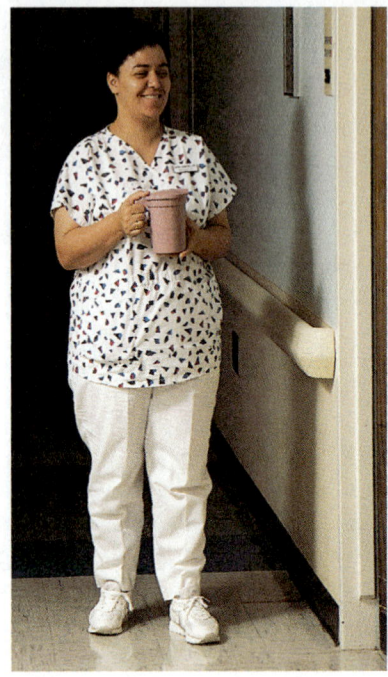

FIGURE 32-15
Provide fresh water frequently, and assist residents with cups and pitchers, if needed.

- Alternate liquids with solids when feeding meals.
- Encourage the resident to attend activities involving food and fluids.
- Accurately monitor and record intake and output, when ordered.
- Promptly notify the nurse of your observations.

PREVENTING INFECTIONS IN RESIDENTS

There are no additional or special infection control techniques in long-term facilities. Section 4 provides instruction on all infection control procedures performed in nursing homes. Effective and frequent handwashing is the best method of preventing the spread of disease from resident to resident, staff person to resident, or resident to staff person. Standard precautions should be implemented in the care of all persons when contact with blood, body fluids, secretions, excretions, mucous membranes, or nonintact skin is anticipated. Isolation techniques are used for residents with known infectious diseases.

It is important to follow these procedures because it is easy for elderly people to get infections. There are a number of reasons for this:

- Body changes due to aging make older people more susceptible to infection. The skin offers less protection because of its fragility. Any break in the skin, such as a pressure sore or skin tear, can quickly become infected.
- Changes in the urinary system cause the bladder to empty less efficiently. Urine left in the bladder contributes to urinary tract infections.

- The ability to cough and raise secretions is reduced. As a result, there is decreased ability to get rid of bacteria from the lungs.
- Elderly people do not always eat well and may be undernourished.
- Elderly people have less resistance to disease because the immune system becomes less effective with age.
- Resistance to disease is reduced when residents have several chronic health problems.
- The sense of thirst is diminished by aging, and elderly individuals frequently do not take in sufficient fluids.

The elderly do not readily show signs of infection. This means they may be sick for some time before you recognize the problem.

- The elderly do not always develop a fever with an infection. The average temperature for an older person may be one or two degrees less than that of a younger person. Therefore, average temperature may represent an increase or fever.
- Some elderly persons do not feel pain as acutely as younger people. They may feel no discomfort with a bladder infection, for example.
- The elderly do not readily develop signs of inflammatory response. A skin infection usually shows redness, swelling, heat, and pain. These signs may be missing or delayed in the elderly person.
- The elderly do not necessarily have an increase in the white blood cell count. This is usually a sign of infection but is often absent in the elderly.
- Elderly people do not cough as frequently when they have respiratory tract infections.
- Residents who are disoriented may not comprehend or be able to communicate feelings of pain or nausea.

The elderly are also more likely to develop serious complications from infections. A simple urinary tract infection can result in *bacteremia* (blood infection), causing the resident to become acutely ill. Sepsis (presence of pus-forming and other pathogens or their toxins in the blood) is also a serious complication of infection in the elderly. These conditions can be fatal to a person who has little ability to cope with additional health problems.

AGE-APPROPRIATE CARE *Alert*

Elderly individuals may develop mental confusion when infection is present. Those with cognitive impairment may experience a worsening of confusion. The confusion usually subsides when the infection is treated and eliminated. Change in mental status is an important observation to report to the nurse.

Prevention of infection in residents is an ongoing concern. There are some steps you can take to help in this process:

- Assist residents to maintain an adequate fluid intake. This helps prevent urinary tract and respiratory tract infections and keeps the skin healthier.

- Assist residents to maintain adequate nutritional intake. Report to the nurse when residents eat less or refuse food.

- Assist residents to perform exercise programs established by the nurse or physical therapist. Follow positioning schedules and orders for range-of-motion exercises and ambulation. This increases circulation, thus lowering the risk of pressure ulcers (a frequent source of infection). Exercise also improves breathing, thereby decreasing the risk of respiratory tract infections.

- Attend to residents' personal hygiene and grooming needs. Regular bathing and oral care help prevent infection. Inspect the body and mouth when performing these procedures.

- Toilet residents regularly who need assistance. This keeps the bladder empty and also assures residents that they will receive help when they need to urinate. Some residents hesitate to drink fluids for fear they will become incontinent. When caring for incontinent residents, be sure to wipe female residents using strokes from front to back. This avoids contaminating the urethra with stool or vaginal excretions.

- Perform catheter care as directed. Avoid opening the closed drainage system. Use aseptic technique when emptying the catheter bag (Figure 32-16).

- Observe residents carefully and report any unusual signs or changes. Urinary tract infections may be discovered from changes in the urine or by incontinence. In some cases, the first sign of any infection is disorien-

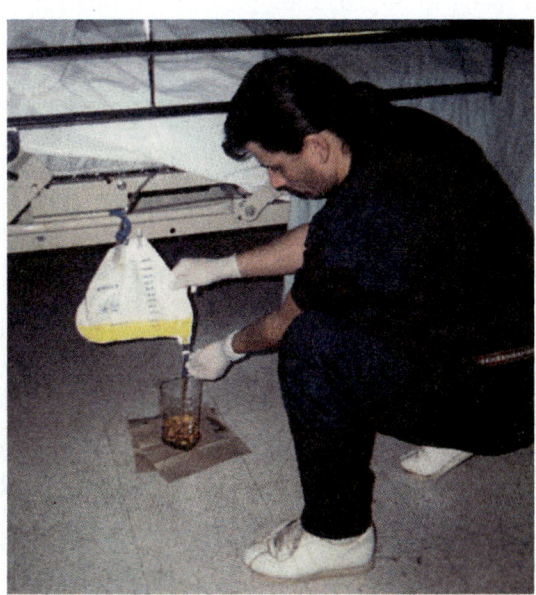

FIGURE 32-16 Use aseptic technique and avoid contamination when emptying the catheter drainage bag.

tation in people who are not usually disoriented. For persons with dementia, a change in behavior may indicate an infection. Incidents of falling often occur in residents with infections.

- You will be asked to collect urine specimens for culture and sensitivity. The specimen should be clean-catch (see Unit 44). You may need help when collecting the specimen. If it is contaminated because of inadequate cleaning or improper collection, the results will be altered.

Fighting infection in the long-term care facility is everyone's responsibility. As a nursing assistant, you can do your part by performing handwashing, universal precautions, isolation techniques, and all principles of medical asepsis on a routine basis. Help new employees to acquire these skills, and assist residents to maintain good personal hygiene practices.

DELIRIUM

Mental confusion is not a normal aging change, and is often caused by reversible conditions. **Delirium** is an acute confusional state caused by reversible medical problems. It is common in the elderly, particularly those over age 75. Delirium is a nonspecific symptom of acute illness and dehydration in the elderly. It may also occur when elderly adults are given anesthesia or some other medications. Sensory losses, including uncorrected vision or hearing, may cause the resident to be unable to interpret the environment correctly. Changes in resident routines and the environment, as well as complications of many different medical conditions, can cause delirium. See Table 32-2 for common causes of delirium. These conditions can occur simultaneously, or can worsen problems in residents with dementia. Because so many factors contribute to delirium, it is often misunderstood, and may be confused with dementia.

Delirium is a very serious condition. Unrecognized and untreated, the mortality rate is high, particularly in residents with chronic disease, mental problems, or dementia. This is unfortunate, because delirium can be reversed if promptly identified and treated.

TABLE 32-2 COMMON CAUSES OF DELIRIUM

- Unfamiliar environment, such as relocation to a new room or being new to the facility
- Vascular insufficiency
- Central nervous system infection
- Trauma
- Tumors or masses, malignancies
- Chemotherapy
- Seizures
- Migraine
- Decreased cardiac output, reduced blood flow, interrupted blood flow
- Urinary retention, urinary tract infection
- Pressure ulcers
- Hypotension
- Inadequate oxygenation
- Pneumonia or other lung infection
- Systemic infections, acute and chronic
- Metabolic disorders
- Anemias
- Decreased renal function
- Endocrine system disorders
- Nutritional deficiencies, malnutrition
- Emotional stress
- Pain
- Surgery, anesthesia
- Alteration in temperature regulation; hyperthermia, hypothermia
- Dehydration, fluid and electrolyte imbalances
- Depression
- Anxiety
- Grief/grieving
- Fatigue
- Sensory/perceptual deficiencies
- Sensory deprivation, isolation, confinement to a restricted area
- Sensory overload
- Immobility, bedrest
- Exposure to toxic substances
- Restraints
- Medication reactions
- Use of invasive equipment such as nasogastric tube or catheter
- Lack of prosthetic devices, including glasses, hearing aid, dentures
- Lack of items that complete body image, such as canes, purses, walkers
- Loss of family contact
- Loss of control over body processes

Signs and Symptoms of Delirium

Delirium develops rapidly. In most cases, the onset is within a few hours or days. Delirium may not be recognized until the resident is critically ill. Staff believe that the resident became ill suddenly, because of the rapid onset of mental changes, but a closer look often reveals subtle changes in the resident's physical or mental condition over the course of several days before the onset of delirium. *Any change in a resident's mental status is significant.*

Residents with acute delirium develop disorientation, behavioral changes, and decreased awareness of the environment (Figure 32-17). Other common signs and symptoms are:

- reduced or fluctuating levels of consciousness
- misinterpretating the environment, misunderstanding or misinterpeting conversations
- hallucinations
- illusions
- delusions
- insomnia and disturbance of sleep-wake cycle
- change in motor activity
- mental confusion and memory impairment

Nursing Assistant Responsibilities

Early identification and careful observation are essential to preventing more serious problems. As a nursing assistant, you will work more closely with residents than other caregivers. This places you in an ideal position to notice subtle changes in mental status and other signs of dehydration, infection, or physical illness that may lead to delirium. You will become familiar with the resident's usual or normal condition. If something differs from the resident's usual condition, do not overlook it. Monitor changes in residents carefully, and report them to the nurse in charge promptly. Keep changes in resident routines and environment minimal. Monitor for and promptly report signs and symptoms of physical illness to the nurse.

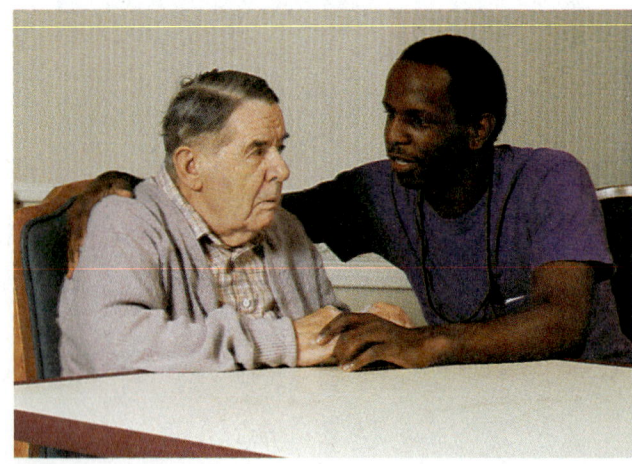

FIGURE 32-17 Residents with delirium develop confusion and decreased awareness of the environment.

KEEPING RESIDENTS SAFE

Each year an estimated 30 to 50% of all nursing home residents fall. The risk and incidence of falls increase with age. Caregivers often recognize these aging changes, but fail to associate them with an increased risk for falls. There are several reasons for this:

- Changes in vision and hearing that most older people experience, which cause a loss of "warning systems."
- Problems with mobility resulting from arthritic changes, loss of flexibility, and endurance.
- Loss of balance related to inner ear changes.
- Reduced reaction time.
- Frequency of urination, leading to fears of incontinence that result in unsafe toileting habits.
- Disorientation and faulty judgment in persons who are mentally incompetent, have delirium or dementia.
- Dizziness that may occur when coming to a standing position too quickly.
- History of falls within previous year.

External factors can also increase the risk of falls:

- Unfamiliar surroundings
- Use of medications that affect mental status, balance, and coordination.
- Unsafe use of assistive mobility devices.
- Poorly planned environment.
- Staff delay in attending to the needs of residents.

In an effort to reduce the number of falls, the environment can be altered to meet the needs of elderly persons:

- Aging changes in the eye cause older people to be more sensitive to glare and to changes in lighting. They also have difficulty seeing colors at the blue-green end of the spectrum. To prevent falls due to faulty vision:
  - Use nonglare wax on floors.
  - Use blinds and curtains to prevent glare from windows.
  - Position or cover mirrors to prevent glare.
  - Use nonglare glass in pictures.
  - Use bright nonglare lighting with constant, even illumination.
  - Use colors that serve as caution reminders to mark the edges of steps and curbs.
  - Use colors in the red and yellow range that increase residents' ability to see changes in walls and floors.
  - Encourage residents to wear sunglasses (if not contraindicated) and hats when they go outdoors.
- Noise increases disorientation and can create anxiety even in alert persons. This increases the risk of falls. Minimizing all noise reduces this risk.
- All tubs and showers should have chairs so residents can remain seated throughout the procedure. Lifts for tubs avoid the needs for the resident to stand in the tub. Avoid using oils that can make the tub bottom slippery.

- Check residents' clothing for fit. Loose shoes and laces, slippers, long robes, and slacks increase the risk of falling.
- Observe ambulatory residents when they get out of bed and chairs, off the toilet, and when they walk.
  - Give instructions to residents who have unsafe habits.
  - Residents who self-propel their wheelchairs may need instruction on how to enter and leave elevators, how to use ramps, and reminders to use the brakes.
  - Dependent residents may benefit by learning self-transfer techniques. Check with the nurse to see if this is possible.
  - When you help dependent residents transfer, always use the method indicated in the care plan.
- Side rails are a frequent cause of falls. Many facilities leave side rails down on one side for residents who can safely transfer without help. In some situations, half rails are more effective.

Review Unit 14 for actions that can reduce the risk of falls and for guidelines regarding the use of restraints.

Other Safety Concerns

Elderly people are at risk for other injuries, such as accidental poisoning, choking, thermal injuries, and skin injuries. These are discussed in Units 14 and 51.

Safety in long-term care facilities is a major concern. Unlike hospitals, residents are given the freedom to move about the facility as they desire. For this reason, the entire building must be free of hazards that contribute to accidents. All employees need to be constantly aware of the residents' safety.

EXERCISE AND RECREATIONAL NEEDS

Residents in long-term care facilities need the stimulation of planned recreation and exercise. The type of activity must be carefully tailored to the needs and abilities of the residents. Health workers in these facilities are often responsible for coordinating this aspect of care.

Recreation

It is important for those who do the activity planning to keep in mind:

- The age and possible physical limitations of the participants.
- The fact that older people have less coordination and are more apt to have hearing and vision deficiencies.
- The fact that recreation with a purpose is considered the most stimulating and enjoyable by mature people.
- That activities planned by the participants are generally the most successful. Shows and skits call for many different talents. Exhibits, sales, and making gifts for others are some other examples of activities that combine recreation with purpose. These types of activities

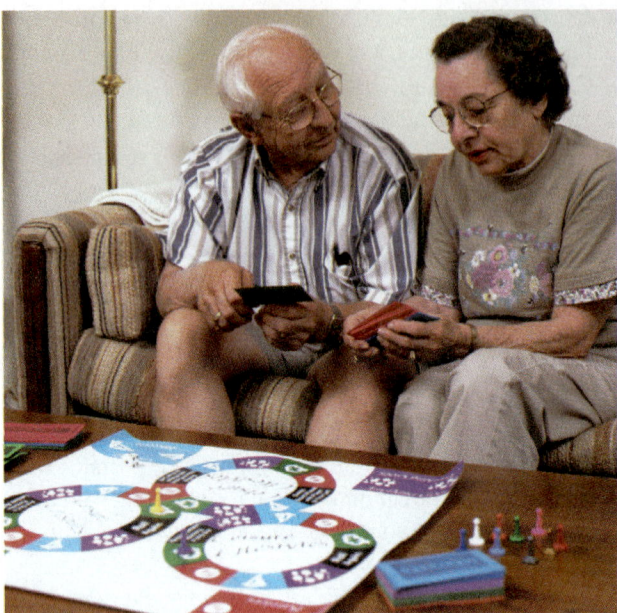

FIGURE 32-18 Playing board games with a friend is enjoyable and maintains coordination and fine motor skills in the fingers. *(Courtesy of Briggs Corporation, Des Moines, IA [800] 247-2343)*

are usually enjoyed by everyone. Most facilities have a special room where out-of-bed residents can gather.

With care, activities that meet special rehabilitation objectives can be planned. For that reason, the occupational therapist is a valuable person who can serve in a consultant capacity, both in care facilities and recreational centers. Recreational planning can thus combine physical and rehabilitative activities with enjoyment.

- Exercising, singing, and clapping hands to music can be enjoyed by bed residents, wheelchair residents, and those who are confused.
- For residents who are ambulatory, dancing can be stimulating as well as enjoyable.
- Handicrafts, games, television, and conversation all offer a measure of entertainment to the less active (Figure 32-18).

GENERAL HYGIENE

Cleanliness of the skin is essential, but a full daily bath for the older person is neither necessary nor advisable. In fact, most elderly are reluctant to bathe daily. Hygiene also includes care of the hands and feet, hair, facial hair, mouth, and observations of the eyes, ears, and nose.

Partial Baths

Although a daily bath is unnecessary, frequent sponging of specific areas is necessary. The face, hands, underarms, perineum, and other body creases need regular cleaning and care. Use standard precautions when cleaning the eyes and genital area.

Skin areas that touch must be kept free from perspiration and should not be allowed to rub together. Whenever moisture, perspiration, urine, or feces are present, skin breakdown and infection are possible. Gently wash and dry local areas.

Total Baths

Bed baths clean the skin, but they are a rather passive activity for the resident. Therefore, a tub or shower bath is desirable two or three times a week to stimulate the resident.

Hand and Foot Care

As we age, fingernails and toenails become thickened and brittle. They split frequently because of decreased peripheral circulation. Fingernails can be cleaned during the morning care period. They should not be neglected.

- A soft brush and blunt-edged orangewood stick will clean the nails without causing injury.
- The hands can be soaked in warm water and the cuticles pushed back gently with a towel.
- Softening creams and olive-oil soaks help to soften the cuticles.
- Fingernails should be cut and filed, following the contour of the fingertips (check your facility policy).
- Care should be taken not to injure the corners; improper cutting of fingernails and toenails is the biggest single cause of infections.

Foot care should also be a routine part of morning care. This should include:

- Careful washing and drying of the foot (Figure 32-19).
- Close inspection for any abnormalities.
- Application of olive oil, lanolin, cocoa butter, hand cream, or lotion to dry, scaly skin.
- Application of a very light dusting of powder to perspiring feet.

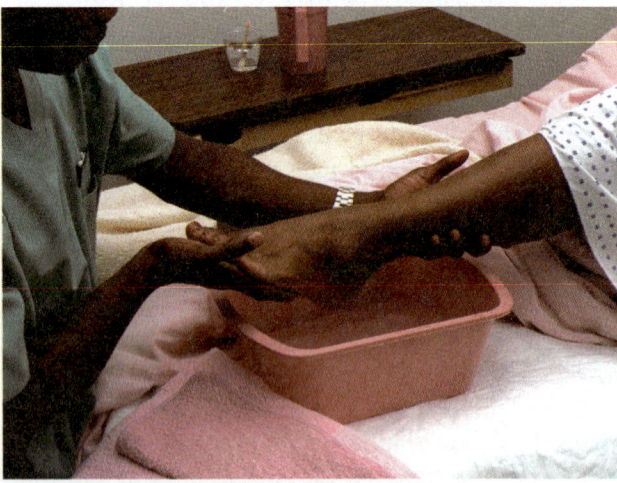

FIGURE 32-19 Foot care is an important part of personal hygiene.

guidelines *for*

Bathing the Elderly

- Some soaps may be drying. Superfatted soaps are less drying and less irritating.
- The skin of an elderly resident is easily damaged and takes a long time to heal because of inefficient general circulation, so care must be taken in handling the skin.
- Dry the skin by patting gently rather than by rubbing. All contact with the skin must be gentle. Even pulling a sheet from under a resident too rapidly can cause trauma.
- Lotions should be applied to dry areas to protect them. Bath oils lubricate the skin, but they are dangerous because they make the bath tub slippery. It is better to use spray-on dry oil or to apply lotions directly to dry areas of skin. Make sure you cover the floor with a towel or bath blanket while spraying cosmetics. The spray tends to get on the unprotected floor, making it slippery.
- General safety factors and the resident's physical limitations should be considered before giving a tub or shower bath. Placement of hand rails, and availability of tub and shower seats or hydraulic lifts (Figure 32-20), should be checked. Be sure you know how to use the hydraulic lift before trying to use one with a resident.
- Warm baths may decrease cerebral circulation. This can lead to confusion. Warm baths may be best just before the resident retires.
- Elderly people tend to be sensitive to deodorants, so care should be used when applying them.
- Inspect the resident's skin over bony prominences for signs of skin breakdown, including redness, warmth, and ischemic pallor.

- The skin should be carefully observed for abnormalities and care must be taken not to disturb them. Any change in color, size, or texture should be reported immediately. Cancer of the skin, often seen in the elderly, has an excellent cure rate (93%) when treated early. This is because skin cancer tends to grow slowly and the cells tend not to spread. These lesions are usually painless. All skin lesions are suspect. You must immediately report any changes noted in a resident's skin.

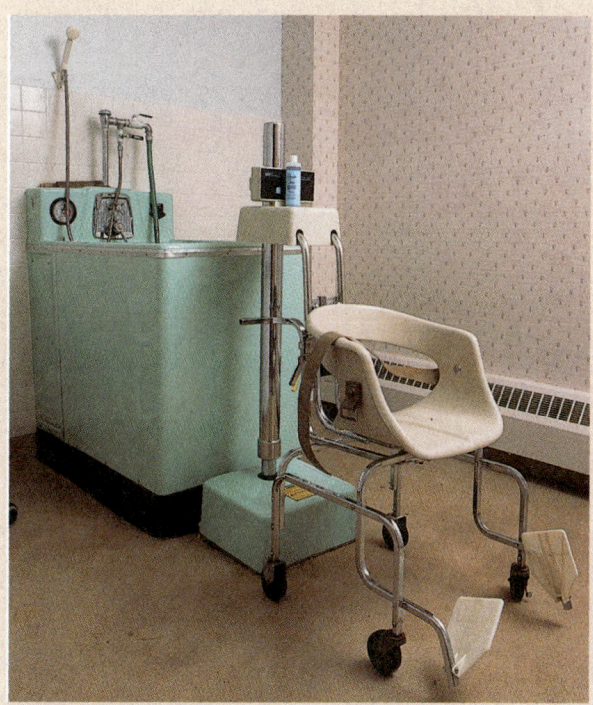

FIGURE 32-20 Check shower chairs and hydraulic lifts before using them. Always fasten the seat belt on the lift chair when moving the resident into and out of the tub.

- Cutting toenails straight across (check your facility policy). Thickened nails, which are difficult to cut, or nails of diabetic residents that must be cut should always be reported to your supervisor.
- Providing slippers or shoes that fit well and are in good repair.

 Note: Check facility policy regarding nail and foot care for diabetic residents.

Hair Care

Hair changes in amount and color as a person ages. These changes are part of the normal aging process. Graying or loss of **pigmentation** (color) is usual. Some graying may be evident as early as the second or third decade of life.

- Genetics probably plays an important role in the change rate. As more and more pigment is lost, the hair becomes white.
- Decreased oil makes the hair dull and lifeless.
- The amount of hair may be reduced in both males and females, and the texture becomes coarser in other areas such as the eyebrows and face.
- Balding is an aging characteristic that first appears at widely varying ages. Again, genetics has a strong influence.

Hair care is important in maintaining the resident's overall personal appearance.

- Hair should be styled and neatly arranged (Figure 32-21).
- Hair is commonly washed when the resident is showered. Check the care plan for specific instructions.
- Dry shampoos are also available. They simplify shampoos for residents confined to bed.
- A mild conditioning shampoo is best.
  - A dryer will dry the hair quickly, decreasing the chance of chilling.
  - The resident must be kept out of drafts while the hair is being washed and dried.
- Hair care may be provided by a beautician or barber, if available, or by a family member or nursing assistant.

AGE-APPROPRIATE CARE *Alert*

Style the residents' hair in age-appropriate styles. Avoid juvenile hairstyles, which can be demeaning to elderly individuals.

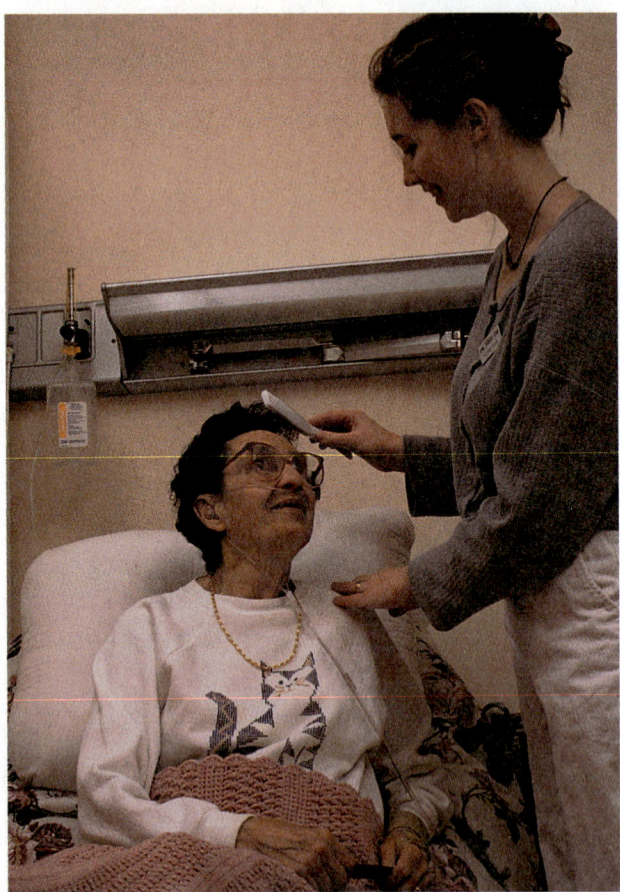

FIGURE 32-21 An attractive hairstyle is important for resident self-esteem.

Facial Hair

Elderly women tend to have an increase in the growth and coarseness of the hair on their chins and upper lips. These can be removed:

- with tweezers.
- by electric needles used by a professional.
- by shaving.
- with a depilatory.

Facial hair may also be lightened by mildly bleaching it.

Elderly men need to be shaved regularly, usually daily. You may need to:

- only provide the equipment.
- use a safety razor or electric razor to shave the resident yourself.
- assist the person to obtain barbering services.

Mouth Care

The condition of the teeth affects the aged person's total health. Hygienic routines and observations are your responsibility when an individual is no longer able to do these things for himself. See Unit 25 for specific care procedures.

Natural Teeth. Poor oral hygiene can result in loss of appetite and weight, and may be the focus of any infection. Even if teeth are missing, the remaining teeth should be cleaned regularly. Dental checkups should be done as often as in younger years.

Dentures. False teeth, called *dentures*, must be cleaned daily (see Procedure 71 in Unit 25).

- Check the mouth and gums routinely for signs of irritation. Use a soft brush to clean mouth and gums.
- Teeth should be checked and polished during periodic dental examinations.

Mouth care is especially important for the bed resident who has lost teeth and is no longer able to keep dentures in the mouth. Check the mouth and gums for irritation. Dentures should be inspected for cracks, rough edges, and broken parts.

- A commercial mouthwash, a warm wash of saline solution, or baking soda should be used before and after meals.
- Glycerine and lemon, applied with applicators between meals, are very refreshing.
- Lips should be inspected for excessive dryness or fissures.
- Creams, petroleum jelly, or lip balm applied to the lips can prevent fissures from developing into deep sores and infections.

Eyes, Ears, and Nose

Eyes, ears, and nose should also be observed daily for any signs of irritation, redness, drainage, or excessive dryness of the skin that could lead to breaks and fissures. Observations of this nature by staff members should be part of routine care.

MENTAL CHANGES

Mental deterioration is not a normal part of aging. However, as people age, the risk of mental deterioration increases. Mental deterioration may stem from physical (organic) or emotional causes. A combination of both may occur in the residents in your care. Periods of mental confusion are often temporary. They may be due to unusual stress, such as an infection; sudden injury, such as a fracture; or transfer to an unfamiliar environment. In some situations, the changes may signify a progressive deterioration of mental abilities. The term dementia refers to any disorder of the brain that causes deficits in thinking, memory, and judgment.

CARING FOR RESIDENTS WITH DEMENTIA

You will care for many residents with dementia in the long-term care facility. Dementia is not a disease in itself, but is a group of symptoms seen in a number of different diseases. You will recall that delirium is a temporary condition, caused by medical illness. Dementia is a permanent condition that is not related to acute physical problems. Residents who have dementia may also develop delirium when they become acutely ill. In such cases, their confusion worsens. It returns to baseline when the medical problem is resolved. Alzheimer's disease is the most common form of dementia. Other types of dementias are related to cardiovascular disease, Parkinson's disease, and Huntington's disease and are listed in Table 32-3. The term dementia is used here when referring to symptoms, behavior, and nursing actions that are appropriate for people with any dementia. Alzheimer's is used when the information is specific to that dementia.

Alzheimer's Disease

Alzheimer's disease can begin during middle age, but is more common in older persons. The disease affects people of all races, levels of intelligence, education, and financial status. It is progressive and cannot be cured. It has been called a "slow death of the mind." In the past, the term senility was used to describe these symptoms. We know now that it is a disease of the brain cells and is not normal aging. The cause of Alzheimer's is unknown. There is no diagnostic test. When symptoms appear, the person should have a medical workup to rule out other diseases. Nutritional problems, depression, medications, and metabolic diseases can all cause similar symptoms. However, these conditions can be reversed with treatment.

In Alzheimer's, changes occur in both the structure and function of the brain. The brain shrinks and becomes smaller. If an autopsy of the brain is performed after death, changes are noted in the brain cells. These changes are called neuritic plaques and neurofibrillary tangles.

Individuals with Alzheimer's often live as long as 20 years after the onset of the disease. Their bodies can be surprisingly healthy. Families and friends have difficulty believing

TABLE 32-3 DESCRIPTION OF MAJOR FORMS OF DEMENTIA		
Disease	**Features**	**Course**
Alzheimer's disease	Lack of chemical in brain causing neurofibrillary tangles, neuritic plaques	Onset age: 60–80 Slowly progressive
Multi-infarct dementia	Interference with blood circulation in brain cells due to arteriosclerosis or atherosclerosis	Onset age: 55–70 Outcome depends on rate of damage to brain cells
Huntington's disease	Inherited from either parent who has gene for the disease	Onset age: 25–45 Average duration 15 years
Parkinson's disease	Deficiency of chemical in brain (dopamine)	Onset age: 55–60 Several years duration
Creutzfeldt-Jakob disease	Noninflammatory virus causes changes in brain	Onset age: 50–60 Rapidly progressive
Syphilis	Spirochete (bacteria) causes brain damage	Occurs 15–20 years after primary infection
AIDS dementia	HIV-1 infection	Symptoms sometimes precede diagnosis of AIDS

that the person is ill. There is much that is unknown about this disease. Caregivers can increase the quality of life for those who have the illness.

The disease generally has three stages, with symptoms becoming progressively worse. The best learned skills tend to remain the longest. An English teacher, for example, may maintain verbal skills longer than usual. However, once a skill is lost, it is lost forever.

Stage I: Mild Dementia.
During the first stage, most people remain at home if they have a supportive family to provide assistance. They are usually physically capable and can attend to the activities of daily living with supervision. Characteristics of Stage I include:

- Short-term memory loss
- Personality changes with loss of spontaneity and indifference (Figure 32-22)
- Decreased ability to concentrate and shortened attention span
- Disorientation to time and space
- Poor judgment
- Lack of safety awareness
- Carelessness in actions and appearance
- Anxiety, depression, and agitation
- Delusions of persecution—the person thinks that others are conspiring to do him harm

Stage II: Moderate Dementia.
Symptoms of this stage are:

- Increased short-term memory loss and deterioration of memory for remote events.
- Complete disorientation.
- Wandering and pacing.
- Sundowning, which is confusion and restlessness that occur during the late afternoon, evening, or night.
- Sensory/perceptual changes. The person is unable to recognize and use common objects, such as eating utensils, combs, and pencils. Also, the person is unable to distinguish between right and left, up and down, hot and cold.
- Perseveration phenomena. This refers to repeating an action. Examples are repeating the same word or phrase, lip licking, chewing, or finger tapping.
- Problems with walking.
- Problems with speech, reading, writing.
- Good eating habits continue.
- Incontinent of bowel and bladder.
- Catastrophic reactions, hallucinations, delusions. A catastrophic reaction is the response of a person with dementia to overwhelming stimuli (Figure 32-23).

Most people with Alzheimer's are admitted to long-term care facilities during the second stage. Although they may still be healthy physically, they require constant care. Most families do not have the emotional resources and physical energy to cope. Admission may be traumatic to families. Families are vital members of the interdisciplinary team. They can provide staff with valuable information about the resident and how to deal with the problems.

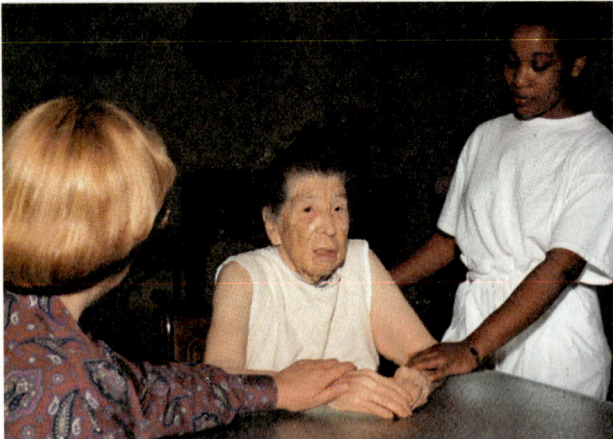

FIGURE 32-22 People with dementia exhibit indifference and loss of spontaneity.

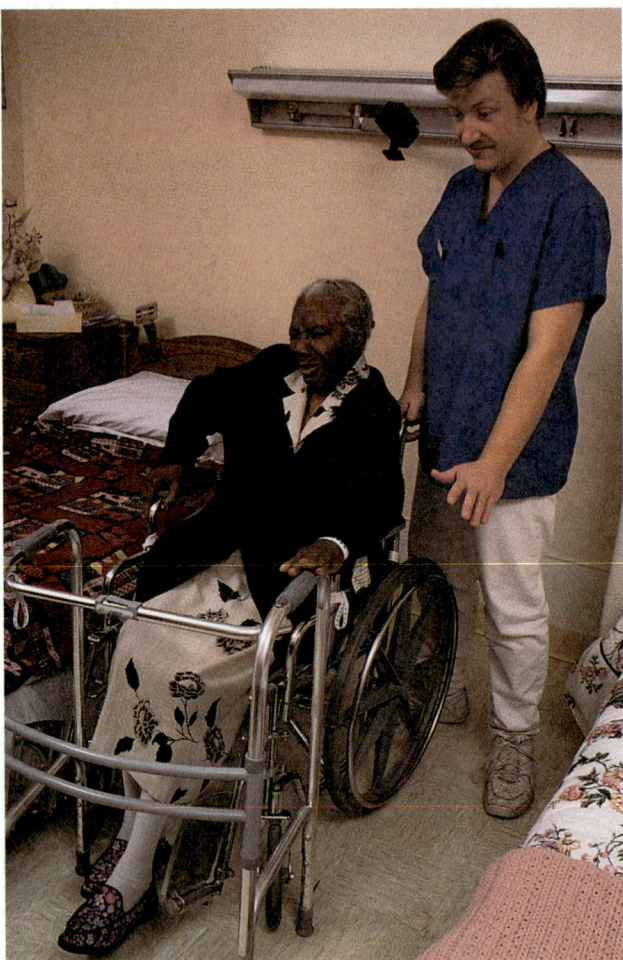

FIGURE 32-23 Catastrophic reactions can occur when the person with dementia feels overwhelmed.

Stage III: Severe Dementia. The person in Stage III:

- is totally dependent.
- is verbally unresponsive.
- may have seizures.

Work with residents who have Alzheimer's disease or any dementia is challenging, rewarding, and gratifying. Caregivers must be compassionate, patient, calm, and have a sense of humor.

When you are caring for residents with dementia, remember to:

- protect residents from physical injury.
- allow residents to maintain independence as long as possible.
- provide physical and mental activities within residents' abilities.
- support residents' dignity and self-esteem.

To meet these goals, the care must be:

- consistent.
- provided with a structured but flexible routine.
- given in a peaceful, quiet environment that is simple, uncluttered, and unchanged.

It is helpful to:

- Make eye contact with residents.
- Use appropriate body language. Residents with dementia can "read" the staff. Therefore, residents' behavior will reflect the mood of the staff (Figure 32-24).

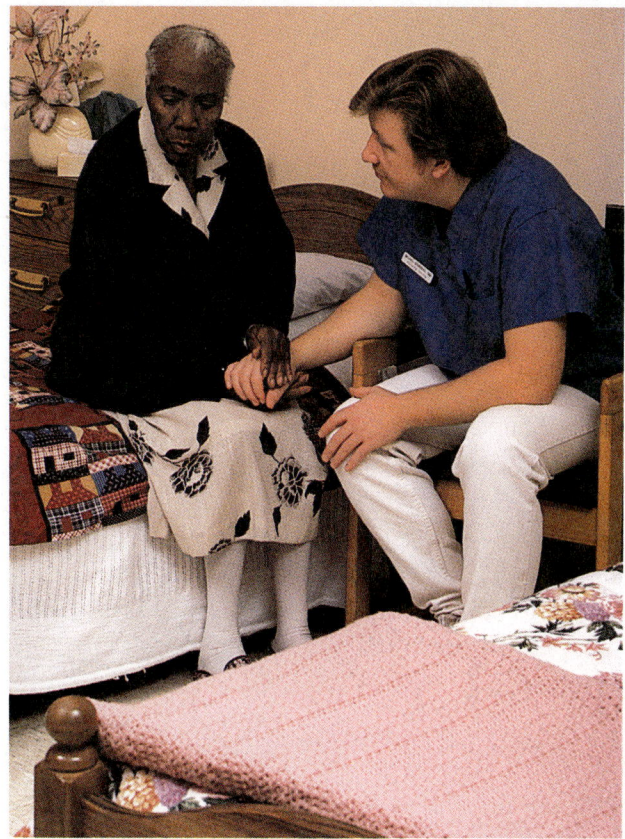

FIGURE 32-24 Residents with dementia are attuned to the body language of caregivers.

guidelines *for*

Activities of Daily Living for Residents with Dementia

- Allow the resident to do as much as possible.
  - Use the hand-over-hand technique for personal care and eating. The **hand-over-hand technique** means that the resident's hand is placed around an object, such as a glass. The caregiver then places a hand over the resident's hand and guides the object to the resident's mouth.
  - Give only one short, simple direction at a time.
- Observe the resident's physical condition. People with dementia are usually unaware of signs of illness.
- Assist residents to maintain a dignified, attractive appearance by helping them with grooming and dressing.
- Monitor food and fluid intake.

- – Too many foods at once are confusing.
- – Place one food at a time in front of the resident.
- – Do not use plastic utensils that can break in the resident's mouth.
- – Provide nutritious finger foods when the resident is unable to use utensils.
- – Avoid pureed foods as long as possible.
- – Check food temperatures.
- – Prepare foods for eating by buttering bread, cutting meat, and opening cartons.
- – Check the resident's mouth after eating for food. "Squirreling" food (hoarding food in the cheeks) can cause aspiration.
- – Weigh residents regularly to detect patterns of weight gain or loss.

continues

guidelines *continued*

- The dining area should be quiet and calm.
- Persons with dementia eventually lose bowel and bladder continence. Taking residents to the bathroom every 2 hours keeps residents dry and prevents skin breakdown.
- Residents with dementia need activities geared to their abilities.
  - Avoid large groups or competitive activities.
  - In later stages, use sensory stimulation with quiet music, soft touching, and calm talk.
  - Holding puppies or kittens (pet therapy) brings pleasure to severely impaired residents.
- Daily exercise should be planned according to residents' habits and abilities (Figure 32-25). The resident who wanders throughout the day may only need range-of-motion exercises.

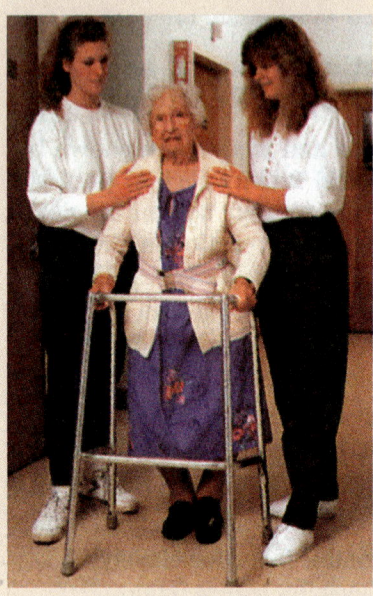

FIGURE 32-25
Daily exercise is important to maintain physical health and well-being.

- Be able to "tune" into and accept residents without being judgmental or critical.
- Use touch appropriately. This can be soothing. But if a resident is surprised by the body contact, it can result in a catastrophic reaction.
- Avoid using logic, reasoning, or lengthy explanations.
- Remember that when the ability to use speech is lost, communication occurs through nonverbal means.
  - Biting, scratching, and kicking may be the only way the resident can express displeasure.
  - Watch for facial expressions and body language for clues to feelings and moods.
  - Learn what triggers agitation or anger. Work on preventing those situations.
- Use techniques of diversion and distraction. For example, calmly take the resident by the hand and walk together or direct the resident's attention to another activity. These techniques work well because of the shortened attention span.
- Realize that people with dementia are not responsible for what they do or say.
  - Their behavior is not intentional, and they cannot change.
  - They are not aware of what they are doing.
  - They lose the ability to control their impulses.
  - Avoid confrontations and always allow them to "save face"—that is, keep their dignity.
  - No one really knows what is happening in the minds of people with dementia.

SPECIAL PROBLEMS

Wandering and Pacing

Persons with Alzheimer's may wander or pace for hours at a time. No one knows why this occurs. Some reasons may be:

- They are looking for companionship, security, or loved ones.
- It is a way to handle stress.

The resident may not know where he is, but knows he does not want to be there. He is seeking a state of mind, not a physical location. Ask the resident his intended destination. A man may tell you he is going to work. A woman may say she is going home to cook dinner for the children. Avoid arguing and providing reality orientation. These techniques will probably agitate the resident. Instead, use reminiscence (Figure 32-26). Talk about the resident's activities, work, meal preparation, or cooking. Make appropriate comments, such as, "That must be very interesting work," or "You must have been a very good cook." Ask the resident about his former work routines. This approach restores the state of mind the resident seeks, reducing stress and the risk of **eloping** (wandering away from the facility).

Many different things trigger wandering behavior. The facility may keep a log to help identify the resident's wandering triggers. You will record information such as the resident's behavior, staff on duty, and temperature and noise in the environment on the log. The nurse uses this information to develop a plan of care. Several studies have shown that noise increases wandering . Health care facilities can be very noisy at times. Loud talking, using the intercom, loud

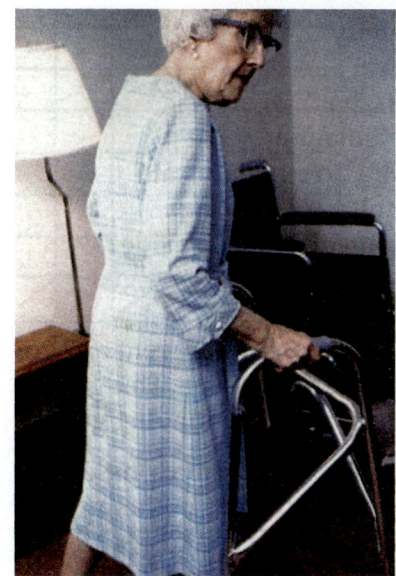

FIGURE 32-26
Some residents with Alzheimer's disease wander continually. They must be reminded to rest, to eat, and to drink.

televisions, and residents calling out for help can be very upsetting to wanderers. Hot or cold environmental temperature may also be a problem. If the resident is uncomfortable, he may wander to escape. Other common wandering triggers are:

- boredom
- unmet physical needs
- feeling stressed
- pain
- hunger
- thirst
- needing to use the bathroom

Other, less common wandering triggers are dehydration, illness, inadequate coping mechanisms, medications, and an unfamiliar environment.

Nursing Assistant Approaches. Allow the resident to wander. Using restraints increases anxiety and frustration, worsening the problem. Walk with the resident whenever possible. Adapt the environment to the wandering resident, to ensure that it is safe and secure. Keeping the resident's stress as low as possible is important because if he feels overwhelmed, he may wander to elope. If the resident's stress is not relieved, he may have a catastrophic reaction. As a rule, try to meet the resident's needs for hunger, thirst, and elimination. If you meet the need, the wandering will cease.

Thinking is a very complex process. If someone tells you *not to think* of a purple dog, you will think of it, then have to unthink it. "Unthinking" is a complex process for a cognitively impaired resident. Avoid saying, "Don't go outside," or "Don't go in that room," because that will cause the resident to think about doing exactly what you told him not to. A better approach is to say, "Stay inside," or "Stay here." Communication is best if it is concrete and does not require abstract thinking.

Remember that nonverbal communication can have a powerful effect on residents. Confused residents are very sensitive to the moods and body language of staff members. Send the right message through facial expressions and body language. Approach the resident in a calm, nonthreatening manner (Figure 32-27). Avoid forcing your own agenda on the resident, which will cause agitation and worsen the behavior. Instead, use gentle persuasion. Avoid making too many demands on the resident during ADLs and direct care. Keep instructions simple and brief. As the resident completes one task, give him another. Be patient, calm, and reassuring. Tell him he is in the right place, safe, and you will help him. Compliment him for his successes, even if they are small. The resident will probably not remember the compliment, but will feel good about himself. He will be more cooperative and less likely to act out or wander.

Seeing items associated with going outdoors may trigger wandering. Remove purses, hats, coats, shoes, or other outerwear from sight. There is no single effective approach for all wandering behavior. Use the approaches listed here and see if they work. If you discover an effective approach, inform your charge nurse so he or she can add it to the care plan. Remember that identifying and modifying the resident's agenda, feelings, and unmet needs will usually modify or stop the behavior. Effective management is individualized to the resident. It is often the result of trial and error. Other approaches that may be listed on the care plan are:

- Taking the resident to the bathroom frequently.
- Adjusting room temperature and ensuring that the resident is wearing appropriate clothing for the temperature and season.
- Reducing environmental noise and stimulation; check residents yelling, television, intercom announcements, and other sources of noise in the facility.

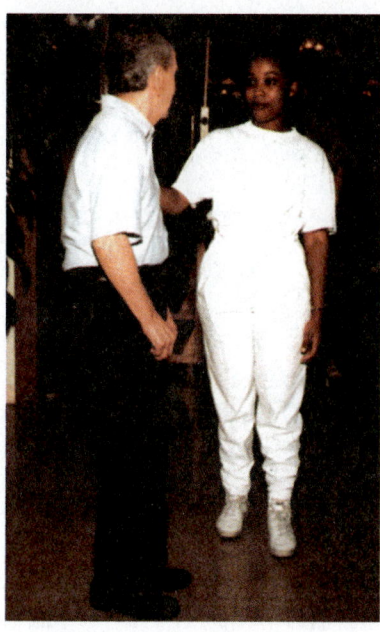

FIGURE 32-27
Your demeanor has a powerful effect on residents. Approach the resident slowly, calmly, and in a nonthreatening manner.

- Providing something to eat or drink.
- Informing the nurse if the the resident complains of pain; he or she may not admit to having "pain," but may admit to having pressure, discomfort, or another unpleasant sensation.
- Providing a magazine, newspaper, book, or picture album (Figure 32-28).
- Visiting with the resident.
- Escorting the resident to activities.
- Having the resident fold towels and washcloths, perform a repetitious task, or sort other harmless items.
- Providing a stereo with earphones and playing soft, soothing music, or the resident's favorite type of music, if known. This approach is often effective when others fail.
- Placing an identifying object, such as a bow, hat, or gender-appropriate decoration on the door of the resident's room and directing him to it.
- Making sure the resident wears glasses and hearing aids, as appropriate. Wandering may worsen if the resident misinterprets environmental signals.
- Avoiding clutter and safety hazards in the environment.

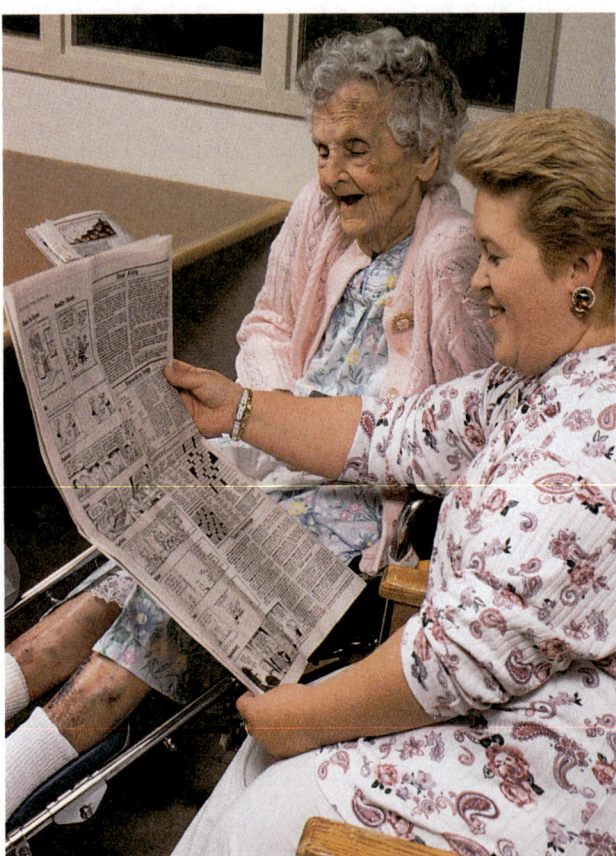

FIGURE 32-28 Some residents with Alzheimer's wander in their wheelchairs. Showing the resident a newspaper will distract her and provide an opportunity to rest.

- Ensuring that chemicals and potential hazards are stored properly.
- Providing a nightlight at night, or leaving the bathroom light on.
- If nighttime wandering is a problem, avoid letting the patient nap during the day. Limit caffeinated food and beverages after the evening meal.
- Avoiding the use of side rails. This resident may climb the rails and suffer a serious fall.
- Attaching the call signal cord to the resident's clothing so the cord will pull from the wall and turn the signal on when he rises. Other types of tab signals or magnetic sensor systems may be used to alert staff if the resident rises or attempts to leave the facility through an exit door.
- Responding promptly to door alarms, bed, or other alarms that alert you to a problem with a wandering resident.
- Covering elevator buttons with soft fabric or duct tape to disguise them. The soft material permits staff and visitors to push the buttons, but wandering residents will usually not recognize them.
- Avoiding restraints, which often worsen agitation.
- Always knowing what the resident is wearing. Write this information down at the beginning or end of each shift. Wanderers are often discovered missing at meal time, when staff cannot find the resident to deliver the tray. This is commonly a problem for second-shift staff. Day shift dresses the resident. Staff on second shift may not know what she is wearing.
- Checking on the resident frequently to note her whereabouts. If you will be tied up with another resident for a prolonged period of time, inform the charge nurse so that another worker can be assigned to monitor the wandering resident in your absence.

Remember that residents who wander will burn extra calories and are at risk for weight loss. Some are so busy wandering they will not sit long enough to eat a meal. Give them finger foods and walk with them, if necessary. Follow the plan of care to ensure that the resident takes in enough nutrients.

Residents who wander may become physically exhausted. They have forgotten how to sit down and may need reminders. Special reclining chairs (Figure 32-29) and beanbag-type chairs may be used to allow residents to rest. Again, the care plan will specify the method to use.

Agitation, Anxiety, and Catastrophic Reactions

Agitation and anxiety are shown by an increase in physical activity, such as pacing, or the perseveration behaviors described for Stage II. If appropriate interventions are not

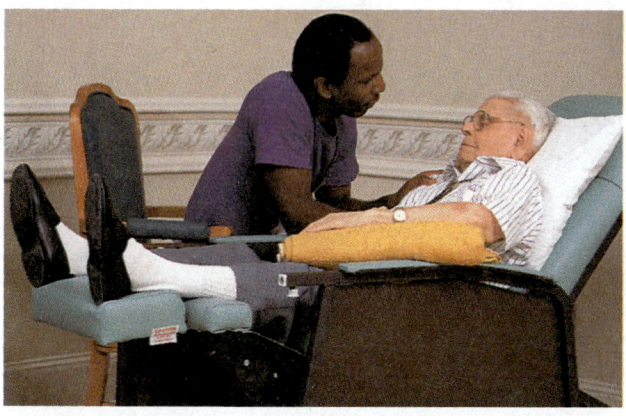

FIGURE 32-29 Some residents will wander until they are physically exhausted. Seating the resident in a recliner enables him to rest.

implemented in time, a catastrophic reaction will likely occur. You may note any or all of the following.

- Increased physical activity
- Increased talking or mumbling
- Explosive behavior with physical violence

To avoid catastrophic reactions:

- Monitor behavior closely.
- Watch for signs of increasing agitation.
- Check to see if the resident:
  - Is hungry
  - Needs to go to the bathroom
  - Is too hot or too cold
  - Is overtired or in pain
  - Has signs of physical illness
- Check the environment for:
  - Too much noise
  - Too many people
  - Staff anxiety
  - Television programs. People with dementia cannot distinguish fiction from reality.
- People with dementia cannot make decisions. For example, the question "What do you want to wear today?" may be more than they can handle.

When agitation or catastrophic reactions occur:

- Do not use physical restraints or force in any attempt to subdue the resident. This increases agitation and can result in injury to the resident or staff.
- Avoid having several staff persons approach the resident at the same time. This is frightening to the resident.
- Use a soft, calm voice. Do not try to reason with the resident. Using touch may or may not be appropriate. Some residents respond to smooth stroking of the arms or back. Others may react violently if they are already agitated.

Sundowning

As previously mentioned, *sundowning* means that the resident has increased confusion and restlessness during the late afternoon, evening, or night. It is sometimes prevented by avoiding too much activity before bedtime and by establishing a consistent bedtime routine.

- Overfatigue can cause sundowning. Encourage the resident to nap or rest in the early afternoon.
- Try to prevent the resident from sleeping too much during the day.
- The evening meal should be eaten at least 2 hours before bedtime. Eliminate caffeine from the resident's diet.
- Involve the resident in quiet evening activities, soft music, or interactions with a caregiver or family member.
- Provide a light bedtime snack that is easily chewed and digested.
- Take the resident to the bathroom. Allow sufficient time for bladder and bowel elimination.
- Give a slow back massage.
- Check with family members and continue the resident's established habits, such as wearing socks to bed, using two pillows, or having a night light.
- Check the lighting of the room. Shadows and reflections are disturbing.
- If the resident awakens during the night, repeat the bedtime routine. If this is ineffective and the resident does not remain in bed, try a recliner or Alzheimer's chair.

Pillaging and Hoarding

These events do not present a major problem unless residents collect items from other residents' rooms or they hide things that are difficult to find.

- Label all residents' belongings.
- If a missing item is located, note where it was found. The resident probably will choose the same hiding place the next time.
- Check the room daily for stale food.
- Keep the resident's hands busy. Activities like folding washcloths or "fiddling" with keys on a ring may help.
- Provide a "rummaging" drawer or box for the resident.

Reality Orientation

Reality orientation (R.O.) is used to help disoriented residents regain connections to the environment, to time, and to themselves. When it is used appropriately, it decreases anxiety in the resident. R.O. may be effective in the first stage and the early part of the second stage of Alzheimer's disease. In later stages it is meaningless and increases agitation.

guidelines *for*

Reality Orientation

- Always treat residents as adults, with respect and dignity, no matter how confused they are.
- Speak clearly and directly. Avoid the temptation to speak louder when they do not understand you.
- Give simple, brief instructions and responses.
- Establish and maintain a structured routine.
- Be polite and sincere.
- Give residents adequate time to respond.
- Allow residents to be independent as long as possible.
- Set residents' watches to the correct time.
- Make sure residents have clean eyeglasses and effective hearing aids if they need them.
- Place large numbered calendars in rooms and cross off the days as they pass.
- There should be clocks with large numbers around the facility.
- Signs with large letters and color codes on walls, floors, and equipment help residents find their way around the facility.
- Call residents by name. Disoriented residents usually respond to their first name more quickly.
- Tell residents your name—do not expect them to remember you.
- Use R.O. in conversation with the residents, for example, "It's only March 5 today but it is warm outside."

When using R.O.:

- Do not put residents on the spot. For example, do not ask, "Do you remember who I am?" or "Do you know what day this is?" If you need to verify orientation, ask "What are your plans for today?"
- Answer questions honestly but avoid confronting the residents with information they are unable to handle. If a resident whose husband is deceased asks, "Is my husband coming today?" it is cruel to answer by saying, "Remember, your husband died two years ago." This response will likely trigger a catastrophic reaction. It is better to answer by asking another question, such as, "Tell me about your husband, Emma." She will receive pleasure from reminiscing and will probably work up to present time on her own.
- Never argue with a resident's reality. When a resident has a delusion, arguing increases the individual's anxiety and agitation. Many delusions are based on past experiences. Because the resident is disoriented, the experience seems to be happening now.
- Do not reinforce the resident's disorientation.
- Remember that a pleasant facial expression, relaxed body language, and a caring touch are the most important aspects of caring for confused residents.

Reminiscing

Reminiscing (remembering past experiences) is a natural activity for people of all ages. We tend to reminisce when we see old friends or get together with families.

- Past experiences are remembered and enjoyed as we think of pleasant times from the past.
- As people age, the tendency to reminisce increases, and the activity becomes more important.
- It is an appropriate activity for residents with dementia if long-term memory is still intact (Figure 32-30).
- Reminiscing may serve as a life review. Elderly people often review the past experiences of their lives. This can bring back unpleasant memories. If these experiences are resolved, peace of mind can be found.
- Reminiscing can help people adapt to old age. It helps to maintain self-esteem. It allows them to work through personal losses.

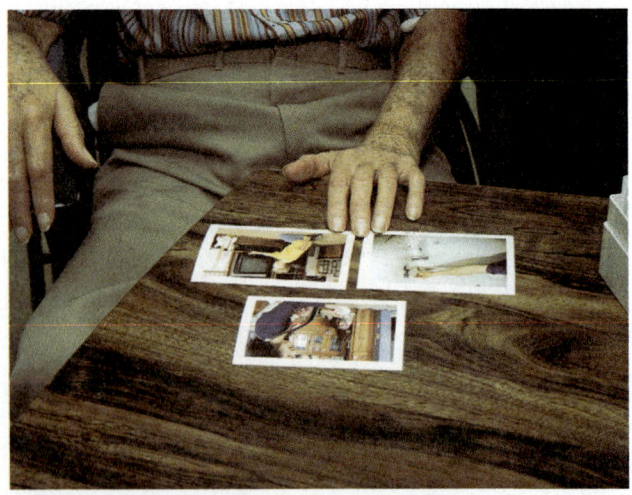

FIGURE 32-30 Residents with dementia retain long-term memory even though short-term memory is lost. Looking at family pictures is an excellent way to reminisce.

- When we listen to residents reminisce, we understand them better.
- Reminiscing therapy can be a group activity if done with a leader who is skillful and sensitive to the feelings of the members.

Validation Therapy

Validation therapy was developed by Naomi Feil. **Validation therapy** is a technique that tries to maintain the disoriented person's dignity by acknowledging the person's memories and feelings.

It is based on these ideas:

- Maintain the identity and dignity of the residents.
- Help disoriented people with dementia feel good about themselves.
- There is a reason for all behavior. What seems like confused behavior may be an acting-out of memories from long ago.
- Acknowledge feelings and memories.
- Disoriented people have the right to express feelings when they can no longer be oriented to reality.
- Living must be resolved in order to prepare for dying.
- Sometimes elderly persons have experienced so many losses during a lifetime that they have no coping abilities left.
- To live in reality is not the only way to live.
- Disoriented elderly have worth. We can give them joy by allowing them to express themselves.
- Within each confused person is a human being who was once a child and later an adult with hopes, joys, sadness, failures, and successes. They deserve to be cared for and loved in their final years.

When using validation therapy, allow residents to express their feelings. Reassure them that the feelings are worthwhile. Use a calm, nonthreatening manner. Speak in a loving tone of voice. When the resident describes an emotion, assure him or her that it is okay. Using validation is an excellent way to communicate with elderly persons. It is also effective for residents with Alzheimer's disease and cognitive impairments. The program is based on the belief that developmental tasks from earlier years must be resolved. If they were not resolved, they will emerge in old age. The elderly person may display many emotions in trying to conclude them. Feil's research has shown that using validation reduces the need for restraints. It helps residents regain feelings of dignity and self-control. Resident response to this therapy can be very encouraging. Seeing positive responses is very rewarding to staff.

Music Therapy

Music therapy is an allied health service similar to occupational therapy and physical therapy. Although it is an enjoyable activity, it is not done strictly for fun and games. Music therapy consists of using music therapeutically to address physical, psychological, cognitive, and social functioning. Music therapy is used successfully with people of all ages and disabilities.

Music therapy dates back to ancient Greece. In that culture, music was part of medical treatment. Think about the effect music has on your own life. Children learn the alphabet by singing the letters. We listen to "oldies" and remember events from our past. You remember the words to songs you have not heard in many years.

Restorative music therapy is used for relieving stress. It can be a planned, formal activity or a spontaneous, informal activity. Singing with residents during bathing and range-of-motion work can be therapeutic and fun for both the resident and the nursing assistant. Studies have shown that participating in music has various mental and physical benefits, including:

- increased metabolism
- increased muscle flexibility
- improved circulation
- increased lung capacity and improved respirations
- improved memory, which contributes to reminiscence and satisfaction
- improvement in mood and emotional states
- feeling a sense of control over life
- increased self-awareness
- anxiety reduction
- stimulation
- opportunities to interact socially with others

Sometimes music therapy is part of a planned exercise program. Playing music during exercise makes the activity fun. Music motivates the residents and singing and clapping relieve stress and anxiety. Music teleprompters make it easy for residents to participate even if they do not know the words (Figure 32-31). For relaxation therapy, a portable player and headset may be used.

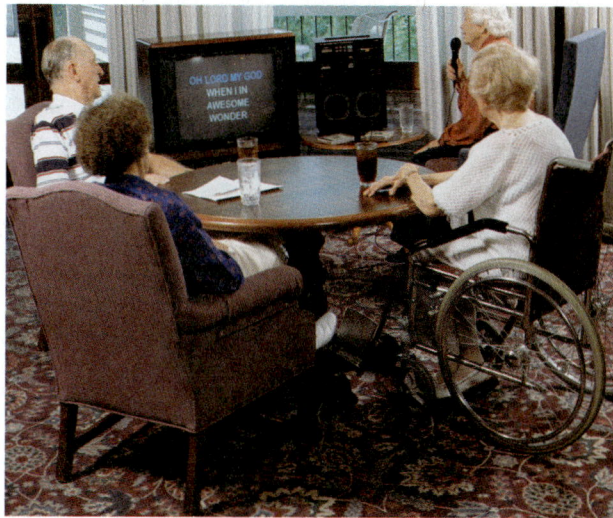

FIGURE 32-31 A teleprompter can be used so residents can sing along even if they don't know the words. *(Courtesy of Briggs Corporation, Des Moines, IA [800] 247-2343)*

The activities department may present music activities for other purposes. A professional music therapist may visit the facility regularly to work with residents. Regardless of whether music is used formally as a form of therapy, or informally for recreation, residents respond well to it. Music is a pleasurable activity that maintains or improves the residents' physical, mental, social, and emotional functioning. The sensory and intellectual stimulation of music help maintain the residents' quality of life.

Animal-Assisted Therapy

Animal-assisted therapy is also called *pet therapy*. Pets have been used in many different ways in the health care environment. Formal programs are developed in which the handler and health care provider consult on specific goals and plan how to accomplish them. With informal pet therapy, an animal is taken to visit residents periodically. Visiting with animals can reduce feelings of loneliness and depression. Some people become more active and responsive because of visits from pets. The pet may make it easier for the resident to talk. He or she may express thoughts, feelings, and memories. Stroking a dog or cat may reduce a person's blood pressure, and encourages good range of motion of the hands and arms. Animals used in pet therapy must have a health certificate. Some formal groups offer special certifications to pets and handlers based on the experience of the animal/human team and complexity of the working environment. Dogs are commonly used for pet therapy, but other types of animals may be used as well.

REVIEW

A. True/False.

Mark the following true or false by circling T or F.

1. T F Older people have the same emotional needs for good mental health as young people.

2. T F Frustration is an emotion often experienced by the elderly.

3. T F As people age, they become less interested in sexuality.

4. T F Elderly people may not be aware of their need for fluids.

5. T F Infections are not a major cause of concern in the elderly.

6. T F The resident's mouth should be carefully inspected and cleaned each time the dentures are cleaned.

7. T F One of the best approaches when working with persons with dementia is to reason with them and use logic.

8. T F Calories should generally be increased in the diet of the elderly.

9. T F Elderly persons are generally fearful of death.

10. T F Daily tub baths or showers are not usually necessary or recommended for elderly residents.

B. Matching.

Choose the correct item from Column II to match each word or phrase in Column I.

Column I	Column II
11. ____ dementia	a. weakening
12. ____ validation therapy	b. remembering past experiences
13. ____ reminiscing	c. deficits in thinking, memory, judgment
14. ____ debilitating	d. tries to maintain disoriented person's dignity
15. ____ sundowning	e. wakefulness of person with Alzheimer's during evening and night

C. Multiple Choice.

Select the one best answer for each of the following.

16. One characteristic of the nursing assistant that is especially important while caring for older adults includes
   a. logical reasoning ability.
   b. kindness.
   c. technical skill.
   d. advanced certifications and training.

17. Characteristics of the elderly include
   a. increased vitality.
   b. decreased night sleep.
   c. increased appetite.
   d. increased mobility and agility.

18. Which of the following nutrients should be increased in the diet of elderly persons?
    a. Fats
    b. Vegetables, fruits, and whole grains
    c. Calories
    d. Sugar

19. Which statement is true in regard to catastrophic reactions?
    a. They are unavoidable in persons with dementia.
    b. They may be precipitated by too much sensory stimulation.
    c. Providing activity will subdue the catastrophic reaction.
    d. They are always expressions of violence.

20. An appropriate approach to reality orientation is to
    a. ask the resident if he knows your name.
    b. ask the resident what his plans are for the day.
    c. ask the resident if he knows the date.
    d. tell the resident what day it is.

21. Residents in assisted living facilities
    a. need 24-hour nursing care.
    b. require supervision with ADLs.
    c. need skilled rehabilitation.
    d. have mental health needs.

22. Residents in skilled nursing facilities
    a. need 24-hour nursing care.
    b. are acutely ill.
    c. require subacute care.
    d. are independent with ADLs.

23. The OBRA regulations
    a. are guidelines that all hospitals follow.
    b. mandate all health care facilities to promote "aging in place."
    c. require facilities to maintain residents at the highest possible level.
    d. do not apply to nursing assistants.

24. Malnutrition
    a. is a risk in certain residents in long-term care facilities.
    b. is a chronic condition in most elderly individuals.
    c. frequently occurs in residents who eat less than all of their meals.
    d. is not a concern for the elderly.

25. When a resident is being tube fed, the head of the bed must be elevated at least:
    a. 10° to 15°.
    b. 25° to 40°.
    c. 30° to 45°.
    d. 50° to 70°.

26. Residents who are at risk of dehydration
    a. drink 6 cups of fluid each day.
    b. are always confused.
    c. have straw-colored urine.
    d. often have difficulty holding a cup.

27. Sepsis is
    a. a serious complication of infection.
    b. a reversible mental illness.
    c. seldom a concern in the elderly.
    d. a complication of malnutrition.

28. Signs and symptoms of delirium are
    a. abdominal pain and nausea.
    b. mental confusion and memory impairment.
    c. catastrophic reaction and reminisence.
    d. headache and sore throat.

29. A resident tells you she is going home to prepare dinner for her children, then proceeds to go toward the front door. Your best response is to walk with her and say
    a. "Don't go outside."
    b. "Your children live in another state."
    c. "Stay inside. What do you like to cook?"
    d. "Your children are spending the night at a friend's house."

30. Validation therapy
    a. helps residents maintain dignity and self-control.
    b. is necessary in physical rehabilitation programs.
    c. orients residents to the season, time, date, and day.
    d. uses music to help residents relax and relieve stress.

D. Nursing Assistant Challenge.

Mr. Delgotti, 83 years old, is one of your assigned patients. Think about the changes that occur with aging and answer these questions.

31. What changes occur in the integumentary system?

32. Because of these changes, what complications could occur during his hospital stay?

33. What actions can you take to avoid these complications?

34. What possible complications can occur in the digestive system?

35. What observations are especially important for all the body systems because of Mr. Delgotti's age?

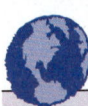

EXPLORING THE WEB

Description	Location
Consumer information about long-term care	http://www.longtermcareliving.com
Nursing care of the older client	http://www.delmarhealthcare.com/olcs/white/pnotes.asp (see Chapter 28)
Administration on Aging	http://www.aoa.gov
Advance for Post Acute Care	http://www.advanceforpac.com
American Geriatrics Society	http://www.americangeriatrics.org
American Medical Directors Association	http://www.amda.com
Eden Alternative	http://www.edenalternative.com
Elder Web	http://www.elderweb.com
Long-Term Care Nursing Leadership	http://ltcnurseleader.umn.edu
LTC-Resources	http://www.ltc-resources.com
National Association of Directors of Nursing in Long Term Care	http://www.nadona.org
National Association of Geriatric Nurse Assistants	http://www.nagna.org
Nursing Home Administrators	http://www.nursinghomeadministrators.net
Nursing Home Compare	http://www.medicare.gov
Nursing Home Quality Initiative	http://www.cms.hhs.gov/providers/nursinghomes/nhi
Nursing Homes Magazine	http://www.nursinghomesmagazine.com
Skilled Nursing/Assisted Living (SNALF)	http://www.snalf.com

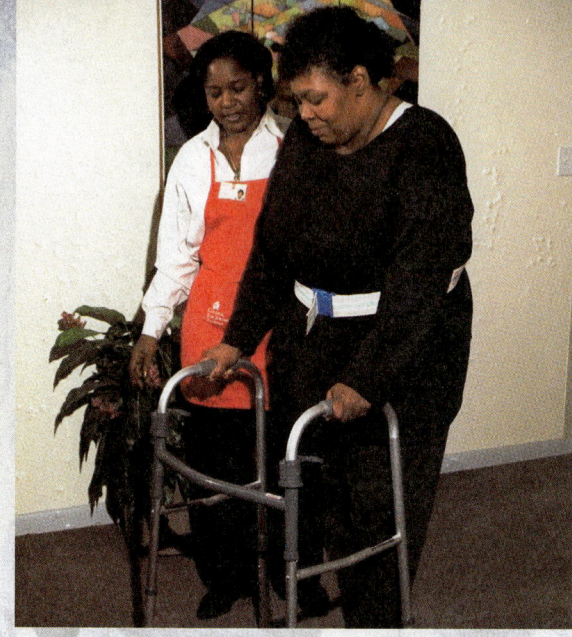

The Organization of Home Care: Trends in Health Care

objectives

After completing this unit, you will be able to:

- Spell and define terms.
- Briefly describe the history of home care.
- Describe the benefits of working in home care.
- Identify members of the home health team.
- List guidelines for avoiding liability while working as a home health assistant.

- Describe the types of information a home health assistant must be able to document.
- Identify several time management techniques.
- List ways in which the home health assistant can work successfully with families.

vocabulary

Learn the meaning and the correct spelling of the following words and phrases:

client care records	intermittent care	time/travel records

INTRODUCTION

The health care of persons (clients) in their own homes is an age-old tradition. It was not until the middle of the twentieth century that there was a massive trend to move patient care out of the home and into the community health care facility. The late nineteenth century saw the growth of medical schools and the licensing of physicians. Schools of nursing soon followed. Hospital staffing slots were filled with students enrolled in these programs. Although the permissive laws of the early 1900s gave requirements for nursing licensure, the laws did not restrict nursing practice. There were few legal restrictions for people who provided care in patients' homes. Almost anyone could hire out to provide such care. A few years later, laws were passed to control nurse education. These laws specifically stated the acts that a nurse could and could not perform. Anyone practicing nursing without a license could be held liable.

World War II brought with it:

- A gradual increase in the need for more technical care, as procedures and equipment became more complex.
- Introduction of antibiotics and better techniques of infection control. (Availability of antibiotics was very limited and most were reserved for use in treating individuals in the military.)
- Growth of a new, supplementary force of workers (nursing assistants) to assist in providing nursing care.
- Construction of many new health care facilities.
- Hospital care of sick people.

Today, the pendulum has swung back once more toward treating acutely ill people in hospitals and providing alternative care (such as home care, day care, or long-term care) for all others (Figure 33-1). Factors that foster this interest in home care include:

- Expensive high technology (Figure 33-2)
- Introduction of diagnosis-related groups (DRGs), resulting in earlier discharge from hospitals
- Growing population of chronically ill people
- The establishment of hospice care, enabling terminally ill people to choose to stay at home during their last months of life
- The preference of the health care consumer to remain at home if possible

PROVIDERS OF HOME HEALTH CARE

Because of the increasing demand for home care, there are many different types of home care providers:

- Government-sponsored agencies controlled by city or county governments
- Private agencies; some are for-profit and others are nonprofit

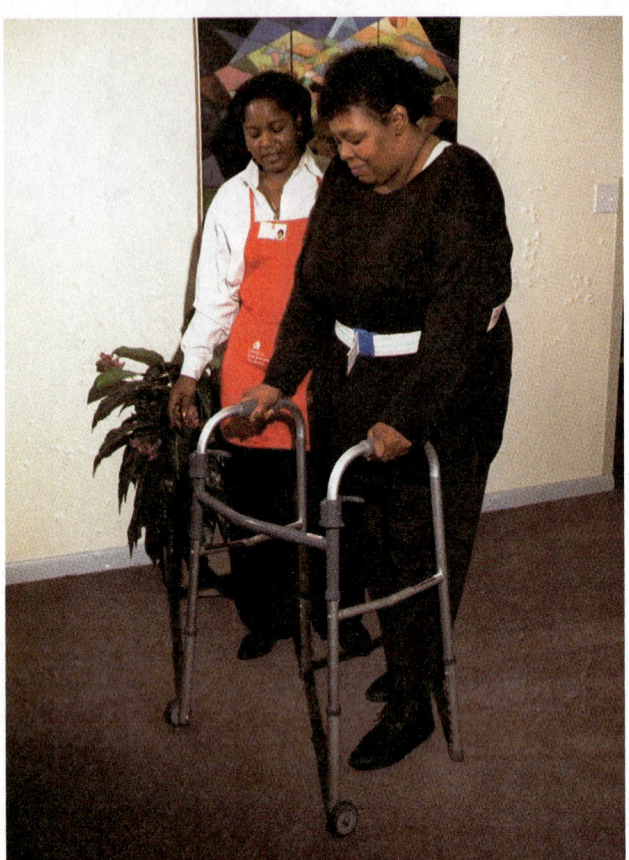

FIGURE 33-1 The trend toward home care is growing in response to increased numbers of people requiring continuing care.

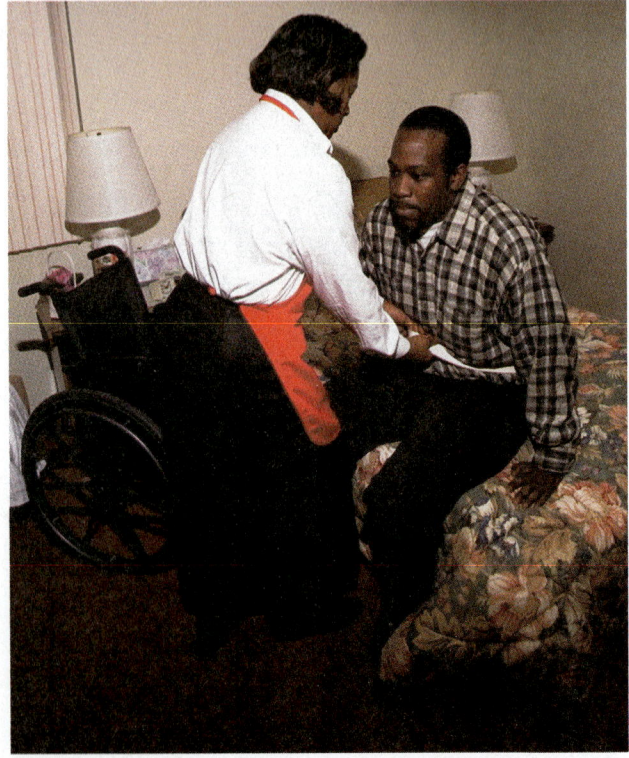

FIGURE 33-2 High technology has increased hospital costs, making home care a practical alternative.

- Hospital-sponsored agencies

These providers employ several types of health care workers, including nurses, nursing assistants, therapists, and social workers. Each employer has personnel policies that regulate job descriptions, salaries, and benefits. The employer provides new employees with an orientation to the agency and to their responsibilities.

In addition to working in clients' homes, home care workers may also visit residents in assisted living facilities (ALF). These facilities do not usually provide nursing services. Residents who become ill or injured may need temporary or short-term nursing care. Rather than moving them from their home in the assisted living facility to a facility that provides a higher level of care, home health care workers visit the resident in the ALF to provide necessary services. Using home care workers in this manner promotes the "aging in place" philosophy of the assisted living facility and enables residents to remain in a familiar environment while they recover.

BENEFITS OF WORKING IN HOME HEALTH CARE

After you have completed your nursing assistant class, you may choose to join a group that provides home health care. There are advantages to working in such agencies:

- Satisfaction of giving complete care to one client at a time
- Satisfaction of caring for the same client over a period of time (Figure 33-3)
- Opportunity to work with greater independence
- Part-time employment, if desired

The person working in home care must have dependable transportation to the homes of the clients. In small towns and rural areas, the worker needs to have a car to get from one client to the next. In larger cities, the worker may be able to use public transportation.

SOURCE OF REFERRAL

Most persons using home care are patients being discharged from a hospital or skilled care facility. The health care team at the discharging facility completes a discharge plan and evaluates the person's need for continuing care at home. The physician must then write an order for home health care. The discharge planner at the hospital or long-term care facility provides the patient and family with a list of agencies from which to choose the home care provider (Figure 33-4). (In some areas of the country, only one agency may be available.) The selected agency is given medical information about the patient and then begins to plan care.

PAYMENT FOR HOME HEALTH CARE

Home health care may be paid for by:

- Medicare, for persons over 65 years of age or for those who have been disabled for 2 or more years
- Medicaid (in some states)
- Private insurance companies
- Client's personal funds

Government programs and most insurance companies will only pay for home care that is considered "skilled" and is provided as intermittent care. This means that the nursing assistant or other caregiver goes to the home, performs certain procedures or treatments, and then leaves. If a family or client needs a caregiver for several hours a day, they will probably have to pay for the services with their own money. Because this is very costly, most home care is given on an intermittent basis.

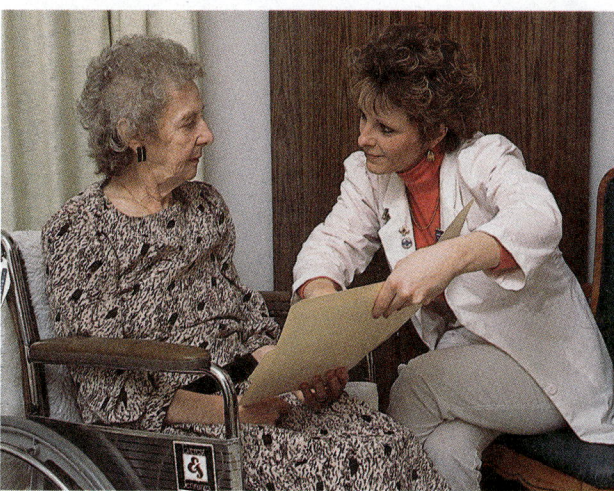

FIGURE 33-3 Caring for the same client over a period of time provides great satisfaction.

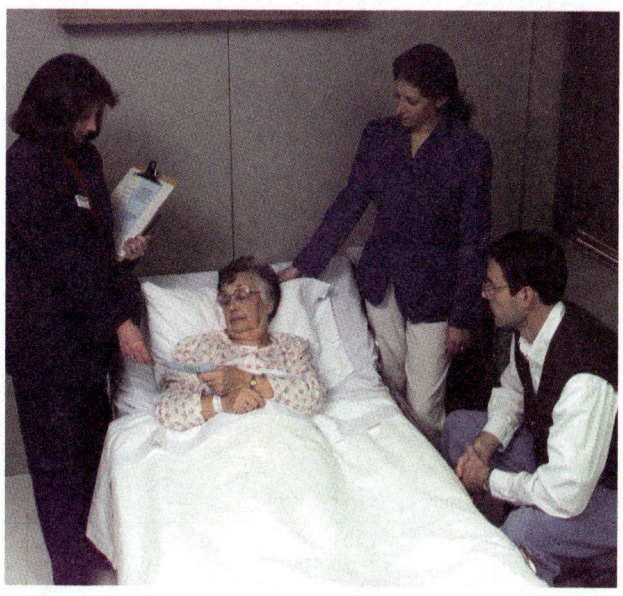

FIGURE 33-4 The patient and family select a home health agency.

AGE-APPROPRIATE CARE *Alert*

Clients receiving home care vary widely in age. They are not all elderly. Many are children with serious illness or disabilities. Some will need temporary care, but others will need lifetime care. The needs of some clients are complex, placing great demands on family caregivers. Caregiving can be difficult for family members and loved ones. Having outside caregivers come to the home assists them to maintain the quality of their own lives, and gives them time to take care of their personal affairs.

THE HOME HEALTH CARE TEAM

The home health care team consists of the:

- Client (the person in need of care)
  - Clients are of various ages.
  - They need differing levels of nursing and physical care.
  - They may have chronic, progressive ailments.
  - They may be recovering from acute illness, surgery, or childbirth.
  - They need assistance with activities of daily living.
  - They usually require skilled services.
- Family
  - Family members may act as alternate caregivers.
  - They may live in the client's home.
  - They may or may not be supportive of the client.
- Nursing assistant
  - Provides direct client care (Figure 33-5).
  - Provides for the client's safety and comfort.
  - Makes observations and reports them to the nurse.
  - Documents observations and care that was given.
- Supervising nurse
  - Completes periodic client assessments.
  - Plans the care.
  - Teaches and supervises nursing assistants.
  - Coordinates care and members of the home care team.
- Physician
  - Writes orders and acts as a consultant and guide.
- Other specialists, such as:
  - physical therapist (Figure 33-6)
  - occupational therapist
  - speech therapist
  - social worker
  - dietitian

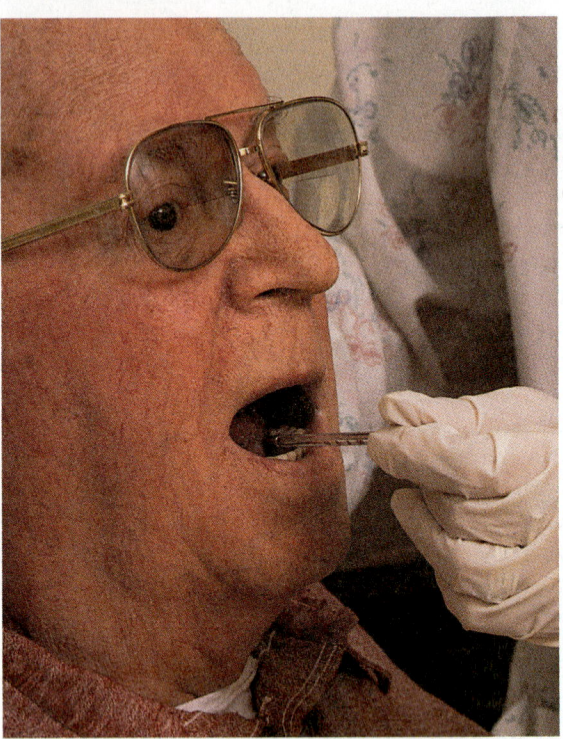

FIGURE 33-5 The home health assistant provides direct client care.

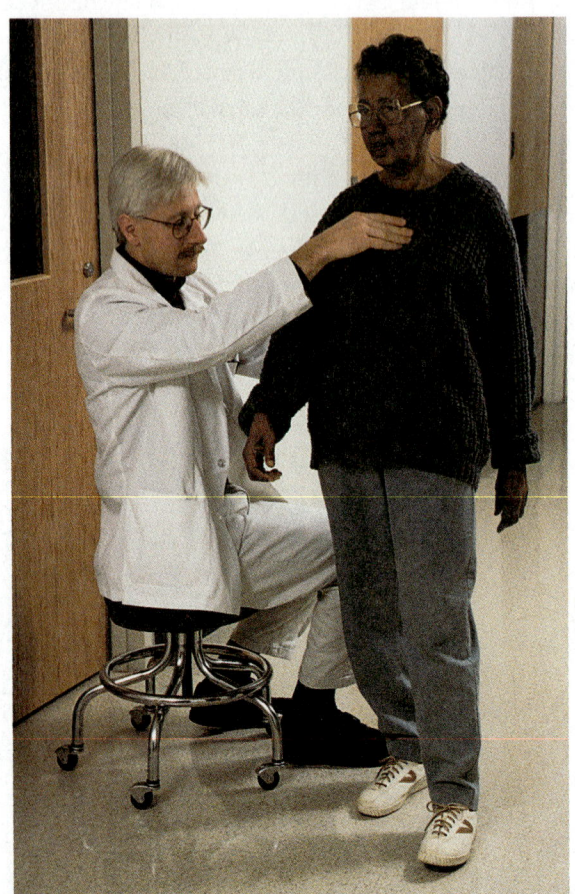

FIGURE 33-6 Many disciplines work together to meet the client's needs. The physical therapist makes home visits several times a week.

THE ASSESSMENT PROCESS

The nurse does an assessment of the client during the first visit. Other health care professionals assigned to the case also complete assessments. After the assessments are finished, the nurse and other team members:

- Identify the client's problems
- Determine approaches to resolve the problems
- Establish goals for the client
- Evaluate the home situation for safety concerns
- Determine the amount of time needed for each visit and the length of time the services may be required

The nurse discusses the plans with the client. The nurse includes the client's wishes as much as possible within the available payment plan. The nurse then develops the assignment for the nursing assistant. You may be assigned to care for several clients or a particular client for a:

- Specified number of hours daily
- Specified period two or three days per week
- Long-term period
- Brief period

LIABILITY AND THE NURSING ASSISTANT

You need to be aware of the responsibilities involved in home care and how to avoid legal problems associated with caregiving.

RECORDKEEPING

Be sure you know exactly what documentation you are expected to do, what types of records you should keep, and the forms you need to use. All documentation must be accurate, complete, and up-to-date. Medicare and insurance companies frequently audit these records to decide whether to pay for the services.

Two types of records are compiled by the nursing assistant giving home care. They are time/travel records and client care records.

Time/travel records (Figure 33-8) are a record of how you spend your time in the client's home. The information recorded includes:

- Time of arrival

guidelines *for*

Avoiding Liability

- Be sure you are given a job description upon employment that lists your specific duties and responsibilities. In some areas, home health assistants are only allowed to do certain assigned tasks if they or the employing agency are working with an insurance company or Medicare. Auditors check the tasks assigned and confirm what is actually done in the client's home.
- Carry out procedures carefully and do them as you were taught.
- Always keep safety factors in mind and be on the lookout for possible hazards.
- Be familiar with client's rights.
- Ask for assistance if you are assigned to a procedure that you have never performed before.

Make sure the procedure is within the legal boundaries of nursing assistant practice.

- Do only those tasks that are assigned to you.
- Know how to contact the supervising nurse for questions and issues related to the care of your client. Do not overstep your authority.

- Know how and when to contact emergency services for the client (Figure 33-7).
- Document your care and observations carefully and completely.
- Participate in care conferences with the other team members.

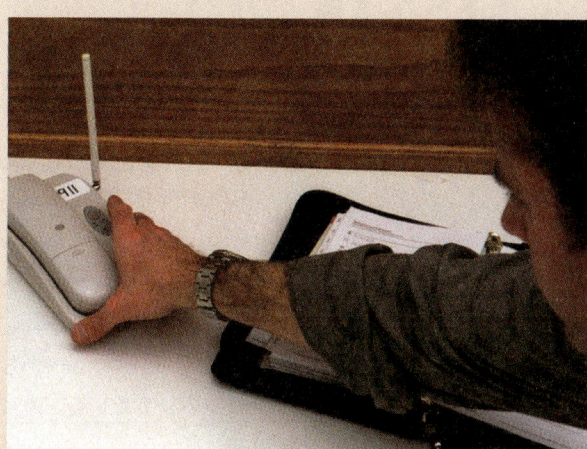

FIGURE 33-7 Home health workers must know how to contact emergency services.

RIVERVIEW HOME HEALTH SERVICE
8987 Walkman Ave
Parkhurst, Nebraska
Time and Travel Log

CARE GIVER NAME ___Siadto, Laura CNA___ TITLE ___Home Health Assistant___ EMPT. NO. __62718__ DATE __Aug. 29__

CLIENT NAME/ADDRESS (Last, first)	SERVICE PROVIDED	VISIT CODE	NON BILL CODE	TIME IN	TIME OUT	CLIENT CONTACT TIME	ODOMETER READING	MILES
Volheim, Eleonore	Bedbath, Shampoo	4		8^{15}	9^{05}	50 min	From: 45,061 To: 45,068	7 miles
Jaronello, Sharri		1		9^{30}	9^{45}	15 min	From: 45,068 To: 45,083	15 miles
Doyle, Kindra	Enema, bedbath, amb	4		10^{10}	11^{30}	1 hr. 20 min.	From: 45,083 To: 46,001	18 miles
Hammond, Rachel	Ass't c colostomy cath care, bath, ROM	4		11^{50}	1^{20}	1 hr. 30 min.	From: 46,001 To: 46,017	16 miles
Minzey, Aimee		2		1^{30}	1^{35}	—	From: 46,017 To: 46,025	8 miles
Galloway, Rosa		5		1^{50}	2^{00}	10 min	From: 46,025 To: 46,028	3 miles
							From: To:	

Total Visits __6__   Total Mileage __67__   Parking Fees __—__

Visit Code
1 IE Initial Eval & Rx
2 FV Follow Up Visit
3 DV Discharge Visit
4 HC Home Care
5 Hospital/Hospice
6 MC Maternal/Child

Nonbill Code
1. Refused Care
2. Patient Not Home
3. Non-Bill
4. Expired
5. Delivered Supplies

Supervising Nurse: __Bruce Davenport R.N.__

FIGURE 33-8 Example of a time/travel record.

LEGAL *Alert*

For your own protection and peace of mind, you should insure your vehicle. You should also check with your employer to find out about auto insurance if you are driving your car to and from work, as well as to homes of various clients throughout the work day. You may be surprised to learn that the employer's insurance does not cover 100% of the time. For example, the policy does not cover you if you have an accident while traveling to or from work and your home. However, it may cover you if you have an accident during the course of your normal work day, when you are visiting clients' homes. Knowing exactly when your employer's insurance policy covers your automobile is important. You should also find out if you will be expected to transport clients in your personal vehicle. If so, investigate whether your insurance or the employer's insurance will cover the client if you are in an accident. Likewise, find out if you will be expected to drive the client's car. If so, you must learn whose insurance will be responsible in the event of an accident.

- Time of departure
- Length of time required for specific activities
- Travel time if working in more than one home
- Mileage or transportation costs

Keeping a time/travel record requires accuracy and some calculations. Fill in the record as you complete each assignment. Do not wait until the end of the day or your assigned time and then try to rely on your memory.

To compute mileage (round off to the nearest full mile):

- Record the car odometer reading before starting to your assignment.
- Record the odometer reading when you arrive at the client's home.
- Subtract the starting odometer reading from the arrival reading.
- Record this difference as the mileage.

For example, if the reading on your car odometer before starting was 45,061 and upon arrival at the client's home it is 45,068, the mileage should be recorded as 7 miles (45,068 – 45,061).

Client care records (Figure 33-9) are a record of:

- Care given, such as bathing, positioning, range-of-motion exercises
- Client responses to care
- Housekeeping tasks completed, if assigned to you by the nurse
- Observations:
  - Condition of skin
  - Vital signs
  - Elimination; bowel and urine
  - Food and fluid intake
  - Appetite
  - Incidents such as client falls
  - Any observation that indicates a change in the client's health status
  - Mental status: orientation, alertness, mood, and behavior

You may be expected to keep reports that cover a longer period of time. For example, you may need to keep a weekly or monthly record of daily blood testing results for a client with diabetes. The physician may change the schedule of insulin based on your long-term report.

TIME MANAGEMENT

As a home health care assistant, you are responsible for planning your assignment and completing the client's care within a certain amount of time. You may have several clients to see during your shift. They will be expecting you at a specific time of the day. There are several actions you can take to make the best use of your time:

- Be sure you have everything you will need for your assignments before you leave home. This might include a thermometer, watch with second hand, stethoscope, blood pressure cuff, forms for documenting, pen.
- Have a work plan in mind before you arrive at the client's home. For example, will you give the client a bath first or help him with his exercises first?
- Organize your supplies before you begin your assignment. Gather together the linens, client clothing, and other items you will need.
- Avoid being distracted by the family. There are many things you may need to discuss with the family, but you probably will not have time for lengthy conversations.
- Call your next client if you find you will be arriving later than expected.
- Avoid getting bogged down in tasks that you are not expected to perform.

WORKING WITH FAMILIES

Clients may have a spouse or other family members who reside in the home. For other clients, their families may live elsewhere but stop in periodically. In some situations family members may live so far away that they can seldom visit. Family members may call or visit while you are there, seeking information on the client's condition. It is best to let the client speak with them directly if possible. If the client cannot do this, then remember to be objective in your comments. If you do not know the answer to a question, be honest and say so rather than providing false information. Refer all medical questions to the physician or the nurse.

Remember that as a home health assistant, you are a guest of the family and client. You may be assigned to clients who have values and cultural beliefs that are vastly different from yours. It is not your role to try to change this. Report to your supervisor if you feel that there are family practices that are detrimental to the client's well-being and health. Families can be an excellent resource for you. They may be able to give you additional information about the client that will help you to give better care. This can avoid frustration for both you and the client. The family may also be able to tell you how they have cared for the client in the past.

Tact and courtesy are important when communicating with the family. They may wish to be involved in the caregiving, but it is important that you complete the tasks to which you have been assigned. The family has a right to know the progress the patient is making, but there may be some information that the client does not wish you to tell the family. You may need to discuss this issue with your supervisor. Families may feel overwhelmed and discouraged at times, particularly if the client has had a long illness. They need your support, so you must be realistic yet hopeful (Figure 33-10).

RIVERVIEW HOME HEALTH SERVICE
8987 Walkman Ave
Parkhurst, Nebraska
Client Care Plan / Progress Notes

HOME HEALTH ASSISTANT YOLANDA BROWN, CNA

CLIENT NAME NICHOLAS FRENCH   CLIENT ID # 72824C

ADDRESS: 529 MAPLE AVE.   PARKHURST, NEBRASKA

ACTIVITY

Time	Activity
0800	Arrived, Determined needs, planned activities Client seemed fatigued "Slept poorly". On nasal O_2 2.5L
0830	Circumoral pallor noted. Vital signs checked. Dyspneic on exertion.
0900	Put laundry into washing machine. Started breakfast. Client ate 1 sl. toast, 8 oz oatbran cereal / milk 6oz orange juice
0930	Prepared equipment for A.M. care – complete bath, shave and denture care.
1000	Asst to commode, soft brown formed stool.
1030	Made comfortable in easy chair. Reading newspaper. Nasal O_2 Cleaned kitchen including refrigerator
1100	Linen changed – dusted and dust mopped bedroom. Vacuumed living room.
1130	Prepared lunch.
1200	Client ate 1/2 chicken sandwich, 8 oz. tea, chocolate pudding, 8 oz. tomato soup.
1230	Client returned to bed for nap
1300	Cleaned lunch dishes and prepared salad, jello for evening meal
1330	Put washed laundry into dryer.
1400	Cleaned bathroom, washed kitchen floor Put bed linen into washer.
1430	Made out shopping list for A.M.
1500	Client awake. Assisted into living room. Watching T.V. Ordered O_2 tank replacement.
1530	Folded and put clean laundry away. Put washed linens in dryer.
1600	Client seems more rested. Color improved. Resp. easier. Notified supervisor of client's progress.
1630	Left client's home @ 3²⁵ P.M.

Y. Brown CNA

VITAL SIGNS	T	P	R	B/P
	97⁴	92	26	116/74
INTAKE	486 ml			
OUTPUT	730 ml			

SUP. SIGNATURE _____

FIGURE 33-9 Examples of client care records. *continues*

RIVERVIEW HOME HEALTH SERVICE
8987 Walkman Ave
Parkhurst, Nebraska
Client Care Plan / Progress Notes

WT. <u>146</u> TEMP. <u>98</u> BP <u>114/80</u> P <u>70</u> R <u>14</u> MD CONTACT <u>C. Boylston</u>

HOMEBOUND DUE TO <u>Spinal Cord Injury – Paraplegia</u> MEN. STATUS <u>Alert – Coherent</u>

PROBLEMS	INTERVENTIONS	TIME	PLAN	OUTCOME
① Potential altered	Maintain high-calorie, low-residue, high protein diet		Morning Care	Tol. Well
nutrition: less than	Reduce high calcium and gas-producing foods.	0700	Breakfast	ate entire meal
body requirements	Provide balanced meals and supplements morn'ng and even'ng	0815	Commode	soft formed stool
		0900	Bath, Cath Care,	
		0945	ROM	
			up in wheelchair	Tolerated well
② Potential for disuse	Exercise to tolerance Avoid fatigue ROM	1030	6oz High Cal drink	
syndrome related to	Turn and reposition q 1 hr.	1045	Returned to Bed	
effects of immobility	Up in wheelchair B.I.D.	1130	Positioned on Rt. Side	
	Encourage self-care activities to tolerance		Positioned on Back	
③ Alteration in bowel	Stool Softener, Glycerine	1230	Lunch	½ tuna sand/tea
elimination: constipation	Suppositories, enemas, PRN.			
	Check for BM q 3 day		up in wheelchair	
		1330	Returned to Bed	
④ Potential for infection	Routine catheter care	1430	Positioned on left side	
related to indwelling	Change per routine schedule		Watching T.V.	
Foley catheter		1500		
⑤ Self-concept disturbance	Encourage verbalization of feelings and fears.			
related to effects of	Encourage independence. Be positive and reassuring.			
limitations				

DAILY SUMMARY

Diet and supplements taken fairly well. Activity tolerated. Muscles soft but some tone. Soft formed stool.

Expressed frustration during transfers from bed to wheelchair. Enjoys reading and watching T.V.

Seems to be gaining some confidence in transfer activities.

Visit Date _____   Pt. Last Name,   Employee

Nursing Supervisor Report   First Initial ___ <u>Mitchell, D.</u> ___   Signature <u>Ruthy Chek, CNA</u>

Joint Visit in Home _____   Patient's personal care and comfort measures by home assistant are:

Conference _____   superior _____ ; good _____ ; satisfactory _____ ; need improvement _____ ;

Services provided were appropriate _____ ; inappropriate _____ .

Comments

FIGURE 33-9 *continued*

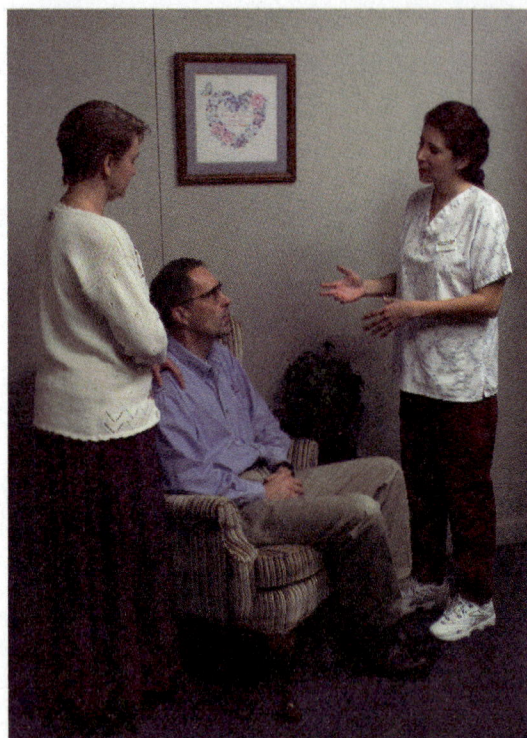

FIGURE 33-10 You must be realistic yet hopeful with families.

If you are spending an entire shift with the client, remember that you are getting paid to spend this time giving care. If all procedures are completed, take your cue from the client or family as to what activities you should complete for the rest of your tour of duty. Some clients may wish to be left alone to read (Figure 33-11) or watch television. Others may seek your companionship for visiting or playing cards. If you are working through the night, ask the client or family if you may read or do quiet activities such as needlework

while the client is sleeping. Family members may ask you to do something that is not part of your assignment. Whether you can meet their request depends on:

- The nature of the request
- The time involved in filling the request
- The policies of the home care agency
- Whether you are assigned to intermittent visits to the client or assigned to work a full shift

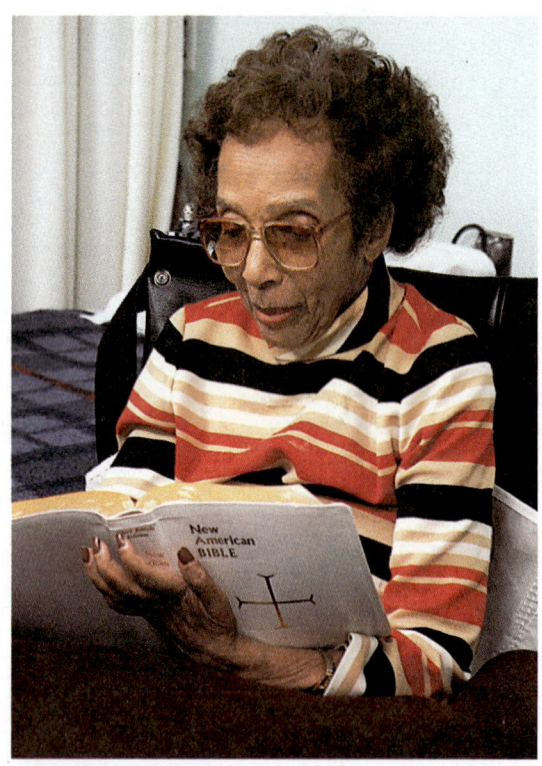

FIGURE 33-11 Some clients may prefer to be left alone to pursue their own interests.

REVIEW

A. True/False.

Mark the following true or false by circling T or F.

1. T F World War I stimulated the enrollment of students in hospital-based nursing programs.

2. T F Many new hospitals were built after World War II.

3. T F Only nurses and nursing assistants are employed for home health care.

4. T F The physician acts as care coordinator for the client's home care.

5. T F Home health assistants are expected to provide direct client care.

6. T F Documentation is an important responsibility of the home care assistant.

7. T F The demand for home care has decreased within the last few years.

8. T F The client may receive the services of a physical therapist.

9. T F The home health care assistant may have the opportunity for part-time employment.

10. T F The home health assistant is responsible for completing periodic assessments of the client.

B. Multiple Choice.

Select the one best answer for each of the following.

11. World War II brought about
    a. an increase in the need for more technical care.
    b. widespread use of antibiotics.
    c. a limited supply of health care workers.
    d. construction of hundreds of nursing homes.

12. Home care is increasing because
    a. hospitals are overcrowded.
    b. there are fewer physicians.
    c. people like being cared for in their own homes.
    d. families can do some of the nursing care.

13. The person receiving home health care is called the
    a. client.
    b. patient.
    c. resident.
    d. recipient.

14. Members of the home care team include
    a. housekeepers.
    b. the family.
    c. laundry workers.
    d. gardeners.

15. Time management is important because
    a. you can get home earlier.
    b. you may have more than one client to care for during your shift.
    c. the client may have other business to tend to.
    d. the agency will make more money if you work faster.

16. Home care assistants must be able to:
    a. know how to care for family pets.
    b. make accurate observations.
    c. manage the household bills.
    d. drive the client's car.

C. Nursing Assistant Challenge.

You are almost finished with your nursing assistant course and you are thinking about employment. You have been offered jobs in a home health agency and in a hospital and are having trouble making a decision. Your instructor advises you to think about both the advantages and disadvantages of working for each employer. Make a two-column list for each, labeling the columns "advantages" and "disadvantages."

EXPLORING THE WEB

Description	Location
Home Accessible Home	*http://www.advancefornurses.com* (see past articles July 1, 2002)
Home Based Primary Care Improves Quality of Life	*http://www.advancefornurses.com* (see past articles January 22, 2001)
Home Healthcare Nurses Association	*http://www.hhna.org/home.html*
Thou Shalt Honor Caregiving Resources	*http://www.thoushalthonor.org*
Visiting Nurse Association	*http://www.vnaa.org*

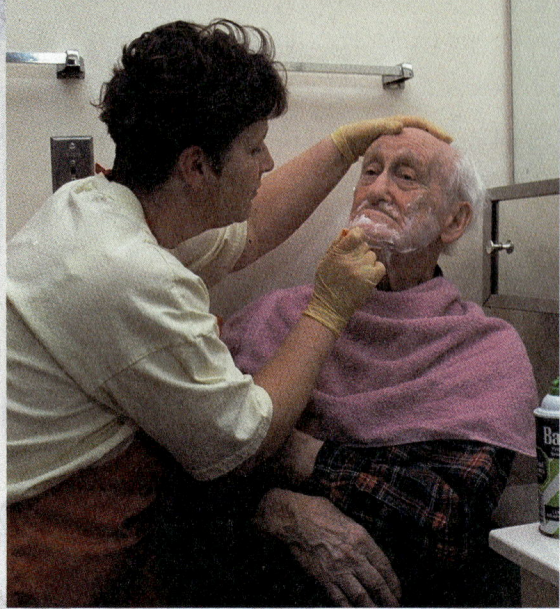

The Nursing Assistant in Home Care

objectives

After completing this unit, you will be able to:

- Spell and define terms.
- Describe the characteristics that are especially important to the nursing assistant providing home care.
- List at least 10 methods of protecting your personal safety when working as a home care assistant in the community.

- Describe the duties of the nursing assistant who works in the home setting.
- Describe the duties of the homemaker assistant.
- Carry out home care activities needed to maintain a safe and clean environment.

vocabulary

Learn the meaning and the correct spelling of the following words and phrases:

home health assistant   homemaker aide   homemaker assistant

THE HOME HEALTH CAREGIVER

In the last unit you learned about the structure of home health care. In this unit you will learn more about the responsibilities of the nursing assistant (home health assistant) working in the client's home.

The nursing assistant is an important part of the health team in the acute hospital and in the long-term care facility. The nursing assistant is part of an equally important team that provides home care.

The nursing assistant may be called:

- **Home health assistant** or home health aide, whose primary role is to provide assistance with nursing care.
- **Homemaker assistant** or **homemaker aide** when the primary role is to do housekeeping chores. The homemaker assistant carries out general household tasks, prepares meals, and runs errands such as food shopping.

The nursing assistant providing health care services may be asked to carry out homemaker assistant duties in some cases.

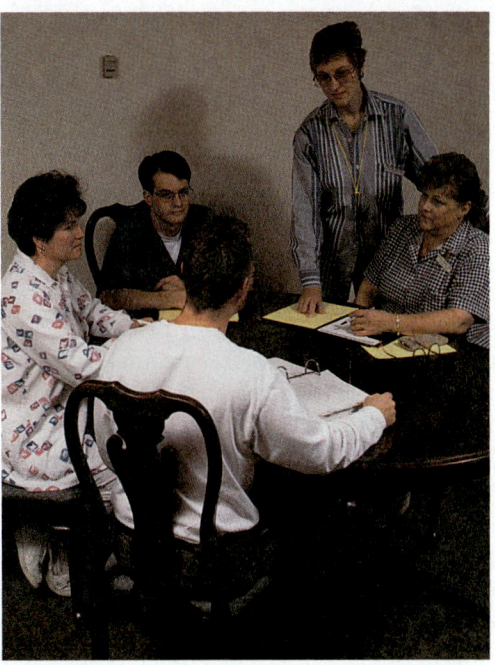

FIGURE 34-1 The home health assistant contributes to the client's care plan.

THE HOME HEALTH ASSISTANT AND THE NURSING PROCESS

You are part of the nursing process. During:

- *Assessment*, your observations and careful reporting can make a valuable contribution to the objective and subjective data from which the analysis of the client's needs is made. Make note of:
  - The client's response to your care
  - The interactions between family members and friends that could lead to stress on the client
  - Support services that may be needed
- *Planning*, you contribute as you actively share in care conferences (Figure 34-1).
- *Implementation*, you spend the most time with the client. You are therefore responsible for seeing that the plan is carried out.
  - Report any difficulties in carrying out the plan.
  - Develop ways to organize your work to make the plan more efficient.
- Evaluation, you once more contribute to the nursing process when you share your observations about the success or lack of success of the care.
  - Be accurate and concise in your reporting.
  - Be honest in your appraisal of the client's progress and the point at which your services are no longer needed.

CHARACTERISTICS OF THE HOME CARE NURSING ASSISTANT AND HOMEMAKER ASSISTANT

The home care nursing assistant and homemaker assistant must have a full measure of the characteristics you have already come to associate with a successful hospital-based assistant. However, some characteristics should be particularly strong in an assistant who works in clients' homes.

Remember that you will be working directly with the client and her personal possessions, without a supervising nurse constantly with you. This means you must demonstrate:

- Honesty, as you handle the client's possessions and shopping money. Treat the possessions with care and respect. Keep an accurate record of all money spent and receipts received.
- Self-starter ability. You must know and carry out your assigned tasks promptly and efficiently without needing someone to remind you.
- Self-discipline. Do not allow yourself to waste time on activities such as smoking, chatting with friends on the phone, and drinking coffee just because there is no supervisor to constantly check on your progress.
- Accuracy and attention to details, so that each task is performed exactly as you were taught.
- Organization, so that you plan your activities to make the best use of your in-home time. Plan your activities around the client's schedule, not your own.

- Maturity, so that judgment and assessments can be made properly.
- Insight that gives you the ability to see the client as a whole person who is an interactive member of a family unit and community.
- Observational skills. Be able to recognize and report abnormal signs and symptoms.
- Adaptability. Although you will need all the physical, emotional, and communication skills you learned and practiced in the clinical setting, you must be creative in adapting them to the home situation. For example, a cut-open plastic bag covered with a towel may be substituted for the bed protectors used in the hospital. Housekeeping chores may be performed as the client rests.
- Acceptance of clients and their home environments. Remember, your clients will be of all ethnic and religious groups and economic levels.
- Ability to perform independently, making decisions within the limits of your responsibilities and the scope of the assignment.

PERSONAL SAFETY

Personal safety is always a concern for home care workers. Be alert to conditions and people around you. Inform your employer promptly if you believe unsafe conditions exist. Thousands of nursing personnel make daily home care visits, and incidents of violence are few. However, you must trust your own instincts. If something does not feel right, it probably is not.

Other ways of protecting your own safety are:

- Map out the route in advance so you know where you are going.
- Inform the patient what time you will be arriving.
- Lock your purse in the trunk of your car at the beginning of your day. Use pockets or a belt-type (fanny) pack for essentials such as driver's license and pens.
- Wear scrubs or clothing that identifies you as a nursing caregiver. Wear your namebadge.
- In potentially dangerous areas, ask your agency if you can make joint visits with a coworker or use an escort.
- If neighbors, relatives, or others become a safety problem, make visits when they are away from the home.
- If a patient suggests that a family member escort you, accept the offer, but never get into someone else's car.
- Keep your gas tank full.
- Avoid parking on deserted streets or in dark areas.
- Keep your car windows up and doors locked at all times.
- Attend classes on personal safety and self-defense.
- Consider purchasing a cellular telephone.

HOME HEALTH CARE DUTIES

The duties of the home health care assistant are planned around the family routine. These duties may include:

- Helping with the activities of daily living
- Giving special treatments, such as prescribed exercises
- Providing comfort measures, such as positioning and special mouth care
- Maintaining a safe environment
- Bathing the client
- Changing linen
- Interacting with family members

Homemaker duties may include:

- Light housekeeping
- Shopping for meals (Figure 34-2)
- Preparing meals

You may also have to transport the client to clinic or therapy visits (Figure 34-3). You must have specific permission from your agency to perform activities outside of the home. The homemaker duties *do not* include:

- Doing heavy housework such as washing windows, waxing floors, or moving heavy furniture
- Making decisions about food purchases, unless the client is unable to do so
- Becoming involved in family disputes by offering opinions or taking sides

The skills you learned in the clinical setting can be adapted to the home environment (Figure 34-4). For example:

- Ice bags can be replaced by plastic bags sealed and wrapped in a towel.

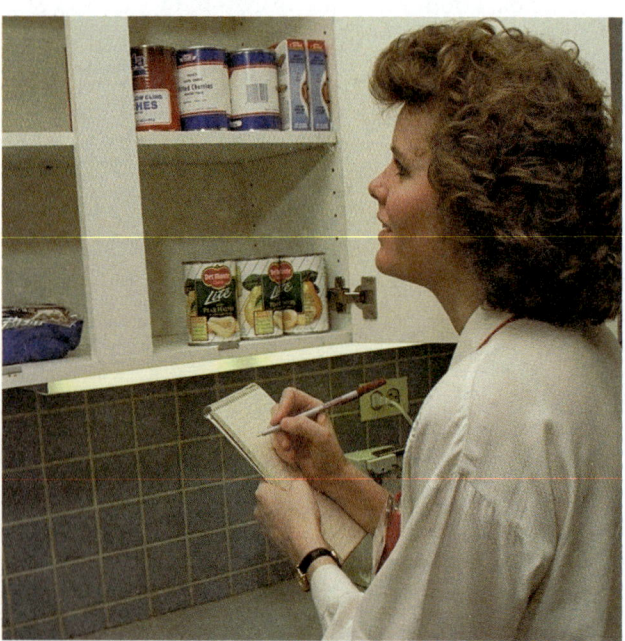

FIGURE 34-2 Homemaker duties may include grocery shopping. Prepare a shopping list before going to the store to make sure you get everything.

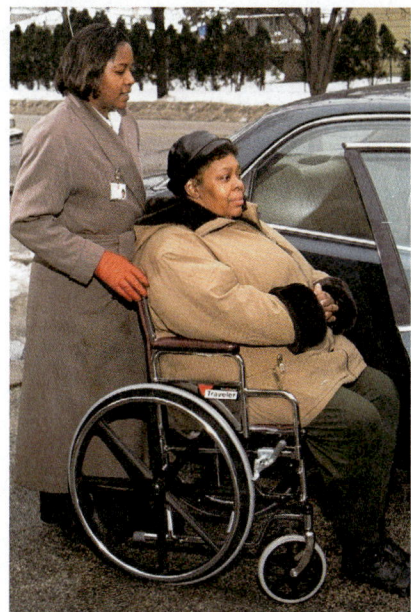

FIGURE 34-3 The home health assistant may have to transport clients to clinics for additional care and therapy.

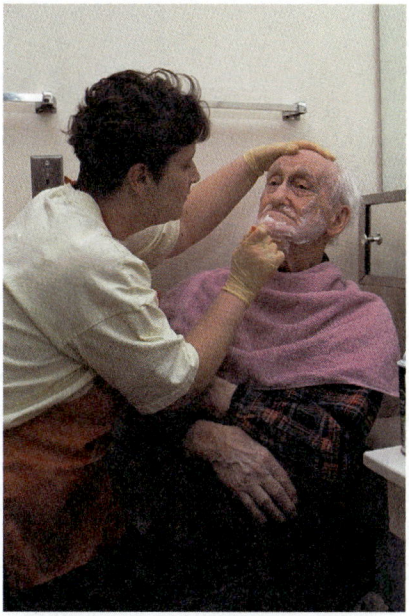

FIGURE 34-4 The skills you have learned may be adapted for care in the home.

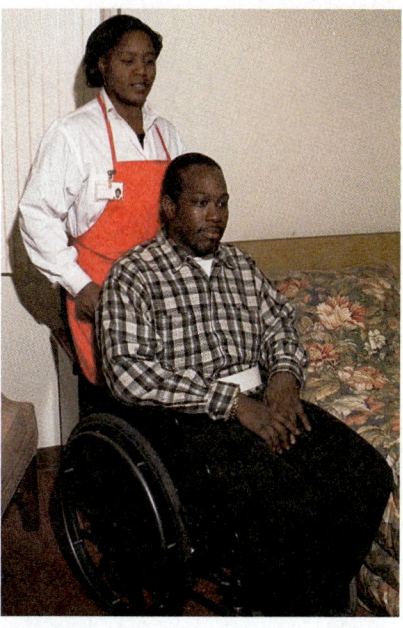

FIGURE 34-5 Equipment may be rented or borrowed from other organizations or agencies.

- Reusable enema equipment can be substituted for disposable enema equipment.
- Extra pillows can be used to support position changes if the bed position cannot be changed.
- Some equipment may be rented from equipment rental companies (Figure 34-5) or borrowed from church groups or other organizations.
- The entire bed can be raised on blocks, to make caregiving easier if the patient is not ambulatory.
- A cotton blanket or lightweight spread can be used for a bath blanket.
- Plastic covered with a twin-size sheet can be used in place of a drawsheet.
- Apply the principles of standard precautions if contact with blood, body fluids, mucous membranes, or nonintact skin is likely.
- A cardboard box can be cut, taped, and padded for use as a back rest (Figure 34-6A).
- Two lightweight pieces of wood nailed at right angles can be padded and used as a footrest to hold bedding off the toes (Figure 34-6B).
- A bed tray can replace an overbed table for eating and activities.
- A paper bag can be taped to the bed springs to dispose of soiled tissues (Figure 34-6C). The entire bag can then be closed and properly handled for disposal.
- A shoe bag tucked under the mattress and hanging by the bedside (Figure 34-6D) can provide compartments for the patient's personal articles.
- A pillowcase hung on the back of a chair can serve as a laundry bag.

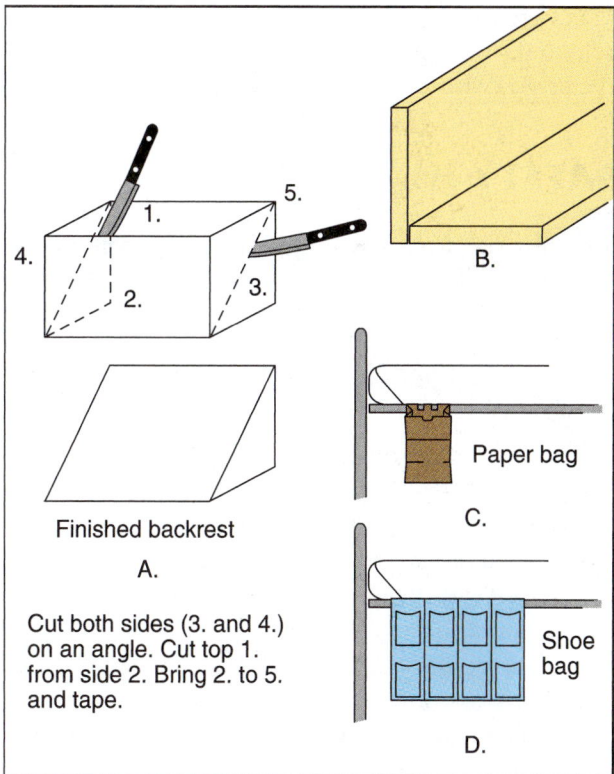

FIGURE 34-6 You can make equipment using readily available materials.

Most home health assistants carry kits that contain:

- Plastic aprons
- Disposable gloves
- Observational equipment such as stethoscope, blood pressure cuff, and thermometers

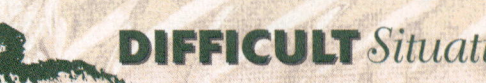

DIFFICULT *Situations*

If the client or a family member informs you of new problems with any of the following when no home care worker is on duty, notify your supervisor: eating, getting in or out of bed, maintaining continence or using the toilet, bathing, or dressing. Clients with new problems related to these activities require further nursing assessment.

SAFETY *Alert*

Pay close attention to safety risks in the following areas, which are the most common locations of injury in the home: stairs and steps, bathroom(s), kitchens, and basements. If you feel there are hazards or other safety or security risks, inform your supervisor promptly. If conditions in the home should be modified, an occupational therapist may be asked to make a home visit to make recommendations. Do not attempt to make mechanical or environmental modifications yourself.

THE HOME ENVIRONMENT

You are responsible for maintaining a safe and comfortable environment for the client. This means you must:

- be alert to unsafe situations.
- control the spread of infection.
- care for and maintain the client's furnishings, supplies, and appliances.
- learn the locations of items that may be needed in an emergency (such as a flashlight or fire extinguisher).

SAFETY IN THE HOME

Your first visit to the home gives you an opportunity to check for safety factors. Tell a family member or supervising nurse about safety problems. For example, things to call to the attention of your supervisor include:

- Furniture or other items that obstruct the client's walkway
- Electrical cords that could cause the client to fall
- Stair railings and stair treads that need repair
- Unstable or lightweight chairs
- Highly polished floors that may be slippery
- The need to lock up specific items if the client is disoriented:
  - chemicals such as household cleaning supplies, paints, insecticides, and cleaning fluids
  - medications, both prescription and over-the-counter
  - aerosol cans
  - small appliances like toasters or irons that can be plugged in and used inappropriately
  - power tools
  - weapons or anything that could be used as a weapon
  - fragile, breakable, or valuable items
  - smoking materials that should only be used with supervision
  - electrical outlets that require covering

- thermostats that may need guards over them
- stove knobs
- Loose scatter rugs, which might cause a fall as the client ambulates
- Electric cords that are under rugs, creating a fire hazard
- Lack of smoke detectors and a fire extinguisher
- Overloaded electrical outlets, which might cause a fire when you use equipment such as an electric lift
- Ambulatory aids that need repair or replacement, such as broken straps on braces or worn rubber tips on walkers, canes, and crutches
- Family or client smoking when oxygen is being used in the home

Your job is not to reorganize the client's home but to ensure a safe environment. Discuss with the nurse any other conditions you feel are unsafe. For example, the client may need:

- Handrails installed by the toilet or the bathtub
- A commode to use if the bathroom is not easily accessible
- A raised toilet seat
- A trapeze to assist with bed mobility
- A mechanical lift for transferring out of bed

These items are readily available from durable equipment providers, and most insurance companies and Medicare will pay for equipment that is required for client care. However, the nurse must consult with the physician and an order must be written for the equipment.

Keep a list of emergency numbers close to the telephone. The list should include the:

- Agency
- Supervising nurse
- Physician
- Family member
- Emergency number 911 (in areas where this number is in use)

If the 911 number is not used in your area, you will need numbers for the:
- Ambulance
- Hospital
- Police department
- Fire department

You should find out if the patient:
- uses a medical alert bracelet or necklace.
- has out-of-hospital code papers or a living will.
- has a special storage place in the house for important medical information that would be needed in an emergency. Some people keep these in the refrigerator so they can be easily located.

Assisting with Medications

The physician may prescribe medications for clients receiving home health care. Nursing assistants are not legally responsible for giving medications. However, you may have to supervise the client as she self-administers the medications. The client may need assistance in opening the container. There are many types of containers available that will hold a week's doses in individual sections labeled for the days of the week. These containers simplify the process and it is easy to determine whether the medications have been taken.

guidelines *for*

Supervising Self-Administration of Medications

- The medicine must be taken at the correct time. Note whether it should be taken before meals, with food, or after meals.
- Check the expiration date to be sure the medicine is not outdated.
- Note whether the client is also taking over-the-counter medications (nonprescription) and check with your supervisor to find out whether these medications will interact with the prescription drugs.
- Perform any monitoring activities required, such as checking the pulse, the blood pressure, or the blood sugar, *before* the drug is taken.
- Note how much medication is left in the container. Follow your instructions for getting the prescription refilled so that the patient does not run out.

ELDER ABUSE

As a home health assistant, you may observe clients who might possibly have been abused. Unit 4 describes the various types of abuse that may be inflicted by staff members, family members, or other residents. These situations may also occur in the home:

- Some families provide loving, capable care for older, dependent relatives for many years without assistance. They may be emotionally stressed and may have also depleted their financial resources.
- In some cases there has been a long family history of one spouse abusing the other.
- Self-abuse may occur when a disabled person is unable to adequately carry out activities of daily living and is unwilling to accept help.

It is not the responsibility of the nursing assistant to determine if an individual has been abused or what type of abuse has been inflicted. It *is* the nursing assistant's responsibility to report to the nursing supervisor any signs or symptoms that might be the result of abuse. This includes:

- Statements of the client that reflect neglect or abuse
- Unexplained bruises or wounds
- Signs of neglect such as poor hygiene
- A change in personality

Remember, these indications do not necessarily mean that the person is being abused. However, they may signal a need for further investigation by your supervisor.

INFECTION CONTROL

Some of the methods used in daily cleaning help to control the spread of infection. Other requirements are:
- Washing your hands (Figure 34-7)

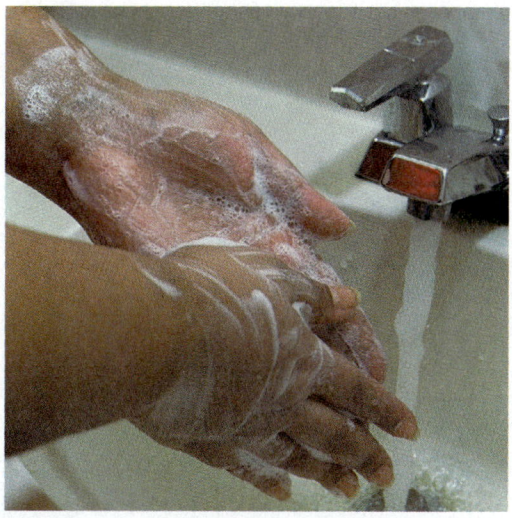

FIGURE 34-7 Handwashing is the most important infection control technique in health care. All handwashing rules and guidelines used in facilities also apply to home care.

- Keeping the kitchen and bathroom clean
- Caring for food properly
- Disposing of tissues and other wastes properly
- Cleaning up dirty dishes
- Dusting daily
- Not allowing clutter to accumulate
- Wearing a plastic apron
- Wearing latex gloves for patient care if contact with blood, body fluids, mucous membranes, or nonintact skin is likely.
- Wearing utility gloves when cleaning environmental surfaces or doing laundry contaminated with blood, body fluids, secretions, or excretions.

HOUSEKEEPING TASKS

In some cases, the homemaker assistant (aide) will perform the housekeeping tasks. In other cases, the home health care nursing assistant may be assigned some or all of these duties.

Cleaning the Client's Room

Keeping the client's room clean is a way to prevent infection. It also helps raise the client's morale. Remember that you are not to rearrange the client's things without permission.

- Pick things up so clutter will not accumulate.
- Keep cleaning equipment in one place so you do not waste time gathering it for each job as you move from room to room (Figure 34-8).
- Clean and put equipment away as soon as you have finished with it.
- Dust the room daily.
- Damp-dust noncarpeted floors weekly or vacuum carpeted floors.

- Remove used dishes and glasses when finished and rinse right away.
- Put clean clothes away after laundering. Hang up robes when not in use.
- Line each wastepaper basket with a plastic bag and empty them regularly.

Cleaning the Bathroom

The bathroom can be a source of infection, so you must be careful and thorough in your daily cleaning (Figure 34-9). Use a disinfectant solution (family's choice) to clean the:

- Inside and outside of the toilet
- Shower or tub after each use
- Sink and faucets
- Countertops
- Floor; if carpeted, vacuum daily

Be sure dirty towels are put into the laundry. Replace them with clean towels and washcloths. Use a deodorant to keep the bathroom smelling fresh and clean.

Cleaning the Kitchen

The kitchen is another area that requires special attention. An unclean kitchen can be the source of infection.

- Clean up after each meal.
- Clean up dirty dishes immediately. Do not allow them to accumulate in the sink.
  - Rinse them and wash by hand in detergent and hot water.
  - Wash glasses first, then silverware, then dishes.

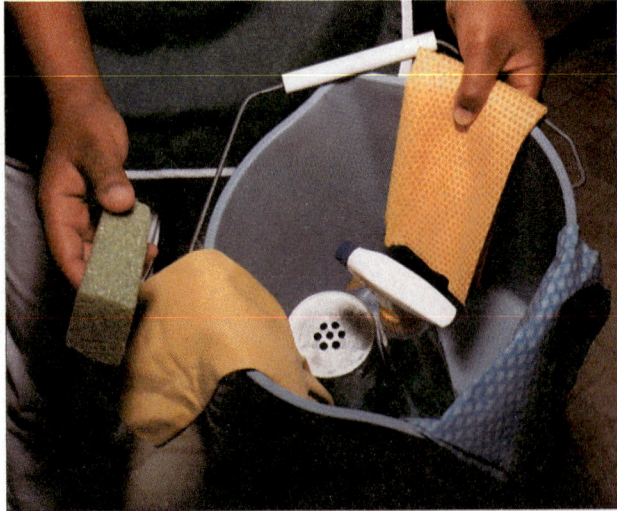

FIGURE 34-8 Keep cleaning equipment together for good organization and efficient time management.

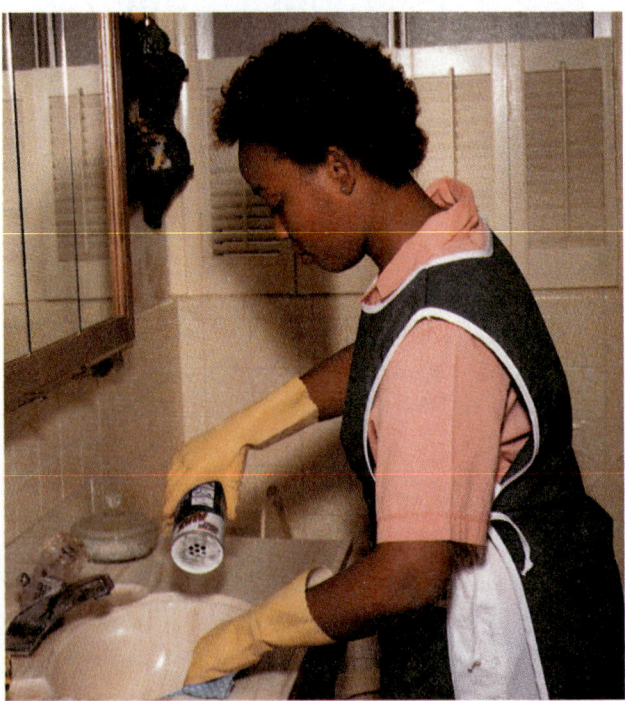

FIGURE 34-9 Clean the bathroom daily.

- Rinse with hot water and allow to dry in drainer.
- Put away when dry.
- You may wash them in the dishwasher by:
  - Rinsing well.
  - Adding recommended detergent to the dishwasher.
  - Loading washer; but do not run the dishwasher until it is full.
- Wash pots and pans by hand; most are not dishwasher-safe.
- Clean sink, countertops, and stove.
- Dispose of garbage properly. It may be put in an in-sink disposer if one is available. Do not include bones. Wrap those tightly in newspaper and put them in the trash (or compactor if available).
- Sweep the floor after each meal.
- Place leftover foods in small covered containers and refrigerate. Use or discard within a few days.
- Keep the refrigerator clean and keep food covered. Clean spills in the refrigerator immediately (Figure 34-10).
- Keep the microwave oven clean (Figure 34-11). Use a damp cloth to wipe up spills immediately and to clean after each use. Make sure you heat food in microwave-safe dishes only. Do not use metal of any kind in a microwave oven. For example, dishes with metallic trim are *not* used.
- Wash the kitchen floor weekly, or more often if necessary.

Ask the client or a responsible family member for instructions on operating appliances before using.

Other Duties

Two other tasks are frequently your responsibility in the home situation. They are food management and laundry.

Food Management. Plan food purchases with the client or a family member. If consultation is not possible, keep these guidelines in mind:

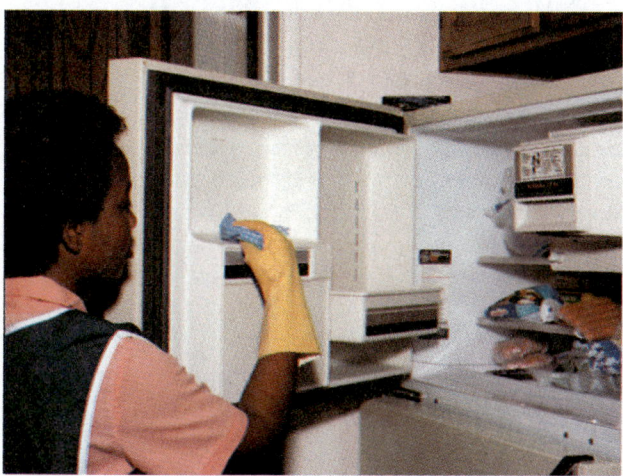

FIGURE 34-10 Wipe up spills immediately.

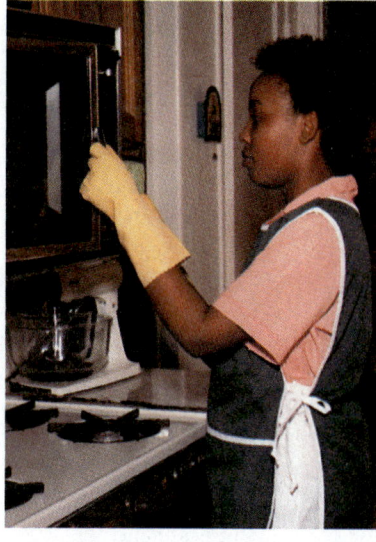

FIGURE 34-11 Wipe the microwave after each use.

- Plan menus a week in advance. Base them on good nutrition.
- Take into consideration the client's preferences, cultural background, and any religious prohibitions.
- Spend only what the client's budget allows.
- Buy only what you need and what can be used. Large quantities are not a bargain if much of it goes unused or is wasted.
- Look for quality bargains.
- Keep track of all money spent and a list of items purchased; keep receipts.
- Make an accounting of all money handled.

Using the weekly menu, prepare foods in such a way that the client's dietary needs are met. Also:

- Wash fresh fruits and vegetables that are to be used soon and store in the refrigerator; store them unwashed if they are not to be used right away. Remember to wash them before use.
- Keep dairy products and meats refrigerated until use.
- Allow frozen meats to thaw in the refrigerator before use.
- Take into consideration the client's ordered diet, any digestive problems, and preferences.
- Keep dried and canned foods in cabinets.

Laundry. Carefully launder the client's clothes. They represent a sizable investment. This may have to be done daily. Always:

- Read labels before laundering. Some clothes must be dry-cleaned or washed at special temperatures.
- Use the client's choice of detergent and read the label for instructions on amount to use.
- Wear gloves when sorting clothing and loading the washing machine if contact with blood, body fluids, secretions, or excretions is likely.
- Separate light and dark fabrics and wash them separately.

- Wash drip-dry fabrics separately so they can be hung and dried or folded.
- Be sure clothes can be dried in a dryer, and use the proper setting.
- Hang clothes after wiping off the clothesline, if a dryer is not available.

- After laundering, fold, iron, or hang clothes.
- Check for needed repairs and do mending before storing clothes.
- Ask the client or a responsible family member for operating instructions before using washer or dryer.

REVIEW

A. True/False.

Mark the following true or false by circling T or F.

1. T F The home health care nursing assistant may be responsible for both nursing care and household tasks.

2. T F The home health care nursing assistant makes no contribution to the nursing process, because care is given at the client's home and not in the hospital.

3. T F Self-discipline is an important characteristic of the nursing assistant who works in a home.

4. T F When washing dishes, wash the plates first, then the pots and pans, and then the glassware.

5. T F As a home health assistant, your primary role is to do the housework and cooking.

6. T F Your observations are important for monitoring the client's progress.

7. T F Because the client is your responsibility, you need not be concerned with the client's family.

8. T F If the client smokes, it is permissible for the home health assistant to smoke with the client.

9. T F Adaptability is an important characteristic for home health assistants.

10. T F You should clean the bathroom daily.

B. Multiple Choice.

Select the one best answer for each of the following.

11. A special characteristic needed by a home health care nursing assistant working in a home is
    a. self-discipline.
    b. being a follower.
    c. being a fast worker.
    d. being able to take shortcuts.

12. Which household tasks would the home health care nursing assistant *not* be required to do?
    a. Shop for food.
    b. Move heavy furniture.
    c. Carry out nursing procedures.
    d. Prepare food for the client.

13. Home health assistant responsibilities include all but which of these?
    a. Washing windows
    b. Cleaning the bathroom daily
    c. Documenting the care given
    d. Shopping for the client

14. The home health assistant should carry a kit that contains
    a. a change of clothes.
    b. thermometers, stethoscope, blood pressure kit.
    c. gardening gloves.
    d. a policy amd procedure manual.

15. Daily tasks may include
    a. sweeping the floor after each meal.
    b. watering the lawn and shrubs.
    c. shampooing the carpets.
    d. washing windows.

C. Nursing Assistant Challenge.

You are working for a home health agency and Mrs. Fernandez is one of your clients. She has had a stroke and needs assistance with all activities of daily living. Your assignment includes: a bath, personal care, dressing, making the bed, making her breakfast, making her lunch so she can have it after you are gone, cleaning the bathroom, and general "picking up" around her apartment. She asks if you will go to the drugstore before you leave to get her prescriptions refilled. Make a work plan that includes all of these tasks, as well as any other routine tasks you need to complete.

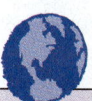

EXPLORING THE WEB

Description	Location
Choosing In-Home Assistance	*http://www.ec-online.net*
Directory of Home Care Resources	*http://www.providerconsult.com*
Hiring a Home Care Aide	*http://www.aoa.gov/wecare/hire.html*
Home Care Aide Association of America	*http://www.nahc.org*
Home Care for Patients Receiving TPN	*http://www.advancefornurses.com* (see past articles December 4, 2000 and December 18, 2000)
How Do I Hire a Home Care Employee?	*http://www.agingkansas.org*
How to Find a Home Care Service	*http://www.mayoclinic.com*
Iowa Association for Home Care	*http://www.iowahomecare.org*
National Association for Home Care	*http://www.nahc.org*
National Family Caregivers Association	*http://www.nfcacares.org*
Oxygen Use in Home Care	*http://www.advancefornurses.com* (see past articles August 14, 2000)
Thou Shalt Honor	*http://www.thoushalthonor.org*
Types of Home Care Agencies	*http://cancerresourcecenter.com*

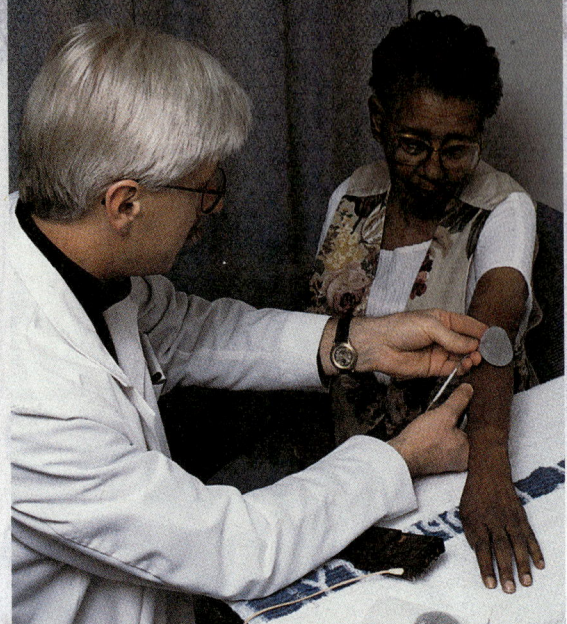

Subacute Care

objectives

After completing this unit, you will be able to:
- Spell and define terms.
- Describe the purpose of subacute care.
- List the differences between acute care, subacute care, and long-term care.

- Describe the responsibilities of the nursing assistant when caring for patients receiving the special treatments in subacute care.
- Demonstrate the following procedures:
  - Procedure 95 Checking Capillary Refill
  - Procedure 96 Using a Pulse Oximeter

vocabulary

Learn the meaning and the correct spelling of the following words and phrases:

alopecia
anorexia
capillary refill
central venous
  catheter (CVC)
chemotherapy
continuous
  ambulatory
  peritoneal dialysis
  (CAPD)

dialysis
epidural catheter
exacerbation
fistula
graft
hemodialysis
hypoxemia
infiltration
Kelly [clamp]

multisensory
  stimulation
narcotic
oncology
patient-controlled
  analgesia (PCA)
peripheral
  intravenous central
  catheter (PICC)
peritoneal dialysis

piggyback
pulse oximetry
radiation therapy
spasticity
subacute care
tracheostomy
transcutaneous
  electrical nerve
  stimulation (TENS)
transitional care

DESCRIPTION OF SUBACUTE CARE

Subacute care is comprehensive, goal-oriented care for individuals with acute illness, injury, or exacerbation (worsening) of a chronic medical condition. It is provided instead of, or immediately after, hospitalization, at a lower cost than the acute care facility. Subacute units can be located in freestanding facilities, or may be specialized units within a hospital or skilled nursing facility. The patients in the subacute unit do not need hospital services, but their needs are greater and more complex than the skilled nursing facility can provide. Thus, subacute care provides a transitional level of care from one setting to another. For this reason, subacute units may be called transitional care units. When the patient reaches his goals, he is transferred out of the subacute care unit. The subacute unit bridges the gap between the acute care hospital and the chronic care setting or the patient's home.

The emphasis and philosophy of subacute is slightly different from those of long-term care. Subacute care focuses primarily on managing new or acute problems, whereas long-term care is designed to manage chronic problems. (Subacute care also manages chronic conditions affecting patient recovery.) The subacute unit is not a permanent place for patients to live. In contrast, nursing facility placement may be permanent.

Patients in the subacute care unit require frequent nursing assessment. Frequent evaluation and adjustment of the overall plan of care are also necessary. The recurring assessment and adjustment continue until the patient's condition stabilizes and treatment goals are met.

On a subacute care unit, there are:

- more medications and treatments to administer than on a regular skilled unit.
- more frequent physician's visits than in a skilled care unit.
- more sophisticated types of equipment than in a skilled care unit.

Types of Care Provided in a Subacute Care Unit

Most subacute care units provide specialized care in one or two areas. Some examples are:

- Rehabilitation—all therapies are provided and the patient participates in rehabilitation for 5 hours a day, 6 or 7 days a week (Figure 35-1).
- Peritoneal dialysis—a method of ridding the body of wastes for a person who has kidney failure.
- Ventilator weaning and tracheostomy care for persons who have been unable to breathe without the help of a ventilator
- Cardiac monitoring for persons who have a myocardial infarction or acute heart failure

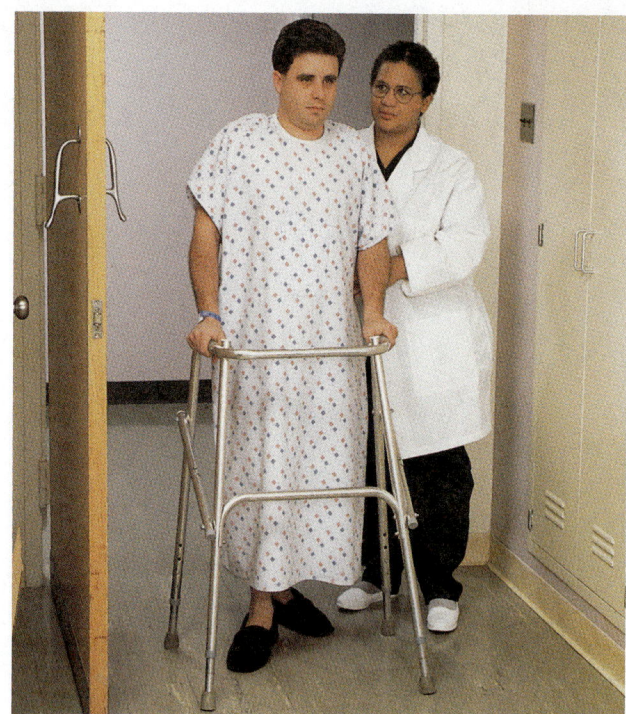

FIGURE 35-1 Some patients have intensive rehabilitation needs to recover from the effects of trauma.

- Pain management and control for persons who have acute or chronic pain
- Oncology—the care of persons with cancer who are receiving treatments such as radiation or chemotherapy
- Wound management for persons with stage 3 or stage 4 pressure ulcers, ulcers related to peripheral vascular disease, or burns
- Specialized care for persons who have suffered brain damage resulting from trauma or stroke
- AIDS care
- Hospice care
- Postoperative care for persons who have other complicating conditions such as chronic obstructive pulmonary disease or diabetes
- Infusion therapy for persons needing ongoing intravenous fluids, nutrition, medications, or antibiotic therapy
- Pre- and posttransplant care—the care of persons waiting for an organ transplant, and management and stabilization of patients after a major organ transplant
- Coma care—weaning off drugs and tubes, multisensory stimulation (intense stimulation of sight, sound, touch, smell, pressure, and pain to help the patient awaken and use previously unused portions of the brain), and management of patients in a coma who have respiratory, nutritional, skin and eye care, contracture prevention, and elimination needs

Types of subacute care units and examples of the services provided in each are listed in Table 35-1.

TABLE 35-1 TYPES OF SUBACUTE CARE UNITS			
Type of Subacute Facility	**Description**	**Typical Medical Problems of Patients Admitted**	**Goals of Care**	**Average Length of Patient's Stay**
Transitional Subacute Unit	• A less expensive setting than the acute care hospital • Provides 24-hour-a-day RN coverage • RNs in this unit have special acute care education, experience, and certifications • Rehabilitation therapies are 7 days a week • Respiratory therapy is available 24 hours a day • A registered dietitian is regularly available	• Severe wounds or stage III or IV pressure ulcers • Strokes • Patients who have had open heart surgery, heart attack, acute congestive heart failure, or other heart conditions • Patients with tracheostomy who require respiratory management • Cancer, including chemotherapy and radiation therapy • Patients who require intensive rehabilitation programs • Medically complex patients with diabetes, digestive problems, or renal disorders	• Manage care and therapy in a less expensive setting than the acute care hospital • Discharge patient to home, an assisted living facility, or a skilled nursing facility	5–40 days
General Medical/Surgical Subacute Unit	• Care for patients with complex medical care and monitoring needs, rehabilitation therapy, nursing assessment and intervention • RN coverage is provided 24 hours a day • RNs working in this unit have special acute care education, experience, and certifications • Rehabilitation therapies are available seven days a week • Respiratory therapy is available 24 hours a day • A registered dietitian is regularly available	• Patients requiring long-term IV therapy for infection, nutrition, or other medical problems without other significant complications • Patients with stable medical problems, including cardiac, digestive, renal, or diabetes • Patients who have had strokes that require 1 to 3 hours of therapy (PT, OT, and/or speech) daily • Patients with neurologic or orthopedic conditions requiring 1 to 3 hours of therapy each day • Patients with HIV disease/AIDS	• Manage care and therapy in a less expensive setting than an acute care hospital in a cost-effective manner • Discharge patient to home, an assisted living facility, or a skilled nursing facility	7–21 days
Chronic Subacute Unit	• Care for patients with little hope of recovery or return to functional independence • RN on duty at least 8 hours a day • If an RN is not on duty, an LPN or LVN is in charge • Restorative nursing care is provided for comfort and to prevent deformities, maintain self-esteem • A registered dietitian is regularly available	• Patients who are dependent on ventilators for breathing • Long-term comatose patients • Patients with progressive neurologic conditions • Patients requiring restorative care from nursing staff with guidance, teaching, or assistance from therapy personnel	• Provide care in the most cost-effective manner, considering medical problems and needs	60–90 days

continues

TABLE 35-1 *continued*

Type of Subacute Facility	Description	Typical Medical Problems of Patients Admitted	Goals of Care	Average Length of Patient's Stay
Chronic Subacute Unit *continued*	• Physical, occupational, speech, and respiratory therapies are available			
Long-Term Transitional Subacute Unit	• Care for medically complex patients and those who depend on an acute ventilator • Many different types of physician specialists must be available to care for patients in this type of unit • Unit director is a highly skilled, educated, and qualified RN with acute care experience • Patients require a high degree of RN intervention because of their acute medical problems • Respiratory therapists usually provide daily services • A registered dietitian is available, if needed	• Acute ventilator-dependent patients who require complex daily care and management of respiratory problems • Medically complex patients with at least two medical or surgical diagnoses requiring special medical services and daily RN assessment and intervention	• Manage care and therapy in a less expensive setting than an acute care hospital	More than 25 days
Specialized Subacute Unit	• Care of specialized groups of patients, such as pediatric patients • Many different types of physicians and other specialists must be available to care for patients in this unit • Unit director is a highly skilled, educated, and qualified RN with experience in the unit specialty • Patients often require a high degree of RN intervention because of their acute medical problems • RN staffing determined by the specialty nature of the unit. Most provide RN services 24 hours a day • Patients require daily RN assessment and intervention • Respiratory therapists usually provide daily services • Rehabilitation therapies are available 7 days a week • A registered dietitian is available, if needed	• Medically complex patients grouped together according to need or medical diagnosis	• Manage care and therapy in a less expensive setting than an acute care hospital • Discharge patient to home, an assisted living facility, or a skilled nursing facility	Varies with the type of unit; commonly 60–90 days

Nursing Assistant Responsibilities

If you work on a subacute care unit, you will participate in special staff development classes to prepare you to meet the needs of patients in your care. A nursing assistant on a subacute unit is expected to:

- work closely with registered nurses who are specialists in critical care or in a specific area of nursing, such as rehabilitation or wound care.
- have extensive knowledge of the types of patients in the unit.
- care for patients receiving complicated treatments.
- have excellent observational skills, because of the complex conditions of the patients.
- be a member of an interdisciplinary team that includes professionals in physical therapy, occupational therapy, speech therapy, respiratory therapy, and social services.

It is important that the staff on a subacute care unit be able to provide for the patients' emotional well-being. Many of these patients will be able to return to their own homes. For them, this is a time of rejoicing and for making plans for the future. These patients may still have concerns if they will have to rely on community services or family members to meet some of their needs. Some of the patients will have an uncertain future. For example:

- Will the patient receiving dialysis receive a kidney transplant in time?
- Will the cancer be cured in the patient receiving oncology treatments?
- Will the patient on a ventilator be able to be weaned off the ventilator, or will it be a lifelong need?
- Will the patient receiving rehabilitation recover enough independence to be able to go home?

SPECIAL PROCEDURES PROVIDED IN THE SUBACUTE CARE UNIT

You will be assigned to care for patients who are receiving special treatments because of their health problems. These treatments may require the use of equipment that is unfamiliar to you. As a nursing assistant, you will not be expected to be responsible for these procedures. However, you will be providing the same personal care and procedures that you would with any patients.

Taking Vital Signs in the Subacute Unit

Patients in the subacute unit require close monitoring of their vital signs. When taking vital signs on patients, remember:

- Avoid taking blood pressure on the side affected by a stroke.

- Avoid taking blood pressure in the arm with a dialysis graft or shunt.
- Avoid taking blood pressure in an arm with an IV.
- Avoid taking blood pressure in the arm on the side where a patient recently had a breast removed.
- Avoid taking an oral temperature on patients with tubes in the nose or mouth.
- Report abnormal vital signs to the nurse immediately.
- If patients are connected to electronic devices for vital sign monitoring, respond to alarms immediately.

Caring for Patients Connected to Special Equipment

Patients in the subacute unit are frequently connected to electronic monitoring and caregiving devices. Many of these devices are used by patients 24 hours a day and cannot be disconnected while personal care is provided. The nursing assistant must be careful not to accidentally move, bump, or disconnect the equipment. Avoid bending, kinking, or placing traction on tubes entering surgical incisions or body cavities. In most cases, you will not be permitted to adjust or regulate the equipment. If an alarm on a piece of equipment sounds, respond immediately. Notify the nurse without delay.

Rehabilitation

Patients may require intense rehabilitation because they have had:

- a stroke that affected their mobility, their ability to complete the activities of daily living, or their speech.
- orthopedic surgery or an amputation (Figure 35-2).

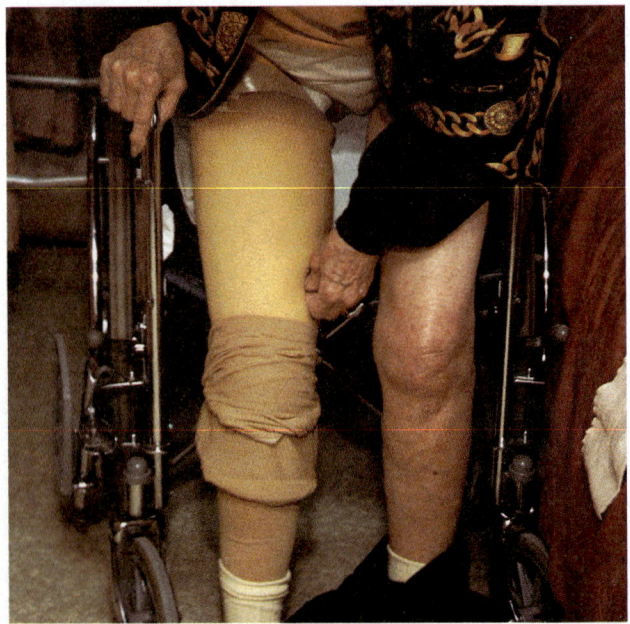

FIGURE 35-2 Some patients are admitted to learn how to apply and use a prosthesis following an amputation.

- an accident that resulted in neurological or orthopedic problems.

All caregivers working with these patients must have a knowledge of rehabilitation as well as a knowledge of the underlying condition (stroke, brain injury, etc.). You need to know what the goals are for the patients and what approaches you will be using to help the patients reach their goals. Consistency is the key to successful rehabilitation.

Intravenous Therapy

Intravenous (IV) therapy refers to medication or solutions administered directly into a vein. Standard intravenous therapy is given into a peripheral vein (a large vein in the arm). This is called an IV. The IV may consist of a single bag of solution connected to simple tubing with a needle or small catheter on the end. Sometimes an additional small bag of fluid is attached to tubing that is connected to the main (primary) tubing. This is called a **piggyback**. The small bag contains medication such as an antibiotic that is intermittently dispersed into the vein (Figure 35-3).

The nurse will immobilize the IV insertion site to prevent the catheter from moving (Figure 35-4). Movement is

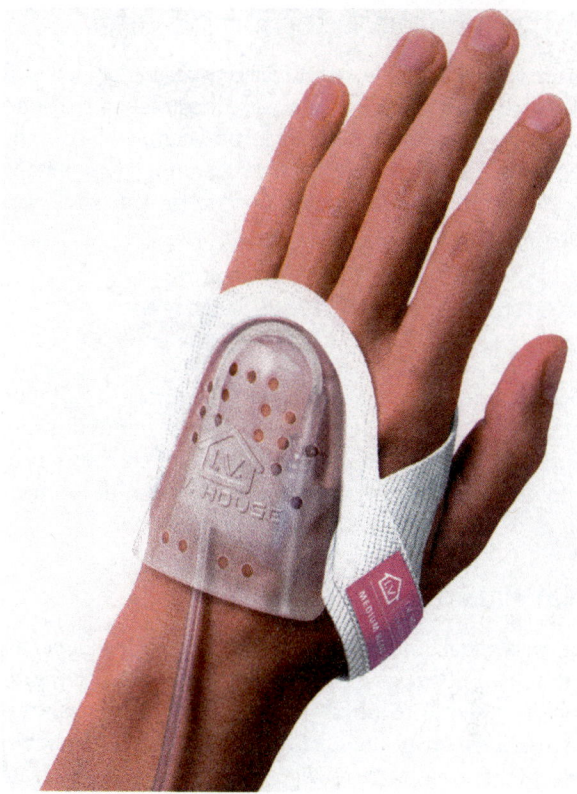

FIGURE 35-4 The nurse will secure the IV insertion site with a transparent dressing or device to prevent movement. Look through the transparent material to check the skin for signs of infiltration. *(Photo courtesy of I.V. House, Inc., St. Louis, MO [800] 530-0400)*

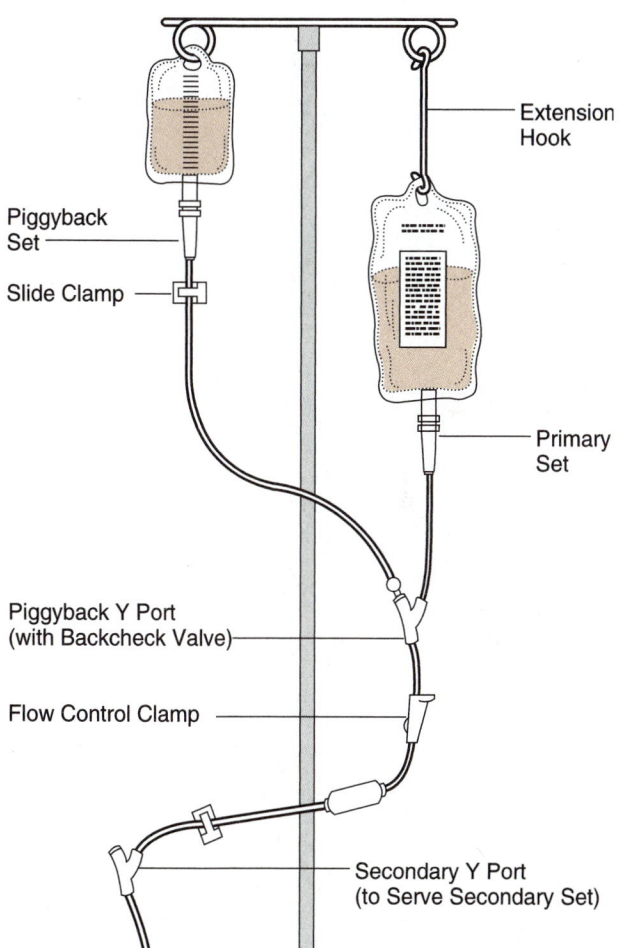

Extension Hook

Piggyback Set

Slide Clamp

Primary Set

Piggyback Y Port (with Backcheck Valve)

Flow Control Clamp

Secondary Y Port (to Serve Secondary Set)

FIGURE 35-3 The large bag contains intravenous fluid that flows continuously into the vein. The small bag (piggyback) contains medication that is given for a short period of time.

uncomfortable and increases the risk of catheter dislodgment. The nurse is responsible for the intravenous infusion. However, you must monitor the intravenous site and tubing each time you are in the room.

The most common problem of IV therapy is **infiltration**. This occurs when the catheter or needle comes out of the vein and fluid flows into the surrounding tissue. If an IV infiltrates, the drip rate often slows or stops. Monitor the needle insertion site for swelling, cool skin temperature, and a white or pale skin color. The patient may complain of burning or pain. If the patient experiences these problems, or if you are unsure of the infiltration status of the IV, promptly notify the RN. If infiltration occurs, he or she will discontinue it and restart it in another area. The nurse may instruct you to apply warm compresses to the area of infiltration.

Use caution when moving the patient to avoid dislodging the intravenous line. When caring for the patient, avoid pulling on, kinking, or otherwise obstructing the tubing. Avoid positioning the patient with the tubing under the body. If possible, position the arm with the IV at heart level when the patient is in bed. When the patient is ambulating, instruct him or her to place the arm with the IV across the abdomen. Advise the patient not to comb hair or brush the teeth using the arm with the IV. Notify the nurse immediately if an alarm sounds on an intravenous pump.

Central Venous Insertion

IV therapy can also be administered through a **central venous catheter** (**CVC**). A special catheter is inserted into a vein near the patient's collar bone (Figure 35-5). The catheter tip ends in or near the heart chamber. CV therapy is used to administer medications or to provide total parenteral nutrition.

Peripheral Intravenous Central Catheter Line

A **peripheral intravenous central catheter** or **PICC** line (Figure 35-6) consists of a catheter that is inserted into a peripheral vein and threaded upward through the vein to the jugular or subclavian vein. It is used to administer medications or to provide total parenteral nutrition.

Total Parenteral Nutrition

Total parenteral nutrition (TPN) is also called hyperalimentation. TPN is given to a patient whose bowel needs complete rest. All required nutrients (carbohydrates, proteins, and fats) are given directly into the vein so the bowel does not have to work to digest food. Patients receiving TPN may need to be weighed daily or every other day. This should be done at the same time of day with the patient

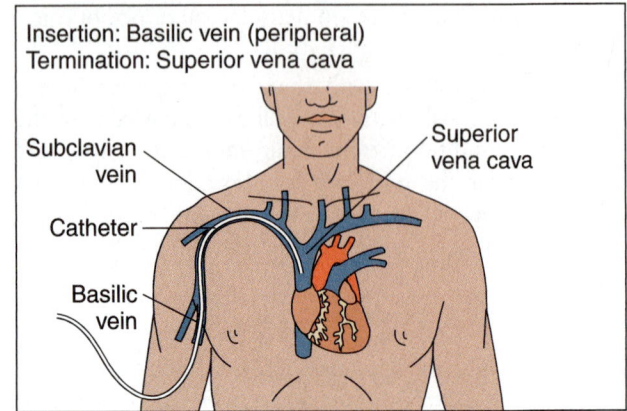

FIGURE 35-6 The peripherally inserted central catheter (PICC) is usually inserted into the upper arm. The long catheter is threaded to the superior vena cava of the heart.

wearing the same type of clothing. The patient may be gradually switched over to enteral feedings. With an enteral feeding, liquid nourishment is administered through a tube inserted into the patient's stomach (Figure 35-7).

TPN feedings bypass the organs of the digestive system entirely, allowing them to rest and heal. The RN will care for the insertion site. Be sure the tubing is not obstructed or kinked. Be very careful to avoid dislodging the tubing when moving or caring for patients. Many health care facil-

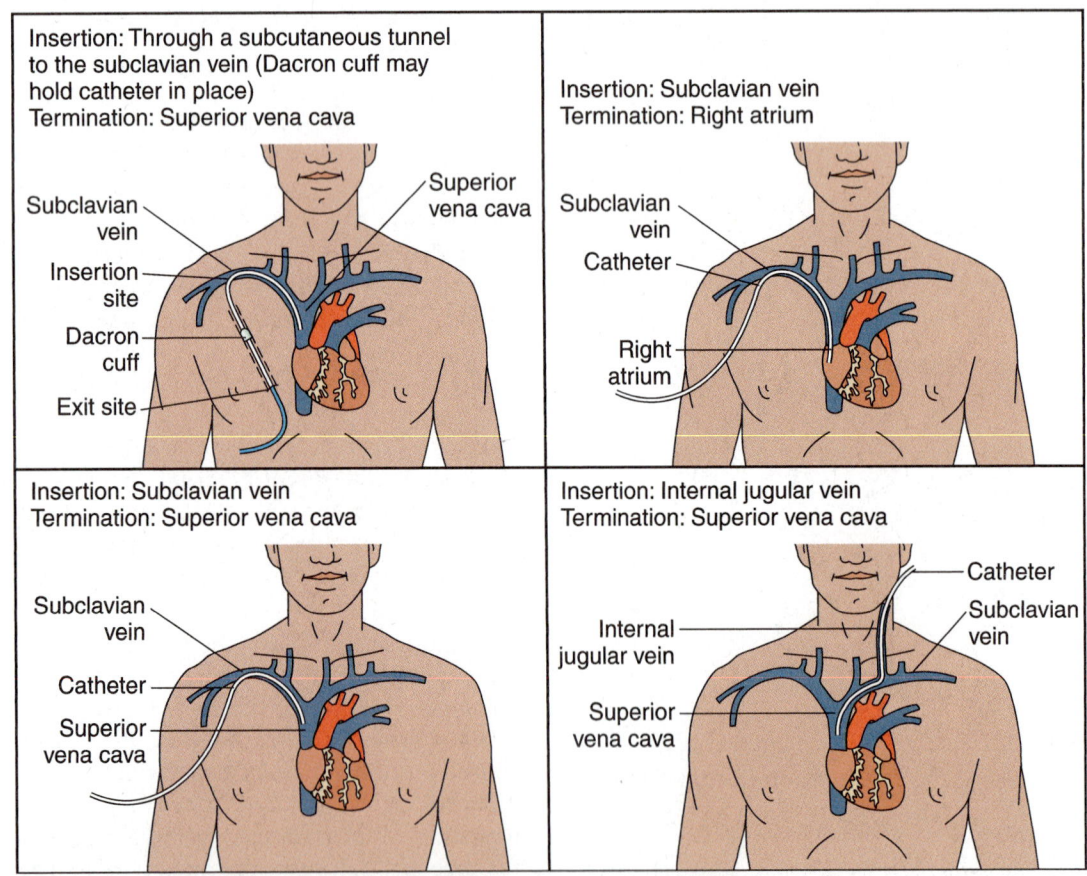

FIGURE 35-5 Locations for central venous catheter insertion. Infection is a high risk with a central catheter. Sterile technique is used to care for the insertion site.

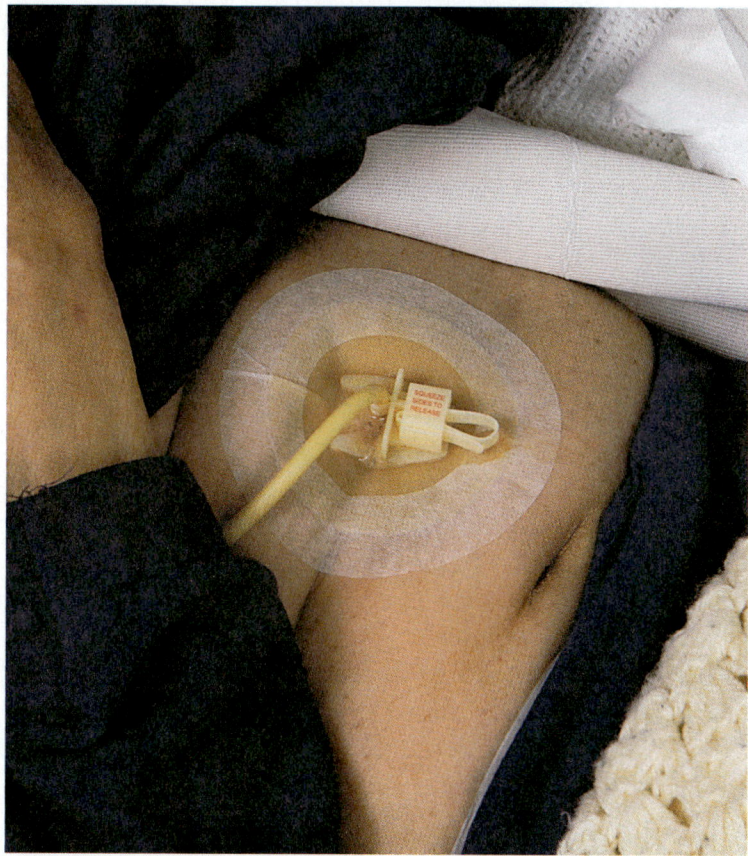 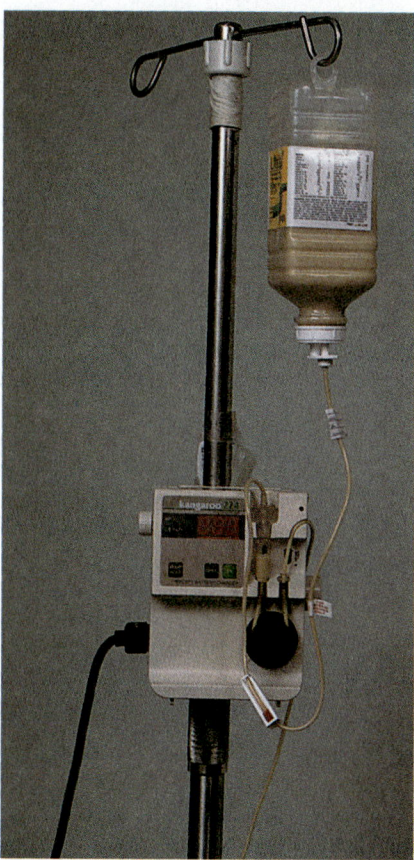

FIGURE 35-7 Liquid nutritional supplements are commonly given through a gastrostomy tube that is surgically inserted through the abdominal wall directly into the stomach.

ities keep a special clamp, called a **Kelly** (Figure 35-8) at the bedside of patients with intravenous lines in the subclavian vein. Serious complications occur if the tubing breaks or becomes dislodged. The Kelly is used to clamp the tubing close to the patient's body if the line breaks or is accidentally pulled loose. If air is allowed to enter the line, it could be fatal. The Kelly should be readily available and visible at all times. Avoid storing it in a drawer or removing it from the room.

SAFETY *Alert*

The Kelly should be sealed in a package or covered in plastic. Taping the package next to or over the head of the bed keeps it from being misplaced, and leaves it visible to all if needed in an emergency.

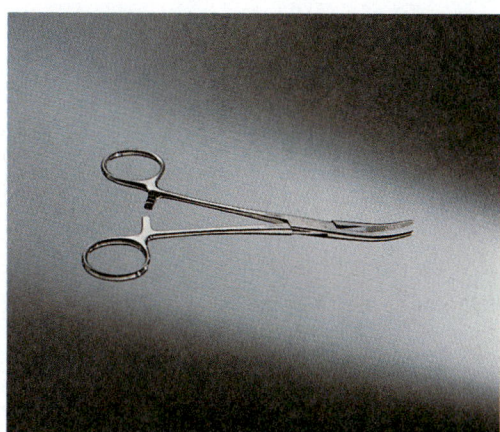

FIGURE 35-8 The Kelly is used to clamp a broken central line to prevent air from entering the patient's venous system. *(Courtesy of Medline Industries, Mundelein, IL [800] MEDLINE)*

You may be required to assist the RN with sterile dressing changes over the intravenous infusion site. When caring for patients with a central venous catheter, notify the nurse immediately if:

- you see blood in the intravenous tubing
- the patient has an elevated temperature or experiences chills
- you observe swelling or redness around the collarbone or near the infusion site
- the patient complains of pain in the neck or chest
- the patient becomes short of breath, develops elevated blood pressure, or edema
- the catheter is broken or cracked
- the alarm sounds on the intravenous infusion pump

guidelines *for*

Caring for Patients with Intravenous Lines

- Make sure the solution is flowing. Know the drip rate in the drip chamber. Notify the nurse if the rate changes or the drip chamber is full.
- Avoid pulling or twisting tubing. Make sure the patient does not lie on the tubing.
- Observe the area of needle insertion for signs of swelling, redness, or warmth.
- Note signs of moisture that may indicate the tubing is leaking.
- Make sure all junctions in the tubing are securely connected.
- Always keep the intravenous solution above the needle insertion site.
- Report immediately to the nurse:
  - Signs of dyspnea, cyanosis, chest pain, or back pain
  - If the alarm sounds on an intravenous pump
  - Blood backing up into the intravenous tubing
  - Redness, swelling, or complaints of pain or burning at the needle insertion site
  - Wetness or moisture at the insertion site or where the tubing connects to the intravenous catheter
  - If the solution in the intravenous bag or bottle is empty or low. The container should never run dry
  - If the intravenous is not dripping, seems to be dripping too fast, or if the drip chamber is completely full

- If the needle becomes dislodged
- If the tubing pulls apart from the needle
- If the solution appears to be leaking
- When caring for patients with any type of IV therapy, NEVER:
  - Change the drip rate
  - Disconnect any tubing
  - Manipulate the needle or tubing. If the tubing or needle accidentally separate, put firm pressure on the needle insertion site with a gloved hand and call for the RN immediately.
  - Remove, change, or manipulate any dressing over the site
  - Adjust the clamps on the tubing
  - Take a blood pressure in the arm with an intravenous infusion
  - Turn off an alarm on an IV pump or other infusion equipment

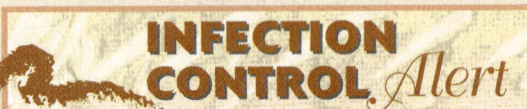

INFECTION CONTROL *Alert*

Remember that all IV procedures are sterile. If you are assisting a nurse with any of these procedures, you must never contaminate the sterile field or supplies.

PAIN MANAGEMENT PROCEDURES

Pain management may be the major reason why some patients are in a subacute unit. Other patients may be undergoing pain management related to conditions such as recent surgery or cancer. Both drug and nondrug treatments can be successful in helping to prevent and control pain. Various types of relaxation techniques are also used for pain management.

Patient-Controlled Analgesia

Patient-controlled analgesia (PCA) is used for acute, chronic, or postoperative pain. *Analgesia* means pain relief. A device is inserted into the patient's vein. It is connected to a solution that contains a narcotic. A narcotic is a drug such as morphine that is used for pain relief. The dosage is controlled by equipment that has been preset by the nurse. The patient pushes the PCA button at times of discomfort (Figure 35-9). The pump has preset controls to prevent accidental medication overdose. Report to the nurse if you note any change in the patient's:

- Level of consciousness
- Rate and pattern of respirations
- Pupil size
- Skin color

Other complications of this therapy that you should report to the nurse are:

- Nausea and/or vomiting
- Inability to urinate or difficulty urinating

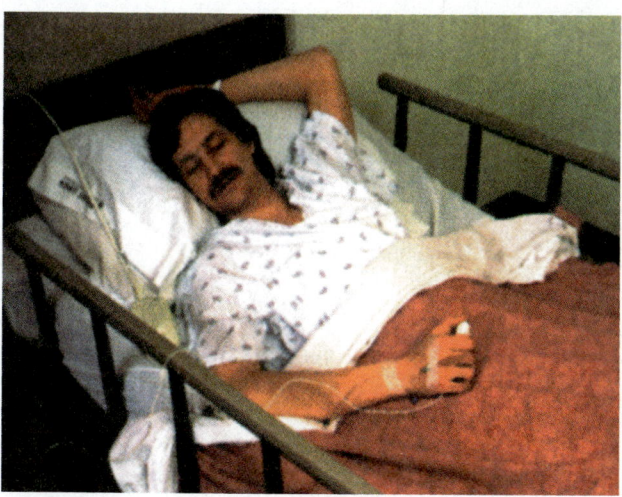

FIGURE 35-9 The patient pushes the button when he needs pain medication. The pump is preset to reduce the risk of overdose.

- Excessive drowsiness
- Confusion
- Itching
- Preset pump alarm sounds

Constipation is a common side effect of narcotic medications. Problems can become serious if not carefully monitored. Encourage patients to eat fiber foods on trays, drink liquids, and be as active as possible in keeping with the plan of care. Carefully monitor and document the patient's bowel activity. Report patient complaints or signs of constipation to the nurse.

Pain Management with an Epidural Catheter

Continuous medication infusion may be used to manage pain after major thoracic, abdominal, and orthopedic surgery. This therapy works by blocking transmission of pain at the spinal cord. Patients receiving continuous epidural analgesia receive stable, consistent doses of pain medication rather than experiencing the peaks and valleys associated with most other control methods. Patients are more willing to participate in their care plans when they are not having pain, and are usually satisfied with their care.

An **epidural catheter** is implanted beneath the patient's skin. It is inserted into the epidural space near the spinal cord (Figure 35–10). Medication is administered either intermittently or continuously through the catheter into

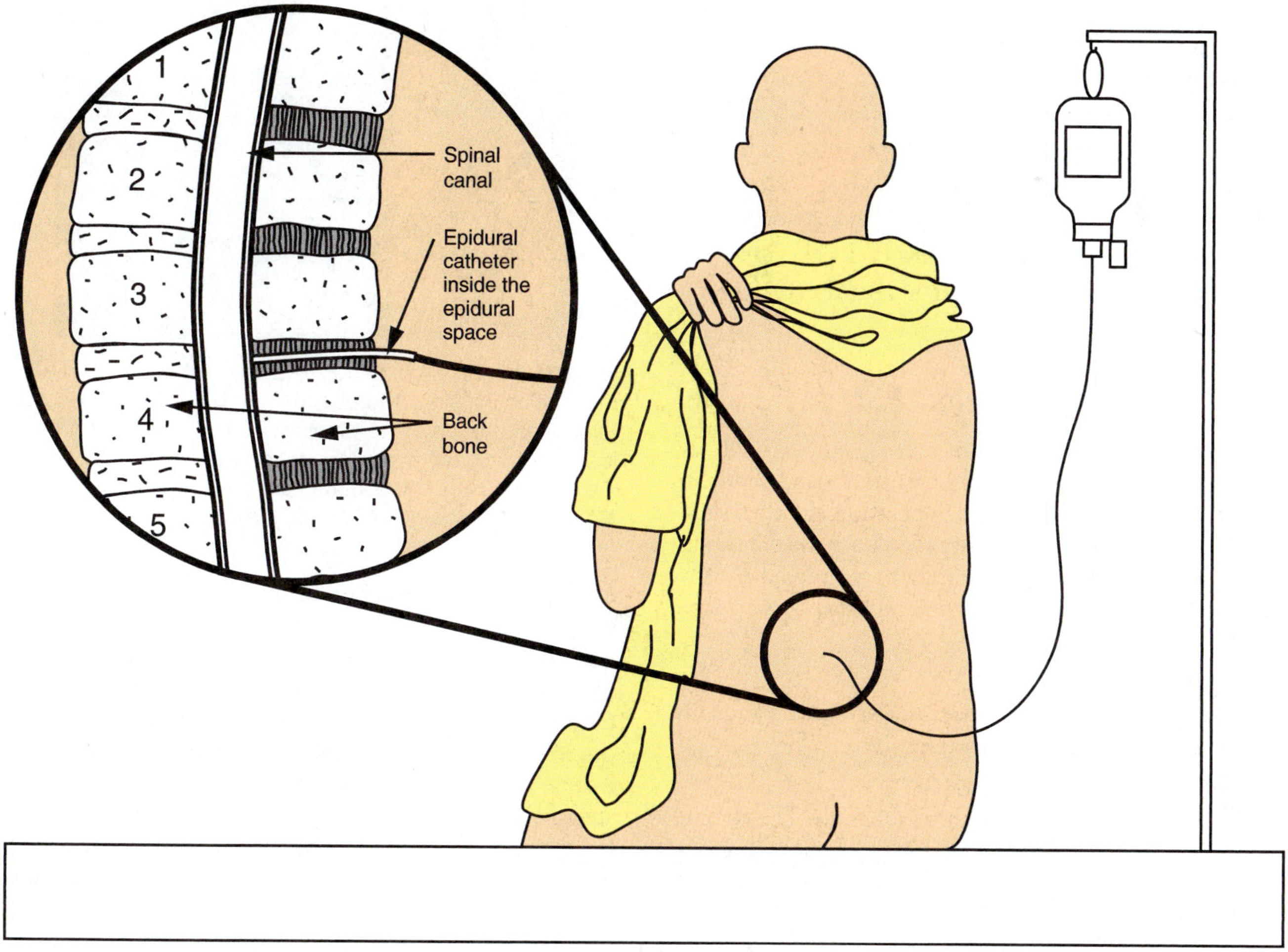

Spinal canal

Epidural catheter inside the epidural space

Back bone

1

2

3

4

5

FIGURE 35-10 The epidural catheter is used for intermittent or constant pain medication.

the epidural space. Narcotic pain-relieving medications and local anesthetics are usually given together, but either drug can be given individually. The patient may have leg numbness and weakness for the first 24 hours after the catheter is inserted. Limited mobility in areas not affected by the medication and decreased blood pressure when rising from bed are also common reactions. Instruct the patient to call for assistance when getting out of bed. Elevate the head of the bed 30° or 40°. You may be assigned to monitor the patient's vital signs frequently. The blood pressure and pulse are checked at least every hour for the first 2 hours after the catheter is inserted, then every 2 hours. Respiration is checked every hour for the first day, then every 2 hours. Report to the nurse at once if:

- the catheter becomes dislodged from the insertion site.
- you note changes in respiration rate and pattern.
- the patient complains of itching.
- the patient vomits or complains of nausea.
- dressings covering the catheter become wet from leaking or an external cause.
- respirations decrease to 12 or below.
- oxygen saturation drops below 90%.
- the patient's level of consciousness decreases.
- there is urinary retention; the patient complains of a need to urinate, but cannot.
- there is low blood pressure (hypotension).
- hives appear.
- there is rapid pulse (tachycardia).
- there is redness, warmth, tenderness, swelling, itching, or drainage at the catheter insertion site.
- the patient complains of inability to move her legs.
- the patient complains of severe low back pain.
- the patient complains of change in sensation or motor function.

Implantable Medication Pumps

Implantable medication pumps are sometimes used for long-term medication delivery in both adults and children. The pumps are surgically placed under the abdominal skin. A tiny catheter is threaded under the skin from the pump to the spine (Figure 35-11). Medications are infused directly into the cerebrospinal fluid. This type of therapy has become common for patients with:

- chronic, severe pain
- severe spasticity (sudden, frequent, involuntary muscle contractions that impair function)
- treatment for some types of cancer

The medication pump is implanted surgically. The patient will have two surgical sites, one on the abdomen and a smaller one near the spine. A physician or specially trained nurse will use a computer (Figure 35-12) to adjust the medication dose over a period of time until the desired response is achieved.

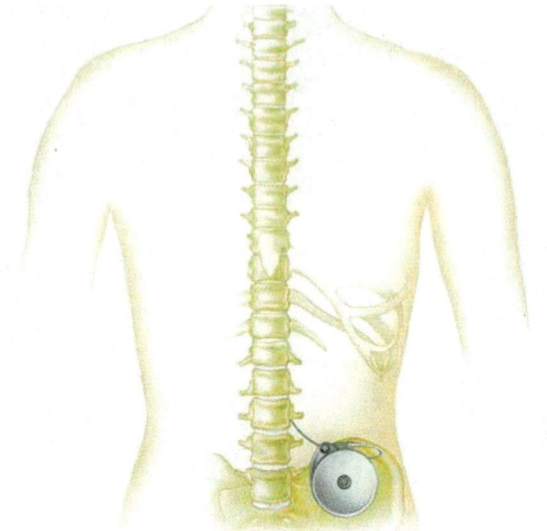

FIGURE 35-11 The implantable medication pump delivers medication directly into the cerebrospinal fluid. *(Courtesy of Medtronic, Minneapolis, MN [800] 505-5000)*

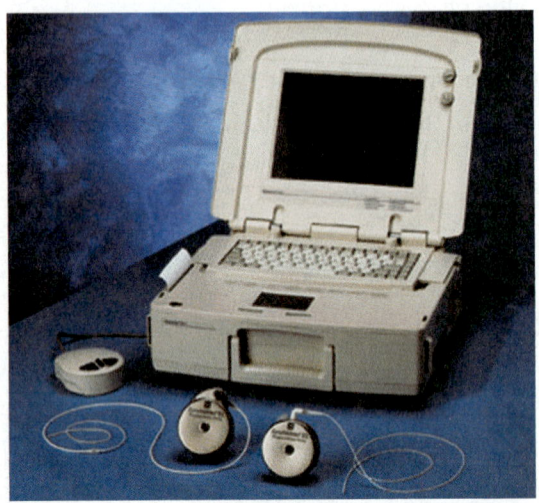

FIGURE 35-12 A computer sets the dosage and time for medication infusion. The dosage can be varied or constant throughout the day. The computer shows how much medication is left in the pump, and when it needs to be filled. An alarm will sound if the pump volume is low. *(Courtesy of Medtronic, Minneapolis, MN [800] 505-5000)*

The patient may remain on bedrest for 2 to 20 hours after surgery, depending on physician preference and patient response. An abdominal binder (Unit 29) may be used after surgery. The nurse may instruct you to apply a cool application or ice pack (Unit 27) to the site where the catheter tunnels under the skin. Some physicians permit patients to resume normal activity immediately, if they are able. If you are assisting the patient with transfers, avoid using a transfer belt until the surgical site is fully healed (usually several months after surgery, according to physician order and facility policy). In some facilities, a wide transfer belt is used for these patients, to prevent pressure on the pump or surgical site.

Patients with newly implanted medication pumps may have a complicated medication regimen in which they slowly withdraw from oral medications and depend increasingly on medications administered through the pump. Notify the nurse if the patient:

- has decreased responsiveness.
- has respirations of 12 or below.
- has a temperature over 100°F orally.
- complains of headache.
- experiences fluid leakage.
- develops a collection of blood or fluid under the skin at the insertion site.
- has redness, warmth, tenderness, swelling, itching, or drainage at the surgical sites.
- complains of a feeling of tightness over the pump site.
- is unable to move the legs.
- has sudden loss of bowel or bladder control.

Transcutaneous Electrical Nerve Stimulation

Transcutaneous electrical nerve stimulation (**TENS**) is a nondrug method of pain relief. Mild, harmless electrical current stimulates nerve fibers to block the transmission of pain to the brain. Electrodes are taped to the patient's skin. The location of the electrodes depends on the areas related to the pain. The electrodes are attached to wires that are in turn attached to a control box (Figure 35-13). The intensity of the stimulation is set on the control box by the nurse.

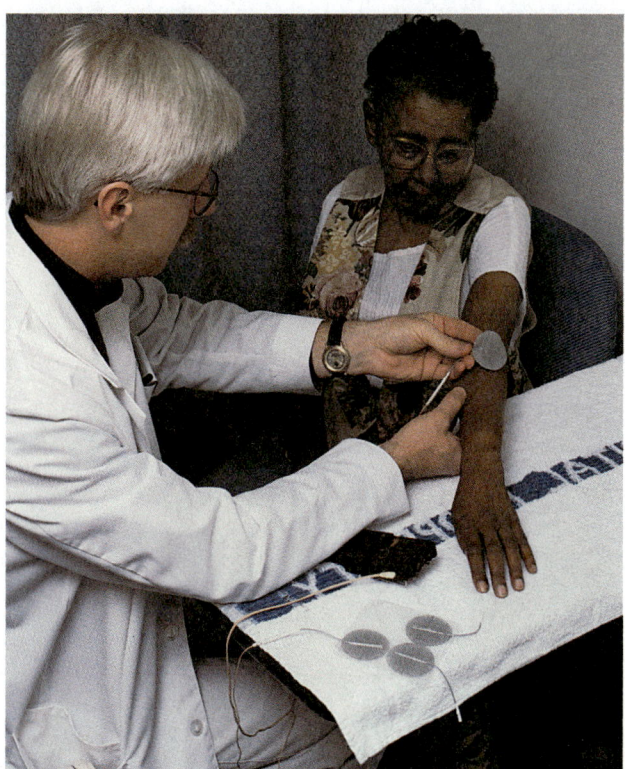

FIGURE 35-13 A TENS unit is used to relieve pain.

CARING FOR SUBACUTE PATIENTS WITH RESPIRATORY CONDITIONS

Many patients are admitted to the subacute unit with problems related to the respiratory system. Some conditions are caused by diseases within the lungs. Some patients experience respiratory problems as a result of complications of other conditions. Attention to the patient's oxygenation is a very important responsibility.

The human body eliminates three main waste products. You have learned about problems with urinary and bowel elimination. The third important waste product is carbon dioxide (CO_2). Every cell in the body produces carbon dioxide. It is transported in venous blood. When it reaches the lungs, it is exhaled into the atmosphere. When the body does not eliminate carbon dioxide, chemical reactions cause an acid buildup. Death will result if levels of acid and carbon dioxide become too high. Signs and symptoms that may indicate problems with oxygen use are:

- Unusual skin color, such as dusky, pale, blue, or gray
- Unusual color of the lips, mucous membranes, nail beds, lining or roof of the mouth
- Cool, clammy skin
- Slow, rapid, or irregular breathing
- Shortness of breath or difficulty breathing
- Noisy breathing
- Gasping for breath
- Wet respirations, rattling in the lungs
- Choking on secretions
- Changes in mental status, including decreased responsiveness, drowsiness, sleepiness for no apparent reason, restlessness, increased confusion
- Tachycardia

Patients at Risk of Poor Oxygenation

Certain patients have a known high risk of developing **hypoxemia**. This is a condition in which there is insufficient oxygen in the blood. It can occur in anyone, and is not a disease. Patients who are immobile and those on bedrest have an increased risk of hypoxemia. Other high-risk conditions are:

- Cardiac disease
- Pulmonary disease (Figure 35-14)
- Being a postoperative patient
- Sleep apnea
- Decreased level of consciousness
- Neuromuscular diseases
- Morbid obesity
- Severe kyphoscoliosis (curvature of the spine)

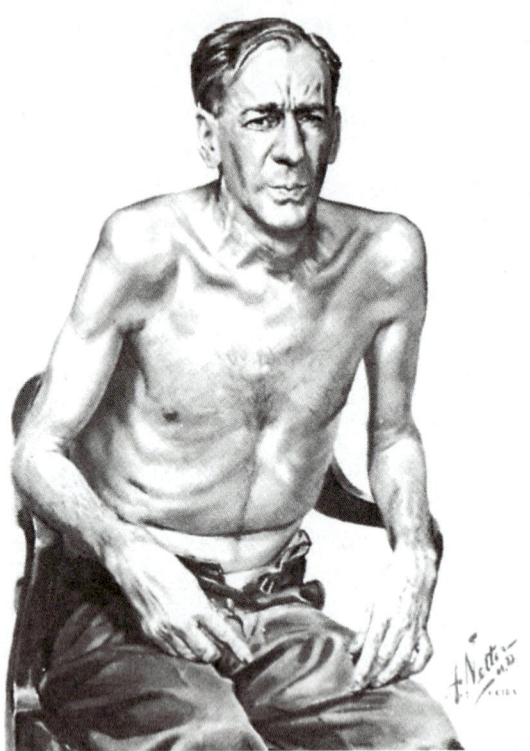

FIGURE 35-14 Patients with chronic obstructive lung disease commonly have a barrel chest. They may lean forward to increase lung capacity, making it possible to take in a little more air. *(Copyright © 1968, CIBA-GEIGY Corporation. Reproduced with permission, from the* Clinical Symposia, *illustrated by Frank H. Netter, M.D. All rights reserved.)*

Capillary Refill

Checking capillary refill is a quick, easy, painless test to evaluate how well oxygen gets to the body tissues. **Capillary refill** is an indication of the patient's peripheral circulation and shows how well the tissues are being nourished with oxygen. In a light-skinned person, skin should be pink, indicating an adequate supply of oxygen. The nail beds, mucous membranes in the mouth, and lips are also an indication of how well the patient's body is using oxygen. The color of these areas should also be pink. In a dark-skinned person, you must look at the nail beds, oral mucous membranes, and lips to determine how well the person is using oxygen, because you cannot evaluate the skin. If the skin, nail beds, mucous membranes, or lips are cyanotic, this indicates a problem with oxygen delivery. This may be due to lack of oxygen in the blood or poor circulation.

The capillary refill test will help you determine the patient's oxygenation. Delayed capillary refill indicates a problem with oxygen delivery. Perform a capillary refill check on all four extremities, or according to facility policy. Although capillary refill varies with age, skin color should return to normal within 2 to 3 seconds in all patients. The color should be restored to the nail bed in the length of time it takes to say the words *capillary refill.* (Refer to Procedure 95.)

Nail Polish. Several procedures involve using and evaluating the patient's fingernail beds. The color of the fingernails is a good indication of how much oxygen is in the blood. Nail polish will interfere with the ability to evaluate

---

PROCEDURE 95

CHECKING CAPILLARY REFILL

1. Carry out beginning procedure actions.
2. Inspect the nails, noting the color.
3. Press the nail for a few seconds, until the skin underneath blanches, or turns white (Figure 35-15A).

4. Release the nail and evaluate the time it takes for the skin to return to its normal color. With normal oxygenation, this will occur within 2 to 3 seconds (Figure 35-15B).
5. Carry out procedure completion actions.

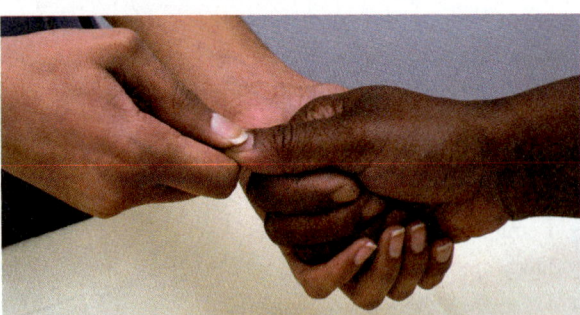

FIGURE 35-15A Inspect the color of the patient's hand, then pinch the thumb.

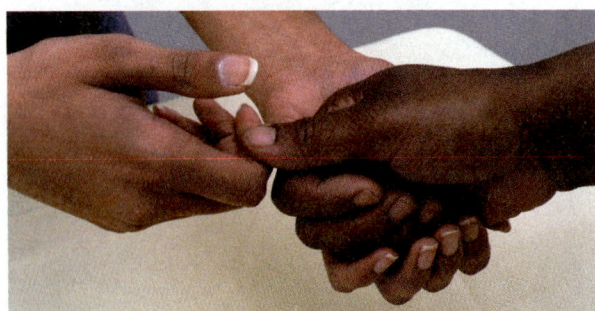

FIGURE 35-15B Observe the color again after releasing the thumb.

the patient. Follow your facility policy for removing polish. Some facilities remove polish from one finger only. Other facilities remove all nail polish. If a female patient has acrylic or sculpted nails, remove the polish with a non-acetone polish remover. Some facilities completely remove the acrylic material from one nail. Know and follow your facility policy.

You can check capillary refill at any time when you are taking vital signs or caring for the patient. If the capillary refill time is greater than 3 seconds, inform the nurse of your findings.

The Pulse Oximeter

Pulse oximetry (Figure 35-16) is another simple, painless test to determine how well oxygen is being carried in the body. The pulse oximeter is an instrument that measures the level of saturation of the patient's hemoglobin with oxygen. Hemoglobin is the part of the blood that carries oxygen to the cells to nourish them. The pulse oximeter measures how full the hemoglobin molecules are with oxygen. The measurement is usually done continuously, but can be intermittent. Having these data readily available enables the nurse to treat the patient quickly. Pulse oximetry will detect critical changes in the patient's oxygen levels before the skin color changes. This makes it a valuable tool that provides details about changes in the patient's condition immediately, as soon as they occur. The patient's outcome is usually better when early treatment is provided. Before applying the pulse oximeter, check the patient's oxygen, if being used. Document the liter flow.

The pulse oximeter is attached to the patient's skin with a sensor. Several different sensors are available. These can be placed on the finger (Figure 35-17A), toe, earlobe, foot, forehead, or the bridge of the nose (Figure 35-17B). The tip of the finger and the earlobe are most commonly used. In these areas, a clothespin-like sensor is attached to both sides. The finger and toe sensors work best with dark-skinned patients. Poor circulation interferes with use of the pulse oximeter.

The unit has two light-emitting diodes (LEDs). One is red, the other is infrared. The sensor contains a photodetector that measures the light as it passes through the tissue. This measures the amount of oxygen in the patient's arterial blood (Figure 35-18). The pulse oximeter converts this into

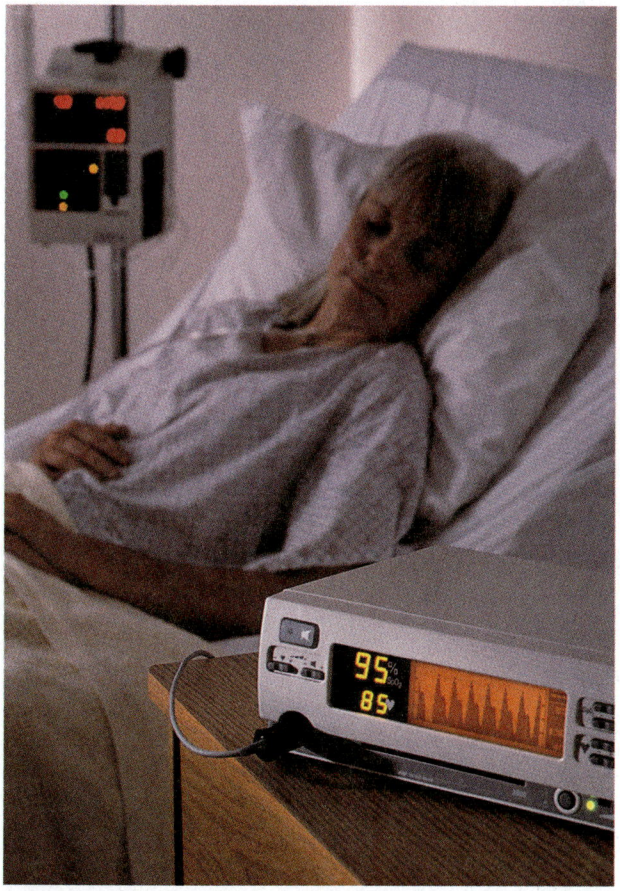

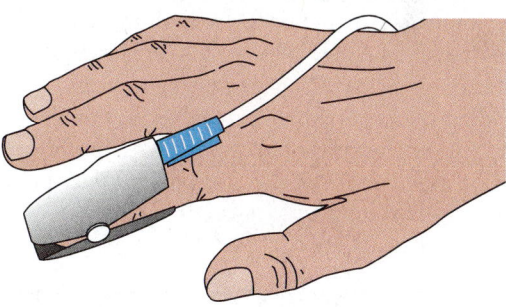

FIGURE 35-17A The finger-clip sensor should be rotated at least every 2 hours.

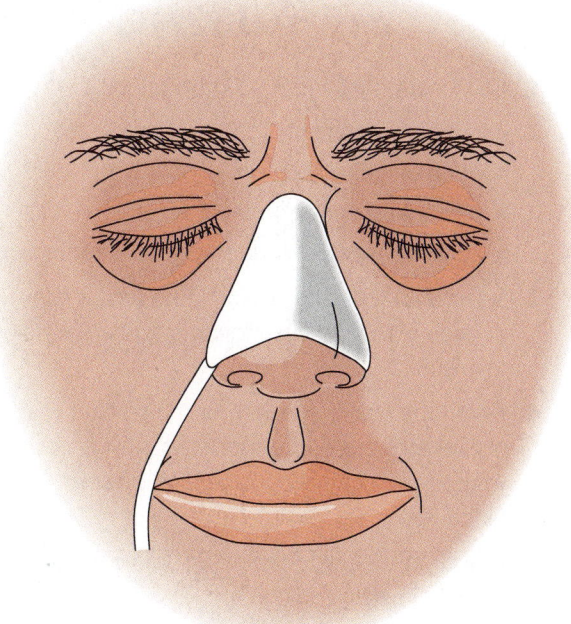

FIGURE 35-16 The pulse oximeter shows the oxygen saturation of the patient's blood as a percentage on the display. *(Courtesy of Ohmeda, Louisville, CO)*

FIGURE 35-17B The nasal sensor.

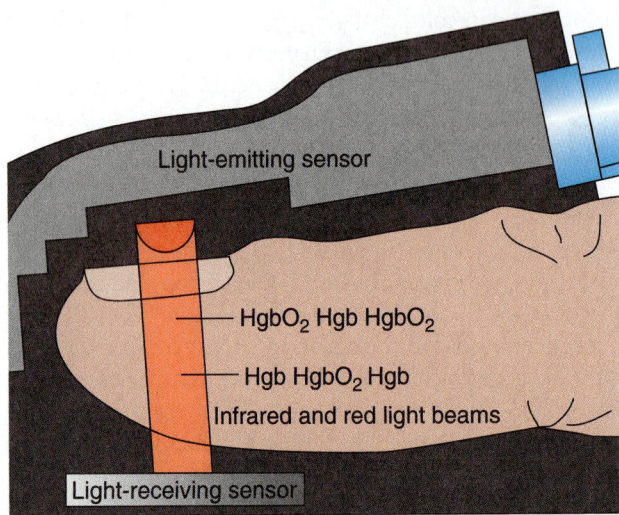

FIGURE 35-18 The pulse oximeter uses light to measure the amount of oxygen in the arterial blood.

a percentage, which can be viewed on the digital display. The physician will order what he or she wants the minimum oxygen saturation to be. The RN will give you this information. A measurement of 95% to 100% is considered normal. Readings below 90% suggest complications. When the reading reaches 85%, there may not be enough oxygen for the tissues. Readings below 70% are life-threatening. The pulse oximeter is not used for patients with known or suspected carbon monoxide poisoning.

The pulse oximeter has an alarm, which is usually preset by the manufacturer to normal limits for adults and children. The RN will advise you if the alarm settings must be changed. This is done by turning a knob or pressing a button. If you turn the unit off, then back on, the oximeter resets itself to the default values. Before leaving the room, make sure that the alarm is in the "on" position, and is set as ordered. Never turn the alarm off. (Refer to Procedure 96.)

Monitoring the Patient. You must monitor the patient regularly when a pulse oximeter is being used. Reporting to the nurse is part of your procedure completion actions. In this case, make sure to report the patient's initial pulse oximeter reading and vital signs. This is important information on which the nurse will act. He or she will further assess the patient and provide care for abnormal values. The nurse must know the initial values as a basis for comparison.

If the patient's vital signs or appearance change significantly from your baseline values, notify the nurse promptly. Also inform the nurse immediately if the patient's pulse oximetry value is less than the level ordered by the physician. Monitor the patient's oxygen, if used, each time you are in the room. Make sure it is set at the liter flow ordered by the physician.

Rotate the position of the finger sensor at least every 4 hours. A spring-clip sensor should be moved every 2 hours. Rotating the location of the sensor reduces the risk of skin breakdown and complications related to pressure. If adhesive tape is used to secure the sensor, monitor for signs and

---

PROCEDURE 96

USING A PULSE OXIMETER

1. Carry out beginning procedure actions.

2. Assemble equipment:
   - pulse oximeter unit
   - sensor appropriate to the site
   - adhesive tape, if needed, to secure the sensor

3. Select and apply the sensor. If the sensor has position markings, align them opposite each other to ensure an accurate reading.

4. Fasten the sensor securely, or the reading will not be accurate. Make sure the sensor is not wrapped so tightly with tape that it restricts blood flow.

5. Attach the sensor to the patient cable on the pulse oximeter.

6. Turn the unit on. You will hear a beep with each pulse beat. Adjust the volume as desired. Some units also have light bars, indicating the strength of the pulse. Note the percentage of oxygen saturation. Inform the nurse and document according to facility policy.

7. Monitor the patient's pulse rate, if the unit provides this reading. Compare with the patient's actual pulse to make sure the unit is picking up each beat. Inform the nurse and document according to facility policy.

8. Monitor the patient's respirations and general appearance. Inform the nurse and document according to facility policy. If the patient's general condition changes at any time, notify the nurse.

9. Carry out procedure completion actions.

symptoms of a reaction to the tape. If a rash, itching, or other signs of tape allergy occur, move the sensor to a different location. Apply a spring-clamp sensor, or attach the sensor with hypoallergenic tape.

Oxygen Therapy

Oxygen is necessary for life. Humans take in oxygen from the air during breathing. Some diseases and conditions prevent the body tissues from getting enough oxygen, so supplemental oxygen is administered. Some patients have normal oxygen levels, but are given oxygen because they are at increased risk of hypoxemia. Oxygen is a prescription item, and a physician's order is necessary to administer it to a patient. The physician will order additional oxygen to be given through an oxygen delivery system. He or she will specify how much oxygen to use and the method of oxygen delivery. Depending on your facility policy, it may also be given at the nurse's discretion, according to protocol or clinical practice guidelines. You should not start, stop, or change the flow rate of oxygen.

The nursing assistant's responsibilities for oxygen administration are determined by facility policy. Most subacute units have a respiratory care practitioner (RCP) on staff to administer oxygen therapy. Nursing personnel monitor patients using oxygen, and notify the RCP as needed. He or she will see the patient one or more times each shift. Although an RCP may be responsible for the patients' oxygen needs, you still must have a working knowledge of oxygen administration. Portable cylinders are used for transporting patients from one area to another, and may be used in emergencies in hallways or other areas without a piped-in oxygen source. You must know where oxygen cylinders are stored, how to assemble them, and how to transport them safely.

Caring for a Patient Who Is Receiving Oxygen Therapy. Elevate the head of the bed when the patient is receiving oxygen. This will make it easier to breathe. A patient using an oxygen mask cannot eat meals while wearing the mask. The physician may order a nasal cannula at meal time. Follow the instructions on the care plan or critical pathway for patient care measures.

Being unable to breathe is very frightening. Patients who are receiving oxygen may need reassurance and emotional support. Check on the patient frequently and spend as much time in the room as possible. Difficulty in breathing also makes it hard to talk. The patient may be unable to hold a normal conversation. Just being with the patient without talking is very reassuring.

You will care for patients using different devices for the administration of oxygen. Carefully check the skin under the device. Make sure it does not become red or irritated from the elastic that holds it in place. Pad the straps with cotton, if necessary. Report problems to the nurse. Because oxygen is drying, patients receiving oxygen will need extra liquids to drink. However, if the patient is short of breath, he or she may be unable to suck on a straw. Assist the

SAFETY *Alert*

When using cylinder oxygen, identify the contents of the cylinder. Oxygen cylinders are always colored green in the United States. Read the label listing the contents as a double-check. Transport oxygen cylinders carefully. They should be chained to a carrier during transport. Cylinder oxygen should be secured in a base or chained to a carrier or the wall. Avoid dropping the tank. Cylinders can explode if the tank is dropped and the cylinder valve is damaged.

patient by holding the glass, if necessary, and helping him to drink the liquid. Patients who use oxygen will also need frequent care of the mouth and nose. Sometimes patients will feel warm and perspire heavily. Extra bathing and linen changes may be necessary. You may need to adjust the temperature in the room and help the patient change into a hospital gown. Cover him or her with a sheet. The care plan or critical pathway will provide information on patient preferences and needs.

Use of Oxygen in an Emergency. There are several differences between routine oxygen use and use of oxygen in an emergency. In an emergency, high concentrations of oxygen are necessary. Cylinders (Figure 35-19), liquid oxygen, or piped-in oxygen are used. Avoid using an oxygen concentrator, because it cannot supply the high liter flows

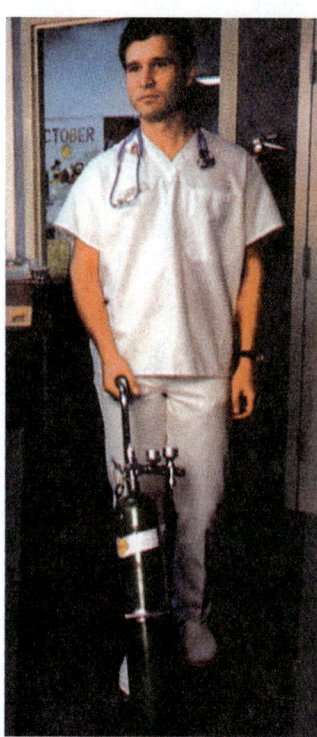

FIGURE 35-19 A portable oxygen tank may be used in an emergency or when the patient is out of the room. No humidification is necessary.

necessary for emergency care. Some facilities use humidifier bottles when routine oxygen is administered, but this is not necessary. Oxygen may be delivered dry. Do not take the time to search for a humidifier. In an emergency, the patient requires high liter flows of oxygen quickly.

Caring for Patients with Tracheostomies

A **tracheostomy** is a tube that is inserted into a surgical opening in the patient's trachea (windpipe). A tracheostomy is performed when the patient is unable to breathe in air through the nose. The tube allows the patient to breathe, as air goes directly into the trachea and then into the lungs. A person who is on a ventilator for a long time will have a tracheostomy that is connected to the ventilator. The patient may have secretions coming from the chest and through the tube. The nurse will use suction to remove these secretions.

The tube may be made of plastic or metal. Tracheostomy tubes consist of an inner, removable tube called a *cannula* and an outer tube called a *neckplate* that is held in place with neck ties. The neckplate rests between the clavicles (breastbones). There is a slot on each side. Tracheostomy ties are inserted here to secure the tube in place (Figure 35-20). Patients with tracheostomies can usually take a bath or shower but must keep the water from entering the opening. Avoid using powders, sprays, or shaving cream around the tube. When you care for a patient with a tracheostomy, observe for:

* changes in respiratory rate, depth, and quality.
* changes in mental status, such as confusion, restlessness, or irritability, that indicate the patient's brain is not getting adequate oxygen.

Report to the nurse immediately if the:

* Tube becomes dislodged from the opening
* Patient is having trouble breathing
* Patient needs suctioning
* Alarm sounds on the respirator

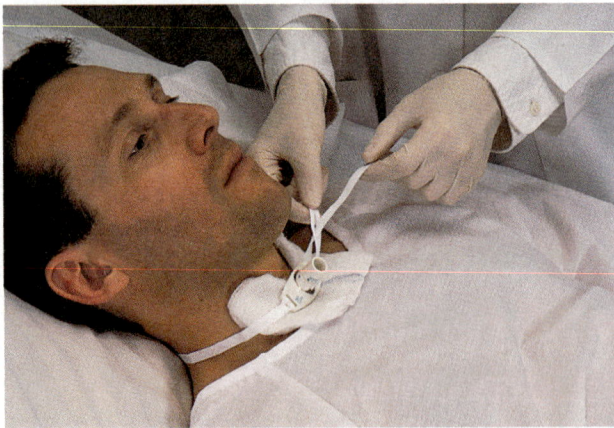

FIGURE 35-20 A tracheostomy tube is held in place with ties. Avoid getting lint, dust, powder, or water in the tracheostomy.

Be sure you know how the patient communicates. The opening in the trachea interferes with the patient's ability to talk. Additional information on caring for patients with tracheostomies and other respiratory conditions is found in Unit 38.

CARING FOR THE PATIENT RECEIVING DIALYSIS TREATMENTS

Dialysis is a process by which the blood is artificially cleansed of liquid wastes when the kidneys are unable to remove the wastes. This procedure is needed when a person has kidney failure. Without dialysis, the person would die as the waste products accumulate in the bloodstream. Dialysis is usually considered a temporary treatment that is used until a suitable organ is found for a kidney transplant. The two types of dialysis are hemodialysis and peritoneal dialysis.

Hemodialysis

During **hemodialysis** treatment, the patient's blood is circulated outside of the body into an artificial kidney machine. In the dialysis machine, the blood is cleansed with a liquid substance called dialysate. After the waste products have been removed, the blood is returned to the patient's body. Most persons needing hemodialysis are treated in a dialysis center. However, you may care for patients in the subacute unit who go as outpatients to the dialysis center for their treatments. Dialysis is usually done three to four times a week and each treatment takes several hours.

To do dialysis, a connection must be made between the patient's circulatory system and the artificial kidney machine. Minor surgery is done to create either a fistula or a graft. The **fistula** (Figure 35-21A) is created by attaching a vein to an artery, either in an arm or a leg. When a **graft** is used (Figure 35-21B), synthetic material is inserted to form a connection between an artery and a vein. Two needles are inserted for treatment with either a fistula or a graft. The needles are connected to tubes that go to and from the artificial kidney machine.

As a nursing assistant, you are not expected to care for the fistula or the graft. You need to be aware that the patient on dialysis will:

* Have fluid restrictions
* Have dietary restrictions for calories, sodium, protein, potassium, calcium, and phosphorus
* Need all fluid intake and output measured accurately and recorded
* Need to be weighed regularly at the same time of day and with the same type of clothing
* Need to be monitored and have vital signs taken frequently after dialysis. Remember that blood pressure should not be taken in the arm used for dialysis. Patients may be weak when they return from dialysis.

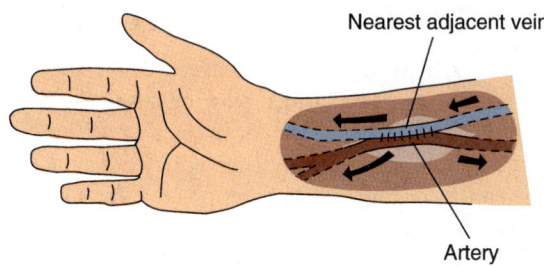

Nearest adjacent vein

Artery

Edges of incision in artery and vein are
sutured together to form a common opening.

FIGURE 35-21A The arteriovenous fistula.

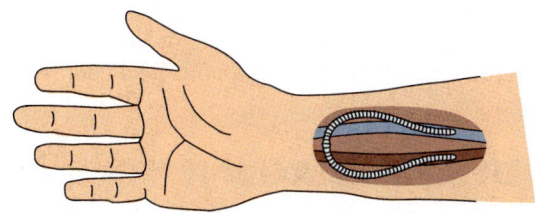

Ends of natural or synthetic graft sutured
into an artery and a vein.

FIGURE 35-21B The arteriovenous vein graft.

Monitor them closely when they ambulate. Watch for dizziness and loss of balance.

Report to the nurse if the patient has:

- Swelling (edema) of the hands, feet, or face
- Changes in vital signs
- Changes in weight
- A change in intake or output measurements
- Shortness of breath
- Complaints of pain at the site of the fistula or graft

Peritoneal Dialysis

Peritoneal dialysis is also a process of cleansing the blood. In peritoneal dialysis, the process takes place within the patient's body in the peritoneal (abdominal) cavity, rather than outside the body in a machine. During dialysis, the dialysate is introduced into the abdominal cavity, allowed to stay in for some time, and then drained out (Figure 35-22). As blood flows through the vessels in the peritoneum, waste

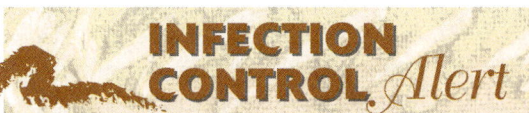

INFECTION CONTROL *Alert*

Caring for the dialysis catheter is a sterile procedure. All personnel in the room should wear masks when the system is open or entered.

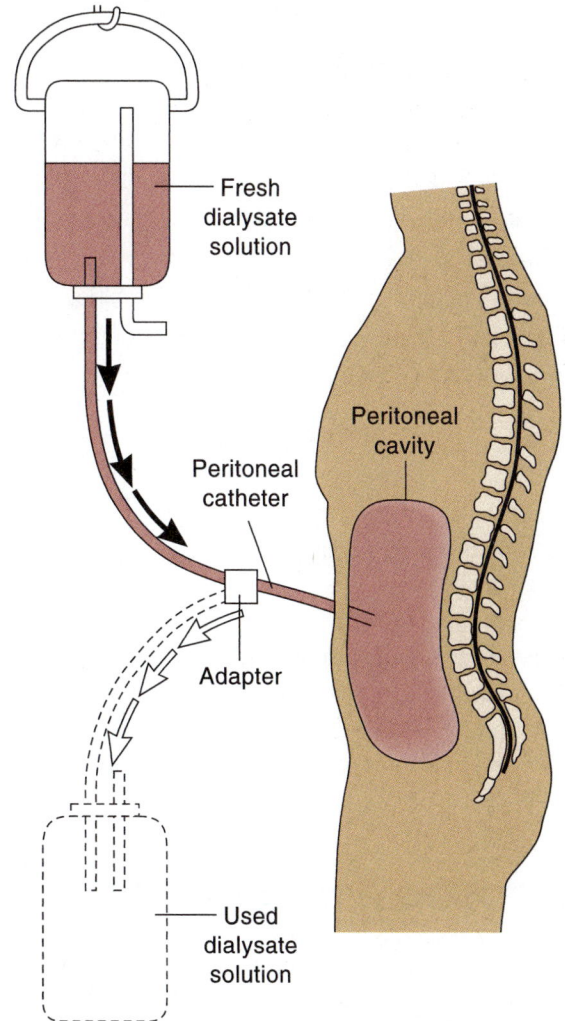

Fresh
dialysate
solution

Peritoneal
cavity

Peritoneal
catheter

Adapter

Used
dialysate
solution

FIGURE 35-22 Waste products and excess fluid are removed as the dialysate flows out of the peritoneal cavity.

products are filtered and excess fluids are removed. The nurse instills the dialysate through a catheter that is surgically implanted through the wall of the abdomen into the abdominal cavity. This is done using sterile technique. You may be asked to assist the nurse with sterile dressing changes. The type of dialysis used in the subacute care unit is usually **continuous ambulatory peritoneal dialysis (CAPD)**.

Nursing assistants are not expected to administer peritoneal dialysis. You may be responsible for monitoring the patient's vital signs every 10 to 15 minutes for the first 1 to 2 hours after a treatment and then every 2 to 4 hours. Notify the nurse if there are any changes in vital signs.

Other signs and symptoms to report to the nurse are:

- The dialysate that returns appears bloody or has blood clots in the solution
- The patient complains of abdominal pain
- The dressing becomes wet or soiled
- Fluid leaks around the insertion site
- The tubing or catheter is disconnected

- The solution does not appear to be running, or is running very slowly
- The drainage container is almost full
- The patient is weak or unsteady
- The patient has low blood pressure or complains of dizziness
- The patient is short of breath or complains of difficulty breathing

ONCOLOGY TREATMENTS

Oncology is the care and treatment of persons with cancer. Cancer may be treated with surgery, radiation, chemotherapy, or a combination of any of these.

Radiation Therapy

Patients receiving radiation therapy in a subacute care unit may be transported to a special cancer treatment center or to a hospital to receive this therapy as outpatients. Radiation therapy is the use of high-energy radiation to kill cancer cells. It is considered a local therapy because it kills only the cancer cells in the area being treated. Patients receiving radiation may complain of fatigue and lack of appetite. When caring for patients receiving radiation therapy:

- report signs of redness, pain, or peeling of the skin in the area being treated.
- do not remove markings made on the skin for treatment purposes.
- do not use any heat or cold treatments on the area being treated.
- wash the area only with tepid water and a soft washcloth; do not apply any soaps, powders, deodorants, perfumes, makeup, lotions, or skin preparations to the area.
- instruct the patient to avoid wearing tight clothing over the area.

Chemotherapy

Chemotherapy is the use of drugs to kill cancer cells within the body. The drugs may be given by mouth (orally), through the vein (IV), or in the muscle (intramuscular [IM]). The nurse or physician administers the drugs. The person receiving chemotherapy may have side effects including nausea, vomiting, anorexia (loss of appetite), or alopecia (loss of hair). Modern treatment techniques have minimized the side effects of chemotherapy, but loss of hair is still common. However, the hair usually comes back after treatments are completed. Some persons prefer to wear wigs during this time. Respect the patient's wishes regarding personal appearance. Assist with modesty, head coverings, caps, or scarves as the patient desires. Patients receiving chemotherapy may fear the outcome of their disease and need a great deal of emotional support. Be a good listener.

WOUND MANAGEMENT

Some patients require wound management for severe pressure sores, burns, or surgical wounds. The nurse or physical therapist will perform frequent dressing changes on these areas using sterile technique. You may be required to assist with dressing changes, so a basic knowledge of sterile technique (Unit 50) is necessary. The patient may have special positioning needs related to the injured area of the skin, or may be on a low-air-loss therapy or another type of specialty bed. You may be required to position the patient hourly, and use special positioning devices and props to promote healing of the injured area. Notify the nurse if any of the following occur:

- The wound appears red, swollen, or has increased drainage
- The dressing becomes saturated with drainage from the wound
- Wound drainage has a foul odor
- The patient complains of increased pain in the wound
- The wound dressing becomes wet, soiled, or falls off
- The wound dressing accidentally becomes contaminated with urine or stool

DOCUMENTATION OF CARE IN THE SUBACUTE UNIT

Reimbursement for care in subacute units is often provided by insurance companies and managed care organizations. In some situations or facilities, reimbursement is based on documentation. The main purpose of documentation is to provide a record of patient care. However, the medical record may also be used to evaluate the level and value of services the facility provides to each patient. The information on the record is used to set payment to the facility.

Payment may be denied if the documentation does not support the care given or what the patient required. The agencies that pay the bills will only pay for care that matches the treatment plan prescribed for the patient. Documentation must reflect the patient's progress toward stated care plan goals and response to treatment provided. You will be responsible for documenting the services you provide. You may also be required to document the patient's response to these services. If you are working with patients on special restorative nursing or therapy programs, you may be required to document additional information. Avoid subjective terms such as good, fair, or poor. Generally, documentation about patient response to services or progress toward care plan goals must be stated in measurable terms, such as:

- "Ambulated 50 feet in hallway with walker."
- "Ate 90% of breakfast meal."
- "Consumed 975 mL of fluid orally this shift."

The facility and its staff depend on payment for services for survival. This is what pays the bills and meets payroll. Therefore, documentation is important for many reasons. Documentation requirements change as reimbursement changes.

Complete, accurate documentation proves that workers have complied with physician orders, complied with the law, and met legal standards of care. It shows that the patients received good care. Properly completed records will show that the patients' risks and needs were identified, and that care was given to meet those needs. You will care for several patients each day, and remembering each small detail is difficult. Make notes if necessary, so you do not forget important information (Figure 35-23). Documenta-

tion is an important communication tool for all workers who care for the patient. Missing, inaccurate, or absent information may cause problems with communication, reimbursement, facility inspections, or legal actions. Accurate, complete documentation protects both the facility and the individual workers. Your facility will provide instruction on special documentation requirements related to subacute care and reimbursement in the subacute unit.

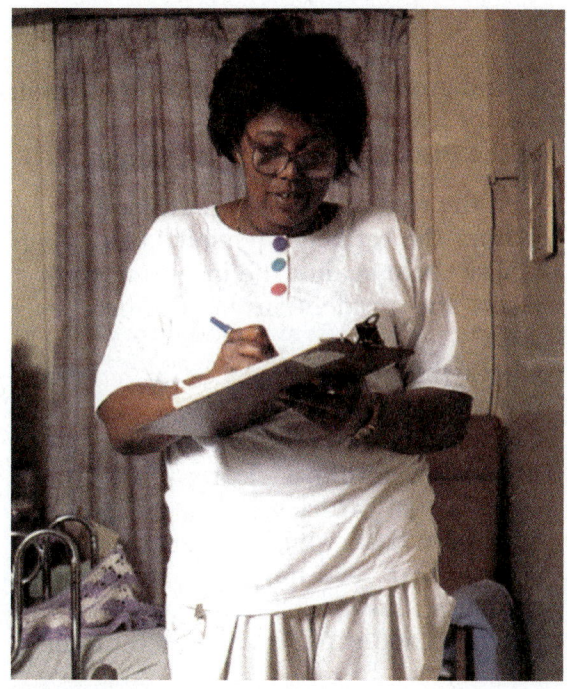

FIGURE 35-23 Accurate records are important for communication and reimbursement.

REVIEW

A. Multiple Choice.

Select the one best answer for each of the following.

1. Subacute care is given to persons who
   a. have been acutely ill.
   b. have had a long, progressive illness.
   c. require only custodial care.
   d. require intensive care.

2. The purpose of subacute care is to
   a. increase the population of long-term care facilities.
   b. discharge patients as quickly as possible.
   c. provide the care a person needs at a lower cost.
   d. provide care to unstable patients.

3. Patients treated in subacute care include persons
   a. who are critically ill.
   b. requiring routine long-term care.
   c. receiving complex wound care.
   d. receiving obstetrical care.

4. A nursing assistant working in subacute care would need to
   a. learn how to start intravenous feedings.
   b. have excellent observational skills.
   c. learn how to administer chemotherapy.
   d. instruct patients in pain management techniques.

5. If you accept a position in a subacute care unit, you may need to learn
   a. how to administer medication.
   b. your responsibilities for patients receiving dialysis.
   c. how to prepare special therapeutic diets.
   d. to care for unstable patients.

6. The procedure to measure the level of oxygen in arterial blood is called
  a. hemodialysis.
  b. pulse oximetry.
  c. total parenteral nutrition.
  d. intravenous therapy.

7. A central venous catheter is inserted into
  a. a vein in the patient's foot.
  b. an artery in the patient's arm.
  c. the jugular or subclavian vein.
  d. the epidural space.

8. Total parenteral nutrition (TPN) is used for patients
  a. who need to lose weight.
  b. who are unconscious.
  c. who refuse to eat.
  d. whose bowel needs complete rest.

9. The nursing assistant's responsibility for caring for patients with intravenous feedings is to
  a. insert the needle into the vein.
  b. add medication to the bag of fluid.
  c. observe for complications.
  d. change the drip rate if it is going too fast or too slow.

10. Patient-controlled analgesia is used
  a. for acute, chronic, or postoperative pain.
  b. for oral medications.
  c. to administer medication every 4 hours.
  d. for medication delivery on a fixed schedule.

11. An epidural catheter is used for
  a. pain management.
  b. administering nutrition.
  c. emptying the bladder.
  d. intravenous feedings.

12. When caring for patients with tracheostomies, you should
  a. not allow the patient to bathe or shower.
  b. observe for changes in respiratory rate, depth, and quality.
  c. maintain the patient on a liquid diet.
  d. be responsible for changing the tracheostomy tube.

13. Dialysis is a procedure for
  a. cleansing the blood of liquid wastes.
  b. relieving postoperative pain.
  c. administering oxygen.
  d. giving total parenteral nutrition.

14. A patient on dialysis will routinely have
  a. a regular diet.
  b. hourly vital signs taken.
  c. frequent weights taken.
  d. physical therapy.

15. When caring for patients on dialysis, you should observe for
  a. edema of the face, hands, and feet.
  b. diarrhea.
  c. constipation.
  d. thirst.

16. Oncology is the care and treatment of patients with
  a. severe wounds.
  b. kidney failure.
  c. cancer.
  d. terminal illness.

17. When caring for patients receiving radiation therapy, you should
  a. remove the markings made on the skin for treatment purposes.
  b. apply cold treatments to the area.
  c. avoid applying soaps, powders, lotions, or deodorants to the treated area.
  d. wrap the treatment area with an elastic bandage.

18. The nursing assistant should avoid taking blood pressure
  a. on a stroke patient's unaffected arm.
  b. with an electronic blood pressure unit.
  c. on an arm with an intravenous infusion.
  d. on the arm with the identification band.

19. Always keep the bag or bottle of intravenous solution
  a. below the needle insertion site.
  b. exactly 6 feet off the floor.
  c. parallel to the needle insertion site.
  d. above the needle insertion site.

20. If the intravenous tubing accidentally becomes separated from the needle, the nursing assistant should
  a. apply firm pressure to the needle insertion site with a gloved hand.
  b. quickly plug the tubing back into the needle or intravenous catheter.
  c. wrap the area with a pressure bandage and call the nurse.
  d. apply a dressing over the open intravenous catheter and call the nurse.

21. Constipation is a common side effect of
  a. spasticity.
  b. narcotic medications.
  c. peritoneal dialysis.
  d. hypoxemia.

22. Do not use a transfer belt for a patient with a
   a. tracheostomy.
   b. dialysis shunt.
   c. central intravenous catheter.
   d. newly implanted medication pump.

23. Capillary refill is used to evaluate
   a. how much oxygen is in the venous blood.
   b. how well oxygen gets to body tissues.
   c. the percentage of oxygen saturation.
   d. the strength of the pulse.

24. The normal capillary refill time is
   a. 10 to 12 seconds.
   b. 5 to 7 seconds.
   c. 2 to 3 seconds.
   d. less than 1 second.

25. The normal oxygen saturation is
   a. 95% to 100%.
   b. 85% to 95%.
   c. 80% to 90%
   d. 70% to 80%.

B. Word Choice.

Choose the correct word or phrase from the following list to complete each statement in questions 26–39.

dialysis	transitional care
enteral	multisensory stimulation
hyperalimentation	exacerbation
piggyback	spasticity
pulse oximetry	Kelly
transcutaneous electrical	hypoxemia
nerve stimulation	CAPD
narcotic	

26. Subacute care is also called _____.

27. A procedure for removing liquid wastes from the blood is called _____.

28. _____ is used for measuring the oxygen level in arterial blood.

29. A _____ refers to a small bag of fluid containing intravenous medication that is connected with a tube to the primary tubing.

30. Total parenteral nutrition (TPN) is also called _____.

31. A feeding administered through a tube into the patient's stomach is called an _____ feeding.

32. A _____ is a potent drug used for pain relief.

33. The use of electrical current to treat pain is done with a procedure called _____.

34. Using various methods of sight, sound, touch, smell, pressure, and pain to help the patient awaken from a coma is called _____.

35. Worsening of the patient's condition is called _____.

36. A patient with severe _____ has sudden, frequent, involuntary muscle contractions that impair function.

37. A _____ is a curved clamp that is used to occlude central intravenous lines in an emergency.

38. _____ is a condition in which there is insufficient oxygen in the blood.

39. The most common type of dialysis used for subacute patients is _____.

C. Nursing Assistant Challenge.

You have completed your nursing assistant course and have been working the night shift for three months in a skilled care facility. The director of nursing calls you into her office and asks you if you would like to work the day shift in the new subacute care unit of the facility. You tell her you would like to think about it for a day and then give your decision. Consider the types of care that are given in subacute care and then answer these questions.

40. What would your duties be in the new unit?

41. You feel confident of your nursing assistant skills. However, you know you will need to learn some new things to care successfully for subacute care patients. What new information or skills will you need to acquire?

42. How do you plan to go about obtaining this education?

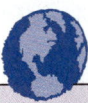 **EXPLORING THE WEB**

Description	Location
Subacute care booklet	*http://www.ltcinfo.net*
Cancer	*http://www.cancer.org*
Cancer nursing	*http://www.ons.org*
Coma recovery	*http://www.comarecovery.org*
Dialysis	*http://www.cdc.gov/ncidod/hip/Dialysis/dialysis.htm*
Implantable medication pumps	*http://www.medtronic.com*
Intravenous therapy	*http://www.ins1.org*
Pain	*http://www.pain.com*
Parenteral/enteral nutrition	*http://www.clinnutr.org*
Respiratory care	*http://www.aarc.org*
Vascular access	*http://www.navannet.org*
Advance for Post Acute Care	*http://www.advanceforpac.com*
JCAHO Subacute Care Programs	*http://www.jcaho.org*
National Association Subacute/Postacute Care	*http://www.nsca.net*
What Is Subacute Care?	*http://www.ahca.org*

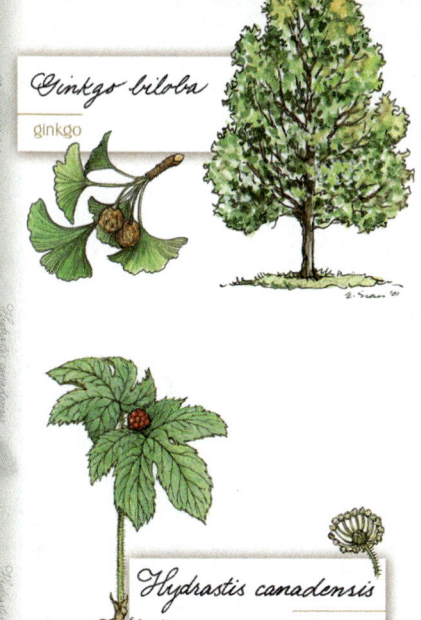

Ginkgo biloba
ginkgo

Hydrastis canadensis

Alternative, Complementary, and Integrative Approaches to Patient Care

objectives

After completing this unit, you will be able to:

- Spell and define terms.
- Define alternative medicine.
- Differentiate alternative practices from complementary and integrative practices.

- List five categories of alternative and complementary therapies.
- Define holistic care.
- List at least three ways in which the nursing assistant supports patients' spirituality.

vocabulary

Learn the meaning and the correct spelling of the following words and phrases:

acupuncture
alternative
alternative medical
  systems
Anthroposophically
  Extended
  Medicine (AEM)
aromatherapy
art therapy
Ayurveda
biofeedback
biological therapy
body-based therapy
chelation therapy
chiropractic care
color therapy

complementary
  medicine
complementary/
  alternative
  medicine (CAM)
cupping
dance therapy
Doctor of
  Osteopathy (D.O.)
electromagnetic
  therapy
energy therapy
guided imagery
herbal therapy
herbs
holistic care

homeopathy
hypnotherapy
integrative
  (integrated)
  health care
light therapy
massage therapy
meditation
mind-body therapy
modalities
movement therapy
moxibustion
Naturopathic
  medicine
nutrition therapy

osteopathic
  manipulative
  treatment (OMT)
prayer
qigong
reflexology
Reiki
relaxation
supplements
therapeutic touch
  (TT)
traditional Chinese
  medicine (TCM)
visualization
yoga

ALTERNATIVES TO MAINSTREAM HEALTH CARE

When most people in Western society think of medical care, they think of medical, surgical, pharmaceutical, and technological treatment of patients. In the United States, these practices and techniques are the accepted, traditional, mainstream approaches to patient care and healing of illness. Throughout history, people have actively sought out other forms of healing the sick. Drawings in caves show early humans practicing healing. Egyptian society (Figure 36-1) was particularly advanced in medical practices. Indian tribes had medicine men. Healing of the sick is mentioned in the Bible. These practices were considered mainstream before twentieth-century advances in technology, research, and medicine. In many ancient cultures, religion and medicine were closely connected. In the Middle Ages, medicine was the concern of either the church or the state. Because of this, many people used folk remedies that involved using herbs (Figure 36-2). Other religious customs and charms were also used for healing. These methods were more readily available and affordable than medical treatments.

Today, some people prefer natural and spiritual treatments for illness. Others are afraid of the technology, drugs, and surgical procedures of today. Some patients believe that conventional medical treatments are worse than the discomfort of disease. They prefer using other methods of relieving symptoms and eliminating sickness. Because of this, many people use alternative health care practices and products to prevent and treat illness. Alternatives are

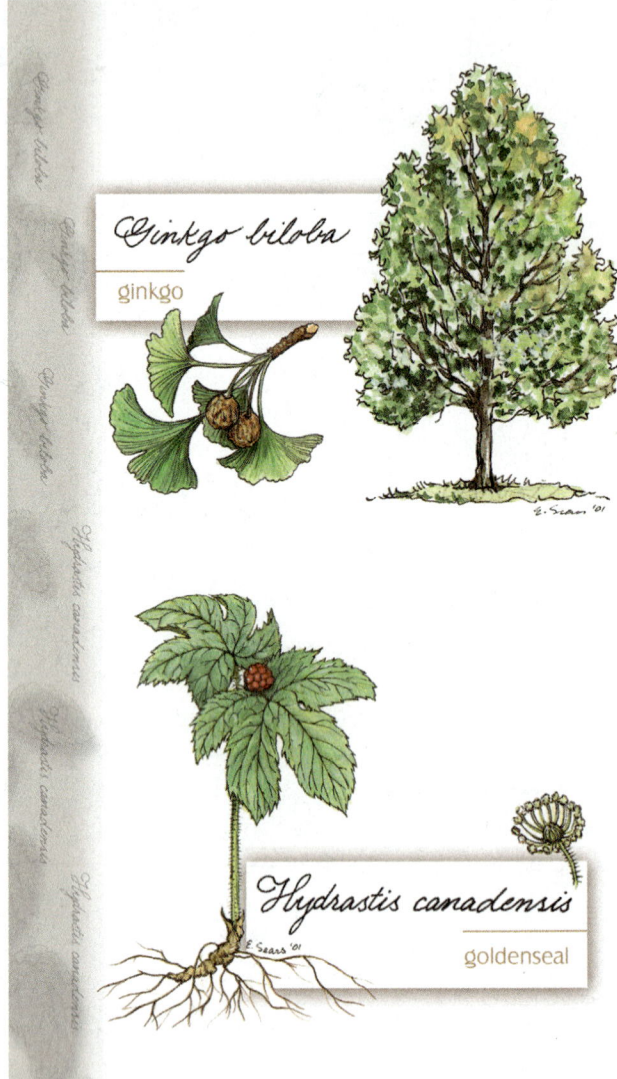

FIGURE 36-2 Herbs are potent natural substances with medicinal properties.

options that are used instead of conventional health care. Most alternative strategies use natural products rather than those derived from chemicals. Alternative therapies are used to treat every imaginable symptom and condition, from pain to menopause. Some people use natural products and practices to prevent illness (Figure 36-3). Most towns have at least one health food store that sells alternative products. Many books and magazines are available describing natural alternatives to health care. Some nontraditional practices have proven effective. Others have shown no real benefit, but this is a popular trend. The use of alternative therapy is not a passing fad; it is here to stay.

Many old remedies, practices, and traditions have been rediscovered and are being used today. Different forms of nontraditional healing are accepted by the public and many medical professionals. These nontraditional methods are called complementary/alternative medicine (CAM). CAM is a group of diverse systems, practices, and products that

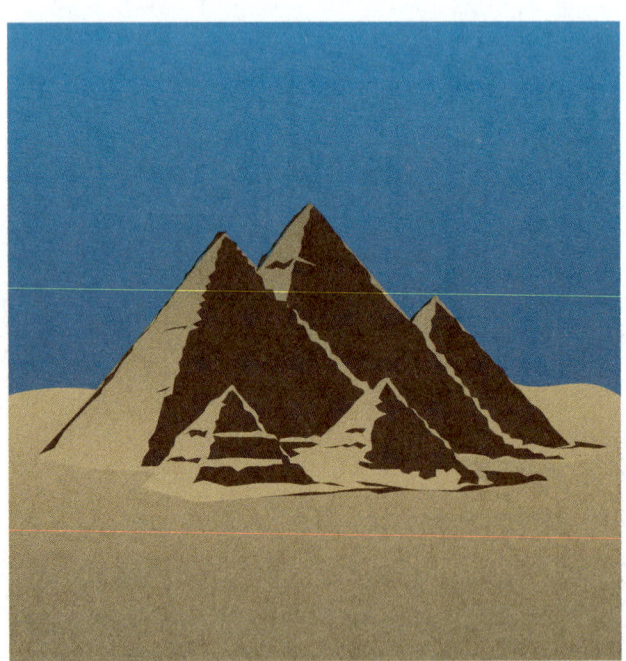

FIGURE 36-1 The ancient Egyptians used many natural substances and medical practices that were advanced for their time.

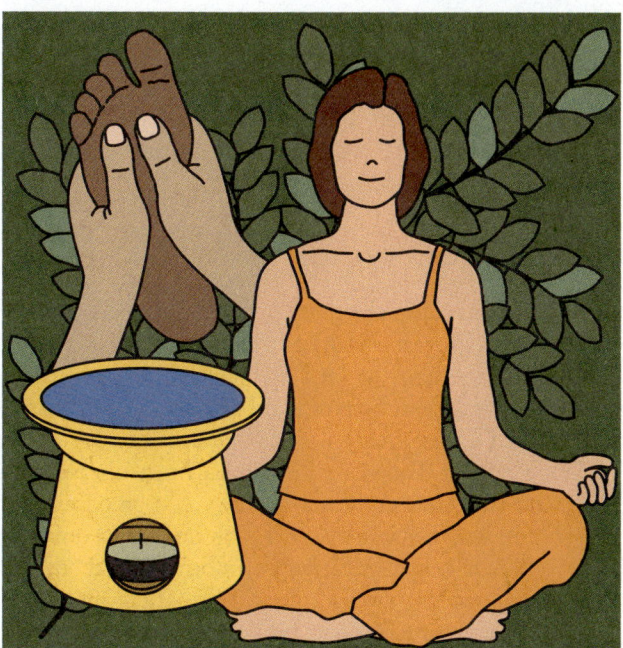

FIGURE 36-3 Many people use natural substances and practices as an alternative to traditional health care, believing that this is more healthful for the body.

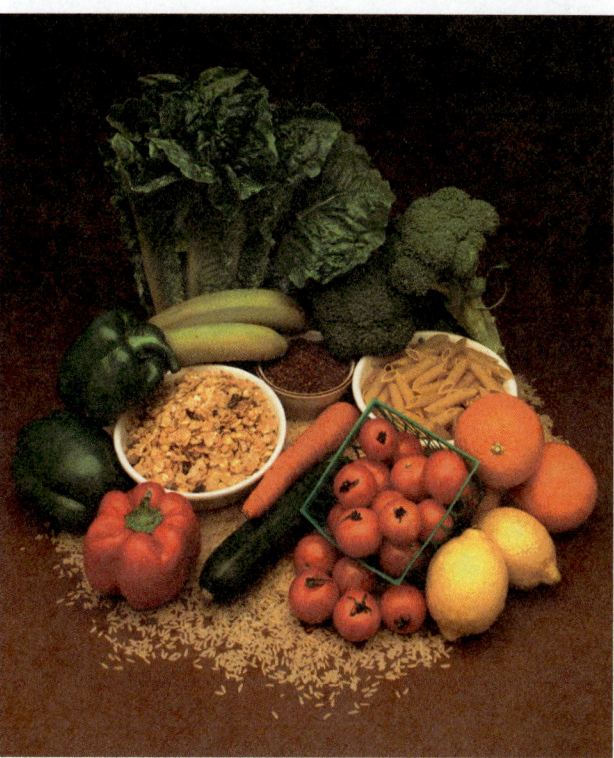

FIGURE 36-4 Natural foods are grown and processed without chemicals and pesticides. The heat used in food processing destroys some of the nutrients. Many natural products are processed with low or limited heat.

are not presently considered part of conventional medicine. This is an area of much research and scientific study. Because of this, practices listed as CAM change continually. Safety is always a great concern in health care. Some CAM practices have been proven unsafe or ineffective and are no longer used. Others have proven safe and effective and have moved into mainstream health care. For safety, a CAM program should always be supervised by a physician or other health care practitioner. New practices and techniques are always emerging.

Complementary and Alternative Practices

Hundreds of different alternative therapies are used instead of traditional medicine. For example, patients use **herbs** (medicines made from plants), **supplements** (nutritional substances used to make up a deficiency or strengthen the whole), and diet (Figure 36-4) to treat cancer instead of surgery, chemotherapy, and radiation therapy. Nutritional products are usually slow to work and no immediate effect is seen when patients take them. The patient may have to take the preparation for a minimum of three to six months before seeing results.

A degree of caution is necessary when using nutritional preparations. Some are toxic or harmful when taken in large quantities. Some have negative interactions with other medications and foods. Some nutritional products contain combinations of vitamins and nutrients. Taking several combination products increases the risk that the patient will exceed the safe dosage range. An example is vitamin A,

which is necessary for good eyesight and night vision. However, when taken excessively, vitamin A can cause blindness. Water-soluble preparations are excreted from the body. Fat-soluble preparations are stored in the tissue for a period of time. Some preparations interfere with drugs and therapies given for other medical conditions. Several have caused serious liver and kidney damage.

Complementary medicine is a treatment regimen in which alternative practices are combined with conventional health care. For example, magnets may be used with medications to relieve pain. Various sound and music therapies are used to reduce complications, relieve stress, make patients feel better, and increase their sense of well-being. **Aromatherapy** (using natural scents and smells to promote health and well-being) (Figure 36-5) is used by chemotherapy patients to relieve nausea. Some people use **guided imagery** in combination with cancer treatment. People who use imagery believe that focusing on and visualizing positive changes causes these changes to occur. **Energy therapies** (Figure 36-6) work with the energy field that allegedly surrounds and penetrates the body. (The existence of this energy has not been confirmed scientifically.) **Relaxation** (techniques and methods of reducing stress) and **meditation** (calming and quieting the mind by focusing attention) are used in combination with heat and medications to relieve pain. Thousands of different treatments and therapies fall under the CAM umbrella. These **modalities** (forms of treatment or uses of therapeutic

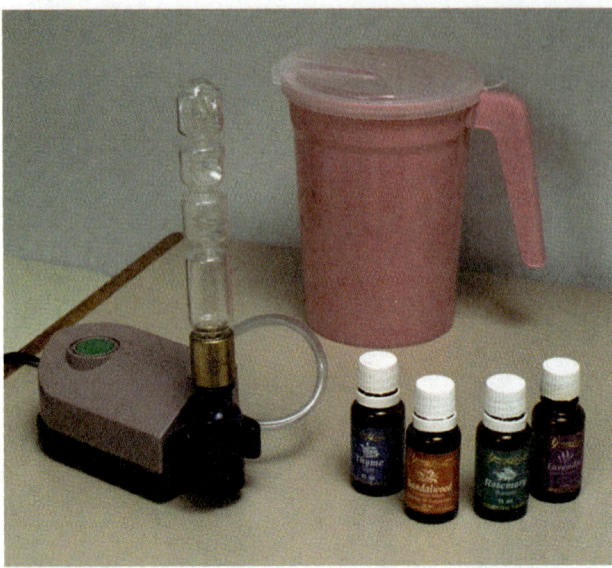

FIGURE 36-5 Aromatherapy is an ancient practice that uses fragrances to produce a reaction in the body. Certain scents are believed to change brain waves, breathing rates, and mood, among other things.

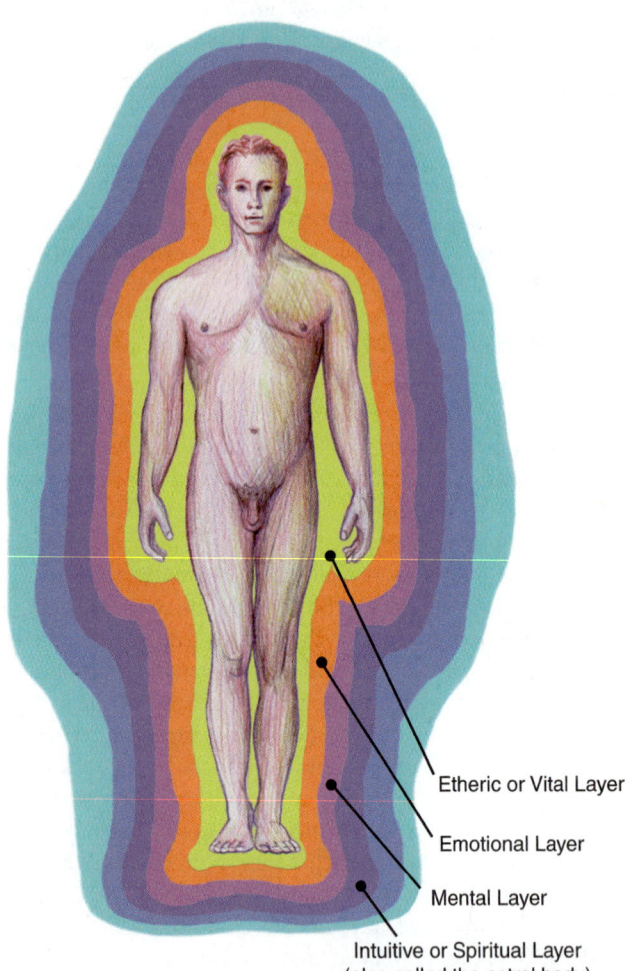

Etheric or Vital Layer

Emotional Layer

Mental Layer

Intuitive or Spiritual Layer
(also called the astral body)

FIGURE 36-6 The energy field that surrounds the body.

agents or regimens) can be placed into five broad categories, which are listed in Table 36-1. Most of these practices can be used alone or combined with more conventional treatment. When used alone, they are called *alternative treatments*. When used with other mainstream practices, they are called *complementary therapies*.

Using CAM

Alternative and complementary practices have become very popular in recent years. Many of these therapies are thought to stimulate the body to heal itself. They are also used to strengthen weak body systems, and reduce or eliminate the discomfort of some medical signs and symptoms, such as pain and nausea. Patients with cancer, heart disease, diabetes, and HIV disease commonly use CAM practices. The decision on whether to use CAM is an important one that must be made based on accurate information about the benefits and risks of the treatment. The patient must look beyond advertisers' claims to find reliable, credible information about the method being considered. Authoritative information is difficult to find for some treatments because little research has been done. When evaluating the negatives and positives, ask:

- What are the advantages, disadvantages, risks, side effects, expected results, and length of treatment?
- What is the safety record of the treatment? Are specific safety precautions necessary?
- Is the treatment effective in circumstances similar to mine? Is it harmful in circumstances similar to mine?
- What are the qualifications of the individual providing the treatment (if applicable)?
- Will the CAM therapy interfere with the conventional treatment or medication being used for an acute or chronic medical problem?
- Can I comfortably comply with the directions for using this treatment?

People use alternative therapies and programs for many different purposes. Many do this on their own, without medical supervision. Potential drawbacks of an unsupervised alternative treatment program are:

- potential for toxicity of herbs and nutritional products
- self-diagnosis is not always accurate
- self-treatment does not always work
- the self-treatment regimen may not be appropriate even if the diagnosis is correct
- the regimen may delay necessary medical treatment
- the program may interfere with prescription drugs
- self-treatment may cure the symptoms, but aggravate other health problems

If you decide to pursue an alternative program, do so under medical supervision. Seek medical help if the condition you are treating does not respond within a week, if the original symptoms worsen, or if new symptoms develop.

TABLE 36-1 COMMON COMPLEMENTARY AND ALTERNATIVE MEDICINE CATEGORIES

Category	Description	Example
Alternative Medical Systems	Therapeutic or preventive health care practices that do not follow generally accepted methods and may not have a scientific explanation for their effectiveness. These treatments are usually based on complete systems of medical practice. Many were developed in other countries and have been used for centuries, predating conventional medical practices.	• Traditional Chinese medicine (TCM) • Ayurveda • Homeopathy • Naturopathy
Mind-Body Therapy	Practices that employ various techniques to enhance the mind's ability to affect bodily function and symptoms (mind-over-matter principle). Many have been accepted by the medical community and are part of integrative health care practices and treatments.	• Meditation • Art therapy • Music therapy • Dance therapy • Patient support groups • Cognitive therapy • Prayer • Guided imagery
Biological Therapy	Biologically based practices using natural substances, such as vitamins, herbs, and foods. Other natural products, such as shark cartilage, are also used.	• Herbs • Nutritional products • Dietary supplements
Body-Based Therapy (may also be called manipulation, or manipulation therapy)	Practices that are based on direct body contact, including manipulation or movement of one or more parts of the body.	• Chiropractic adjustments • Osteopathic manipulation • Massage therapy
Energy Therapy	The study of how living organisms interact with electromagnetic energy fields. Although some practitioners believe touch is necessary for healing, others believe they can effect healing by placing the hands within the field. Two types of energy therapy are commonly used. *Biofield* therapies work by laying hands on the body or through its energy field to transfer a healing force. The biofield may also be called an *aura*. The energy field is believed to permeate the body and extends outward for several inches. *Biomagnetic-based* therapy is a form of energy therapy in which the hands are placed in or through the energy field to apply pressure on the body.	• Reiki • Therapeutic touch • Magnet therapy and use of magnetic fields • Pulsed current fields • AC and DC current fields

INTEGRATIVE (INTEGRATED) HEALTH CARE PRACTICES

Some researchers estimate that at least 50% of the American public uses at least one form of alternative or complementary treatment. Because of this, many hospitals have opened specialized units and clinics in which integrative (integrated) health care is practiced. Integrative health care involves using both mainstream medical treatments and CAM therapies to treat the patient. Approximately 20% of the hospitals in the United States offer some type of integrative medical services. Most integrative health care programs have two components. The wellness component helps participants stay well and prevent disease. The illness management component helps eliminate uncomfortable symptoms and strengthens the body to overcome the effects of illness. Many patients in the illness track also use approaches from the wellness track to prevent worsening of their conditions. Thus, patients who are well can participate to prevent illness, and those who are ill can participate to aid in their recovery.

Usually, the CAM method is used to enhance mainstream treatment, or to relieve signs and symptoms. Some services combine drug therapy with nutrition, diet, exercise, or other nontraditional therapies. CAM practices that promote relaxation (Figure 36-7) and relieve pain are some of the most commonly used in integrative care. This is based on the belief that when the mind and body are relaxed, pain and unpleasant symptoms decrease, and a healing environment is established within the body. Professionals who practice integrative care are very cautious, and CAM treatments are usually selected only when there is solid evidence of safety. If there is a high risk of harm to the patient, the treatment combination is not used.

Some patients practice integrative care on their own, without the knowledge of their health care provider. This can be dangerous, because some therapies increase the risk of complications when combined with some medical treatments and medications. For example, Mrs. Rosenberg has a strong family history of Alzheimer's disease. She fears she will contract this condition. She has taken herbs regularly for several years, as a preventive measure. Mrs. Rosenberg is hospitalized for a routine surgical procedure. She does not tell the doctor about the herbs, because they are nonprescription, natural products. During surgery, she experiences a large, unexpected blood loss and requires a blood transfusion. Mrs. Rosenberg did not know that the herbs she takes have a blood-thinning effect. Because the physician did not know of the herb use, he did not take measures before surgery to reduce the increased risk of bleeding.

The use of herbs in pregnancy can also be risky. In fact, herbs are very powerful substances that should be treated with caution and respect. They interact with many different prescription and nonprescription medications. Patients should always inform their health care provider if they are using alternative products. If a patient advises you that he or she uses alternatives, always inform the nurse. He or she will notify the physician.

Holistic Care

Standard medical care focuses on treating single body parts or systems. Most integrative medicine practitioners believe in using **holistic care** (practices that consider the whole person, including mind, body, and spirit). Holistic care (Figure 36-8) is designed to nourish, balance, and vitalize the whole individual. The patient's strengths are used to overcome weaknesses. Nursing care, in its purest form, has always been guided by principles of holistic care. In nursing, we look at the whole person. We know that one weakness can affect the patient's overall health and well-being. By supporting and strengthening all body systems, holistic medical care provides additional tools with which to fight disease.

Practitioners of holistic care also consider the effect that disease has on the patient's family dynamics and relationships. This reaches beyond curing a disease. Holistic care considers the entire person as a complex being with many problems and needs. The patient is an active member of the health care team, not a passive participant. Besides standard medical care, consideration may be given to:

- food and nutrition
- fluid balance
- elimination of body wastes
- getting adequate rest and sleep
- stress-relieving strategies
- exercise
- recreation
- avoidance of unhealthy practices and substances
- loving relationships and support systems

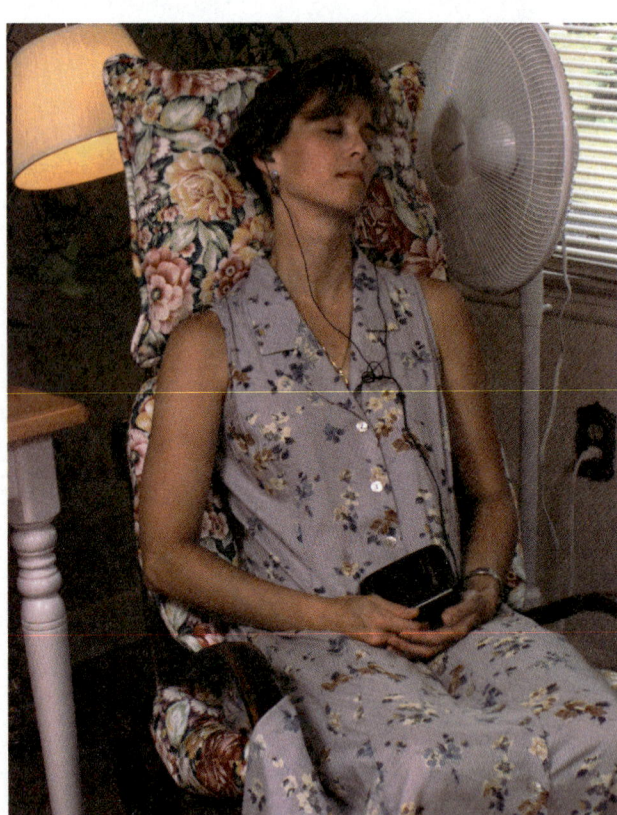

FIGURE 36-7 Some people use music during relaxation and meditation.

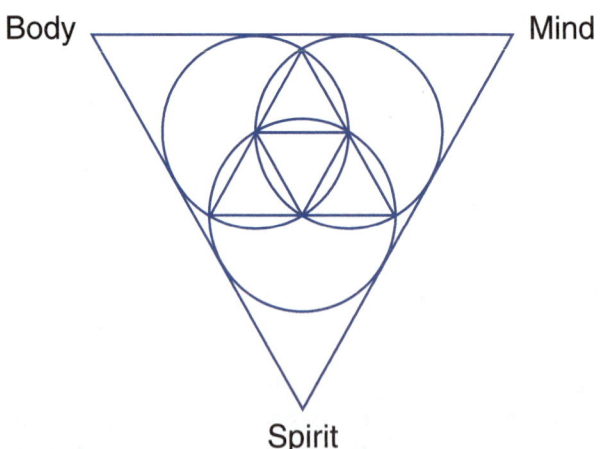

FIGURE 36-8 Holistic care looks at the patient as a person. Practitioners believe mind, body, and spirit must be balanced for health and wellness.

- inner strength
- creative expression
- spiritual expression and well-being

CAM Practices and Holistic Care

When the patient and physician agree to consider an integrated approach to treatment, the assessment process begins. Integrative health care is based on certain principles:

- Each individual can be empowered to bring greater wellness and healing into his or her own life.
- Complementary therapies can be used to support and strengthen overall health. Some therapies promote healing. Others relieve symptoms, such as pain and nausea.
- The mind affects the healing process.
- Every person is unique and no single set of recommendations will be right for everyone. The integrative program must be individualized to meet the patient's needs and circumstances. More than one supportive therapy may be necessary.

The assessment for a holistic integrative care program will consist of:

- evaluating the nature of the patient's medical and nursing problems
- determining if further diagnostic tests are needed (and obtaining tests, if necessary)
- evaluating the patient's coping resources
- identifying the patient's goals and expectations
- evaluating the patient's knowledge about his or her disease
- evaluating the patient's knowledge about CAM
- identifying patient teaching needs and developing a patient teaching plan
- agreeing with the patient on treatments to use and goals of therapy
- developing an individualized integrative treatment plan
- making referrals, consultations, and appointments, if necessary

Patient teaching is done so the patient can make informed decisions about his or her care. You may be asked to contribute information to the assessment. You may also reinforce patient teaching when you are caring for the patient. Always follow the plan of care. Teaching is an ongoing process during treatment. The patient's response to treatment will be evaluated frequently, and the treatment plan adjusted as often as necessary to achieve a positive response.

COMMON CAM THERAPIES

Many CAM therapies are being used in health care facilities today. The following lists modalities that are commonly used in integrative practice in hospital units and clinics:

- **Acupuncture** (Figure 36-9) is an ancient practice dating back thousands of years. Acupuncture is used to

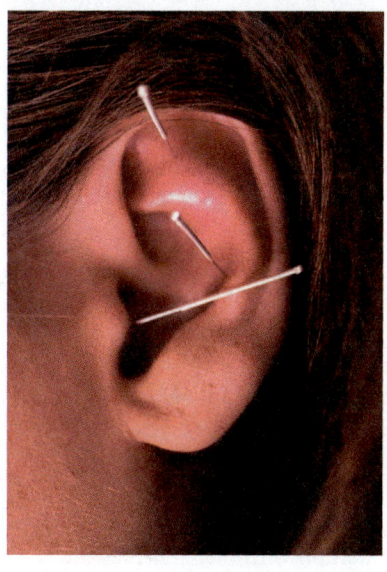

FIGURE 36-9
Acupuncture is used to treat many different conditions by correcting energy imbalances throughout the body. The needles are usually left in place from 5 to 20 minutes.

treat many acute and chronic conditions. Tiny, thin needles are placed in various parts of the body to correct imbalances in energy. It is safe and painless when done by a trained and qualified practitioner.

- **Anthroposophically Extended Medicine (AEM)** is a holistic Western system of natural medicine. AEM treats the whole person and not just the disease or symptoms. Practitioners consider the human being as far more than a physical machine. Treatment is designed to harmonize the relationship of body, mind, and spirit. AEM practitioners may use herbal and homeopathic preparations to support and guide the natural healing processes in the body.
- *Aromatherapy* involves using essential oils to stimulate the patient's sense of smell. Smelling the oils stimulates the olfactory nerve, sending messages to the brain. Although this treatment has many uses, it is commonly used to promote relaxation, relieve pain or nausea, and boost the immune system.
- **Art therapy**, **dance therapy**, and music therapy all focus on use of the senses. Each helps the patient express himself. They provide distraction and stress reduction. Art therapy helps the patient deal with emotional conflict, increase awareness, and express unspoken concerns. Dance therapy uses dance to decrease body tension, reduce pain, improve body image and self-esteem, decrease fear, and express anger. Music therapy has many therapeutic purposes and can be used alone or as part of other programs for relaxation, pain relief, and improved self-esteem.
- **Ayurveda** is a natural system of medicine that originated in India more than 3,000 years ago. Translated, *ayurveda* means "knowledge of life." This system is based on the belief that disease is due to an imbalance in the individual's consciousness. Practitioners encourage certain lifestyle interventions, natural therapies, and regaining a balance between the body, mind, and the environment. It begins with an internal purification

process, followed by a special diet, herbal remedies, massage therapy, yoga, and meditation. It is commonly used to treat high blood pressure, reduce stress, and reduce blood cholesterol.

- **Biofeedback** is a method of retraining your mind to control various physical problems and stresses that you would normally not be aware of.

- **Chelation therapy** involves intravenous (IV) injection of an amino acid by a licensed professional. It is commonly used to treat serious circulatory problems and reduced blood flow in the legs because of a buildup on the walls of the blood vessels. The amino acid injection bonds with substances within the blood vessels and removes them into circulation, where they are excreted in the urine. Although chelation therapy is usually considered safe, side effects range from mild to serious. It is usually used in combination with diet and exercise.

- **Chiropractic care** is a common, accepted CAM treatment that many people consider part of the mainstream medical system. Health insurance and Medicare pay for chiropractic visits; they do not pay for treatments for which effectiveness has not been proven. Chiropractic treatment has proven effective in relieving some types of pain, headaches, and menstrual cramps. Chiropractic care is based on the premise that the nervous system must function properly for good health. Because the nerves run through the spinal cord, chiropractic adjustments are done to keep the vertebrae in good alignment. This relieves pressure on nerves, muscles, and joints. Most chiropractors also promote exercise, diet, and good nutrition for overall health.

- Many studies have been done on how color affects the human mind. Some of these have also shown that color affects the body. Color is believed to stimulate many different senses and emotions. Marketing experts and advertisers use color to affect your moods and decisions. The color scheme on the packaging of most products is carefully designed to encourage you to buy. Past due bills are usually pink, which is associated with being very important. Red and orange color themes in restaurants are designed to increase your appetite. Many different alternative health care practices involve the use of **color therapy**. Color therapy is commonly used to affect mood, emotions, relationships, and sense of well-being. Color can be meditated on, gazed at, worn, or beamed in with various lights. Spiritual light and color are used for healing the body and mind. Color is also used for deepening meditation and creating specific effects on the body's energy field.

- **Electromagnetic therapy** is based on the belief that electric and magnetic energy exist within the body. Treatment is given to correct imbalances in the electrical and magnetic fields, which are believed to cause illness and disease. Different forms of electrical energy are used to correct imbalances. Mainstream medicine has adopted many electromagnetic approaches, such as

using a defibrillator to start the heart or a TENS unit to relieve pain.

- **Herbal therapy** is used throughout the world for its medicinal effect. Many food products we use today are herbs. Herbs are medicines made from plants that provide a different way of treating pain and illness. However, herbs are generally very strong, and some can be very toxic. The use of herbs as medicine should be supervised by a trained and qualified practitioner.

- **Homeopathy** is a practice of medicine that uses a wide range of natural (plant and mineral) substances to stimulate the body's immune system to fight disease. Homeopathic medicines are given to stimulate natural healing abilities of the body.

- **Hypnotherapy** is used to create an altered state of consciousness in which the patient is more open to the power of suggestion. It has many different applications, but in health care it is commonly used to relieve pain, anxiety, depression, addiction, and insomnia.

- **Light therapy** is used to treat mood and sleep disorders, jet lag, and depression. Treatment involves exposing patients to special lights covered with a plastic screen to block ultraviolet rays. The most common treatment involves sitting in front of a light box with the eyes open, but not looking directly into the light. Treatment time is progressively increased up to 90 minutes a day. One treatment involves shining a light behind the patient's knees. Research is being done on using light in the treatment of many conditions, including obesity and premenstrual syndrome.

- **Massage therapy** (Figure 36-10) is provided by licensed massage therapists. Massage stimulates and improves circulation, providing relaxation and pain relief. It is believed to stimulate the immune system to fight disease. Massage increases feelings of well-being and reduces stress and fatigue.

- *Meditation* is a form of body and mind relaxation. It has various applications, ranging from stress relief to

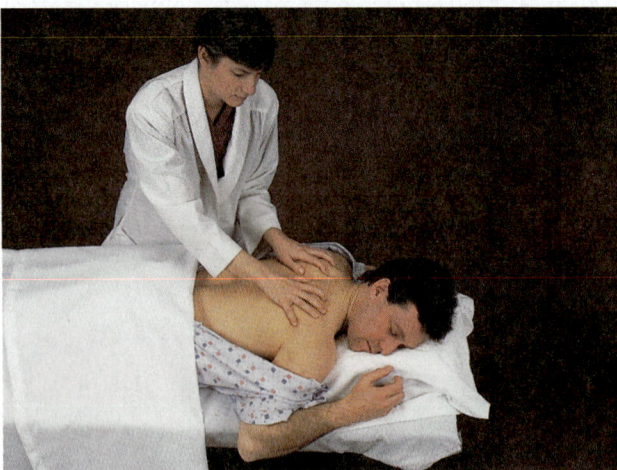

FIGURE 36-10 The massage therapist manipulates various areas of the body to stimulate tissues and promote healing.

pain relief. Meditation is an intensely personal and spiritual experience for most people. To meditate is to turn inward, to concentrate on the inner self. Meditation is a three-step process involving preparation, concentration, and merging with the object of concentration. It is commonly used for personal growth and developing tolerance. Meditation is said to channel awareness into a more positive direction by transforming one's state of mind.

- **Movement therapy** is a form of nonaerobic exercise and breath control that gives patients an awareness of how the body moves. Practitioners learn to alter posture and motion to reduce pain and stress. It is useful in chronic neurological disorders, such as Parkinson's disease, multiple sclerosis, and stroke. It has been used for increasing self-esteem.

- Doctors of **Naturopathic medicine** receive extensive education at one of five schools in North America. Naturopathic care focuses on whole-person wellness, emphasizing prevention and self-care. The doctor looks for the cause of illness, rather than strictly treating symptoms. Naturopathic practitioners cooperate with and refer patients for medical diagnosis and treatment when necessary. They use nontoxic, natural medications that are compounded and individualized to the patient's needs.

- **Nutrition therapy** evaluates the patient's diet to ensure that it contains optimal nutrition for health, wellness, and healing. This may mean eliminating some foods and adding others. Vitamins, minerals, and nutritional supplements may be added for wellness promotion or healing, such as calcium to prevent osteoporosis, or vitamin C to promote pressure-ulcer healing.

- **Prayer** (Figure 36-11) is a CAM technique that is used alone and in combination with other treatments. Some people use it with meditation. Patients have many different religious rituals and activities. Prayer is a connection with a person's higher power. One large study showed that patients who received prayer recovered faster after surgery than patients who were not the recipients of prayer. Many of the study patients were not aware that others were praying for their recovery.

- Practitioners of **qigong** believe that everyone is born with a life force energy, called *qi* or *chi*. This treatment involves physical and mental activities to teach the patient to channel the chi, thereby improving health. It is used to treat a variety of problems, including arthritis, gastric ulcers, insomnia, headaches, allergies, and high blood pressure.

- **Reflexology** (Figure 36-12) is an ancient form of healing used to reduce stress and treat illness. Certain reflex areas in the hands and feet are stimulated. The stimulation affects other parts of the body, reducing stress, stabilizing body functions, and correcting health problems.

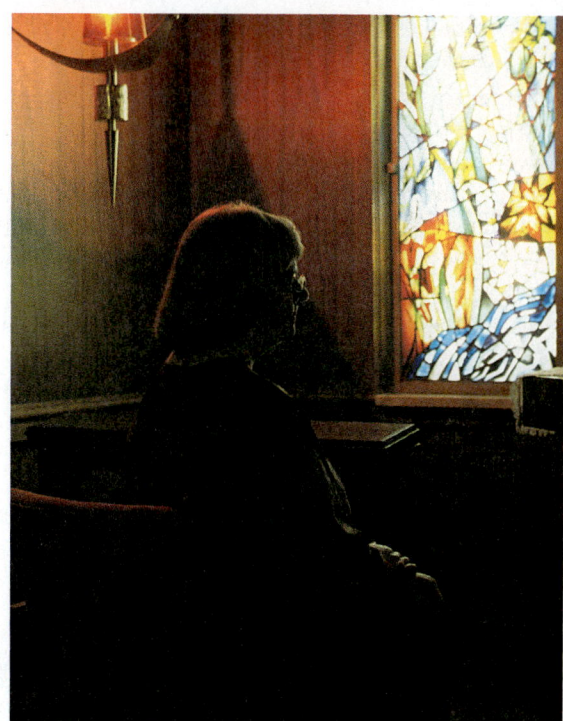

FIGURE 36-11 Prayer is a means of connecting with one's higher power.

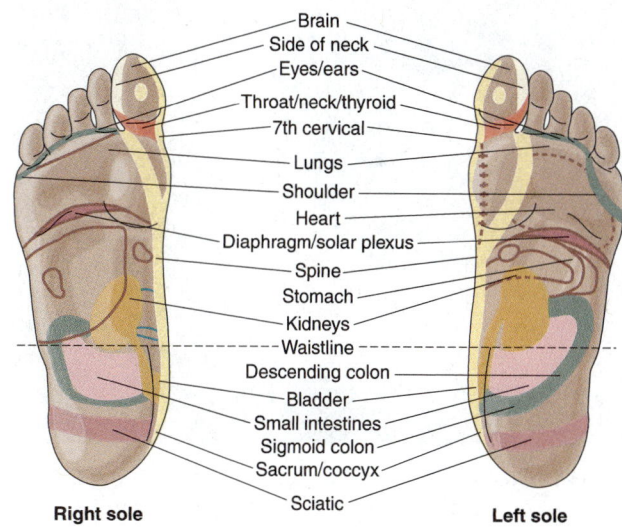

- Brain
- Side of neck
- Eyes/ears
- Throat/neck/thyroid
- 7th cervical
- Lungs
- Shoulder
- Heart
- Diaphragm/solar plexus
- Spine
- Stomach
- Kidneys
- Waistline
- Descending colon
- Bladder
- Small intestines
- Sigmoid colon
- Sacrum/coccyx
- Sciatic

Right sole   **Left sole**

FIGURE 36-12 Practitioners of reflexology believe that they can heal many areas of the body by manipulating the feet. This is based on the principle that different areas of the foot are connected to different areas of the body, from the internal organs to the ears.

- **Reiki** uses touch on various areas of the body to promote health and well-being. The hands are placed in various positions, beginning with the head and working down. The hands are held in place on each area for 3 to 5 minutes. Practitioners believe that sickness drains a person's physical and emotional energy. Reiki is applied to restore energy, enhancing the body's natural healing ability. Reiki practitioners receive special training. It is used to promote spiritual and mental well-being, relieve stress, relieve pain, and promote relaxation.

- **Therapeutic touch (TT)** is a term commonly used to describe touching patients in a caring manner. However, in this context, it is a CAM treatment that involves using the hands to exchange energy and stimulate healing (Figure 36-13A). Therapeutic touch practitioners believe that when energy is unbalanced, disease occurs. TT restores the energy field in the body to create a healing environment. The hands do not touch the patient (Figure 36-13B). The goal is to align the mind, body, and spirit for good health. TT is commonly used in the care of patients with AIDS, chronic pain, anxiety, and high blood pressure.

- **Traditional Chinese medicine (TCM)** is a complete health care system that is thousands of years old. It has changed little over the centuries. The basic idea is that a vital life force surges through the body. Any imbalance in the life force can cause illness. Disease is caused by an imbalance in the opposite and complementary energies that make up the life force, called *yin* and *yang*. The TCM doctor treats disease by restoring the balance between the internal body organs and the external elements of earth, fire, water, wood, and metal. Treatment may involve acupuncture, **moxibustion** (burning herbal leaves on or near the body), **cupping** (use of warmed glass jars to create suction on certain points of the body), massage, herbal remedies, movement, and concentration exercises.

- **Visualization** is one of the practices involved in guided imagery. This technique involves using the imagination to visualize something. Creating images in the mind helps reduce stress, pain, and symptoms associated with many medical conditions. The patient sets health goals and objectives. He or she is guided to visualize and work toward the goals. Two methods are commonly used. Visualization of colors is done to reduce stress. Another method involves visualizing the elimination of health care problems; for example, the patient may imagine a PacMan gobbling up cancer cells in the body.

- **Yoga** (Figure 36-14) means the union between mind and body. Yoga involves a combination of breath control, postures, relaxation, and meditation. It is used to improve lung function and circulation, decrease pain, and reduce anxiety.

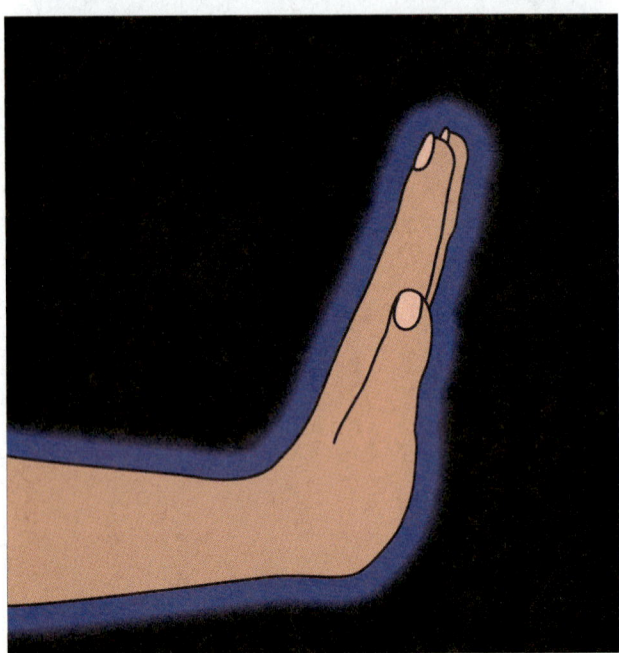

FIGURE 36-13A Therapeutic touch imparts healing energy from the practitioner's hands to the patient's body.

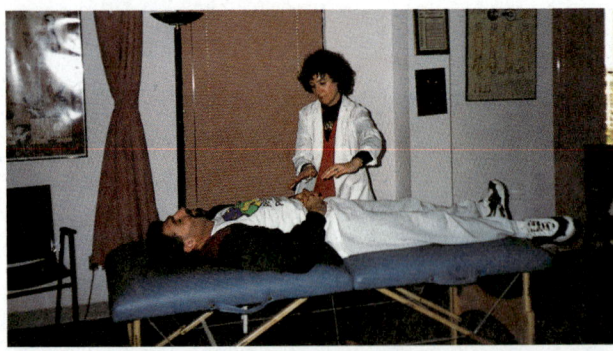

FIGURE 36-13B The therapeutic touch practitioner does not touch the patient.

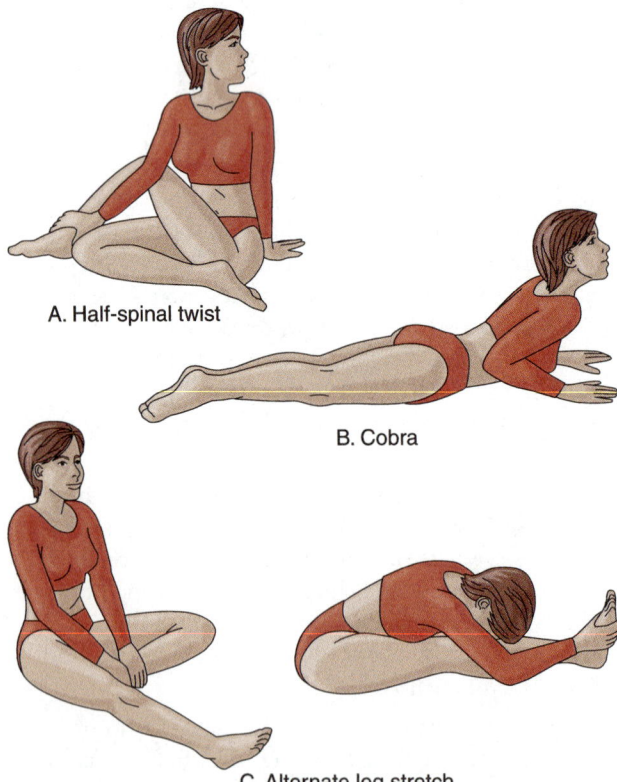

A. Half-spinal twist

B. Cobra

C. Alternate leg stretch

FIGURE 36-14 Many different yoga positions are used, but the focus is on breathing, which is supposed to awaken the consciousness.

Osteopathic Medicine

Some individuals consider osteopathic medicine to be an alternative practice, but over the years, this branch of medicine has been accepted as a form of mainstream medicine. The Doctor of Osteopathy (D.O.) has preparation similar to that of a medical doctor (M.D.). A D.O. receives a complete medical education. He or she receives additional training in osteopathic manipulative treatment (OMT), a passive, thrusting motion similar to the chiropractic adjustment. OMT is used to restore normal body movement, in combination with regular medical treatment. For example, a D.O. treats a patient with an infection of the foot by prescribing antibiotic therapy. Additionally, he provides an OMT treatment to enhance blood and oxygen flow through the body. This is based on the belief that the antibiotic will be more effective in eliminating the infection if the circulation to the foot is not impeded.

Osteopathic Medicine versus Chiropractic Care.
Some people believe that chiropractic and osteopathic treatments are identical, but they are not. Chiropractic care focuses mainly on the spine and involves many very fine maneuvers. The chiropractor focuses on preventing interruptions in nerve flow. The osteopathic physician focuses on how tight muscles and joints affect the function of all body systems. The emphasis is on ensuring proper movement of air (oxygen) and fluid within the body. This is based on the belief that the body works most effectively when:

- all tissues are nourished with oxygen
- wastes can be removed in body fluids
- the body is in an optimum state of health; healing will occur when it is nourished with oxygen and wastes have been removed

The osteopathic physician uses OMT with regular medical treatment, whereas the chiropractor uses only spinal manipulation. Because of this, the D.O. can treat many conditions that do not respond to chiropractic care.

SPIRITUALITY

Spirituality and religion also have a place in nontraditional health care practices. Many people believe that spirituality and religion are the same thing, but they are not. Spirituality is more of an umbrella that defines:

- our perceptions of our place in the universe (Figure 36-15)
- a higher power (if any)
- our responsibilities to others
- our fears and beliefs about living and dying

The need for spirituality may be fueled by experiences, relationships, opportunities that provide the motivation for deeper healing, and growth throughout life. Illness can be a powerful motivator for eliminating emotional, mental, and physical patterns that limit and restrict spiritual growth. A key to caring for patients' spiritual needs is respecting

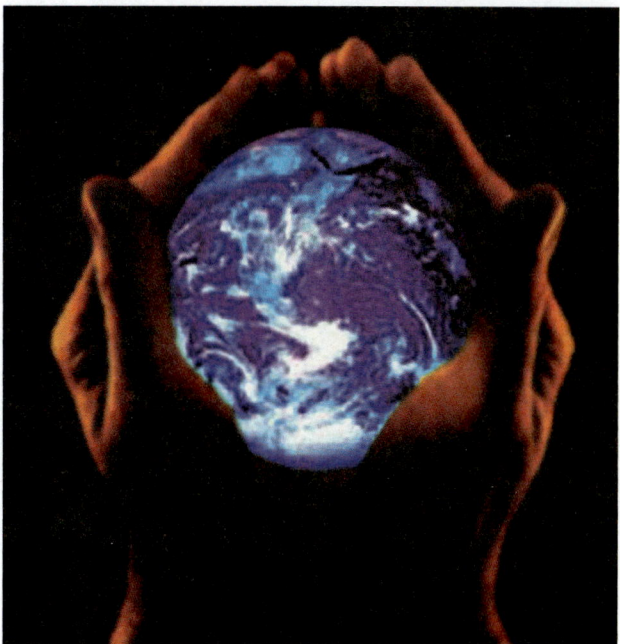

FIGURE 36-15 Spirituality defines our perceptions of our place in the universe and our responsibilities to others.

each patient as an individual, and appreciating that no two people are alike.

When patients use spirituality for healing, they allow the power of the spirit to work more fully in their lives, leading to greater harmony and balance. It is usually a quiet time for introspection and questioning. Healing may require making changes. It involves blending of the physical, mental, emotional, and spiritual aspects of self. When a person experiences deep physical or emotional healing, all parts of the self are changed. Physical problems often involve thoughts and emotions. Patients sometimes have surprises during periods of intense spirituality. They may release a great emotional burden instead of experiencing a physical recovery. The lifting of the emotional burden brings a great sense of inner peace.

Nursing Assistant Actions

The nursing assistant must recognize that all humans are spiritual beings, although we all choose different paths. Be sensitive to the patients' paths and choices. Avoid making judgments about patients' religious, spiritual, ethnic, and cultural practices and choices in health care treatment. Although spiritual beliefs are usually considered a private concern, the need for spiritual caring is fundamental when serious health problems occur. The patient may question the meaning and purpose of life, her ability to hope, belief in herself, belief in caregiver's ability, belief in the physician's ability, and belief in a higher power.

Health care personnel are privileged to have a role in these very personal times of significant stress and turmoil in patients' lives. Pay attention to what the patient is saying. Your role is to listen, to reflect, and to clarify information. Never try to interpret or define spiritual meaning or truth to the patient. Avoid imposing your beliefs on the patient. Avoid pat, uncaring answers to questions. Never give patients false hope. Never use problem-solving techniques to analyze spiritual truths for patients. Admitting that you do not know an answer is all right.

Remember that caring for patients during very private moments is a privilege. Do not be so distracted with your workload or the environment that you fail to show sensitivity when patients express spiritual concerns. Provide privacy and support while they work through challenges to their health and well-being. Inform the nurse or social worker of the patient's concerns. He or she may be able to provide assistance, intervention, or referrals to other sources of help.

REVIEW

A. True/False

Mark the following true or false by circling T or F.

1. T F Alternative practices are unapproved therapies that are used as part of mainstream health care treatment.

2. T F Complementary therapies are used instead of traditional medical treatments.

3. T F Safety is a major concern when considering complementary and alternative methods.

4. T F Some CAM therapies involve manipulation of the body with the hands.

5. T F Herbs are medications made from plants.

6. T F Imagery involves focusing on and visualizing positive changes.

7. T F An osteopathic physician and a chiropractor have similar education and practice.

8. T F The nursing assistant should assist patients in interpreting spiritual issues.

9. T F Complementary therapies have no place in health care.

10. T F Integrative health care involves a combination of mainstream medicine and alternative health care treatments.

11. T F Biofeedback involves training the mind to control physical problems.

12. T F Chiropractic adjustments are done to relieve pressure on nerves.

B. Matching

Choose the correct phrase from Column II to match the words in Column I.

Column I

13. _____ hypnotherapy

14. _____ homeopathy

15. _____ acupuncture

16. _____ Reiki

17. _____ movement therapy

18. _____ meditation

19. _____ aromatherapy

20. _____ therapeutic touch

21. _____ yoga

22. _____ Ayurveda

23. _____ qigong

24. _____ massage

Column II

a. stimulating sense of smell

b. concentrating on inner self

c. creates awareness of how body moves

d. rubbing body to stimulate circulation, promote relaxation

e. views disease as an imbalance in a person's consciousness

f. activities to teach the patient to channel chi

g. alters the state of consciousness

h. uses natural substances to stimulate immune system

i. begins with hands on head, working down over body

j. restores energy field so healing can occur

k. uses thin needles

l. union between mind and body

C. Multiple Choice

Select the one best answer for each of the following.

25. Holistic care includes
   a. meditation and biofeedback.
   b. using strengths to overcome weaknesses.
   c. freeing nerves from entrapped vertebrae.
   d. focus on the disease process.

26. An integrative care program always begins with

    a. patient teaching.

    b. goal-setting.

    c. assessment.

    d. assisting the patient to cope.

27. Cognitive therapy is a form of

    a. mind-body therapy.

    b. energy therapy.

    c. manipulation.

    d. biological therapy.

28. Chelation therapy is used to

    a. cleanse the mind.

    b. promote rest and relaxation.

    c. relieve stress.

    d. cleanse blood vessels.

29. Yin and yang are concepts used in

    a. Ayurveda.

    b. traditional Chinese medicine.

    c. qigong.

    d. Reiki.

D. Nursing Assistant Challenge

Your patient, Mrs. Matassarin, has been diagnosed with colon cancer. She has chosen an integrative medicine program to treat her illness. She meditates and prays several times each day. The care plan states you are to assist her in preparing to meditate at 3:15 PM each day. You are running a little late. You enter the room at 3:22 PM and find the patient deep in meditation.

30. What nursing assistant action should you take if the patient is meditating? Why?

31. What actions can you use in the future for assisting the patient with the meditation care plan?

32. If you are unsure of what actions to take, how will you find out?

33. Based on your knowledge of integrative health practices, what effect will the meditation have on Mrs. Matassarin?

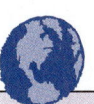

EXPLORING THE WEB

Description	Location
Alternative/complementary health care practices	http://www.delmarhealthcare.com/olcs/white/pnotes.asp (see Chapter 13)
Alternative and complementary therapies	http://www.delmarhealthcare.com/olcs/whiteduncan/pnotes.asp (see Chapter 8)
Herbal links and resources	http://www.delmarhealthcare.com/olcs/libster/links.asp
Holistic health	http://www.delmarhealthcare.com/olcs/white/pnotes.asp
Acupuncture	http://acupuncture.com
Animal-assisted therapy	http://www.dog-play.com/therapy.html
	http://www.superdog.com/therapy.htm
Aromatherapy	http://www.aromaweb.com
	http://www.naha.org
Ayurveda	http://www.ayurveda.com
Biomagnetic therapy	http://www.biomagnetic.org
Chiropractic care	http://www.chiro.org
Dance therapy	http://www.adta.org
Music therapy	http://www.musictherapy.org
Naturopathic medicine	http://www.naturopath.org
Osteopathic medicine	http://www.aacom.org
	http://www.aoa-net.org

continues

EXPLORING THE WEB   *continued*

Description	Location
Qigong	*http://www.qi.org*
Reflexology	*http://www.reflexology.org*
Reiki	*http://www.reiki.org*
Traditional Chinese medicine	*http://www.actcm.org*
Alternatives to Pain	*http://www.advancefornurses.com* (see past articles October 1, 2001)
American Music Therapy Organization	*http://www.musictherapy.org*
Entering the World of Healing Plants	*http://www.delmarhealthcare.com/pdf/0766827100_01.pdf*
Getting the Most from Holistic Healing	*http://www.holisticmed.com*
Getting to the Point	*http://www.advancefornurses.com* (see past articles April 2, 2001)
Herbal Option	*http://www.advancefornurses.com* (see past articles October 29, 2001)
Herbs and the Common Cold	*http://www.advancefornurses.com* (see past articles August 14, 2000)
Love, Medicine, and Miracles	*http://www.advancefornurses.com* (see past articles September 25, 2000)
National Institutes of Health	*CAM http://nccam.nih.gov/health*

Body Systems, Common Disorders, and Related Care Procedures

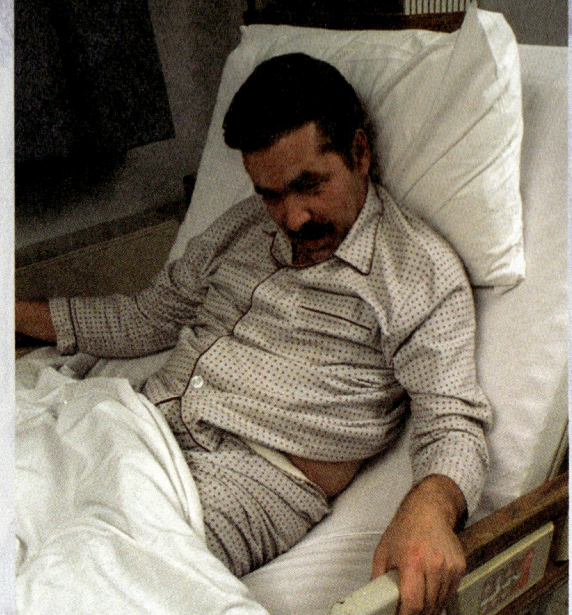

Integumentary System

objectives

After completing this unit, you will be able to:
- Spell and define terms.
- Review the location and function of the skin.
- Describe some common skin lesions.
- List three diagnostic tests associated with skin conditions.
- Describe nursing assistant actions relating to care of patients with specific skin conditions.
- Identify persons at risk for the formation of pressure ulcers.
- Describe measures to prevent pressure ulcers.
- Describe the stages of pressure ulcer formation and identify appropriate nursing assistant actions.
- List nursing assistant actions in caring for patients with burns.

vocabulary

Learn the meaning and the correct spelling of the following words and phrases:

abrasion	dermis	mites	senile purpura
allergen	epidermis	necrosis	shearing
allergies	eschar	nodules	skin tears
anaphylactic shock	excoriation	obese	subcutaneous tissue
contraindicated	friction	pallor	sudoriferous gland
contusion	hematoma	papule	tepid
crust	integument	pediculosis	vesicle
cyanotic	Kaposi's sarcoma	pressure ulcer	wheal
debride	lesion	pustule	
decubitus ulcer	macule	rubra	
dermal ulcer	malodorous	sebaceous gland	

INTEGUMENTARY SYSTEM STRUCTURES

The integumentary system (Figure 37-1) includes:

- Skin
- Hair
- Nails
- Sweat glands
- Nerves
- Oil glands

The outermost layers of the skin make up the epidermis. The dermis lies under the epidermis. The subcutaneous tissue that attaches the skin to the muscles lies under the dermis.

The nails are horny cell structures found on the dorsal, distal surfaces of the fingers and toes. They protect the sensitive fingers and toes. The teeth are formed from the tissues of the integument (body shell).

Epidermis

The epidermis consists of dead outer cells that are constantly shed as new cells move upward from the dermis. There are no blood vessels in the epidermis, so injury to this layer does not cause bleeding. Nerve endings reach into this outer layer. The nerves are sense organs that keep us in contact with changes in the environment. Nerve endings called *receptors* receive information about:

- Heat
- Cold
- Pain
- Pressure

Dermis

The dermis contains blood vessels, nerve fibers, and two kinds of glands:

- Sweat glands (sudoriferous glands)
- Oil glands (sebaceous glands)

Sweat Glands

The sweat glands produce perspiration that reaches the skin surface through tubes or ducts that end in openings called pores. Heat from deep in the body is brought to the skin by blood vessels. This heat is transferred to the perspiration. At the skin surface, the perspiration and the heat are lost through the pores to the air. The heat of the body is controlled by changes in the size of the blood vessels in the skin.

- When the central opening of a blood vessel becomes enlarged (dilated), more heat is brought to the body surface.
- When the central opening of a blood vessel becomes smaller (constricted), less heat is brought to the body surface.

Oil Glands and Hair

Oil glands lubricate and keep flexible the hairs found in the skin. Hair covers almost all body surfaces except for the palms of the hands and the soles of the feet.

SKIN FUNCTIONS

The skin has many functions that are critical to the well-being of the body:

- Protection—forms a continuous membranous covering for the body and regulates body temperature
- Storage—stores fat and vitamins
- Elimination—loses water, salts, and heat through perspiration
- Sensory perception—contains nerve endings that keep us aware of environmental changes

The skin tells us much about the general health of the body.

- A fever may be indicated by hot, dry skin.
- Unusual redness—rubra, or flushing of the skin—often follows strenuous activity.
- Pallor, which is less color than normal, is a sign associated with many conditions.
- The oxygen content of the blood can be noted quickly by the color of the skin. When the oxygen content is very low, the blood is darker and the skin appears bluish or cyanotic.

AGING CHANGES

As a person ages, changes become evident in the skin and its elements. These changes include:

- Glands that are less active

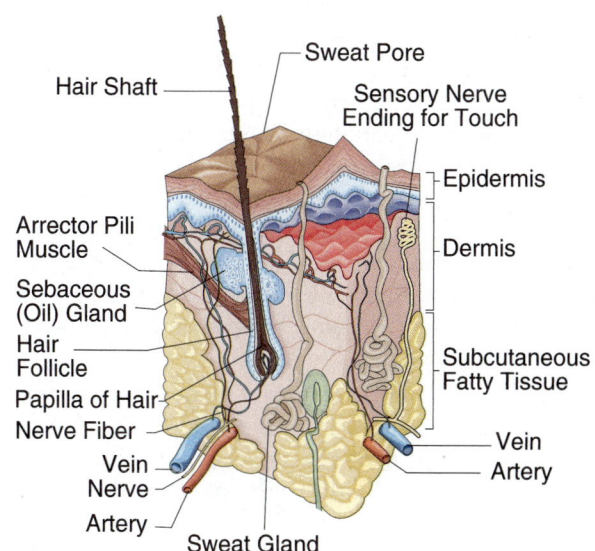

FIGURE 37-1 Cross-section of the skin.

Labels:
Hair Shaft
Sweat Pore
Sensory Nerve Ending for Touch
Epidermis
Arrector Pili Muscle
Dermis
Sebaceous (Oil) Gland
Hair Follicle
Subcutaneous Fatty Tissue
Papilla of Hair
Nerve Fiber
Vein
Vein
Artery
Nerve
Artery
Sweat Gland

- Decreased circulation
- Dryness, thinning, and scaling
- Thickening of fingernails and toenails
- Loss of fat and elasticity
- Loss of hair color
- Development of skin irregularities such as skin tabs, moles, and warts

SKIN LESIONS

Injury or disease can cause changes in skin structures. These changes are called **lesions**. The lesions may be caused by disease, trauma, wear, or the aging process. When caring for patients with skin lesions, standard precautions are followed. Some of the most common skin lesions or eruptions are:

- **Macules**—flat, discolored spots, as in measles (Figure 37-2)

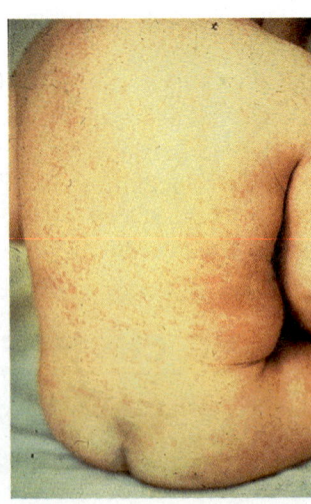

FIGURE 37-2 The macules of German measles. *(Courtesy of the Centers for Disease Control and Prevention [CDC], Atlanta, Georgia)*

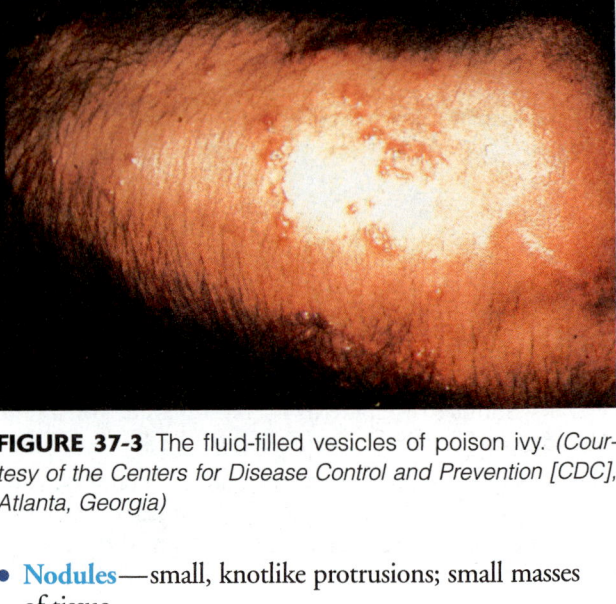

FIGURE 37-3 The fluid-filled vesicles of poison ivy. *(Courtesy of the Centers for Disease Control and Prevention [CDC], Atlanta, Georgia)*

- **Nodules**—small, knotlike protrusions; small masses of tissue
- **Papules**—small, solid, raised spots, as in chickenpox
- **Pustules**—raised spots filled with pus, as in acne
- **Vesicles**—raised spots filled with watery fluid, such as a blister (Figure 37-3)
- **Wheals**—large, raised, irregular areas frequently associated with itching, as in hives
- **Excoriations**—portions of the skin appear scraped or scratched away
- **Crusts**—areas of dried body secretions, such as scabs

Skin lesions may be a result of systemic responses:

- Communicable disease—diseases that are easily transmitted, directly or indirectly, from person to person. Measles and chickenpox are two such diseases. Each has characteristic skin lesions called *skin eruptions* or *rashes*.
- Immune system problems—Persons whose immune systems are depressed, such as those suffering from HIV infection, may develop a specific type of cancer called **Kaposi's sarcoma** (Figure 37-4). It appears as lesions in the skin and eventually in other organs. The skin lesions begin as macules, papules, or nodules that gradually become bigger and darker. The lesions are reddish-purple to dark blue in color. In addition to persons with HIV disease, Kaposi's sarcoma (Figure 37-4A and Figure 37-4B) is most common in men over 60 years of age. Recent research suggests that it is caused by a herpes virus, and may be spread by kissing an infected person. Kaposi's lesions can also appear in the mouth and internal organs. Progression of the disease may be slow or rapid.
- **Allergies**—also called *sensitivity reactions*, may have associated skin lesions. The vesicles of poison ivy are well known. The material causing the sensitivity is called an **allergen**. Individuals respond to allergens in different ways.
- **Anaphylactic shock**—a severe, sometimes fatal, sensitivity reaction.

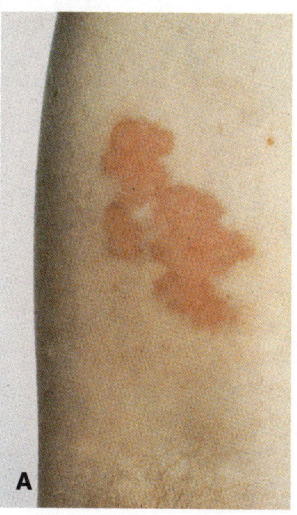
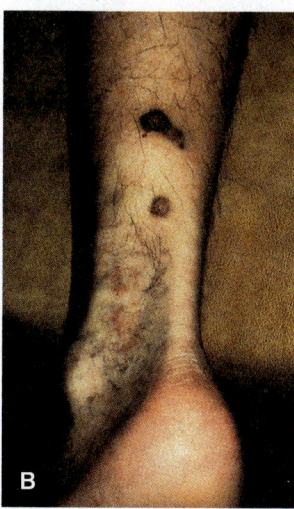

FIGURE 37-4 A. Typical lesions of Kaposi's sarcoma. B. Raised lesions of Kaposi's sarcoma. *(Both courtesy of Daniel J. Barbaro, MD, Fort Worth, Texas)*

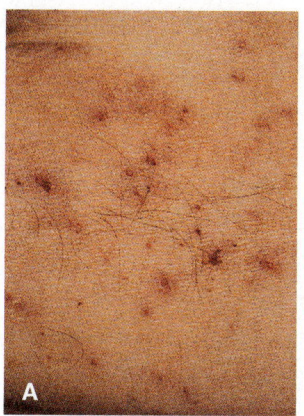
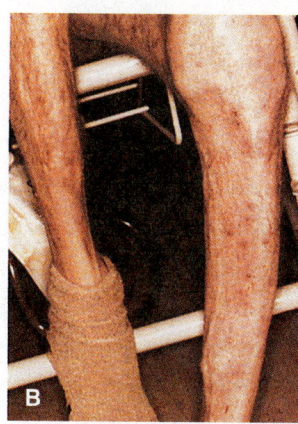

FIGURE 37-6 A. Scabies rash on the back. B. Scabies rash on the knees and lower legs. *(Both courtesy of L.E. Morris and Donna J. Lewis, "Management of Chronic, Resistive Scabies: A Case Study," Geriatric Nursing 16 (Sept./Oct. 1995): 230–37)*

- **Pediculosis** (body lice) and scabies **mites**—these tiny parasites are difficult or impossible to see (Figure 37-5). The patient usually complains of intense itching. The skin may have a rash-like appearance. The rash of scabies usually follows the blood vessels. It commonly appears in the webs of the fingers, inside the wrists, outside the elbows, in the underarm, at the waist, and in the nipple area (Figure 37-6A). It is also sometimes seen in the genital area in men, and around the knees (Figure 37-65B) and lower buttocks. One type of scabies causes scaling of the skin on the palms of hands and soles of feet. Lice and scabies are highly infectious and are spread by direct and indirect contact with an infected person or object.

Some lesions commonly occur when the skin is injured:

- **Abrasions** are injuries that result from scraping the skin.
- **Contusions** are mechanical injuries (usually caused by a blow) resulting in hemorrhage beneath the unbroken skin.
- An ecchymosis is a bruise.
- A **hematoma** is a localized mass of blood that is confined to one area.
- Lacerations are accidental breaks in the skin.
- **Senile purpura** are dark purple bruises on the forearms and backs of hands. These are common in elderly individuals.

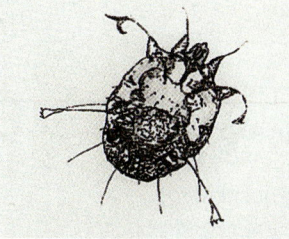

FIGURE 37-5 The scabies mite cannot be seen with the eye. *(Courtesy of L.E. Morris and Donna J. Lewis, "Management of Chronic, Resistive Scabies: A Case Study," Geriatric Nursing 16 (Sept./Oct. 1995): 230–37)*

- **Skin tears** are shallow injuries in which the epidermis is torn. The shape is often irregular. These injuries are also common in elderly individuals.

Observation of the skin and accurate descriptions of what you see must be carefully charted.

Diagnosing Skin Lesions

Your careful observations and accurate description of any skin lesions provide valuable information about the patient's condition. Several diagnostic tests may be ordered by the physician to help establish the cause of a lesion. These tests include:

- Studying scrapings from the skin lesion under the microscope.
- Culturing the skin lesion if an infection is suspected.
- Performing skin testing if sensitivities are suspected, by introducing small quantities of substances (allergens) known to bring about an allergic (hypersensitivity) reaction in humans. Allergens include pollens, foods, dust, animal dander, and medications.

Care of Skin Lesions

When skin lesions are present, certain general nursing care is indicated. Take the following precautions when caring for these patients.

- Closely observe the patient's skin on admission, but do not remove any dressings. Any changes noted should be reported immediately and described accurately.
- Soap and water and rubbing lotions are often **contraindicated** (not permitted). Check the nursing care plan before bathing the patient or giving a backrub.
- Special products may be used for bathing or soaking the skin, such as *colloidal oatmeal*. This product is used for many different skin conditions to relieve irritation, reduce itching, and moisturize, soften, and protect the skin. When bathing the patient, you may be instructed

to use **tepid** (lukewarm) water instead of hot water. Make sure that the patient does not get the treated bath water in the eyes. The product may make the tub slippery. Instruct the patient to use the hand rail when rising from the tub, and provide assistance as needed.

- Wear gloves when contact with blood, body fluids (including drainage from blisters or skin lesions), or nonintact skin is likely.
- Do not attempt to remove any crusts from skin lesions without special instruction from your supervisor.
- Handle the patient gently. Avoid rubbing the skin.
- Special bed linen may be used, such as sterile linen, linen that has been washed in special detergent, or disposable linen. Special bedding will be listed on the care plan.
- A bed cradle (Unit 25) may be placed on the bed to prevent the sheet from contacting the open skin areas.
- Notify the nurse if the:
  - skin lesions are draining
  - nature of the drainage changes
  - amount of drainage increases
  - drainage becomes **malodorous** (having a bad or foul odor)
  - drainage changes in color

Pressure Ulcers (Dermal Ulcers)

Pressure ulcers, commonly called bedsores or **dermal ulcers**, may occur in patients of any age. You may also hear them called **decubitus ulcers**. This is an older term that continues to be used. It is not as accurate as *pressure ulcers*. Pressure ulcers are open areas that develop on the skin over a bony prominence as the result of pressure. If there is pressure on the skin for a prolonged period, ulceration can occur, regardless of the patient's position. *Decubitus* is Latin for lying down. Because ulcers can occur when a patient is not in bed, the descriptive terminology was changed to

"pressure ulcer" for accuracy. They are particularly common in patients who are:

- Elderly
- Very thin
- Overweight (**obese**)
- Unable to move
- Incontinent
- Debilitated
- Poorly nourished (eats less than half of meals and snacks)
- Confined to bed or wheelchairs
- Disoriented
- Dehydrated
- In prolonged contact with moisture
- Circulation-impaired
- Has discolored, torn, or swollen skin
- Subjected to shearing

Shearing (Figure 37-7) occurs when the skin moves in one direction while the structures under the skin, such as the bones, remain fixed or move in the opposite direction. This can happen when patients are dragged rather than lifted up in bed, when positions are changed, or when patients slide down in bed or in a wheelchair (Figure 37-8). Blood vessels become twisted and stretched, causing the tissues being served to lose essential oxygen and nutrients, leading to breakdown. In addition, shearing may cause actual tears in fragile skin. These skin tears are painful, a portal of entry for infectious pathogens, and commonly lead to further breakdown. **Friction** (rubbing the skin against another surface,

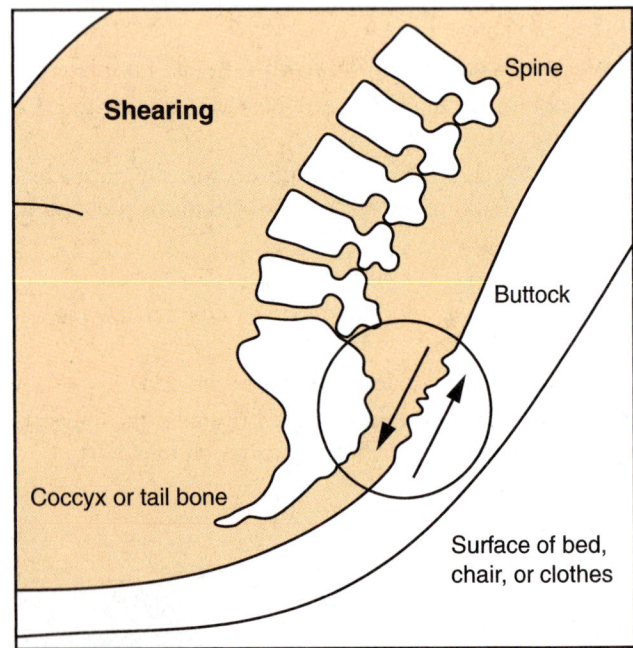

FIGURE 37-7 Shearing occurs when the skin is stretched in one direction and the underlying structures move in the opposite direction.

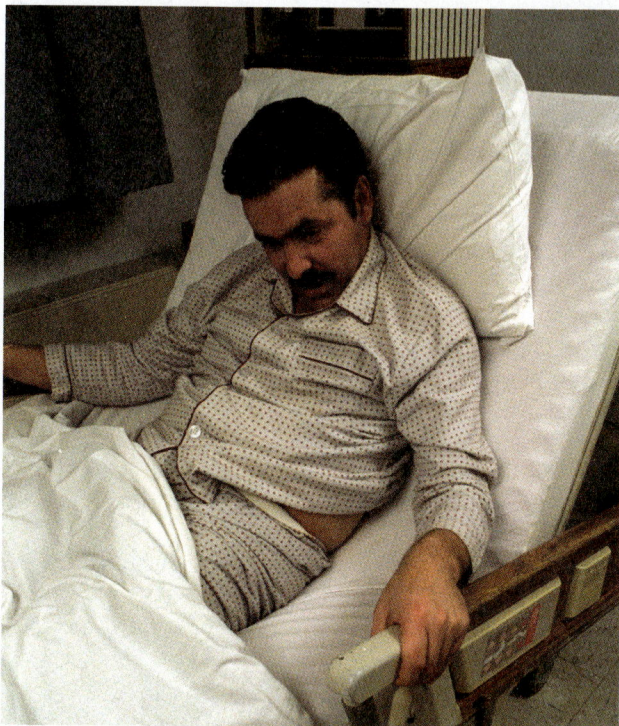

FIGURE 37-8 Shearing occurs when a patient slides down or is improperly pulled up in bed.

such as bed linen) also contributes to pressure ulcer formation. It usually occurs when the patient is being moved.

Pressure ulcers are caused by prolonged pressure on an area of the body that interferes with circulation. The tissue first becomes reddened. As the cells die (undergo *necrosis*) from lack of nourishment, the skin breaks down and an ulcer forms. The resulting pressure ulcers may become large and deep.

Pressure ulcers occur most frequently over areas where bones come close to the surface. The most common sites (Figure 37-9A and 37-9B) are the:

- Elbows
- Heels
- Shoulders
- Sacrum, coccyx
- Hips
- Buttocks
- Ankles
- Ears
- Knees (inner and outer parts)
- Toes

Patients tend to develop pressure ulcers where body parts rub and cause friction. Common sites are:

- Between the folds of the buttocks
- Legs
- Under the breasts
- Abdominal folds

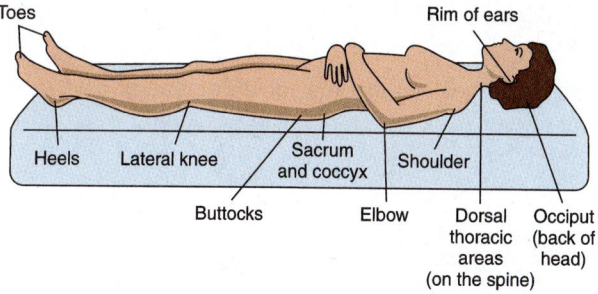

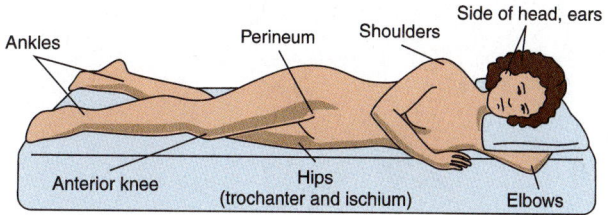

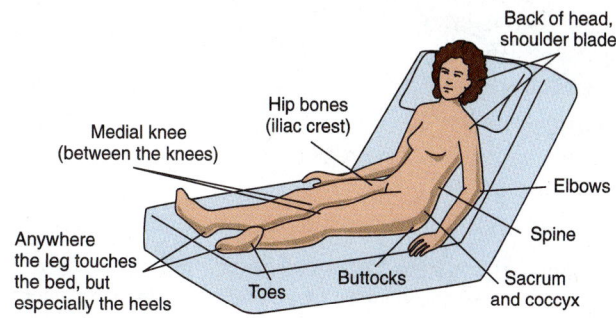

FIGURE 37-9A Potential areas of pressure when a patient is in bed.

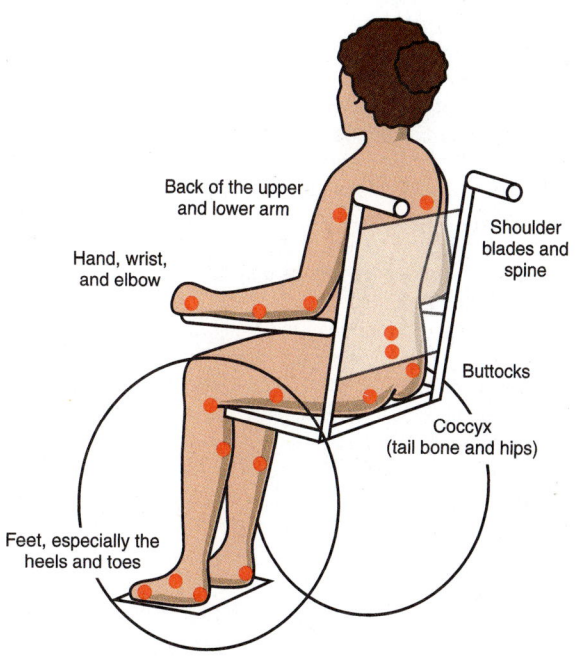

FIGURE 37-9B Potential areas of pressure when a patient is in a chair or wheelchair.

- Ankles
- Knees

The rubbing of tubing and other equipment used in the care of patients over a long period can also cause pressure sores (Figure 37-10).

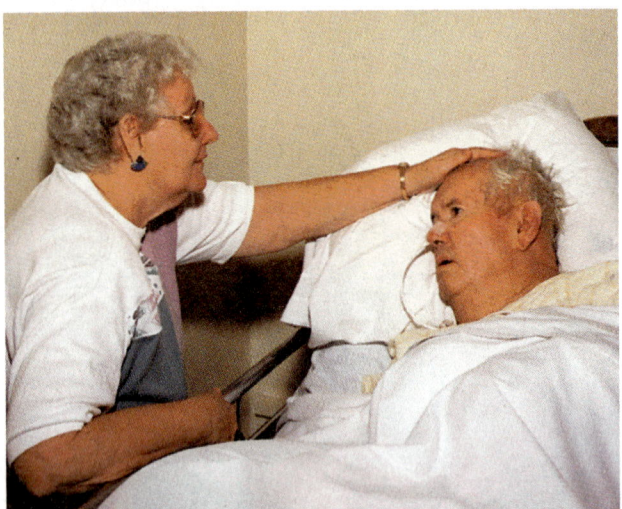

FIGURE 37-10 Rubbing and pressure from tubes can cause irritation and skin breakdown.

Preventing Pressure Ulcers. Because pressure ulcers are far easier to prevent than to cure, everyone participating in the patient's care has a responsibility to prevent skin breakdown.

When a patient is admitted, the nurse will assess the patient's current status and potential for skin breakdown. This assessment gives a baseline against which all future assessments may be measured. The assessment may be described on the patient's chart in words, pictures, diagrams, or as a score (Figures 37-11A and 37-11B). If a nursing diagnosis of actual or "risk for impaired skin or tissue integrity" is made, every staff member must make extra efforts to prevent skin breakdown, limit any breakdown that has already occurred, and promote the healing process.

Development of Pressure Ulcers

Tissue breakdown occurs in four stages. Nursing intervention at each stage can limit the process and prevent further damage. Remember to continue all preventive measures throughout care.

Stage I. In Stage I, the skin develops a redness (Figure 37-12A and 37-12B) or blue-gray discoloration over the pressure area. In dark-skinned people, the area may appear drier, or it may appear dark blue or black. The redness or

---

PATIENTS AT RISK TO DEVELOP PRESSURE SORES: Identify any patient at risk to develop pressure sores by assessing the seven clinical condition parameters and assigning a score. Any patient with intact skin, but scoring **8 or greater** should have nursing diagnosis **"Potential Impairment of Skin Integrity"** identified.

Clinical Condition Parameters—Risk of Pressure Sores

Clinical Condition Parameters	Score	Clinical Condition Parameters	Score
General Physical Condition (health problem)		**Mobility (extremities)**	
Good (minor)	0	Full active range	0
Fair (major but stable)	1	Limited movement with assistance	2
Poor (chronic/serious not stable)	2	Moves only with assistance	4
		Immobile	6
Level of Consciousness (to commands)		**Incontinence (bowel and/or bladder)**	
Alert (responds readily)	0	None	0
Lethargic (slow to respond)	1	Occasional (≤ 2 per 24 hours)	2
Semi Comatose (responds only to verbal		Usually (> 2 per 24 hours)	4
or painful stimuli)	2	No Control	6
Comatose (no response to stimuli)	3		
Activity		**Nutrition (for age and size)**	
Ambulant without assistance	0	Good (eats/drinks adequately ³/₄ of meal)	0
Ambulant with assistance	2	Fair (eats/drinks inadequately—at least ¹/₂ of meal) .1	
Chairfast	4	Poor (unable/refuses to eat/drink—less than ¹/₂) . .	2
Bedfast	6		
		Skin/Tissue Status	
		Good (well nourished/skin intact)	0
		Fair (poorly nourished/skin intact)	1
		Poor (skin not intact)	2
		Total	

FIGURE 37-11A Assessing risk of pressure ulcers. *(Courtesy of Artistic Press, Los Angeles, CA)*

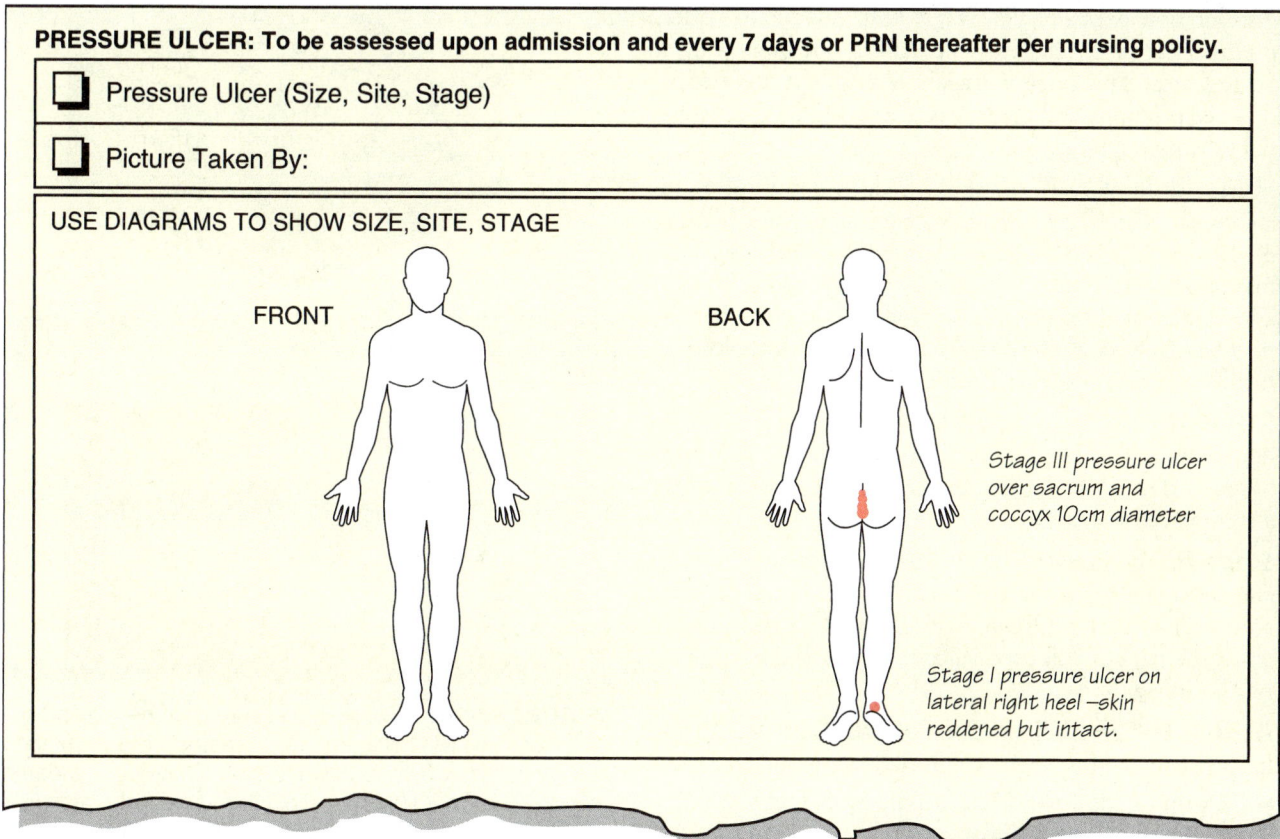

PRESSURE ULCER: To be assessed upon admission and every 7 days or PRN thereafter per nursing policy.

☐ Pressure Ulcer (Size, Site, Stage)

☐ Picture Taken By:

USE DIAGRAMS TO SHOW SIZE, SITE, STAGE

FRONT

BACK

Stage III pressure ulcer over sacrum and coccyx 10cm diameter

Stage I pressure ulcer on lateral right heel —skin reddened but intact.

FIGURE 37-11B Words, pictures, and diagrams are used to document pressure ulcers.

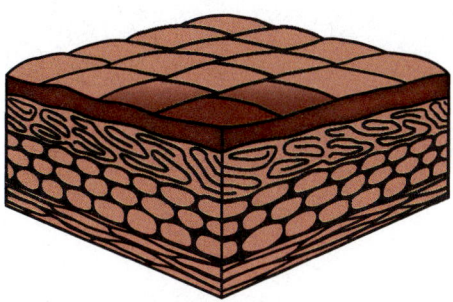

FIGURE 37-12A Cross-section of skin showing damage from Stage I pressure ulcer.

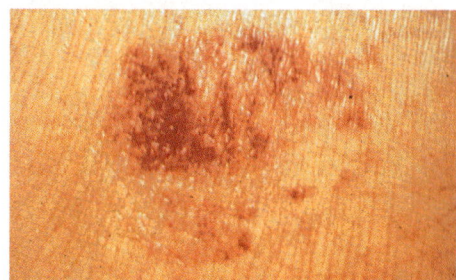

FIGURE 37-12B A Stage I pressure ulcer has nonblanchable erythema (redness) of intact skin, the lesion that precedes skin ulceration. In individuals with darker skin, discoloration of the skin, warmth, edema, induration, or hardness may also be indicators. *(Permission to reproduce this copyrighted material has been given by the owner, Hollister, Inc.)*

LEGAL *Alert*

Pressure ulcers are always easier to prevent than to treat. They can worsen rapidly and become seriously infected. Most health care facilities conduct a pressure ulcer risk assessment upon admission, so that patients who are at high risk become known immediately. Once identified, these patients should receive special attention in preventive skin care. Patients who have pressure ulcers are always at high risk of developing additional ulcers. However, patients who are normally healthy, but suddenly become sick and dehydrated, are also at great risk. These patients may be overlooked because of their age or overall good health. They may be fine one day and the next day have a pressure ulcer without warning. Pressure ulcers are a leading cause of lawsuits against health care facilities and providers. Take your responsibility for preventing pressure ulcers very seriously.

discoloration does not go away within 30 minutes after pressure has been relieved. The skin is not broken in a Stage I area. This stage is usually reversible if the area is detected promptly and pressure is relieved. It has the potential to worsen rapidly.

Stage II. In Stage II, the skin is reddened and there are abrasions, blisters, or a shallow crater at the site (Figure 37-13A and 37-13B). The area around the breakdown site may also be reddened. The skin may or may not be broken. The epidermis alone or both the epidermis and the dermis may be involved. If this stage of involvement is neglected, further and deeper damage occurs.

Stage III. In Stage III, all the layers of the skin are destroyed and a deep crater forms (Figure 37-14A and 37-14B). The nurse documents the size of the lesion using a commercial scale.

Stage IV. In Stage IV, the ulcer extends through the skin and subcutaneous tissues, and may involve bone, muscle, and other structures (Figure 37-15A and 37-15B). At this stage, the patient will experience fluid loss and is at great risk for infection.

Actions to Take When Breakdown Occurs. Nursing assistant actions when skin breakdown occurs include:

- Performing the actions listed in the guidelines to prevent further breakdown
- Following the care plan exactly

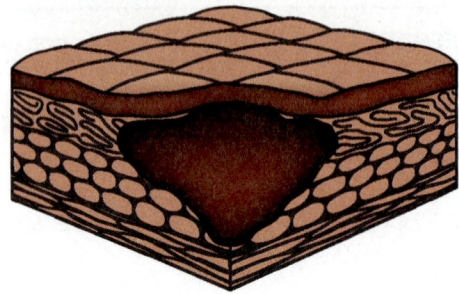

FIGURE 37-14A Cross-section of skin showing damage from Stage III pressure ulcer.

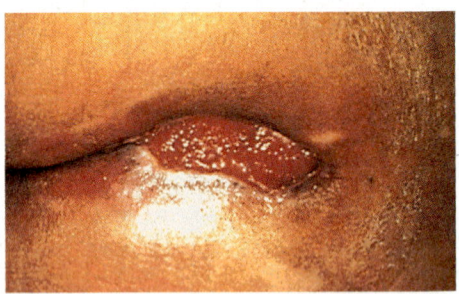

FIGURE 37-14B A Stage III pressure ulcer has full-thickness skin loss involving damage to or necrosis of subcutaneous tissue that may extend down to, but not through, underlying fascia. The ulcer presents clinically as a deep crater with or without undermining of adjacent tissue. *(Permission to reproduce this copyrighted material has been given by the owner, Hollister, Inc.)*

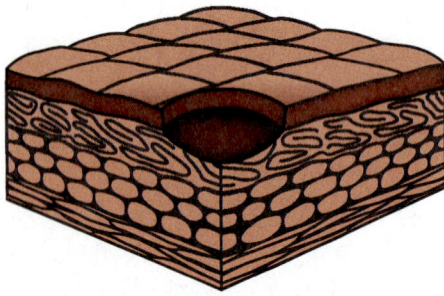

FIGURE 37-13A Cross-section of skin showing damage from Stage II pressure ulcer.

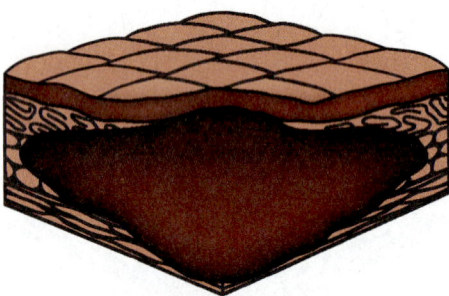

FIGURE 37-15A Cross-section of skin showing damage from Stage IV pressure ulcer.

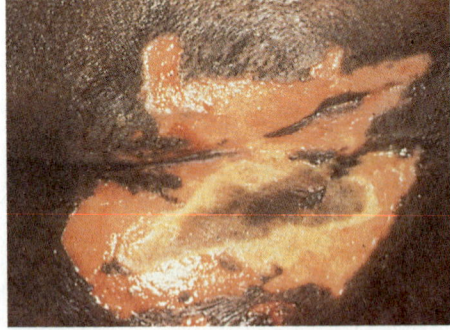

FIGURE 37-13B A Stage II pressure ulcer has partial-thickness skin loss involving epidermis, dermis, or both. The ulcer is superficial and presents clinically as an abrasion, blister, or shallow crater. *(Permission to reproduce this copyrighted material has been given by the owner, Hollister, Inc.)*

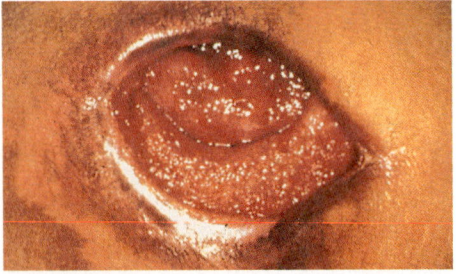

FIGURE 37-15B A Stage IV pressure ulcer has full-thickness skin loss with extensive destruction, tissue necrosis, or damage to muscle, bone, or supporting structures (e.g., tendon, joint capsule). Undermining and sinus tracts may also be associated with Stage IV pressure ulcers. *(Permission to reproduce this copyrighted material has been given by the owner, Hollister, Inc.)*

guidelines *for*

Preventing Pressure Ulcers

Nursing assistant actions are vital in identifying potential causes of breakdown and eliminating or minimizing them. The following care should be given:

- Change the patient's position at least every 2 hours. Some patients will require positioning more often. A major shift in position is required. When positioning a patient, be careful to avoid friction, such as sliding the patient over bedclothes or against equipment. Use lifting devices to avoid dragging. The care plan for each patient must be followed carefully. The turning schedule will be posted in the care plan and in the room. Figure 37-16 shows an example of the sequence of turns.

- Encourage patients sitting in geri-chairs or wheelchairs to raise themselves every 10 minutes to relieve pressure, or assist patients to do so.

- Encourage proper nutrition and adequate intake of fluids. Breakdown occurs more readily and healing is delayed when the patient is poorly nourished. Proper nutrition may require tube feedings with enriched high-protein and high-vitamin supplements. Patients who are able to eat should be encouraged to do so. Adequate fluids are a requirement.

- Immediately remove feces or urine from the skin, because they are very irritating. Wash and dry the area immediately.

- Whenever giving personal care to patients, carefully inspect areas where pressure ulcers commonly form. Report any reddened areas immediately.

- Inspect skin daily and report the condition.

- Keep the skin clean and dry at all times.

- Keep linen dry and free from wrinkles and hard objects such as crumbs and hairpins.

- Bathe patient frequently. Pay particular attention to potential pressure or friction areas. Avoid hot water and friction.

- Keep the skin supple and well-lubricated with lotion. Do not massage directly on the ulcer site and do not use alcohol. Apply moisturizers on dry skin by patting. Do not rub vigorously.

- Do not use lotion on broken skin.

- Separate body areas that are likely to rub together, especially over bony prominences, by using pillows or foam wedges according to the care plan.

- Use mechanical aids, such as foam padding, sheepskin, or an alternating-pressure mattress, to relieve pressure, friction, and shearing.

- Protect areas at risk, such as heels and elbows.

- Use a turning sheet to move dependent patients in bed.

- Elevate the head of the bed no higher than 30 degrees, to prevent a shearing effect on the tissues.

- Carry out range-of-motion exercises at least twice daily to encourage circulation.

- Check for improperly fitted or worn braces and restraints.

- Check nasogastric tubes and urinary catheters to be sure they are positioned so as not to be a source of irritation. Keep the nasal and urinary openings clean and free of drainage. These areas must be checked frequently and carefully.

- Use sheepskin and foam cushions between patients and bottom linen, wheelchair backs, or wheelchair seats where excess pressure may be expected.

- For patients sitting in geri-chairs or wheelchairs, use foam, gel, or air cushions to reduce pressure on buttocks and sacrum. Routinely monitor such patients for skin problems.

- For patients in bed, relieve pressure on heels by supporting feet off the bed. Use a pad between the legs when the patient is on her side.

- Report signs of infection, such as fever, odor, drainage, inflammation, or bleeding, to the nurse.

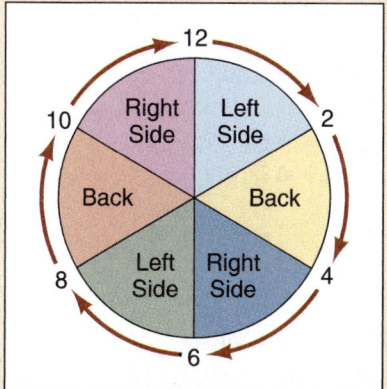

FIGURE 37-16 Sample turning schedule.

- Reporting indications of infection, such as fever, odor, drainage, bleeding, and changes in size
- Keeping the area around the breakdown clean and dry
- Assisting with whirlpool baths, if ordered, to keep the area clean

The nurse or physician may perform other procedures to care for areas of skin breakdown. For example:

- The area may be covered with a dry, sterile dressing (DSD). Holding a DSD in place without causing additional injury is not easy. The skin of some patients may be sensitive to regular tape. In this case, silk tape, paper tape, cellophane tape, or other hypoallergenic tape may be used. To prevent injury when removing the tape for a dressing change, a saline solution is applied to loosen the tape.
- Patients may be placed on low-air-loss mattresses or pressure-reducing mattresses or beds.
- In some facilities, open lesions are packed loosely with gauze soaked in a wound gel. The gel keeps the lesions moist, breaks down dead cells, and promotes healing.
- The area may be protected and kept moist by using special dressings. These dressings have a clear plastic covering that permits air to reach the tissues, but also keeps them moist to promote healing. The dressing must extend beyond the wound edge. It is held in place with a frame of either paper or silk tape. The dressing must be changed every three to five days unless there is leakage or according to facility policy.
- The wounds may be cleaned by the nurse or physician with saline solution and debrided (dead tissue removed) using instruments and proteolytic enzymes (substances that react with skin proteins).
- Antiseptic sprays, antibiotic ointments, and dressings are used to control infection.
- Surgery may be needed to close the ulcerated area in severe cases.

Patients are encouraged to participate to whatever extent is possible in their own care. Attentive nursing care is essential in preventing skin breakdown. Remember that it is far easier to prevent pressure ulcers than to heal them!

Blood Circulation to Tissues. Ensuring adequate circulation to tissues is a major factor in preventing skin breakdown. This can be accomplished by:

- Positioning the patient properly
- Using mechanical aids
- Giving backrubs
- Performing active or passive range-of-motion exercises

Positioning. Five basic in-bed positions are used to relieve pressure as the patient's condition permits. Each position must be supported for comfort. The nursing assistant must remember that not all patients are able to assume the full range of positions, because of disabilities such as arthritis, contractures, and breathing limitations. Patients who sit in geri-chairs or wheelchairs for long periods of time must also change position to relieve pressure.

Patients with special problems require extra care when they are positioned in bed. For example:

- Be sure the patient can breathe properly.
- Remember that a fractured hip is never rotated over the unaffected leg.
- If the patient had a stroke, elevate the weak arm to reduce edema.
- Always maintain proper body alignment.
- The patient with a recent stroke is turned on the unaffected side.

The five basic positions patients assume in bed are:

- Supine position
- Semisupine position
- Lateral position
- Semiprone position
- Fowler's position

Protecting the Feet. Bedfast patients are at very high risk of developing pressure ulcers on the feet and ankles. Patients with hip fractures are at great risk. The skin in the feet and lower legs is thin, and there is little fatty padding. A shallow injury or pressure ulcer can become a deep Stage IV ulceration very quickly. The heels and ankles are at greatest risk of ulceration, although occasionally ulcers develop on the toes and the sides of the foot. Foot ulcers are easy to prevent by propping the calves on pillows positioned lengthwise. This suspends the heels over the surface of the bed, relieving all pressure. Follow the patient's care plan and use the pressure prevention measures listed in the guidelines for pressure ulcer prevention. Other measures to prevent pressure ulcers on the feet and ankles are:

- Keep the skin well-lubricated with lotion (but avoid the area between the toes)
- Protect the feet from injury
- Make sure the patient is wearing properly fit footwear when out of bed. The patient should always wear socks under shoes. He or she should never ambulate barefoot or wearing only socks on the feet.
- Make sure bed linen is not too tight on the feet. Use a bed cradle to keep the bedding away from the skin.
- Make sure footwear is not too tight; if footwear fits tightly, notify the nurse.
- Monitor the skin on the feet and ankles daily and report abnormalities promptly.

Mechanical Aids

Mechanical aids are used to prevent pressure ulcers. Examples are

- Sheepskin pads (or artificial sheepskin)
- Foam pads and pillows
- Protectors for areas such as heels (Figure 37-17A) and elbows (Figure 37-13B) that are subject to friction as the patient moves in bed. Heel protectors prevent friction and shearing, but they do not relieve pressure.

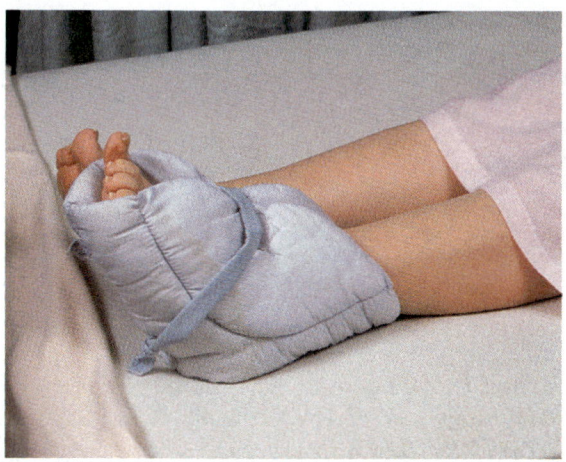

FIGURE 37-17A Heel protector. *(Courtesy of J.T. Posey Company, Arcadia, CA)*

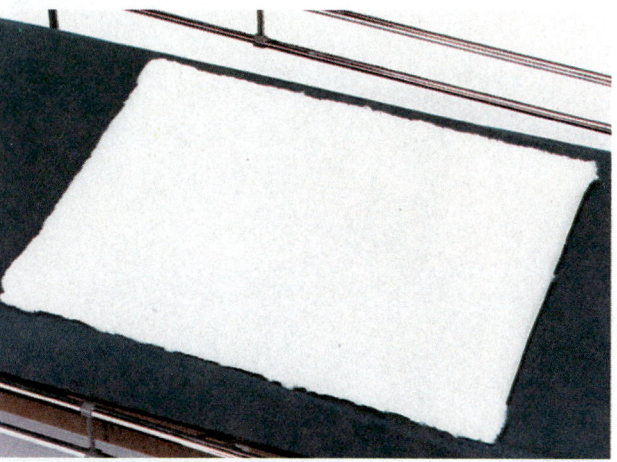

FIGURE 37-17C A synthetic sheepskin pad prevents friction. It does not relieve pressure.

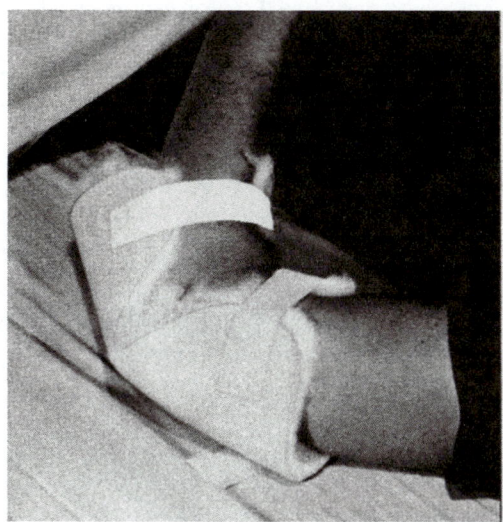

FIGURE 37-17B Elbow protector. *(Courtesy of J.T. Posey Company, Arcadia, CA)*

- Bed cradles
- Alternating-pressure mattresses
- Flotation mattresses
- Air mattresses
- Pillows
- Gel-filled mattresses
- Low-air-loss beds and other therapeutic beds or mattresses

Sheepskin Pads (or Artificial Sheepskin). These absorb moisture and reduce friction and shearing when placed under the patient (Figure 37-17C). They do not relieve pressure.

Foam Pads and Pillows. These are used to bridge areas to reduce pressure. Watch patients for signs of disorientation that might be caused by the feeling of weightlessness. Adequate fluid intake to prevent urinary stasis must be provided and conscientious range-of-motion exercises must be carried out.

Bed (Foot) Cradles. Cradles can lift the weight of bedding but must be carefully positioned and may be padded, because injury can occur if the resident strikes them.

Alternating-Pressure Mattress. This type of mattress is used in some facilities. Air pressure is reduced in a different area of the mattress on an alternating basis. The air-pressure alteration reduces pressure against the body so that no skin area is continuously subjected to pressure.

Low-Air-Loss Therapy Beds and Mattress Overlays. A low-air-loss bed (Figure 37-17D) provides pressure relief for patients who have pressure ulcers, those who are at risk of pressure ulcers, and some patients with burns. Low-air-loss therapy beds relieve pressure and keep the patient cooler and drier than other types of beds. Some beds are designed with many special features, such as an instant deflate switch in the event that CPR is necessary. Some are equipped with bed scales. A low-air-loss mattress overlay (Figure 37-17E) is also available. The overlay is used to replace the mattress on a regular hospital bed. Low-air-loss beds reduce pressure on the patient's skin, and reduce friction

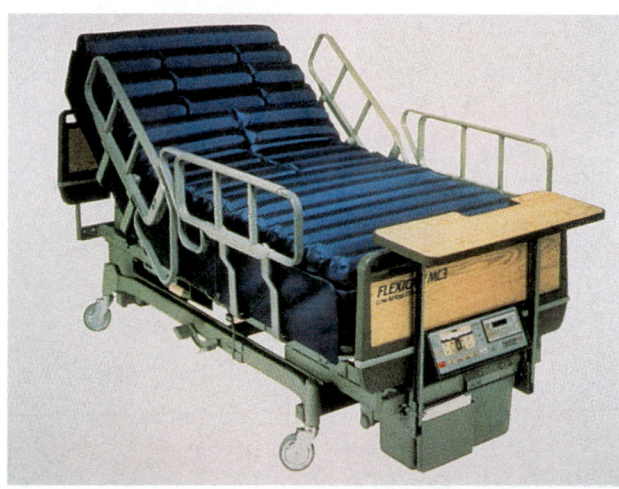

FIGURE 37-17D The low-air-loss bed. *(Courtesy of Hill-Rom, Charleston, SC)*

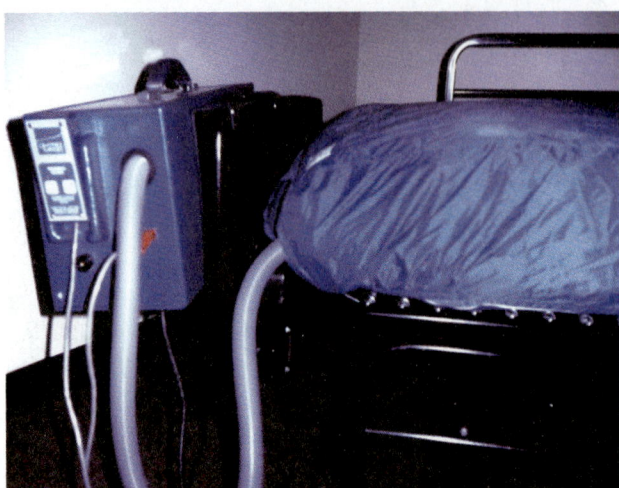

FIGURE 37-17E A low-air-loss mattress overlay can be used in place of a regular mattress.

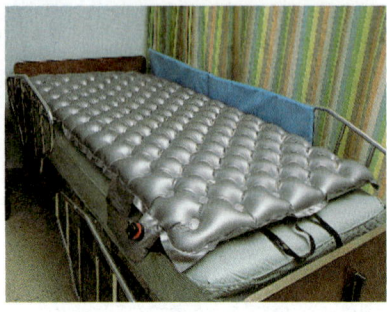

FIGURE 37-17G A water-filled mattress helps to minimize pressure on bony prominences.

and shearing, which are contributing factors to skin breakdown. These beds use a system of air-filled pillows in which inflation pressure can be adjusted so the characteristics of the support surface are matched to those of the body being supported. The pillows can be inflated and deflated to adjust the level of pressure relief. The design of the bed allows slight air escape upon movement, which reduces pressure.

Patients using a low-air-loss bed must be turned and positioned regularly to prevent skin breakdown, which can occur despite the pressure-reducing mattress. Avoid tucking the bottom sheet in tightly, as this increases pressure on the patient's skin. If used, a flat sheet should be loosely applied. Some facilities use these beds with nylon covers only, without sheets. The nylon cover (Figure 37-17F) reduces friction and shearing. Most facilities have several extra covers for each bed, to allow for washing and air-drying. (The nylon cannot withstand the heat of some commercial dryers and must be air-dried.) Special disposable underpads are used with the low-air-loss bed. Follow the care plan and facility policies.

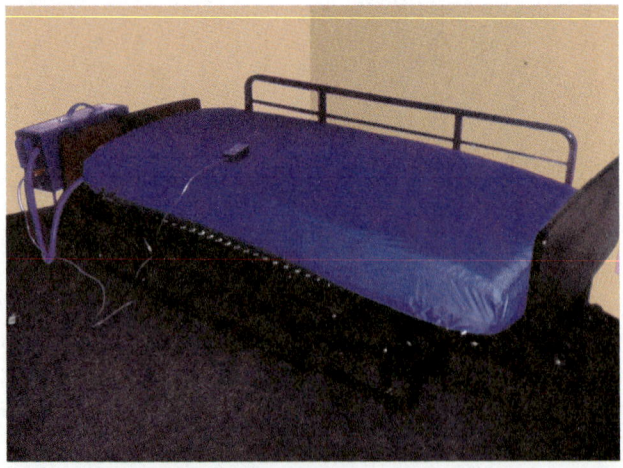

FIGURE 37-17F The nylon cover for the low-air-loss bed is used without sheets in some facilities.

Flotation Mattress. This is a water bed with controlled temperature (Figure 37-17G). The weight of the patient's body displaces water so that pressure is consistently equalized against the skin. Sheets should not be tucked tightly over a flotation mattress because this will restrict its function.

Special Equipment. Specialized beds or overlays are available for patients who need continuous pressure relief. One type is the Clinitron® bed. It is filled with a sandlike material. Warm, dry air circulates through the material to maintain an even temperature and support the body evenly.

Gel-Filled Mattress. The gel in this type of mattress has a consistency similar to body fat. It allows a more equal distribution of body weight because it conforms to the body contours.

Pillows. Pillows are used in a technique called *bridging*. In bridging, body parts are supported by pillows so that spaces are left to relieve pressure on specific areas.

Burns

Whenever large sections of skin are destroyed, the body loses fluids and chemicals called electrolytes, and is vulnerable to infection. Burns are a common cause of loss of large amounts of skin.

Classification. The temperature and length of exposure determine the severity of a burn. Prognosis is based on the extent of the burns. Burns are commonly classified as first-, second-, and third-degree. Burns may also be classified according to the depth of tissue involvement:

First-degree burns (partial thickness)
– Epidermis. When only the epidermis is involved, the skin is pink to red. There may be some temporary swelling and pain. There is usually no permanent damage or scarring.

Second-degree burns (partial thickness)
– Dermis. When both epidermis and dermis are involved in the burn, the color may vary from pink or red to white or tan. There is blistering and pain and some scarring.

Third-degree burns (full thickness)
– When the epidermis, dermis, and subcutaneous tissue are involved, the tissue is bright red to tan and brown. The area is covered with a tough, leathery coat (eschar). There is no pain initially because

nerve endings have been destroyed. Later, pain and scarring will result from this injury.

When the epidermis, dermis, subcutaneous tissues, muscles, and bones are involved, the tissue appears blackened. Scarring will be extensive.

Management of Burns. Once a burn patient is in the medical facility, the care will involve:

- Assessment of the burn damage
- Analgesia for pain
- Management of fluids and electrolytes
- Prevention of infection
- Clean technique using cap, gown, mask, and gloves
- Complete reverse isolation technique in some cases
- Monitoring the patient for respiratory distress, shock, and anemia
- Cleaning of the burned areas and removal of all debris
- Application of topical antibiotics
- Emotional support

Some hospitals have established burn centers where specially trained personnel care for burn cases. One of two approaches is in common use:

- Open method—the burns are left uncovered. Sterile technique is used to care for the patient.
- Closed method—the burns are covered by special ointments, wrapped in layers of gauze. The part is checked for circulation distal to the dressing and maintained in proper alignment.

New techniques, such as keeping the patient submerged in a silicone solution, are also being used. Each method has its advantages and disadvantages. There are four goals of treatment, whatever method is selected:

1. Replacement of lost fluids and electrolytes to combat shock.
2. Relief of pain and anxiety.
3. Prevention of contractures, deformities, and infections. A *contracture* is a shortening of a muscle, which limits motion and causes deformities. Plastic surgery may also be required.
4. Provision of emotional support and motivation.

Nursing Assistant Care. Special care emphasizes:

- Reporting pain so that appropriate analgesics may be prescribed and given.
- Maintaining proper alignment.
- Gentle positioning, as ordered, to prevent contractures.

Note: The burn patient may be on a CircOlectric® bed, Stryker frame, or Clinitron® bed to permit frequent rotation to relieve pressure.

- Encouraging a high-protein diet.
- Carefully measuring intake and output.
- Giving emotional support and encouragement.
- Carrying out procedures that prevent infection.
- Applying the principles of standard precautions and wearing gloves if contact with burned skin areas is likely.

REVIEW

A. True/False.

Mark the following true or false by circling T or F.

1. T F Obesity is a predisposing cause of pressure ulcer formation.
2. T F The sacrum is a common site for the development of pressure ulcers.
3. T F To avoid pressure ulcers, change the patient's position at least every 2 hours.
4. T F If an area is reddened, massage directly over the area.
5. T F The nails and hair are part of the integumentary system.
6. T F When only the epidermis is damaged by burning, the patient experiences no pain.
7. T F The skin stores carbohydrates and minerals.
8. T F When both the dermis and epidermis are damaged by burns, blisters are apt to form.
9. T F Prevention of infection is an important consideration when caring for a patient with burns.
10. T F The patient with burns needs great emotional support.
11. T F Friction and shearing do not contribute to pressure ulcer development.
12. T F A sheepskin is an excellent pressure-relieving device.
13. T F A Stage I pressure ulcer will fade when pressure is relieved for more than 30 minutes.
14. T F Cover the low-air-loss bed tightly with a sheet to reduce pressure.
15. T F Nodules are small tissue protrusions.
16. T F When assisting with a colloidal oatmeal bath, instruct the patient to keep the solution out of the eyes.

B. Matching.

Choose the correct item from Column II to match each question in Column I.

Column I	Column II
17. _____ redness	a. pressure ulcer
18. _____ skin	b. rubra
19. _____ thick leathery covering that forms in severe burns	c. tactile sense
	d. necrosis
20. _____ bedsore	e. integument
21. _____ feeling	f. obese
22. _____ flat, discolored spots, as in measles	g. eschar
	h. crusts
23. _____ raised spots filled with watery fluid	i. excoriations
	j. vesicles
24. _____ large, raised areas associated with itching, as in hives	k. papules
	l. macules
25. _____ areas of dried body secretions such as scabs	m. wheals
26. _____ areas where skin seems to be scraped or scratched away	

C. Multiple Choice.

Select the one best answer for each of the following.

27. Flat, discolored spots such as those seen in measles are called
    a. pustules.
    b. macules.
    c. papules.
    d. vesicles.

28. Raised spots filled with fluid, such as blisters, are called
    a. pustules.
    b. macules.
    c. papules.
    d. vesicles.

29. Anaphylactic shock is
    a. a severe sensitivity reaction.
    b. never fatal.
    c. a communicable disease.
    d. associated with partial-thickness burns.

30. When caring for patients with skin lesions,
    a. rub the skin vigorously.
    b. use soap and water when bathing.
    c. do not attempt to remove any crusts.
    d. use rubbing lotion.

31. To help ensure adequate circulation to prevent skin breakdown, you could
    a. change the patient's position frequently.
    b. position the patient on bony prominences.
    c. rub red areas well.
    d. apply rubbing alcohol to the skin after bathing.

32. Scabies and body lice are commonly spread by
    a. air and droplets.
    b. direct and indirect contact.
    c. fomites and common vehicles.
    d. viruses and bacteria.

33. When assisting a patient with a colloidal oatmeal bath, the nursing assistant should
    a. use tepid water.
    b. give a bedbath.
    c. use very hot water.
    d. scrub the skin well.

34. Safety precautions to follow when assisting a patient with an oatmeal bath include
    a. using sterile water to prevent infection.
    b. scrubbing the lesions well with a sponge.
    c. stirring the water well so the oatmeal will dissolve.
    d. advising the patient to use the hand rail to prevent slipping.

35. In a dark-skinned patient, a Stage I pressure ulcer may appear
    a. red or pink.
    b. gray or green.
    c. blue or black.
    d. shiny and oily.

36. Patients using low-air-loss beds
    a. do not require repositioning, as the bed relieves pressure.
    b. should be turned and positioned at least every 2 hours.
    c. should be turned and positioned twice each shift.
    d. should be turned and positioned every 30 to 45 minutes.

D. Completion.

Complete the statements by filling in the correct word(s).

37. Three nursing assistant actions related to the care of patients with skin lesions are:
    a. _____   c. _____
    b. _____

38. Three diagnostic tests used to identify skin-related lesions are:
    a. _____   c. _____
    b. _____

39. Five types of patients at risk for the development of pressure ulcers are:

   a. _____   **d.** _____

   b. _____   **e.** _____

   c. _____

40. Name five common sites of pressure ulcer formation.

   a. _____   **d.** _____

   b. _____   **e.** _____

   c. _____

41. It is especially important to encourage proper nutrition and fluids in patients who have ulcers because _____.

E. Nursing Assistant Challenge.

Agnes Finlay has been transferred to your facility from a long-term care facility. She uses a wheelchair but fell and fractured her arm. You notice a reddened area around the base of her spine. Answer the following by selecting the correct word.

42. People sitting in wheelchairs should raise themselves every _____ minutes.

(20) (10)

43. The head of the patient's bed should not be elevated more than _____ degrees.

(30) (40)

44. While she is in bed, Ms. Finlay's position should be changed at least every _____ hours.

(three) (two)

45. Range-of-motion exercises should be carried out at least _____ a day.

(once) (twice)

EXPLORING THE WEB

Description	Location
Decubitus ulcer information	*http://www.ldhpmed.com*
Pressure sore dangers	*http://www.mdausa.org*
Wounds	*http://www.woundsresearch.com*
ConvaTec Connection	*http://www.convatec.com/en_US*
DermIS	*http://129.206.95.15*
Dermis.net	*http://dermis.multimedica.de*
Hill-Rom Wound and Skin Care Solutions	*http://www.hill-rom.com*
National Decubitus Foundation	*http://www.decubitus.org*
Tempur·Med	*http://www.tempurmed.com*
3M Healthcare Skin Health	*http://www.3m.com/us*
World Wide Wounds	*http://www.worldwidewounds.com*
Wound Care Information Network	*http://www.medicaledu.com*
The Wound Care Institute	*http://www.woundcare.org*
Wound Care Strategies	*http://www.woundcarestrategies.com*
Wound Consultants, Inc.	*http://www.woundconsultant.com*
Wound, Ostomy, & Continence Nurses Society	*http://www.wocn.org*
WoundHeal.com	*http://www.woundheal.com*
Wounds1.com	*http://www.wounds1.com*

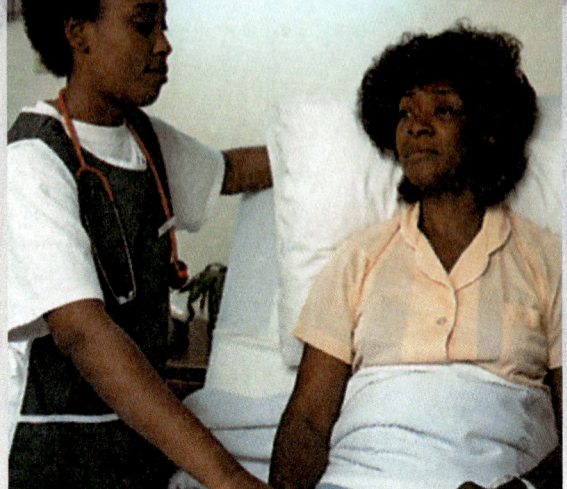

Respiratory System

objectives

After completing this unit, you will be able to:
- Spell and define terms.
- Review the location and function of the respiratory organs.
- Describe some common diseases of the respiratory system.
- List five diagnostic tests used to identify respiratory conditions.
- Describe nursing assistant actions related to the care of patients with respiratory conditions.
- Identify patients who are at high risk of poor oxygenation.
- Describe the care of patients with a tracheostomy, laryngectomy, and chest tubes.
- List five safety measures for the use of oxygen therapy.
- Demonstrate the following procedures:
  - Procedure 97 Attaching the Humidifier to the Oxygen Flow Meter or Regulator
  - Procedure 98 Collecting a Sputum Specimen

vocabulary

Learn the meaning and the correct spelling of the following words and phrases:

alveoli	continuous positive	nebulizer	sputum
asthma	airway pressure	orthopneic position	stoma
biopsy	(CPAP)	oxygen	trachea
bronchi	dyspnea	oxygenation	tracheostomy
bronchioles	emphysema	oxygen concentrator	tripod position
bronchitis	expectorate	oxygen mask	upper respiratory
cannula	high Fowler's	pharynx	infection (URI)
carbon dioxide	position	pleura	ventilation
chest tubes	humidifier	pleural effusion	vocal cords
chronic obstructive	incentive spirometer	pneumonia	
pulmonary disease	larynx	respiratory care	
(COPD)	nasal cannula	practitioner (RCP)	

INTRODUCTION

Life cannot be maintained without oxygen, and carbon dioxide must be eliminated from the body. Diseases of the respiratory tract that interfere with this vital exchange of oxygen and carbon dioxide bring acute distress. Nursing care is directed toward making breathing easier and preventing transmission of infection.

STRUCTURE AND FUNCTION

The respiratory system (Figure 38-1) is sometimes called the lifeline of the body. It extends from the nose to the tiny air sacs (**alveoli**) that make up the bulk of the lungs.

The organs of the respiratory system include the:

- Nose
- Pharynx (throat)
- Larynx (voice box)
- Trachea (windpipe)
- Bronchi
- Lungs

The sinuses, diaphragm, and intercostal muscles between the ribs are called auxiliary structures.

Air is warmed, moistened, and filtered as it passes through the nasal cavities, which are separated by the nasal septum. The air passes through the **pharynx**, a passageway for both air and food, into the larynx and trachea. It then passes into the **bronchi** to join the upper respiratory tract to the lungs. Within the lungs, the bronchi branch into smaller and smaller divisions called **bronchioles**. The *alveoli* are tiny air sacs that extend from the bronchioles. It is at the level of the alveoli that the exchange of gases takes place (Figure 38-2).

The alveoli, bronchioles, and the important pulmonary blood vessels form the lungs. The way in which oxygen and

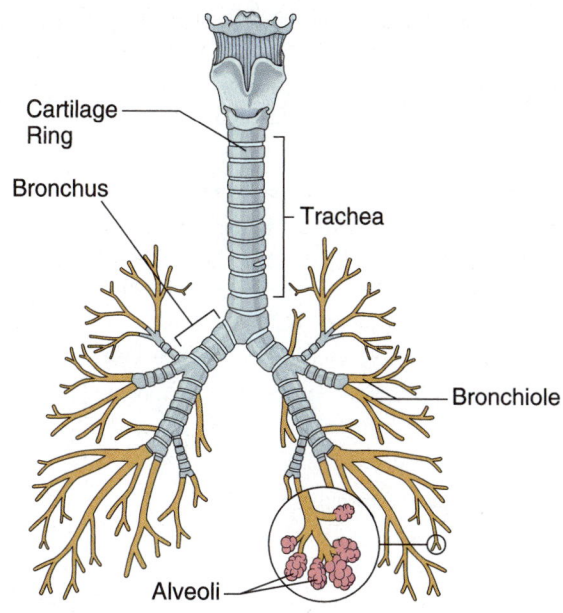

FIGURE 38-2 The lower respiratory tract.

carbon dioxide are exchanged between the alveoli and the capillaries is shown in Figure 38-3.

The purpose of this system is to bring **oxygen** (O_2) into the body to meet cellular needs and to expel carbon dioxide (CO_2). **Carbon dioxide** is a gaseous, metabolic waste produced by the cells.

Each cell in the body must have a constant supply of oxygen. The oxygen is used to produce the energy for cellular activity.

Nutrients + oxygen yields energy + water + CO_2

There is a close connection between the respiratory and circulatory systems. Oxygen is delivered throughout the body by means of the bloodstream. Every cell in the body produces carbon dioxide. It is transported in venous blood. When it reaches the lungs, it is exhaled into the atmosphere. When the body does not eliminate carbon dioxide, it creates chemical reactions causing an acid buildup. Death

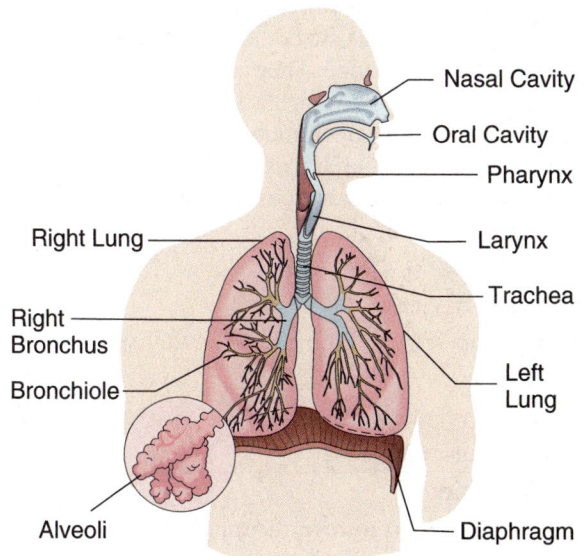

FIGURE 38-1 The respiratory system.

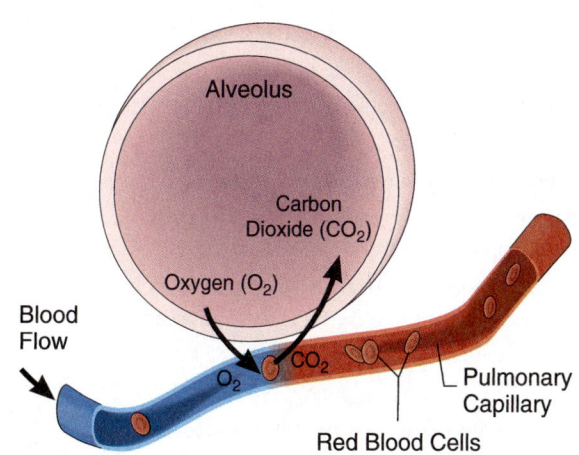

FIGURE 38-3 Oxygen and carbon dioxide are exchanged in the alveoli.

will result if levels of acid and carbon dioxide become too high. Signs and symptoms that indicate problems with oxygen use are listed in Table 38-1. Observations to report promptly to the nurse are listed in Table 38-2.

TABLE 38-1 SIGNS AND SYMPTOMS OF DECREASED OXYGENATION

- Respiratory rate below 12 or above 20
- Unusual skin color, such as dusky, pale, blue, or gray
- Unusual color of the lips, mucous membranes, nail beds, lining or roof of mouth
- Cool, clammy skin
- Slow, rapid, or irregular breathing
- Shortness of breath or labored breathing
- Noisy breathing
- Gasping for breath
- Changes in mental status, including decreased responsiveness, drowsiness, sleepiness for no apparent reason, restlessness, increased confusion.
- Tachycardia
- Cheyne-Stokes respirations
- Wheezing
- Coughing (dry or moist/productive)
- Retractions

TABLE 38-2 SIGNS AND SYMPTOMS OF INADEQUATE BREATHING TO REPORT TO THE NURSE IMMEDIATELY

- Movement in the chest is absent, minimal, or irregular.
- Breathing movement appears to be in the abdomen, not the lungs.
- Air movement cannot be detected by listening and feeling for breath sounds on your cheek and ear.
- Respiratory rate is too slow or rapid.
- Respirations are irregular, gasping, very deep, or shallow.
- Respirations appear labored.
- Patient is short of breath.
- Patient's skin, lips, tongue, ear lobes, mucous membranes, or nailbeds are blue or gray.
- Patient is unable to speak at all, or cannot speak in sentences because he or she is short of breath.
- Respirations are noisy.
- Nasal flaring is present during inspiration.
- The muscles below the ribs and/or above the clavicles retract inward during respiration.

The Act of Respiration

Two lungs are located in the thorax. Each lung is surrounded by a double-walled membrane called the **pleura**. Between the layers of the pleura is a small amount of fluid that reduces friction as the lungs alternately expand and contract, filling with and then expelling air.

The size of the thorax depends on the contraction of the diaphragm and intercostal muscles. As the muscles contract, the thorax enlarges, expanding the lungs. Air carrying oxygen enters the lungs. When the muscles relax, the thorax becomes smaller. Air carrying carbon dioxide leaves the lungs and is breathed out.

- *Inspiration* (or inhalation) is the act of drawing air into the lungs.
- *Expiration* (or exhalation) is the act of expelling air.
- **Ventilation** is the combination of these two actions.
- **Oxygenation** is the movement of oxygen from the lungs and into the blood to be carried to the cells.

Voice Production

The **larynx**, or voice box, is part of the respiratory tract. It is important in voice production. Two membranes called the **vocal cords** stretch across the inside of the larynx. As air moves upward through the larynx, it passes through an opening in the vocal cords. Changes in the shape of the vocal cords and the size of the opening permit controlled amounts of air to reach the mouth, nasal cavities, and sinuses, where specific speech sounds are made when formed by the teeth, lips, and tongue.

PATIENTS AT RISK OF POOR OXYGENATION

Hypoxemia is a condition in which there is insufficient oxygen in the blood. Many of the patients who are at high risk for developing hypoxemia are not in the intensive care unit where monitoring is routine. They are on medical and surgical units, in the long-term care facility, or in other patient care areas. Patients who are immobile and those on bedrest have an increased risk of hypoxemia. When hypoxemia develops, immobility makes a positive outcome less likely. Other high-risk conditions are:

- cardiac disease
- pulmonary disease
- being postoperative (for up to a week after surgery)
- sleep apnea
- decreased level of consciousness
- neuromuscular diseases
- morbid obesity
- kyphoscoliosis (curvature of the spine)
- trauma

Checking capillary refill (Unit 35) is a quick means of evaluating how well oxygen is getting to body tissues. You may also use the pulse oximeter (Unit 35) for monitoring patients with high-risk conditions.

Respiratory Care

Patients with respiratory disorders have many needs that require highly skilled care. The respiratory care practitioner (RCP) is a licensed professional who specializes in the care of patients with disorders of the cardiopulmonary system, respirations, and sleep disorders that affect the patient's breathing. The RCP will be highly involved in the care of the patient and the specialized equipment used for treatment.

UPPER RESPIRATORY INFECTIONS

An upper respiratory infection (URI) follows invasion of the upper respiratory organs by microbes. The upper respiratory organs include the nose, sinuses, and throat. A common cold, which is caused by a virus, is an example of an upper respiratory infection. It is one of the most ordinary illnesses found in people. Symptoms include:

- Elevated temperature (fever)
- Runny nose
- Watery eyes

This usually self-limiting disease is best treated by:

- Use of a drug to reduce fever, such as acetaminophen
- Rest
- Increased fluid intake

Patients with respiratory infections should be taught to:

- cover the nose and mouth with a tissue when coughing or sneezing.
- dispose of soiled tissues by placing them in a plastic or paper bag to be burned.

OSHA *Alert*

We all know that respiratory infections are spread by the airborne and droplet methods of transmission. Handwashing is an often overlooked means of preventing the spread of respiratory infection. Secretions containing pathogens make their way to the environment. You pick up these pathogens on your hands. Good handwashing is the best method for preventing infection, including respiratory infection.

- turn the face away from others when coughing or sneezing.
- wash their hands after handling soiled tissues.

You must take special note of and report the following:

- Dyspnea (difficult breathing)
- Changes in rate and rhythm of respiration
- Presence and character, color, and amount of respiratory secretions
- Cough
- Changes in skin color, such as pallor or cyanosis

URIs sometimes move down into the chest and develop into bronchitis or even pneumonia.

Pneumonia

Pneumonia is a serious inflammation of the lungs. It can be caused by a variety of infectious organisms. Three common causes of pneumonia are:

- Viruses
- Bacteria
- Protozoa

Pneumocystis carinii is most often seen in patients who have poorly functioning immune systems. Today, most pneumonias, though serious and potentially life-threatening, respond favorably to antibiotic therapy.

CHRONIC OBSTRUCTIVE PULMONARY DISEASE

Chronic obstructive pulmonary disease (COPD) is also called chronic obstructive lung disease (COLD). This term refers to conditions that result in chronic blockage or obstruction of the respiratory system that is not reversible. Several conditions constitute COPD, including:

- Emphysema
- Chronic bronchitis
- Bronchiectasis

It can be very difficult to differentiate asthma from COPD, particularly in older patients.

Asthma

Asthma is a breathing disorder resulting from:

- Constriction of the muscles of the bronchioles
- Swelling of the respiratory membranes
- Production of large amounts of mucus that fill the narrowed passageways

A person having an asthma attack has labored breathing and frequent coughing. An attack may result when the person contacts an allergen. Respiratory infections can also cause an asthma attack. Common allergens are:

- Pollen

- Medications
- Dust
- Feathers
- Foods such as peanuts, eggs, or chocolate

If a patient has known allergies (hypersensitivity to specific items), they should be marked in the patient's health record. Long-term treatment consists of determining the allergen and eliminating it. To relieve the attack, the patient is given medication to decrease the swelling and dilate the bronchioles. Low levels of oxygen may also be given.

Chronic Bronchitis

Chronic bronchitis is prolonged inflammation in the bronchi due to infection or irritants. Signs and symptoms include:

- Swollen and red bronchial tissues, resulting in narrowed bronchial passageways
- Persistent cough
- Sputum production
- Respiratory distress

Treatment includes:

- Antibiotics to fight the infection
- Drugs to loosen secretions deep in the respiratory tract
- Techniques to improve ventilation and drainage
- Adequate fluid intake to keep secretions thin so they can be coughed up

Emphysema

Emphysema develops after chronic obstruction of the air flow to the alveoli. The air sacs:

- Become distended
- Lose their elasticity and recoil ability
- Finally become nonfunctional
- Lose the ability to exchange gases

The patient can bring air into the lungs, but it becomes more difficult to expel air from the lungs (Figure 38-4). As a result, there is less and less room for air to reenter.

Risk factors for emphysema are:

- Genetic
- Airways that are very responsive to irritants
- Exposure to tobacco smoke
- Exposure to dust and chemicals in the workplace
- Exposure to indoor and outdoor air pollution
- Repeated lung infections

Emphysema alone (without chronic bronchitis, which often accompanies it) is a dry disease. There is no sputum production. However, patients with emphysema are at high risk of developing pneumonia. This condition also causes the heart to work harder. The most common sign of respiratory problems in a patient with emphysema is headache.

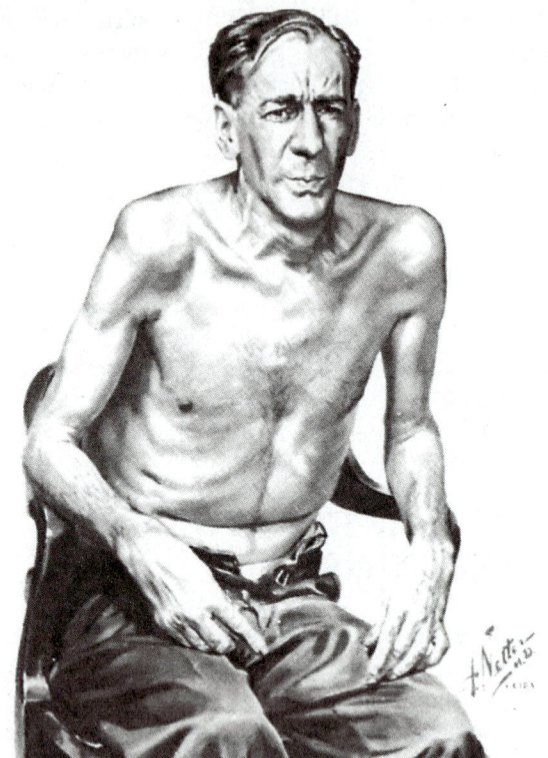

FIGURE 38-4 Typical posture for a patient with emphysema. The patient leans forward on the arms and purses his lips. *(Copyright © 1968, CIBA-GEIGY Corporation. Reproduced with permission, from the Clinical Symposia, illustrated by Frank H. Netter, M.D. All rights reserved.)*

This is caused by increasing carbon dioxide levels in the blood. Other signs and symptoms of emphysema are:

- fatigue
- chronic oxygen deprivation
- difficulty breathing
- loss of appetite and weight loss

General Care. The care of the emphysema patient includes all the care required of any patient with COPD:

- Assisting with the proper breathing techniques, such as pursed-lip breathing
- Encouraging breathing exercises
- Positioning to improve ventilation
- Assisting with postural drainage (this therapy is not commonly used for emphysema)
- Providing care during low-flow oxygen therapy
- Assisting with and encouraging good nutrition
- Treating infections with antibiotics and drugs to loosen and thin respiratory secretions
- Encouraging fluid intake
- Taking annual flu shots and the pneumonia vaccine at the frequency specified by the health care provider
- Encouraging patients to avoid crowds, especially during the flu season
- Encouraging patients not to smoke

Tips: When caring for patients with COPD, pace activities. Help them to conserve energy as much as possible. Minimize activities in which the patient must raise the arms over the head. Avoid exposing patients to aerosol sprays.

Wear gloves if your hands may contact the patient's respiratory secretions. Wear a gown, goggles or face shield, and a surgical mask if the patient is coughing and spraying respiratory secretions into the air.

SURGICAL CONDITIONS

Most respiratory problems are not treated with surgery. However, several problems require surgical correction to ensure uninterrupted air flow.

Tracheostomy

A tracheostomy (Figure 38-5) is done for some patients who have had head and neck surgery, and some victims of serious trauma. It may also be done for patients who:

- have required a ventilator to support their breathing for a long time
- need suctioning to clear airway secretions

A tracheostomy may be temporary or permanent. The external opening on the skin surface is the stoma. Eventually, the stoma will heal and remain permanently open. A tube is inserted through the stoma to maintain patency until the stoma has healed open. This tube is the cannula. An outer and inner cannula are used. Several types of outer cannulae are available. The most common has an inflatable cuff (Figure 38-6). It seals or reduces the air flow to the nose and throat, so virtually all breathing is done through the tracheostomy. The cuff also helps reduce the risk of aspiration of feedings. Care of the cuff is not a nursing assistant responsibility. The nurse or RCP will inflate and deflate the cuff periodically. The cuff must be inflated before feeding the patient or providing mouth care. A cuffless tube may also be used, but this is less common. Patients with a cuffless tube are able to breathe through the

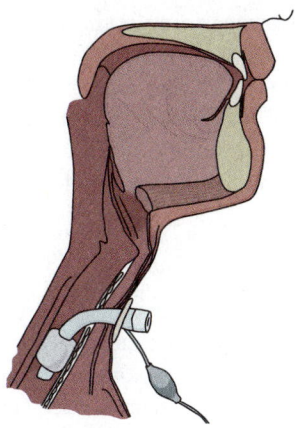

FIGURE 38-6 A tracheostomy with the cuff inflated.

nose, mouth, and trachestomy. The outer cannula has a flat plate, with a flange on each side that is fastened to twill tape or Velcro fastener that encircles the patient's neck. The tape helps hold the device securely in place. The inner cannula has an adapter on the distal end that can be attached to the manual resuscitation bag. The parts of the tracheostomy apparatus are shown in Figure 38-7.

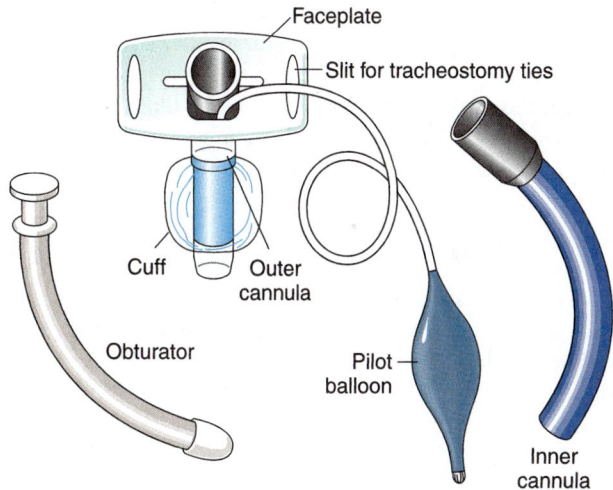

FIGURE 38-7 Parts for the tracheostomy.

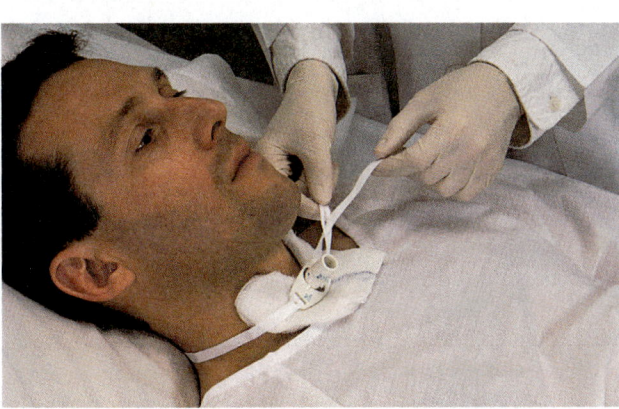

FIGURE 38-5 The tracheostomy stoma is a surgical opening in the trachea. The cannula keeps the stoma open.

INFECTION CONTROL Alert

The nasal hairs and tonsils filter pathogens and other substances from the air, preventing them from reaching the lungs. A patient with a tracheostomy does not have this advantage. The stoma provides a direct, unfiltered passageway to the lungs for irritating foreign substances and pathogens. Practice good infection control techniques when caring for patients with a stoma.

Caring for the tracheostomy is the nurse's responsibility. Notify the nurse immediately if the ties are loose or any part of the device comes apart or is removed. The ties can also be too tight. You should be able to slide your finger underneath the tie on either side of the neck. If you cannot, it is too tight, and you should notify the nurse immediately.

Malignancies

Malignant tumors can develop in any part of the respiratory tract. Although the exact causes of malignancy are not fully understood, cigarette smoking and exposure to cancer-producing agents in the environment are known to be contributing factors. Lung cancers are treated by surgery, radiation, or chemotherapy, or a combination of all three therapies.

Cancer of the Larynx

Cancer of the larynx may require removal of the larynx, resulting in loss of the voice. The patient breathes through an artificial opening in the neck and trachea. When the larynx is removed, there is no longer a connection between the upper and lower airways (Figure 38-8).

A patient with a laryngectomy (removal of larynx) breathes through a permanent opening in the neck and trachea, called a **stoma**. A laryngectomy stoma is a special kind of opening in the neck. Though it may look like a regular tracheostomy, it is very different. If you are caring for a patient with a stoma, you must know whether it is a tracheostomy stoma or a laryngectomy stoma. If the patient has a tracheostomy, the passageway from the mouth and nose through the trachea remains intact. Patients can still smell odors, blow their noses, and suck on a straw. If a patient has had a laryngectomy, the larynx (voice box) has been removed. The upper airway is no longer connected to the trachea. The patient will not be able to talk, smell, blow his nose, whistle, gargle, or suck on a straw.

Loss of voice is a major trauma for anyone. Just think for a moment of how frustrated you would feel if you could no longer use your voice to communicate your thoughts, feelings, wants, and needs to others.

Postsurgical care is given in the acute care hospital. At this time, writing is the major form of communication available to such patients. Later, the patient may be taught new ways to speak through esophageal speech or electronic speech.

Esophageal Speech. The patient learns to swallow air and then bring it back up through the esophagus into the mouth. Here the air is formed by the teeth and tongue into words, as it would be if it were being exhaled from the lungs. Esophageal speech is difficult to learn, but motivated patients can succeed.

Electronic Speech. Patients who cannot use esophageal speech may be able to use an electronic artificial larynx to create speech. Some patients may use a combination of both techniques.

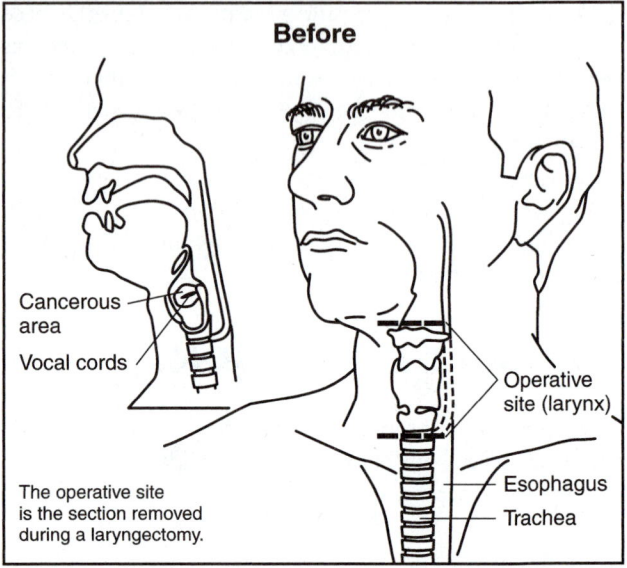

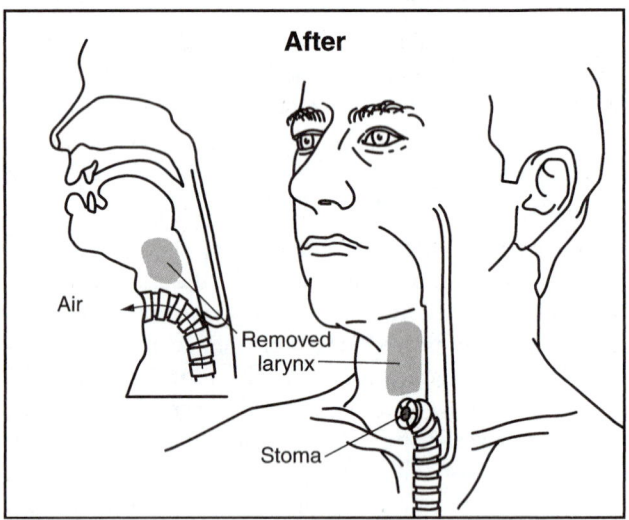

FIGURE 38-8 The anatomy of the face and neck before and after laryngectomy surgery.

Patients with laryngectomies need patience and understanding from all health care providers. Communication is possible, but the voice does not sound normal. More time is needed by the patient to formulate the sounds. A difficult psychological adjustment must be made by the patient. The loss of one's voice requires an adjustment similar to that experienced when grieving for the loss of a loved one. Expect periods of depression, anger, and hostility.

Caring for a Patient with a Tracheostomy or Laryngectomy Stoma. When people breathe normally, the structures in the nose and mouth capture microbes and other foreign particles, preventing them from entering the airway. In addition, the body moistens and warms air before it enters the lungs. Inhaling cold, dry air is very uncomfortable, and it irritates the lungs. Because the tracheostomy bypasses the normal breathing structures, the patient's body cannot use its normal protective mechanisms to warm, moisten, and filter the air. Thus, care is designed to replace these body functions. Warm, humidified oxygen may be administered to patients with a tracheostomy.

The stoma now provides a direct passageway into the lungs. Because of this, some patients wear a mask similar to a surgical mask over the opening. The risk of inhaling a foreign particle is greatly increased. Inhaling small objects or water (such as during a shower) can cause serious complications. Check with the nurse or care plan for precautions to take when showering the patient. Avoid getting powder, lint, dust, water, or other objects near or in the stoma.

Likewise, the opening in the neck provides an open pathway for bacteria to enter, causing infection. Use standard precautions and frequent handwashing when caring for a patient with a tracheostomy. Secretions may be expelled from the tracheostomy when the patient coughs. The patient has no control over this. If he or she is expelling secretions, you will also need to wear a gown, mask, and eye protection when caring for the patient.

The stoma in the patient's neck is the primary airway. If the tube becomes blocked, dislodged, disconnected, or otherwise disrupted, the patient's airway will be seriously compromised. Be especially careful when turning and bathing the patient. Monitor the patient's skin color closely. Watch for cyanosis, changes in color of the nailbeds or mucous membranes, or respiratory distress.

Chest Tubes

Chest tubes (Figure 38-9) are sterile, plastic tubes that are inserted through the skin of the chest, between the ribs and into the space between the pleural membrane that covers the lung and the pleural membrane that lines the chest wall. They are used after surgery to drain any bloody fluid drainage from the chest. These tubes also allow air to escape if there is a leak of air at the suture line after lung surgery.

In subacute care, patients are most likely to have chest tubes for two reasons: one is an air leak after lung surgery that is slow to heal, and the other is to drain fluid that collects around the lungs (often seen in patients who have cancer). This fluid is called a pleural effusion.

The chest tube is always attached to a drain of some sort (Figure 38-10). The nurse will manage the system. To help

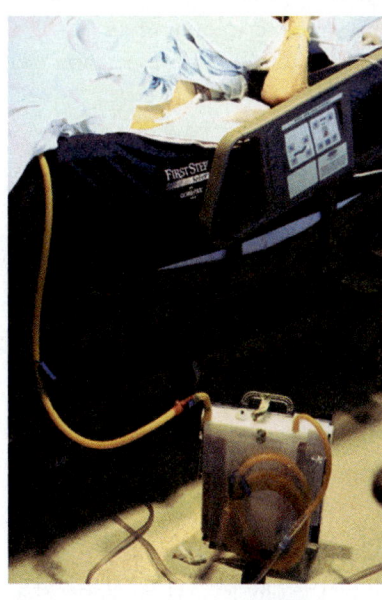

FIGURE 38-10
Make sure the tubing is not obstructed and that the bottle is lower than the patient's heart.

monitor and care for the patient, make sure that nothing pulls on the tube that comes out of the chest. Position the drainage system in an upright position, below the level of the heart at all times. Reposition the patient every 2 hours, or as instructed. Make sure the chest tube is never twisted, kinked, or obstructed. The tubing that connects the chest tube to the drain should be coiled on the bed the same way you would position tubing for a Foley catheter.

If the drain is connected to a vacuum regulator, check with the nurse before you disconnect it to take the patient to the bathroom, for example. Do not hesitate to get the patient up in a chair and to keep him mobile if his condition allows, even though he has a chest tube. The patient with a chest tube should always have oxygen and suction set up at the bedside. A tray of emergency equipment will also be kept in the room. Never remove these items.

Notify the nurse promptly if the:

- vital signs change
- pulse oximeter alarm sounds
- dressing on the chest wall is loose
- color or amount of drainage from the chest tube changes
- patient coughs up blood
- patient becomes short of breath or cyanotic
- patient develops new swelling on the torso, neck, or face that "crackles" when you touch it
- the tube comes out of the chest wall

DIAGNOSTIC TECHNIQUES

Some techniques used to diagnose problems of the respiratory system include:

- Tissue biopsy (microscopic examination of a specimen of tissue removed from the patient)
- Cultures of secretions

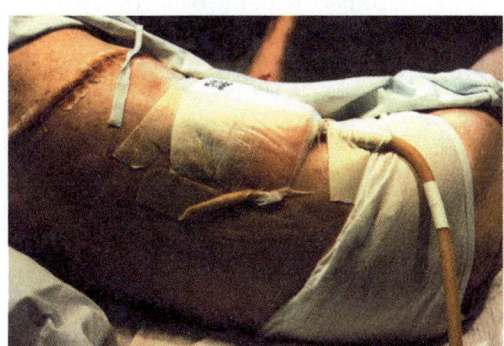

FIGURE 38-9 The chest tube is securely covered with dressings.

- Volume studies that measure the amount of air entering or leaving the lungs during various respiratory movements
- Radiographic techniques such as x-rays, CT scans, and MRIs
- Direct visualization procedures such as bronchoscopy

SPECIAL THERAPIES RELATED TO RESPIRATORY ILLNESS

Nursing assistants aid patient breathing by proper positioning and by helping provide moisture and oxygen. They also are assigned to collect sputum specimens for examinations.

Oxygen Therapy

Oxygen is often ordered by the physician. Remember that when oxygen is in use, special precautions are required to prevent fires and to administer the oxygen safely. Information about general fire control is presented in Unit 14.

Special safety measures must be emphasized in areas where oxygen is being used:

- Be certain that there are no open flames and that no one smokes or has matches.
- Post "no smoking" or "oxygen-in-use" signs.

Hospitals have a centralized source of oxygen piped to wall units in the patient's room (Figure 38-11). In some facilities, the oxygen is stored in a tank that is brought to the patient's room when therapy is ordered. The amount of oxygen (rate of flow measured in liters) is ordered by the physician. Oxygen is a prescription item, and changing the flow rate is the responsibility of a licensed nurse or RCP.

Caring for a Patient Who Is Receiving Oxygen Therapy. The care plan may instruct you to elevate the head of the bed when the patient is receiving oxygen. This will make it easier to breathe. Patients using oxygen masks cannot eat meals while wearing the mask. The physician may

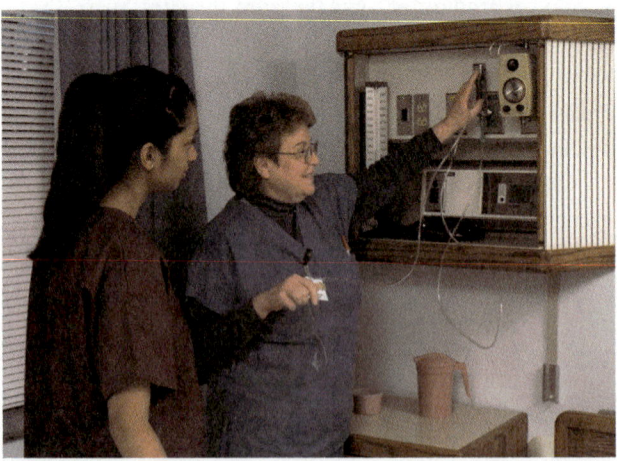

FIGURE 38-11 Oxygen is usually piped to each unit through a central delivery system.

order a nasal cannula at meal time. Follow the instructions on the care plan or critical pathway for patient care measures. Being unable to breathe is very frightening. Patients who are receiving oxygen may need reassurance and emotional support. Check on the patient frequently and spend as much time in the room as possible. Difficult breathing makes it hard to talk. The patient may be unable to hold a normal conversation. Just being with the patient without talking is very reassuring. If the patient is having trouble breathing, try to ask questions that can be answered "yes" or "no" so it is easier for the patient to communicate with you.

You will care for patients using different devices for the administration of oxygen. Carefully check the skin under the device to make sure it is not red or irritated from the elastic that holds the oxygen device in place. Report any skin problems to the nurse. Oxygen is drying, so patients who are receiving oxygen may need extra liquids to drink. They also need frequent care of the mouth and nose. Sometimes patients feel warm and will perspire heavily. Extra bathing and linen changes may be necessary. You may need to adjust the temperature in the room and help the patient change into a hospital gown. Cover him or her with a sheet. The care plan or critical pathway will provide information on patient preferences and needs. When caring for a patient who uses oxygen, you should:

- wear gloves and apply the principles of standard precautions if contact with the patient's oral or nasal secretions is likely.
- know the oxygen flow rate that was ordered and set for your patient.
- be able to read the flow meter for the rate of oxygen delivery if instructed to check the rate by the nurse.
- notify the nurse immediately if there is a change in the flow rate.
- check that the tubing is not obstructed in any way that would prevent oxygen from reaching the patient.
- check for proper position of the catheter, cannula, or mask and that the elastic band around the head is snug but not constricting.

- check whether straps, cannula, or mask are causing skin irritation.
- provide frequent mouth care.
- use a portable tank to transport the patient to other areas of the hospital. Do not remove the oxygen without permission from the RCP or RN.

If a tank is used as the source of oxygen, be sure that:

- there is sufficient oxygen in the tank. Check the gauge each time you visit the patient (Figure 38-12).
- the oxygen is on.
- an additional tank is available to exchange for the tank in use when it is empty.
- empty tanks are marked and stored according to facility policy.
- the tank is upright and secure on the carrier or in the stand.

Humidifiers. In some facilities, a **humidifier** (Figure 38-13) is attached to the oxygen administration equipment if the patient's liter flow exceeds 5 liters. Use of oxygen humidifiers is a controversial subject. Humidification is not necessary in liter flows below 5. Humidifiers are not used at all in some facilities.

The humidifier is a water bottle that moistens the oxygen for comfort and prevents drying of the mucous membranes in the nose, mouth, and lungs. The bottle screws into a male adapter on the flow meter. Oxygen passes through the water in the humidifier, picking up moisture, before it reaches the patient. The delivery device plugs into a male adapter on the side of the humidifier. The respiratory care practitioner usually cares for the humidifier, but this is a nursing assistant responsibility in some health care settings. If this is the case, you will be responsible for checking or changing the humidifier. Sterile distilled water is always used in the humidifier. Avoid tap water. Inhalation of tap water

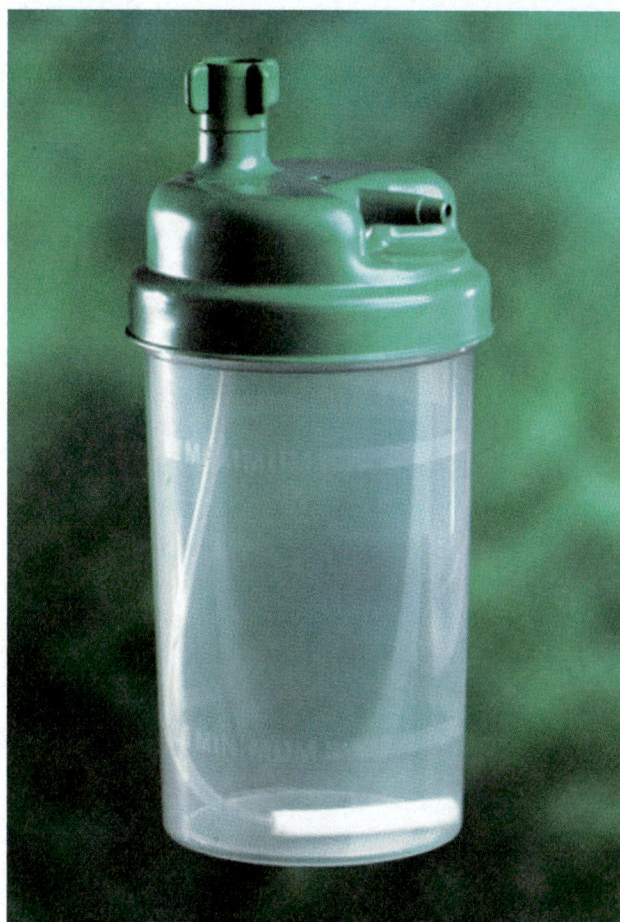

FIGURE 38-13 A humidifier. *(Courtesy of Hudson RCI, Temecula, CA, USA)*

is associated with an increased incidence of Legionnaire's disease. The water level in the humidifier should always be at or above the "minimum fill" line on the bottle.

When the oxygen delivery system is functioning correctly, the water in the humidifier will bubble. Oxygen will not exit the tubing into the mask or cannula if the tubing is kinked or obstructed. If this occurs, pressure builds up in the unit and discharges through a pressure relief valve. When setting up a humidifier, check this valve by turning the oxygen on and pinching the connecting tubing.

Two types of humidifiers are used. The *prefilled* type of humidifier is commonly used in acute care hospitals. This unit is usually changed once a week, when it is empty, or according to the manufacturer's directions or facility policies and procedures. Discard the bottle after replacing it with a new one. Your facility may require you to attach a sticker to the bottle listing the date and time it was changed, and your initials.

Refillable humidifiers are washed with soap and water or 2% alkaline gluteraldehyde solution every 24 hours. They are rinsed well, then sterilized. Refill the sterile bottle with sterile distilled water. Never add water to a partially filled humidifier. A sticker may be attached to this bottle showing the date and time it was changed (refer to Procedure 97).

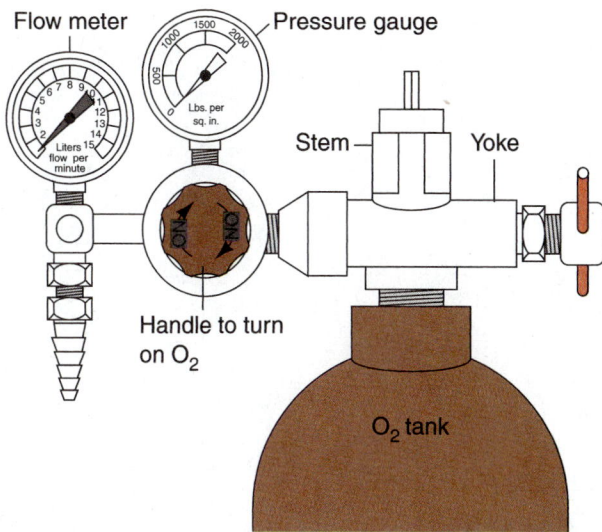

FIGURE 38-12 The flow meter shows the amount of oxygen being delivered. The pressure gauge shows the amount of oxygen remaining in the tank.

PROCEDURE 97

ATTACHING A HUMIDIFIER TO THE OXYGEN FLOW METER OR REGULATOR

1. Carry out beginning procedure actions.

2. Assemble equipment:
   - sterile disposable or refillable humidifier bottle
   - sterile distilled water for refillable humidifier

3. Open the humidifier package and remove the bottle.

4. If a refillable humidifier is used, obtain a fresh bottle that has been washed and sterilized. Unscrew the lid, and place it with the clean inside up on the table. Fill the bottle with sterile distilled water, then replace the lid. Do not touch the inside of the bottle or lid with your fingers.

5. Connect the female adapter in the top of the humidifier bottle to the male adapter on the flow meter. Tighten the nut securely.

6. Connect the tubing on the cannula or mask to the male adapter on the side of the humidifier bottle.

7. Turn on the flow of oxygen. Pinch the connecting tubing to ensure that the safety valve pops off.

8. Affix a sticker with the time and date of change, and your initials, according to facility policy.

9. Carry out procedure completion actions.

Methods of Oxygen Delivery. Oxygen may be delivered to the patient by several different methods. The same basic care is required for each method, with modifications.

- *Nasal cannula:* Delivery of oxygen by nasal cannula is the most common method used today. The oxygen is delivered through a tube that has two small plastic prongs or nipples (Figure 38-14). The prongs are placed at the entrance to the patient's nose. A strap around the patient's head holds the prongs in place.
   - Make sure the strap is secure but not too tight.
   - Check for signs of irritation where the prongs touch the patient's nose.
   - Check that mucus has not blocked the prong openings. Clean if necessary.

   - Make sure the cannula is stored when not in use in such a way that it is not contaminated.

- *Mask:* The oxygen mask is a cuplike mask held in place by straps around the head The oxygen mask fits over the patient's nose, mouth, and chin. A small tube connects the mask to the oxygen source. Masks are available in adult and pediatric sizes. Several different face masks are used, depending on the patient's oxygen needs (Figure 38-15). A special mask fits over a tracheostomy (Figure 38-16). Using an oxygen mask is necessary when high liter flows of oxygen are ordered.

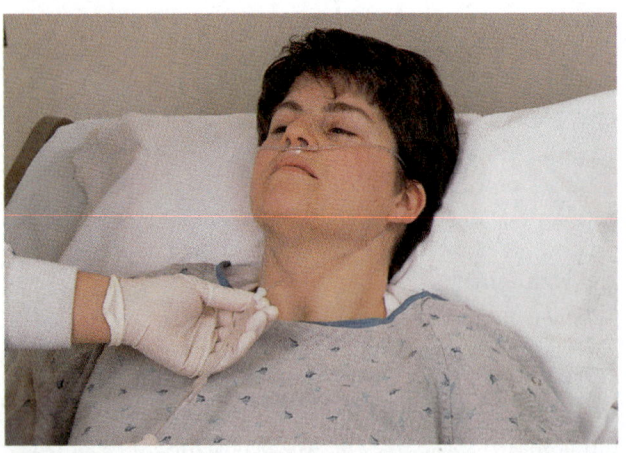

FIGURE 38-14 Oxygen being administered by nasal cannula.

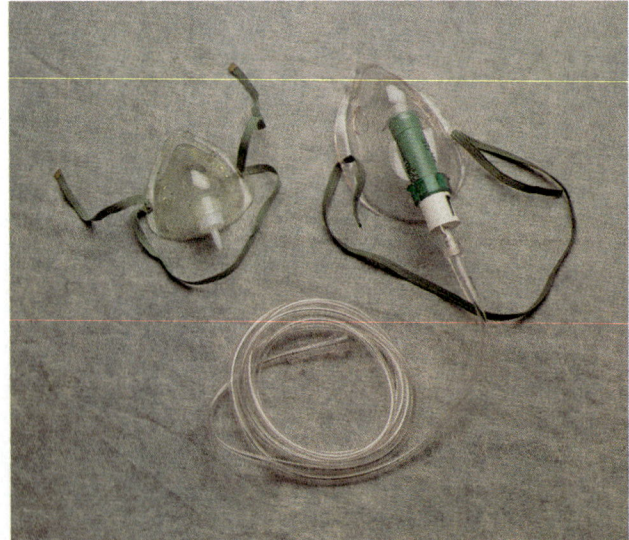

FIGURE 38-15 Various types of oxygen masks.

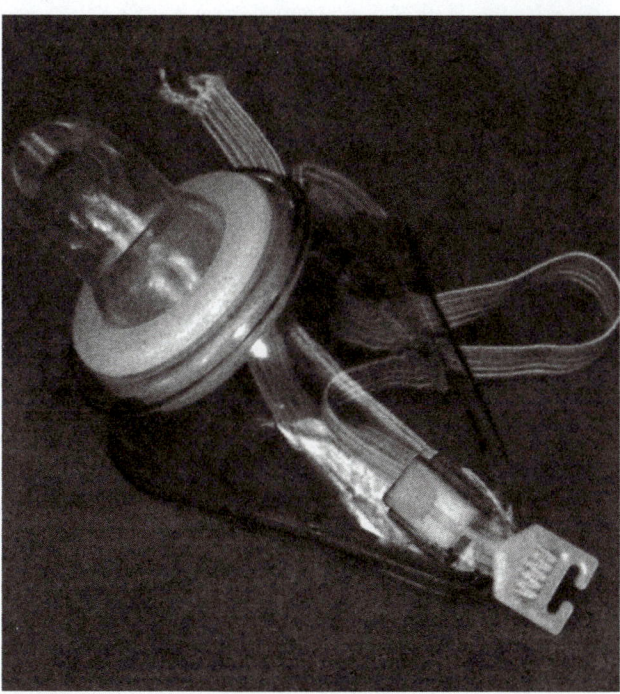

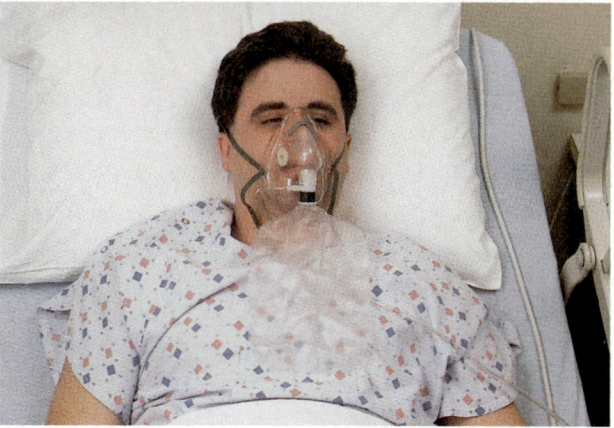

FIGURE 38-17 The nonrebreathing mask is used for severe hypoxemia. The patient's exhaled air escapes through the one-way flaps on the sides, but room air cannot enter because of the one-way design. The bag at the bottom increases the amount of oxygen delivered to the patient. It should not collapse more than halfway when the patient inhales.

FIGURE 38-16 An adult tracheostomy mask.

Masks may also be used for individuals who breathe through their mouths. A mask is never used with liter flows under 5 because it will cause rebreathing of exhaled carbon dioxide, and has a smothering effect. An elastic strap that slips over the back of the head holds the mask in place.

- Place the mask over the patient's nose and mouth.
- Adjust the fit by pulling on the ends of the elastic next to the mask so the fit is snug, but not too tight.
- Adjust the metal tab over the bridge of the nose, if needed for comfort.
- Periodically remove the mask. Wash the area under it and dry carefully.
- Some masks have inflatable bags at the bottom (Figure 38-17). The combination of bag and mask increases the amount of oxygen delivered to the patient. The bag should be inflated at all times. Notify the nurse if the bag collapses more than halfway during inspiration. This type of mask provides very high amounts of oxygen and should not be used for more than 24 hours without an evaluation by a health care provider.
- *Tent:* An example of a tent is a Mistogen® unit (croupette). A *croupette* is a small, portable unit.

Oxygen Concentrator

An oxygen concentrator (Figure 38-18) takes in room air and removes impurities and gases other than oxygen, allowing the oxygen to become concentrated in the unit. The air delivered to the patient from the concentrator is more than

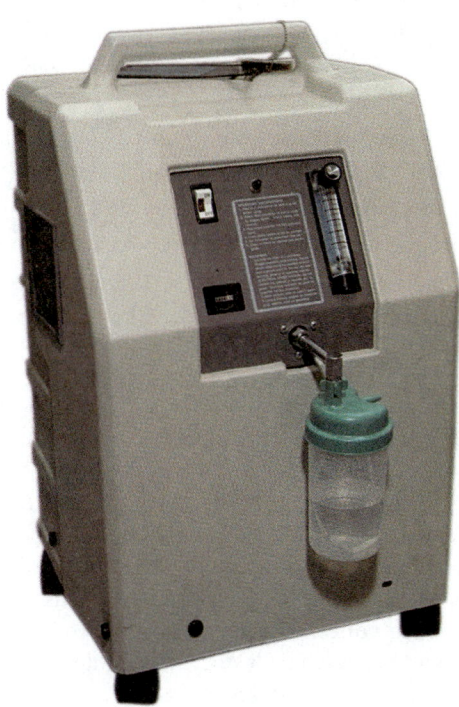

FIGURE 38-18 The oxygen concentrator delivers low liter flows. Most concentrators have an attachment for a humidifier, but humidification is not necessary at low liter flows.

90% oxygen. It is delivered by tubing attached to a nasal cannula or mask. The flow rate is usually 2 liters per minute (L/min).

General Oxygen Concentrator Precautions. Follow these precautions when a concentrator is used to supply oxygen to a patient:

- Place the concentrator at least 5 feet away from any heat source and at least 4 inches away from the wall.

- Smoking is not permitted in the same room.
- Be sure the unit is plugged in and grounded.
- Do not use an extension cord with the concentrator.
- Never change the flow-meter setting.
- Notify the nurse if the alarm sounds.
- A mask is not used with a concentrator because the exhaled carbon dioxide cannot be expelled with low liter flows of oxygen.
- Wipe the cannula daily with a damp cloth (do not use alcohol- or oil-based products).
- Clean concentrator surfaces using a damp cloth only.
- Remove the filter weekly. Wash in warm soapy water, rinse, squeeze dry, and replace.

Liquid Oxygen

Oxygen also comes in a liquid canister (Figure 38-19). Liquid oxygen is made by cooling the oxygen gas. As it cools, it changes to a liquid form. One advantage is that large amounts of liquid oxygen can be stored in small, more convenient containers. These can be filled from the larger unit. However, liquid oxygen cannot be stored for a long period of time because it will evaporate. The canister delivers higher oxygen concentrations than a concentrator, and is portable and convenient. It does not require electricity to operate. The canister is quiet compared with a concentrator, which has an electric motor and makes a humming noise. It is more expensive than using a concentrator.

Safety Precautions for Liquid Oxygen. Liquid oxygen is nontoxic, but will cause severe burns upon direct contact. Avoid opening, touching, or spilling the container. If your skin or clothing contacts the liquid oxygen, flush the area immediately with a large amount of water. When liquid oxygen is used, high concentrations of oxygen build up quickly. Some materials are very flammable when saturated with oxygen. Follow all safety precautions for preventing sparks and fires (Unit 14). Never seal the cap or vent port on the liquid oxygen. Doing so will increase pressure within the system, creating a potentially dangerous

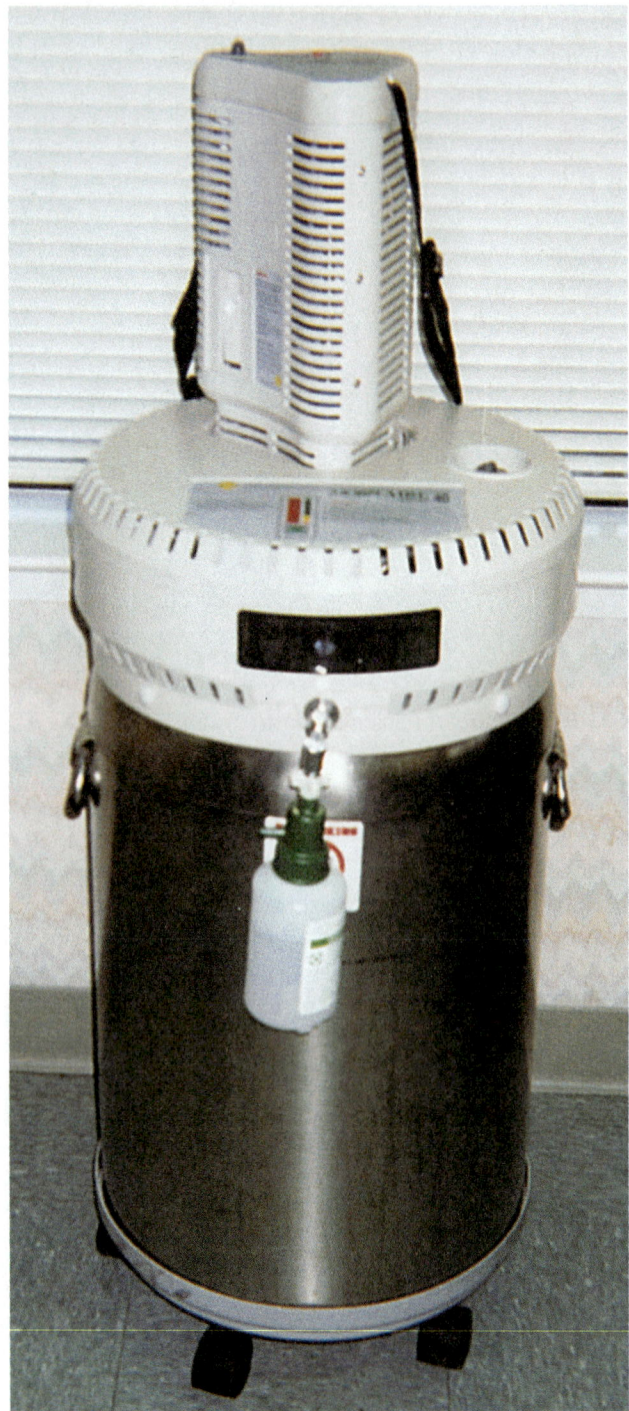

FIGURE 38-19 The liquid oxygen canister. The portable tank on top is filled from the large tank, then detached.

situation. If a bottle falls or tips, evacuate yourself and the patient from the room and close the door. Follow facility policies for getting assistance in this type of emergency.

Respiratory Positions

Positioning of the patient to permit expansion of the lungs and a straightened airway is helpful to patients with respiratory distress.

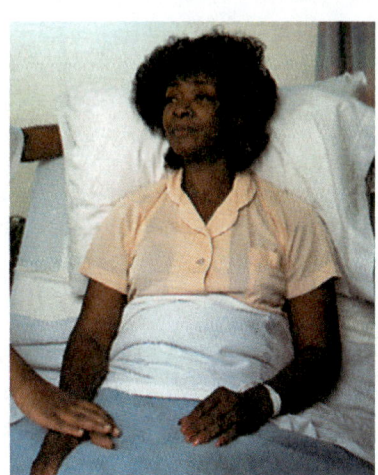

FIGURE 38-20 The patient is in the high Fowler's position.

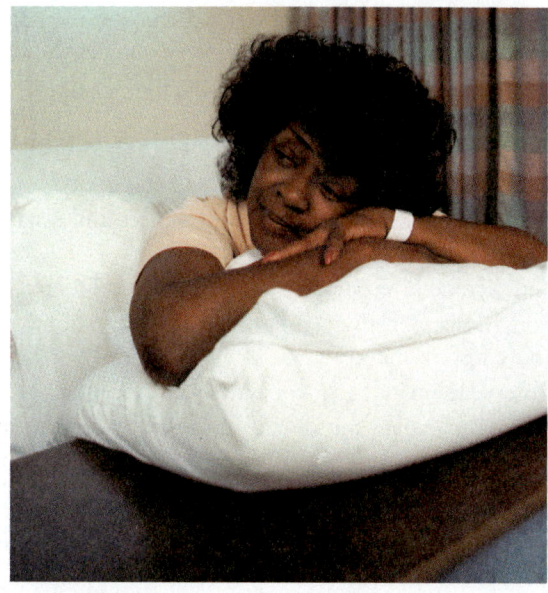

FIGURE 38-22 The tripod position enlarges the chest cavity, making breathing easier.

High Fowler's Position. In the high Fowler's position, the patient is sitting up with the back rest elevated (Figure 38-20).

- Position three pillows behind the patient's head and shoulders. Adjust the knee rest.
- Keep the feet in proper position.
- Check for signs of skin breakdown over the coccyx from shearing forces.

Orthopneic Position. The orthopneic position (Figure 38-21) may be used as an alternative to the high Fowler's position. *Orthopneic* means "needing to sit up to breathe comfortably." The patient sits as upright as possible and leans slightly forward, supporting herself with the forearms. This position makes the thorax larger on inspiration, enabling the patient to inhale more air. The tripod position (Figure 38-22) is another alternative to improve ventilation.

- The head of the bed is upright, as far as it will go.
- The bedside table is brought across the bed and a pillow or two are placed on top.
- The patient leans forward across the table with arms on or beside the pillows.

- Another pillow is placed low behind the patient's back for support.

Another alternative to improve ventilation is to seat the patient on the side of the bed, with the bed in the lowest horizontal position. Make sure the patient's legs are supported on a floor or a stool. The patient can lean across an overbed table, if desired, for additional support.

Incentive Spirometer

The physician may write orders for use of an incentive spirometer (Figure 38-23) to help the lungs expand fully. This prevents atelectasis (collapse of the alveoli) and also helps prevent pneumonia.

This procedure may be carried out with the patient in bed, with head and shoulders well supported, if permitted. The procedure usually is taught before surgery.

- The patient is instructed how to use the incentive spirometer by a respiratory care practitioner or nurse.

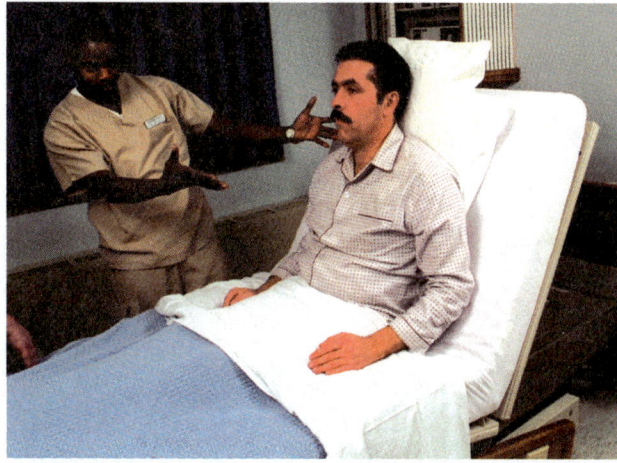

FIGURE 38-21 The patient in the orthopneic position sits straight up, supported on the arms.

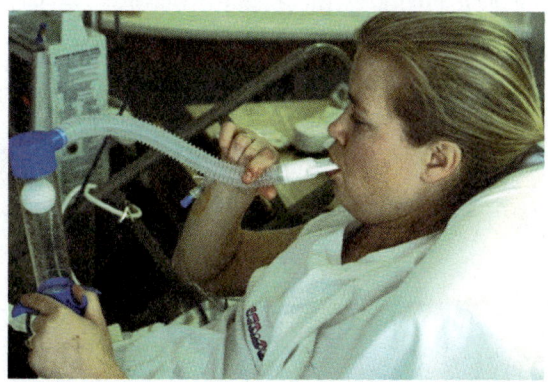

FIGURE 38-23 The patient inhales through the mouth, raising the level of the balls inside the plastic chambers.

- The patient exhales normally and then, with the lips placed tightly around the mouthpiece, inhales through the mouth strongly, enough to raise the balls in the chambers.
- The deep breath should be held as long as possible (or as ordered), thereby keeping the balls suspended.
- The patient then removes the mouthpiece and exhales normally.
- The exercise is repeated as many times as is ordered.

Although this procedure is started by the professional, you too have responsibilities:

- Observe the patient for correctness of procedure.
- Advise the patient not to take in too many deep breaths in a row, as this will cause dizziness.
- Be sure the patient does not become overly fatigued.
- Encourage the patient to cough and clear the respiratory passages.
- Report to the nurse if the patient seems overly fatigued during the procedure.
- Carefully observe and report any unusual responses such as pain, dizziness, or throat and airway irritation.
- When patient has completed the pulmonary exercise, wash the spirometer mouthpiece in warm water, dry it, replace it in the plastic bag, and leave it at the bedside.
- Provide mouth care as needed or desired.

Tips: The incentive spirometer is usually left at the bedside. The patient will be prompted to use it throughout the day. He or she is instructed to take four to five slow, deep breaths using the spirometer, or as ordered. If the patient becomes dizzy or complains of tingling in the fingers, he or she may be breathing too fast. Have the patient relax and breathe normally until the sensation passes. Monitor the patient's breathing before and after the treatment. Report your observations to the nurse.

- Patients should be praised for their efforts. Many times this encourages greater effort the next time the incentive spirometer is used.

Other Techniques

Aerosol Therapy. Nebulizers deliver moisture or medication deep into the lungs. Drugs that dilate the bronchi are often prescribed. Small-volume nebulizers (Figure 38-24)

turn liquid medicine into a mist that can be breathed in by the patient. Typically, drugs are ordered to open up obstructed airways for patients with COPD and asthma. The nebulizer may be powered by oxygen or compressed air. After a nebulizer treatment is given, the patient should be encouraged to cough and assessed by the nurse for improvement after medication delivery.

Continuous Positive Airway Pressure (CPAP)

Some patients stop breathing periodically while they sleep. This condition is called *sleep apnea*. It is commonly caused by a blockage or obstruction in the patient's airway that occurs when the patient falls asleep and the muscles relax. Patients with sleep apnea may stop breathing hundreds of times a night, and they snore loudly when they start to breathe again. This interrupts their sleep, and they are often very tired during the day. Treatment in many cases consists of use of a device that delivers pressure to the airway while the patient sleeps; this pressure holds the airway open.

The device is called CPAP (pronounced see-pap) which stands for continuous positive airway pressure (Figure 38-25). A mask is placed on the patient's face and held in place with a head strap. Large-diameter corrugated tubing connects the mask to a device (sometimes called a blower) that creates low levels of pressure. Because there is always pressure in the system, the mask must fit tightly against the face. Pressure is usually controlled by an adjustment on the device. The amount of pressure can range from approximately 2 cm H_2O to 20 cm H_2O. This level is ordered by the physician. The device is usually initially set up by a respiratory care practitioner, who works with the patient to determine which type of mask is most effective and most comfortable.

Many patients will put on their own masks at bedtime. Remind them to wash and dry the face thoroughly before putting the mask on so that less skin oil will get on the mask. You should help monitor the patient while he is connected to a CPAP machine. Check to make sure the mask is comfortable. Air leaks around the top can allow air to blow into the patient's eyes, which is very irritating. If this happens,

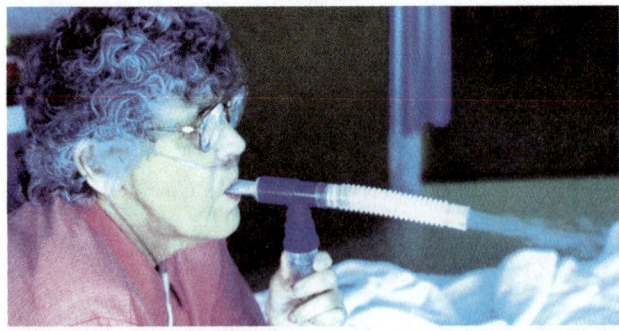

FIGURE 38-24 A hand-held, small-volume nebulizer.

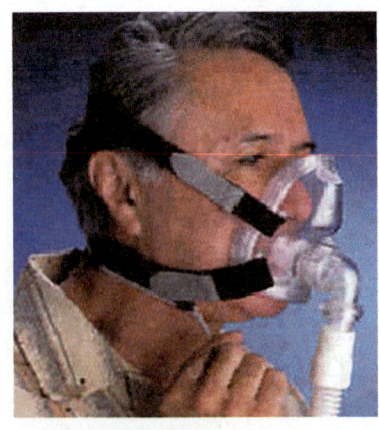

FIGURE 38-25 The CPAP mask applies pressure to keep the airway open while the patient sleeps, preventing sleep apnea.

you can adjust the mask to see if you can reduce the leak. However, if the mask is too tight, the patient may feel pain or there may be redness or skin breakdown on the nose.

If the patient complains of excessive dryness in his nasal passages, the nurse will check with the RCP to see if a humidifier can be added to the CPAP system. The nurse may also get an order for saline spray or nosedrops to reduce the irritation. It is important not to use petrolatum products with respiratory devices. If a patient swallows a lot of air from the mask, belches frequently, and feels pressure in the abdomen, elevate the head of the bed to see if this reduces air swallowing.

Wash the mask each morning, after the patient takes it off. Wash it with soap and water, or according to facility policy. Store the dry mask in a clean plastic bag until use at bedtime.

COLLECTING A SPUTUM SPECIMEN

You may need to collect a sputum specimen from the patient. **Sputum** is matter that is brought up (**expectorated**) from the lungs. A culture of the specimen identifies the cause of an infection.

You must be sure that the specimen comes from the lungs and is not saliva from the mouth.

If the patient cannot expectorate sputum, suctioning may be needed to obtain the specimen. (The nurse performs this procedure.) It is easier to collect the specimen when the patient wakes up in the morning and after taking two or three deep breaths. (Refer to Procedure 98.)

PROCEDURE 98

COLLECTING A SPUTUM SPECIMEN

1. Carry out beginning procedure actions.

2. Assemble equipment:
   - disposable gloves
   - sterile container and cover for specimen
   - glass of water
   - label, including:
     - patient's full name
     - room number
     - patient number
     - date and time of collection
     - physician's name
     - examination to be done
     - other information as requested
   - tissues
   - emesis basin
   - biohazard specimen transport bag
   - laboratory requisition

3. Wash your hands and put on disposable gloves.

4. Ask the patient to rinse her mouth with water and spit into the emesis basin.

5. Ask the patient to breathe deeply and then cough deeply to bring up sputum. The patient spits the sputum into the container.
   a. While coughing, have the patient cover her mouth with a tissue to prevent the spread of infection.
   b. Collect 1 to 2 tablespoons of sputum unless otherwise ordered.
   c. Do not contaminate the outside of the container.
   d. Avoid touching the inside of the container or lid. Instruct the patient not to touch the inside of the container or lid.

6. Remove your gloves and discard them according to facility policy.

7. Wash your hands.

8. Cover the specimen container tightly and attach a completed label.

9. Place the specimen container in a biohazard transport bag and attach a laboratory requisition.

10. Carry out procedure completion actions.

11. Follow facility policy for transporting specimens to the laboratory.

REVIEW

A. True/False.

Mark the following true or false by circling T or F.

1. T F In asthma, there is increased production of mucus, which blocks the respiratory tract.
2. T F Drugs to reduce fever fight infection.
3. T F An allergen causes a sensitivity reaction.
4. T F URI stands for underrated respiratory injections.
5. T F The use of the incentive spirometer can help prevent pneumonia.
6. T F Always post a sign when oxygen is in use.
7. T F The oxygen flow rate is ordered by the physician.
8. T F Immobility is a risk factor for hypoxemia.
9. T F When oxygen is administered by mask, make sure the straps are very tight.
10. T F In the high Fowler's position, the patient leans forward across the overbed table.

B. Matching.

Choose the correct word from Column II to match each the phrase or statement in Column I.

Column I	Column II
11. _____ inflammation of the lungs	**a.** emphysema
12. _____ an example of COPD	**b.** sputum
13. _____ difficult breathing	**c.** pneumonia
14. _____ cough up	**d.** dyspnea
15. _____ material brought up from lungs	**e.** spirometer
	f. expectorate

C. Multiple Choice.

Select the one best answer for each of the following.

16. Patients with respiratory disease should
    a. cover the nose and mouth when coughing.
    b. turn the face toward others when sneezing.
    c. wash their hands only after toileting.
    d. dispose of soiled tissues by dropping them in the nearest trash can.

17. When tank oxygen is in use,
    a. mark empty tanks and store them in the patient's room.
    b. attach the tank to the patient's bed.
    c. make sure additional tanks are available.
    d. check the gauge indicating the amount in the tank once each shift.

18. Nursing care for a male patient who is using oxygen includes
    a. keeping the head of the bed elevated 10 degrees.
    b. shaving the patient with an electric razor.
    c. covering the patient with a wool blanket for warmth.
    d. providing frequent mouth care.

19. When your patient is receiving oxygen, you should
    a. monitor intake and output.
    b. know the ordered rate.
    c. check the flow rate once each shift.
    d. check the flow rate every 3 hours.

20. When administering oxygen by mask, in addition to routine care and precautions, you should
    a. pull the straps until they are very tight.
    b. provide emotional support and reassurance.
    c. make sure mask covers only the mouth.
    d. remove the mask for bathing and meals.

D. Nursing Assistant Challenge.

Mrs. Harvey has had asthma all her life. She is sensitive to many allergens. She is admitted to your facility for emphysema. She is receiving respiratory assistance with an oxygen concentrator. Complete the following questions related to her care.

21. The flow rate of the concentrator is usually _____. (10 L/min) (2 L/min)

22. Smoking in the same room _____ permitted. (is) (is not)

23. The flow meter on a concentrator _____ be changed by the nursing assistant. (may) (may not)

24. The concentrator should be placed at least _____ from a heat source. (2 feet) (5 feet)

25. The concentrator filter should be cleaned _____. (daily) (weekly)

EXPLORING THE WEB

Description	Location
Breathing disorders	*http://www.breathingdisorders.com*
Pulse oximetry	*http://www.utmb.edu*
American Association for Respiratory Care	*http://www.aarc.org*
American Lung Association	*http://www.lungusa.org*
American Sleep Apnea Association	*http://www.sleepapnea.org*
American Society for Asthma, Allergy, and Immunology	*http://allergy.mcg.edu*
Breathin' Easy	*http://www.breathineasy.com*
Campaign for Tobacco-Free Kids	*http://www.tobaccofreekids.org*
Canadian Society for Respiratory Therapy	*http://www.csrt.com*
Emphysema Foundation for Our Right to Survive	*http://www.emphysema.net*
Global Initiative for Chronic Obstructive Lung Disease	*http://www.goldcopd.com*
National Association for Medical Direction of Respiratory Care	*http://www.namdrc.org*
Pulmonary Education and Research Foundation	*http://www.perf2ndwind.org*
PulmonaryChannel.com	*http://www.pulmonarychannel.com*
Respiratory Infection Tracker	*http://www.rtialert.com*
Respiratory Therapy Society of Ontario	*http://www.rtso.org*
Society of Thoracic Surgeons	*http://www.sts.org*

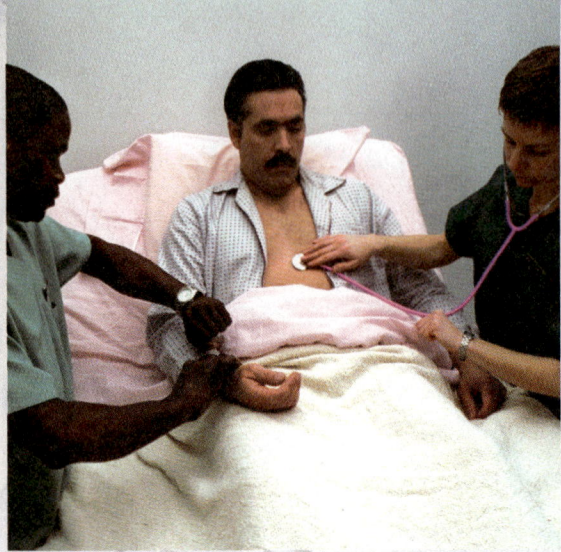

Circulatory (Cardiovascular) System

objectives

After completing this unit, you will be able to:
- Spell and define terms.
- Review the location and functions of the organs of the circulatory system.
- Describe some common disorders of the circulatory system.
- Describe nursing assistant actions related to care of patients with disorders of the circulatory system.
- List five specific diagnostic tests for disorders of the circulatory system.

vocabulary

Learn the meaning and the correct spelling of the following words and phrases:

anemia	congestive heart	infarction	phlebitis
angina pectoris	failure (CHF)	ischemic	plasma
artery	coronary embolism	leukemia	stent
ascites	coronary occlusion	leukocytes	sympathectomy
atheroma	coronary thrombosis	lymph	TED hose
atherosclerosis	diuresis	lymphatic vessel	thrombocytes
atrium	dyscrasia	myocardial infarction	thrombus
capillary	embolus	(MI)	transient ischemic
cardiac cycle	endocardium	myocardium	attack (TIA)
cardiac	erythrocytes	orthopnea	varicose vein
decompensation	heart block	pacemaker	vein
compensate	hypertension	pericardium	ventricle
	hypertrophy	peripheral	

INTRODUCTION

The circulatory system may be thought of as a transportation system. It takes nourishment and oxygen to the cells and carries away waste products. The closed system is kept in motion by the force of the heartbeat. Diseases that attack any part of this system interfere with overall body function. Long-standing diseases of the cardiovascular system eventually affect the pulmonary system as well.

STRUCTURE AND FUNCTION

The organs of the cardiovascular system include:

1. Heart—a central pumping station
2. Blood vessels
   a. **Arteries**—tubes that carry blood away from the heart. They
      - have muscular, elastic walls with smooth linings.
      - branch to form arterioles with thinner walls. Arterioles then become capillaries.
      - carry blood with a high concentration of nutrients and oxygen to the body cells.
   b. **Veins**—tubes that carry blood toward the heart. They
      - have thinner muscular walls.
      - carry blood back to the heart.
      - carry blood with a lower concentration of oxygen, more carbon dioxide, and more waste products.
      - have cuplike valves that help move the blood.
   c. **Capillaries**—tubes that connect arteries and veins. They
      - have walls only one cell thick.
      - are the site of exchange of nutrients and oxygen from the blood to the cells, and carbon dioxide and waste products from the cells to the blood.
3. **Lymphatic vessels**—tubes that carry lymph or tissue fluid to the bloodstream. Fluid from the bloodstream passes into the tissue spaces, where it is called *tissue fluid*. Some of the tissue fluid returns to the bloodstream by way of the capillaries. Some of it is first drawn off into the lymphatic vessels, where it is called **lymph**. Eventually the lymph is returned to general circulation and once more becomes part of the blood.
4. Lymph nodes—masses of lymphatic tissue along the pathway of the lymph. They filter the lymph.
5. Spleen—a lymphatic organ. The spleen produces some of the blood cells and helps destroy worn-out blood cells. It acts as a blood reservoir or blood bank.
6. Blood—a connective tissue made up of a liquid (plasma) and cellular elements.

The Blood

Blood is a red body fluid composed of plasma and cellular elements. The body contains 4 to 6 quarts (liters) of blood. Fifty-five percent of the blood is formed of the liquid plasma. **Plasma** is a watery solution containing:

- Antibodies (gamma globulin)—chemicals to fight infection
- Nutrients—such as glucose, amino acids, fats, salts
- Gases—such as oxygen and carbon dioxide
- Waste products—such as urea and creatinine

The blood cells are produced in the bone marrow and lymphatic tissues of the body. The bone marrow, liver, and spleen destroy worn-out blood cells. (See Unit 5.) The blood cells include red blood cells, white blood cells, and thrombocytes.

- Red blood cells (RBC)—**erythrocytes**—carry most of the oxygen and small amounts of carbon dioxide. There are 4.5 to 5 million RBC per cubic millimeter (mm³).
- White blood cells (WBC)—**leukocytes**—fight infection. There are 7,000 to 8,000 WBC/mm³.
- **Thrombocytes** (or platelets)—are not whole cells but only parts of cells. They seal small leaks in the walls of blood vessels and initiate blood clotting. There are 200,000 to 400,000 thrombocytes/mm³.

The Heart

The heart is a hollow muscular organ about the size of a fist (Figure 39-1). It is divided into a right and left side by a muscular wall called the *septum* and into four chambers. There are three layers in the heart wall. The **endocardium** lines the heart chambers. The **myocardium** is the muscle layer. The **pericardium** is a membranous outer covering.

The four chambers are:

1. The right **atrium** (RA)—(right upper heart chamber) receives blood from all over the body. This blood has a low oxygen content and a relatively high carbon dioxide level. It is called *deoxygenated blood*.
2. The right **ventricle** (RV)—(right lower heart chamber) receives blood from the right atrium and sends it out to the lungs through the pulmonary artery to pick up oxygen and get rid of the carbon dioxide.
3. The left atrium (LA)—(left upper heart chamber) receives oxygenated blood from the lungs and sends it to the left ventricle.
4. The left ventricle (LV)—(left lower heart chamber) receives blood from the left atrium and sends it out through the aorta to the entire body.

Valves separate the chambers. They also guard the exit of the pulmonary artery and aorta to prevent backflow and maintain a constant forward motion. The pulmonary artery carries blood to the lungs. The aorta is the largest blood vessel in the body. The valves are located as follows:

- Tricuspid valve—between right atrium and right ventricle

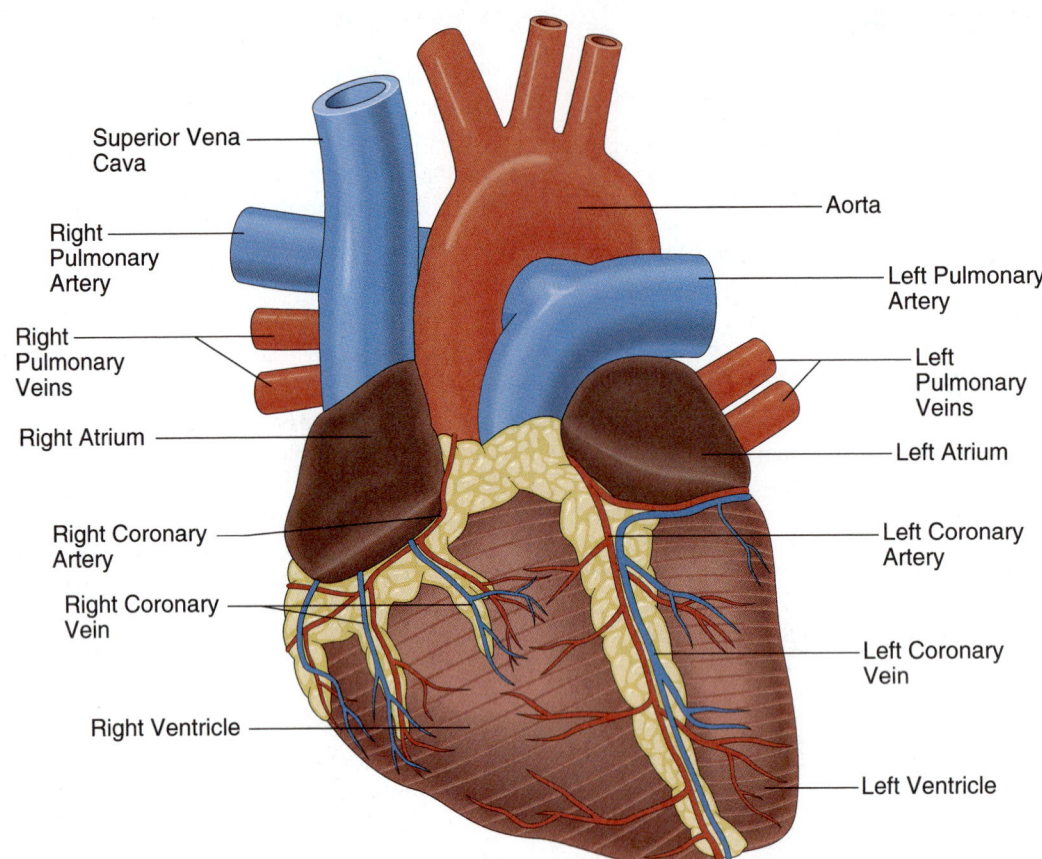

FIGURE 39-1 The heart and blood vessels.

- Bicuspid (mitral) valve—between left atrium and left ventricle
- Pulmonary semilunar valves—between right ventricle and pulmonary artery
- Aortic semilunar valve—between left ventricle and aorta

Nerve impulses make the heart contract regularly according to body needs. For example, when you run, your body cells need more oxygen. The cells signal the brain that they need more oxygen. The brain sends a signal to the heart through the nerves, telling it to supply more blood. These nerve impulses cause the heart to beat faster. Thus, more oxygenated blood is pumped to the body cells to supply the oxygen required. These impulses cause the heart to beat faster.

The Cardiac Cycle. The heart pumps blood through the body by a series of movements known as the **cardiac cycle**. First, the upper chambers of the heart, called *atria*, relax and fill with blood as the lower chambers contract, forcing blood out of the heart through the aorta and pulmonary arteries. Next, the lower chambers relax, allowing blood to flow into them from the contracting upper chambers. Then the cycle is repeated (Figure 39-2). Each cycle lasts about 0.8 second. This happens about 70 to 80 times per minute.

The pulse you feel at the radial artery corresponds to ventricular contraction. The sounds you hear when listening to the heart and when taking a blood pressure are the sounds made by the closing of the valves during the cardiac cycle.

The rate and rhythm of the cardiac cycle are regulated by the conduction system. The conduction system is made up of special neuromuscular tissue that sends out impulses. The impulses eventually reach the myocardial cells, which respond by contracting.

- The impulses begin at the S-A node in the right atrium and spread across the two atria.
- The atria contract.
- Impulses from the S-A node reach the A-V node in the right atrium.
- Messages from the A-V node then spread through the bundle of His in the septum. From there they go through the Purkinje fibers to the walls of the ventricles.
- The ventricles contract, forcing the blood forward.

An electrocardiogram, called an ECG or an EKG, is a test that traces the electrical impulses of the heart. Heart disease may be detected with this test.

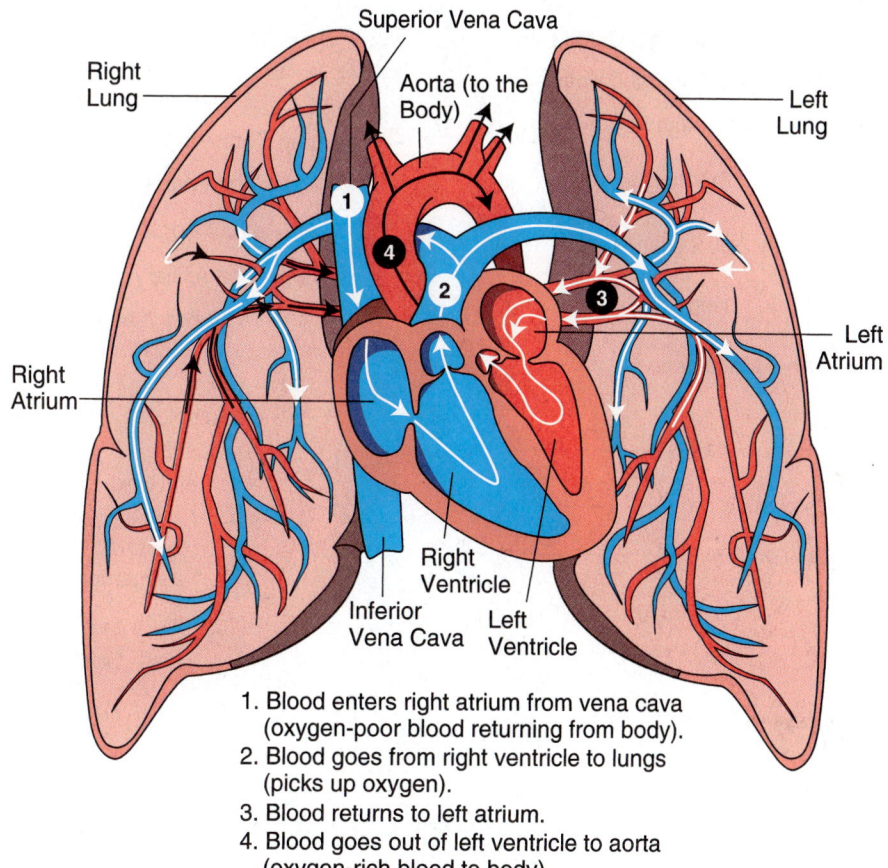

Superior Vena Cava
Right Lung
Aorta (to the Body)
Left Lung
Right Atrium
Left Atrium
Right Ventricle
Inferior Vena Cava
Left Ventricle

1. Blood enters right atrium from vena cava (oxygen-poor blood returning from body).
2. Blood goes from right ventricle to lungs (picks up oxygen).
3. Blood returns to left atrium.
4. Blood goes out of left ventricle to aorta (oxygen-rich blood to body).

FIGURE 39-2 Flow of blood from the heart to the lungs, to the body, and back to the heart to begin the cycle again.

Blood Vessels

Many large arteries and veins take their names from the bones they are near or from the part of the body they serve. For example, the femoral artery and vein run close to the femur (thigh bone). The subclavian arteries and veins are found under the clavicle. The axillary arteries and veins are found in the axillary (armpit) area. Figure 39-3 shows the arterial system that distributes blood from the heart. Figure 39-4 shows the venous system that returns blood to the heart.

COMMON CIRCULATORY SYSTEM DISORDERS

Common disorders of this system include:

- Diseases relating to the blood vessels
- Diseases of the heart
- Blood dyscrasias (abnormalities); these diseases can involve the bone, bone marrow, liver, or spleen.

Observations the nursing assistant is to report in patients with disorders of the circulatory system are:

- Color change, pallor or cyanosis, redness
- Cool to touch
- Hot to touch
- Changes in pulse rate or rhythm
- Changes in blood pressure
- Edema
- Disorientation

PERIPHERAL VASCULAR DISEASES

The blood vessels that serve the outer parts of the body, particularly those of the hands and feet, are referred to as peripheral (toward the outer part) blood vessels. Diseases of these vessels affect the parts of the body through which they pass. The health of these vessels also influences heart function.

Peripheral vascular diseases that affect the arteries diminish the flow of blood to the extremities. Tissues through which the narrowed arteries pass may not get the nourishment they need. Areas affected are the extremities: the arms, legs, and brain. The signs and symptoms associated with decreased peripheral circulation are:

- Burning pain during exercise
- Hair loss over feet and toes

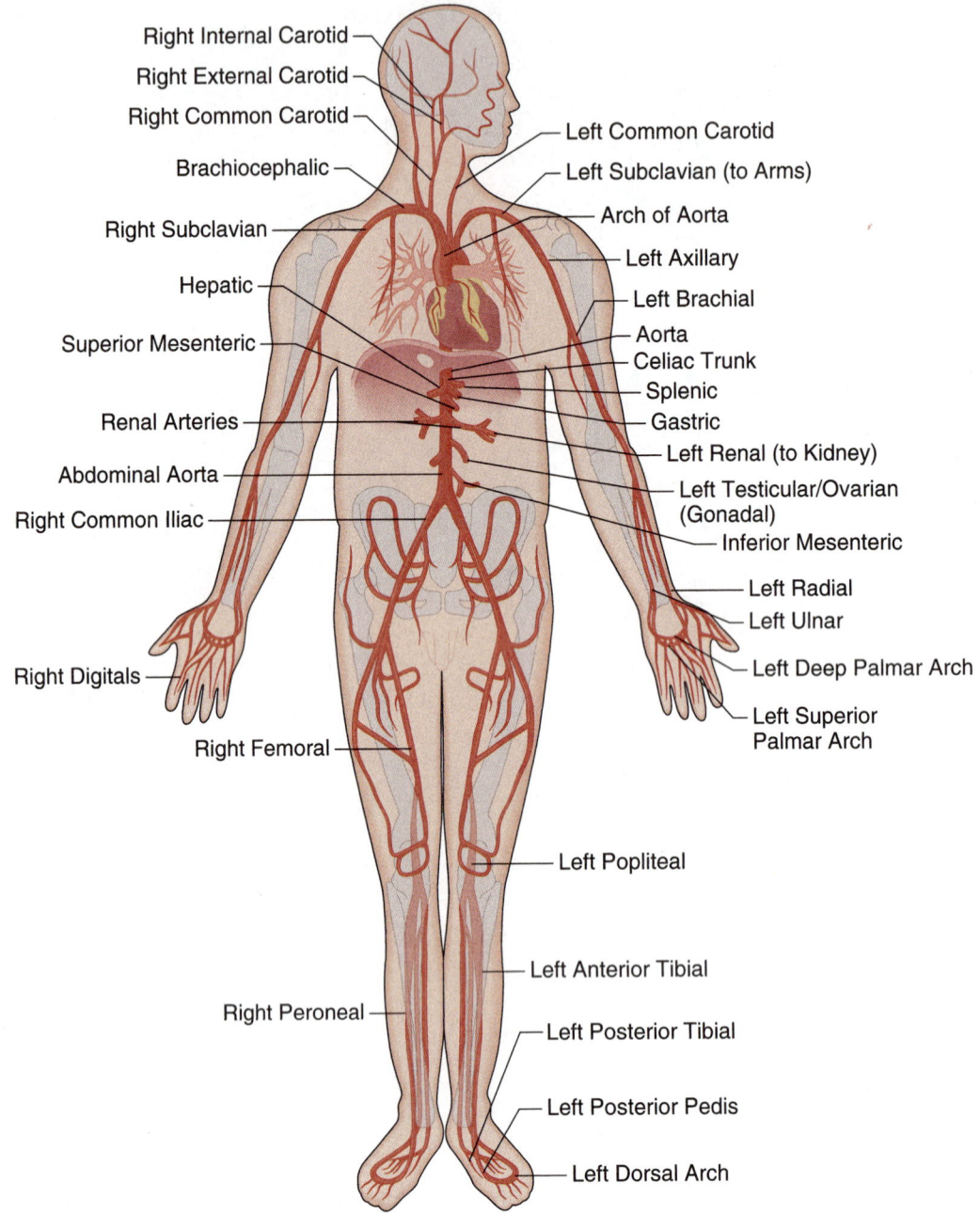

FIGURE 39-3 Arteries of the body.

- Thick and rigid toenails
- Dusky red skin or cyanotic, brownish skin
- Dry and scaly or shiny skin
- Chronic edema of the feet and legs
- Cool skin temperature of feet and legs
- Difficulty with ambulation

When the arteries are affected, the blood flow may be seriously interrupted. This condition requires immediate medical treatment. Vascular ulcers may occur. These are sores that start because of the poor circulation of the blood in the legs. These ulcers are difficult to treat and may take months to heal.

Treatment is aimed at:

- Increasing local circulation
  - Positioning and specific prescribed exercises can promote arterial flow and venous return.
  - Sometimes an oscillating (rocking) bed is employed to improve the circulatory flow. The oscillating bed rocks up and down in cycles, raising the patient's feet 6 inches above his head and then lowering them 12 to 15 inches. The steady rhythm provides both passive exercise for the patient and some circulatory stimulation.
  - Nothing that would hamper the patient's circulation is permitted.
- Preventing injuries that may heal poorly.

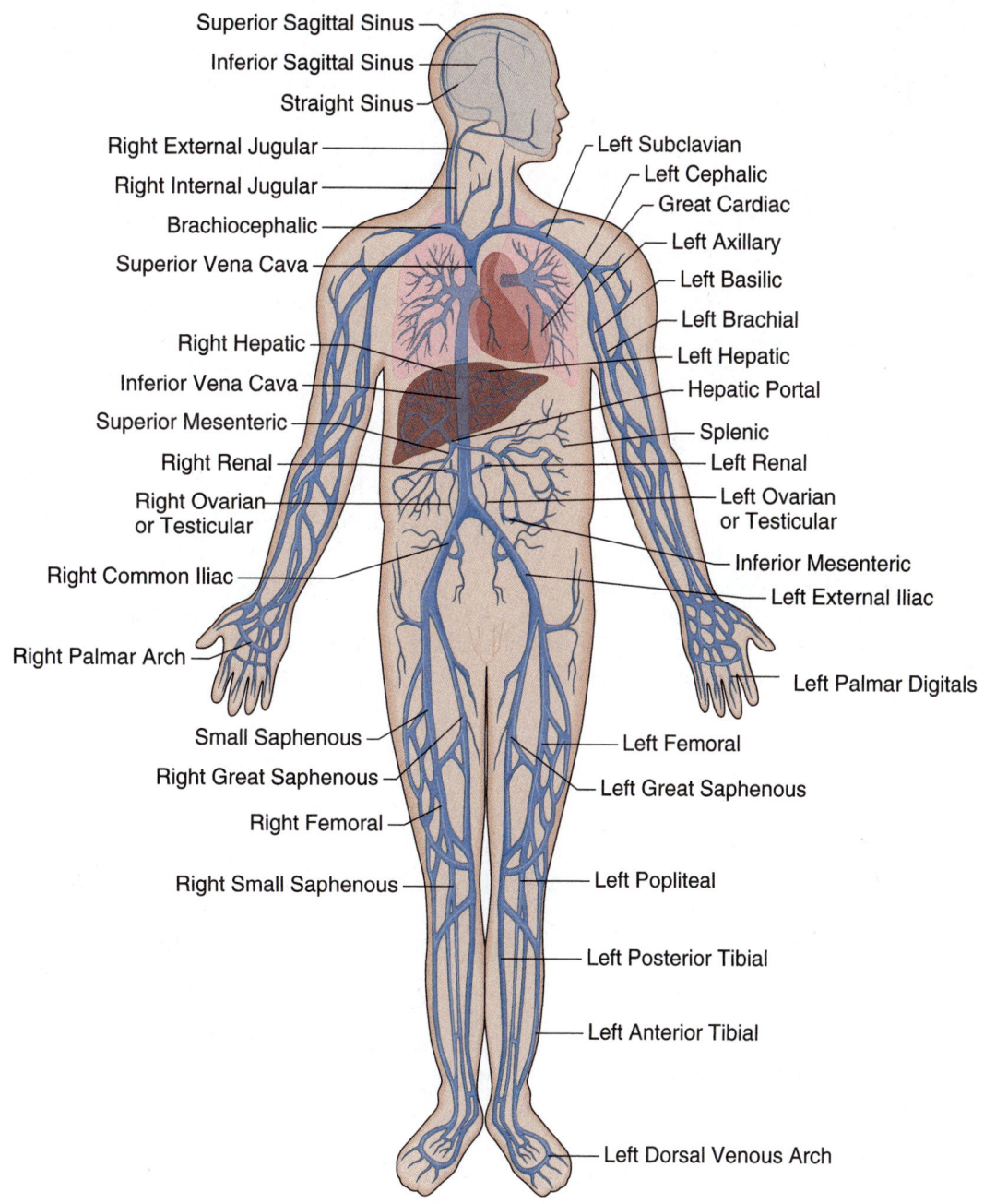

FIGURE 39-4 Veins of the body.

Protecting the Feet. Patients with impaired circulation are at great risk of ulceration, gangrene (Figure 39-5), and eventual amputation due to pressure or injuries to the feet and ankles. A small injury or ulcer can lead to major complications. Nursing assistant care for patients with peripheral vascular disease includes:

- Checking the feet and legs daily and reporting abnormalities to the nurse promptly.
- Protecting the feet from injury.
- Making sure the patient is wearing properly fit footwear when out of bed. The patient should always wear socks under shoes. He or she should never ambulate barefoot or wearing only socks on the feet.

- Not cutting toenails; this is a licensed health care provider responsibility. Avoid using sharp objects such as a nail file on the toes.
- Making sure bed linen is not too tight on the feet. Use a bed cradle, if ordered.
- Checking the skin under support hose regularly. Remove the hose periodically, according to the care plan.
- Making sure footwear is not too tight; if footwear fits tightly, notify the nurse.
- Propping bedfast patients' calves on pillows that are positioned lengthwise so that the heels are elevated from the surface of the bed. You may also position the

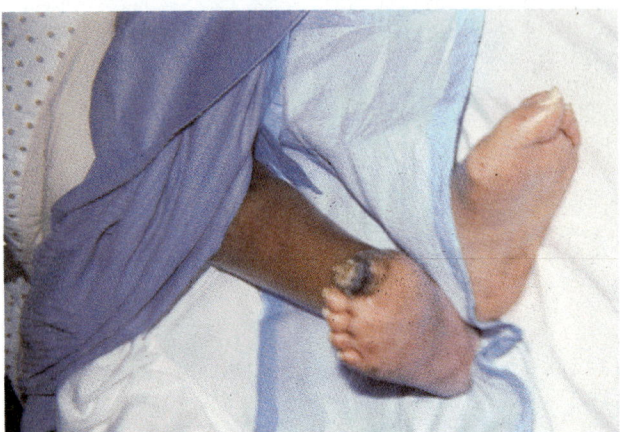

FIGURE 39-5 The big toe is gangrenous. The toe was eventually amputated, but the foot was saved.

patient so that the heels hang over the end of the mattress, with the soles of the feet against a footboard. Do not position the pillow width-wise under the calves. Heel protectors are excellent for preventing friction and shearing, but they do not prevent pressure on the heels.

Other devices are available to keep the heels off the surface of the bed to relieve pressure. Follow the care plan and the nurse's instructions.

- Making sure the feet are supported on footrests when the patient is using a wheelchair; avoid dragging them across the floor.

Atherosclerosis

Atherosclerosis is a common form of vascular disease.

- Roughened areas known as **atheromas**, which are growths developed over deposits of fatty materials, form on the inner walls of the arteries and narrow the vessels.
- The vessels of the heart and brain, and those leading to the legs from the body, are often affected.
- The atheromas gradually grow larger until they eventually block blood flow to the parts and organs served by the affected vessels (Figure 39-6).
- Sometimes clots that have formed over the irregular areas in the vessel walls break off and travel as emboli to block distant vessels.

guidelines *for*

Caring for Patients with Peripheral Vascular Disease

- Elevate the feet when the patient will be sitting in a chair for a long time. When the feet are not elevated, make sure that the patient's feet are flat on the floor. If they are not, support the feet with a footstool. Discourage the patient from crossing the legs when sitting. Discourage the patient from using circular garters.
- Discourage smoking—it interferes with circulation.
- Avoid using the knee gatch of the bed.
- Avoid using heating pads or hot water bottles. The patient may not feel temperatures that are too hot.
- Maintain body warmth. Make sure the patient has warm clothes, including socks that fit well. Provide blankets for the bed.
- Prevent injury to the feet:
  - Instruct the patient to wear shoes when out of bed.
  - Check to see that the shoes are in good repair and that they fit well.
  - Avoid pressure to the legs and feet from any source.

- Inspect the feet carefully when you bathe the patient or if the patient complains of any discomfort in the feet. Promptly report any signs of inflammation, injury, or circulatory problems:
  - Broken skin
  - Color change (redness, whiteness, or cyanosis)
  - Heat or coldness
  - Cracking between toes
  - Corns or calluses
  - Swelling
  - Pain
  - Loss of function
  - Drainage
- Bathe the feet regularly.
  - Dry thoroughly and gently between the toes.
  - Use a moisturizing lotion on the feet and legs if the skin is dry.
- Do not cut the toenails of patients who have peripheral vascular disease.

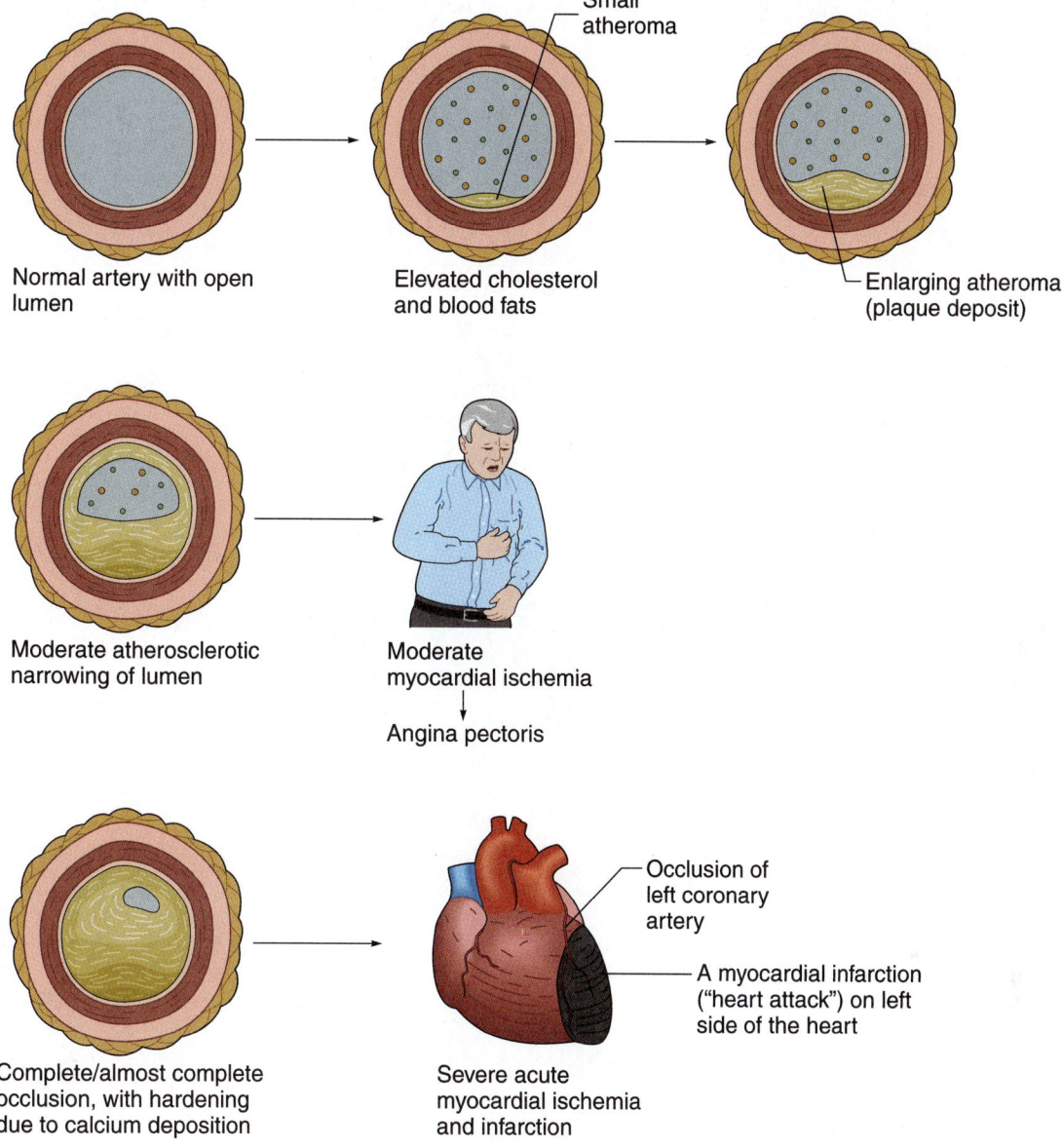

Small atheroma

Normal artery with open lumen

Elevated cholesterol and blood fats

Enlarging atheroma (plaque deposit)

Moderate atherosclerotic narrowing of lumen

Moderate myocardial ischemia

Angina pectoris

Complete/almost complete occlusion, with hardening due to calcium deposition

Severe acute myocardial ischemia and infarction

Occlusion of left coronary artery

A myocardial infarction ("heart attack") on left side of the heart

FIGURE 39-6 Cross-sections through a coronary artery that is undergoing atherosclerotic changes.

- The narrowing of vessels can lead to serious complications, such as:
  - Formation of blood clots
  - Angina pectoris
  - Myocardial infarction (MI)
  - Strokes (CVA) (also known as brain attacks)
  - Gangrene

Refer to Figure 39-7.

The exact cause of this vascular disease is unknown, but several factors seem to increase the risk that a person will develop it. These factors include:

- Hypertension
- Diabetes mellitus
- Overweight
- Heredity
- Smoking
- Stress
- Lack of exercise
- Diets high in cholesterol and fats

Treatment includes:

- Exercise
- Proper diet
- Reduction of stress
- Control of smoking and obesity

AFFECTED SITE   **COMPLICATION**

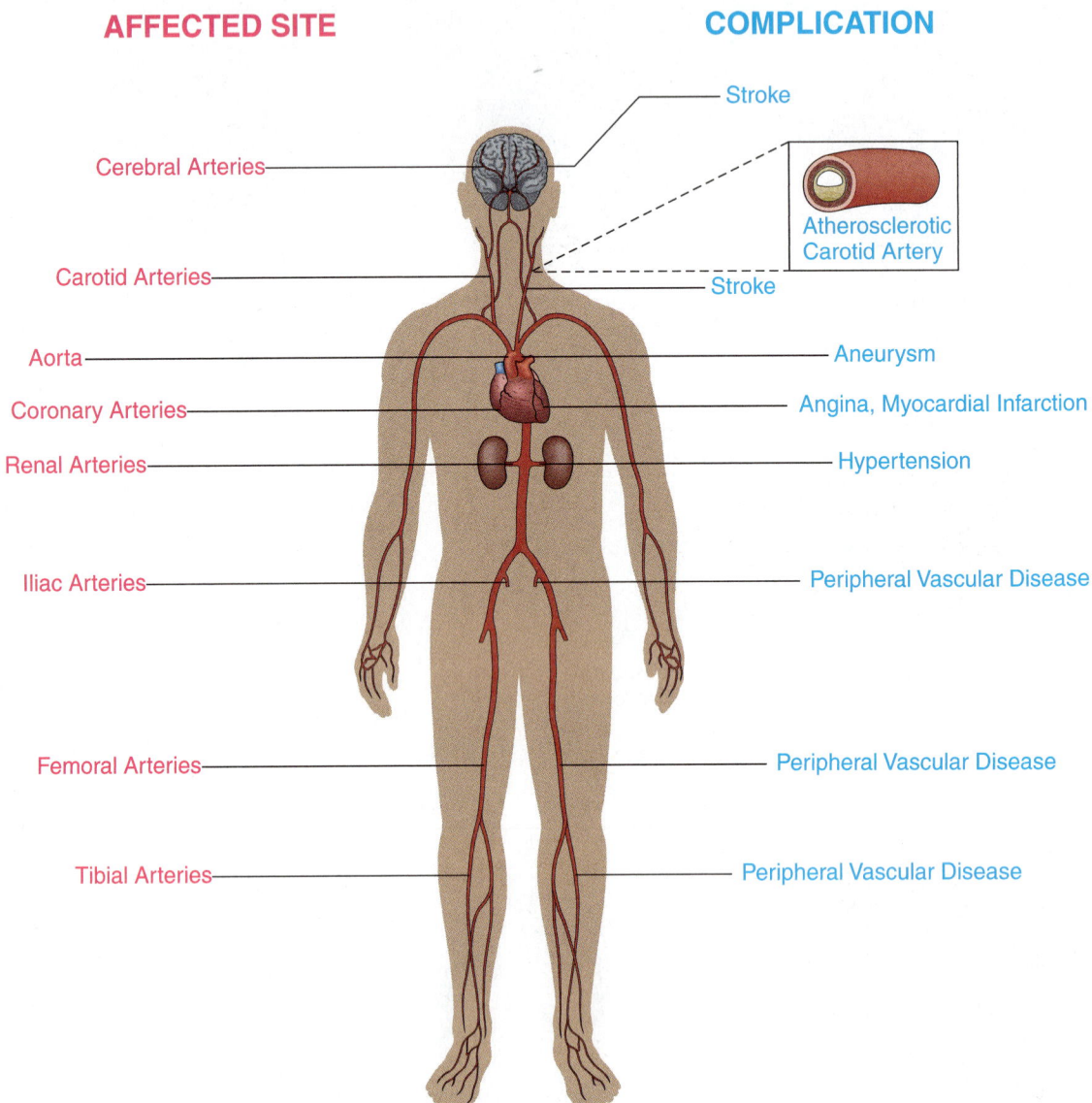

FIGURE 39-7 Atherosclerosis can cause disease in many parts of the body.

Varicose Veins

The veins can also cause problems. **Varicose veins** form when the valves in the veins in the legs become weakened (Figure 39-8). This means:

- The blood does not flow through the veins as it should.
- The veins become distended and visible through the skin.
- The veins may become inflamed (**phlebitis**).
- A blood clot may form in the vein.

Report the following signs:

- Pain or aching in the legs
- Signs of inflammation (warmth and redness)

Remember that you *never* rub or massage the area of a varicose vein.

Transient Ischemic Attack

Transient ischemic attack (**TIA**) is a temporary interruption of the blood flow to part of the brain. The patient may experience:

- Weakness or paralysis of any extremity or the face
- Vision problems
- Difficulty with speech
- Difficulty with swallowing

These symptoms come on quickly and may last from just a few minutes to 24 hours. There are no permanent effects. However, a TIA is usually a warning that a brain attack will occur at some time. If a patient has any of the symptoms listed, report them to the nurse immediately.

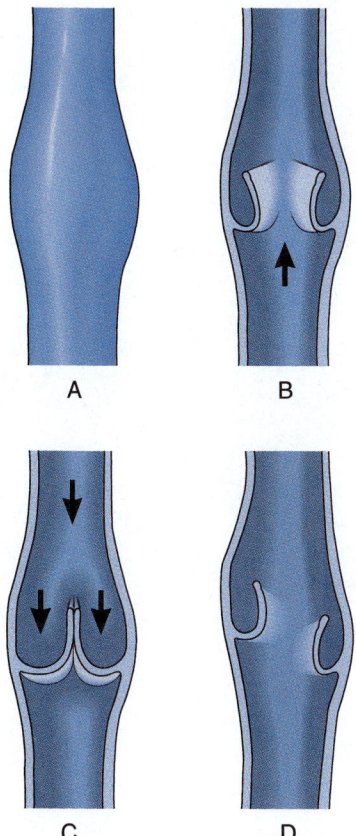

FIGURE 39-8 Veins contain valves to prevent the backward flow of blood. A. External view of the vein shows wider area of valve. B. Internal view with the valve open as blood flows through. C. Internal view with the valve closed. D. Vein with weakened valve that causes a varicose vein.

Hypertension

Hypertension is another name for high blood pressure. It may have no known origin, or it may follow illnesses that affect such organs as the:

- Blood vessels
- Kidneys
- Liver

High blood pressure:

- Promotes the development of atherosclerosis, which further narrows the vessels. This increases the blood pressure even more.
- Increases the stress on the heart.
- Increases the damage to the blood vessel walls, so they are more apt to rupture.
- Further limits the blood flow to the organs of the body.

Treatment may consist of:

- Drugs that lower the blood pressure
- Diet low in sodium
- Diet that promotes weight loss
- Regular exercise program
- Quitting smoking

- Surgical **sympathectomy** (a procedure in which the nerves that cause blood vessels to constrict are cut. When the nerves are cut, the blood vessels dilate.)
- Moderation in lifestyle
- Biofeedback techniques to lower the blood pressure

Report immediately any of the signs and symptoms of hypertension:

- Flushed face
- Dizziness
- Nosebleeds
- Headaches
- Changes in speech patterns
- Blurred vision

HEART CONDITIONS

Heart disease may sometimes be due to an infection, but most heart disease develops because of changes in the blood vessels. As the openings of the blood vessels become smaller, the heart must work harder and harder to do its job of pumping blood to the body.

Tips: Always take patient complaints of chest pain seriously. If a patient complains of chest pain, assist him or her to stop all activity and assume a comfortable position. Notify the nurse promptly.

Angina Pectoris

Angina pectoris is known as cardiac "pain of effort." You will recall that the blood vessels nourishing the heart are the coronary arteries. These vessels often are the site of atherosclerotic changes. In an angina attack, the vessels are unable to carry enough blood to meet the heart's demand for oxygen. This may develop:

- gradually over a period of time as atheromas develop.
- suddenly, as the vessels constrict.

Factors that precipitate (bring on) an attack include:

- Exertion
- Heavy eating
- Emotional stress

The signs and symptoms of angina pectoris that you should immediately report include:

- Pain when exercising or under stress. Stress causes a need for an immediate increase in coronary circulation. The pain is described as dull, with increasing intensity. It is usually centered under the breast bone (sternum), spreading to the left arm and up into the neck.
- Pale or flushed face.
- Patient who is freely perspiring.

Signs and symptoms may differ with individuals, but the symptoms are usually the same each time a person experiences an attack.

Treatment of angina pectoris consists of:

- Diagnosing hidden causes. A treadmill stress test is one method of doing this.
- Teaching the patient to avoid stress and sudden exertion.
- Drugs that relax the coronary arteries.
- Coronary artery bypass surgery.
- Angioplasty, a surgical procedure to open the vessels.

You may assist the patient who has angina pectoris by:

- helping the patient to avoid unnecessary emotional or physical stress.
- encouraging the patient not to smoke.
- reporting any signs or symptoms of an attack to the nurse at once.

Myocardial Infarction (Coronary Heart Attack)

The term **myocardial infarction** (**MI**), or heart attack, refers to a period in which the heart suddenly cannot function properly. There are different kinds of heart attacks. They differ in their severity and prognosis (expected outcome). Remember that the heart is muscle tissue and may become tired just as any muscle may tire. The cells of the heart require nourishment and oxygen like all other cells.

An acute myocardial infarction occurs when the coronary arteries, which nourish the heart, are blocked. Part of the heart muscle supplied by these vessels becomes **ischemic** (loses its blood supply). Unless circulation is restored quickly, the cells die (**infarction**). If too much tissue dies, the person cannot survive. Coronary heart attack is also called:

- **Coronary occlusion**—blockage of coronary arteries
- **Coronary thrombosis**—when a **thrombus** (stationary blood clot) forms at the site, blocking the blood flow
- **Coronary embolism**—when a moving clot or insoluble particle (**embolus**), which originated elsewhere and has moved, becomes lodged in the artery

Signs and Symptoms. The signs and symptoms of a heart attack include:

- Pain—may resemble severe indigestion. It is often described as "crushing" chest pain that radiates to the jaw and left arm (Figure 39-9).
- Nausea/vomiting.
- Irregular pulse and respiration.
- Perspiration (diaphoresis).
- Feelings of anxiety and weakness.
- Indications of shock, which include drop in blood pressure and pallor.
- Shortness of breath.
- Syncope (fainting).
- Restlessness.
- Cyanosis or gray skin color.

The signs and symptoms of a heart attack vary with the individual. The pain may be in the chest in some patients,

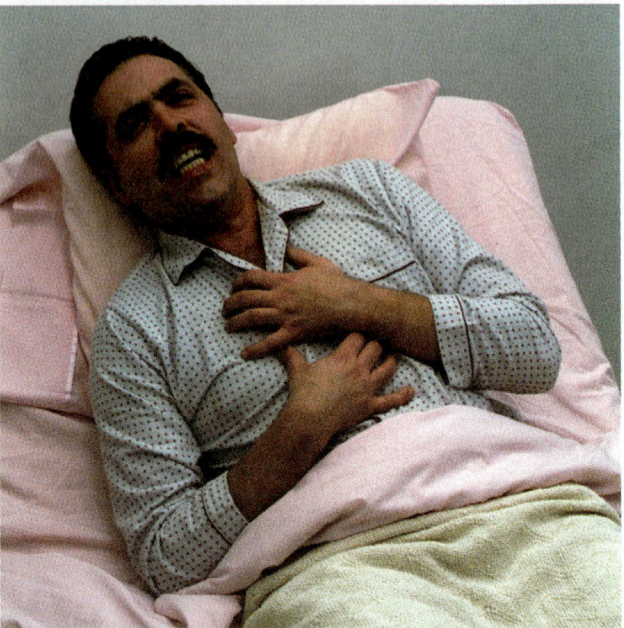

FIGURE 39-9 The patient having a heart attack usually experiences crushing chest pain that is described as, "the worst pain I've had in my life," or "It feels like an elephant is standing on my chest."

and radiate to the jaw or either arm. If a patient has chest pain combined with any other signs or symptoms, he or she should be evaluated by a health care professional. Have the patient stop any activity immediately and assume a comfortable position. Stay with the patient and call for assistance.

Immediate treatment has saved many people. The treatment is directed toward:

- Relieving the pain
- Reducing heart activity
- Altering the clotting ability of the blood
- Administering drugs to dissolve the clot

Nursing Care. During the acute stage, heart attack patients require professional care. Many hospitals provide intensive cardiac care units for these patients. Nursing care supports the therapy ordered. Special attention must be given to:

- Noting signs of a recurrence and reporting immediately to the nurse
- Watching for bleeding and reporting immediately
- Assisting with activities of daily living
- Monitoring vital signs
- Patient teaching to eliminate risk factors

Congestive Heart Failure (CHF)

The heart, like any other muscle, will enlarge and tire if it has to work against increasing pressure. When blood vessels narrowed by atherosclerosis increase the resistance to blood flow, and when there is severe damage to major organs like the liver and spleen, it is more difficult to maintain the circulation. The heart is not pumping well enough to meet the body's demands for oxygen. The heart muscle may also have been damaged and weakened by myocardial infarction. Other common causes are heredity, longstanding high blood pressure, alcohol abuse, and a virus. The heart must pump harder to maintain the internal flow of blood.

At first, the heart enlarges (**hypertrophy**) and makes up (**compensates**) for the additional workload. Eventually, however, it reaches a point when it can no longer compensate. Heart failure follows.

This form of heart disease is known as **congestive heart failure** (**CHF**) or **cardiac decompensation**. The condition got its name because of *failure* of the *heart* to pump efficiently, which results in *congestion* of the lungs. The heart tries to compensate for the problem, but this worsens the condition.

Signs and Symptoms. The signs and symptoms are the result of the heart being unable to pump the blood with sufficient force.

- Hemoptysis (spitting up blood)
- Cough
- Dyspnea (difficulty breathing)
- **Orthopnea** (difficulty in breathing unless sitting upright)
- **Ascites** (fluid collecting in the abdomen)
- Neck vein swelling
- Fatiguing easily
- Hypoxia (inadequate oxygen levels)
- Confusion
- Edema (swelling), which develops in dependent tissues and slows blood flow, congesting the vessels and allowing more fluid to enter the body spaces and tissues. It is most common in the abdomen, ankles, and fingers.
- Waking up at night with breathlessness
- Being unable to lie flat at night
- Fluid accumulation in the lungs
- Cyanosis, which occurs because fluid in the lungs makes gas exchange less efficient
- Irregular and rapid pulse.
- High blood pressure
- Palpitations (galloping heartbeat)
- Kidney malfunction in later stages
- Liver malfunction

Treatment. Treatment involves:
- Drugs to help the heart beat more strongly and regularly and to increase the output of fluids (**diuresis**) by the kidneys.
- Minimally invasive procedures may be done to open the arteries. These involve inserting a long tube into an artery in the groin. The tube is threaded through the system to the heart. A balloon on the tube is inflated to open blocked arteries (Figure 39-10A). The balloon-tipped catheter is removed and replaced with a **stent** (Figure 39-10B), a device that keeps the arteries open.

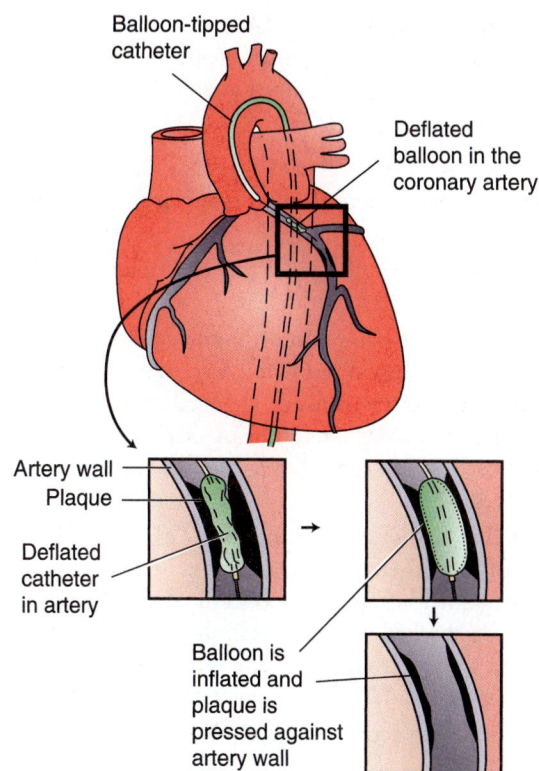

FIGURE 39-10A The balloon presses the plaque against the wall of the artery, making the vessel larger.

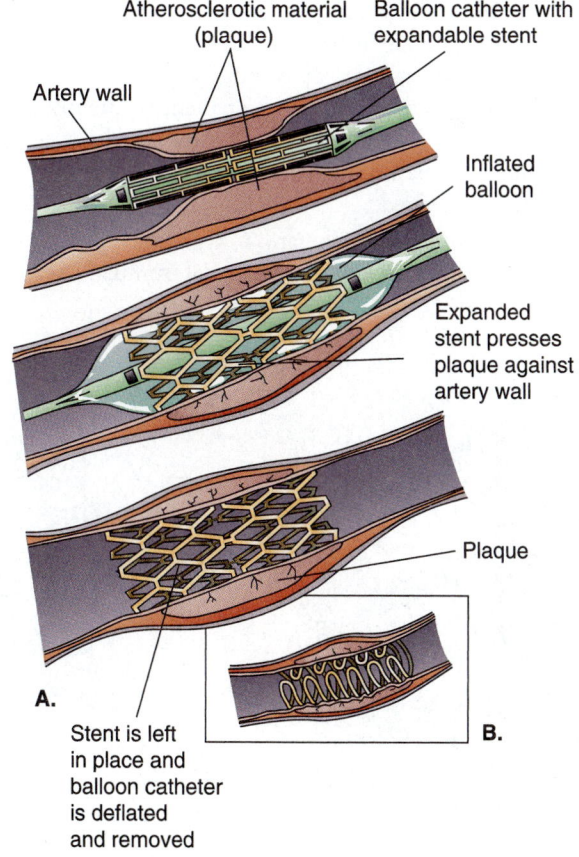

FIGURE 39-10B The stent is left in place to keep the artery open and the balloon is removed.

This procedure pushes the fatty deposits back against the artery walls, making more room for blood to flow through and preventing heart attack.

- Low-sodium diet.
- Restriction of fluids, if ordered.
- Weighing the patient daily to monitor level of fluid retention.
- Monitoring the apical pulse and observing for pulse deficit (Figure 39-11).
- Positioning the patient in orthopneic position or high Fowler's supported by pillows, or supported in a chair. The position must be changed frequently, but changes in position should be made slowly. Padded footboards help keep the weight of the bedding off the toes.
- Applying elasticized stockings or **TED hose**. TED hose are elastic anti-embolism stockings. TED hose and Ace bandages help channel blood to the deeper vessels. They must be checked often and reapplied every 6 to 8 hours. Check the extremities carefully for adequate circulation. The skin should be normal color and warm.
- Assisting with activities of daily living as needed.
- Attending to general hygiene. Complete bathing is tiring, but partial baths can stimulate circulation and provide comfort. Special attention must be given to the skin because the combination of position, edema, and poor circulation contributes to tissue breakdown. Allow the patient to be as independent with bathing as possible, unless you are instructed otherwise. Bathing is not normally a strenuous activity, but the patient with CHF may tire easily. Check the patient frequently while he or she is bathing. Be prepared to take over and complete the bath if the patient becomes short of breath or too tired.
- Assisting with oxygen therapy. Oxygen therapy may be provided either by face mask or nasal cannula. Because

cardiac patients often breathe through the mouth, the mouth tends to be very dry. Special mouth care may be needed.

- Providing for elimination. A bedside commode is convenient. The use of a commode is less tiring for the patient than using a bedpan for elimination.
- Encouraging adequate nutrition. Small, easily digested meals should be provided. You may need to assist in feeding the patient to prevent fatigue.
- Monitoring and recording fluid intake. Patients with acute heart failure may be given drugs that increase the output of urine and alter the heart rate. Measuring the intake and output and taking daily weights are ways of determining if fluid is being retained. The patient may be on fluid restriction (Unit 26) in the acute phase of the illness.
- Regularly checking vital signs. Sometimes the force of heart contraction, which propels the blood forward into the blood vessels, does not have enough strength to make the vessels expand.
- Keeping the feet elevated when the patient is up in a chair or wheelchair.
- Encouraging regular rest periods throughout the day.
- Assisting with exercise, as specified on the care plan.

Heart Block

Heart block is a condition that develops due to interference in the electrical current through the heart. (The flow of electrical current through the heart muscle makes the normal cardiac cycle possible.)

An electronic device called a **pacemaker** (Figure 39-12) is implanted under the chest muscles or in the abdomen. An electrode carries electrical current from the pacemaker directly into the heart muscle to replace the lost control. The electrical current signals the heart to contract. Some pacemakers send messages only if normal messages carried by the conduction system are delayed. This type of pacemaker is called a *demand pacemaker*. Other pacemakers send regular signals to keep the heart contracting at a preset rate.

When caring for a patient who has a pacemaker:

- count and record the pulse rate.
- report any irregularities or changes below the present rate.
- report any discoloration over the implant site.
- report hiccupping, because this may indicate problems.
- keep the patient away from microwave ovens and cellular phones, because they may disrupt the function of the pacemaker.

Patients usually function very well with pacemakers so long as they are adequately monitored.

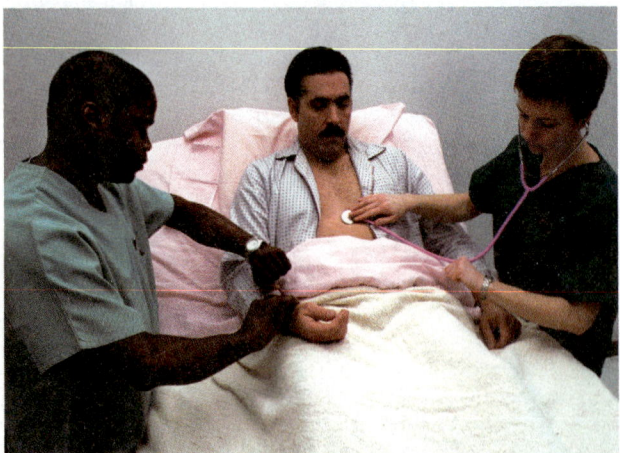

FIGURE 39-11 Ineffective heart contractions may cause a pulse deficit.

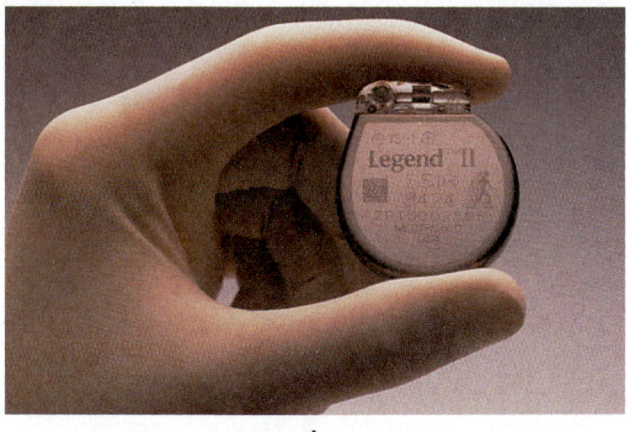

A

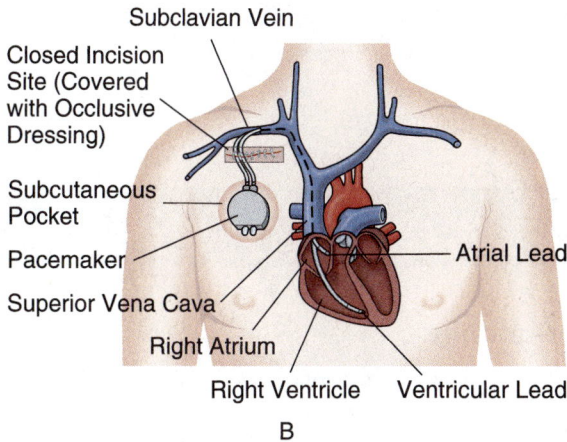

B

FIGURE 39-12 The electronic pacemaker sends electrical impulses to the heart muscle, causing it to contract. A. A typical pacemaker. B. The pacemaker is inserted under the skin with the electrode placed inside the heart, resting on the heart muscle. *(Photo courtesy of Medtronic, Inc.)*

BLOOD ABNORMALITIES

Blood abnormalities are often called *blood dyscrasias.*

Anemia

Anemia is a condition that results from a decrease in the quantity or quality of red blood cells. There are several causes, such as:

- Poor diet
- Low production of new red blood cells
- Blood loss, as in hemorrhage

Types of anemia include:

- Pernicious—inability to absorb vitamin B_{12} (most often seen in the elderly). Vitamin B_{12} is required by the body to produce red blood cells.
- Sickle cell—inability to form normal hemoglobin. Sickle cell anemia is transmitted genetically. It is seen most often in African Americans.

- Deficiency—inadequate intake of iron, inability to absorb iron, or excessive loss of iron.
- Dietary—inadequate intake of iron or vitamins in diet.

Signs and Symptoms. The person with anemia may:

- have little energy.
- be pale or jaundiced.
- have dyspnea.
- experience digestive problems.
- have a rapid pulse.
- complain of light-headedness.
- feel cold.
- experience dizziness.
- have an increased respiratory rate.

Treatment. Treatment is aimed at:

- Improving the quantity and quality of the blood by giving iron supplements
- Eliminating the basic cause of the disease
- Giving blood transfusions as needed
- Providing nutrients and nutritious meals

Leukemia

Leukemia is sometimes called cancer of the blood. The causes of the many forms of leukemia are not known. This disease may strike young or old. The number of white blood cells increases, but the white blood cells may be of poor quality. The number of erythrocytes and platelets decreases. Patients with leukemia are highly susceptible to infection. During the course of the disease, even minor trauma causes bleeding.

Treatment. Treatment is aimed at:

- Easing symptoms and keeping the patient comfortable.
- Maintaining normal blood levels. Transfusions may be needed to combat the anemia that accompanies the condition.
- Combating infection by using antibiotics.
- Slowing the production of abnormal white cells through chemotherapy and/or radiation therapy.

INFECTION CONTROL *Alert*

Patients with leukemia are at high risk of infection. Conscientiously apply the principles of standard precautions in all patient care. Notify the nurse promptly if signs or symptoms of infection are present.

Special Care

Patients who have cancer or anemia require special care. You must:

- Check vital signs
- Encourage rest
- Handle the patient very gently
- Encourage good nutrition
- Give special mouth care, because the mouth and tongue become sensitive
- Be sure to report any signs of bleeding, such as bruises or discolorations, because further blood loss makes the condition worse
- Keep patient warm
- Protect patient from falls that may result from dizziness or weakness
- Change the patient's position often, at least every 2 hours
- Provide emotional support

DIAGNOSTIC TESTS

Some techniques used to diagnose problems of the cardio-vascular system include:

- Blood chemistry tests, such as electrolyte panels
- Complete blood cell count (CBC)
- Electrocardiogram (ECG or EKG)
- Cardiac catheterization and angiogram—introduction of catheter and dyes into the vascular system under fluoroscopy
- Ultrasound—sound waves are bounced against tissues to reflect variations in tissue density

REVIEW

A. True/False.

Mark the following true or false by circling T or F.

1. T F The person with atherosclerosis is encouraged to smoke.
2. T F The treadmill test is done to detect hidden cardiac stress.
3. T F When warmth is needed by someone with peripheral vascular disease, a heating pad should not be used.
4. T F Another name for a heart attack is coronary infarction.
5. T F In leukemia, there is an increase in white cells.
6. T F The heart muscle shrinks as it undergoes hypertrophy.
7. T F An embolus is a moving blood clot.
8. T F Anemia is an example of a blood dyscrasia.
9. T F Hypertension is best treated with a high-sodium diet.
10. T F The person with CHF should be monitored for pulse deficit.

B. Matching.

Choose the correct word from Column II to match each phrase in Column I.

Column I	Column II
11. ____ inflammation of a vein	a. hypertension
12. ____ death of the heart muscle	b. edema
13. ____ another term for stroke	c. myocardial infarction
14. ____ high blood pressure	d. plasma
15. ____ blocking of the blood supply to the heart	e. phlebitis
	f. CVA
	g. hypotension
	h. coronary occlusion

C. Multiple Choice.

Select the one best answer for each of the following.

16. Which of the following is not a predisposing cause of atherosclerosis?
    a. Emboli
    b. Diabetes mellitus
    c. Heredity
    d. Stress

17. You suspect the patient needs immediate attention for a possible heart attack because the person
    a. has chest pain.
    b. complains of not feeling well.
    c. has ankle edema.
    d. has pink nailbeds.

18. Nursing care of the patient with anemia might include
  a. blood letting.
  b. good nutrition.
  c. pacemaker.
  d. chemotherapy.

19. The patient with anemia has a
  a. high energy level.
  b. pink, rosy skin.
  c. low energy level.
  d. slower than normal respiratory rate.

20. An attack of angina pectoris could be brought about by
  a. bathing in the evening.
  b. resting in bed.
  c. emotional stress.
  d. walking in the hallway.

D. Completion.

Complete the statements in the spaces provided.

21. Five specific tests used to diagnose cardiac, vascular, or blood abnormalities are:
  a. _____   **d.** _____
  b. _____   **e.** _____
  c. _____

22. Six predisposing factors for atherosclerosis are:
  a. _____   **d.** _____
  b. _____   **e.** _____
  c. _____   **f.** _____

E. Nursing Assistant Challenge.

Mrs. O'Brien is only 38 years old, but has been diagnosed with hypertension. Recently she experienced dizziness and weakness and had difficulty speaking for a short period. The doctor suspects she had a TIA. Complete the statements in questions 23–30 by choosing the correct word from the following list.

blurred vision	low
brain	permanent
discouraged	potassium
encouraged	sodium
exercise	stroke
high	temporary
hypertension	

23. Hypertension means this patient has _____ blood pressure.

24. The TIA means there was a _____ interruption of the blood flow to the _____.

25. The diet for this patient should be low in _____.

26. Smoking should be _____.

27. The TIA indicates that a _____ will probably occur at some time.

28. Treatment for hypertension includes regular _____.

29. _____ is a sign that should be reported immediately.

30. Nosebleeds are a danger sign for people with _____.

EXPLORING THE WEB

Description	Location
General cardiology information, Peripheral vascular disease	*http://cardio-info.com* *http://www.footcare4u.com*
American Heart Association, Heart Profilers	*http://www.americanheart.org*
Cardiovascular Institute of the South	*http://www.cardio.com*
Combined Health Information Database	*http://chid.nih.gov/subfile/subfile.html*
CVNet	*http://www.cvmg.com/cv-net*
Guide to Heart Disease	*http://heartdisease.miningco.com*
Heart Center Online	*http://www.heartcenteronline.com*
National Heart, Lung, and Blood Institute	*http://www.nhlbi.nih.gov*
Preventive Health Center	*http://www.md-phc.com*
Women's Heart Institute	*http://www.womensheartinstitute.com*

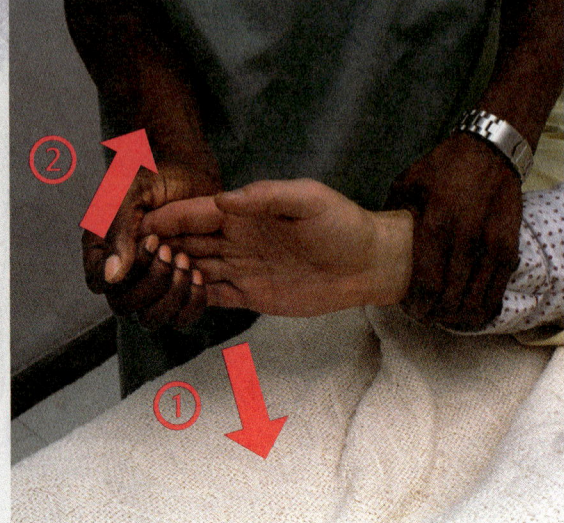

Musculoskeletal System

objectives

After completing this unit, you will be able to:

- Spell and define terms.
- Describe the location and functions of the musculoskeletal system.
- Describe some common conditions of the musculoskeletal system.
- Describe the nursing assistant actions related to the care of patients with conditions and diseases of the musculoskeletal system.

- List seven specific diagnostic tests for musculoskeletal conditions.
- Demonstrate the following procedures:
  - Procedure 99 Applying an Arm Sling
  - Procedure 100 Procedure for Continuous Passive Motion
  - Procedure 101 Performing Range-of-Motion Exercises (Passive)

vocabulary

Learn the meaning and the correct spelling of the following words and phrases:

abduction	compression fracture	insertion	radial deviation
abduction pillow	continuous passive	inversion	range-of-motion (ROM)
adduction	motion (CPM)	involuntary muscle	exercises
amputation	countertraction	laminectomy	remissions
arthritis	degenerative joint	ligament	rheumatoid arthritis (RA)
atrophy	disease (DJD)	nucleoplasty	rotation
avulsion fracture	depressed fracture	oblique fracture	spica cast
bursae	dorsiflexion	open (compound)	spiral fracture
bursitis	ecchymosis	fracture	stimulus
cardiac muscle	eversion	open reduction/	supination
cartilage	exacerbation	internal fixation	tendon
cervical traction	extension	origin	total hip arthroplasty
closed (simple)	fibromyalgia	osteoarthritic joint	(THA)
fracture	flexion	disease (OJD)	transverse fracture
comminuted fracture	fracture	osteoporosis	trapeze
compartment	fusion	pathologic fracture	ulnar deviation
syndrome	gout	pelvic belt traction	vascular
complete fracture	greenstick fracture	phantom pain	vertebrae
compound (open)	impacted fracture	plantar flexion	visceral muscle
fracture	incomplete fracture	pronation	voluntary muscle

THE MUSCULOSKELETAL SYSTEM

The bony frame of the body is called the *skeleton*. Tissue that is made up of contractile fibers (fibers that contract and relax) or cells that produce movement are called *muscles*. Together, the skeleton and muscles are termed the musculoskeletal system.

The musculoskeletal system includes:

- Skeletal muscles
- Bones
- Joints
- Tendons
- Ligaments

The system functions to:

- Give shape and form to the body
- Protect and support delicate body parts
- Permit movement
- Produce some blood cells
- Store calcium and phosphorus

When muscles, bones, or joints have been injured, a long period of rest and inactivity may be required for the part to heal. During this period, it is important that all other mov-ing parts get sufficient exercise. Bones that are not stressed lose calcium and become less functional.

Structure and Function

Bones. It will be helpful for you to learn the names and general location of the bones of the body. To learn the names, study the skeleton in Figure 40-1A and the skull in Figure 40-1B. Note that the same number and kinds of bones are found on one side of the midline as on the other.

The bones:

- Number 206
- May share the same name. For example, there are:
  - 24 ribs helping to form the chest
  - 56 phalanges, the finger bones
  - 2 femurs, the thigh bones
  - 31 bones (vertebrae) in the spinal column. Small discs or pads of cartilage with soft, gel-like centers between the vertebrae help to cushion these bones. The anterior (front) of the vertebrae support the head and body. The posterior (rear) portions form a tunnel that surrounds the delicate spinal cord and nerves.
- Are of different shapes and sizes, such as
  - long, like the femur, humerus, ulna, and radius

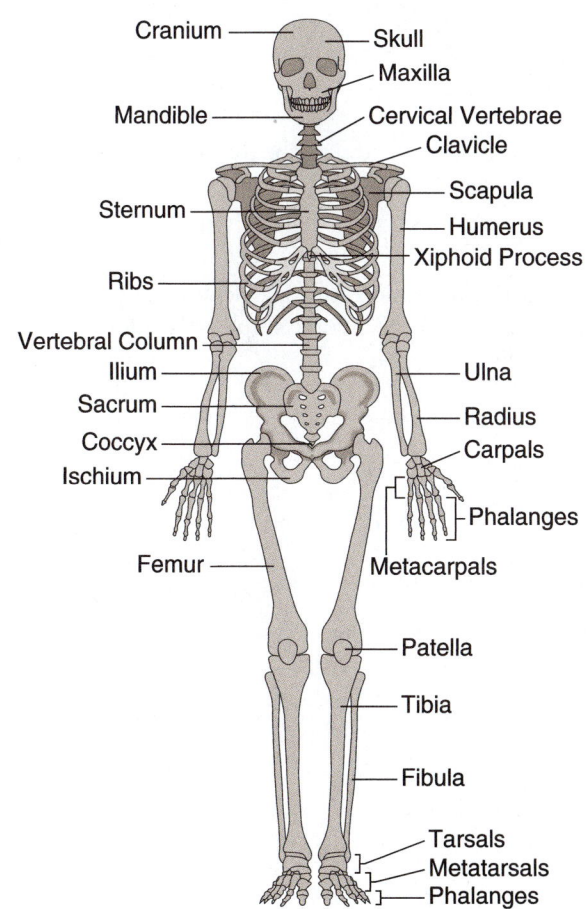

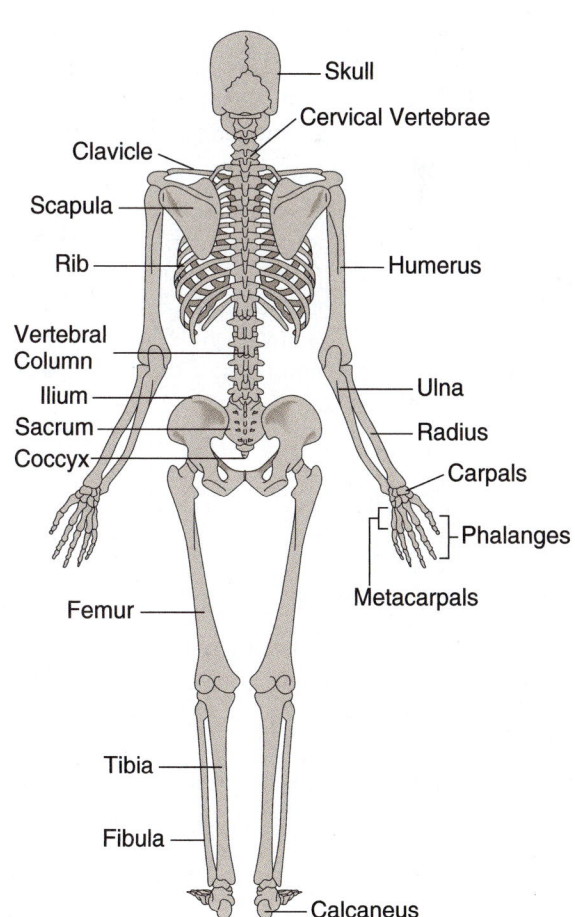

FIGURE 40-1A The human skeleton.

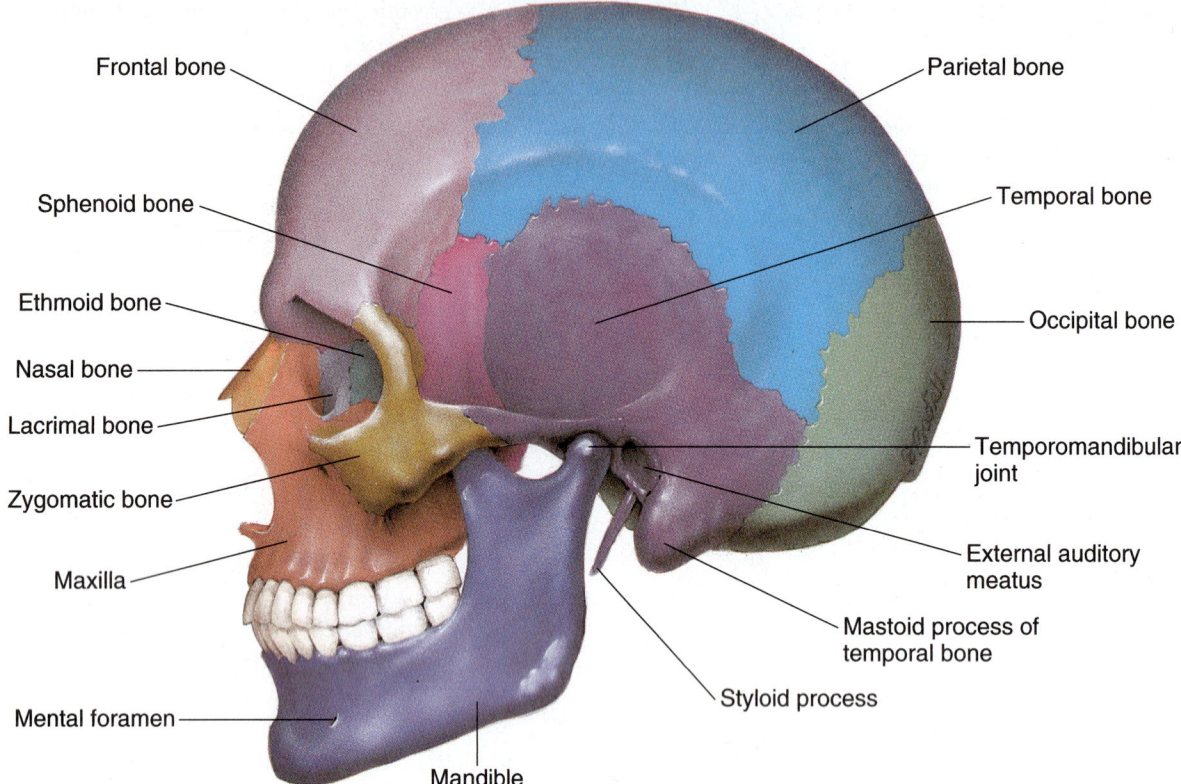

FIGURE 40-1B Bones of the skull.

- short, like the phalanges, carpals, and tarsals
- flat, like the scapula and cranial bones
- irregular, like the vertebrae and mandible
- Meet one another to form joints

Joints. Joints are points where bones come together and there is the possibility of movement. Without movable joints, walking, bending, lifting, and sitting would not be possible. Joints are capable of different movements depending upon the type of joint (Figure 40-2). **Ligaments** are strong bands of fibrous tissues that hold the bones together and support the joints. **Bursae** are small sacs of synovial fluid that are located around joints and help reduce friction.

Special terms are used to describe the different movements in a diarthrotic joint.

- **Flexion**: Decreasing the angle between two bones (Figure 40-3A). For example, bending the elbow.
- **Extension**: Increasing the angle between two bones (Figure 40-3B). For example, straightening the elbow.

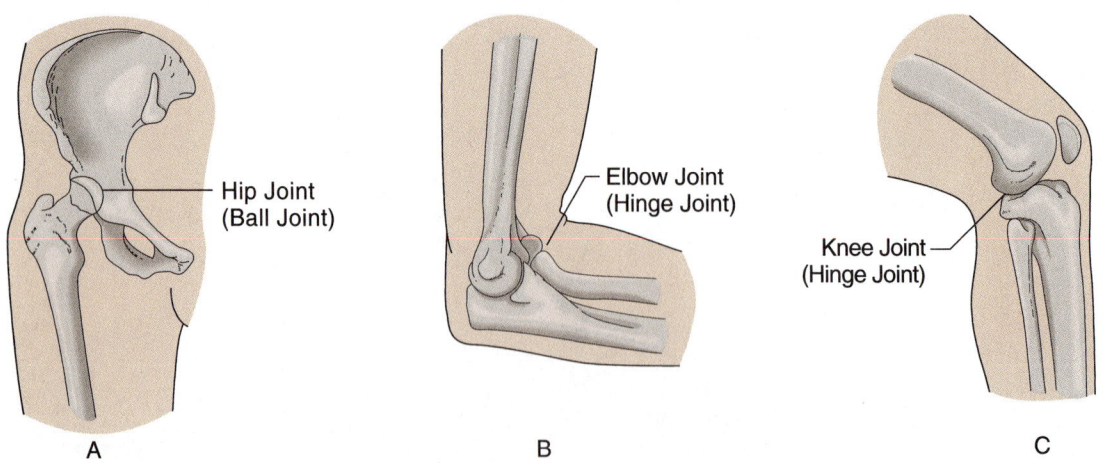

A   B   C

FIGURE 40-2 Types of joints: A. Ball joint. B. and C. Hinge joints.

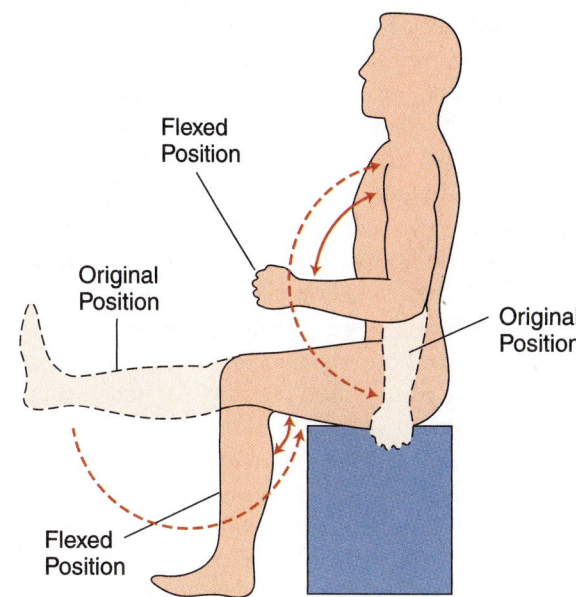

FIGURE 40-3A Flexion—bending a joint.

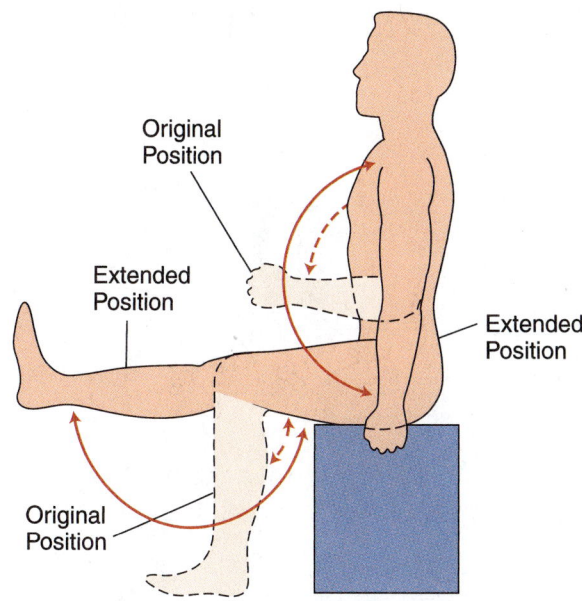

FIGURE 40-3B Extension—straightening a joint.

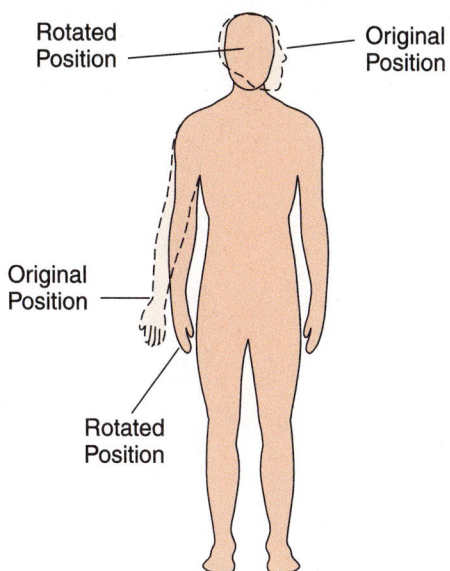

FIGURE 40-3C Rotation—moving a joint in a circular motion.

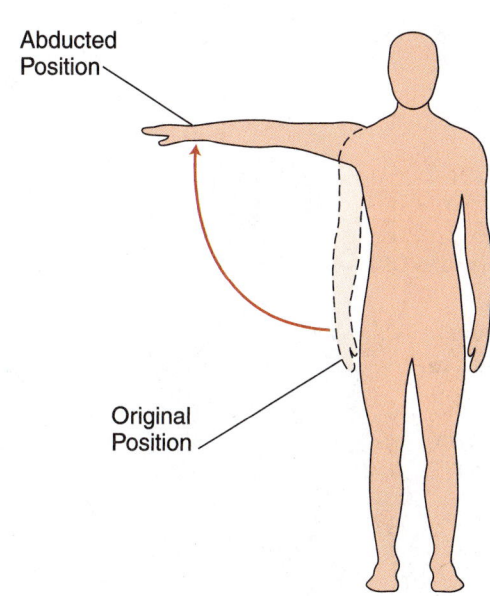

FIGURE 40-3D Abduction—moving an extremity away from the body.

- **Rotation**: Circular motion in a ball-and-socket joint (Figure 40-3C). For example, the shoulder and hip joints, which can move in all directions.
- **Abduction**: Moving away from the midline (Figure 40-3D).
- **Adduction**: Moving toward the midline (Figure 40-3E).

Muscles. There are more than 500 muscles in the body (Figures 40-4A and B). The muscles work in groups. There are three kinds of muscles:

1. **Cardiac muscle** forms the wall of the heart.
2. **Voluntary muscles** are skeletal muscles that are attached to bones. When we wish to pick up

something, for instance, we can make our muscles contract and perform the necessary movements.
3. **Involuntary** or **visceral muscles** form the walls of organs. These muscles operate without our conscious control.

Muscles receive their names in three ways:

1. Their location. For example, rectus femoris near the femur
2. Their shape. For example, trapezius—trapezoidal shape
3. Their action. For example, flexors—bring about flexion

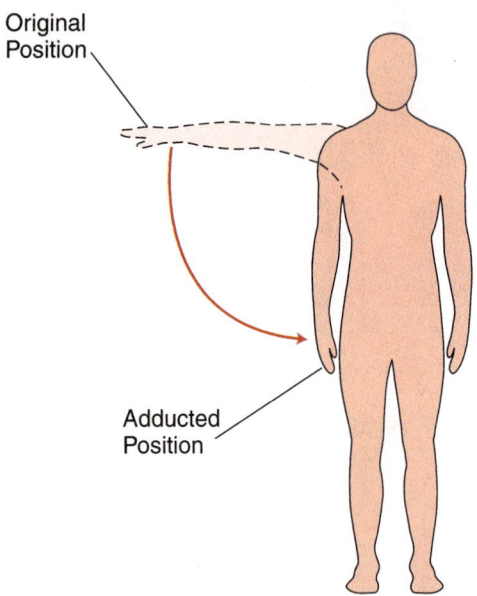

FIGURE 40-3E Adduction—moving an extremity back toward the body.

You can easily locate the major muscle groups responsible for an activity if you remember that:

- Muscles can only shorten (contract) and lengthen (relax). Contraction occurs when nerves bring the message (**stimulus**) to the muscle cells. Muscles relax when there is no stimulus.

- Muscles have two points of attachment to the bone. As they stretch from one point (**origin**) to the other (**insertion**), they cross over one or more joints.

- Muscles are not inserted directly into bones. Rather, they are connected to the bone by strong, fibrous bands of connective tissues called **tendons**. Ligaments support bones at joints.

- As muscles contract, they shorten, pulling their points of origin and insertion closer together. For example, bending the forearm at the elbow takes place when the biceps muscle contracts. The biceps muscle is on the anterior arm and extends from the shoulder to below the elbow. At the same time, the triceps muscle relaxes. This muscle is attached to the posterior shoulder and to the arm below the elbow. To straighten the arm at the elbow, the triceps contracts and the biceps relaxes.

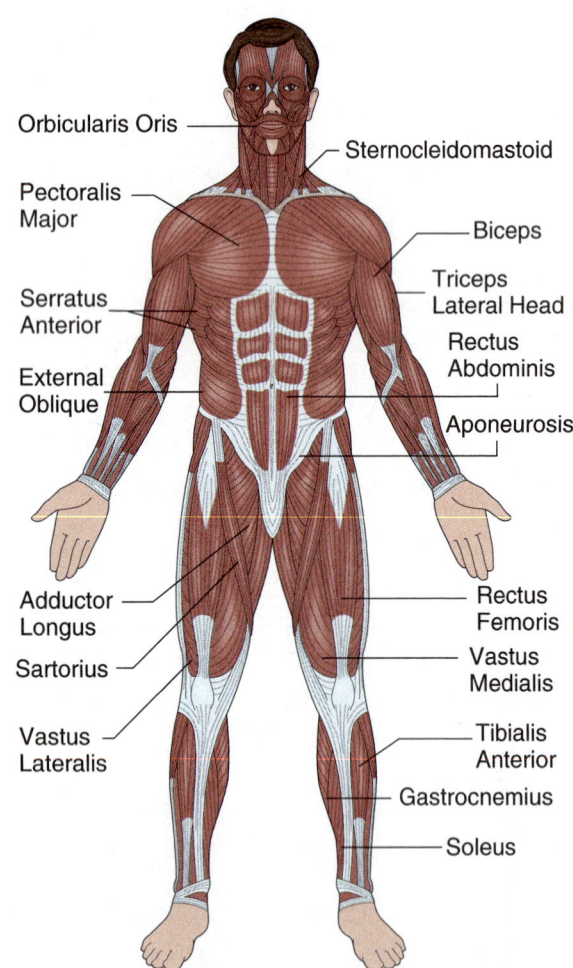

FIGURE 40-4A Major muscles of the body, anterior view.

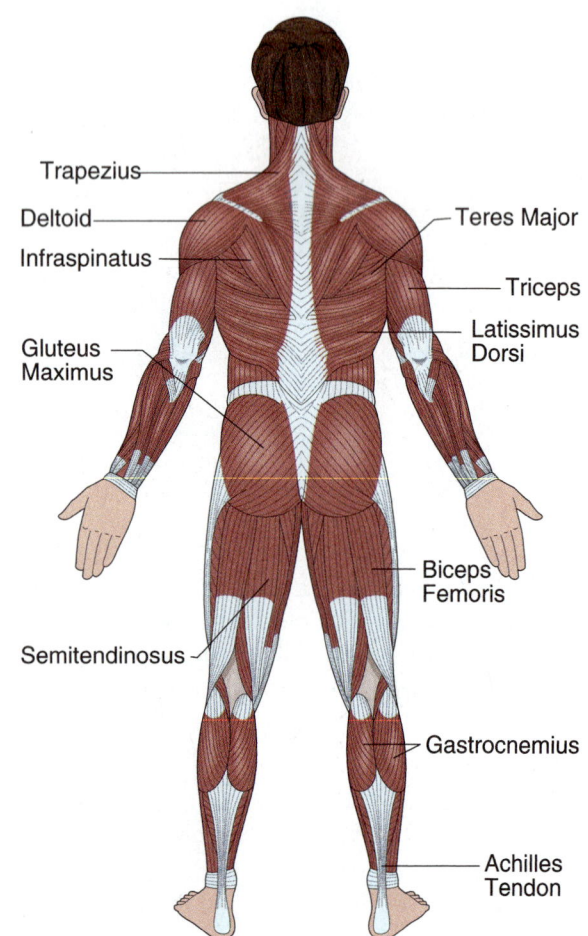

FIGURE 40-4B Major muscles of the body, posterior view.

- The more muscles are used, the more powerful they become. The less muscles are used, the weaker they become.

COMMON CONDITIONS

Many conditions can affect the bones, muscles, tendons, ligaments, and joints. Often, when one of these structures is diseased or injured, the surrounding tissues are also involved.

Bursitis

Bursae are small sacs of fluid found around joints. They help to reduce friction when muscles move. At times, the bursae can become inflamed and the tissues around a joint may become painful. This condition is known as bursitis. Treatment of bursitis includes:

- Applications of heat to promote healing
- Immobilization so that the joint cannot move, to relieve pain around the joint
- Removal of excess fluid from the joint by aspiration with a needle
- Administration of steroids

Arthritis

The term arthritis (Figure 40-5) means inflammation of the joints. It may develop following an acute injury, or it may be chronic and progressive. The most common forms of chronic arthritis are:

1. Rheumatoid arthritis (RA) affects the joint tissues and the joint lining, and can affect any other body system. It is a serious form of arthritis that can occur in persons of any age. The cause is not specifically known. It is believed to be an autoimmune response. It usually follows an intermittent course. RA has

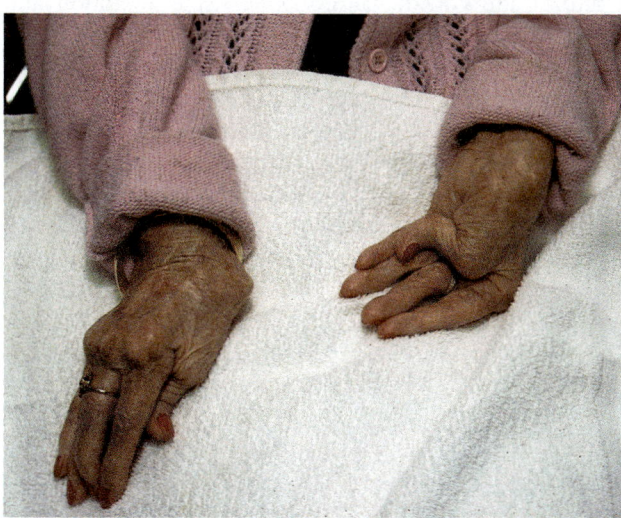

FIGURE 40-5 These deformities, caused by rheumatoid arthritis, make hand movement difficult.

exacerbations, or times in which the condition seems to worsen, and remissions, or times in which the disease appears stable. The involved joints may feel hot to touch. The condition causes reduced joint function and deformities. These can be severe and disabling.

2. Osteoarthritic joint disease (OJD) or degenerative joint disease (DJD) affects the cartilage covering the ends of the bones that form a joint. Cartilage breaks down and the ends of the bones rub together, causing pain and deformity. The joints most often affected are the weight-bearing joints. Several factors seem to contribute to the disease process, including:

   - Aging
   - Trauma
   - Obesity

   The most common symptom of osteoarthritis is pain. This is usually described as a deep, aching pain that occurs after exercise, weight bearing, or exertion. It is often relieved by rest. Changes in the weather may also cause pain. Other symptoms include limited ability to move and stiffness, particularly upon arising in the morning. This also may occur after strenuous exercise or physical overactivity. In some individuals, an audible grating sound can be heard in the joints during movement. Osteoarthritis may cause redness and swelling in the joints. Conditions such as obesity and stress aggravate the symptoms.

3. Gout (gouty arthritis) is a metabolic disease that can be severely disabling. It is caused by increased uric acid in the bloodstream, which deposits in the joints and forms crystals that cause pain. It can occur in any joint, but is most common in the feet and legs. The great toe is often the first joint affected. Gout also follows a course of remission and exacerbation. It can lead to complete disability, hypertension, and chronic renal disease. The cause is unknown, but it is thought to be caused by a genetic defect in the ability to metabolize uric acid. The affected joints may be red or cyanotic in appearance. The patient may have a low-grade fever during this time. After the initial, painful period, symptoms subside. The condition goes into remission and the patient will be pain-free for a period of time. The next attack is usually more painful and severe than the first. Eventually, chronic disease sets in. It is marked by constant pain, tenderness, and swelling in the joints. Other body systems may be affected in this stage. Dietary restrictions are used to reduce the uric acid level in the blood. The dietitian will plan a diet that restricts the amount of red meat and foods rich in purines.

Arthritis can cause mild discomfort to severe deformities and disability. Patients with arthritis are at high risk of contractures (Figure 40-6). If permitted by your facility, place patients with this condition in the prone position periodically. This reduces the risk of contractures of the hips and

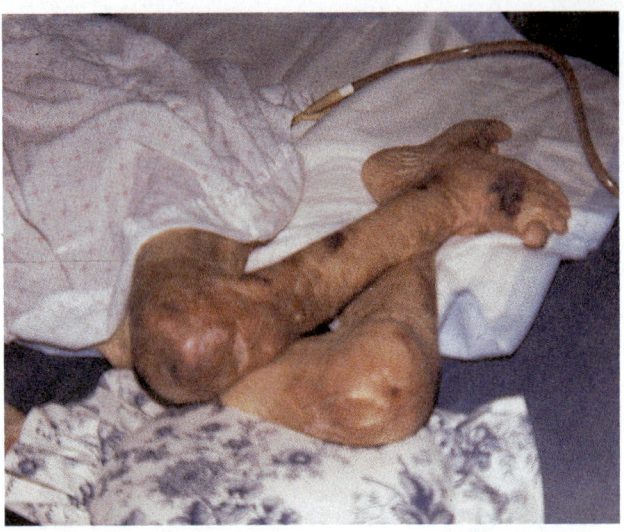

FIGURE 40-6 This patient has many problems with her legs, including arthritic deformities and contractures.

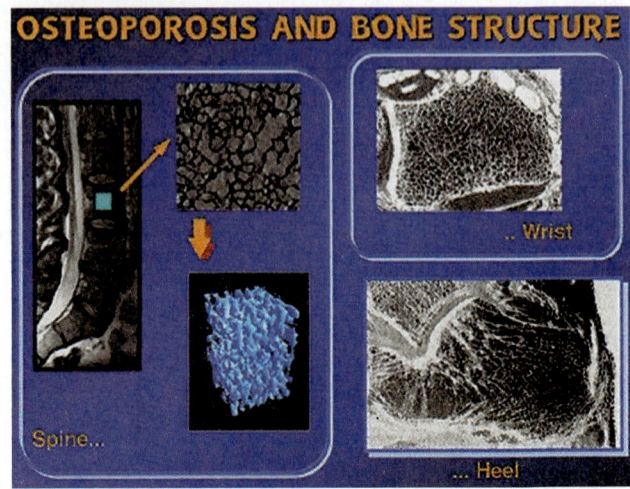

FIGURE 40-7 Bone loss from osteoporosis causes painful, disabling fractures in both sexes. About 40% of women and 13% of men will suffer a bone fracture due to osteoporosis in their lifetime. (*Courtesy of Sharmila Majumdar, Ph.D., Professor, University of California, San Francisco*)

knees. Avoid placing pillows under the knees or elevating the knee area of the bed. Using a small, flat pillow under the head and neck is best. A large pillow pushes the neck into a position of flexion. You may be assigned to perform range-of-motion exercises on patients with arthritis. Be very gentle. Avoid moving joints past the point of resistance.

Treatment of arthritis includes:

- Relief of pain
- Balance of rest and exercise
- Joint immobilization where there is pain
- Weight control to relieve pressure on the joints
- Medication to relieve pain and reduce the inflammation
- Physical therapy when inflammation subsides, to maintain joint mobility
- Replacement of badly damaged joints by surgery
- Use of splints, braces, and adaptive equipment to enable the patient to get the most range of motion from injured joints
- Exercise of arthritic joints in warm water (with or without whirlpool action) to maintain function and relieve pain
- Prevention of deformities and contractures

Osteoporosis

Osteoporosis is a metabolic disorder of the bones. It is most common in elderly females, but can occur in males. Bone mass is lost, causing bones to become porous and spongy (Figure 40-7). Because of this, affected bones are at very high risk for fracture. Fractures can occur spontaneously, such as when the patient is walking. They can also occur by moving or turning the patient in bed or during transfers.

The cause of osteoporosis is unknown. It is thought to result from years of inadequate calcium intake. Other potential causes are declining adrenal function, faulty protein metabolism, estrogen deficiency, and lack of exercise or activity.

Signs and Symptoms. The first sign of osteoporosis is usually a fracture. Commonly, the patient moves or lifts something and hears a "pop" or snapping sound in a bone. This frequently occurs in the lower back or hip. The patient who is walking may suddenly fall. In this case, the fall is the *result* of the fracture; in most falls, the opposite is true. After the initial incident, the area is very painful, particularly upon movement. Sometimes the onset of osteoporosis begins with a curvature of the spine and loss of height. The back progressively weakens, straining the neck, hips, and low back. Spontaneous fractures may occur during movement or as a result of a minor injury.

Treatment. The goals of treatment are to prevent further fractures and control pain. Gentle range-of-motion and other exercises may be ordered. Splints, braces, and other devices may be ordered to support weakened bones. Patients are given estrogen replacement and other drugs to replace calcium and bone mass. You must handle the patient very gently. If you are assigned to perform range-of-motion exercises, do so slowly and carefully. Avoid stretching the joint past the point of resistance. Use a mechanical lift for transfers whenever possible. This is less traumatic than pulling on the patient. Make sure you have extra help for all procedures in which you will be moving or positioning the patient. Follow the care plan exactly in the care of the patient.

Fibromyalgia

Fibromyalgia is a common chronic pain syndrome for which there is no known cause or cure. It affects more women than men. The area between the shoulder blades and the bottom of the neck is often painful. The pain is described as either a general soreness or a gnawing ache, and stiffness is usually worst in the morning. Although this is a common problem, it is very controversial. Some physicians believe that there is no physical cause, and that psychiatric problems or sleep disorders are responsible for the patient's symptoms. The condition can be very painful and interfere with the patient's quality of life and daily activities. To be diagnosed with this condition, the patient must meet certain criteria, such as:

- having pain on both sides of the body
- having pain both above and below the waist
- having pain upon palpation in at least 11 of 18 specified body sites (Figure 40-8)

Signs and Symptoms. Signs and symptoms of fibromyalgia are:

- pain and stiffness
- feeling abnormally tired
- waking up tired
- pain upon touch in certain areas of the body

Treatment. Treatment involves pain medications and exercise. Muscle-relaxant medications and antidepressants are sometimes used. Some patients use alternative and complementary therapies to relieve pain and stiffness. The most common complementary therapies used to treat this condition are:

- massage
- biofeedback
- acupuncture
- hypnosis
- relaxation, meditation, and other forms of stress management

Because the cause of fibromyalgia is not known, there is no prevention or cure for this condition. Fibromyalgia complicates treatment for many other medical problems because of the underlying pain and difficulty in assuming some positions necessary for examination and treatment.

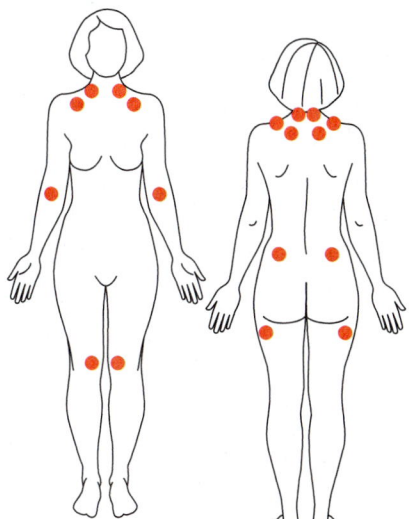

FIGURE 40-8
The patient must have pain at 11 of 18 specific areas of the body for a diagnosis of fibromyalgia.

Tips: Most patients with fibromyalgia are middle-aged women. They are often very deconditioned because pain and fatigue have caused them to limit movement and stop exercising. The pain and fatigue of fibromyalgia often improve with mild exercise, and the physician will usually order some type of exercise program. Encourage the patient to adhere to the program, but not to push to the point of exhaustion. Patients should start exercising slowly, and should not try to keep the same exercise pace as they did before the fibromyalgia developed. A restful night's sleep will improve comfort and mood. Be attentive to the patient's needs for uninterrupted sleep. Plan your care to allow the patient to sleep for prolonged periods without interruption.

Fractures

A fracture is any break in the continuity of a bone. Falls are the most common cause of fractures. If the bone breaks through the skin, the injury is called an *open compound fracture*. If the bones do not break through the skin, the fracture is known as *closed*.

Fractures (Figure 40-9) are classified by the type of break in the bone and whether or not the skin is broken:

- A complete fracture involves a break across the entire cross-section of the bone. It is often displaced, or improperly aligned, and must be reduced and straightened.
- An incomplete fracture involves only part of the cross-section of bone.
- A closed or simple fracture (Figure 40-9A) occurs when the skin is intact and not broken.
- An open or compound fracture (Figure 40-9B) occurs when the skin over the fracture is broken. The bone may or may not protrude.
- A pathologic fracture is a fracture in a diseased bone. It occurs as a result of osteoporosis, a tumor, or cancer.

The pattern of a fracture describes the manner in which the bone is broken:

- A greenstick fracture (Figure 40-9C) occurs when only one side of the bone is broken and the other side is bent. This fracture is common in children, whose bone growth is incomplete. The bones tend to bend like young trees; hence the name "greenstick" fracture.
- A transverse fracture (Figure 40-9 D), breaks completely across the bone.
- An oblique fracture (Figure 40-9E) runs at an angle across the bone.
- A spiral fracture (Figure 40-9F) twists around the bone.
- A comminuted fracture (Figure 40-9G) involves shattering and splintering of the bone into more than three fragments.
- A depressed fracture (Figure 40-9H) is seen only in fractures of the skull and face. This type of fracture depresses the bone and drives fragments inward.

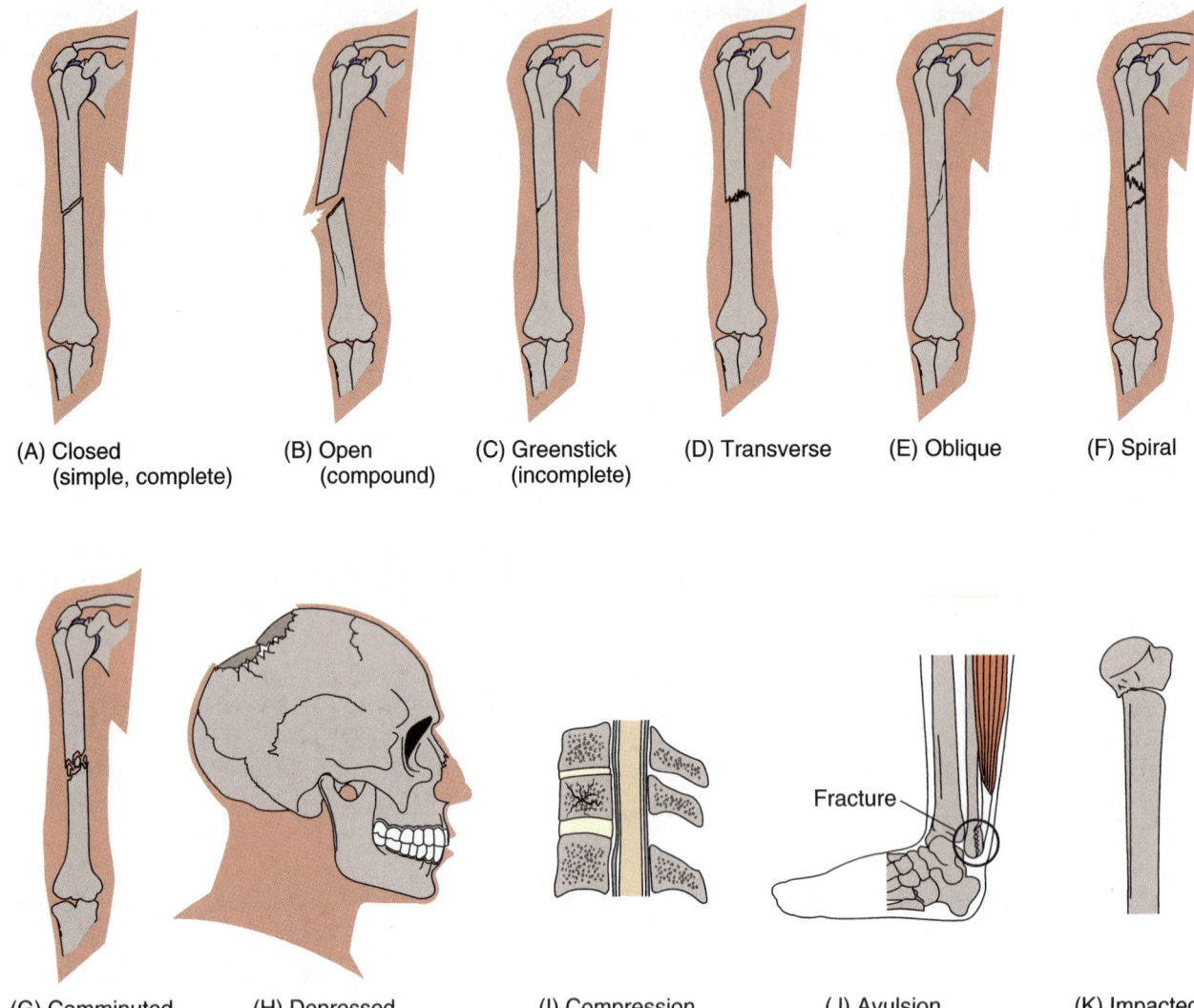

FIGURE 40-9 Types and patterns of fractures.

- A **compression fracture** (Figure 40-9I) is seen only in the vertebrae of the spine. This type of fracture collapses the bone inward.
- An **avulsion fracture** (Figure 40-9J) occurs when a bone fragment is pulled off at the point of ligament or tendon attachment.
- An **impacted fracture** (Figure 40-9K) occurs when the fragment from one bone is wedged into another bone.

Signs and Symptoms. Signs and symptoms of fractures will vary with the type of fracture and location. Fractures are painful conditions. Movement is limited, or the patient may be unable to move the injured area. The skin surrounding the fracture may appear deformed. Edema is common. **Ecchymosis**, or bruising, may occur. Some parts of the body, such as the area over the femur, are very **vascular**. Areas that are vascular contain many blood vessels. They bleed readily under the skin. An ecchymosis the size of an adult's fist over the femur indicates loss of approximately one pint of blood.

Treatment. A new fracture is usually treated in the hospital emergency department. Admission for surgical correction of the fracture may be necessary. The immediate goals of care are to:

- control pain
- prevent complications of immobility
- prevent or reduce edema
- keep the fracture in good alignment
- keep the fractured extremity immobile

Fractures of any kind are treated by keeping the part that is injured immobilized in proper position until healing takes place. Injured bones take from several weeks to several months to heal. Immobilization is achieved through the use of:

- Pins (Figure 40-10)
- Screws
- Splints
- Bone plates

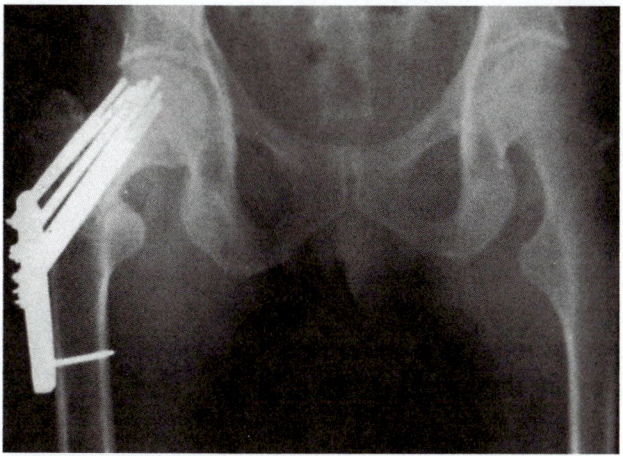

FIGURE 40-10 Certain fractures are repaired using plates, pins, or screws.

- Casting
- Traction

Special beds and attachments are used to make nursing care easier. The patient may be placed on a Stryker frame or the CircOlectric® bed.

Be sure you know how to operate each bed and attachment before attempting care. In many facilities, an RN must be present when the bed is turned. Know and follow the policy of your facility.

You will assist patients who have fractures with range-of-motion exercises several times each day. Check with the nurse or care plan for specific instructions. In most cases, you will not exercise the fractured extremity. You may be assigned to exercise the patient's joints above and below the cast to keep them mobile. For fractured arms and legs, you may be permitted to exercise fingers and toes. Exercising the rest of the patient's body is important. The exercise prevents complications related to immobility and inactivity.

You may also assist the patient with coughing and deep breathing exercises to prevent pneumonia. When working with patients with fractures, encourage adequate fluid intake. The increased fluid liquefies secretions that accumulate in the lungs. Coughing and deep breathing exercises are the same as those used in postoperative care. A trapeze (Figure 40-11) may be attached to the bed to assist the patient with movement. Your supervisor will teach you how to move and reposition the patient without interfering with the traction. The casted extremity is elevated on pillows if traction is not used.

Treatment for patients with fractures begins soon after admission. The type of treatment is determined by the location and type of fracture, and method of fracture reduction. Patients with fractures will be evaluated by the physical and occupational therapists. Therapists will design rehabilitation programs to meet the patients' needs and help them to regain as much mobility as possible.

Care of Patients with Casts. Two types of cast materials are commonly used:

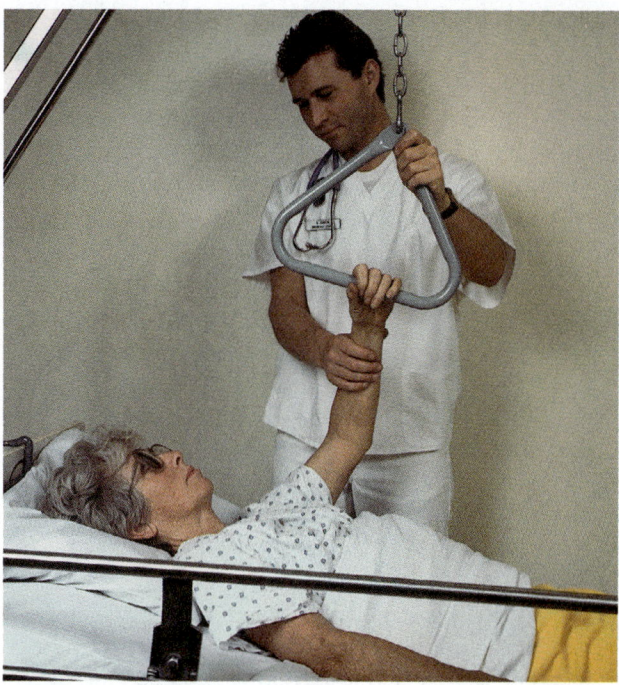

FIGURE 40-11 The overhead trapeze is a helpful adjunct that enables the patient to move in bed. The trapeze is not used for some patients with back injuries and back surgeries, because independent positioning can worsen the condition or cause further injuries.

1. Plaster of Paris, which can take up to 48 hours to dry completely
2. Fiberglass, which dries very rapidly

Cast material is wet when it is applied. During the drying period, the cast gives off heat. Special care for the newly casted patient includes:

- Supporting the cast and body in good alignment with pillows covered by cloth pillowcases, and keeping the cast uncovered.

SAFETY *Alert*

A fiberglass cast dries immediately. A plaster arm or leg cast will take 24 to 48 hours to dry completely. A plaster body or spica cast will take 48 to 72 hours to dry. Proper positioning of the cast is essential during the drying period to prevent depressions that can cause pressure and edema. Never use a table or hard object to support the cast during the drying period. Avoid rubber or plastic pillows, which increase heat under the cast. When the cast is dry, it will look white and shiny. It will not appear soft or damp.

- Elevating the casted extremity on a pillow as instructed. When positioning a patient with a leg cast, elevate the foot higher than the hip. The fingers should be higher than the elbow. Avoid placing the cast on a flat surface. Avoid placing anything plastic under a wet cast. Check the skin distal to the cast frequently for signs of poor circulation.

- Turning the patient frequently to permit air circulation to all parts of the cast. Maintain support. Use the palm of your hand, not your fingers, to support the wet cast.

- Not positioning the cast against the footboard or side rail. Leaving the cast open to air until it dries is best. If the patient is cold, cover the cast loosely with a sheet. Avoid tucking the sheet under the mattress. A bed cradle may be used, if necessary. The greatest area of heat loss is the head. Covering the upper body and back and top of the head with a blanket may help keep the patient warm.

- Closely observing the uncasted areas of the extremities, such as the fingers and toes, for signs of decreased circulation. Report coldness, cyanosis, swelling, increased pain, numbness, or tingling immediately.

- Closely observing skin areas around the cast edges for signs of irritation (Figure 40-12). Rough edges should be covered with adhesive strips to prevent skin irritation.

Recall the following key of reportables when checking the patient:

- C = color
- M = motion
- E = edema
- T = temperature

Special Care After Cast Is Dry. After the cast has completely dried:

- Turn the patient to the noncasted side. This is particularly important in moving a patient with a body cast (**spica cast**) (Figure 40-13) because turning to the casted side may crack the cast.

- Always support the cast when turning or moving a patient.

- Encourage use of a trapeze to assist the patient in helping herself.

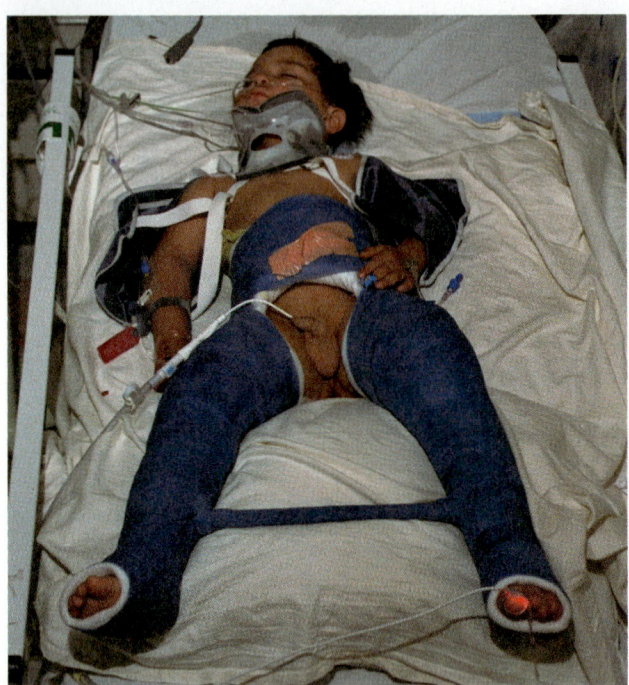

FIGURE 40-13 The spica cast is a full-body cast that is commonly used to treat hip fracture and after hip surgery in children.

- Tape edges of casts to prevent pressure and abrasive areas, if edges were not covered when the cast was applied.

- Use plastic to protect cast edges that are near the genitals and buttocks, to help prevent soiling during toileting.

After the cast dries, you may observe changes that indicate infection or ulceration under the cast:

- odor from the cast
- drainage through the cast

The care plan may instruct you to keep the casted extremity elevated to prevent edema. A sling (Figure 40-14) may be used to elevate an arm cast when the patient is out of bed. (Refer to Procedure 99.) A wheelchair with an elevated leg rest is used for patients with leg casts. Cover the cast with plastic during bathing. Keep small objects from

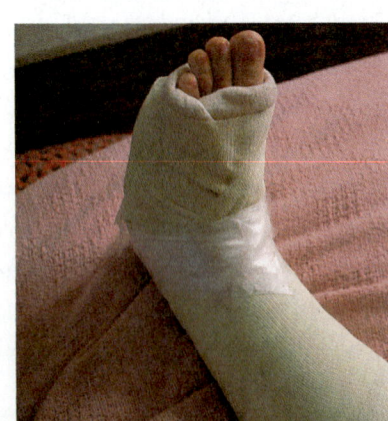

FIGURE 40-12 Check the skin around the edges of the cast regularly for signs of irritation. Check the circulation in the toes.

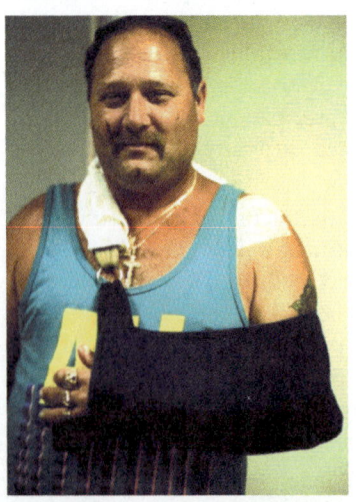

FIGURE 40-14 A sling may be ordered to elevate the hand and wrist.

PROCEDURE 99

APPLYING AN ARM SLING

1. Carry out beginning procedure actions.

2. Gather equipment:
- arm sling or triangular bandage
- padding for neck, if needed

3. Position the affected arm at a 90° angle.

4. Apply the sling:
- If a triangular bandage is used, place one end of the triangle over the unaffected shoulder. Position the point of the triangle under the affected elbow. Bring the other end of the triangle over the shoulder on the affected side, covering the arm. Adjust the bandage so the fingers are elevated, and tie the ends of the bandage in back. Position the knot slightly to the side so it is not directly over the spine. Pad the skin under the knot to prevent pressure and irritation. Fold the extra fabric over at the elbow. Secure it on the inside with pins or tape.
- If a commercial sling is used, support the affected arm. Guide the sling up over the hand until the elbow is covered and the fingers are exposed. Wrap the strap around the patient's neck, then fasten it to the buckle on the sling. Adjust the strap so the fingers are elevated. Pad the strap under the neck (Figure 40-15) to prevent pressure and irritation.

5. Carry out procedure completion actions.

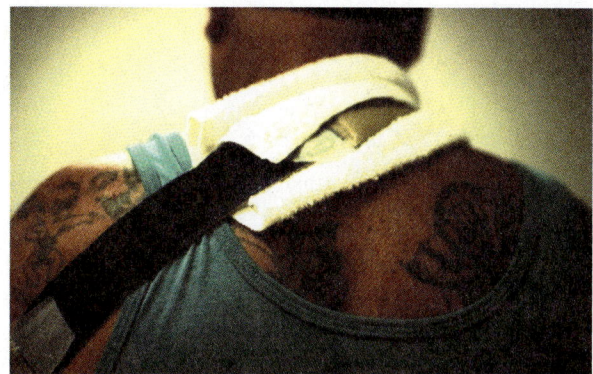

FIGURE 40-15 Pad the neck strap of the sling to prevent pressure and irritation from the weight of the cast.

SAFETY *Alert*

If the patient has an arm sling, monitor the skin at the back of the neck for irritation and breakdown from the strap. Monitor the skin under the arm daily for redness and breakdown. Make every effort to keep the underarm area clean and dry.

---

getting inside the cast. The patient may complain of an itching sensation under the cast. Discourage him or her from placing objects down the cast to scratch. This could cause a skin injury and infection. Report complaints of itching to your supervisor.

Care of Patients in Traction. Traction is designed to pull two body areas slightly apart to:
- relieve pressure.
- help tightly contracted (spasmodic) muscles relax.
- keep them in proper position as healing takes place.

Traction is of two types:
- Skin traction, where traction is applied to the skin or outside of the body (Figure 40-16)
- Skeletal traction, where traction is applied through the skin to the bone

Traction is applied by attaching weights to a part of the body above or below the area to be treated. The patient's body weight serves as **countertraction** by pulling in the direction opposite to the traction. Belts, head halters, or tapes may be applied to the patient's skin to hold the traction. Traction may be applied continuously or intermittently.

Skeletal traction (Figure 40-17) uses tongs or pins placed into bones with weights applied to the tongs or pins. Skeletal traction is always continuous once applied. The weights for skeletal traction must not be lifted or removed until the traction is to be discontinued.

When patients are in traction:
- Review the correct placement of straps and weights with the therapist or nurse. Get instructions for moving the patient up in bed and turning to the sides, as ordered.

- Do not disturb the weights or permit them to swing, drop, or rest on any surface. Avoid moving, dropping, or releasing the weights. They should not touch the bed, swing back and forth freely, or rest upon any

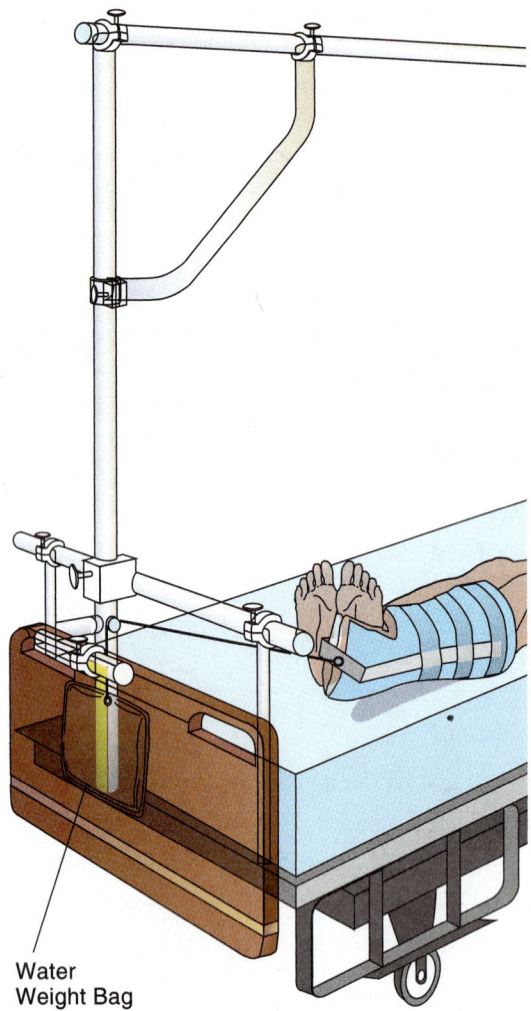

Water Weight Bag

FIGURE 40-16 Buck's traction is a type of skin traction that may be used for a hip fracture.

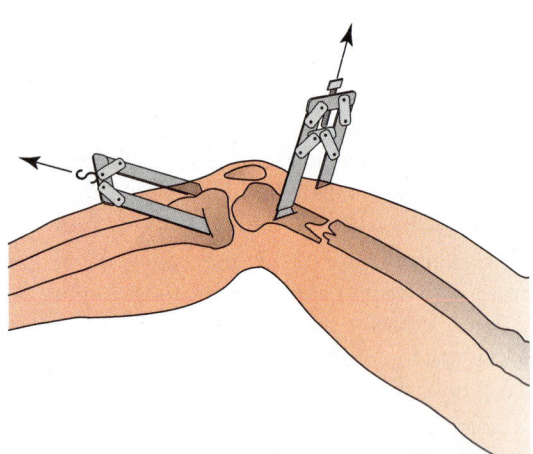

FIGURE 40-17 Skeletal traction immobilizes a body part by attaching weights directly to the patient's bones with pins, screws, wires, or tongs.

object or surface. The water bag or weight hangs motionless at the end of the bed.

- Keep the patient in good alignment in the center of the bed. Make sure that the body is acting properly as countertraction by keeping the head of the bed low. The feet should not rest against the end of the bed.
- Check under straps and belts for areas of pressure or irritation.
- Make sure straps and belts are smooth, straight, and properly secured.
- Keep bed covers off ropes and pulleys.

Not all patients remain in traction continually. If **pelvic belt traction** (Figure 40-18), or **cervical traction** with a head halter (Figure 40-19), is to be discontinued, take the following steps:

- Slowly raise the weights to the bed. Avoid abrupt or jerking movements, as this may cause the patient pain. If two sets of weights are being used, raise them at the same time and rate.
- Remove the weight holder and weights from the connection with the halter or belt and place them on the floor. Remove the head halter or pelvic belt.
- To reapply traction, reverse the procedure.
- Remember never to jerk or drop the weights quickly or lower them unevenly. Always apply weights smoothly to avoid causing the patient pain.

Bedmaking. Bedmaking for orthopedic patients varies according to the type of traction.

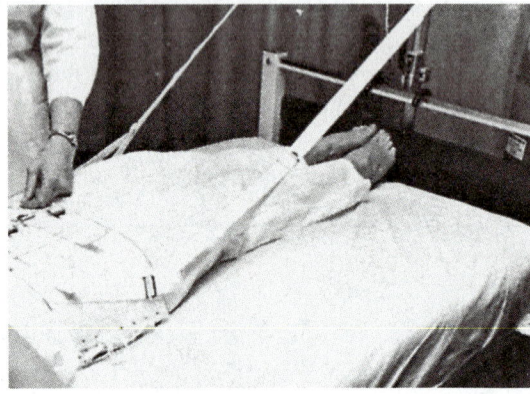

FIGURE 40-18 Pelvic belt traction. A bag filled with water is used as a weight.

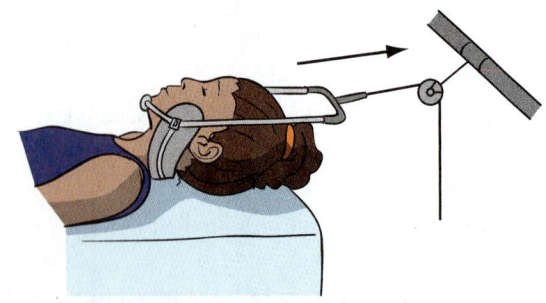

FIGURE 40-19 Cervical traction.

- Two half sheets are often used in place of a large sheet for the bottom.
- Bottom linens may be changed from top to bottom rather than side to side.
- The top linen is arranged according to the patient's special needs. Half sheets and folded bath blankets can be worked around the traction to keep the patient covered and comfortable.

Fractured Hip

Hip fractures are the most common type of fracture in the elderly. It is not unusual for a patient to be admitted to the hospital for treatment of another problem, then fall and break a hip. The most common cause of hip fractures is falls, but fractures may also occur because of osteoporosis. In this case, the patient may hear a popping sound in the bone, then fall. An x-ray will reveal a fracture. The term "hip fracture" really is not accurate. This term refers to a fracture anywhere in the upper third or head of the femur.

Signs and Symptoms of Hip Fracture. A patient with a fractured hip is usually found on the floor. He or she will be unable to get up or move the injured leg. The leg on the affected side may be shortened and in a position of external rotation. In this position, the toes point outward. The shortening and rotation occur because the strong muscles in the upper leg contract. This causes the bone ends to override each other.

The patient will complain of severe pain in the hip. The pain of a hip fracture is usually localized in the hip. Some patients complain of pain in the knee. This may be confusing or misleading. Edema and ecchymosis may be present in the hip, thigh, groin, or lower pelvic area.

Emergency Care. Avoid moving the patient until you are instructed to do so by a nurse. You will use a sheet, backboard, or other device to move the patient. Avoid excessive movement, which can worsen the injury. Moving a patient with a hip fracture requires four or five individuals. The patient is logrolled onto the lifting device. The device is lifted to the bed or stretcher. You may be assigned to monitor the patient's vital signs and check for signs of shock. Some patients are treated with Buck's traction.

Open Reduction/Internal Fixation. The most common treatment for a fractured hip is a surgical procedure called **open reduction/internal fixation**. This means the surgeon makes an incision, manipulates the fractured bone into alignment, and then inserts a device such as a nail, pin, or rod to hold the ends of the fractured bone in place. If you are assigned to a patient who has had this surgery, you must:

- Know how to position the patient in bed. It is important to avoid adduction and internal and external rotation of the affected hip.
- Know the correct procedure if the patient is allowed to ambulate. The patient is usually not allowed to bear weight on the affected side for a few weeks after surgery.

DIFFICULT *Situations*

A patient who has had hip surgery will probably have physician orders for antiembolism hosiery and an incentive spirometer. A pressure-relieving mattress may be ordered. Following hip surgery, the patient will be at high risk for pressure ulcer development, particularly on the heels. Take active measures to prevent pressure. Follow the care plan. Check the skin regularly for redness, irritation, and breakdown.

Total Hip Arthroplasty

Total hip arthroplasty (**THA**), or insertion of a hip prosthesis (artificial body part), is a common procedure. This surgery is done because the patient:

- has fractured a hip and the bone cannot be set by traditional methods
- has degenerative arthritis that has caused the hip joint to deteriorate

The patient's hip joint is surgically removed and a metal or synthetic ball and socket are inserted (Figure 40-20). There are specific body positions that the patient must avoid to prevent damage to the new joint.

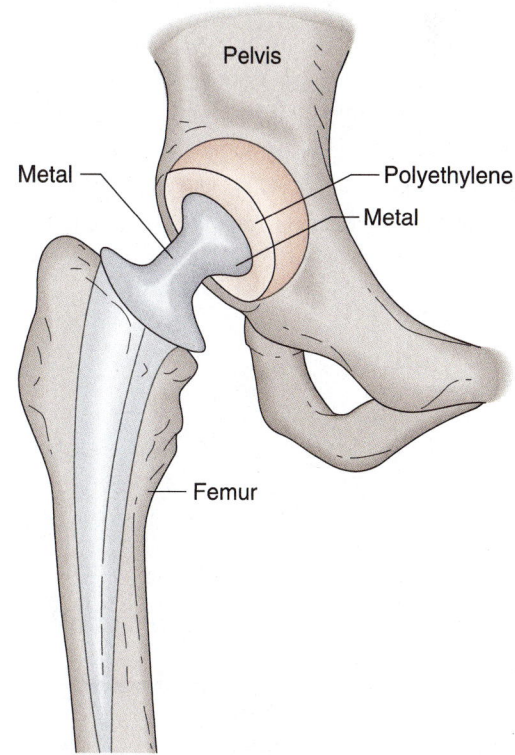

FIGURE 40-20 A hip prosthesis replaces the ball of the femur and the socket when the patient has a total hip arthroplasty.

Caring for the Patient with Hip Surgery. After hip surgery, the following general procedures are commonly ordered:

- A trapeze is attached to the bed to assist with movement. The patient is instructed not to press down on the foot of the affected leg when using the trapeze.
- Antiembolism stockings are applied.
- A fracture bedpan is used initially for elimination. When the patient is able to use the toilet, an elevated toilet seat is used.
- The head of the bed is not elevated more than 45 degrees without a specific order.
- Avoid acute flexion of the hip and legs. The physician will give directions for positioning and the degree of flexion permitted.
- Patients who have had hip replacement surgery will usually have a special pillow, called an abduction pillow, to keep the legs apart (Figure 40-21). This is

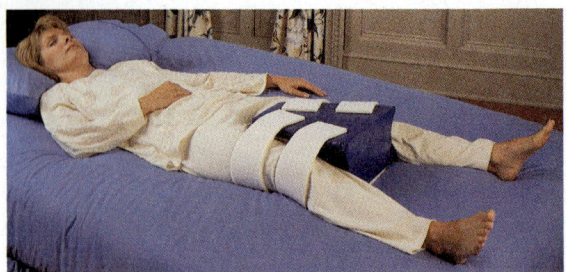

FIGURE 40-21 An abduction pillow is commonly used after hip surgery to keep the legs from adducting or crossing at the ankles.

particularly important when the patient is turned on the side. The patient will be instructed to avoid crossing the legs, which can cause a dislocation.

The physician will specify how long the patient must avoid weight bearing after surgery. The physical therapist will work with the patient to restore mobility. Some patients are

guidelines *for*

Caring for Patients with THA

The patient should **not**:

- Flex the hip more than 90 degrees (Figure 40-22A).
- Cross the affected leg over the midline of the body, whether in bed or sitting in a chair (Figure 40-22B).
- Internally rotate the hip on the affected side (Figure 40-22C).

Never do passive range-of-motion exercises on a joint that has had surgery, unless you are specifically instructed to do so—and then only if you have been given instructions as to which actions can safely be performed.

The patient will have limited weight bearing on the affected leg for several days or weeks after surgery.

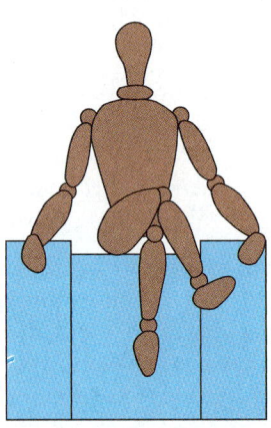

FIGURE 40-22B The patient with a new hip prosthesis should never cross the affected leg over the midline of the body.

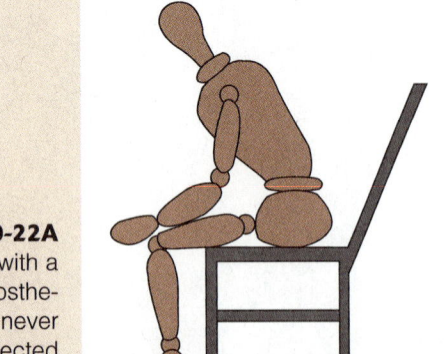

FIGURE 40-22A The patient with a new hip prosthesis should never flex the affected hip more than 90 degrees.

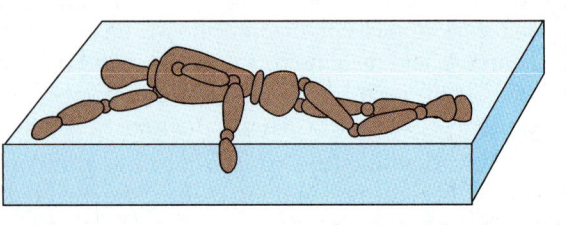

FIGURE 40-22C The patient with a new hip prosthesis should never internally rotate the hip on the affected side.

able to ambulate soon after surgery. A walker, crutches, or cane are commonly used for a period of time after surgery. Some physicians do not permit full weight bearing for as long as four to six weeks. Initially, you will assist with procedures to prevent the complications of immobility. These include range-of-motion exercises of the unaffected extremities, turning and repositioning, and coughing and deep breathing exercises. Patients with hip surgery are at very high risk of developing heel pressure ulcers. Follow the care plan and get specific instructions from the nurse for positions and techniques to use for turning and repositioning the patient. Relieve pressure from the heels and check the patient's skin carefully each day for signs of red or open areas.

Total Joint Replacement

Sometimes joints are completely replaced because of arthritis or severe damage to the joint. The goal of joint replacement surgery is to relieve pain, which is often so severe that the patient avoids using the joint as much as possible. This weakens the muscles and worsens the problem. Hip and knee replacements are the most common, but joint replacement surgery can be done on the ankle, foot, shoulder, elbow, and fingers. Postoperative care will vary with the surgical procedure. General care for joint replacement surgery includes:

- preventing infection
- preventing blood clots
- administering anticoagulant medication to thin the blood
- applying antiembolism hosiery (Unit 29)
- doing exercises to increase blood flow in the leg muscles, if not contraindicated
- using sequential compression therapy (Unit 29)

DIFFICULT *Situations*

A patient who has had hip replacement surgery may usually have the head of the bed elevated up to 45 degrees for comfort. Never elevate the head more than this without specific permission from the nurse. Some physicians will permit greater elevation. Try to limit elevation of the head to 30 minutes at a time, if possible. In any event, do not let the patient remain in a position of hip flexion for more than 90 minutes, because longer periods increase the risk of prosthesis dislocation. Positioning the patient in the supine position, with the affected leg in extension, for 1 hour three times a day will help prevent contractures of the hip joint.

Continuous Passive Motion. Continuous passive motion (CPM) therapy (Figure 40-23) may be ordered following joint replacement and other orthopedic procedures. Moving a joint is painful for most patients postoperatively. If the patient fails to move the joint, stiffness and limited range of motion will occur. Months of physical therapy will be necessary for the patient to fully recover. CPM therapy prevents stiffness by delivering a form of passive range-of-motion exercise so the joint is moved without the patient's muscles being used. CPM therapy is effortless for the patient. A machine moves the affected joint through a prescribed range of motion for an extended period of time. CPM therapy:

- enhances circulation, which lowers the risk of blood clots
- reduces edema
- promotes collagen formation within the joint, which enhances healing
- reduces scarring
- decreases stiffness
- improves range of motion (which decreases postoperatively without movement)
- reduces the risk of complications in the joint, such as contractures and adhesions
- helps reduce pain

Many orthopedic surgeons prescribe CPM therapy following knee replacement and other surgical procedures. CPM devices are available for the knee, ankle, toes, jaw, shoulder, elbow, wrist, and hand. Indications for using CPM therapy are:

- Crush injuries of the hand without fractures or dislocations
- Burn injuries
- Stable fractures
- Joint and tendon repair
- Surgical release of contractures
- Knee or hip replacement

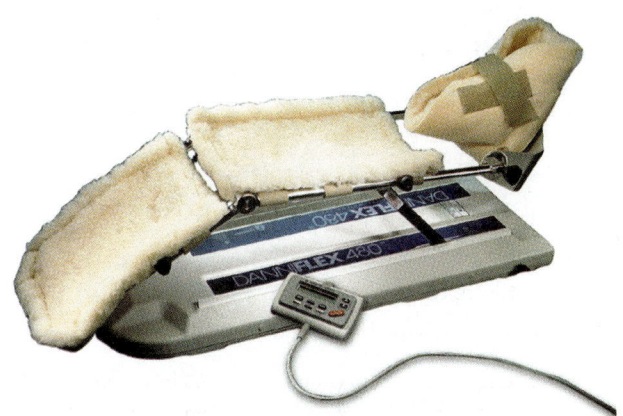

FIGURE 40-23 The continuous passive motion (CPM) machine performs passive range-of-motion exercises on the affected joint without straining the patient's muscles. *(Courtesy of OrthoRehab, Inc.)*

- Reconstructive surgery on bone, cartilage, tendons, and ligaments
- Prolonged joint immobilization

The physician prescribes how the CPM unit should be used. He or she orders the settings on the CPM unit that control the speed, duration of use, range of motion, pause settings, hours of use per day, and rate of increase of motion. The directions for use will vary slightly depending on the body area being treated, the type of CPM machine used, and physicians' orders. In some facilities, this procedure is done only by licensed nurses. In others, the nursing assistant can set up the unit, but the nurse must check the settings for accuracy. This is a key step. Improper settings can damage reconstructive work in the joint. Follow your facility policies and procedures. (Refer to Procedure 100.)

Contraindications for CPM therapy include:

- untreated infections
- unstable fractures
- known or suspected blood clots (deep vein thrombosis)
- hemorrhage

If the patient develops any of the following signs or symptoms upon using the device, stop the unit and inform the nurse promptly:

- fever
- increasing redness or irritation
- increasing warmth
- edema
- bleeding
- increased or persistent pain

Do not proceed with treatment until the nurse informs you that the physician has approved continued use of the device.

Check the patient periodically when using the CPM machine. Each time the settings are changed, stay with the patient for several cycles to be sure she tolerates the change. Check the skin every 2 hours for signs of redness, irritation, or breakdown. Report problems and abnormalities to the nurse.

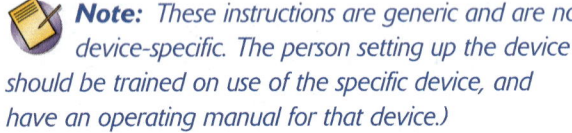

PROCEDURE 100

PROCEDURE FOR CONTINUOUS PASSIVE MOTION

 Note: *Be sure this is a nursing assistant procedure at your facility.*

 Note: *These instructions are generic and are not device-specific. The person setting up the device should be trained on use of the specific device, and have an operating manual for that device.)*

1. Carry out beginning procedure actions. Apply the principles of standard precautions during this procedure if contact with wound drainage or nonintact skin is likely.

2. Gather equipment:
   - CPM unit
   - soft goods kit, if available OR
   - sheepskin foot pad
   - tibia/femur sling
   - hip pad
   - Velcro fasteners

3. Check the unit for safety and stability. Make sure that the attachments are tight, the frame is stable, and the electric controls work. Have the nurse adjust the settings according to the doctor's orders, or follow facility policy for setting the speed and degree of flexion. (In some facilities, assistants are permitted to adjust the settings. If this is the case, have the nurse check the settings before proceeding.) Stop the machine in full extension.

4. Raise the side rail on the side of the bed where you will be placing the unit.

5. Position the CPM unit on the bed and secure the attachment, depending on the type of device being used.

6. Fasten the foot pad to the foot plate with a Velcro fastener.

7. Attach the tibia/femur sling (wide section toward the footrest). Fasten the Velcro closures under the sling.

8. Apply the hip pad to the hinge area of the adjustment bar. Position the femur sling straps over the hinges, then fasten underneath with Velcro.

9. Fit the CPM machine to the patient's leg length by lengthening or shortening the frame.

continues

PROCEDURE 100

continued

10. Align the knee joint with the knee hinge, then position the knee approximately 1 inch below the knee joint line (Figure 40-24A).

11. Center the leg on the unit. Avoid pressure on the side and middle of the knee joint.

12. Adjust the foot pad so the patient's foot is comfortable and well supported (Figure 40-24B). The leg should be lifted at the thigh with no pressure on the foot. Secure the Velcro straps across the thigh and top of foot (Figure 40-24C).

13. When the leg is in the proper position, give the patient the control (Figure 40-24D). Instruct the patient to start the unit. Instruct the patient to turn the unit off and use the call signal if the exercise causes extreme pain, or the unit malfunctions.

14. Stay with the patient for at least two full cycles to make sure she tolerates the procedure.

15. Return to check on the patient frequently when the unit is in use. Some devices have compliance monitors that allow you to check usage of the device. After the patient is experienced in the use of the CPM machine, he or she may be instructed to keep a record of the times the unit is used, or you may be required to document this information.

16. Carry out procedure completion actions.

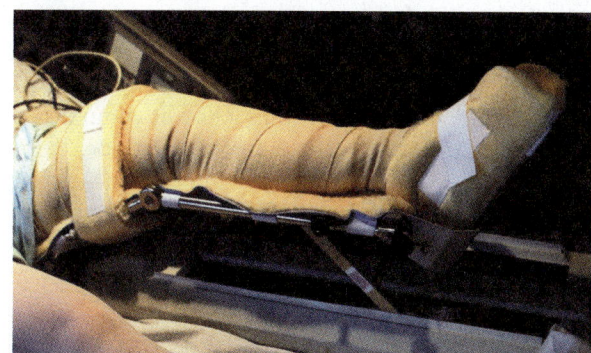

FIGURE 40-24C Secure the straps across the leg and foot. Make sure the strap is not too tight.

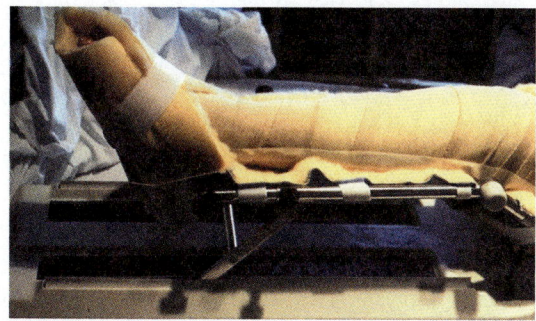

FIGURE 40-24A Position the leg straight, with the toes upright. Line the knee up with the marking at the hinge.

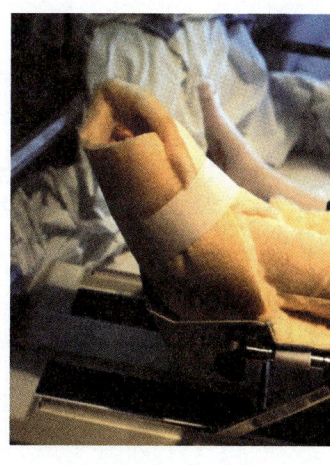

FIGURE 40-24B
Make sure the foot is comfortable and well supported. Add padding if needed for patient comfort.

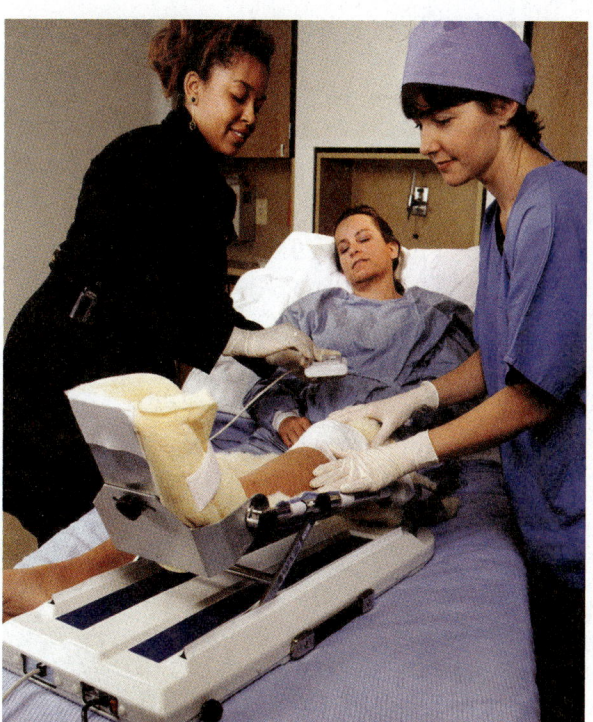

FIGURE 40-24D Show the patient how to turn the unit on, then give her the switch. Stay in the room until the machine goes through at least two cycles if the unit is being used for the first time. *(Courtesy of OrthoRehab, Inc.)*

Compartment Syndrome

Compartment syndrome is a very painful condition that occurs when pressure within the muscles builds up, preventing blood and oxygen from reaching muscles and nerves. This is a very serious complication that may develop following an injury or surgical procedure. It may also occur following athletic injuries, burns, snake bites, IV infiltration, frostbite, and musculoskeletal conditions in which there is no fracture. Patients of all ages can be affected.

Compartment syndrome is usually seen after a traumatic injury, such as a long bone fracture. It may develop if an injury or surgical site swells after a cast has been applied. A tough membrane, called *fascia*, surrounds the muscles in the arms and legs. Fascia does not expand readily. Compartment syndrome develops gradually over several hours. Bleeding or swelling occurs in the muscle tissue, under the fascia. In some cases, pressure from a cast or compression device also increases the pressure from the outside. If the swelling is not relieved, pressure on the muscles and nerves builds. Eventually, the pressure inside the fascia compartment will exceed the blood pressure, causing the capillaries to collapse. Blood flow to the muscles and nerves stops. If it is not restored promptly, tissue death begins.

Signs and Symptoms. The most common symptom of acute compartment syndrome is severe pain, especially when the muscle is moved. The pain may seem out of proportion to the injury. The patient may also complain of

- severe pain when the muscle is gently stretched
- tenderness when the area is touched gently
- pain during deep breathing
- tingling
- burning
- numbness
- feeling tight or full in the affected muscle
- abnormal sensations in the affected area
- weakness or inability to use the muscle

You may observe:

- The color of the extremity may appear pale, cyanotic, or red
- The skin of an extremity with no cast may feel warm to touch

- The fingers or toes of a casted extremity may feel cool to touch
- Edema (swelling)

Loss of the pulse in the extremity is a late sign. Rapid identification and treatment of this condition is necessary.

Nursing Assistant Responsibilities. Follow the care plan and monitor patients with musculoskeletal injuries and casts frequently. Monitor for changes in the extremity. Check the color and temperature of the extremity distal to a cast. Notify the nurse if the color is abnormal. Ask the patient if he or she is able to move the fingers or toes. Notify the nurse promptly of any unusual findings. If the patient complains of severe pain, or if the pain is not relieved after the patient receives pain medication, notify the nurse promptly. This condition is frightening for the patient. Provide emotional support.

Compartment syndrome is a surgical emergency. The nurse will assess the patient and notify the physician of the findings. If compartment syndrome is suspected, the patient will be taken to surgery quickly to relieve the pressure. Follow facility policies and the nurse's instructions for preparing the patient for surgery.

Ruptured or Slipped Disc

It is possible for a disc to bulge (slip) out of place or for the soft center to rupture. In either case, pressure is placed on the spinal nerves (Figure 40-25). Depending on which disc is injured, the patient may experience, in different parts of the body:

- Pain
- Numbness
- Tingling
- Weakness of one or more muscles

Treatment. Treatment attempts to relieve pressure on the nerve roots. Early treatment is very conservative and includes rest, medication, ice, compresses, physical therapy, and exercise. Some people use complementary and alternative therapies, most commonly:

- acupuncture
- chiropractic
- massage
- yoga
- biofeedback

If conservative attempts to relieve pressure fail, other methods will be used to relieve pressure on the spinal cord. These are:

1. Traction. This is an older treatment that is seldom used nowadays.
2. Surgery to remove the protruding portion of the disc (**laminectomy**). The surgery sometimes includes a fixation (**fusion**) of the vertebral bones.
3. A surgical procedure called **nucleoplasty**. This is a minimally invasive procedure with rapid recovery. In

---

DIFFICULT *Situations*

The most common location of compartment syndrome in adults is in a fractured tibia. The most common location of compartment syndrome in children is the humerus.

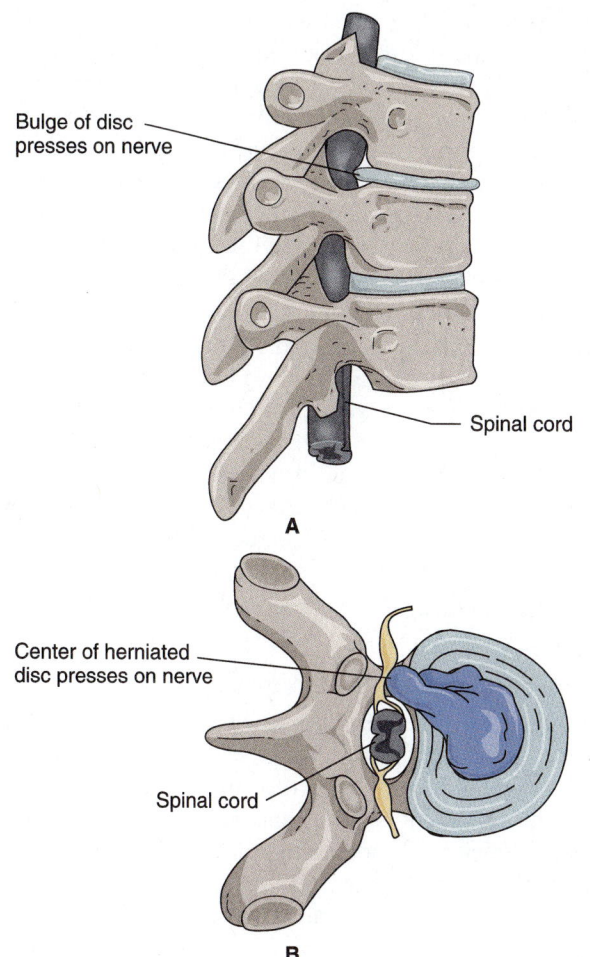

FIGURE 40-25 A. Uneven pressure causes the disc to bulge, putting pressure on the nerve root (slipped disc). B. A herniated (ruptured) disc applies pressure on the nerve root as the gel-like center oozes backward.

this procedure, a tiny wand is inserted through the back into the disc. Tissue is removed through the wand, and the channel is thermally sealed. The wand is then removed. This may be done as an outpatient surgery in some facilities.

Lower Extremity Amputation

You may care for patients who have had one or both legs surgically removed (amputated). A leg may have to undergo **amputation** because of circulatory problems, a malignancy, or an accident in which the leg was severely damaged.

It is common for people to experience **phantom pain** after the removal of a limb. Patients with phantom pain may feel pain or tingling where the limb used to be. These feelings may persist for months. The pain is real, although it is difficult to explain.

When you are positioning a patient who has had an amputation of the lower extremities, remember:

- Avoid abduction and flexion of the patient's hip— because the weight of the lower leg is not there, the hip

on the affected side will quickly become contracted if flexion is allowed.

- If the patient has a below-the-knee amputation (BKA), avoid flexion of the knee, so that a contracture does not form.
- Avoid placing pillows under the amputated extremity. Position the leg flat on the bed.
- Avoid elevating the head of the bed for prolonged periods.
- Keep the legs in a position of adduction. A trochanter roll is helpful. Avoid positioning the patient with pillows between the legs.
- Assist the patient to lie in the prone position twice a day, if permitted.
- Encourage and assist the patient to move in bed frequently.

After the surgery, the patient will either have the stump wrapped with elastic bandage or will wear a stump shrinker. It is important that these be on at all times except during the bath. It is the nurse's responsibility to apply either of these items. If you notice that the bandage or shrinker is loose or needs to be reapplied, notify the nurse. The purpose of these items is to make sure that the stump heals in the appropriate shape.

If you bathe a patient with an amputation:

- Gently wash the stump with soap and warm water, rinse well, and pat dry.
- Observe the stump for:
  - redness
  - swelling
  - drainage from the incision
  - open areas in the incision or anywhere else on the stump
- Do not apply lotion to the stump. Lotion softens the skin, making safe prosthesis use difficult.
- Make sure the skin is protected before applying the prosthesis. Never apply a prosthesis over unprotected skin.

After an amputation, some patients are fitted with an artificial leg (prosthesis). They have to learn how to walk and sit when the prosthesis is worn. A prosthesis is custom-made

SAFETY *Alert*

Make sure that the stump shrinker or wrap is smooth, with no wrinkles or exposed skin. Inform the nurse promptly if the patient complains of throbbing under the stump shrinker. Throbbing is an indication of impaired circulation, a potentially serious complication.

DIFFICULT *Situations*

When the stump is healed and the patient prepares to use the prosthesis, the physician may order special care. This involves not shaving the stump, as shaving increases the risk of rash and irritation. Bathing of the stump may be ordered at bedtime, because warm water may increase swelling, and make application of the prosthesis difficult. The physician may also order alcohol rubs to the stump several times a day to toughen the skin. Avoid powders and lotions, which soften the skin. Monitor the stump for irritation and report to the nurse, if present. The stump sock may require frequent changing to avoid wetness. The socks must be handwashed. Muscle-strengthening exercises will be ordered to prepare the patient to lift the weight of the prosthesis.

for the person who will be wearing it. A special health care professional measures the patient and makes the prosthesis. The physical therapist teaches the patient how to apply the prosthesis and how to use it. If you are responsible for helping a patient put on a prosthesis, be sure you know how to attach and secure it, because each device is different.

Various types of materials are used to make prostheses. They need to be cleaned regularly, and the method of cleaning depends on what materials were used to make the prosthesis. Wipe the inside of the prosthesis daily with a damp, soapy cloth to remove sweat and body oils. Rinse with a second damp cloth. Dry the inside of the socket well. Avoid placing a damp prosthesis on a patient. Never attempt to adjust the prosthesis. Consult your supervisor if you believe an adjustment is necessary.

RANGE OF MOTION

Patients who have been ill or confined to bed are not as active, so joints may not move through the normal range of motion daily. Weakness and muscle wasting from lack of use is called atrophy. Over time, muscles become rigid. The joints do not move as freely as they once did. Joint movement may be painful because the muscles have shortened from lack of use. When the joint moves, the muscle stretches. This causes discomfort or pain, and the patient may move even less because of it.

Contractures and deformities develop when the patient is immobile. *Contractures* are disfigurements caused by muscle shortening. They are serious, painful complications of inactivity. Contractures make caring for the patient more difficult. There is a direct relationship between contractures and pressure ulcers. Patients with contractures of the feet and ankles cannot walk. A footboard should be used with all bedfast patients to prevent contracture development. If permitted, placing patients in the prone position for 15 to 30 minutes daily helps to stretch the muscles. This helps to prevent contractures. Avoiding the sitting position for prolonged periods also helps prevent flexion contractures.

Patients' joints must be moved regularly to prevent complications. If patients cannot move independently, you will be responsible for exercising their joints. All patients should be exercised regularly to prevent deformities. This includes patients with no potential for rehabilitation. Like pressure sores, contractures are much easier to prevent than to reverse. However, they can be reversed, particularly in the early stages. Reversing contractures requires a diligent effort by staff.

Other complications of inadequate exercise are:

- bones lose minerals.
- general body circulation is slowed.

Active range-of-motion exercises are done by the patient during activities of daily living. Passive range-of-motion (PROM) exercises are performed for patients when independent movement is impossible. Passive range-of-motion exercises maintain movement and prevent deformities. They do *not* strengthen the muscles. You will perform PROM for patients with conditions such as:

- paralysis
- contractures
- orthopedic conditions
- neurologic disorders
- severe cognitive impairment

Passive range-of-motion exercises are also ordered when active movement:

- increases spasticity
- causes pain
- creates excessive stress on the heart
- makes patients unable to move joints safely

The patient must be comfortable and relaxed during the exercises. Each joint is taken through the normal range of movement.

The nurse will instruct you as to the type or limitation of range-of-motion exercises to be done. These exercises are usually done during or after the bath and before the bed is made. They may be carried out at other times as well.

Precautions and Special Situations

Patients with certain conditions require special care and handling. Avoid exercising extremities with fractures or dislocations. When assisting patients with healed hip or other joint replacements, avoid internal rotation. Also avoid adduction beyond the midline. Some patients have bones that break easily. Osteoporosis is a condition in which bone mass decreases. This leads to fractures with little or no trauma. You have learned that patients with this condition may develop spontaneous fractures. Check with the nurse and the care plan when your patient has a special situation or osteoporosis. If the patient has a wound or pressure ulcer, check to see if exercise will harm the healing tissue. If a patient is combative or resists exercise, avoid forcing him or her. Gently explain and demonstrate the procedure. Try to coax the patient into participating. Sometimes singing an old song will distract the patient. Encourage the patient to sing along with you. If distracted, he or she may allow you to perform the exercises. The patient may even have fun! Performing range-of-motion exercises in the bathtub or whirlpool may also be an option, if permitted. Notify the nurse if the patient continues to refuse.

Some patients have muscle spasms and rigidity. When exercising patients with these conditions, move the joint slowly and smoothly. Stop at the point of pain or resistance. Apply gentle, steady pressure until the muscle relaxes (Figure 40-26). Avoid rapid, jerking movements. Do not stretch the joint too far. These activities cause pain and worsen the condition. Suspect muscle spasms if resistance progressively increases during exercise. Rigidity presents as resistance to movement in any direction. Slow, continuous, sustained movements help prevent spasticity and rigidity. If rigidity and muscle spasms develop, hold steady, gentle pressure on the muscle. Avoid forcing the muscle past the point of resistance. This should enable you to complete the exercise. Report the problems to the nurse. The nurse or therapist will provide specific instructions.

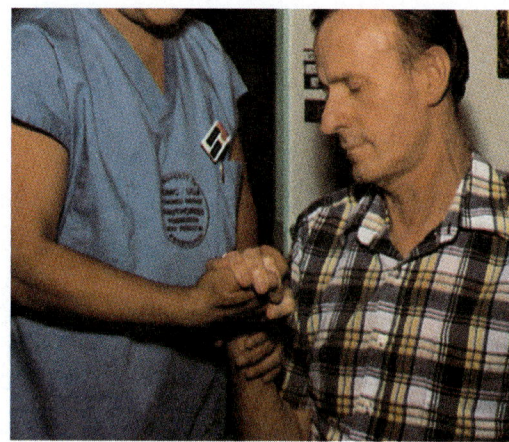

FIGURE 40-26 Apply steady, gentle pressure to reduce spasticity.

guidelines *for*

Assisting Patients with Range-of-Motion Exercises

- Check the care plan or ask the nurse for specific guidelines and limitations.
- Explain the procedure to the patient.
- Before beginning, make sure the patient is comfortable.
- Position the patient in good body alignment, in the supine position, before beginning.
- Elevate the bed to a comfortable working height.
- Use good posture and apply the principles of good body mechanics.
- Encourage the patient to assist, if able, but keep your hands in position to provide support.
- Make sure you have enough space for full movement of the extremities.
- Expose only the part of the body you are exercising.
- Support each joint by placing one hand above and one hand below the joint.
- Move each joint slowly and consistently. Stop briefly at the end of each motion.
- Work systematically from top of the body to the bottom.

- Never push the patient past the point of joint resistance. Move each joint as far as it will comfortably go.
- In many facilities, the neck is not exercised without a physician's order. Know and follow your facility policy.
- Perform each joint motion five times, or according to facility policy.
- Stop the exercise and report to the nurse if the patient complains of pain. Watch the patient's body language and facial expression for signs of pain.
- Be alert for changes in the patient's condition during the activity. If you feel that the activity is harming the patient, stop. Notify the nurse. Changes that suggest a potential problem are pain, shortness of breath, sweating, and change in color.
- Help the patient relax during exercise.
- Use the session as quality time to communicate with the patient.
- For patients who are stiff or combative, consider doing the exercise in the bathtub or whirlpool. Check with the nurse.

PROCEDURE 101

PERFORMING RANGE-OF-MOTION EXERCISES (PASSIVE)

LEGAL *Alert*

Passive range of motion that involves the neck is usually carried out by a physical therapist or a registered nurse. Patients who can exercise this area themselves are encouraged to do so. Check your facility policy regarding ROM neck exercises.

Note: *This procedure may be carried out as an independent procedure or as part of the bath. Repeat each action five times. ROM is described here as an independent procedure.*

1. Carry out beginning procedure actions.

2. Assemble equipment:
   - bath blanket

3. Position the patient on his back close to you.

4. Adjust the bath blanket to keep the patient covered as much as possible.

5. Supporting the elbow and wrist, exercise the shoulder joint nearest you as follows:

   a. Bring the entire arm out at a right angle to the body (horizontal abduction) (Figure 40-27).

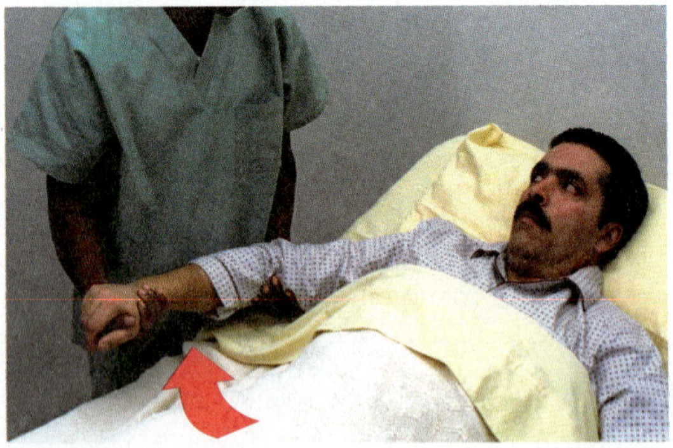

   b. Return the arm to a position parallel to the body (horizontal adduction).

6. a. With the arm parallel to the body, roll the entire arm toward the body (internal rotation of shoulder).

   b. Maintaining the parallel position, roll the entire arm away from the body (external rotation of shoulder).

7. With the shoulder in abduction, flex the elbow and raise the entire arm over the head (shoulder flexion) (Figure 40-28).

8. With the arm parallel to the body (palm up— **supination**), flex and extend the elbow (Figures 40-29A and B).

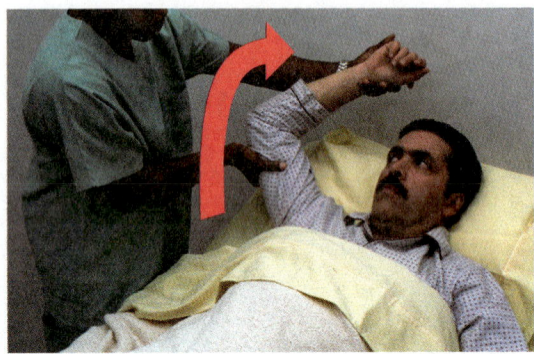

FIGURE 40-28 Shoulder flexion. With the shoulder in abduction, flex the elbow and raise the entire arm over the head.

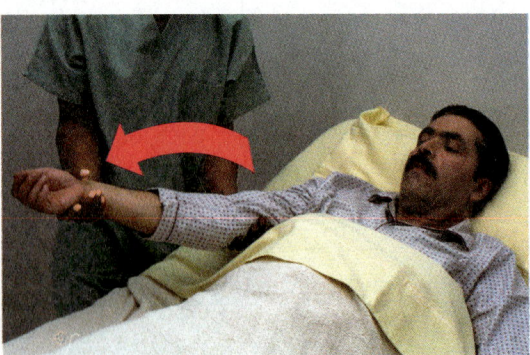

FIGURE 40-29A Elbow extension and flexion. Support the upper arm and wrist, then straighten the elbow.

FIGURE 40-27 Shoulder abduction and adduction. Support the arm at the elbow and wrist, then bring the entire arm out at a right angle from the body.

continues

PROCEDURE 101

continued

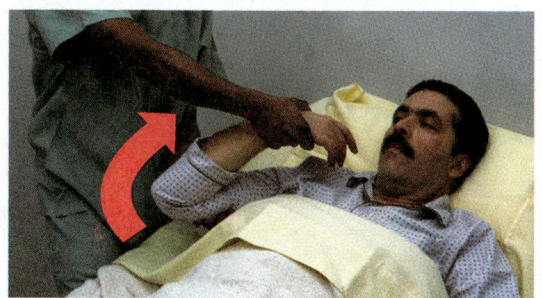

FIGURE 40-29B Flex the lower arm toward the upper arm.

9. Flex and extend the wrist (Figure 40-30). Flex and extend each finger joint (Figure 40-31).

10. Move each finger, in turn, away from the middle finger (abduction) (Figure 40-32A) and toward the middle finger (adduction) (Figure 40-32B).

11. Abduct the thumb by moving it toward the extended fingers (Figure 40-33).

12. Touch the thumb to the base of the little finger, then to each fingertip (opposition) (Figure 40-34).

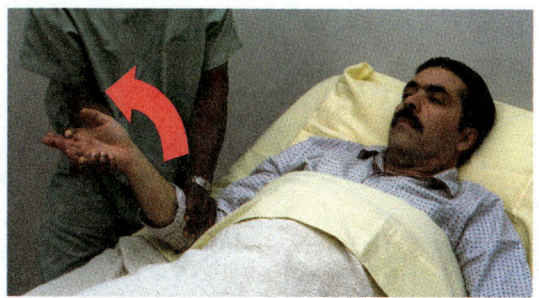

FIGURE 40-30 Wrist extension and flexion. Supporting the arm above the wrist and hand, straighten the wrist.

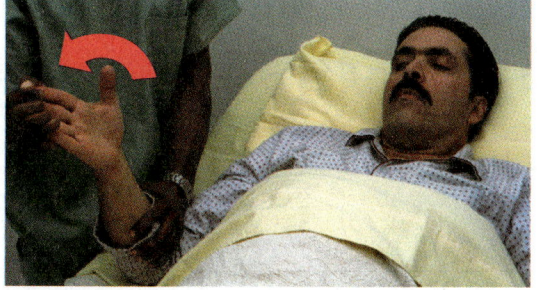

FIGURE 40-31 Finger extension. Slip your fingers over the patient's flexed fingers, then straighten the fingers.

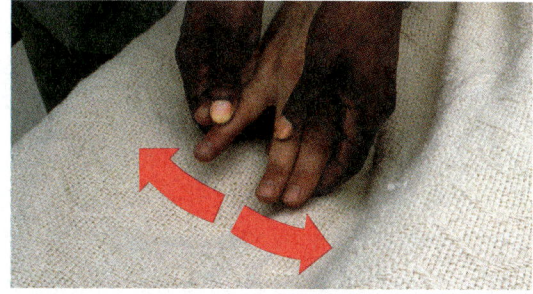

FIGURE 40-32A Abduction of the fingers.

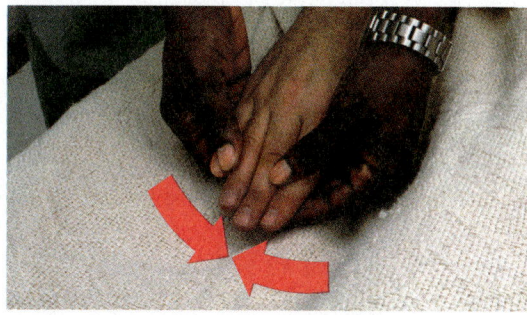

FIGURE 40-32B Adduction of the fingers.

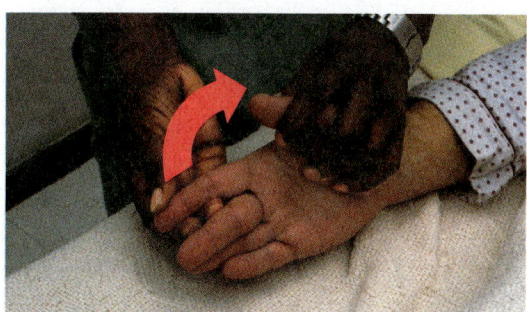

FIGURE 40-33 Abduction and adduction of the thumb and fingers. Supporting the hand, draw the thumb toward and away from the extended fingers.

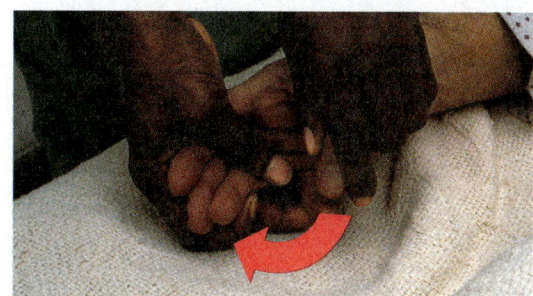

FIGURE 40-34 Thumb opposition. Supporting the hand, touch each finger with the thumb.

continues

PROCEDURE 101

continued

13. Turn the hand palm down (**pronation**), then palm up (supination).

14. Grasp the patient's wrist with one hand and the patient's hand with the other. Bring the wrist toward the body (**inversion**) and then away from the body (**eversion**) (Figure 40-35).

15. Point the hand in supination toward the thumb side (**radial deviation**), then toward the little-finger side (**ulnar deviation**).

16. Cover the patient's upper extremities and body. Expose only the leg being exercised. Face the foot of the bed.

17. Supporting the knee and ankle, move the entire leg away from the body center (abduction) (Figure 40-36) and toward the body (adduction).

18. Turn to face the bed. Supporting the knee in bent position (flexion), raise the knee toward the pelvis (hip flexion) (Figure 40-37A). Straighten the knee (extension) (Figure 40-37B), as you lower the leg to the bed.

19. a. Supporting the leg at the knee and ankle, roll the leg in a circular fashion away from the body (lateral hip rotation).

    b. Continuing to support the leg, roll the leg in the same fashion toward the body (medial hip rotation).

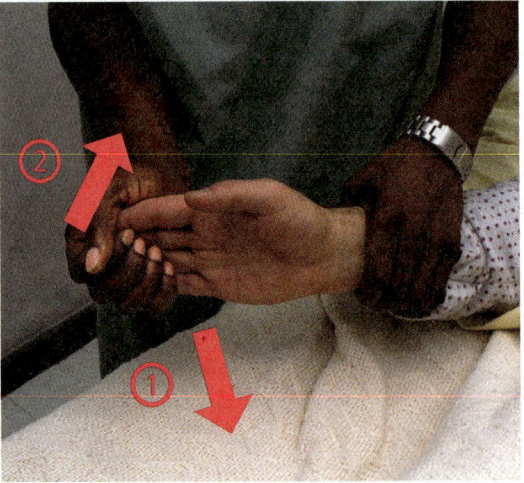

FIGURE 40-35 Wrist inversion (supination) and eversion (pronation). Grasp the patient's wrist with one hand. Grasp the patient's hand with your other hand. Bring the wrist toward the body, then away from the body.

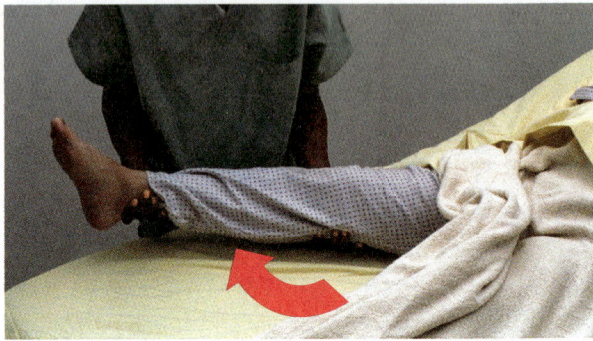

FIGURE 40-36 Abduction of the hip. Supporting the patient's knee and ankle, move the entire leg away from the center of the body.

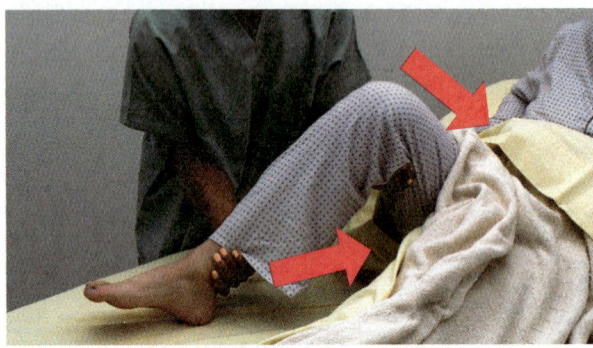

FIGURE 40-37A Hip and knee flexion. Supporting the leg, return toward the center of the body.

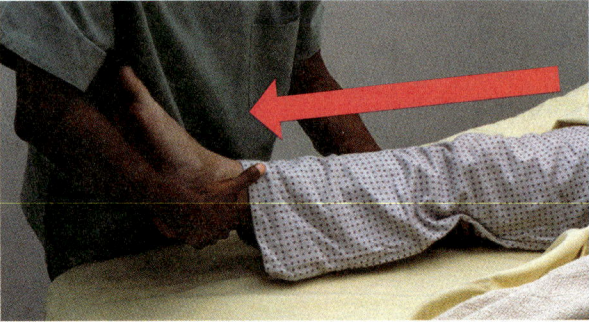

FIGURE 40-37B Knee extension. Supporting the knee and ankle, straighten the leg.

20. Grasp the patient's toes and support the ankle. Bring toes toward the knee (**dorsiflexion**) (Figure 40-38A). Then point the toes toward the foot of the bed (**plantar flexion**) (Figure 40-38B).

 Note: *The patient may be more comfortable if the knee is slightly flexed during this motion.*

continues

PROCEDURE 101

continued

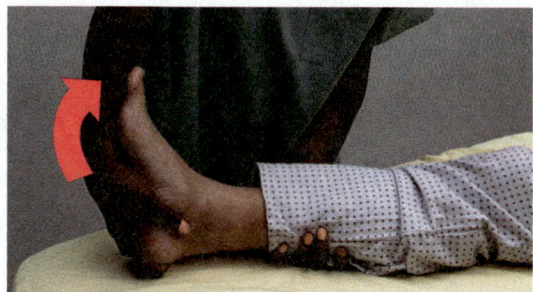

FIGURE 40-38A Ankle flexion. Grasp the patient's heel with one hand, using your upper arm to support the foot. Dorsiflex the ankle by bringing the toes and foot toward the knee.

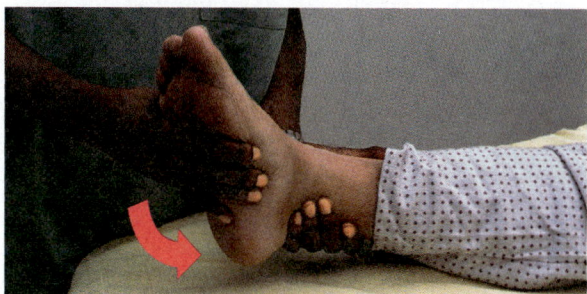

FIGURE 40-39 Foot inversion. Grasp the patient's foot and gently turn it inward.

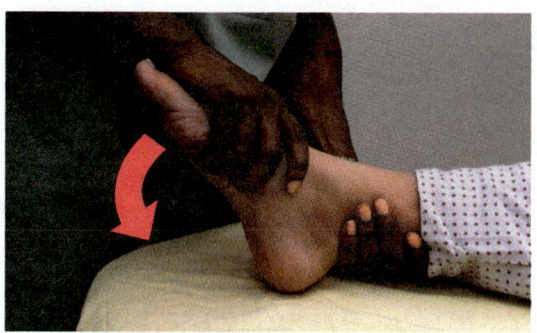

FIGURE 40-38B Plantar flex the ankle by drawing the foot in a downward position.

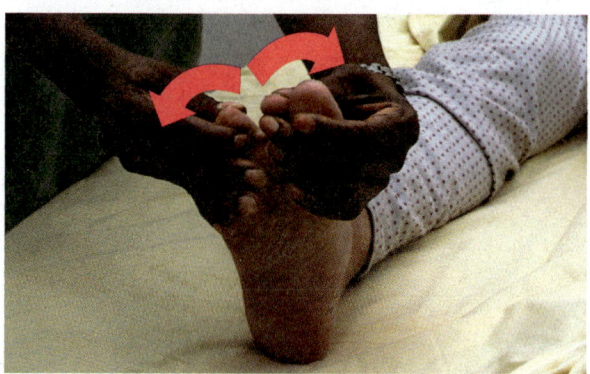

FIGURE 40-40A Toe abduction. Move each toe away from the second toe one at a time.

21. Gently turn the patient's foot inward (inversion) (Figure 40-39) and outward (eversion).

22. Place your fingers over the patient's toes. Bend the toes (flexion) and straighten them (extension).

23. Move each toe away from the second toe (abduction) (Figure 40-40A) and then toward the second toe (adduction) (Figure 40-40B).

24. Cover the leg with the bath blanket. Raise the side rail and move to the opposite side of the bed.

25. Move the patient close to you and repeat steps 5 through 24.

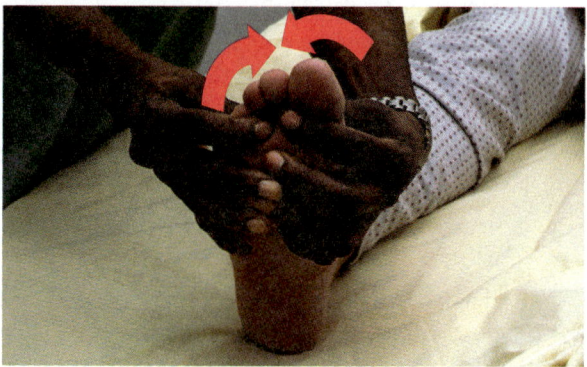

FIGURE 40-40B Toe adduction. Move each toe toward the second toe one at a time.

DIAGNOSTIC TECHNIQUES

Some techniques used to diagnose problems of the musculoskeletal system include:

- Radiographic techniques such as x-ray.
- Electromyography (EMG) test to measure the effectiveness of muscle/nerve interaction.
- Measurements of alkaline and acid phosphatases.
- Bone marrow examination, when a sample of the bone marrow is removed and evaluated.

- CAT scan to check for bone, muscle, and joint conditions.
- Radioisotope scanning, a technique that often can detect early bone and joint changes.
- Arthroscopy for direct visualization of a joint.

- Magnetic resonance imaging (MRI) to show conditions of tissues around bones. This helps to diagnose tumors, a ruptured disc between two vertebrae, and other conditions.

REVIEW

A. True/False.

Mark the following true or false by circling T or F.

1. T F Osteoporosis is a type of arthritis in which joint deformities are common.

2. T F If ROM is not carried out faithfully, the patient's future mobility is threatened.

3. T F When carrying out ROM, always support the parts being exercised at the joint.

4. T F The nursing assistant will carry out special corrective exercises.

5. T F Aging is a contributory factor in osteoarthritis.

6. T F When the patient has a painful arthritic joint, it should be exercised vigorously.

7. T F An overbed bar (trapeze) will assist orthopedic patients to move more easily and enable them to help themselves.

8. T F A fracture is any break in a bone.

9. T F Before operating beds or attachments used with orthopedic patients, the nursing assistant must be sure of her competency to operate this equipment.

10. T F It only takes a few moments for a plaster cast to dry completely.

11. T F Patients recovering from fractured hips are generally not allowed to bear weight on the affected side for several weeks.

12. T F If a patient has an open reduction/internal fixation for a fractured hip, it means a cast will have been applied.

13. T F Phantom pain after an amputation is imaginary and of no concern to caregivers.

14. T F The nursing assistant is responsible for teaching patients with prostheses how to use them.

15. T F It is important to prevent contractures after an amputation.

B. Matching.

Choose the correct word from Column II to match each phrase in Column I.

Column I	Column II
16. _____ correct position	**a.** arthritis
17. _____ small fluid-filled sacs found around joints	**b.** spica
	c. closed
18. _____ name given to a cast covering hips and one or both legs	**d.** bursae
	e. simple
19. _____ fracture where bone breaks through skin	**f.** alignment
	g. open
20. _____ inflammation of joints	

C. Multiple Choice.

Select the one best answer for each of the following.

21. When assigned to perform ROM, you should
   a. exercise every joint.
   b. exercise joints to the point of pain.
   c. check with the nurse for any limitations before starting.
   d. perform each exercise four times.

22. A greenstick fracture
   a. occurs mainly in children.
   b. fragments the bone.
   c. occurs mainly in the elderly.
   d. twists around the bone.

23. While a leg cast is drying,
   a. cover it tightly so moisture will not be lost.
   b. maintaining general alignment is not important.
   c. carefully observe the extremities for circulation.
   d. use only fingertips to handle the cast.

24. When caring for the patient in traction,
   a. maintain proper alignment.
   b. lift the weights rapidly.
   c. allow weights to rest on the floor.
   d. position the patient's feet against the footboard.

25. Your patient has a ruptured disc. You should note and report
- **a.** crossing of the legs.
- **b.** ambulation in the room.
- **c.** numbness and tingling.
- **d.** complaints of feeling tired.

26. The most common symptom of osteoarthritis is
- **a.** swollen joints.
- **b.** pain.
- **c.** redness.
- **d.** limited mobility.

27. Gout is caused by
- **a.** renal disease.
- **b.** hypertension.
- **c.** arthritic changes in aging.
- **d.** elevated uric acid levels in the blood.

28. When positioning a patient with hip replacement surgery, you should
- **a.** elevate the head of the bed at least 60 degrees.
- **b.** cross the legs at the ankles.
- **c.** avoid elevating the head more than 45 degrees.
- **d.** position the hips and knees in complete flexion.

29. Compartment syndrome is a
- **a.** serious surgical emergency.
- **b.** normal side effect of a fracture.
- **c.** chronic condition related to arthritis.
- **d.** side effect of medications.

30. Position the patient with an amputation
- **a.** with the legs in abduction.
- **b.** with pillows between the legs.
- **c.** with the head elevated at least 90 degrees.
- **d.** with the legs in adduction.

Nursing Assistant Challenge.

You are assigned to care for Mrs. Nellie Goldstein, 62 years old, who had a total hip arthroplasty two days ago. She will be starting rehabilitation today and will continue her therapy as an outpatient after she is discharged in three more days. Mrs. Goldstein is a very active person and is eager to be "up and going."

31. What restrictions do you need to be aware of when taking care of Mrs. Goldstein?

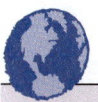

EXPLORING THE WEB

Description	Location
Assessment of Osteoporosis Using MRI	http://www.mrsc.ucsf.edu/bone.html
American Academy of Orthopedic Surgeons	http://www.aaos.org
Arthritis Research Campaign	http://www.arc.org.uk
Back Door Orthopedic and P.T. Links	http://members.aol.com/backbuster
Center for Orthopedics & Sports Medicine	http://www.arthroscopy.com
Combined Health Information Database	http://chid.nih.gov/subfile/subfile.html
Joint Replacement Institute	http://www.jri-oh.com
KneeGuru	http://www.kneeguru.co.uk
Lowbackpain.com	http://www.lowbackpain.com
National Association of Orthopedic Nurses	http://www.orthonurse.org
OrthoGate	http://owl.orthogate.org
OrthoGuide.com	http://www.orthoguide.com
Osteoporosis prevention and treatment	http://www.umassmemorial.org
Preventive Health Center (osteoporosis)	http://www.md-phc.com
Spine-Health.com	http://www.spine-health.com
Spine Universe	http://www.spineuniverse.com
University of Iowa Back Institute	http://www.uihealthcare.com
Wheeless Textbook of Orthopedics	http://www.ortho-u.net
WorldOrtho Electronic Textbook	http://www.worldortho.com

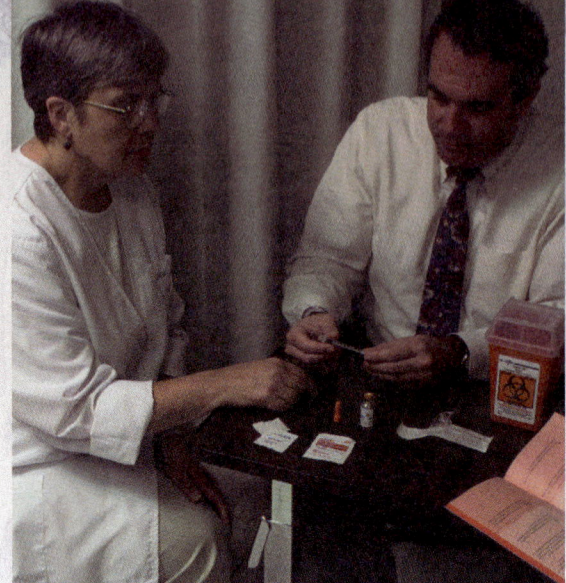

Endocrine System

objectives

After completing this unit, you will be able to:

- Spell and define terms.
- Review the location and functions of the endocrine system.
- List five specific diagnostic tests associated with conditions of the endocrine system.
- Describe some common diseases of the endocrine system.
- Recognize the signs and symptoms of hypoglycemia and hyperglycemia.

- Describe nursing assistant actions related to the care of patients with disorders of the endocrine system.
- Perform blood tests for glucose levels if facility policy permits.
- Perform the following procedure:
  - Procedure 102 Obtaining a Fingerstick Blood Sugar
  - Procedure 103 Testing Urine for Acetone: Ketostix® Strip Test

vocabulary

Learn the meaning and the correct spelling of the following words and phrases:

acetone	gonads	iodine	polyphagia
Addison's disease	hormones	islets of Langerhans	polyuria
adrenal glands	hypercalcemia	lancet	progesterone
assimilate	hyperglycemia	non–insulin-	scrotum
Cushing's syndrome	hypersecretion	dependent	simple goiter
diabetes mellitus	hyperthyroidism	diabetes mellitus	sperm
endocrine glands	hypertrophy	(NIDDM)	testes
estrogen	hypoglycemia	ovaries	testosterone
fingerstick blood	hyposecretion	ovum	tetany
sugar (FSBS)	hypothyroidism	parathormone	thyrocalcitonin
glucagon	insulin	parathyroid gland	thyroid gland
glucose	insulin-dependent	pineal body	thyroxine
glycogen	diabetes mellitus	pituitary gland	
glycosuria	(IDDM)	polydipsia	

STRUCTURE AND FUNCTION

The **endocrine glands** (Figure 41-1):

- secrete hormones.
- control body activities and growth.
- are found as distinct glands or clusters of cells.
- are subject to disease that can result in **hyposecretion** (underproduction) or **hypersecretion** (overproduction) of hormones.

Hormones are chemicals that regulate the body's activities.

Pituitary Gland

Because it controls most of the other glands, the **pituitary gland** is called the master gland.

The pituitary gland has two portions called *lobes*. Each of the lobes secretes more than one hormone.

1. The anterior lobe secretes:
   - STH (somatotropic hormone)—a growth hormone that stimulates the growth of long bones
   - TSH (thyroid-stimulating hormone)—stimulates the thyroid gland
   - FSH (follicle-stimulating hormone)—promotes growth of the ovarian follicle in which the egg develops during the menstrual cycle
   - ACTH (adrenocorticotropic hormone)—stimulates production by the adrenal gland
   - LH (luteinizing hormone)—in females, helps stimulate ovulation during the menstrual cycle
   - ICSH (interstitial cell-stimulating hormone)—stimulates the male testes
   - Lactogenic hormone (LTH)—stimulates milk production in pregnant women
2. The posterior lobe secretes:
   - ADH (antidiuretic hormone)—acts on kidneys to prevent excess water loss
   - Pitocin (oxytocin)—stimulates uterine contractions during childbirth

Pineal Body

The **pineal body** is a small gland that is also located in the skull beneath the brain. Very little is known about this gland. It is thought to be related somehow to sexual growth, because it tends to get smaller at maturity. It produces:

- Glomerulotropin, which influences the adrenal gland

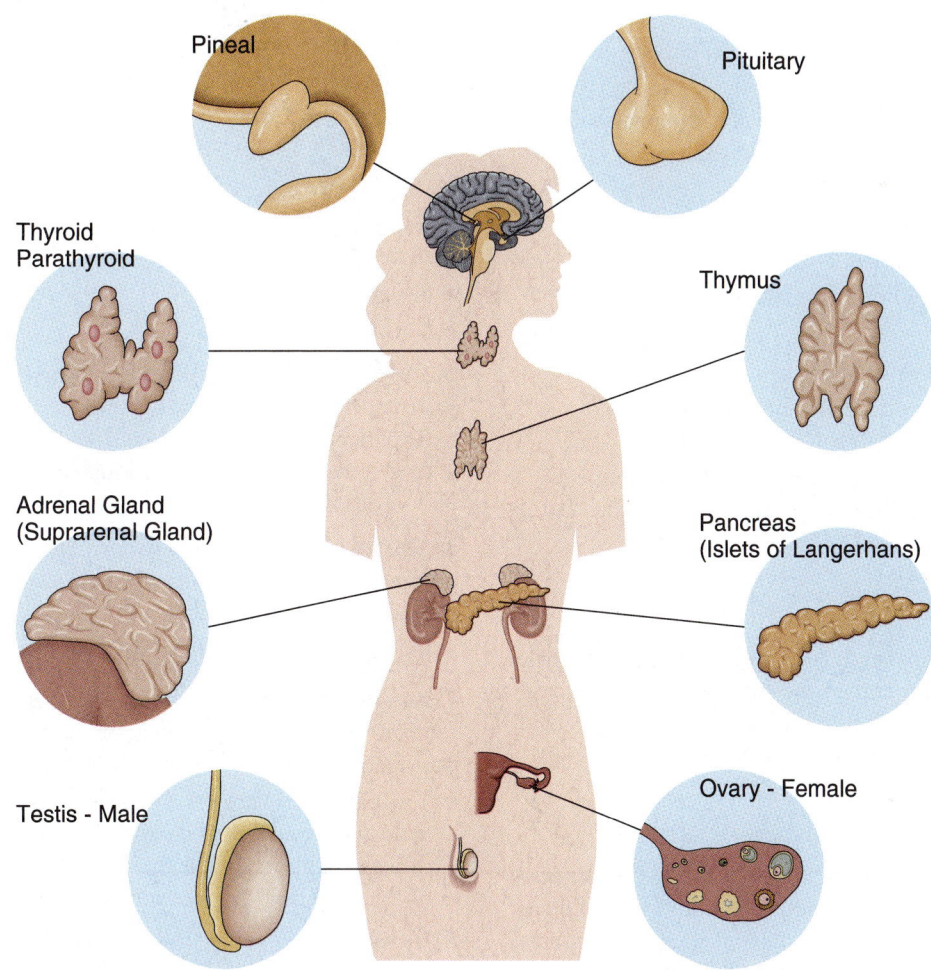

Pineal

Pituitary

Thyroid
Parathyroid

Thymus

Adrenal Gland
(Suprarenal Gland)

Pancreas
(Islets of Langerhans)

Testis - Male

Ovary - Female

FIGURE 41-1 Endocrine system.

- Serotonin, which acts in the brain
- Melatonin, which keeps sexual maturity from occurring too early and may affect the sleep/wake cycle.

Adrenal Glands

There are two adrenal glands. One gland is located on top of each kidney. Each gland has two distinct portions that secrete separate hormones.

1. The adrenal medulla (inside) produces norepinephrine (noradrenalin) and epinephrine (adrenalin), which stimulate the body to produce energy quickly during an emergency.
2. The adrenal cortex (outside) produces:
   - Glucocorticoids—elevate blood sugar levels and control the response of the body to stress and inflammation. They also depress inflammation.
   - Mineral corticoids—manage sodium and potassium levels.
   - Gonadocorticoids—influence both male and female sex hormones.

Gonads

The term gonads refers to the male and female sex glands. The female gonads (two ovaries):

- Are located within the pelvic cavity on either side of the uterus.
- Produce two hormones, estrogen and progesterone. These hormones are responsible for the development of female characteristics such as:
  - Breast development
  - Pubic and axillary hair
  - Onset and regulation of menstruation
  - Pregnancy

The male gonads (two testes):

- Are located on the outside of the body in a pouch called the scrotum.
- Produce the hormone testosterone. This hormone is responsible for secondary male characteristics such as:
  - Muscular development
  - Deepening voice
  - Hair growth

The male and female gonads also produce special cells—in the female, the ovum and in the male, the sperm. These cells unite during fertilization to form the embryo that becomes a new human being.

Thyroid Gland

The thyroid gland has two lobes and is found in the neck, anterior to the larynx. Hormones secreted by this gland are thyroxine and thyrocalcitonin. Thyroxine regulates metabolism. Iodine is an important component of this hormone. Thyrocalcitonin regulates calcium and phosphorus levels.

Parathyroid Glands

The tiny parathyroid glands are embedded in the posterior thyroid gland. The hormone they manufacture is called parathormone. Parathormone helps control the body's use of two minerals, calcium and phosphorus. Insufficient amounts of calcium result in severe muscle spasms or tetany. Untreated tetany can lead to death.

Islets of Langerhans

The islets of Langerhans are small groups of cells found within the pancreas. These cells produce two hormones: insulin and glucagon. Insulin lowers blood sugar. Glucagon elevates blood sugar.

COMMON CONDITIONS OF THE THYROID GLAND

The thyroid gland may secrete too much or not enough hormones. Either situation is treatable. If not treated, severe illness or death will occur.

Hyperthyroidism

Hyperthyroidism, or overactivity of the thyroid gland, results in production of too much thyroxine (hypersecretion). The person shows:

- Irritability and restlessness
- Nervousness
- Rapid pulse
- Increased appetite
- Weight loss
- Sensitivity

Nursing Assistant Actions. When caring for these patients, the nursing assistant must be understanding and have patience. The room should be kept quiet and cool. The patient's increased nutritional needs should be met with foods that are liked.

Treatment. Treatment of hyperthyroidism is designed to reduce the level of thyroxine through:

- Surgical thyroidectomy
- Radiation to reduce the number of functional cells

Thyroidectomy. It may be necessary to treat hyperthyroidism with surgery. You may be assigned to assist in the postoperative care. Following surgery:

- The patient is placed in a semi-Fowler's position, with neck and shoulders well supported. Remember at all times to support the back of the neck. Hyperextension of the neck may damage the operative site.
- Assist with oxygen, if ordered, using all oxygen precautions.
- Give routine postoperative care.

- Check for and report the following:
  - Any signs of bleeding (this may drain toward the back of the neck). The pillows behind the patient should be checked, as well as the dressings.
  - Signs of respiratory distress.
  - Inability of the patient to speak. Initial hoarseness is common, but any increase should be reported.
  - Greatly elevated temperature and pulse, pronounced apprehension, or irritability.
  - Numbness, tingling, or muscular spasm (**tetany**) of the extremities.

Hypothyroidism

Hypothyroidism results in an undersecretion of thyroxine. Recall that iodine is an essential component of thyroxine. A lack of iodine in the diet can result in low thyroxine production.

- The condition is called **simple goiter**.
- The thyroid gland enlarges (**hypertrophies**).
- Secretions produced have low thyroxine content.

Hypothyroidism can usually be successfully managed with thyroxine replacement.

COMMON CONDITIONS OF THE PARATHYROID GLANDS

Parathormone, secreted by the parathyroids, regulates the levels of electrolytes, calcium, and phosphates. Hypersecretion of this hormone results in:

- Excessively high levels of blood calcium (**hypercalcemia**)
- Developmental of renal calculi (kidney stones)
- Loss of bone calcium

Hypersecretion is usually caused by tumors. Tumors can be treated by surgical removal.

Hyposecretion can lead to:

- Abnormal muscle-nerve interaction
- Severe muscle spasm (tetany)

This can be an emergency situation, requiring management of the muscle spasms and administration of calcium. In the chronic state, calcium replacements and increased dietary calcium are prescribed.

COMMON CONDITIONS OF THE ADRENAL GLANDS

The adrenal gland secretions regulate:

- Development and maintenance of sexual characteristics
- Carbohydrate, fat, and protein metabolism
- Fluid balance
- Electrolyte levels of sodium and potassium

Hypersecretion results in **Cushing's syndrome**, which is characterized by:

- Weakness due to loss of body protein
- Increased blood sugar levels (hyperglycemia)
- Edema
- Hypertension
- Loss of potassium and retention of sodium
- Masculinization of a female

Therapy is primarily surgical and supportive.

Hyposecretion results in **Addison's disease**, which is characterized by:

- Loss of sodium and retention of potassium
- Abnormally low blood sugar (hypoglycemia)
- Dehydration
- Low stress tolerance

Addison's disease is treated by hormone replacement therapy and techniques to combat dehydration.

DIABETES MELLITUS

In the United States, 17 million people have diabetes mellitus. Approximately 5.9 million of these have not been diagnosed yet. Diabetes occurs in people of all ages and races, but is most common in African Americans, Native Americans, Latinos, Asian Americans, and Pacific Islanders. The incidence of diabetes increases with age.

Diabetes mellitus is a chronic disease that results from a deficiency of insulin or a resistance to the effects of insulin. The problems with insulin cause the body to be unable to properly process food into energy. The glucose from the food breakdown remains in the blood, resulting in elevated blood sugar. Persistent, elevated glucose levels affect the blood vessels and nerves, making the person with diabetes more likely to develop heart attack, stroke, blindness, renal disease, and other serious complications and conditions.

The reason why diabetes develops is not fully understood. Factors that seem to play a role in the incidence of diabetes are:

- Heredity
- Obesity
- Age
- Diet
- Lack of exercise

All diabetics should wear or carry a Medic Alert® identification so that proper and immediate care can be provided in an emergency. It is also recommended that the diabetic carry food that provides a quick source of carbohydrates.

Disease Mechanism

In diabetes, the normal metabolism of fats, carbohydrates, and proteins is unbalanced. Normally, when carbohydrates are absorbed into the bloodstream, the blood sugar (glucose) level rises. The pancreas responds to an increase of **glucose** by secreting more insulin. Insulin is the hormone primarily responsible for:

- Lowering the blood sugar level by allowing glucose to cross the cell membrane.
- Increasing the oxidation of glucose by the tissues.
- Stimulating the conversion of glucose to glycogen by the liver. **Glycogen** is a storage form of energy.
- Decreasing glucose production from amino acids.
- Stimulating glucose formation into fat for storage.

In diabetes, there is insufficient insulin for these metabolic functions.

- Glucose cannot be properly utilized for energy.
- Fats and proteins are incompletely broken down. This leads to an accumulation of ketone bodies, and nitrogenous waste products.
- The excess glucose is eliminated, along with water and salts, through the kidneys. This causes dehydration and electrolyte imbalance.
- The characteristic symptoms of excessive thirst, hunger, and increased urination are directly related to the loss of fluids, electrolytes, and sugar.

Types of Diabetes Mellitus

Diabetes mellitus is typed and named according to the need for insulin. Examples are insulin-dependent diabetes mellitus (IDDM) and non–insulin-dependent diabetes (NIDDM). IDDM appears more commonly in the young and NIDDM is more common in older people.

Insulin-dependent diabetes mellitus (**IDDM**) (Type I) accounts for approximately 5% to 10% of diabetes. This type tends to run in families. It is most common in children and young adults. Symptoms may mimic the flu in young children. People with Type I diabetes must take daily insulin injections to stay alive. Typical signs and symptoms are:

- **Polyuria** (excessive urination)
- **Polydipsia** (thirst)
- **Polyphagia** (hunger)
- **Glycosuria** (sugar in the urine)

Non–insulin-dependent diabetes mellitus (**NIDDM**) (Type II) is a metabolic disorder that occurs when the body does not make enough insulin, or does not properly use insulin. This is the most common form of diabetes. It accounts for 90% to 95% of all diabetes. It is said to be nearing epidemic proportions due to the high incidence of obesity and sedentary lifestyles. People usually develop Type II diabetes after age 45, but may not be aware they have the condition until symptoms become severe or complications develop. The risk for Type II diabetes increases with age. More than 20 percent of the United States population aged 65 and older has diabetes. Common signs and symptoms of Type II diabetes are:

- Easy fatigue
- Skin infections
- Slow healing
- Itching
- Pruritus vulvae (itching of the vulva)
- Burning on urination
- Vision changes
- Obesity

Often only one or two symptoms are apparent in the elderly person. The older person may:

- complain of constant fatigue.
- have a skin lesion that takes an unusually long time to heal.
- experience vision changes that may be mistakenly attributed to aging.

Care of the diabetic is directed toward maintaining a normal blood glucose level so that complications may be prevented. To regulate blood glucose, the diabetic person must:

- eat a healthful, well-balanced diet as prescribed by the physician.
- exercise regularly in a manner appropriate for the person's age and ability.
- check the blood sugar regularly
- use insulin or oral antidiabetic agents correctly if ordered by the physician.

For some persons this may require lifestyle changes. Nurses and dietitians are responsible for teaching patients who are newly diagnosed with diabetes how to care for themselves. People with diabetes who are knowledgeable about the disease and who are willing to manage their lives accordingly can live happily and productively (Figure 41-2).

Diet

Diet is an important part of diabetic treatment. Physicians do not fully agree as to how strictly a diet must be followed by all patients.

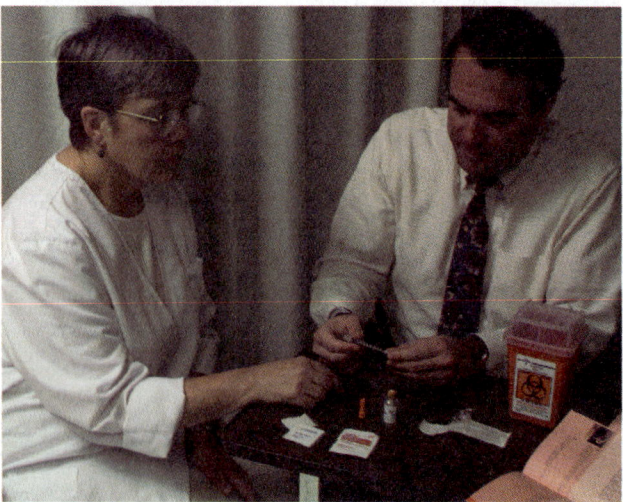

FIGURE 41-2 Patients are taught to manage their diabetes by the nurse.

- Weight reduction is favored.
- Weight reduction alone may be sufficient to bring the condition under control in NIDDM.

Meal Planning. The dietitian is a key member of the health care team for patients with diabetes. The dietitian helps the patient plan meals in keeping with the patient's goals, lifestyle, laboratory values, caloric and nutritional needs, and food preferences. Many diabetics use the diabetic food guide pyramid (Figure 41-3). This is similar to the USDA Food Guide Pyramid, but portion sizes and the total number of portions per day have been adjusted. The dietitian will work with the patient to develop a healthy meal plan.

The goals of the diet include maintaining near-normal blood sugar, optimal fat levels, and adequate calories based on individual needs. Meal plans are flexible. The diet should be well balanced, with sufficient fiber.

The diabetic exchange system of foods was formulated by a committee with representatives from the American Diabetic Association and the diabetic branch of the U.S. Public Health Service. The exchanges are available through the registered dietitian or diabetes educator. Although the exchange list system has been used for years, it is regularly updated to reflect new trends. The lists provide maximum flexibility in planning a healthy diet. The dietitian teaches the patient the importance of reading food labels, and how to interpret them. Common household measures are used to determine portion size.

Exercise

Exercise is an important part of the overall treatment. The amount and type of exercise the patient routinely engages in are balanced by the food intake and insulin or hypoglycemic drug requirements.

Hypoglycemic Drugs

Diabetes mellitus is treated by one of two main drug groups. One is administered subcutaneously or intravenously. The other is given orally.

At present, there are several types of insulin. They vary in their:

- Speed of action
- Duration
- Potency or strength

Insulin is:

- Administered by the nurse. The nurse rotates the administration sites.
- Given by injection.

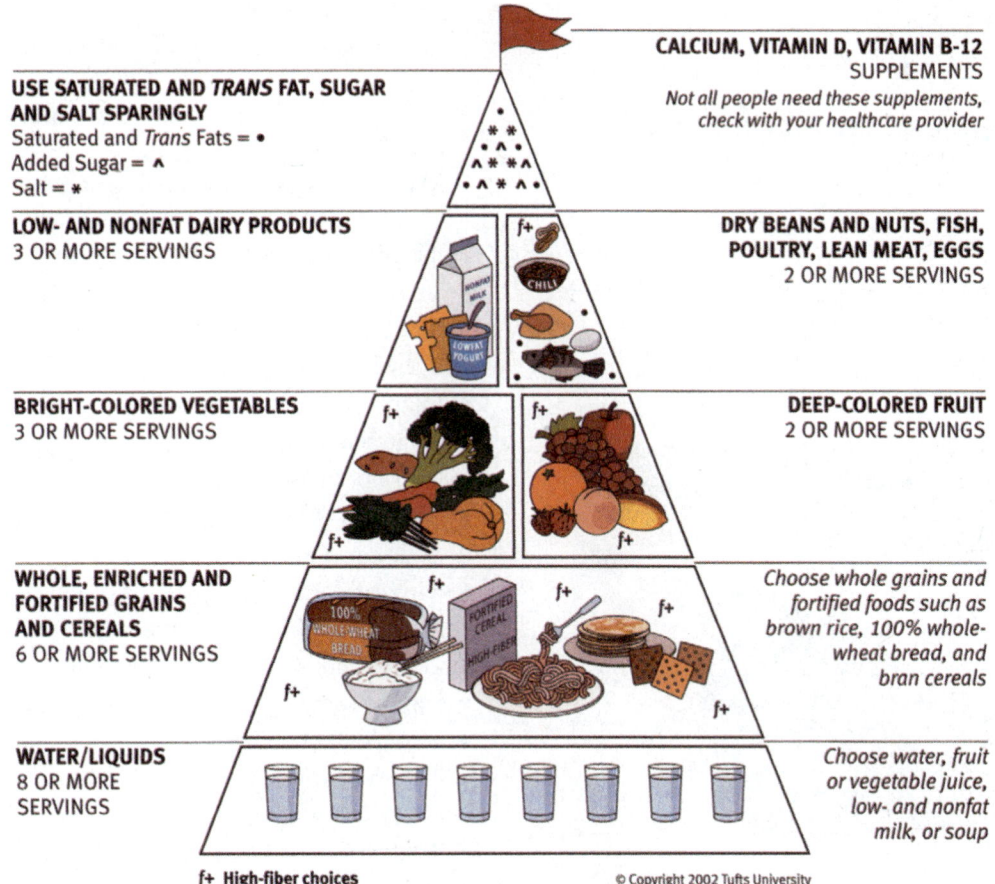

FIGURE 41-3 The diabetic food guide pyramid. *(Copyright 2002 Tufts University)*

- Increasingly given through use of an insulin pump. The insulin pump delivers a prescribed amount of insulin on a regular basis into the patient's body.
- Used to treat IDDM and some patients with NIDDM.

Persons living at home are taught to administer their own insulin.

Note: When insulin is self-administered, it is important to report any missed injections or signs of infection around the administration site.

Oral hypoglycemic drugs are:

- Administered by the nurse.
- Given by mouth.
- Used to treat NIDDM.

Complications

Because persistent, increased glucose levels cause damage to the nerves and blood vessels, the following complications can occur:

- Renal disease
- Circulatory impairments that often result in gangrene (Figure 41-4) and amputation
- Poor healing
- Hypertension
- Cardiovascular problems
- Diabetic coma
- Insulin shock (hypoglycemia)
- Vision problems and blindness

Hypoglycemia (Low Blood Sugar)

Hypoglycemia occurs when the blood glucose level is below normal. It:

- May occur rapidly.
- Is referred to as *insulin reaction* or *insulin shock* when due to an overdose of insulin.

Hypoglycemia can be brought on by:

- Skipping meals

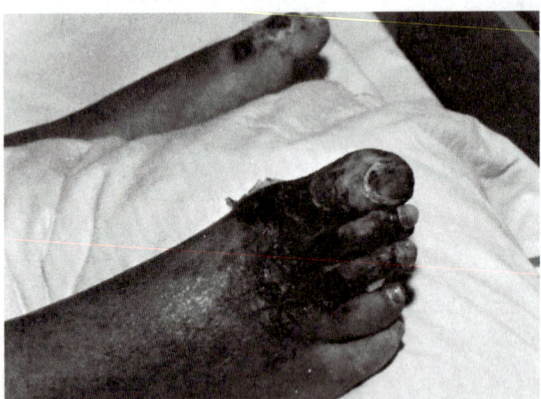

FIGURE 41-4 Gangrene of the feet and toes will require amputation. In most cases, the leg is amputated below the knee.

- Unusual activity
- Stress
- Vomiting
- Diarrhea
- Omission of planned snack or meals
- Interaction of drugs
- Too much insulin or antidiabetic medication

Signs and Symptoms. The signs and symptoms of hypoglycemia include:

- Complaints of hunger, weakness, dizziness, shakiness
- Skin cold, moist, clammy, pale
- Rapid, shallow respirations
- Nervousness and excitement
- Rapid pulse
- Unconsciousness
- No sugar in the urine
- Low blood sugar results from fingerstick test

If the patient is awake and alert, treatment includes intake of orange juice, milk, or another easily absorbed carbohydrate such as hard candy. If the patient is unconscious, the physician or nurse may give glucagon, which causes a rapid elevation of blood sugar.

Hyperglycemia (High Blood Sugar)

Hyperglycemia (diabetic coma):

- Occurs when there is insufficient insulin for metabolic needs.
- Usually develops slowly, sometimes over a 24-hour period.
- May be seen as confusion, drowsiness, or a slow slippage into coma in a patient who is confined to bed.

Hyperglycemia may be brought on by:

- Stress
- Illness such as infection
- Dehydration
- Injury
- Forgotten medication
- Intake of too much food

Signs and Symptoms. The signs and symptoms of diabetic coma include:

- Early headache, drowsiness, or confusion
- Sweet, fruity odor to the breath
- Deep breathing, labored respirations
- Full, bounding pulse
- Low blood pressure
- Nausea or vomiting
- Flushed, dry, hot skin
- Weakness
- Unconsciousness
- Sugar in the urine

• High blood sugar results from fingerstick test
Treatment includes administration of insulin, fluids, and electrolytes.

Other Complications

Persons with diabetes should have regular health monitoring so that complications may be detected early and treated promptly. Health monitoring should include:

- Eye examinations by an ophthalmologist for early detection of diabetic retinopathy, which can lead to impaired vision and eventually blindness.
- Urinalysis and other urological examinations to evaluate the condition of the kidneys.
- Cardiac evaluation; monitoring of heart action and blood pressure.
- Circulatory evaluation.
- Care and treatment of any wounds.
- Blood sugar monitoring.

Nursing Assistant Responsibilities

- Know the signs of insulin shock and diabetic coma.
- Be alert for the signs of diabetic coma or insulin shock and report them immediately to the nurse.
- Know the storage location of orange juice or other easily **assimilated** (absorbed) sources of carbohydrates.
- Keep easily assimilated carbohydrates, such as orange juice, crackers, hard candy, or Karo syrup, available if caring for a diabetic patient at home.
- Make sure you serve the patient proper trays of food.

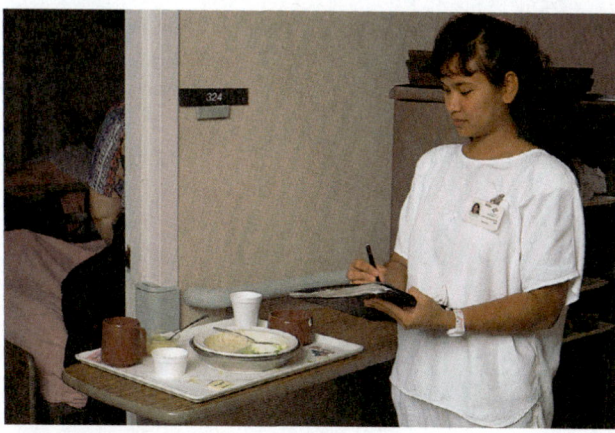

FIGURE 41-5 The amount and type of food consumed by patients with diabetes is closely observed and recorded.

- Do not give extra nourishments without special permission.
- Document food consumption, on the patient's chart.
- Report uneaten meals to the nurse (Figure 41-5).
- Give special attention to care of the diabetic patient's feet.
  - Wash daily, carefully drying between toes.
  - Inspect feet closely for any breaks or signs of irritation.
  - Report any abnormalities to the nurse.
  - Do not allow moisture to collect between toes.
  - The toenails of a diabetic should be cut only by a nurse or a podiatrist, a specialist who is trained in foot care.
  - Shoes and stockings should be clean, be free of holes, and fit well. Anything that might injure the feet or interfere with the circulation must be avoided.
  - Do not allow the patient to go barefoot.

DIAGNOSTIC TECHNIQUES

Techniques used to diagnose problems of the endocrine system include:
- Blood analysis for hormone levels
- Urine analysis for hormone levels
- Radioisotope scanning for thyroid disease
- Radioactive iodine uptake for thyroid function
- Basal metabolic rate (BMR) to measure the speed of oxygen uptake

BLOOD GLUCOSE MONITORING

Bedside glucose testing has become very common in the management of patients with diabetes. Many individuals perform this testing at home several times each day. The antidiabetic medication may be adjusted according to the patient's blood sugar. A blood sample is taken from a capillary. The test meter will display the blood sugar value in

DIFFICULT *Situations*

Attention to personal hygiene, oral care, and cleanliness is particularly important in individuals with diabetes. Diabetics must bathe regularly to prevent localized skin infections. However, they should avoid prolonged soaking in a tub, which can soften the tissues and lead to breakdown. If you observe unusual areas, such as yellowish pimples or boils, on a diabetic patient's skin, or angry-looking red areas in skin folds (such as under the breasts, underarms, or groin), inform the nurse. Assist the patient with toothbrushing and flossing. The teeth have five surfaces, and toothbrushing only reaches three. Flossing effectively cleans the areas that are not accessible with the brush. Good foot care and drying well between the toes are essential. Report signs and symptoms of infection, even if they seem minor.

one minute or less. This is a convenient, accurate method of monitoring the blood sugar. Nursing assistants perform this procedure in some facilities. Know and follow your facility policy.

The physician will order specific times for blood sugar testing. The specimen may be collected at a fixed time, such as before meals. The nurse may administer insulin to the patient based on the blood sugar value. Collect the capillary sample exactly as ordered. Specimens that are not collected at the proper time can cause misinterpretation of the results. Always report the value to the nurse, and document according to facility policy.

If the nurse suspects that a patient is having complications related to diabetes, he or she may ask you to obtain a stat blood sugar. This test must be performed immediately. Report the results immediately.

Fingerstick Blood Sugar

Fingerstick blood sugar (**FSBS**) is checked by collecting a sample of capillary blood with a **lancet**, or tiny needle. The blood is transferred to a reagent strip or other test strip. For most reagent strips, you must place a hanging drop of blood onto the reagent pad. Avoid smearing the strip against the finger. The Multistix® (Figure 41-6) and Chemstrip BG® can be read visually, by comparing the color on the reagent strip with the key on the bottle. The Chemstrip BG® may also be used in the Accucheck® blood glucose meter.

Many new meters do not use a reagent strip. After making the fingerstick, a drop of blood is transferred to the test strip, which is inserted into the meter before beginning. The tiny tube draws blood to the inside on contact. This feature works well with patients from whom it is difficult to obtain a hanging drop of blood. An audible beep informs you when the tube has collected enough blood.

Many different blood glucose meters are available. All are accurate and simple to use. Each meter has its own reagent or test strip. For accuracy, make sure the strip is compatible with the meter you are using (Figure 41-7). Also, check the expiration date on the bottle. Do not use the strips that are beyond the expiration date. Follow the directions for

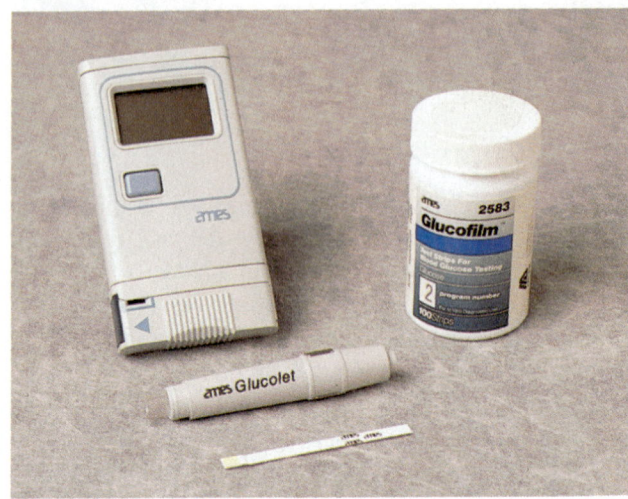

FIGURE 41-7 The reagent strips must be compatible with the glucose meter.

the meter and reagent strips you are using. All are slightly different.

Many different lancets are also available for performing blood glucose checks. Retractable lancets, which are spring-loaded, have the lowest incidence of injury. The needle withdraws after the finger has been punctured, reducing the chance of needlestick injuries. Discard lancets into a puncture-resistant sharps container. Many health care workers have been injured by lancets that were inadvertently dropped in the bed or on the floor.

The normal blood sugar values vary with the health care facility. The normal fasting range in most facilities is somewhere between 65 and 120, with the normal value commonly being 70 to 110. Values below 70 always suggest hypoglycemia. Fasting values above 110 suggest hyperglycemia. Learn the normal values for your facility. Values that are well above or below the normal range suggest serious diabetic problems. Notify the nurse immediately of blood sugar values outside of the normal range or other signs and symptoms of blood sugar problems, such as:

- Inadequate food intake
- Eating food not permitted on diet
- Refusal of meals, supplements, or snacks
- Nausea, vomiting, or diarrhea
- Inadequate fluid intake
- Excessive activity
- Complaints of dizziness, shakiness, racing heart

Some blood glucose meters do not have a wide range. Typically, hand-held blood glucose meters will read a blood sugar value as low as 40. A few measure blood sugars as low as 20. For values below the lowest meter reading, the screen will display the word "low." On the high end, most meters do not read values above 400 or 500. If the fingerstick blood sugar exceeds the meter high reading, the display will read "high." If the screen displays the word *low* or *high*, the patient has the potential for serious complications. His or her condition may deteriorate quickly. Inform the nurse immediately.

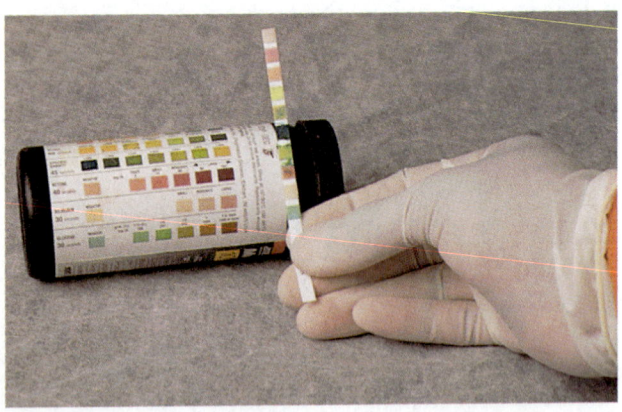

FIGURE 41-6 Multistix® are used for many different blood tests.

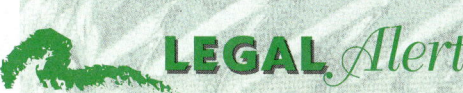

PROCEDURE 102

OBTAINING A FINGERSTICK BLOOD SUGAR

LEGAL *Alert*

Be sure this is a nursing assistant procedure in your facility.

 Note: *This procedure is generic and applies the principles used for most blood glucose meters. Follow the directions for the meter and strip you are using. The operating directions are slightly different for each.*

1. Carry out beginning procedure actions.

2. Gather equipment:
   - disposable exam gloves
   - alcohol sponge
   - lancet
   - blood glucose meter
   - reagent strip or test strip for the blood glucose meter being used
   - sharps container
   - plastic bandage strip
   - plastic bag for used supplies

3. Wipe the patient's finger with the alcohol sponge. Allow the alcohol to dry.

4. Pierce the sides of the middle or ring finger using the lancet (Figure 41-8A).

5. Discard the lancet in the sharps container.

6. Squeeze the sides of the finger gently to obtain a drop of blood.

7. Hold the puncture site directly over the reagent strip, and place a hanging drop of blood onto the reagent pad. If using the capillary tube (straw-like) strips, peel the package back to open it. Hold the package firmly with your thumb and forefinger over the test end (patient end) of the strip. Insert the strip into the meter (Figure 41-8B). Remove and discard the package. Hold the strip next to the puncture site to draw blood into the straw (Figure 41-8C).

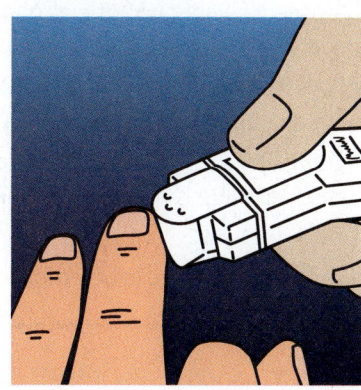

FIGURE 41-8A Pierce the side of the finger with the lancet.

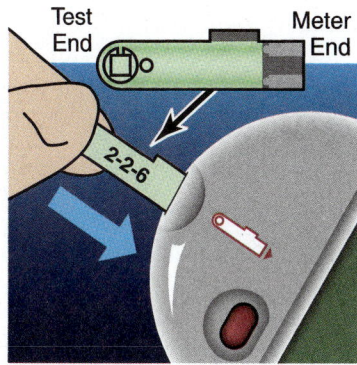

FIGURE 41-8B Insert the strip into the meter.

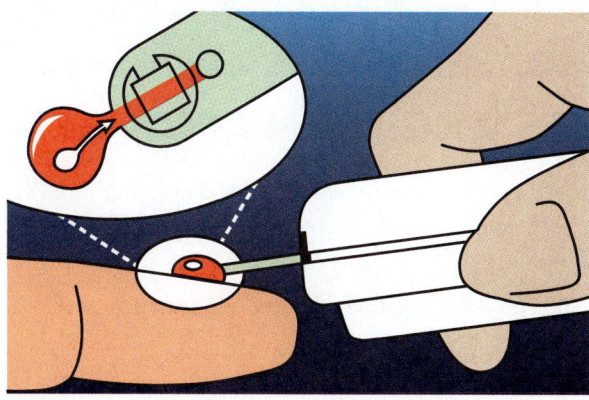

FIGURE 41-8C The strip is like a straw that will draw blood into the meter.

continues

PROCEDURE 102

continued

8. Insert the strip into the meter, if this was not done previously.

9. Wipe the patient's finger with the alcohol sponge and allow to dry. Apply pressure until bleeding stops. Apply a bandage strip, if necessary.

10. Wait the designated period of time for the meter you are using. An audible beep will indicate when the blood sugar value is displayed on the screen (Figure 41-8D).

11. Carry out procedure completion actions.

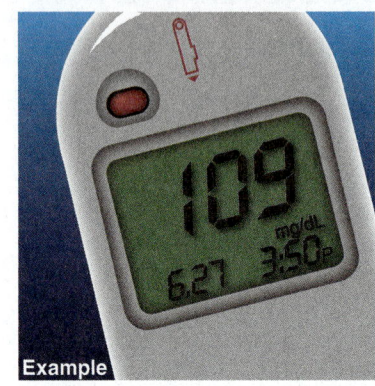

FIGURE 41-8D
Read the meter after the designated period of time.

Acetone Monitoring

You may be expected to test the patient's urine for acetone. **Acetone** is a substance that accumulates in the body when the blood glucose is out of balance. A simple urine test detects the presence of acetone. Some blood glucose meters also check for ketones in the blood. However, urine monitoring is still done when the ketone level must be measured.

DIFFICULT *Situations*

Ketone bodies are created when body fat is burned for fuel instead of sugar. The ketone bodies cause a chemical imbalance, resulting in accumulation of acids and upset of the patient's buffer system. If a patient's blood sugar is over 250 mg/dl, the nurse may instruct you to check the patient's urine for ketones. If the patient is very ill, the nurse may request a ketone test even if the blood sugar is not high.

PROCEDURE 103

TESTING URINE FOR ACETONE: KETOSTIX® STRIP TEST

 Note: *If the results of the blood glucose tests are above normal, the nurse may request that the urine be tested for acetone.*

1. Carry out beginning procedure actions.

2. Assemble equipment:
   - disposable gloves
   - Ketostix® reagent strips
   - sample of freshly voided urine in container

3. Put on disposable gloves.

4. Remove one test strip from the bottle and recap the bottle.

5. Dip one end of the test strip (the end with the reagent areas) into the urine (Figure 41-9A).

continues

PROCEDURE 103

continued

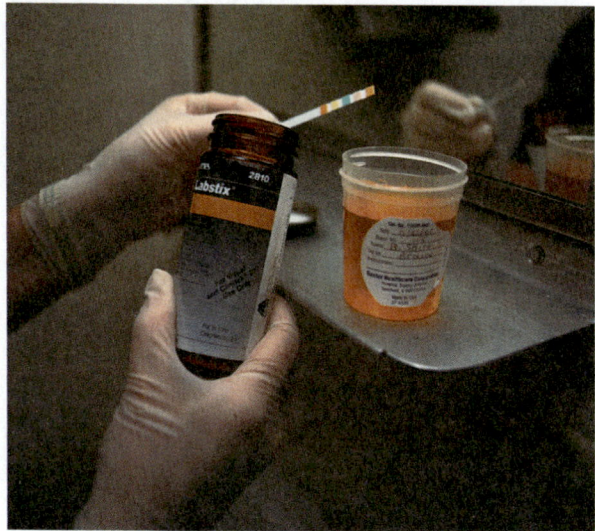

FIGURE 41-9A Remove a strip from the bottle, then recap the bottle tightly. Dip the strip into the fresh urine sample.

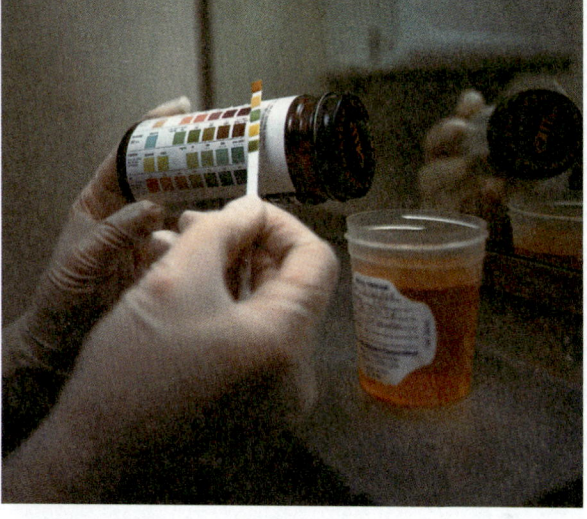

FIGURE 41-9B Compare the strip with the color chart on the bottle. Do not touch the strip to the label.

6. Remove the strip and hold it horizontally.

7. Fifteen seconds later, compare the strip with the color chart on the bottle label (Figure 41-9B). Match it as closely as possible to one of the colors on the chart. Do not touch the wet strip to the bottle label.

8. Dispose of the strip and urine specimen unless orders have been given to save either or both of them.

9. Remove and properly dispose of gloves according to facility policy.

10. Carry out procedure completion actions.

REVIEW

A. True/False.

Mark the following true or false by circling T or F.

1. T F The person with polyphagia has a high urine output.

2. T F In Type II diabetes, the body does not make enough insulin, or does not properly use insulin.

3. T F Glucose is another name for blood sugar.

4. T F The person with hyperthyroidism is slow-moving and lethargic.

5. T F Hyperthyroidism causes people to lose weight.

6. T F You should keep the room of a patient with hyperthyroidism quite warm.

7. T F Obesity may play a role in the incidence of diabetes mellitus.

8. T F If the patient with IDDM appears drowsy and confused, you should suspect the possibility of hyperglycemia.

9. T F Foot care is especially important for the diabetic patient.

10. T F Disposable gloves should be worn when testing urine for sugar.

B. Matching.

Choose the correct item from Column II to match each phrase in Column I.

Column I

11. _____ internal secretion produced by glands

12. _____ diabetic coma

13. _____ excess thirst

14. _____ sugar in the urine

15. _____ produces hormones

16. _____ excess hunger

17. _____ blood sugar

18. _____ overweight

19. _____ master gland

20. _____ located above the kidneys

Column II

a. polydipsia

b. polyphagia

c. polyuria

d. glycosuria

e. endocrine gland

f. hormone

g. obesity

h. glycogen

i. NIDDM

j. insulin shock

k. glucose

l. adrenal glands

m. pituitary gland

C. Multiple Choice.

Select the one best answer for each of the following.

21. Your patient has had a thyroidectomy. You should
  a. keep the patient flat in bed.
  b. watch for and report signs of respiratory distress.
  c. carry out ROM exercises immediately.
  d. position the patient in a left Sims' position.

22. Lack of iodine in the diet can result in
  a. hypothyroidism.
  b. hyperthyroidism.
  c. diabetes mellitus.
  d. ketosis.

23. The pituitary gland is responsible for secreting hormones that
  a. stimulate ovulation during the menstrual cycle.
  b. manage sodium and potassium levels.
  c. control calcium and phosphorus.
  d. regulate blood sugar.

24. Your patient is an insulin-dependent diabetic. You know this
  a. is a stable form of the disease.
  b. affects only older persons.
  c. requires hypoglycemic drugs.
  d. is a less stable form of the disease.

25. Insulin is an important hormone because it
  a. lowers blood sugar.
  b. raises blood sugar.
  c. stimulates the conversion of glycogen to glucose.
  d. breaks fat down to form glucose.

D. Nursing Assistant Challenge.

You are assigned to two patients who both have diabetes. Sally Sakowski is 29 years old and has had diabetes for 10 years. She is considered to be IDDM. Ruth Young is 72 years old and has just been diagnosed with NIDDM. Although these patients both have diabetes, there may be many differences in their signs, symptoms, and problems. Consider these questions:

26. What differences would you see in the signs and symptoms experienced by these two women?

27. What differences would you expect in their treatment?

28. Knowing the difference in their ages, how would you expect the disease to affect the lifestyle of each woman?

29. Hypoglycemia and hyperglycemia may be a complication for either patient. List the differences in the signs and symptoms of both complications.

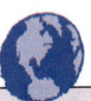

EXPLORING THE WEB

Description	Location
Diabetes public health resources	http://www.cdc.gov/diabetes/index.htm
Directory of diabetes-related organizations	http://www.niddk.nih.gov/health/diabetes/pubs/diaborgs/diaborgs.htm
American Association of Clinical Endocrinologists	http://www.aace.com
American Association of Diabetes Educators	http://www.aadenet.org
American Diabetes Association	http://www.diabetes.org

continues

EXPLORING THE WEB　*continued*

Description	Location
Ask Noah	*http://www.noah-health.org*
Canadian Diabetes Association	*http://www.diabetes.ca*
Combined Health Information Database	*http://chid.nih.gov/subfile/subfile.html*
Diabetes Mall	*http://www.diabetesnet.com*
Diabetes Monitor	*http://www.diabetesmonitor.com*
Doctors' Guide to Diabetes	*http://www.docguide.com*
International Diabetes Federation	*http://www.idf.org*
Medline Plus	*http://www.nlm.nih.gov/medlineplus/diabetes.html*
MedWeb Plus	*http://www.medwebplus.com*
Merck Manual	*http://www.merck.com*
National Diabetes Education Program	*http://ndep.nih.gov*
National Diabetes Fact Sheets	*http://www.cdc.gov/diabetes/pubs/factsheet.htm*
National Institute of Diabetes	*http://www.niddk.nih.gov/health/diabetes/dia/*
Preventive Health Center	*http://www.md-phc.com*
Yahoo Health	*http://dir.yahoo.com/Health*

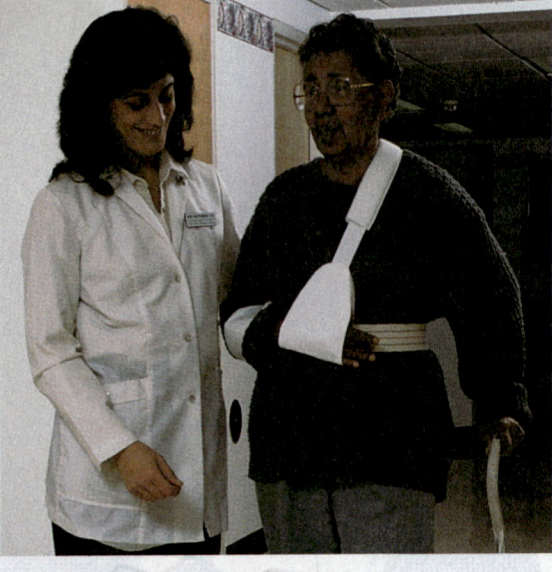

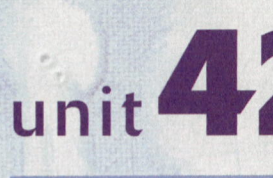

Nervous System

objectives

After completing this unit, you will be able to:

- Spell and define terms.
- State the location and functions of the organs of the nervous system.
- List five diagnostic tests used to determine conditions of the nervous system.
- Describe eight common conditions of the nervous system.
- Describe nursing assistant actions related to the care of patients with conditions of the nervous system.
- Explain the proper care, handling, and insertion of an artificial eye.

- Explain the proper care, handling, and insertion of a hearing aid.
- Demonstrate the following procedures:
  - Procedure 104 Caring for the Eye Socket and Artificial Eye
  - Procedure 105 Warm Eye Compresses
  - Procedure 106 Cool Eye Compresses
  - Procedure 107 Applying a Behind-the-Ear Hearing Aid
  - Procedure 108 Removing a Behind-the-Ear Hearing Aid
  - Procedure 109 Applying and Removing an In-the-Ear Hearing Aid

vocabulary

Learn the meaning and the correct spelling of the following words and phrases:

absence seizure	convulsion	lacrimal gland	post polio syndrome
akinesia	cornea	Lhermitte's sign	(PPS)
amyotrophic lateral	dendrite	macular degeneration	pupil
sclerosis (ALS)	emotional lability	meninges	quadriplegia
aphasia	epilepsy	meningitis	receptive aphasia
aura	eustachian tube	multiple sclerosis (MS)	retinal degeneration
autonomic dysreflexia	expressive aphasia	nerve	semicircular canal
axon	flaccid paralysis	neuron	spastic paralysis
brain attack	generalized tonic-clonic	neurotransmitter	spatial-perceptual deficit
brain stem	seizures	nystagmus	status epilepticus
cataract	Glasgow Coma Scale	ossicle	stroke
cerebellum	glaucoma	otitis media	synapse
cerebrospinal fluid (CSF)	global aphasia	otosclerosis	transient ischemic attack
cerebrovascular accident	grand mal seizure	paralysis	(TIA)
(CVA)	hemianopsia	paraplegia	tremor
cerebrum	hemiplegia	Parkinson's disease	tympanic membrane
cochlea	intention tremor	petit mal seizure	unilateral neglect
cognitive impairment	intracranial pressure	position sense	vertigo
conjunctiva	iris		

STRUCTURE AND FUNCTION

The nervous system controls and coordinates all body activities, including the production of hormones. Special parts of the nervous system are concerned with maintaining normal day-to-day functions. Other parts act during emergency situations. Still others control voluntary activities. Neurological conditions require highly specialized nursing care. You will assist with the less technical aspects of that care.

Neurons

Cells of the nervous system are called **neurons** (Figure 42-1A). They are specialized to conduct electriclike impulses.

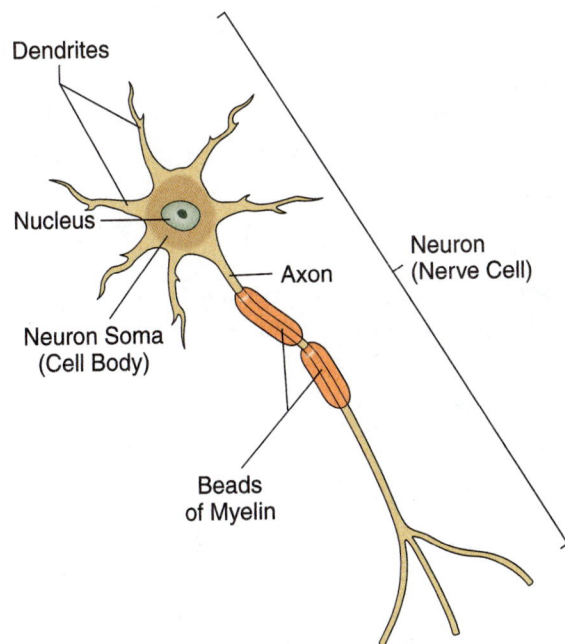

Dendrites

Nucleus

Neuron Soma (Cell Body)

Axon

Neuron (Nerve Cell)

Beads of Myelin

FIGURE 42-1A The neuron.

The neuron has extensions called **axons** and **dendrites**. Impulses enter the neuron only through the dendrites and leave only through the axon.

Although neurons do not actually touch each other, the axon of one neuron lies close to the dendrites of many other neurons. In this way, impulses may follow many different routes. The space between the axon of one cell and the dendrites of others is called a **synapse**. Axons and dendrites in the periphery are covered with *myelin*, which acts as insulation.

Neurotransmitters

Neurotransmitters are chemicals that enable messages (nerve impulses) to pass from one cell to another (Figure 42-1B). If the chemicals are not produced in the right amounts, the message pathway becomes confused or blocked.

Nerves

Some axons and dendrites are long. Others are short. Axons and dendrites of many neurons are found in bundles. The bundles are held together by connective tissue. These bundles resemble telephone cables and are called **nerves**. The cell bodies of the axons and dendrites in these nerves may be found far from the ends of the nerves in clusters called *ganglia*.

Sensory nerves are made up of dendrites. They carry sensations to the brain and spinal cord from the various body parts. Feeling is lost when these nerve impulses are interrupted. Motor nerves carry impulses from the brain and spinal cord to muscles that cause body activity. Paralysis or loss of function occurs when these nerves are damaged.

For easier study, the nervous system can be divided into two parts: the central nervous system (CNS) and the peripheral nervous system (PNS). The CNS is composed of the brain and spinal cord (Figure 42-2). The PNS is composed of the 12 pairs of cranial nerves and 31 pairs of spinal nerves that reach throughout the body (Figure 42-3).

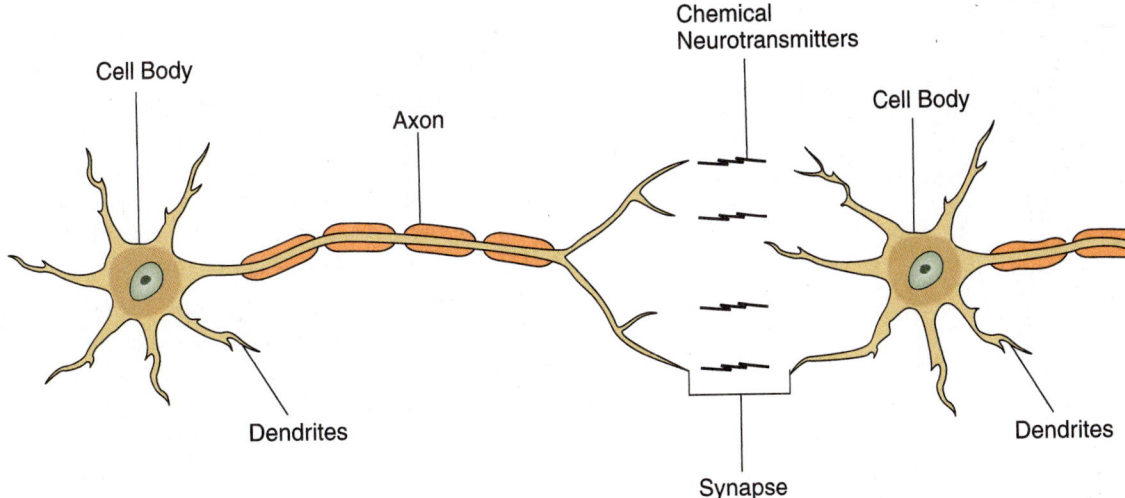

Chemical Neurotransmitters

Cell Body

Axon

Cell Body

Dendrites

Dendrites

Synapse

FIGURE 42-1B Chemicals called neurotransmitters help pass the message across the synapse from one neuron to another.

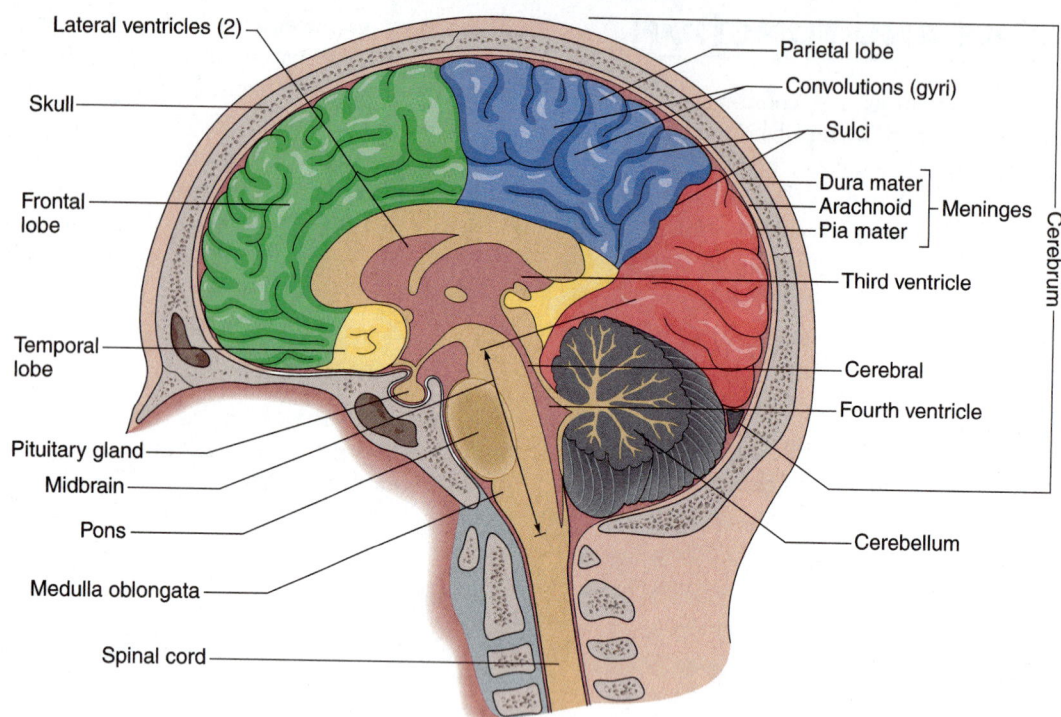

FIGURE 42-2 The central nervous system is composed of the brain and the spinal cord.

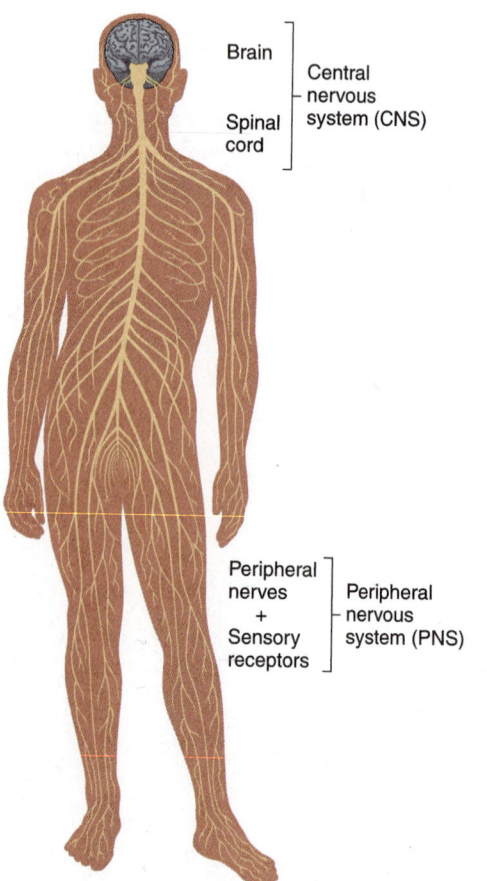

FIGURE 42-3 The peripheral nervous system connects the central nervous system to the various structures of the body. Messages are relayed from these structures back to the brain through the spinal cord.

Remember, though, that the nervous system is one interwoven system, a complex of millions of neurons.

The Central Nervous System

The brain and spinal cord are:

- Surrounded by bone
- Protected by membranes called *meninges*
- Cushioned by cerebrospinal fluid (CSF)

The brain and spinal cord are a continuous structure found within the skull and spinal canal. The spinal cord is about 17 inches long. It ends just above the small of the back. Nerves extend from the brain and the spinal cord.

The Brain

The brain (encephalon) is a large, soft mass of nerve tissue contained within the cranium. It is composed of gray matter and white matter. Gray matter consists principally of nerve-cell bodies. White matter consists of nerve cells that form connections between various parts of the brain.

The brain can be further subdivided into the:

- **Cerebrum**—The largest portion of the brain. The outer portion is formed in folds known as convolutions and separated into lobes. The lobes take their names from the skull bones that surround them (Figure 42-4).

  - The outer portion, the cerebral cortex, is composed of cell bodies and appears gray.
  - The inner portion is composed of axons and dendrites and so appears white.

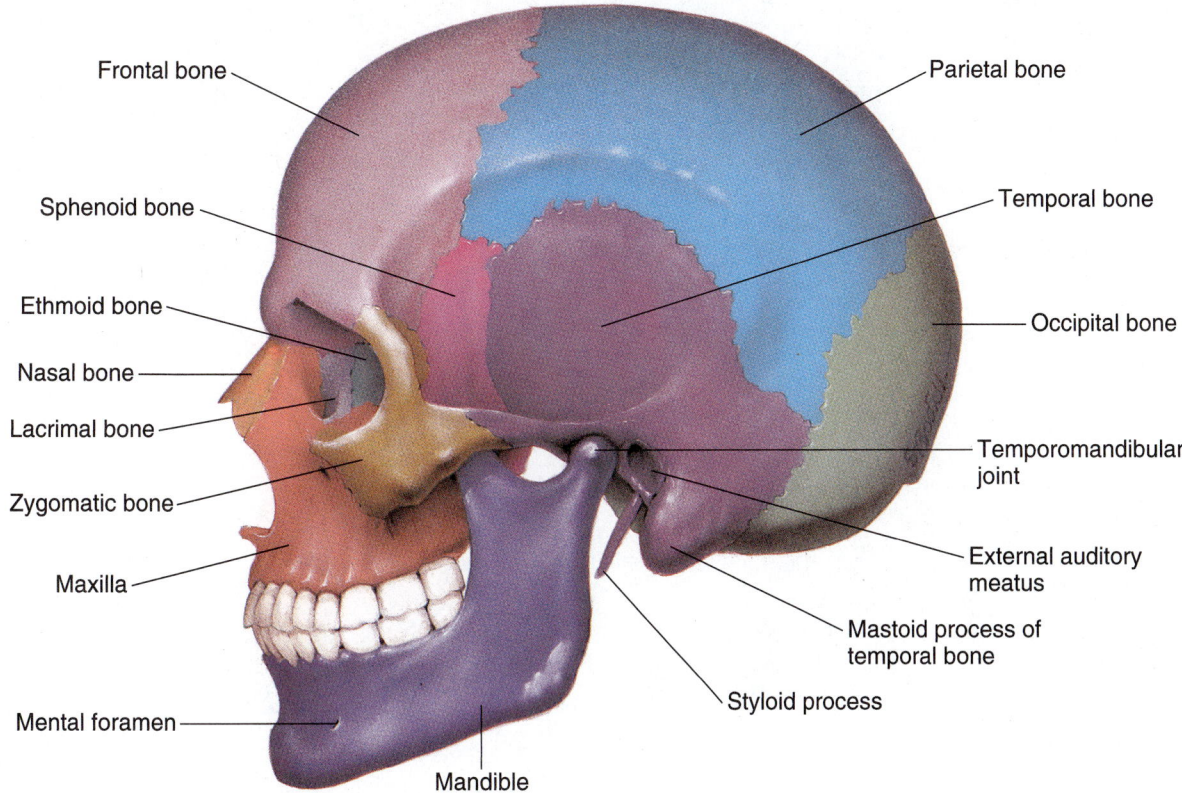

FIGURE 42-4 The lobes of the brain are named according to the skull bones.

- All mental activities—thought, direction of voluntary movements, interpretation of sensations, and experience of emotions—are carried out by cerebral cells (Figure 42-5). Certain activities are centered in each lobe.
- In general, the right side of the cerebrum interprets for and controls the left side of the body and vice versa.
- **Cerebellum**—Found beneath the occipital lobe of the cerebrum. It too has an outer layer of gray cell bodies. This portion of the brain coordinates muscular activities and balance.
- **Brain stem**—The midbrain, pons, and medulla are in the brain stem. They are composed mainly of axons and dendrites. These fibers serve as connecting pathways between the control centers in the cerebrum and cerebellum and the spinal cord. Control centers are found within the brain stem for involuntary movements of such vital organs as the:
  - Heart
  - Blood vessels
  - Lungs
  - Stomach
  - Intestines

The Spinal Cord

The spinal cord (Figure 42-6) extends from the medulla to the second lumbar vertebra in the spinal canal, which is

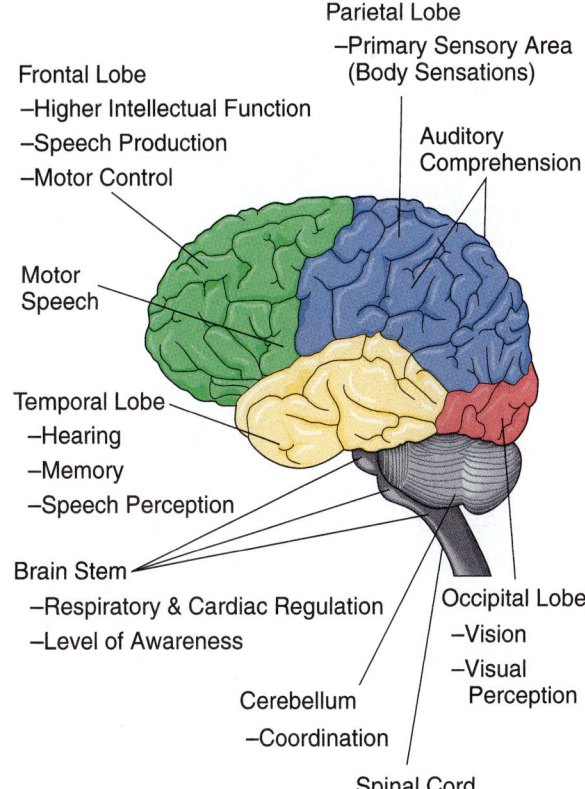

FIGURE 42-5 Each lobe of the brain is responsible for a different function.

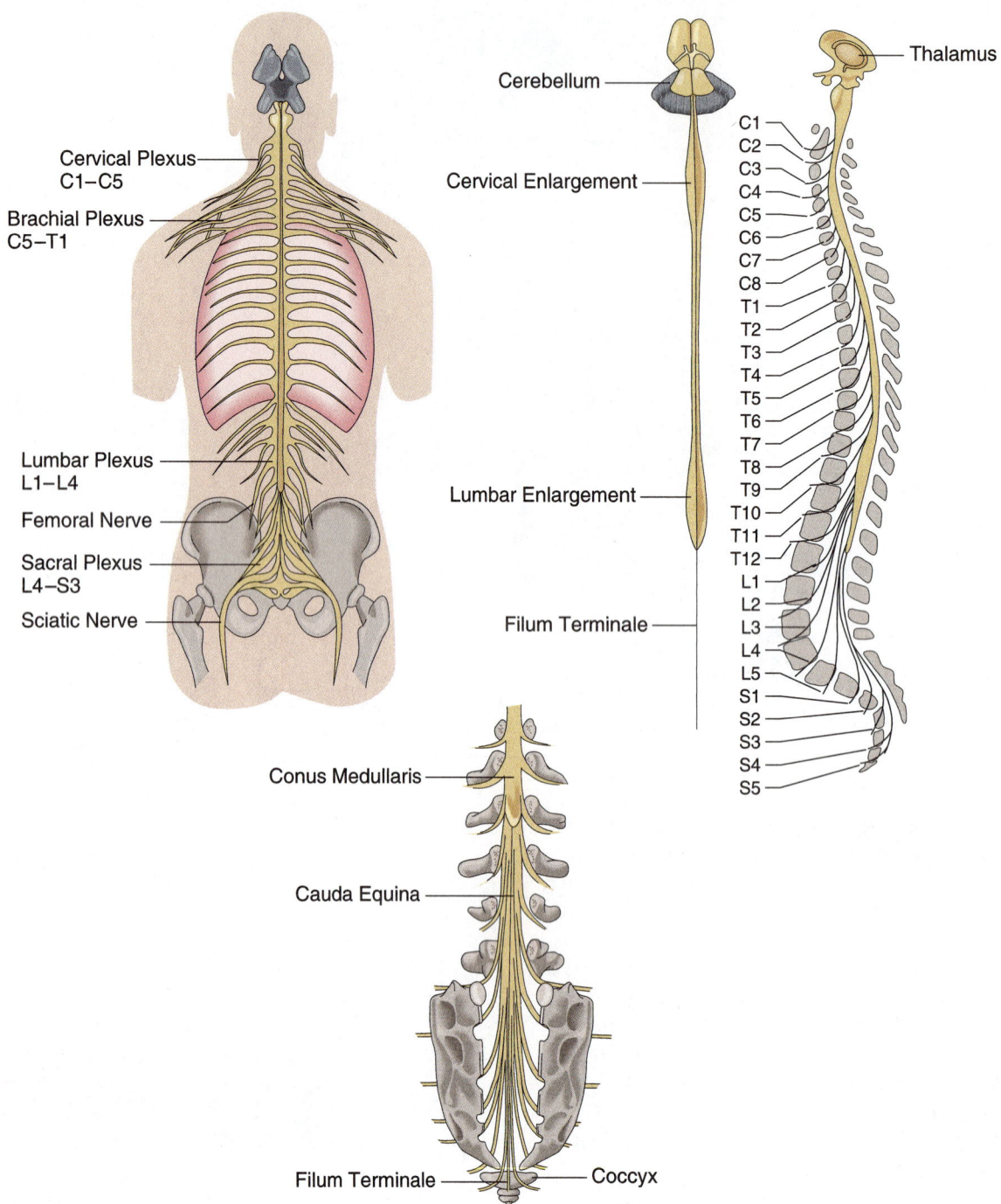

FIGURE 42-6 Spinal cord and nerves.

above the small of the back, a distance of about 17 inches. Nerves entering and leaving the spinal cord carry impulses to and from the control centers. Certain reflex activities performed without conscious thought are controlled within the cord. Pulling your hand away from something hot is an example of this type of reflex activity (Figure 42-7).

The Meninges

Three membranes, called **meninges**, surround both the brain and the spinal cord. They are the dura mater, the arachnoid mater, and the pia mater.

The dura mater is the tough outer covering. The arachnoid mater is the middle, loosely structured layer. It is filled with cerebrospinal fluid. The pia mater is the innermost, delicate layer. It is very vascular (contains many blood vessels) and clings to the brain, spinal cord, and nerve roots.

Cerebrospinal Fluid

Ventricles are cavities within the cerebrum that are lined with highly vascular tissue. These tissues produce **cerebrospinal fluid** (**CSF**), which flows around the brain and the spinal cord. The cerebrospinal fluid bathes the central nervous

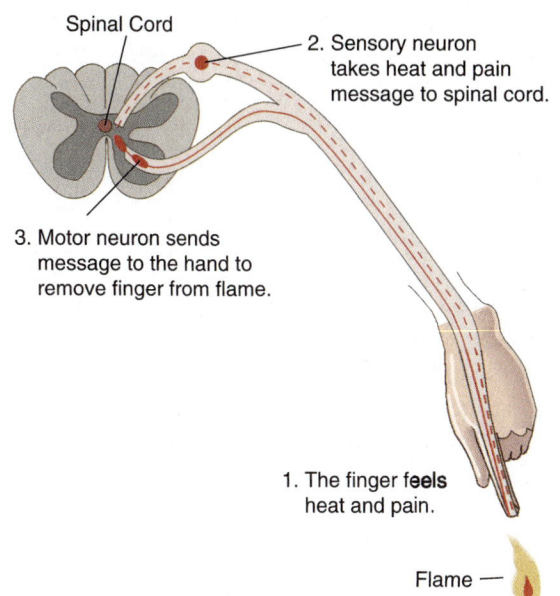

FIGURE 42-7 Reflex arc.

Spinal Cord

2. Sensory neuron takes heat and pain message to spinal cord.

3. Motor neuron sends message to the hand to remove finger from flame.

1. The finger feels heat and pain.

Flame

system as tissue fluid and cushions it against shock and possible injury.

Special Relationships: The Autonomic Nervous System

The phrase *autonomic nervous system (ANS)* refers to special pathways that travel in cranial and spinal nerves (Figure 42-8). The control center is in the brain stem. The pathways begin in the CNS and reach out to the glands, smooth muscle walls of organs, and heart.

The autonomic nervous system consists of two parts: sympathetic fibers and parasympathetic fibers. Sympathetic fibers stimulate activities that prepare the body to deal with emergency situations. It is called the mechanism of "fight or flight." Parasympathetic fibers control the usual functions of moderate heartbeat, digestion, elimination, respiration, and glandular activity.

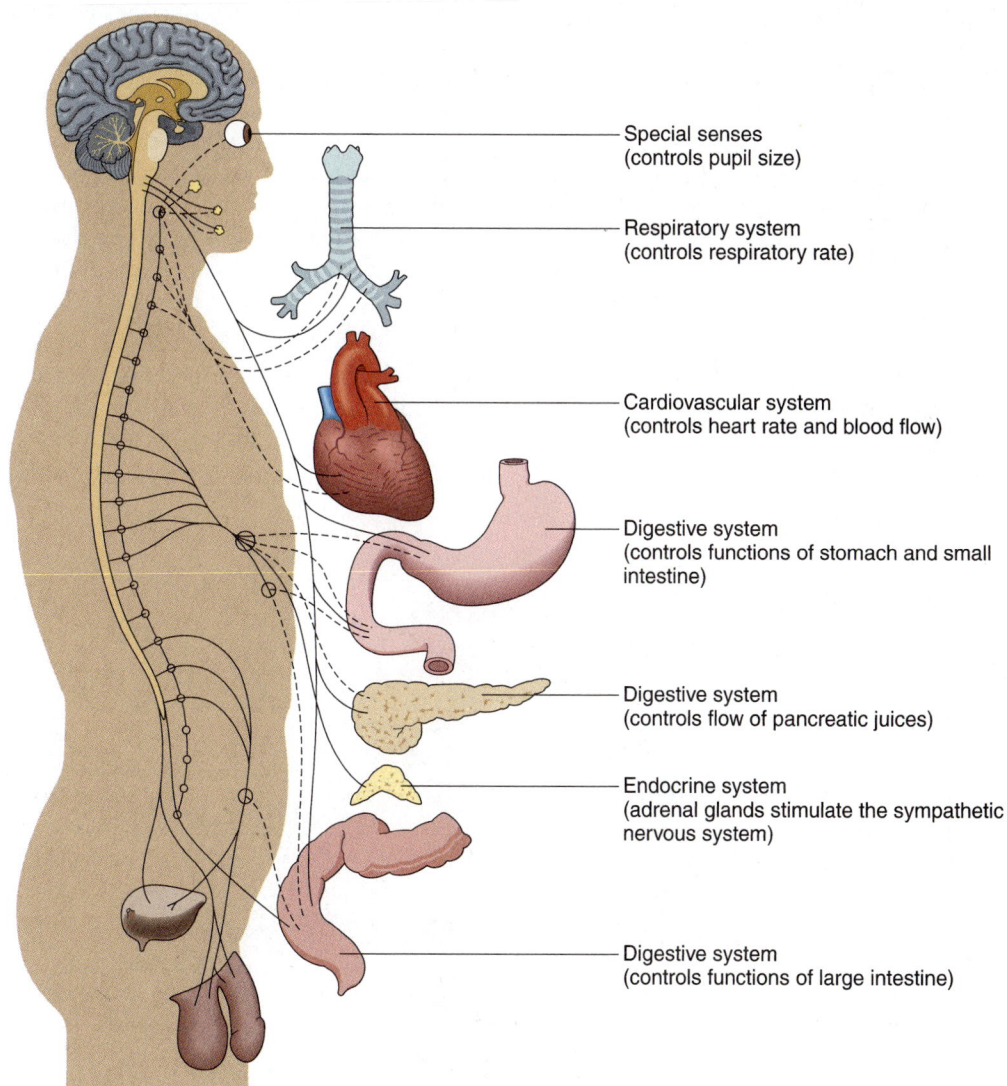

Special senses
(controls pupil size)

Respiratory system
(controls respiratory rate)

Cardiovascular system
(controls heart rate and blood flow)

Digestive system
(controls functions of stomach and small intestine)

Digestive system
(controls flow of pancreatic juices)

Endocrine system
(adrenal glands stimulate the sympathetic nervous system)

Digestive system
(controls functions of large intestine)

FIGURE 42-8 Autonomic nervous system.

Sensory Receptors

The ends of the dendrites carrying sensations to the central nervous system are found throughout the body.

- Some begin in joints and bring information about body positions to the brain.
- Others in the skin carry sensations of pain, heat, pressure, and cold.
- Those in the nose carry the sense of smell.
- The dendrites in the tongue carry the sense of taste.

Sensory dendrites also receive stimulation through two very special end organs, the eye and the ear. All of these structures are called sensory receptors because they carry information about the outside world to the brain. The brain interprets and processes the information.

The Eye

The eye (Figures 42-9A and B) is a hollow ball filled with two liquids called the *aqueous humor* and the *vitreous humor*. The wall of the eye is made up of three layers:

- The sclera: A tough, white outer coat that is protective. The cornea is the transparent portion in the front. Light rays pass through the cornea into the eye.
- The choroid: The nutritive layer found beneath the sclera. The choroid nourishes the eye tissues through its large number of blood vessels.
- The retina: The innermost layer is made up of neurons that are sensitive to light. The neurons join together and their axons leave the eye as the optic nerve. The two nerves cross beneath the brain and carry their impulses to the occipital lobe of the cerebrum to let us know what we are seeing.

Seeing. We see as light enters the eye through the cornea. The amount of light entering the eye is controlled by the iris. The iris is the colored portion of the eye. It is found behind the cornea. Fluid between the cornea and iris helps to bend the light rays and bring them to focus on the retina. The opening in the iris is called the pupil. The pupil appears black because there is no light behind it. Directly behind the iris is the lens. Small muscles pull on either side of the lens to change its shape. The changing shape of the lens makes it possible for us to adjust the range of our vision from far to near or from near to far.

The eye is:

- Held within the bony socket by muscles that can change its position.
- Covered by a mucous membrane, called the conjunctiva. The conjunctiva lines the eyelids and covers the eye.

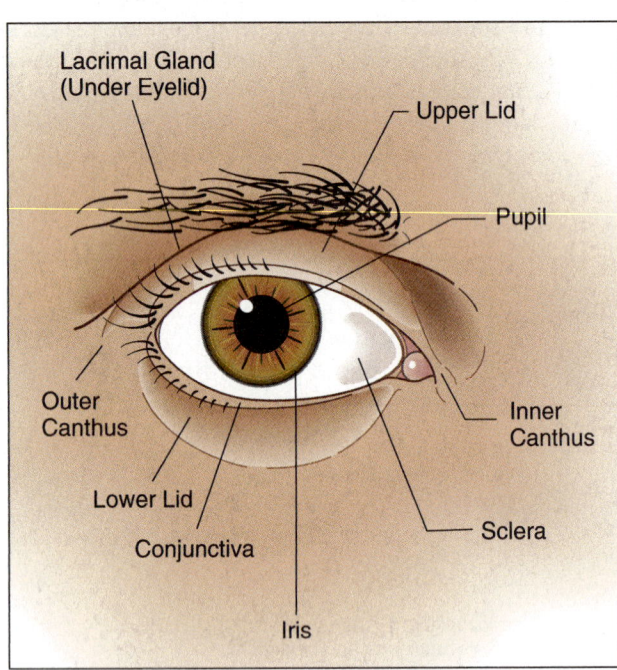

FIGURE 42-9A External view of the eye.

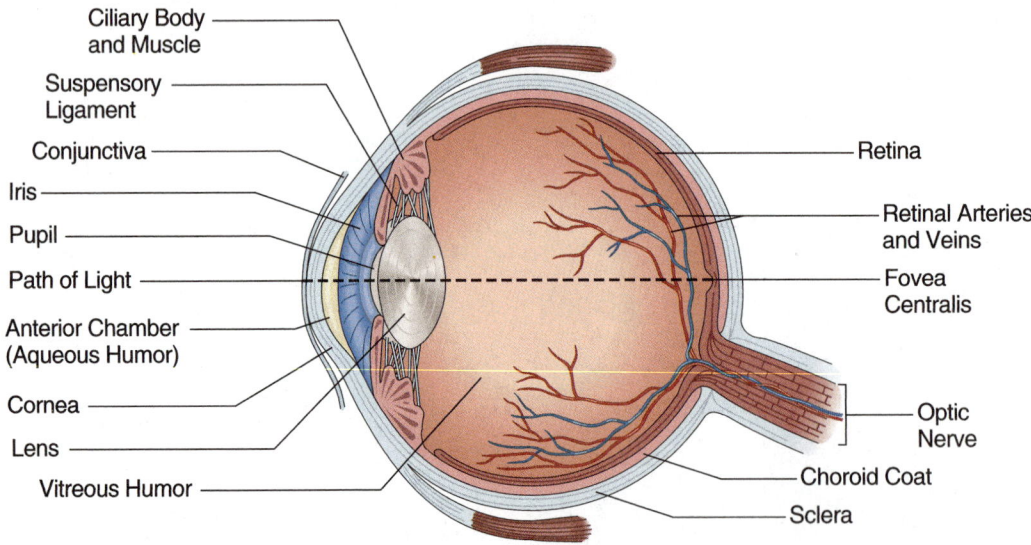

FIGURE 42-9B Internal view of the eye.

- Protected by the eyelids and eyelashes. Tears are manufactured by the lacrimal glands found beneath the lateral side of the upper lid. Tears protect the eye as they wash across the eye, keeping it moist, and then drain into the nasal cavity.

The Ear

Just as the eye is sensitive to light, the ear is sensitive to sound (Figure 42-10). The ear functions in hearing and equilibrium (balance). The ear has three parts: the outer ear, the middle ear, and the inner ear. The outer ear consists of the visible external structure known as the *pinna* and a canal, which directs sound waves toward the middle ear. At the end of the canal is the eardrum, or tympanic membrane. Sound waves cause the eardrum to vibrate.

The middle ear is made up of three tiny bones called ossicles. The ossicles form a chain across the middle ear from the tympanic membrane to an opening in the inner ear. These bones are known as the:

- Incus or anvil
- Malleus or hammer
- Stapes or stirrup

Small tubes, called the eustachian tubes, lead from the nasopharynx into the middle ear to equalize pressure on either side of the eardrum. Sound waves pushing against the tympanic membrane cause the ossicles to vibrate and push against the opening of the inner ear. This motion starts fluid moving in the inner ear.

The inner ear is a very complex structure. It has two main parts: the cochlea and three semicircular canals. The cochlea looks somewhat like a coiled snail shell. Within the cochlea are the tiny dendrites of the hearing or auditory nerve.

Fluid covers the dendrites. When the fluid is set in motion by the vibration of the middle ear bones, it stimulates the dendrites with sound sensations. The auditory nerves, one from each ear, carry the sensations to the temporal lobe of the cerebrum to let us know what we are hearing.

The three semicircular canals also contain liquid and nerve endings. When these nerve endings are stimulated, impulses about the position of the head are sent to the brain. This helps us keep our balance.

COMMON CONDITIONS

The nervous system usually remains healthy. However, injury or disease to the brain, spinal cord, or nerves requires appropriate treatment.

Increased Intracranial Pressure

The structures within the skull normally exert a certain amount of pressure, called the intracranial pressure. The pressure is due to:

- Nervous tissue
- Cerebrospinal fluid
- Blood flowing through cerebral vessels

Any change in the size or amount of these components changes the pressure. Increased intracranial pressure can result from:

- Head injury. Bleeding from damaged blood vessels and edema puts pressure on the delicate nervous tissue.
- Inflammation or infection plus edema.
- Intracranial bleeding due to ruptured blood vessels. This is called a cerebrovascular accident (CVA).

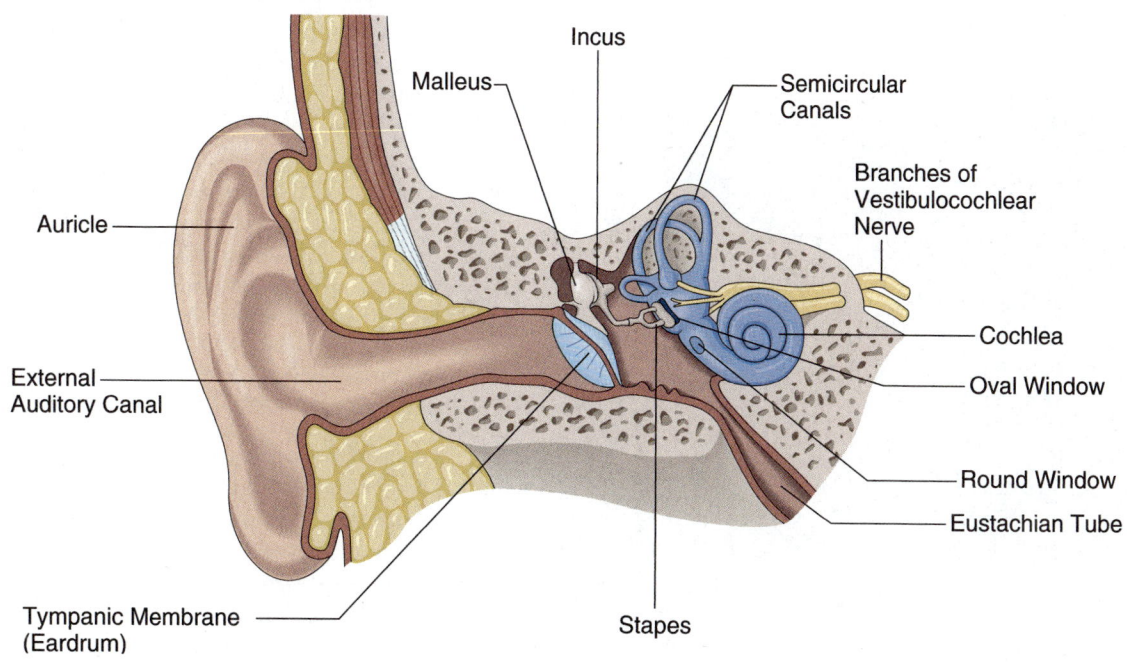

FIGURE 42-10 Internal view of the ear.

- Toxins.
- High temperature.
- Blockage of the normal flow of cerebrospinal fluid.
- Tumors.

Signs and Symptoms. Indications of increased intracranial pressure include:

- Alteration in pupil size and response to light. In the normal eye, the pupil becomes smaller when a flashlight is directed at each eye. The equality of the pupils and their ability to react to light is an important observation when a head injury occurs.
- Headache.
- Vomiting.
- Loss of consciousness and sensation.
- Paralysis—loss of voluntary motor control.
- Convulsions (seizures)—uncontrolled muscular contractions that are often violent.

How long all or part of the symptoms remain depends on the extent and cause of damage to the brain cells. Remember also that paralysis is not always accompanied by sensory loss.

Specific Nursing Care. Patients who are acutely ill with head injuries or increased intracranial pressure require skilled nursing care (Figure 42-11). The nurse is responsible for monitoring the patient's:

- Level of consciousness
- Degree of orientation to time and place
- Reaction to pain and stimuli
- Vital signs

If you note any change in the patient's response or behavior as you are assisting in care, bring it to the nurse's attention immediately. Changes that might be very significant include:

- Incontinence
- Uncontrolled body movements

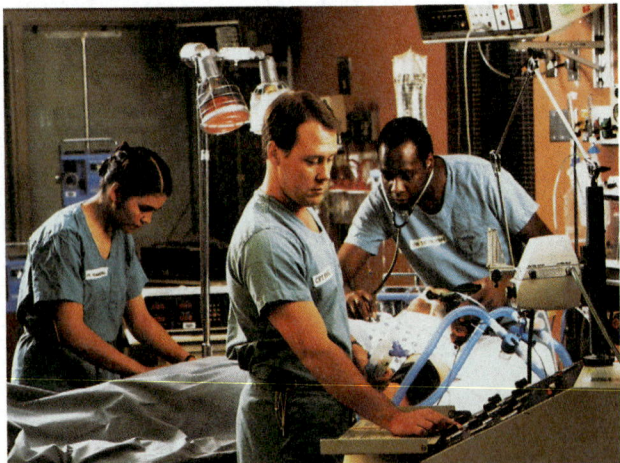

FIGURE 42-11 Critical care nursing. "Be All You Can Be." *(Courtesy United States Government, as represented by the Secretary of the Army)*

- Disorientation
- Deepening or lessening in the level of consciousness
- Dizziness
- Vomiting
- Alterations in speech
- Change in ability to follow directions

Once improved, the patient may be moved from a critical unit to an intermediate unit. From there, the patient may go to a long-term care facility for a possibly long period of convalescence. The patient may require extensive rehabilitation to regain functional skills. The nursing measures first established in the critical care unit must be maintained throughout this extended period.

Loss of sensation and decreased mobility make these patients more prone to pressure sores, infection, and contractures. You must continue to:

- Give special skin care.
- Carry out range-of-motion exercises.
- Check skin over pressure points frequently.
- Change the patient's position regularly.
- Report early signs of infection.
- Monitor elimination. Loss of muscle tone and inactivity may lead to constipation and impaction.
- Check drainage tubes such as indwelling catheters. They must receive careful attention.
- Provide reality orientation as needed.
- Be alert to any signs of mood change and plan extra time to provide essential support. Patients recovering from these illnesses often experience anxiety and depression.
- Keep a careful check on vital signs of any patient with a head injury. A special record (neurological monitoring record) may be kept for recording all observations.
- The Glasgow Coma Scale (Figure 42-12) is used to monitor neurologic problems after trauma, stroke, and other illnesses and injuries. The examiner determines the best response the patient can make to stimuli. The score is determined by adding the total of all three categories. Higher point values are assigned to responses that indicate increased awareness and arousal. A score of less than 8 indicates a neurological crisis. A score of 9–13 indicates moderate dysfunction, and a score of 13–15 indicates moderate to minor dysfunction.

Transient Ischemic Attack

A transient ischemic attack (TIA) is a temporary period of diminished blood flow to the brain. The attack comes on rapidly and may last from 2 to 15 minutes or for as long as 24 hours. Symptoms are similar to those of a stroke but are temporary and reversible. Transient ischemic attacks may occur once or several times in a lifetime. Persons experiencing TIAs are at risk for eventually suffering a stroke.

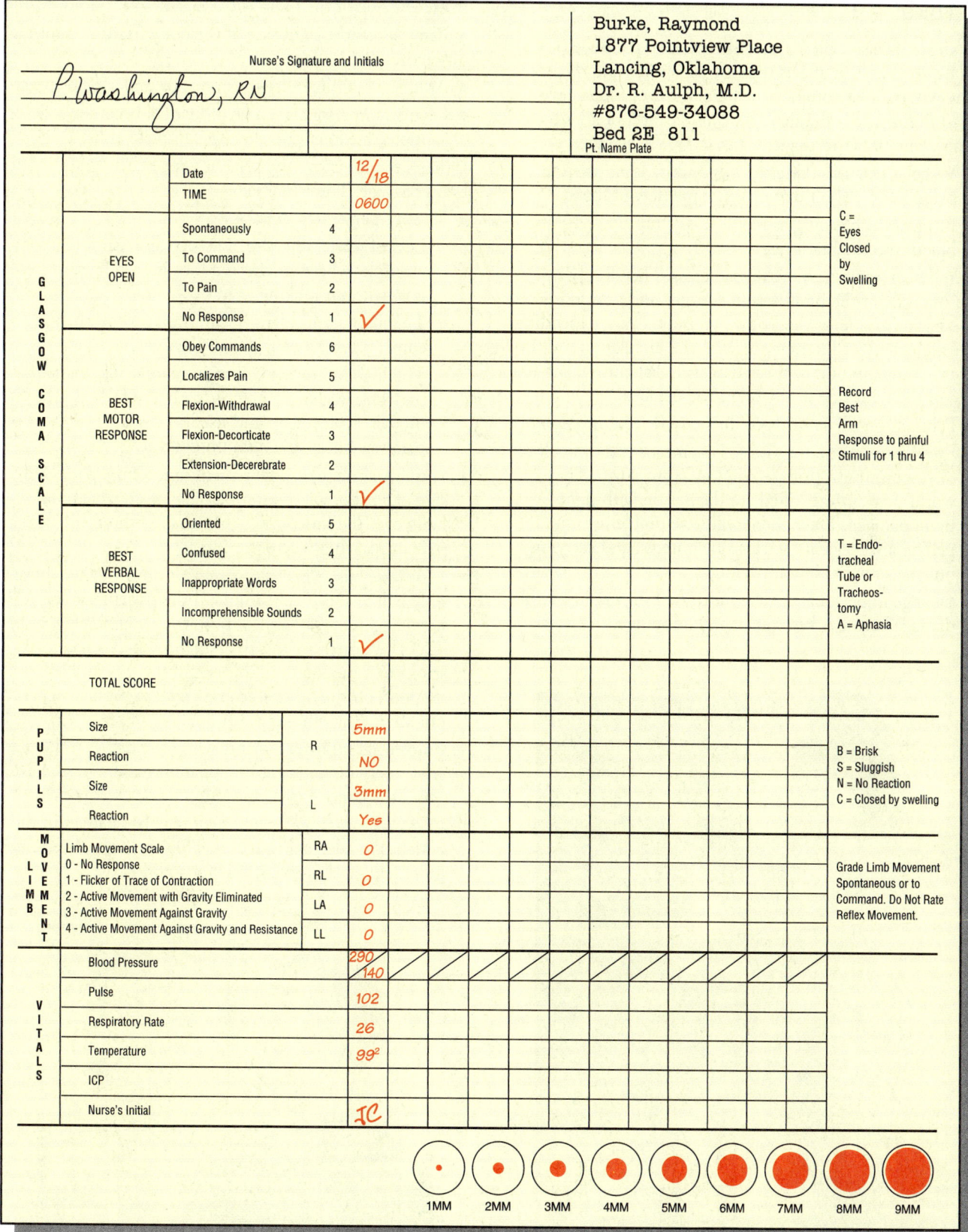

					12/18									C = Eyes Closed by Swelling
G L A S G O W C O M A S C A L E		Date			12/18									
		TIME			0600									
	EYES OPEN	Spontaneously	4											
		To Command	3											
		To Pain	2											
		No Response	1		✓									
	BEST MOTOR RESPONSE	Obey Commands	6											Record Best Arm Response to painful Stimuli for 1 thru 4
		Localizes Pain	5											
		Flexion-Withdrawal	4											
		Flexion-Decorticate	3											
		Extension-Decerebrate	2											
		No Response	1		✓									
	BEST VERBAL RESPONSE	Oriented	5											T = Endo-tracheal Tube or Tracheos-tomy A = Aphasia
		Confused	4											
		Inappropriate Words	3											
		Incomprehensible Sounds	2											
		No Response	1		✓									
		TOTAL SCORE												
P U P I L S		Size	R		5mm									B = Brisk S = Sluggish N = No Reaction C = Closed by swelling
		Reaction			NO									
		Size	L		3mm									
		Reaction			Yes									
L I M B M O V E M E N T		Limb Movement Scale 0 - No Response 1 - Flicker of Trace of Contraction 2 - Active Movement with Gravity Eliminated 3 - Active Movement Against Gravity 4 - Active Movement Against Gravity and Resistance	RA		0									Grade Limb Movement Spontaneous or to Command. Do Not Rate Reflex Movement.
			RL		0									
			LA		0									
			LL		0									
V I T A L S		Blood Pressure			290/140									
		Pulse			102									
		Respiratory Rate			26									
		Temperature			99²									
		ICP												
		Nurse's Initial			JC									

Nurse's Signature and Initials

P. Washington, RN

Burke, Raymond
1877 Pointview Place
Lancing, Oklahoma
Dr. R. Aulph, M.D.
#876-549-34088
Bed 2E 811
Pt. Name Plate

1MM 2MM 3MM 4MM 5MM 6MM 7MM 8MM 9MM

FIGURE 42-12 Typical documentation for a patient with a neurological injury. The top part is the Glasgow Coma Scale. The bottom records routine neurological checks.

Stroke

A **stroke** is also called a **cerebrovascular accident** (**CVA**) or **brain attack**. It affects the vascular system and the nervous system. The complete or partial loss of blood flow to the brain tissue is frequently a complication of atherosclerosis or brain hemorrhage. Causes of CVA include:

- Vascular occlusion due to a thrombus, atherosclerotic plaques, or emboli that obstruct the flow of blood
- Intracranial bleeding as blood vessels rupture, releasing blood into the brain tissue

Remember, most nerve pathways cross. Therefore, damage on one side of the brain results in signs and symptoms on the opposite side of the body. Symptoms vary depending on the extent of interference with the circulation and on the area and amount of tissue damaged. Patients with damage to the right side of the brain will exhibit:

- Paralysis on the left side of the body (left **hemiplegia**).
- **Spatial-perceptual deficits**. This means it is difficult to distinguish right from left and up from down. The world may appear "tilted" to the person with right-brain damage. The patient will have problems propelling a wheelchair, setting down items, and carrying out the activities of daily living.
- Change in personality. The individual with right brain damage becomes very quick and impulsive.

If the left side of the brain is damaged, you will note:

- Paralysis on the right side of the body (right hemiplegia) (Figure 42-13).
- **Aphasia**—an inability to express or understand speech.
- Change in personality. The individual becomes very cautious, anxious, and slow to complete tasks.

Other symptoms may be present with either right- or left-brain damage. These include:

- Sensory-perceptual deficits
  - Loss of **position sense**. The person cannot tell, for example, where an affected foot is or what position it is in without looking at it.
  - The inability to identify common objects such as a comb, a fork, a pencil, or a glass.
  - The inability to use common objects. The patient may know what an item is, such as a fork, but be unable to pick it up and use it. This is not a result of paralysis but is due to brain damage.
- **Unilateral neglect**. The patient ignores the paralyzed side of the body. For example, the affected arm may hang over the side of the wheelchair without the patient realizing where the arm is.
- **Hemianopsia**. This is impaired vision. Both eyes have only half vision. For example, if the patient has left hemiplegia, the left half of both eyes is blind (Figure 42-14). Remember this if a patient who has had a stroke eats the food on one side of the tray and leaves the food on the other side. The patient probably cannot see it. Turn the tray around.
- **Emotional lability**. Patients who have had a stroke may start to cry or laugh for no apparent reason. They have very little control over this and may be embarrassed.
- **Cognitive impairments**. There may be changes in the patient's intellectual function. This may affect memory, judgment, and problem-solving abilities.

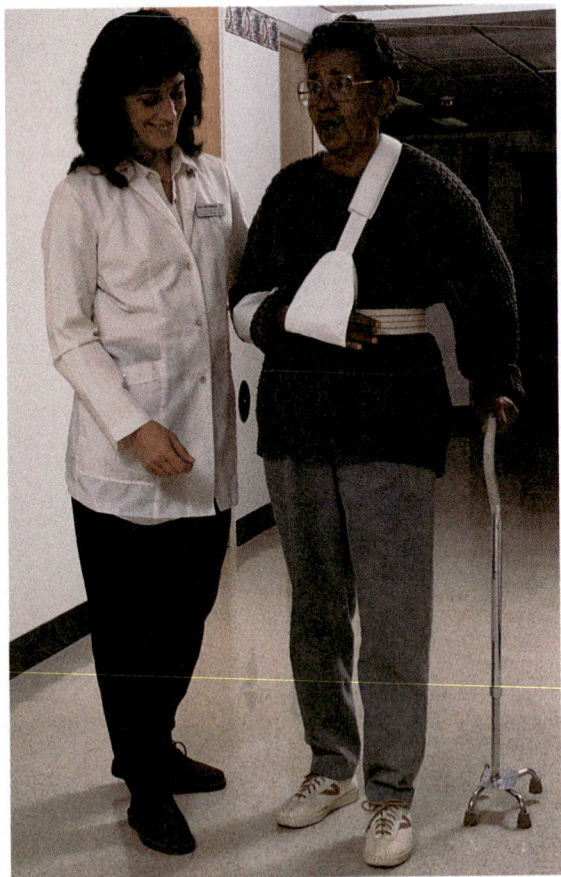

FIGURE 42-13 Right hemiplegia.

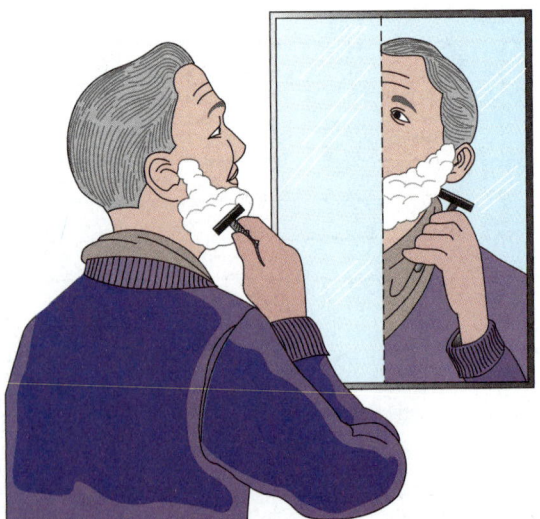

FIGURE 42-14 Hemianopsia is a common problem after a stroke.

Nursing Care. The goals of poststroke care include:

1. Maintaining the skills and abilities that the patient has left.
2. Preventing complications caused by immobility:
   - Contractures
   - Pressure ulcers
   - Pneumonia
   - Blood clots
3. Helping the patient regain functional abilities:
   - Activities of daily living (Figure 42-15)
   - Bowel and bladder control
   - Mobility
   - Communication skills

During Recovery. Recovery from a stroke is often a very frustrating experience for the patient. Caregivers must be patient. In your approach to the patient, remember two things:

1. The patient has more than enough frustration for both of you, so be careful not to let yours show. The last thing the patient needs is your silent reinforcement of his helplessness.
2. The degree and speed of recovery are directly related, in most cases, to the patience and encouragement of the caregivers with whom the patient has close contact.

Other interventions during recovery include:

- Physical therapy to increase independent mobility: bed movement, getting to the side of the bed, standing by the side of the bed, transferring out of bed and into a chair, and ambulation.
- Occupational therapy to regain the ability to perform the activities of daily living, such as bathing, grooming, dressing, and eating, with little or no assistance.
- Speech therapy to regain or to learn different methods of communication. The speech therapist also works with swallowing problems caused by the stroke.

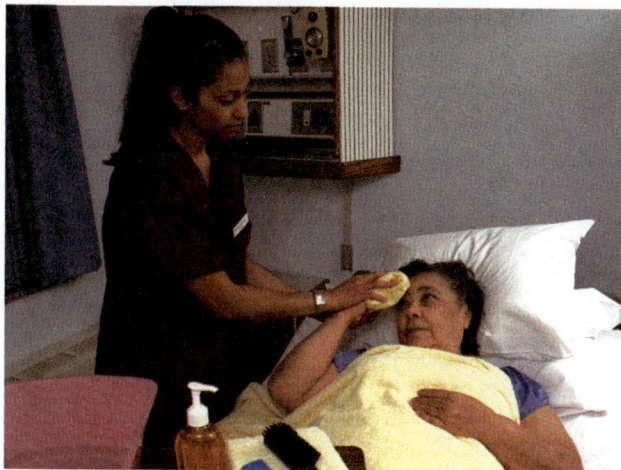

FIGURE 42-15 The patient who has had a stroke may need to relearn activities of daily living.

COMMUNICATION *Highlight*

Try to develop rapport with the patient on your first contact. At times, this is difficult because a stroke often causes mood changes. If the patient is newly dependent, he may also have mood or behavior problems. Be consistent and avoid becoming discouraged. Try to remember that the illness is causing the problem. Find the most effective means of communicating the information you need to convey. Ask yes or no questions whenever possible. Avoid treating the patient like a child and do not correct his speech. If you must repeat yourself, do so quietly and calmly. Use gestures, if necessary.

- Nursing care to:
   - Implement bowel and bladder training programs, or give catheter care if necessary
   - Implement pressure ulcer prevention programs
   - Reinforce the programs provided by the therapists
- Care to prevent contractures by:
   - Positioning the patient appropriately and changing positions at least every 2 hours
   - Performing passive range-of-motion exercises as directed
   - Applying splints or braces as ordered

All staff can help with rehabilitation efforts by:

- Encouraging the patient to communicate
- Maintaining a positive and supportive attitude at all times
- Providing only the assistance that the patient needs
- Following approaches consistently as outlined in the patient's care plan

Convalescence is often long. The nursing care is demanding, requiring much patience and understanding.

Aphasia

Stroke victims often suffer from aphasia or language impairment. They have difficulty forming thoughts or expressing them in coherent ways. This is extremely frustrating and frightening for the patient and family.

- **Receptive aphasia** means that the person cannot comprehend communication.
- **Expressive aphasia** means that the person cannot properly form thoughts or express them coherently.
- **Global aphasia** means that the person has lost all language abilities.

Review Unit 7 for guidelines for communicating with patients with aphasia.

Parkinson's Disease

Parkinson's disease is believed to be caused by not having enough neurotransmitters (dopamine) in the brain stem and cerebellum. The symptoms are progressive over many years. Some people will show minor changes. Others will have much more obvious symptoms (Figure 42-16).

Signs and Symptoms. Signs and symptoms of Parkinson's disease include:

- Tremors (uncontrolled trembling). Tremors of the hands commonly affect the fingers and thumb in such a way that an affected person will appear to be rolling a small object (such as a pill) between them. These tremors occur frequently. They usually begin in the fingers, then involve the entire hand and arm, and finally affect an entire side of the body. Starting on one side, the tremors eventually involve both sides of the body. Tremors are more evident when the person is inactive. A typical posture of a patient suffering from Parkinson's disease is shown in Figure 42-17.

- Muscular rigidity (loss of flexibility). The muscular rigidity is more evident when the patient is inactive. It seems to be lessened when the person sleeps or engages in activities such as walking or other exercises that require large-muscle involvement. The rigidity makes the person with Parkinson's disease more prone to falls and injury.

- Akinesia (difficulty and slowness in carrying out voluntary muscular activities). Persons with advanced Parkinson's typically have:
  - A shuffling manner of walking
  - Difficulty starting the process of walking
  - Difficulty stopping smoothly once walking has started
  - Affected speech, causing words to be slurred and poorly spoken (enunciated)
  - Facial muscles that lose expressiveness and emotional response

- Loss of autonomic nervous control. Because of loss of autonomic nervous control, persons with Parkinson's may:
  - drool.
  - become incontinent.
  - become constipated.
  - retain urine.

- Mood swings and gradual behavioral changes. A patient may appear happy and positive one moment, and then be depressed the next. The depression tends to be progressive. Personality and behavioral changes may occur that cause psychotic breakdowns and dementia in later stages.

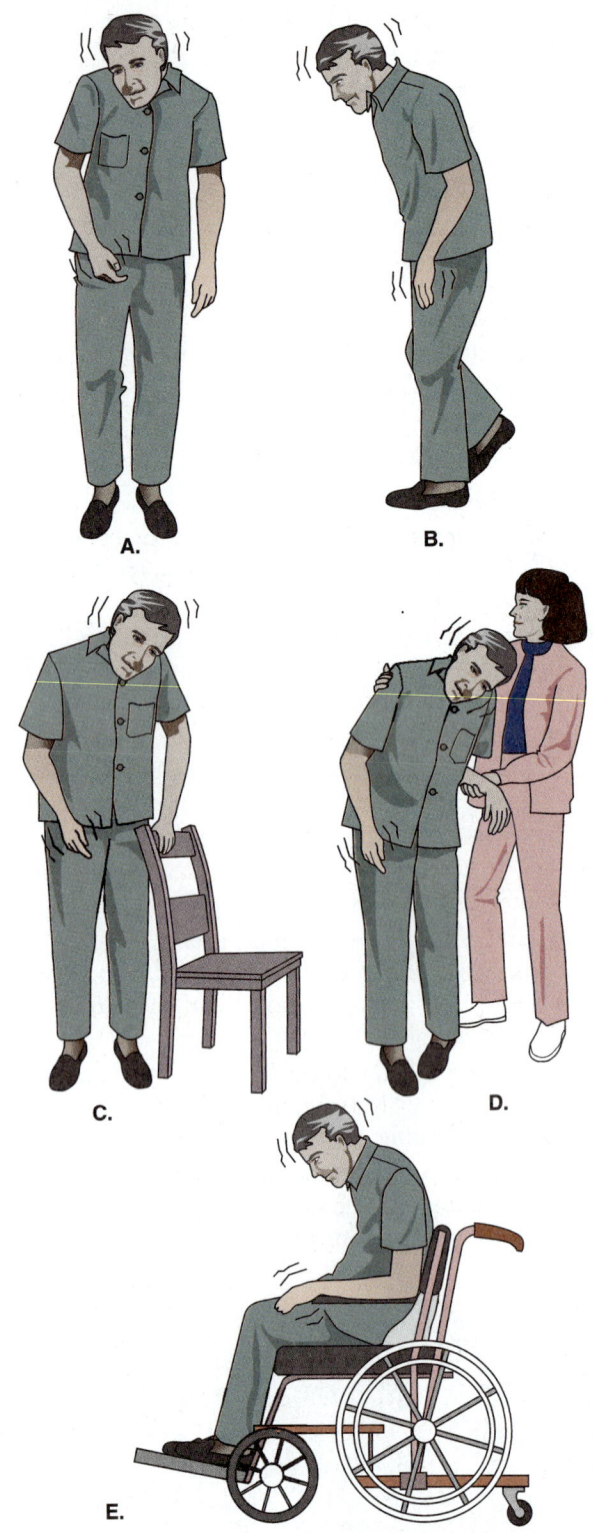

FIGURE 42-16 Progression of Parkinson's disease. A. The patient leans slightly forward and develops flexion of the affected arm. B. The patient stoops forward slightly and walks with a shuffling gait. C. As the disease progresses, the patient needs support to prevent falling. The patient tends to shuffle faster and faster, leaning farther forward until he falls on his face. D. The disease progresses to the point where the patient needs assistance for ambulation. E. The patient has profound weakness and severe tremors. Ambulation becomes impossible.

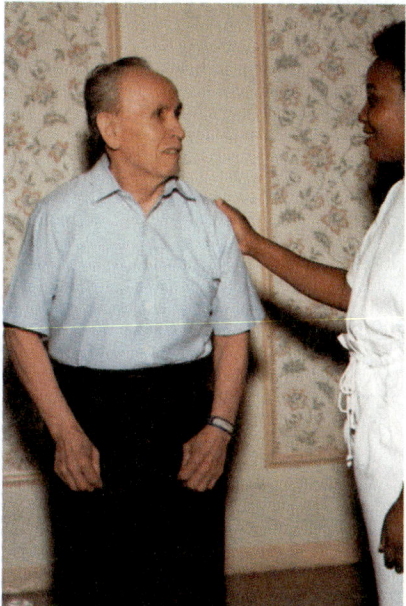

Ventral view

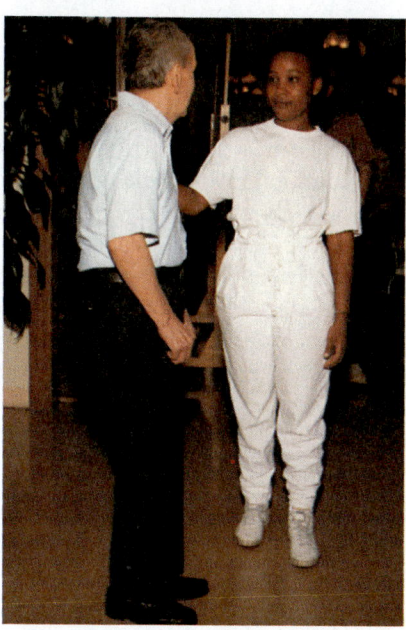

Lateral view

FIGURE 42-17 The typical posture of a patient with Parkinson's disease. In addition to the standing posture, note the patient's hands.

Treatment. The treatment consists of:
- Surgery for some younger persons
- Drug therapy
- Therapy to limit the muscular rigidity and to meet the basic physical and emotional needs

Nursing Care. Nursing care of the person with Parkinson's disease includes:
- Maintaining a calm environment. Symptoms are more intense when the patient is under stress.

DIFFICULT *Situations*

Patients with Parkinson's disease may have inconsistent needs for physical support and assistance. If the patient is tired, he may need more support than when he is rested. When the patient is stressed, the tremors may worsen, increasing the need for hands-on assistance.

- Assisting and supervising the activities of daily living. For example, directing food into the mouth and then keeping it there to be chewed and swallowed is very difficult for many persons with Parkinson's disease.
- Providing emotional support and encouragement.
- Carrying out a program of general and specific exercises.
- Providing protection for patients with dementia.

Multiple Sclerosis

Multiple sclerosis (**MS**) generally occurs in young adults. It is the result of the loss of insulation (myelin) around central nervous system nerve fibers. This interferes with the ability of the nerve fibers to function.

The cause of MS is unknown. Many individuals live the usual life span even though they have this chronic condition. The symptoms are variable and may not be the same for all individuals. Symptoms may include:

- Loss of sensation with regard to temperature, pain, and touch
- Feelings of numbness and tingling
- **Vertigo** (a spinning or dizzy sensation)
- **Lhermitte's sign** (a tingling, shock-like sensation that passes down the arms or spine when the neck is flexed)

Problems with vision occur in almost half of the people who have MS. The problem may be temporary or permanent. Vision symptoms may include:

- Blurriness, color blindness, or difficulty seeing objects in bright light
- Double vision
- **Nystagmus** (jerky eye movements)

Mobility is usually affected:

- Pain in the legs that disappears with rest
- **Paraplegia** (paralysis of both legs) and **quadriplegia** (paralysis of all four extremities) in advanced cases
- Spasticity of muscles
- **Intention tremor** (shaking of the hands that gets worse as the individual tries to touch or pick up an object)

In severe MS, speech is affected because of the weakness of the muscles in the chest, face, and lips. The speech may be slow, with poor articulation. The mind usually remains alert. Incontinence of bowel and bladder are common in advanced cases.

One of the most disabling features of MS is fatigue. The fatigue is very real and is not psychological.

MS may follow one of four courses:

- *Benign course:* mild attacks with long periods of no symptoms.
- *Exacerbating-remitting:* Severe attacks (exacerbations) followed by periods of partial or complete recovery (remissions). Often the periods of exacerbation get longer and more severe with shorter periods of remission.
- *Slowly progressive:* slow, steady deterioration.
- *Rapidly progressive:* deterioration is rapid and progressive and may be life-threatening.

Nursing Care. Nursing care of the patient with multiple sclerosis includes:

1. Implement pressure ulcer prevention program.
2. Implement contracture prevention programs through consistent changes of position and passive range-of-motion exercises. Apply splints correctly, if ordered.
3. Pay careful attention to catheter care if the patient has an indwelling catheter, to prevent bladder infections.
4. Encourage independence. Follow instructions from the nurse or the therapists for specific techniques to use.
5. Help the patient maintain a balanced schedule of rest and activity.
6. Provide emotional support and encouragement.

Treatment. There is no known way to stop the progression of the disease. Treatment consists of maintaining functional ability as long as possible through general health practices and physical therapy.

DIFFICULT *Situations*

A warm bath or shower is often very relaxing to a patient with multiple sclerosis. However, you must make sure that the water is not too hot, which temporarily intensifies some symptoms of MS. Keeping bath water at about 100°F to 105°F is best. Take your responsibility for assisting with range-of-motion exercises seriously. ROM is especially important in patients with MS to maintain joint mobility and muscle tone, reduce spasticity, improve coordination, and boost self-esteem.

Post Polio Syndrome (PPS)

Polio is a very serious neurological disease that has been with us since at least 1350 B.C. This disease is caused by a virus. The virus attacks the motor neurons in the spinal cord. Muscles affected by these neurons no longer function properly, resulting in weakness and paralysis. Some patients had respiratory paralysis, and needed a special ventilator to breathe. Others had speech and swallowing problems. Most had paralysis and weakness in the arms and legs. Many people died as a result of polio. Most of those who survived learned to overcome their disabilities and lead productive lives.

There were large annual outbreaks of polio in the United States every summer. The largest was in 1952. In 1955, an injectable vaccine was developed to prevent polio. Because of the severity of the condition, most children received the vaccination. In 1962, an oral polio vaccine was developed. Both vaccines continue to be used today. Because of the effectiveness of the vaccines, infectious polio has been eliminated in the United States.

Post polio syndrome (**PPS**) is a neurologic condition marked by increased weakness and abnormal muscle fatigue in persons who had polio many years earlier. Estimates are that 30 to 70% of all polio survivors will develop this condition. There are several theories about the cause of PPS. The most common involves the motor neurons. Most polio survivors have about half as many motor neurons as others who were not affected by polio. It is believed that motor neurons that were not destroyed by the initial polio infection compensated by sprouting new connections. Some of the new neurons adapted to innervate areas that are five to seven times larger than normal. These neurons may be slowly dying, perhaps because of years of overuse. As the neurons die, they lose their muscle connections, and muscles stop responding.

Signs and Symptoms. Signs and symptoms of PPS range from annoying to debilitating. Onset may be sudden, following trauma, infection, surgery, a fall, or a stressful event. The new injury puts stress on the remaining motor neurons, causing further reduction in function, pain, and fatigue. Signs and symptoms include:

- fatigue that may be debilitating.
- new joint and muscle pain.
- new weakness in muscles affected by polio; unaffected muscles are also affected. The new weakness may be more prominent on one side of the body.
- new dyspnea and other respiratory problems.
- severe cold intolerance, even with mild cold exposure. This causes the muscle weakness to worsen, the arms or legs to become pale or cyanotic, and the extremities to feel cold to the touch. The patient may say, "It's so cold it hurts."
- muscle spasms and cramps that are sometimes severe and painful.
- difficulty swallowing.

- difficulty falling asleep and waking frequently during the night.

Some PPS patients become anxious when they are hospitalized. Emotional expressions of discouragement and displays of anger are fairly common. The patient may be fearful. Health care practices and attitudes were very different during the era of the polio epidemic. Many PPS patients were children during the original infection. They were in the hospital for a long time, and may have been forcibly separated from their parents. This was traumatic and caused them to feel isolated. Sadly, some were physically, emotionally, and sexually abused by hospital personnel. When a person with PPS is in the hospital, old feelings and fears sometimes return. The patient may experience feelings of fear and powerlessness that she cannot or will not talk about. Provide reassurance and emotional support, and report the patient's behavior to the nurse.

Most PPS patients experience pain daily. Muscle spasms often worsen the pain. Use nursing comfort measures, such as positioning and a backrub, to relieve pain. Inform the nurse of the patient's complaints of pain. Reducing strain and adjusting activities to conserve energy also help relieve pain. You may be asked to provide a heat treatment, which also relieves pain.

Many polio survivors have disturbed sleep because of muscle spasms, pain, or anxiety. Some experience sleep apnea, but are not aware of it. Body positioning is important during sleep to support weakened areas and deformities. Certain positions may be painful for the patient and extra pillows may be needed for support. Observe the patient's sleep at night and manage problems as they arise. Report your observations to the nurse.

Fatigue occurs daily, and can be debilitating. It may worsen as the day progresses. Some require more sleep than others who are not affected by PPS. Encourage the patient to rest and nap periodically throughout the day. Help the patient pace her activities and use measures to conserve energy. Therapy may be ordered to teach the patient to conserve energy.

About one-fifth of all PPS patients have swallowing problems. This increases the risk of choking. Position the patient as upright as possible while he is eating, and for 30 to 60 minutes after meals. Monitor the patient while eating and teach her to avoid talking while eating. Encourage her to alternate food and fluid, and to avoid swallowing when her head is tipped back. Assist with oral care after meals to remove retained food particles.

Patients with PPS have serious problems with cold because the nerves that control blood vessel size were destroyed by the virus. The legs and feet are commonly affected. One theory is that people with PPS function as if it were 20 degrees colder than the actual temperature. Their legs and feet turn bright red following a hot bath. When the patient stands up, she may become dizzy or faint as blood pools in the legs, causing the blood pressure to drop. If the patient complains of cold, assist her with socks or extra blankets.

You may be instructed to soak the feet in warm water, or assist with a warm bath. Caution the patient to call for help before getting out of the tub.

Surgical Procedures. Post polio patients who are admitted for surgery have many special needs. They are much more sensitive to anesthesia than persons who have not had polio. They require less medication and half the anesthesia, yet take twice as long as other patients to recover from the anesthesia. Because of this, the patient with PPS must be monitored closely for other problems. Patients may:

- Shiver violently after surgery. Provide warm blankets.
- Have side effects from common drugs. Monitor closely for abnormalities, and report to the nurse promptly.
- Have problems from blood loss, even a small amount. Monitor the operative site and vital signs carefully and report to the nurse.
- Have respiratory problems because of muscle weakness and lung problems. Encouraging the patient to cough and deep breathe after surgery is very important.
- Be unable to reposition themselves in bed. Assist the patient as needed.
- Have positioning problems because of deformities or discomfort. Do your best to make the patient comfortable. Use pillows and props for comfort and support.
- Vomit. This may cause fainting if the patient is upright. Monitor for choking. Report nausea or vomiting to the nurse.
- Choke on secretions. Position the patient on his side until he is fully awake. Monitor closely.
- Have problems with transfers and ambulation after surgery. Instruct the patient to call when she is ready to get out of bed. Have the patient dangle before rising. Use a transfer belt for safey.

Nursing Assistant Care. Patients with post polio syndrome are usually in the hospital for treatment of another condition. The problems caused by post polio are seldom severe enough to require hospitalization. However, they complicate the care of other conditions and procedures. Remember that these patients have lived with their polio condition for years and have found ways to adapt to it. Overall, they are experts in their own care. Respect their expertise. Coping with the new problems from PPS is often much more difficult than the recovery from the original illness. Be prepared to help with activities of daily living, bed mobility, transfers, and ambulation. Patients with post polio syndrome may have many special needs. They may not complain because most were taught that part of their recovery includes being "normal." They have spent their lives trying to appear normal. Asking for help may be very difficult for these patients.

Most PPS patients have their homes arranged so they can function independently. Temporarily staying in a different environment, such as a hospital, can be very troublesome for the patient. She may need help with tasks that she could do independently at home. Most PPS patients fear becoming dependent on others. The patient may have great difficulty asking for help. Anticipate her needs and ask if assistance is needed. Do not be surprised if the patient refuses your offer of help. Respect the refusal, but advise the patient that accepting assistance is different from being dependent. In fact, assistance may help the patient to remain independent. Even if the patient refuses your help, stand by to see if she can perform the task or procedure safely. Adapt the environment, whenever possible, for optimal independent function. You may do this by moving furniture, or bringing a bedside commode, for example. Most polio survivors are in tune to what their bodies are telling them. If the patient says she cannot do something, pay attention.

Amyotrophic Lateral Sclerosis (ALS)

Amyotrophic lateral sclerosis (**ALS**) is a progressive neuromuscular disease that causes muscle weakness and paralysis. It is a disease of the motor nerves that control voluntary movement. The cause is unknown. There seems to be a familial link in about 10% of the cases. ALS occurs in all races and both genders, although it is more common in men. The most common age of onset is 55, but it can occur in persons of any age. It is a progressive condition for which there is no cure. ALS is almost always fatal. In the United States, ALS is also called Lou Gehrig's disease, after a famous baseball player. Other names may be used in other countries. About half of the patients diagnosed with ALS die within 18 months, although some may live for many years. One drug has been successful in slowing progression of the disease, but there is no known cure. Some medications are used to relieve the symptoms.

Signs and Symptoms. ALS takes months to diagnose because the signs and symptoms are similar to those of other neurologic conditions. Common signs and symptoms of ALS are:

- stumbling, tripping, and falling
- loss of strength and muscle control in hands, arms, and legs
- difficulty speaking
- difficulty swallowing
- drooling
- breathing becoming progressively more difficult
- muscle cramping, shaking, and twitching, progressing to spasticity
- muscle weakness and atrophy
- abnormal reflexes

ALS is not a painful disease, but the effects of ALS often cause pain. These are:

- muscle cramps
- contractures
- constipation
- burning eyes

- swelling feet
- muscle aches
- pressure sores

ALS does not affect the entire body. The patient's mental acuity is intact. Depression is common. The heart, bowel and bladder control, and sexual function are not affected. The eyes are the last muscles affected and are sometimes not affected at all.

Progression of ALS. Progression of ALS varies with the patient. Worsening occurs over several months to several years. A common pattern is:

- Difficulty walking, causing the patient to use a cane, then a walker, then a wheelchair.
- As the legs weaken, the hands and arms also become weaker.
- The patient loses the ability to write and feed herself.
- The patient experiences difficulty speaking, chewing, swallowing, and talking.
- Eventually a feeding tube becomes necessary.
- The patient needs an alternate communication system.
- Chest and diaphragm muscles weaken, causing lung problems.
- The patient needs a ventilator to stay alive.

Nursing Assistant Care. Most ALS patients are cared for at home, with brief hospitalizations to manage complications. Because of this, ALS often involves the whole family. Patients are taught to manage their own illness. Allow the patient to be in control of daily routines, and respect his intelligence. Adaptive equipment is used to maintain independence for as long as possible.

Many ALS patients are not bedridden, despite being completely paralyzed. Special wheelchairs and portable ventilators are often used so patients can get out of bed. Follow the patient's care plan for mobility. If the patient does not get out of bed, reposition and turn her at least every 2 hours, or more often, as instructed.

Nursing care is designed to prevent complications of immobility. The most common problems are constipation, contractures, and pressure ulcers. You will also take measures to prevent choking and infection. Care of the patient is largely determined by the stage of the patient's disease at hospital admission. Follow the care plan and the nurse's instructions. Care of the typical ALS patient involves:

- Attention to positioning. An upright position (such as high Fowler's) may be ordered to ease respirations.
- Range-of-motion and light exercises to prevent deformities and maintain the strength of muscles that are not yet affected.
- Assisting the patient to use the incentive spirometer (Unit 38).
- Having the patient rest before meals to conserve muscle strength and reduce the risk of choking.
- Providing small, frequent feedings.

DIFFICULT *Situations*

ALS is a particularly cruel disease that causes fairly rapid degeneration of the nervous system, making the patient dependent. The mind remains intact and alert, so the patient is aware of each small change and its implications. Strive to develop a good rapport with the patient and provide generous emotional support and compassion.

- Taking swallowing precautions when feeding the patient. The speech therapist may have taught the patient positions and techniques to use to prevent choking. Commonly, the patient is as upright as possible, with the neck flexed slightly forward.
- Not washing solid foods down with liquids. This increases the risk of choking and aspiration in the ALS patient.
- Checking the mouth after meals to make sure that no food particles remain. They can cause choking later. Provide mouth care promptly after each meal.
- Scheduling rest and activities to preserve the patient's strength and energy.
- Using good infection control measures, handwashing, and standard precautions to reduce the risk of infection.

Seizure Disorder (Epilepsy)

Seizure disorder (convulsions, epilepsy) involves recurrent, transient attacks of disturbed brain function. It is characterized by various forms of convulsions called *seizures*. Not all seizures are alike. A seizure occurs when one or more of the following is present:

- An altered state of consciousness, which may be momentary or prolonged
- Convulsive uncontrolled movements
- Disturbances of feeling or behavior

Seizures may develop:

- congenitally, associated with a difficult birth.
- following a head injury.
- as a result of increased intracranial pressure.
- as a result of lesions of the brain such as tumors.
- as a result of cerebrovascular accidents.
- as a result of high fever or infection, especially in infants and children.
- from taking certain medications or street drugs.

Some persons experience an aura just before the seizure occurs. An aura involves one of the senses. The person may smell an unusual odor or hear a sound. The aura is usually consistent and remains the same each time it is experienced. For some people the aura serves as a warning so the person can get to a safe place. Other people may not remember the aura.

Some people have service dogs that warn them of an impending seizure so they can take safety precautions before the seizure begins. A dog's sense of smell is much more sensitive than a human's. It is believed that the dog smells a chemical reaction that signals the onset of a seizure. All states have access laws regarding service animals, but these vary widely. Your facility may have policies regarding the use of service animals while patients are hospitalized.

There are many different types and categories of seizure activity. The most common types of seizure activity are classified as follows:

- Partial seizures
  - There may or may not be loss of consciousness.
    - Seizures generally begin in one part of the body and involve only one side of the body.
- Generalized seizures (Figure 42-18)
  - These include grand mal seizures. These are also called generalized tonic-clonic seizures. There is bilateral generalized motor movement and muscular rigidity. Consciousness is lost and special awareness may or may not precede convulsive movements. The sensory awareness or aura may be in the form of lights, sounds, or aromas and is part of the seizure. When this seizure begins, the patient cries out, then falls to the floor. The muscles stiffen (tonic phase), then the extremities begin to jerk and twitch (clonic phase). The patient may lose bladder control. Consciousness returns slowly. After this seizure, the patient may feel tired, or be confused and disoriented. This state may last from a few minutes to several hours or days. The patient may fall asleep, or gradually become less confused until full consciousness returns.
  - Petit mal seizures are characterized by momentary loss of muscle tone. These are also called absence seizures. The seizure begins without warning, and consists of a period of unconsciousness, in which the patient blinks rapidly, stares blankly, breathes rapidly, or makes chewing movements. The seizure lasts 2 to 10 seconds, then ends abruptly. The patient usually resumes normal activity immediately. Because these seizures are mild, they may go unnoticed. Children with absence seizures may have learning problems if the seizures are not identified and treated.
- Status epilepticus is a seizure that lasts for a long time, or repeats without recovery. It is a serious medical emergency. Death may result if the patient is not treated immediately. Status epilepticus can be convulsive (tonic-clonic) or nonconvulsive (absence). A person in nonconvulsive status epilepticus may become confused or appear dazed. The highest incidence of status

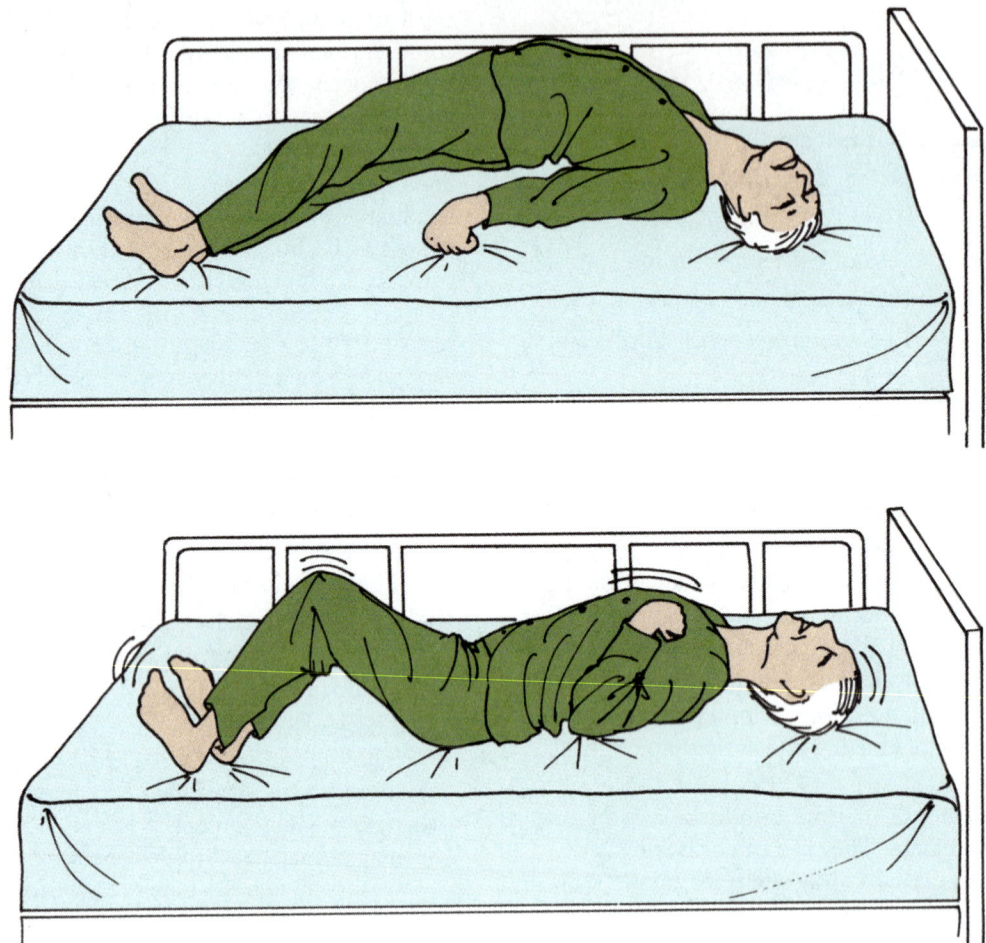

FIGURE 42-18 Generalized tonic-clonic seizures involve the entire body. Side rails should be padded for patients with seizure disorder. The side rails are down in this picture for clarity.

epilepticus occurs during the first year of life and after age 60. In elderly adults, most cases are related to cerebrovascular accidents.

Nursing Care During Seizures. The main nursing focus during a seizure is to:

- Prevent injury by:
  - Staying with the person
  - Assisting the person to lie down, if there is time
  - Making no attempt to restrain the person's movements or to put anything in her mouth
  - Moving away any object the person might hit, to protect the person from injuring herself
- Maintain an airway by:
  - Loosening clothing, particularly around the neck
  - Turning the person's head or body to one side so that saliva or vomitus drains out
  - Opening an airway, if necessary, by lifting the person's shoulders and allowing the head to tilt back

If you find a person who is having a seizure:

- Do not leave the person.
- Do not move the person.
- Do not put anything in the person's mouth.
- Maintain an airway.
- Ring or call for assistance.
- Protect the person from self-inflicted injury.
- Watch the person carefully.

- Apply standard precautions when caring for a patient with seizure activity. There is a high probability of contact with blood, body fluids, secretions, and excretions during the care of this patient.

Observation of the patient should be made during and following the seizure. Breathing should be carefully monitored. Ring for assistance, if possible, but do not leave the patient alone. As much as possible, protect the patient from injuring herself during the seizure.

Nursing Care after a Seizure. When the seizure stops, tell the patient where she is and what happened. Assist her to bed. The patient will be very tired. Allow her to sleep. She may be confused and require periodic reorientation. Leave the patient in a position of comfort and safety with the call signal and needed personal items within reach. Other care includes:

- providing incontinent care, if necessary.
- checking the vital signs as instructed; you may take vital signs frequently until the patient is stable.
- monitoring the patient closely for return of seizure activity.
- assisting the nurse to administer oxygen or suctioning, if needed.

Report to the nurse:

- any change in the patient before the seizure, such as an aura, confusion, or change in behavior.
- a description of the way the seizure looked, including the body parts involved.
- loss of bowel or bladder control, eyes rolling upward, rapid blinking, biting tongue.
- the time the seizure started and stopped, if known.
- condition of the patient after the seizure.
- vital signs.

Spinal Cord Injuries

Injuries to the spinal cord result in loss of function and sensation below the level of the injury. These patients are particularly prone to contractures and pressure ulcers. Special terms have been given to the conditions resulting from such injury:

- Quadriplegia—both arms and legs are paralyzed (paralyzed from the neck area down)
- Paraplegia—lower part of the body is paralyzed

Flaccid paralysis involves loss of muscle tone and absence of tendon reflexes. Some patients have spastic paralysis. These patients have no voluntary movement. The extremities move in an involuntary pattern, similar to muscle spasms. The patient is aware of the movements, but cannot stop them. The type of paralysis is determined by the level of injury. Patients with upper motor injuries are more likely to exhibit spastic paralysis.

Signs and Symptoms. Signs and symptoms of paralysis vary with the level of the injury. The patient will be paralyzed below the level where the spinal cord was damaged.

For example, an injury to the upper vertebrae in the neck will cause respiratory depression. The patient will be unable to move the arms and legs. He or she will lose bowel and bladder control. An injury near the waist will also cause loss of bowel and bladder control. The patient will be unable to move the legs.

Treatment. Treatment depends on the level of injury. Overall, treatment is directed at:

- preventing complications of immobility.
- preventing deformities.
- restoring the patient to the highest degree of independence possible.

Responsibilities of the Nursing Assistant. Patients with spinal cord injury need long-term nursing care, which includes:

- Listening. Many persons with spinal cord injury are taught to give directions to caregivers who are doing for the person what the individual cannot do for himself.
- A consistently calm and patient approach, because the loss of sensory and motor functions often makes self-care difficult.
- Acceptance of the patient's expressions of anger, fear, and depression, as well as clumsy attempts at self-care. Remember that the patient's ability to think is not necessarily impaired. Frustration is even greater because these patients can no longer will their actions.
- Careful skin care, because:
  - Incontinence not only causes the patient embarrassment and discomfort but also makes the skin prone to breakdown
  - The lack of nervous stimulation decreases circulation to the skin
  - Pain and pressure cannot be felt
- Attention to elimination needs. For example, suppositories may be given daily. A catheter may be inserted into the bladder, so catheter and drainage care will be needed. Special pads within plastic incontinence pants may also be used.

OSHA *Alert*

Patients with spinal cord injury can provide limited to no assistance with positioning, moving, and transfers. To prevent injury to your back, never move a patient who has a spinal cord injury by yourself. Make sure that another assistant is available to help you. The use of lift sheets, mechanical lifts, and other adjunctive devices makes moving the patient easier for both the patient and the nursing assistant.

- Avoidance of contractures and deformities, which occur rapidly after the onset of paralysis. When moving and positioning patients with paralysis, move the extremities slowly and gently. Rapid, rough movements will cause spasticity. If a patient's extremities move into a position of flexion, position them in extension. If the extremities move into a position of extension, position them in flexion. Positioning devices may be necessary to maintain position. Attention to proper positioning is very important. This is a major key to preventing contractures and deformities in these high-risk patients.

- Provision of ROM exercises. These will be needed for the rest of the patient's life.

- Proper attention and care to prevent:
  - Respiratory infections
  - Urinary tract infections
  - Pressure ulcers

Autonomic Dysreflexia. Autonomic dysreflexia is a potentially life-threatening complication of spinal cord injury. It usually occurs in patients with injuries above the mid-thoracic area. It indicates uncontrolled sympathetic nervous system activity. Problems that seem minor can trigger this condition. As a rule, injuries that would normally cause pain below the level of spinal injury can set this life-threatening chain of events in motion. For example:

- overfull bladder (this is the most common cause)
- urinary retention
- urinary infection
- blocked catheter
- overfilled urinary drainage bag
- constipation or fecal impaction
- hemorrhoids
- infection or irritation in the abdomen, such as appendicitis or acute abdominal conditions
- pressure ulcers
- prolonged pressure by an object in the chair, shoe, wrinkled clothing, and the like
- minor injury, such as a cut, bruise, or abrasion
- ingrown toenails
- burns, including sunburn
- pressure on skin from tight or constrictive clothing
- menstrual cramps
- labor and delivery
- overstimulation during sexual activity
- fractured bones

Signs and symptoms of autonomic dysreflexia are:
- extremely high blood pressure, over 200/100
- severe headache
- red, flushed face
- red blotches on the skin above the level of spinal injury
- sweating above the level of spinal injury

- stuffy nose
- nausea
- bradycardia (pulse below 60)
- goose bumps below the level of injury
- cold, clammy skin below the level of injury

If you observe any of these signs and symptoms, notify the nurse immediately. Treatment for this condition involves identifying the offending stimulus and removing it. If you believe something has triggered the condition, inform the nurse. Remove tight and constricting clothing and shoes. Check the catheter and drainage bag. Follow the nurses' instructions.

Meningitis

Meningitis is an inflammation of the meninges. It is usually caused by microorganisms.

The signs and symptoms of meningitis are:
- Headache
- Nausea
- Stiffness of the neck
- Seizures
- Chills
- Elevated temperature

This condition is treated with antibiotics. If it is communicable, droplet precautions are used.

Cataracts

Cataracts (Figure 42-19) are the leading cause of vision loss in adults over the age of 55. Because of this, cataract surgery is one of the most common surgeries in the United States today.

Cataracts cause the normally clear lens of the eye to become cloudy. The cloudy (opaque) lens will not allow light rays to pass through. Therefore, the person is no longer able to see.

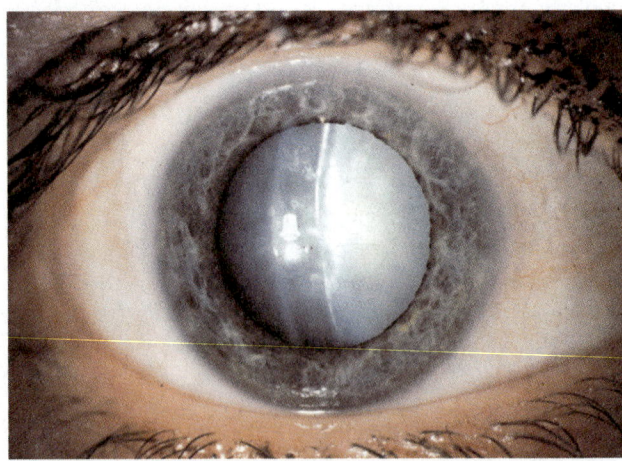

FIGURE 42-19 When the patient develops a cataract, the lens is cloudy instead of transparent. *(Photo courtesy of Linda Jaakobovitch, Cincinnati Eye Institute)*

Treatment. Removal or replacement of the lens permits light rays to enter the eye. Sight is then restored. The lens is needed to adjust vision to different distances. The latest innovations in cataract surgery increase comfort and convenience for the patient. Until recently, most surgery for cataracts involved removing the center (nucleus) of the lens through a larger incision. Currently, most surgeons remove cataracts with a small incision and ultrasound.

The surgery is performed either as an outpatient procedure or in a day surgery center. The patient is admitted to the center in the morning and remains for one to two hours after the surgery, or until vital signs are stable. Eye drops are used to numb the eye. In this surgery, the cataract is removed. A plastic, silicone, or hydrogel lens is usually implanted (Figure 42-20A and 42-20B), and the incision is naturally sealed. Stitches are not used. Some surgeons apply a patch to the eye, but most do not.

Nursing Care. Nursing care of the cataract patient includes:

- Routine postoperative care.
- Relief of pain. Discomfort is usually mild. If pain worsens, the patient complains of sharp pain, or vision decreases, promptly notify the nurse.
- Being sure all needed items, such as signal cords, are within easy reach.
- Taking extra precautions if the patient is confused or restless.
- Checking vital signs until stable.
- Keeping the surgical site undisturbed. After surgery, the patient may feel as if something (such as an eyelash) is in the eye. The patient may complain of itching. Slight

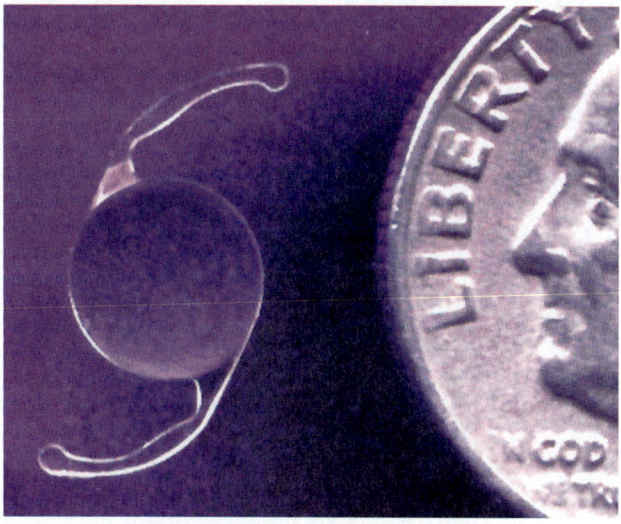

FIGURE 42-20B The lens implant is left in place. The patient cannot feel it after the eye heals. The lens implant is similar to a contact lens and is smaller than a dime. *(Photo courtesy of Linda Jaakobovitch, Cincinnati Eye Institute)*

fluid discharge may be present, and the eye may be sensitive to light and touch. Instruct the patient not to rub or squeeze the eye.

- Helping the patient to adapt to temporarily blurred vision. This is normal due to the bright lights used in surgery and drops used to dilate the eyes. The problem should resolve on its own promptly.
- Assisting the patient with initial ambulation, if needed. Many patients are able to walk without help immediately after surgery.

After the patient is stable, he or she is usually discharged home.

Orders regarding postoperative activity usually include:

- Protecting the eye from injury for the first four weeks.
- Avoid straining activities such as bending over, lifting objects that weigh more than 20 pounds, or strenuous coughing. Bending increases pressure in the eye. The patient can usually walk, climb stairs, and do light housework. The surgeon or nurse will instruct the patient on the level of activity.
- Using medicated eye drops for several weeks to promote healing and control pressure. These may sting a little, but the medication is necessary to promote a successful outcome.
- Wearing an eye shield at night, if instructed by the doctor.
- Informing the physician if there is an increase in pain or loss of vision.

Glaucoma

Glaucoma is a condition of increased pressure within the eye. The most common type of glaucoma is *open angle glaucoma*, a slowly progressive, chronic condition. There are no

Lens Implant Surgery for Cataracts

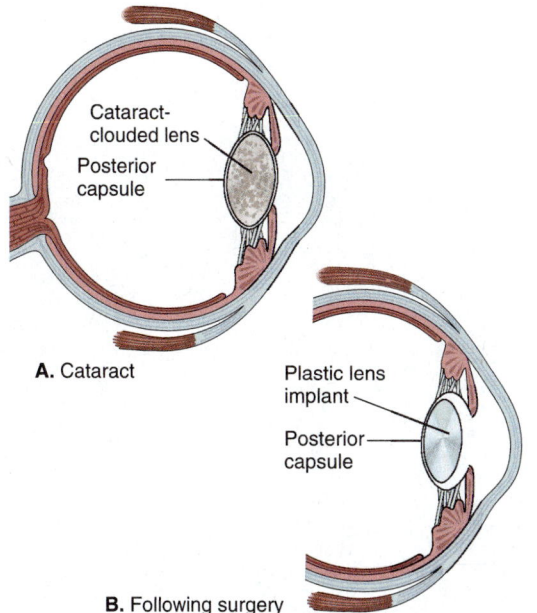

A. Cataract

Cataract-clouded lens

Posterior capsule

Plastic lens implant

Posterior capsule

B. Following surgery

FIGURE 42-20A The lens is removed and the plastic intraocular lens is permanently placed in the eye.

early signs and symptoms. As the problem progresses, the patient begins to experience vision loss. The problem causes gradual loss of peripheral vision. The patient:

- develops eye pain
- has difficulty adjusting to darkness
- may be unable to detect color
- sees halos around lights

Untreated, it progresses to loss of central vision and blindness. The problem is usually detected during a routine eye examination. Untreated, the condition compresses the lens into the vitreous humor. This places pressure on the neurons in the retina, leading to blindness. Open angle glaucoma commonly occurs in both eyes at the same time.

An acute glaucoma, called *closed angle glaucoma*, is less common. This type usually occurs in one eye. When the pressure within the eye increases, the iris will bulge out. The patient usually has severe pain and vision loss in the eye. Other signs and symptoms are:

- nausea and vomiting
- headache
- feeling very tired
- blurred vision
- rainbow-like halos around lights

This is an emergency situation that must be promptly treated.

Care of the Patient with Glaucoma. Glaucoma is treated with medications and special eye drops that reduce pressure. Surgery may be done to drain fluid and relieve pressure. The patient must have regular eye examinations to measure the pressure within the eye. Care of the patient with glaucoma includes:

- monitoring accurate intake and output if the patient is on intravenous medication to reduce eye pressure.
- checking vital signs every two to four hours.
- reporting complaints of eye pain promptly to the nurse.
- arranging needed items so the patient can see them; avoid moving things unless the patient gives permission.
- avoiding strain and exertion that will increase intra-ocular pressure.
- keeping the patient from stooping or lifting.
- avoiding tight and constrictive clothing, which also increases pressure.
- keeping the patient safe, if vision is limited.

Retinal Degeneration

Breakdown of the retina, known as **retinal degeneration** or **macular degeneration**, occurs over a period of months or years. The incidence increases with age. Central vision is progressively lost as the macula (area of acute central vision) is damaged. Subretinal hemorrhages lead to scarring of this important area.

Early treatment with laser therapy can seal the tiny capillaries to prevent further damage to the macula.

Vision Impairment

Cataracts, glaucoma, retinal degeneration, eye infections, and other eye conditions, such as ocular tumors, can cause blindness. Persons who are legally blind may still have partial vision. The degree of visual limitation must be considered when giving care. It is also important to consider the patient's attitude to the limitations. Adjustment to blindness is both a physical and an emotional process.

Allow the person who is blind or nearly blind the opportunity to do as much as possible in personal care and other activities. Many blind people are capable and independent. In fact, most blind people do well with minimal help and support once they are fully oriented to their surroundings. Review Unit 7 for guidelines for working with persons who have visual impairments.

Artificial Eye

Situations such as severe injury to the eye or untreatable cancer may require the surgical removal of an eye. An eye prosthesis (artificial eye) is usually inserted after the surgery. The care plan should provide information if the patient has an artificial eye.

Some patients remove the artificial eye at night. Others prefer not to remove the eye at all. You may be responsible for removing the eye. If the eye is to remain out of the socket, store it in a marked cup in contact lens disinfectant solution (Figure 42-21) (Procedure 104). The socket is usually cleansed and irrigated when the eye is removed. Irrigation of the socket may be a licensed nursing procedure in your facility. Know and follow your facility policy. Apply the principles of standard precautions when caring for the artificial eye and mucous membranes in the eye socket.

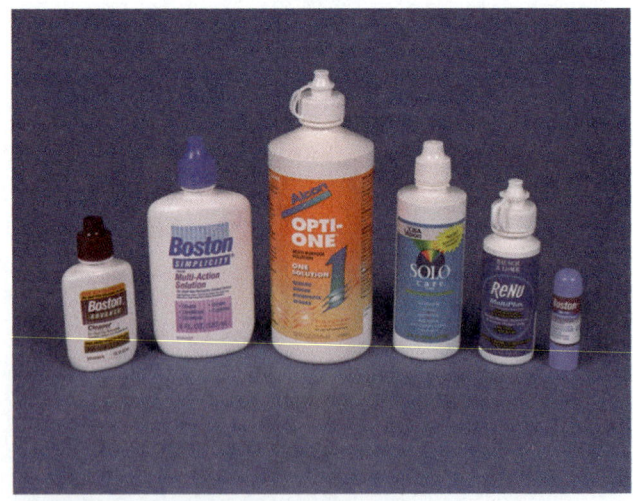

FIGURE 42-21 Many different disinfectant solutions are used to clean the artificial eye.

PROCEDURE 104

CARING FOR THE EYE SOCKET AND ARTIFICIAL EYE

1. Carry out beginning procedure actions.

2. Assemble equipment:
   - eye cup or clean denture cup
   - prescribed solution, if ordered
   - small plastic bag
   - 4 to 6 cotton balls
   - 2 4 × 4 gauze pads
   - emesis basin with lukewarm water
   - disposable gloves
   - towel

3. Place the patient in supine position, if tolerated. Place a towel across the patient's chest.

4. Put on disposable gloves.

5. Moisten cotton balls in lukewarm water in the emesis basin.
   a. Ask the patient to close his eyes.
   b. Wipe the upper lid of the affected eye from the inner corner of the eye to the outer edge. Repeat with a clean cotton ball until the area is clean and free of mucus.

6. Dispose of the used cotton balls in a plastic bag.

7. Place a 4 × 4 gauze pad in the bottom of the eye cup or denture cup.

8. Remove the artificial eye:
   a. Gently pull down the lower eyelid with your thumb (Figure 42-22A). Open the upper lid with your index finger.

b. Grasp the artificial eye as it comes out of the eye socket and place it on the gauze in the cup.

c. Some patients use a small suction cup to remove the eye. Gently hold the eye open with the fingers of one hand. Depress the suction cup between your thumb and index finger (Figure 42-22B). Place the suction cup in the center of the artificial eye. Release the pressure. Gently pull the eye from the socket (Figure 42-22C).

9. Use clean cotton balls moistened with water or solution as ordered and clean the empty eye socket. Dry gently with clean, dry cotton balls. Use a new cotton ball for each wipe. Pat the patient's face dry, as needed.

10. Carry the cup with the artificial eye to the sink. Fill the sink one-third full with lukewarm water.

11. Wash the eye under lukewarm running water, or use the prescribed solution. Use gauze if necessary to loosen and remove any accumulation from the eye.

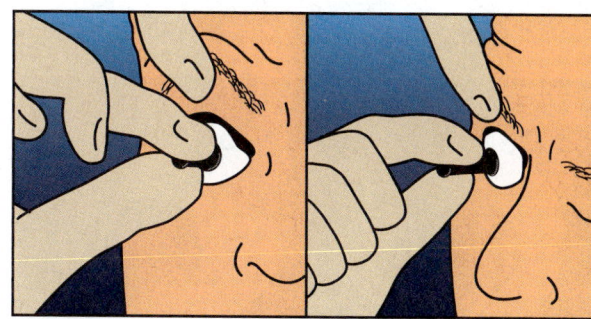

FIGURE 42-22B Squeeze the cup, place it against the eye, then release the suction.

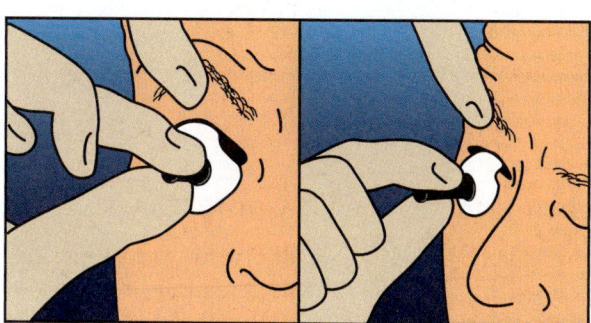

FIGURE 42-22C Pull the eye down gently from the socket.

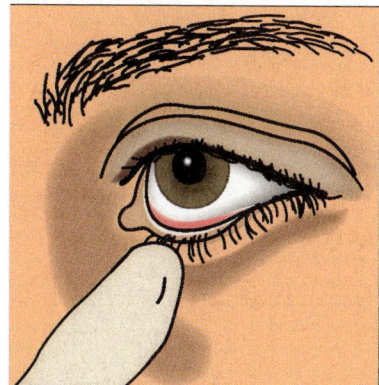

FIGURE 42-22A To loosen the eye, pull the lower lid down, then push back up slightly.

continues

PROCEDURE 104

continued

12. Rinse the eye and place it on a dry 4 × 4 gauze pad, or store the eye in sterile water or the prescribed solution, according to the care plan. (Do not dry an artificial eye.)

13. Discard the water or solution in the eye cup and rinse the cup.

14. Remove your gloves. Wash your hands. Carry the artificial eye to the patient's bedside.

15. Explain to the patient what you are going to do.

16. Insert the artificial eye into the eye socket:

    a. Carry out beginning procedure actions.

    b. Put on disposable gloves.

    c. Clean and rinse the artificial eye with the prescribed solution, if you have not already done so.

    d. Position the notched edge of the eye toward the patient's nose (Figure 42-22D).

    e. Gently open the upper eyelid. Bring the prosthesis up past the lower lid and under the upper lid. Set it flush once it is past the lower lid and touching the upper tissues (Figure 42-22E).

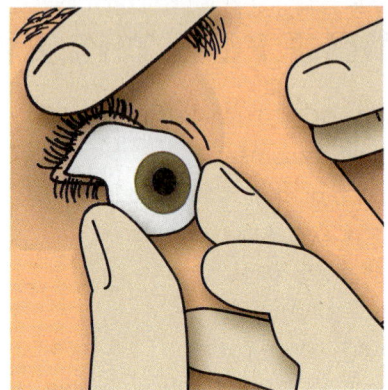

FIGURE 42-22E Gently move the artificial eye up past the lower lid.

    f. Place your index finger on the prosthesis and slip it up under the upper lid (Figure 42-22F).

    g. Release the upper lid.

    h. Draw the edge of the lower lid forward, covering the lower edge of the eye. Press down lightly.

17. Carry out procedure completion actions.

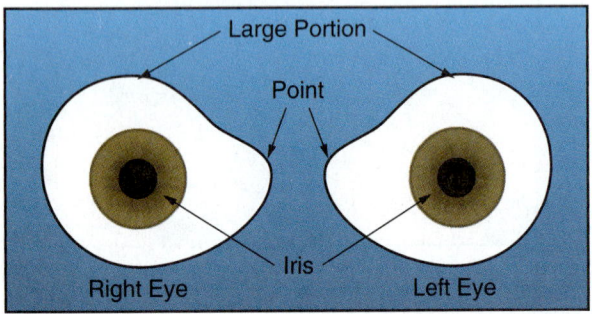

FIGURE 42-22D The notched part of the eye is positioned next to the patient's nose.

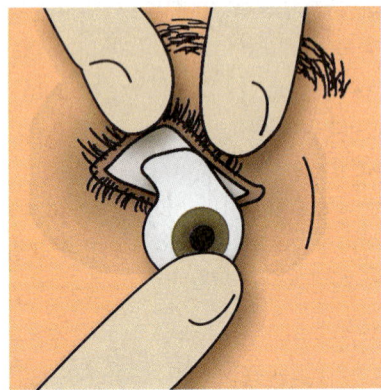

FIGURE 42-22F Using your index finger, push the eye the rest of the way up and under the upper lid.

Warm and Cool Eye Compresses

Many elderly patients have dry, itchy eyes. This may be caused by allergies, irritants, squinting, rubbing, or blinking the eyes. The eyes may appear red, with swollen eyelids. If patients rub or scratch their eyes, they may become infected. Patients with dry, itchy eyes may complain of:

- burning
- scratchy feeling
- itching

- light sensitivity
- difficulty moving eyes
- excess mucus production
- severe pain
- blurred vision
- seeing halos

Observe the patient for:

- drainage from the eyes

- redness of eyelid rims
- scaly, flaky skin around the eyes
- edema of the eyelids

Report your observations to the nurse. You may be instructed to apply warm or cool soaks to the eyelids. Apply the principles of standard precautions when performing this procedure. If an infection is suspected, use separate equipment for each eye. This will prevent the infection from spreading.

PROCEDURE 105

WARM EYE COMPRESSES

1. Carry out beginning procedure actions.

2. Assemble equipment:
   - towel
   - small bottle of sterile saline solution
   - small sterile basin
   - sterile gauze pads
   - disposable gloves
   - plastic bag

3. Position the patient for comfort. For warm compresses, assist the patient to a Fowler's or high Fowler's position, if possible. This helps reduce edema. Cover the neck and shoulders with a bath towel.

4. Heat the bottle of sterile saline under hot running water, or place it in a second bowl of hot water. The solution should become warm, not hot. Check the temperature with a thermometer. It should be approximately 105°F.

5. Pour the heated solution into the small, sterile bowl.

6. Wash your hands.

7. Apply disposable gloves.

8. Place the gauze pads in the bowl.

9. Remove a gauze pad from the bowl and squeeze out the excess solution.

10. Instruct the patient to close her eyes.

11. Apply one compress to the affected eye.

12. Remove a second gauze pad from the bowl and squeeze out the excess solution.

13. Apply the second compress on top of the first.

14. Repeat with the other eye, as directed.

15. If the patient complains that the compress is too hot, remove it immediately.

16. Change the compresses every few minutes for the prescribed length of time. The treatment should not last longer than 15–20 minutes. Check the skin under the compress each time you change it for signs that the solution was too hot.

17. After 15–20 minutes, or as directed, remove the compresses. Discard them in the plastic bag.

18. Use the remaining, clean gauze pads to dry the eye. Wipe from the inner corner to the outer corner. Use each gauze pad one time, then discard it in the plastic bag.

19. Carry out procedure completion actions.

PROCEDURE 106

COOL EYE COMPRESSES

1. Carry out beginning procedure actions.

2. Assemble equipment:
   - towel
   - small bottle of sterile saline solution
   - ice
   - small sterile basin
   - sterile gauze pads
   - disposable gloves
   - plastic bag

3. Position the patient for comfort. The supine position is best for this procedure, as it reduces edema. Turn the patient's head slightly so the affected eye is up. Cover the neck and shoulders with a bath towel.

4. Place some ice chips in the small sterile basin.

5. Pour the saline solution into the basin.

6. Wash your hands.

7. Apply disposable gloves.

8. Place the gauze pads in the bowl.

9. Remove a gauze pad from the bowl and squeeze out the excess solution.

10. Instruct the patient to close his eyes.

11. Apply one compress to the affected eye.

12. Remove a second gauze pad from the bowl and squeeze out the excess solution.

13. Apply the second compress on top of the first.

14. Repeat with the other eye, as directed.

15. If the patient complains that the compress is too cold, remove it immediately.

16. You may be directed to cover the compress with an ice pack. Make a small ice pack by placing ice chips in a sandwich bag or disposable glove. Squeeze the air out, then tie the end. Keep the pack size small. Cover the cool compress with the ice pack, as directed. Remove it immediately if the patient complains of pain.

17. Change the compresses every few minutes for the prescribed length of time. The treatment should not last longer than 15–20 minutes. Check the skin under the compress each time you change it for signs that the solution was too cold. If an ice pack is used, it will be left in place for the duration of the treatment. Check the skin under the pack every 5 minutes for signs of injury.

18. After 15–20 minutes, or as directed, remove the compresses. Discard them in the plastic bag.

19. Use the remaining clean gauze pads to dry the eye. Wipe from the inner corner to the outer corner. Use each gauze pad one time, then discard it in the plastic bag.

20. Carry out procedure completion actions.

Otitis Media

Otitis media is an infection of the middle ear. Infections of the nose and throat can move along the eustachian tube to the middle ear, causing inflammation of the middle ear. Fluid and pus form within the middle ear. This may result in fusion (locking) of the middle ear bones. Increased pressure may cause the eardrum to rupture. Both conditions decrease the ability to transmit sound waves. This condition, which is rare in adults, is common in children.

Antibiotics are usually given. A surgical opening (myringo-tomy) is sometimes made in the eardrum to drain the pus. Small tubes may be inserted for drainage.

Otosclerosis

Otosclerosis is a progressive form of deafness of unknown cause. The process involves the growth of new, abnormal bone in the bony labyrinth. This growth prevents the stapes from vibrating properly.

Hearing is improved by the use of a hearing aid. Surgery (stapedectomy) removes the excess bone and replaces it with a prosthesis.

Hearing Impairment

Some of your patients will be hard of hearing or completely deaf. A hearing aid (Figure 42-23A and 42-23B) will sometimes improve the patient's level of hearing and comprehension. (Refer to Procedures 107 to 109.) Lip reading or sign language may be needed to communicate.

Review Unit 7 for guidelines for working with persons who have hearing impairments.

Caring for Hearing Aids

A hearing aid is a delicate and expensive prosthesis. It requires safe handling and regular care.

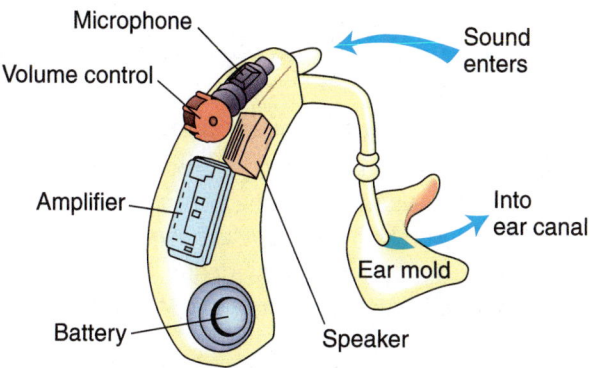

FIGURE 42-23A Parts of a behind-the-ear hearing aid. The ear mold is placed in the ear canal. The rest of the hearing aid is worn outside and over the top of the ear.

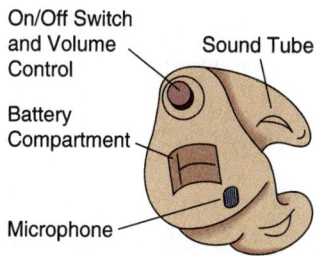

FIGURE 42-23B This hearing aid is worn inside the outer ear canal.

guidelines *for*

Caring for a Hearing Aid

- Store hearing aids at room temperature when they are not being worn. Temperature extremes can damage hearing aids. They should not be worn for more than a few minutes in very cold weather. Avoid exposing them to hair dryers.
- Keep hearing aids dry. If an aid is worn accidentally in the shower, ask the nurse how to dry it. Never try to dry the aid with a hair dryer.
- Store extra batteries in a cool, dry place. Remove the batteries from the hearing aid at night or open the battery compartment. This allows any moisture to evaporate.
- Keep hearing aids safe. They break easily if dropped on a hard surface.
- Remove the hearing aid if hair spray is being used, as the spray may cause damage.
- Turn the hearing aid off when it is not in use. Turn the aid off before removing it.
- Wipe in-the-ear aids daily with a dry tissue.

- Check regularly to make sure the opening of the aid or ear mold is free of wax. In-the-ear types come with a cleaning tool. This should be used only by someone who has been instructed how to use it. Never use a toothpick, paper clip, or other sharp object to clean the hearing aid.
- Insert the hearing aid properly. Sometimes the shape of the ear changes with aging and the hearing aid may have to be refitted. If the patient complains of pain or the aid is difficult to insert, this may be the problem. Advise the nurse if this occurs.
- When communicating with the patient, follow the same guidelines that you use when communicating with a patient who has hearing impairment.
- Check bed linen carefully before placing it in the soiled linen hamper. A hearing aid is small, expensive, and easily lost. It will not survive a trip through the washer and dryer!

guidelines *for*

Troubleshooting Hearing Aids

If the aid is not producing sound, before inserting it in the patient's ear:

- Check to make sure the "+" (positive) side of the battery is next to the "+" inside the hearing aid battery case or compartment.

- Try a new battery—the old one may be dead. Hold the hearing aid in the palm of your hand. Turn the volume all the way up. Cup the aid between your hands. You should hear a loud whistle. A weak or absent sound indicates that the battery is low.

- Before changing the battery, check the position of the old battery so you can put the new one in the same way. When inserting a new battery, place it in the unit gently. If you meet resistance, do not force it. Consult the nurse.

- Check the ear mold to see if it is plugged with wax.

- Make sure the hearing aid is set on "M" (microphone), not "T" (telephone switch).

- If the hearing aid works intermittently or makes a scratchy sound, check for dirt under and around the battery. Also check the volume control and connections. If the hearing aid has a connecting wire, make sure it is plugged in tightly and is not cracked or bent.

If the hearing aid is making squealing sounds:

- If the hearing aid is in the patient's ear and makes a loud, whistling sound, check the position. The aid should be securely in the ear. Make sure that hair, ear wax, or clothing are not interfering with the position. Check the tubing for cracks. Whistling usually indicates an air leak.

- Determine if the ear mold fits properly. It should be completely in the ear. If it does not fit well, report it to the nurse.

- Check the volume on the aid. If it is too high, turn it down until the squealing stops.

- Check the plastic tubing on a behind-the-ear aid. If it is cracked or split, it must be replaced.

PROCEDURE 107

APPLYING A BEHIND-THE-EAR HEARING AID

1. Carry out beginning procedure actions.

2. Assemble equipment:
   - hearing aid

3. Check the appliance to be sure the batteries are working and the tubing is not cracked (Figure 42-24).

4. Check to make sure the hearing aid is off or the volume is turned to its lowest level.

5. Check the patient's ear for wax buildup or any abnormalities.

    Note: If the patient complains that the hearing aid hurts or does not fit properly, it may have to

be refitted; the ear structure changes with age. Report this to the nurse.

6. Handle the aid carefully.
   - Do not drop it.
   - Do not allow it to get wet.
   - Store it carefully with the switch in the off position when it is not in use. Some aids should have batteries removed when being stored.

7. Hand the aid to the patient so that you support the appliance as the patient inserts the ear mold into the ear canal.

continues

PROCEDURE 107

continued

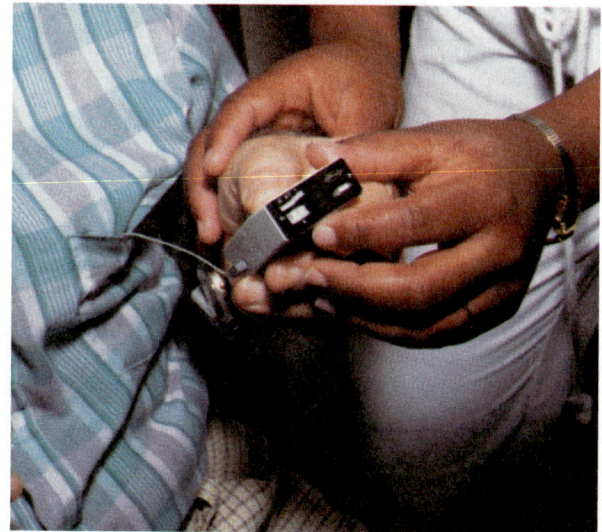 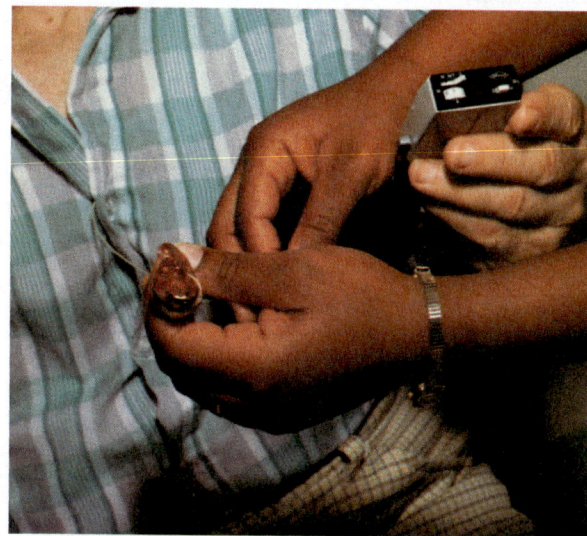

FIGURE 42-24 Check the appliance to make sure the batteries are working and the tubing is not cracked.

Alternate Actions:

8. Place the hearing aid over the patient's ear, allowing the ear mold to hang free.

9. Adjust the hearing aid behind the patient's ear.

10. Grasp the ear mold and gently insert the tapered end into the ear canal.

11. Gently twist the ear mold into the curve of the ear, pushing upward and inward on the bottom of the ear mold while pulling on the ear lobe with the other hand.

12. Turn on the control switch and adjust the volume to a comfortable level.

13. Carry out procedure completion actions.

PROCEDURE 108

REMOVING A BEHIND-THE-EAR HEARING AID

1. Carry out beginning procedure actions.

2. Explain to the patient what you plan to do.

3. Turn off the hearing aid.

4. Loosen the outer portion of the ear mold by gently pulling on the upper part of the ear.

5. Lift the ear mold upward and outward.

6. Make sure the on-off switch is in the off position. Store the hearing aid in a safe area.

7. Carry out procedure completion actions.

PROCEDURE 109

APPLYING AND REMOVING AN IN-THE-EAR HEARING AID

Applying the Hearing Aid

1. Carry out beginning procedure actions.

2. Assist the patient into a comfortable position, with head turned so that the ear needing the hearing aid is closest to you.

3. Turn the hearing aid off and turn the volume down.

4. Make sure you insert the aid in the correct ear.

   a. Grasp the ear mold and gently insert the tapered end into the ear canal (Figure 42-25).

   b. Gently twist the ear mold into the curve of the ear while gently pulling on the ear lobe with the other hand. The hearing aid should fit snugly but comfortably, flush with the ear.

5. Turn on the control switch. To adjust the volume, talk to the patient as you increase the volume. Stop when the patient can hear you.

Removing the Hearing Aid

1. Wash your hands and explain to the patient what you plan to do.

2. Turn off the hearing aid.

3. Loosen the outer portion of the ear mold by gently pulling on the upper part of the ear.

4. Lift the ear mold upward and outward.

5. Store the aid in a safe area. Either remove the batteries and store them in a safe place, or open the battery compartment.

6. Carry out procedure completion actions.

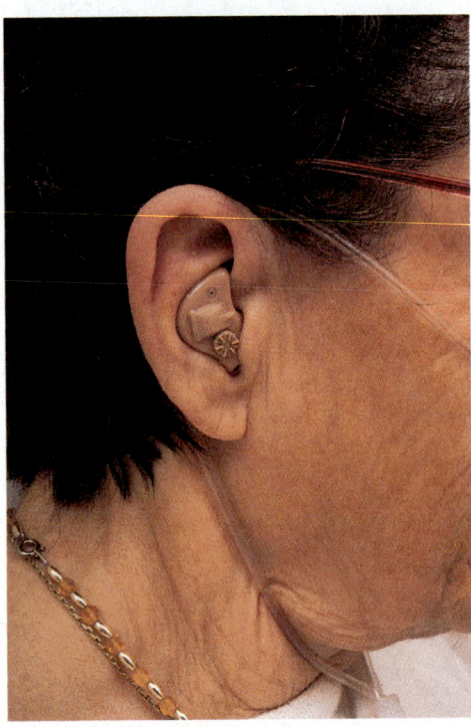

FIGURE 42-25 Gently insert the tapered end of the in-the-ear hearing aid into the ear canal.

DIAGNOSTIC TECHNIQUES

Numerous tests and techniques help physicians diagnose problems of the nervous system. Diagnostic tests include:

- Magnetic resonance imaging (MRI)
- Computerized axial tomography (CAT) scan
- Electroencephalogram (EEG) to measure electrical activity of the brain
- Myelogram, which introduces a traceable dye into the central nervous system
- Tonometry to measure intraocular pressure
- Audiometry to evaluate hearing
- Spinal puncture

Spinal Puncture

Spinal or lumbar punctures are done to withdraw cerebrospinal fluid for examination or to introduce medication or anesthetic into the spinal column. The physician inserts a long, sterile needle between the lumbar vertebrae into the fluid-filled space between the arachnoid mater and pia mater. The pressure of the cerebrospinal fluid is measured. A sample is withdrawn and placed in a sterile test tube. This test may be performed in the patient's room with nurses or nursing assistants helping with the procedure. The patient is placed in a position that will make it easier for the needle to enter the spinal column. It is important that the patient not move during the procedure. The patient may be placed in a lateral position:

- The patient is placed on the side facing away from the physician.
- The knees are drawn up to the abdomen, with the head bent down on the chest.
- The arms are comfortably flexed (Figure 42-26).

The patient may also be placed in a sitting position (Figure 42-27):

- The patient is seated on the edge of the bed facing away from the physician.

- The shoulders are hunched forward.
- The patient may lean on an overbed table for support.
- It is important for someone to steady the table to prevent the patient from falling.

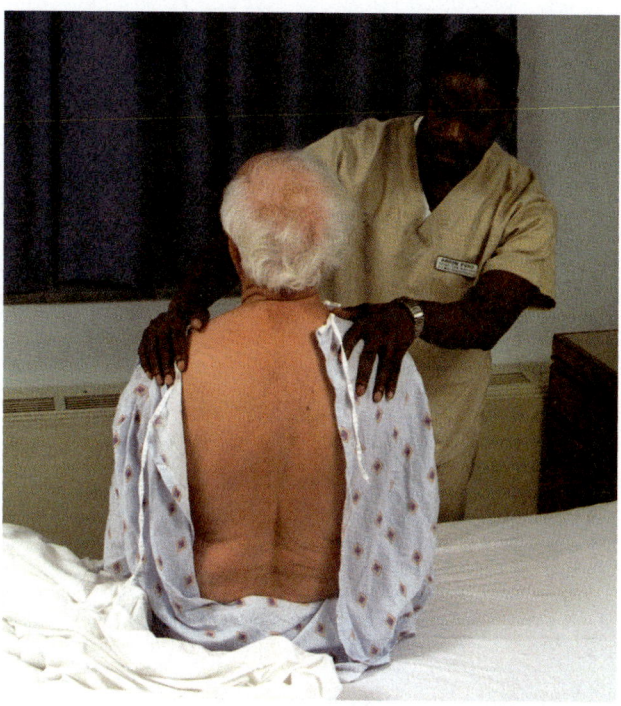

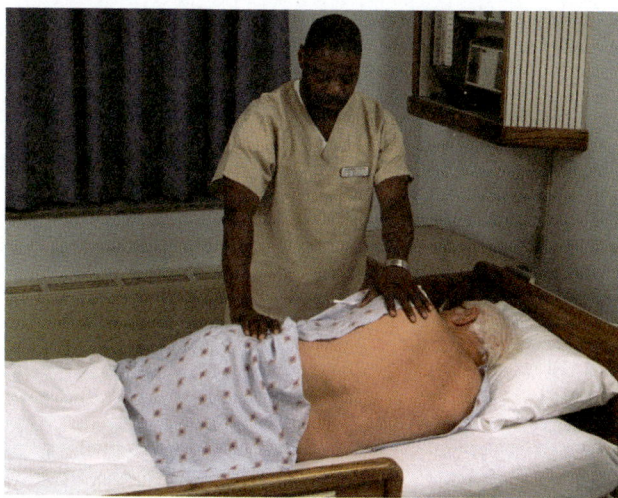

FIGURE 42-26 The patient may be positioned on his or her side with the upper body and legs flexed for a cerebrospinal puncture.

FIGURE 42-27 An alternate position for cerebrospinal puncture.

REVIEW

A. True/False.

Mark the following true or false by circling T or F.

1. T F The patient with right-brain damage will not be able to speak.

2. T F If a patient has aphasia, it is not necessary to speak to him because he cannot understand anyway.

3. T F The patient suffering from a CVA will need assistance in carrying out ROM exercises.

4. T F Hemiplegia is a paralysis on one side of the body.

5. T F The patient with Parkinson's disease characteristically has a "pill-rolling" tremor in the hands.

6. T F Status epilepticus is a serious condition.

7. T F The Parkinson's disease patient often has mood swings.

8. T F The person with quadriplegia is paralyzed on the left side only.

9. T F Fluid may be withdrawn from the spinal canal for examination.

B. Multiple Choice.

Select the one best answer for each of the following.

10. The brain and spinal cord make up the
  a. central nervous system.
  b. peripheral nervous system.
  c. sensory organs.
  d. cerebrospinal fluid space.

11. Neurotransmitters are
  a. neurons.
  b. special nerves.
  c. chemicals that help pass messages.
  d. brain cells.

12. The brain stem controls
  a. voluntary movement.
  b. thinking.
  c. vital functions of the body.
  d. emotions.

13. When the lens of the eye becomes cloudy and impairs vision, it is called
  a. glaucoma.
  b. macular degeneration.
  c. diabetic retinopathy.
  d. cataract.

14. Hearing aids should be kept
  a. wrapped in tissue.
  b. dry.
  c. disassembled.
  d. in the refrigerator when not in use.

15. Persons with Parkinson's disease generally have
  a. pain.
  b. rigidity.
  c. spasticity.
  d. hearing impairment.

16. A person who has had a stroke on the left side of the brain will
  a. have left hemiplegia.
  b. become quick and impulsive.
  c. have aphasia.
  d. have no personality changes.

17. The person who has had a stroke on the right side of the brain will
  a. have left hemiplegia.
  b. have aphasia.
  c. become slow, anxious, and cautious.
  d. have hearing loss in the right ear.

18. Patients with stroke
  a. need proper positioning to prevent contractures.
  b. must be repositioned every 4 hours.
  c. will be unable to speak during the acute phase.
  d. will always be NPO.

19. Multiple sclerosis occurs because
  a. the myelin sheath of the neuron is damaged.
  b. of a hemorrhage in the brain.
  c. of a lack of a certain neurotransmitter.
  d. of muscle damage.

20. Patients with multiple sclerosis may experience
  a. hemiplegia.
  b. no obvious signs or symptoms.
  c. loss of sensation to temperature, pain, and touch.
  d. inability to swallow.

21. Increased intracranial pressure can develop from
  a. Parkinson's disease.
  b. head injuries.
  c. ruptured disc.
  d. post polio syndrome.

22. If you are assisting in the care of a patient with a head injury, you should note and report
  a. blood pressure of 112/74.
  b. pulse rate of 96.
  c. changes in levels of consciousness.
  d. skin warm and dry.

23. You come into a room and find a patient having a seizure. You should
  a. leave and find help.
  b. restrain the patient's movements.
  c. raise the foot of the bed.
  d. remove any object the patient might hit.

24. The patient with post polio syndrome experiences
  a. nausea and vomiting.
  b. visual disturbances and facial droop.
  c. cold intolerance and weakness.
  d. hemiplegia.

25. After surgery, patients with post polio syndrome
  a. often take longer to recover from the anesthesia than other patients.
  b. usually experience bowel and bladder incontinence.
  c. do not feel pain as acutely as other patients.
  d. commonly experience tachycardia for 24 hours.

26. Patients with ALS commonly experience
  a. hemiplegia.
  b. muscle weakness and atrophy.
  c. difficulty hearing.
  d. mental confusion.

27. When caring for a patient with ALS, the nursing assistant should
  a. encourage the patient to feed himself so he does not lose this ability.
  b. allow the patient to set the routines, because his mental clarity is unaffected.
  c. keep the patient in bed and as still as possible.
  d. limit fluids to prevent choking and aspiration.

28. Autonomic dysreflexia can be caused by
  a. hunger.
  b. thirst.
  c. overfull bladder.
  d. drowsiness.

29. Autonomic dysreflexia is
   a. a life-threatening condition.
   b. a minor complication of surgery.
   c. very painful.
   d. common in patients with multiple sclerosis.

30. Cataracts are
   a. a condition caused by very high pressure in the eye.
   b. caused by chemical exposure.
   c. related to retinal degeneration.
   d. a clouding of the lens of the eye.

31. When caring for a patient with glaucoma, the nursing assistant should
   a. apply patches to the patient's eyes at bedtime.
   b. perform tasks that would strain or exert the patient.
   c. apply eye drops to the affected eye.
   d. apply cool eye compresses every 2 hours.

C. Matching.

Choose the correct item from Column II to match each word or phrase in Column I.

Column I

32. _____ uncontrolled trembling

33. _____ CVA

34. _____ difficulty and slowness in carrying out voluntary muscular activities

35. _____ language impairment

36. _____ convulsion

37. _____ aura

38. _____ nystagmus

Column II

a. akinesia
b. aphasia
c. tremors
d. seizure
e. sclera
f. stroke
g. involuntary movement of the eye seen in multiple sclerosis
h. sensation experienced by some persons just before having a seizure

D. Nursing Assistant Challenge.

You are assigned to care for Mr. Johnson, who has had a stroke. You learn from his care plan that he has right hemiplegia and aphasia. Consider these questions:

39. From this information, you know that which part of Mr. Johnson's brain was affected by the stroke?

40. What does right hemiplegia mean?

41. What will you expect from Mr. Johnson's attempts to communicate verbally?

42. What complications is he at risk for? What can you do to prevent these complications?

43. What observations would indicate cognitive impairment?

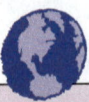 # EXPLORING THE WEB

Description	Location
Stroke	*http://www.stroke.org*
ALS Society of Canada	*http://www.als.ca*
ALS Survival Guide	*http://www.lougehrigsdisease.net*
American Association of Neuroscience Nurses	*http://www.aann.org*
American Epilepsy Society	*http://www.aesnet.org*
American Parkinson's Disease Association	*http://www.apdaparkinson.com*
American Speech-Language-Hearing Association	*http://www.asha.org*
Artificial Eye Clinic	*http://artificialeyeclinic.com*
ArtificialEye.com	*http://www.artificial-eye.com*
Better Hearing Institute	*http://www.betterhearing.org*
Brain Injury Association of America	*http://www.biausa.org*
Cincinnati Eye Institute	*http://www.cincinnatieye.com*
Combined Health Information Database	*http://chid.nih.gov/subfile/subfile.html*
Epilepsy Action	*http://www.epilepsy.org.uk*
Epilepsy Foundation	*http://www.epilepsyfoundation.org*
Gazette International Networking Institute (post polio)	*http://www.postpolio.org*
Harvest Center Post Polio Network	*http://members.aol.com/harvestctr*
International MS Support Foundation	*http://www.msnews.org*
Lincolnshire Post Polio Network	*http://www.ott.zynet.co.uk*
Muscular Dystrophy Association	*http://www.mdausa.org*
National Institute of Neurological Disorders and Stroke	*http://www.biausa.org*
National Parkinson's Foundation	*http://www.parkinson.org*
NeuroExam.com	*http://www.neuroexam.com*
Neurology Algorithms	*http://www.medal.org*
Neurosurgery Online	*http://www.neurosurgery-online.com*
Parkinson's Disease Foundation	*http://www.pdf.org*
Polio.net	*http://www.polionet.org*
Rehabilitation Guidelines for Stroke	*http://www.wrh.org*

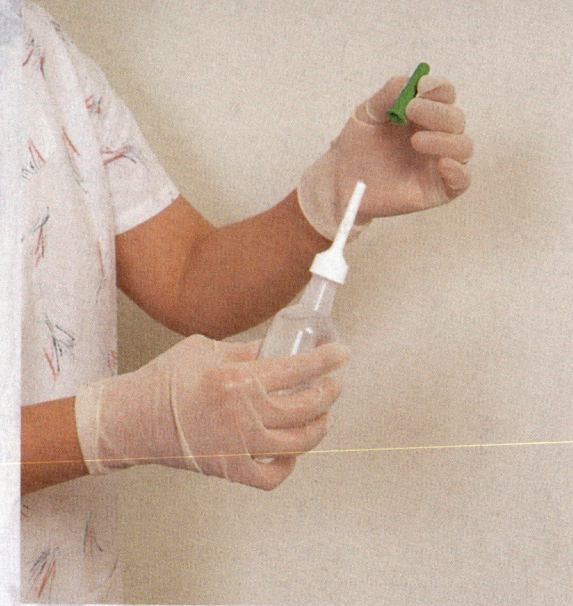

Gastrointestinal System

objectives

After completing this unit, you will be able to:
- Spell and define terms.
- Review the location and functions of the organs of the gastrointestinal system.
- List specific diagnostic tests associated with disorders of the gastrointestinal system.
- Describe some common disorders of the gastrointestinal system.
- Describe nursing assistant actions related to the care of patients with disorders of the gastrointestinal system.

- Identify different types of enemas and state their purpose.
- Demonstrate the following procedures:
  - Procedure 110 Collecting a Stool Specimen
  - Procedure 111 Giving a Soap-Solution Enema
  - Procedure 112 Giving a Commercially Prepared Enema
  - Procedure 113 Inserting a Rectal Suppository
  - Procedure 114 Inserting a Rectal Tube and Flatus Bag

vocabulary

Learn the meaning and the correct spelling of the following words and phrases:

abdominal distention	diarrhea	hernia	pepsin
bile	duodenal resection	herniorrhaphy	peristalsis
bolus	duodenal ulcer	hydrochloric acid	proctoscopy
cholecystectomy	enema	(HCl)	pyloric sphincter
cholecystitis	fecal impaction	ileostomy	sigmoidoscopy
cholelithiasis	fecal material	incarcerated	stool
chyme	flatus	(strangulated)	suppository
colon	gastrectomy	hernia	ulcer
colostomy	gastric resection	nasogastric tube	ulcerative colitis
constipation	gastric ulcer	(NG tube)	urgency
defecation	gastroscopy	occult blood	

INTRODUCTION

The digestive tract extends from the mouth to the anus. It receives the help of the teeth, tongue, salivary glands, liver, gallbladder, and pancreas in breaking food into simpler substances. These substances are used by the body cells to carry on their work of supplying nutrition and eliminating wastes.

STRUCTURE AND FUNCTION

The gastrointestinal system is also called the GI or digestive tract. It extends from the mouth to the anus and is lined with mucous membrane (Figure 43-1). The organs along the length of this system change food into simple forms that can pass through the walls of the small intestine and into the circulatory system. The circulatory system then carries the nutrients to the body cells. The gastrointestinal system includes the:

- Mouth, teeth, tongue, salivary glands
- Pharynx
- Esophagus (gullet)
- Stomach
- Small intestine
- Liver, gallbladder, pancreas
- Large intestine

In the digestive system:

- proteins are changed to amino acids.
- carbohydrates are changed to simple sugars like glucose.
- fats are changed to fatty acids and glycerol.

These changes are brought about by mechanical action and chemicals called *enzymes*. The nondigestible portions of what we eat are moved along the intestines and are finally excreted from the body as feces. Several organs contribute to the digestive process and many disease conditions affect them.

Mouth

In the mouth (Figure 43-2), food is chewed so it can be swallowed easily. The digestive process begins with the help of the:

- Tongue—a skeletal muscle that is covered by tastebuds. The tongue pushes the food between the teeth to be broken up. It assists in mastication (chewing). It propels the food backward toward the pharynx to assist in swallowing. It also aids in speech formation.
- Salivary glands—secrete saliva containing a digestive enzyme called salivary amylase.
  - Salivary amylase begins carbohydrate digestion
  - 1½ quarts of saliva are secreted daily
  - Saliva moistens food to help in swallowing
- Teeth—mechanically break up the food into smaller particles, forming a **bolus** of food. The bolus is then swallowed. There are two natural sets of teeth. The first set (deciduous or temporary) numbers 20. The second set (permanent) numbers 32 and gradually replaces the deciduous set.
- Pharynx—allows the passage of both food and air. It leads to the esophagus.
- Esophagus—a tube 10 to 12 inches long that carries the food to the stomach. Strong muscular contractions called *peristaltic* waves move the food along the tract. These waves begin in the esophagus and continue throughout the intestinal tract.

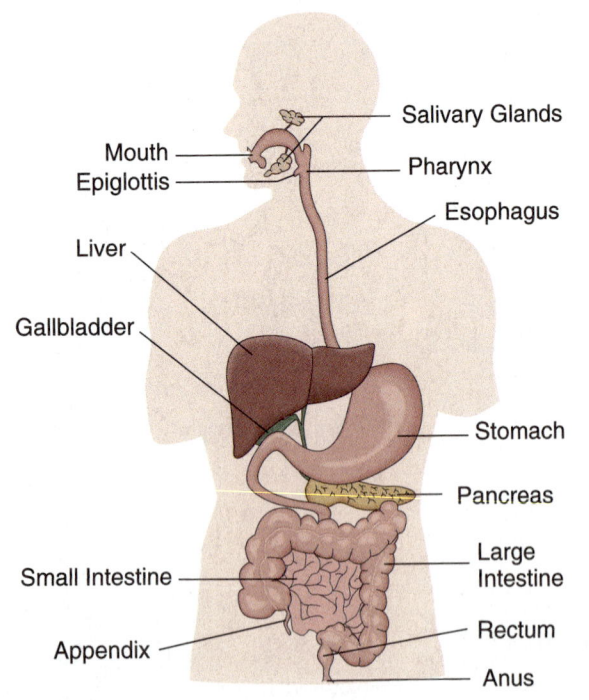

FIGURE 43-1 Digestive system.

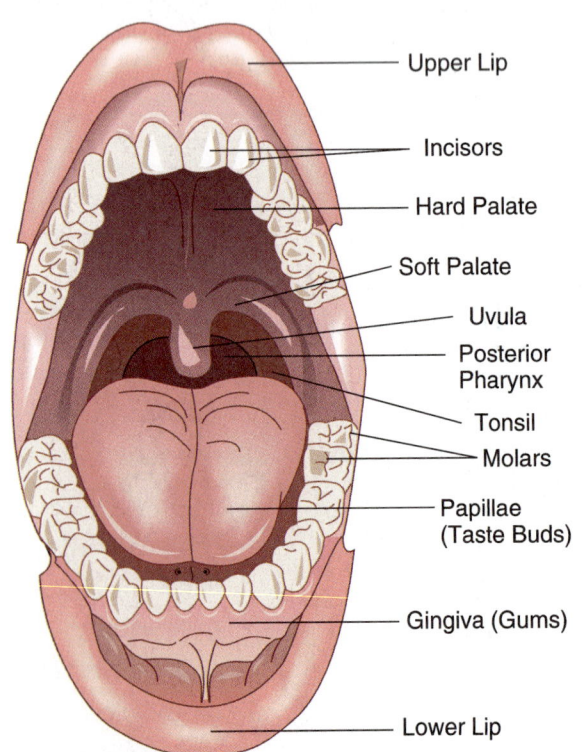

FIGURE 43-2 Mouth.

The Stomach

The stomach

- Is a hollow, muscular, J-shaped organ
- Is found in the peritoneal cavity
- Is two-thirds to the left of the midline
- Is just below the diaphragm
- Has circular muscles at either end that hold the food while it is thoroughly mixed with digestive enzymes
- Begins the chemical process of digestion
- Holds the food between 3 to 4 hours

The stomach has three parts:

1. Fundus—the area above the entrance of the esophagus
2. Body—holds the food
3. Pylorus—the long, narrowly tapered distal end that connects with the small intestines. The muscle guarding this exit point is called the **pyloric sphincter**. Sometimes in babies this muscle is so tight (pyloric stenosis) that milk cannot get through and the muscle must be cut surgically.

The stomach cells produce gastric juice, which contains:

- Proteolytic enzyme (**pepsin**) to begin protein breakdown
- Hydrochloric acid (HCI)
- Intrinsic factor, needed for the absorption of vitamin B_{12}

The Intestines

When food leaves the stomach, it is in a semiliquid form called **chyme**. Chyme enters the small intestine, where any undigested nutrients are broken down by intestinal and pancreatic enzymes and bile from the liver.

Materials continue to be moved through the intestines by waves of **peristalsis**. Food digestion is completed in the small intestine. Most of the nutrients and food the body needs are absorbed into the bloodstream through the walls of the small intestine.

The small intestine is about 20 feet long. It coils within the peritoneum. There are three main portions:

1. The duodenum—about 12 inches long. Has an opening in the back to receive the bile and pancreatic secretions.
2. The jejunum—about 8 feet long.
3. The ileum—the last 12 to 13 feet. Terminates in the ileocecal valve and is connected to the large intestine. The ileocecal valve prevents food from traveling backward into the small intestine.

The large intestine (colon) is 4½ feet long. It is divided into several sections:

- Cecum
- Ascending colon
- Transverse colon
- Descending colon
- Sigmoid colon
- Rectum
- Anus

No digestive enzymes are secreted in the colon. The colon is the place where:

- Some vitamins are absorbed into the circulatory system.
- More complex carbohydrates are acted upon by bacteria.
- Much of the remaining water is absorbed through the walls of the large intestine, changing wastes to a more solid form. In this way, the large intestine helps to maintain the water balance of the body.

Peristalsis continues to move waste through the large intestine until it reaches the rectum. When a certain amount has been collected in the rectum, it is eliminated as feces through the anus. This process is called **defecation**.

The Appendix

The appendix is located in the lower right quadrant, attached to the cecum. Its function is not known. When it becomes inflamed, the condition is called *appendicitis*.

Liver and Gallbladder

The liver is a large gland that has four lobes. It is located just beneath the right diaphragm. It carries on numerous metabolic functions. For example, the liver helps control the amount of protein and sugar in the blood by changing and storing excess amounts. It produces blood proteins such as prothrombin and fibrinogen, which are important factors in the blood clotting process. The liver also produces bile, which is carried directly to the small intestine for use in digestion or to the gallbladder for storage. Bile prepares (emulsifies) fats for digestion.

The gallbladder is a small hollow sac that is attached to the underside of the liver. It holds about two ounces of bile that it receives from the liver. It releases bile into the small intestine to help digest a fatty meal. The presence of bile in the digestive tract gives solid wastes their usual brown color.

The Pancreas

The pancreas is a glandular organ that produces both exocrine secretions (digestive enzymes) and endocrine secretions (insulin and glucagon). It extends from behind the stomach into the curve of the duodenum. It manufactures pancreatic juice. The pancreatic juice is sent into the duodenum to aid in the digestion of foods. The pancreas also produces insulin and glucagon. Both insulin and glucagon are sent directly into the bloodstream.

COMMON CONDITIONS

The tubelike mucus membrane structure of the alimentary canal lends itself to the possibility of malignancies, ulcerations, obstructions, and herniations.

Malignancy

Malignancies (cancers) of the gastrointestinal tract are very common. The symptoms they cause depend on their location. Among the symptoms are:

- Obstruction. Blocking of the passageway is sometimes the first major indication of a long-growing tumor.
- Indigestion.
- Vomiting.
- Constipation.
- Changes in the shape of the stool (bowel movement).
- Flatus (gas).
- Blood in the stool.

Treatment. Malignancies of the intestinal tract are usually treated surgically by removing the affected part. For example:

- Esophagectomy—removal of the esophagus
- Subtotal gastrectomy—removal of part of the stomach
- Colectomy (bowel resection)—removal of a part of the colon (large intestine).
- Colostomy—creation of an artificial opening in the abdominal wall and bringing a section of the colon to it for the elimination of feces
- Ileostomy—creation of an artificial opening in the abdominal wall and bringing a section of ileum through it for the elimination of waste

Ulcerations

An ulcer (sore or tissue breakdown) can occur anywhere along the digestive tract. Common places are the:

- Colon—ulcerative colitis. In colitis, malnutrition and dehydration are brought about by loss of fluids in frequent, watery, foul-smelling stools with mucus and pus.
- Stomach—gastric ulcer.
- Duodenum—duodenal ulcer.

Treatment. Treatment of ulcerative colitis includes:

- Medication to slow peristalsis (the wave-like contractions of the intestines) and reduce patient anxiety.
- Modification of diet to include high protein, high calories, and low residue. The low-residue diet is one in which the foods are almost completely digested. There is little waste with this type of diet.
- Medication (steroids) to reduce inflammation.
- Antibiotics to control infection by the microorganism *H. pylori*.

Patients with gastric or duodenal ulcers have periodic burning pain about 2 hours after eating. Most patients improve when they are placed on a diet in which foods that cause distress are not served. Medications are given to neutralize the hydrochloric acid (HCl), to coat the stomach, and to decrease anxiety. It is sometimes necessary to remove part of the stomach (gastrectomy or gastric resection) or

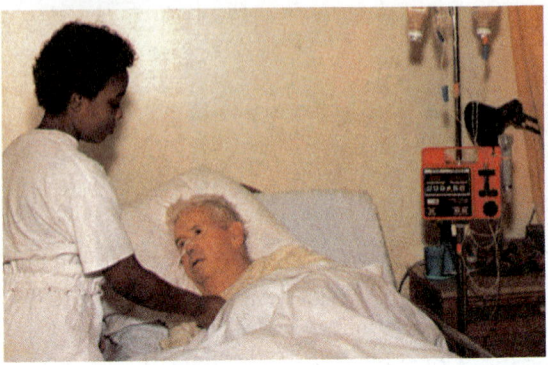

A.

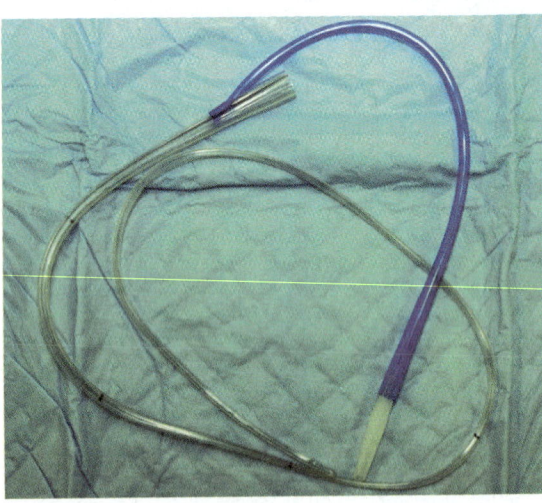

B.

FIGURE 43-3 A. Materials for feeding tube insertion. B. Double-lumen nasogastric tube.

duodenum (duodenal resection). Following such surgery, the patient is:

- Placed on NPO. Special mouth care is therefore needed.
- Placed on gastrointestinal drainage. A nasogastric tube (NG tube) (Figure 43-3A and B) is inserted through the patient's nose and into the stomach. The tube is attached to a drainage bottle. Additional tubes are inserted into the intestinal tract. Be careful not to disturb the tubes. Check frequently to ensure that the drainage is not blocked. If drainage becomes blocked, report it to your supervisor at once. The type and amount of drainage are noted and recorded.

Hernias

A hernia results when a structure such as the intestine pushes through a weakened area in a normally restraining wall. The danger of such abnormal protrusions is that some of the protruding tissue can become trapped in the weakened area. Circulation then becomes limited so that the tissue is in danger of dying. This is called an incarcerated (strangulated) hernia.

Frequent sites of herniation are:

- Groin area (inguinal hernia)

- Near the umbilicus (umbilical hernia)
- Through a poorly healed incision (incisional hernia)
- Through the diaphragm (hiatal hernia)

Hernias are usually repaired surgically with a **herniorrhaphy**.

Gallbladder Conditions

Two common conditions affecting the gallbladder are:

- **Cholecystitis**—an inflammation of the gallbladder.
- **Cholelithiasis**—the formation of stones in the gallbladder. The stones may obstruct the flow of **bile** (fluid that aids digestion), giving rise to signs and symptoms such as:
  - Indigestion
  - Pain
  - Jaundice (yellow discoloration of the skin and whites of the eyes)

Treatment. Cholecystitis and cholelithiasis may be treated by:

- Low-fat diet.
- Surgery to remove the gallbladder and stones. This surgical procedure is called a **cholecystectomy**.
- Laser therapy to break up the stones.

Drains are often placed in the operative areas. Initially, large amounts of yellowish-green drainage may be expected.

In addition to routine postoperative care:

- Position the patient in a semi-Fowler's position.
- Do not disturb drains.
- If you notice fresh blood on the dressing, increased jaundice, or dark urine, report it immediately to your team leader.

COMMON PROBLEMS RELATED TO THE LOWER BOWEL

The frequency of bowel elimination varies with the individual. Some people have more than one bowel movement (BM) a day, but others have a BM every two or three days. **Fecal material** (solid body waste, bowel movement, BM) is normally brown, but the color can be affected by certain foods, medications, and diseases. The bowel movement is normally soft and formed. If it passes through the colon too quickly, it is loose and watery. Multiple watery stools is called **diarrhea**. If stool passes through the colon too slowly, the fecal material becomes hard, dry, or sticky and pasty in consistency. This is referred to as **constipation**. Certain foods, medications, infections, and diseases can cause constipation and diarrhea. As foods move through the gastrointestinal tract by peristalsis, gas is formed. When the gas is expelled from the body, it is called "passing flatus" or flatulence. If the gas is not passed, it accumulates in the intestine. The abdomen will enlarge and appear bloated. This is called **abdominal distention**, and is an important

observation to report to the nurse. Abdominal distention may also be caused by constipation and urinary retention.

Changes in Function of the Gastrointestinal System Associated with Aging and Disease

Change in bowel function may be caused by aging, disease, surgery, diet, and medications. Lack of privacy may also affect the patient's ability to have a bowel movement. As a person ages, movement in the colon is decreased. Food absorption is slowed and fewer digestive juices are produced. Constipation is a common problem. Other factors that affect bowel function are:

- Bedrest
- Inactivity
- Inadequate exercise
- Inability to chew foods properly
- Loose or missing teeth
- Inadequate fluid intake
- Stress
- Change in environment
- Change in diet
- A diet that does not contain enough fiber, fruits, or vegetables

Observations to Make when Assisting Patients with Bowel Elimination

You must observe the amount/quantity, color, odor, character, and consistency of the patient's bowel movement before discarding it. Notify the nurse if the fecal material has an unusual color or odor, if there is an unusual amount, or if there is blood, mucus, parasites, or food particles (except corn and raisins) in the stool. If you think a stool is abnormal, save it for the nurse to assess.

Constipation and Fecal Impaction

Report problems with constipation to the nurse. The patient is probably constipated if he has not had a bowel movement in more than three days, strains, or passes hard, marble-like stools. **Fecal impaction** (Figure 43-4) is the most serious form of constipation. It is caused by retention of stool in the rectum, where water is absorbed. Over time, the stool becomes hard and dry. The patient may be unable to pass it. The dried waste irritates the bowel. Mucus dissolves the hard, outer part of the mass. The rectum becomes so full that the fluid escapes around the impaction and is eliminated from the rectum as diarrhea. The patient may complain of:

- abdominal or rectal pain
- nausea
- loss of appetite
- feeling the need to have a bowel movement, but cannot

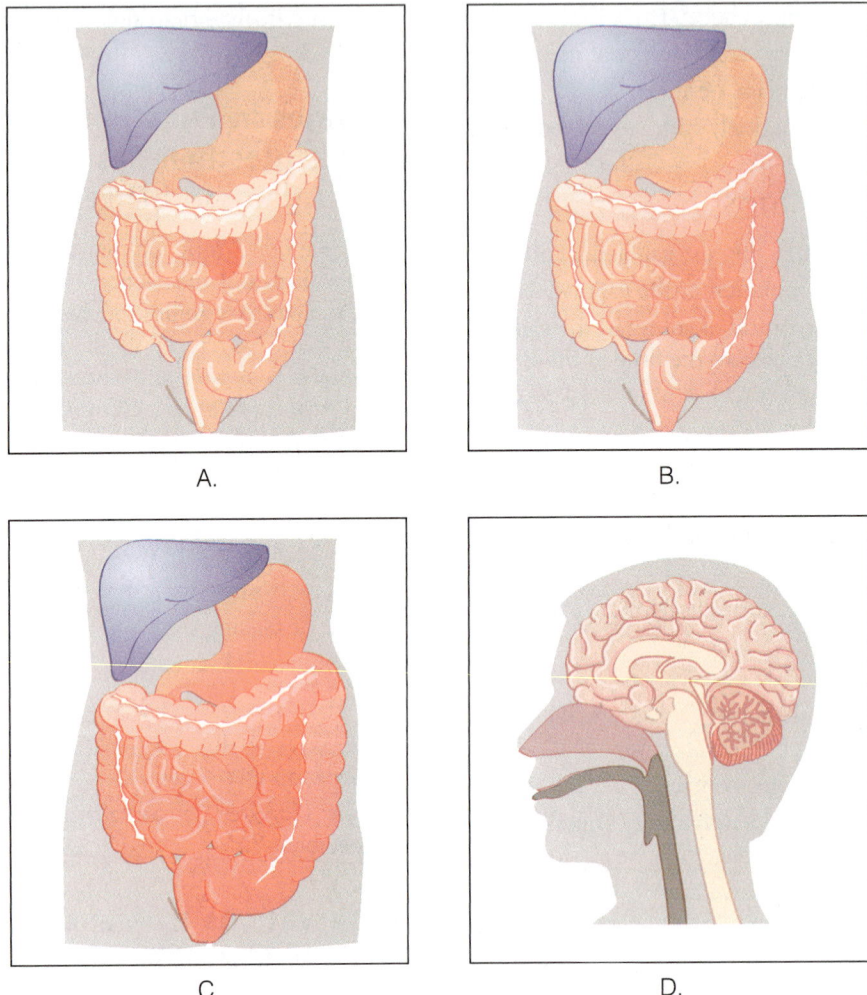

A.

B.

C.

D.

FIGURE 43-4 Progression of a fecal impaction, a life-threatening condition. A. A fecal impaction blocks the rectum. The rectum and sigmoid colon become enlarged. B. The colon continues to enlarge. C. Fecal material fills the colon. Digested and undigested food back up into the small intestines and stomach. The patient has signs and symptoms of acute illness, including lethargy, distention, constipation, and pain that is dull and cramping. D. The entire system is full, and the patient vomits fecal material. The feces are commonly aspirated into the lungs.

Other signs and symptoms of impaction are:

- passing excessive flatus
- bloating and abdominal distention
- frequent urination
- inability to empty the bladder
- leaking around the catheter
- mental confusion
- fever
- liquid stool or mucus seeping from the rectum

Fecal impaction is a very serious condition that is usually treated by manual removal of the mass by the nurse or advanced care provider. Laxatives and enemas are also used to treat fecal impaction. The best thing to do is observe the patient's bowel elimination carefully and prevent fecal impaction from developing.

Diarrhea

Diarrhea occurs when peristalsis in the intestines is very rapid. The need to defecate is usually very urgent if the patient has diarrhea. Some patients may become incontinent because of the force with which the fecal material moves through the intestines. The patient may also complain of abdominal pain and cramping.

Diarrhea can cause dehydration and other serious medical problems if undetected or untreated. Most health care facilities have a definition of diarrhea, such as three or more loose stools within a defined period of time. One loose stool is not diarrhea. Remember to be objective in reporting your observations. When reporting loose stools to the the nurse, report the color, odor, consistency, character, amount, and frequency of stools. Also report any patient complaints of pain or other discomfort.

Bowel Incontinence

Bowel incontinence is involuntary passage of fecal material from the anus. It has many causes, including trauma, neurological diseases, inability to reach the toilet on time, and mental confusion. It is not as common as urinary incontinence. Fecal material is very irritating to the skin, so the patient must be cleansed well after each episode of incontinence. Skin exposed to fecal material will break down quickly. Bowel incontinence may lower the patient's self-esteem. Be professional, compassionate, and understanding when assisting patients with bowel elimination and incontinence.

Patients with bowel incontinence may be placed on a bowel retraining or incontinence management program. If this is ineffective, a fecal incontinence collector (Figure 43-5) may be used.

Role of the Nursing Assistant in Assisting Patients with Bowel Elimination

Assisting with bowel elimination is a very important responsibility. Always apply the principles of standard precautions when assisting with elimination. Avoid contaminating environmental surfaces with your gloves. Wear a gown, eye protection, and face mask if splashing is likely.

COMMUNICATION *Highlight*

Remember that bowel activity is a normal body function. Do not show disgust in your facial expressions or body language when assisting patients with elimination. Documenting bowel activity is a very important responsibility. Unrelieved constipation is a serious, uncomfortable condition. The nurse depends on the accuracy of your documentation in the elimination record. The nurse will use this record to contact the physician, and administer medications and other treatments related to bowel elimination.

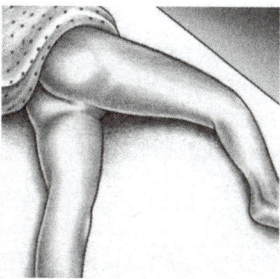
1. Position patient on side.

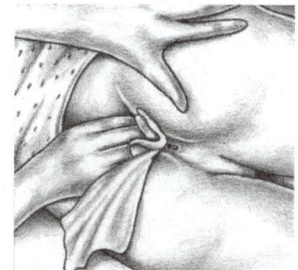
2. Clean and dry skin.

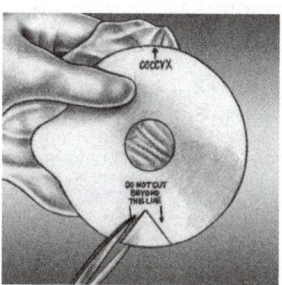
3. Trim barrier, if needed.

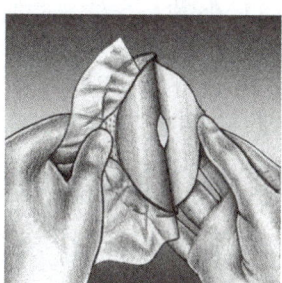
4. Remove release paper.

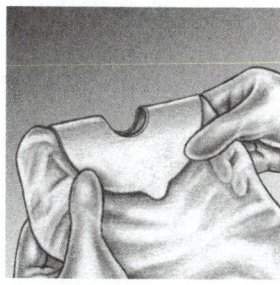
5. Fold barrier.

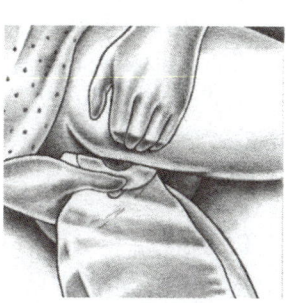
6. Separate buttocks.

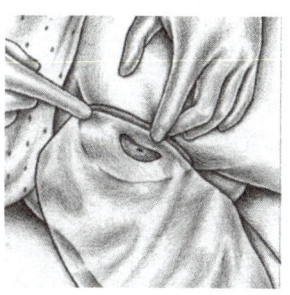
7. Position collector.

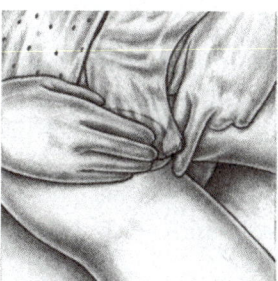
8. Press and seal barrier.

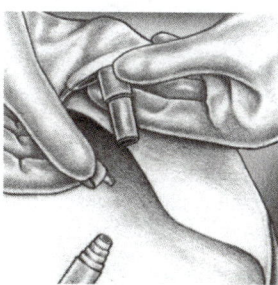
9. Connect to bedside collector.

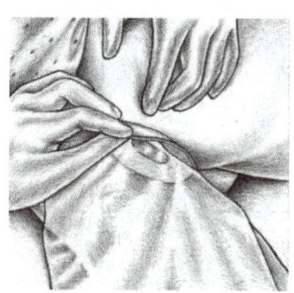
10. Remove.

FIGURE 43-5 Fecal incontinence collection system. *(Permission to reproduce this copyrighted material has been given by the owner, Hollister, Inc., Libertyville, Illinois)*

guidelines *for*

Assisting Patients with Bowel Elimination

- Apply the principles of standard precautions when assisting with bowel elimination. Avoid environmental contamination from your gloves.
- Encourage patients to consume an adequate amount of fluid. Maintaining fluid intake is as important for bowel elimination as it is for urinary elimination.
- Encourage patients to eat a well-balanced diet.
- Allow adequate time for patients to eat meals.
- Encourage patients to chew food well. Cut it into small pieces if necessary. Report chewing problems to the nurse for further assessment.
- If you observe that a patient has not eaten fiber foods, fruits, or vegetables, offer a substitute. The dietitian may visit the patient to discuss likes and dislikes and assure that the patient will eat the foods served.
- Encourage exercise and activity, as allowed and as tolerated.
- Assist patients with toileting at regular intervals and provide privacy.
- Position patients in a sitting position, if allowed, for bowel elimination.
- Use a bath blanket to cover a patient who is using the bedpan or commode, for privacy and warmth.

- Leave the call signal and toilet tissue within reach and respond to the call signal immediately.
- Allow adequate time for defecation.
- Provide perineal care as needed, or according to facility policy. Feces are very irritating to the skin and prolonged contact promotes skin breakdown and infection.
- Assist patients with cleaning the anal area (this may be called the rectal area by some health care providers).
- Assist patients with handwashing and other personal hygiene after bowel elimination.
- Monitor bowel elimination and report irregularities.
- Record bowel movements on the flow sheet or other designated location. If a patient is independent with bowel elimination, ask if she has had a bowel movement each day.
- Report to the nurse: frequent stools, absence of stools, pain, cramping, excessive flatulence, abnormal color or consistency of stool, extremely small amounts of stool, hard, dry stool, or enlargement of the abdomen.
- Specific abnormalities in stools to report are presence of blood, pus, mucus, black or other unusual color, undigested food (except corn and raisins), or presence of parasites.

Stool Specimens

A specimen of stool is a sample of fecal material (solid body waste or bowel movement) collected in a special container. (See Procedure 110.) The specimen is then sent to the laboratory for examination. In the laboratory, stool may be examined for:

- Pathogenic microorganisms (germs)
- Parasites
- **Occult blood** (hidden blood or blood that cannot be seen by the naked eye)
- Chemical analysis

The following advanced procedures are included in Unit 50:

- Testing for Occult Blood Using Hemoccult® and Developer
- Testing for Occult Blood Using Hematest® Reagent Tablets

PROCEDURE 110

COLLECTING A STOOL SPECIMEN

1. Carry out beginning procedure actions.
2. Assemble equipment:

- disposable gloves
- bedpan and cover or collection container

continues

PROCEDURE 110

continued

- specimen container and cover
- biohazard specimen transport bag
- label, including:
  - patient's full name
  - room number
  - date and time of collection
  - physician's name
  - examination to be performed
  - other information required
- toilet tissue
- tongue depressors
- basin

3. Wash your hands and put on disposable gloves.

4. Uncover the container that was used to collect the bowel movement (bedpan or commode receptacle). (If a toilet insert is used, the specimen will be collected from the insert.) If the patient is incontinent of feces, use tongue depressors to obtain a specimen from bed linens, diaper, or protective padding. A specimen may also be obtained from a fecal incontinence collection bag when the bag is changed.

5. Following defecation, the patient washes his hands. Fill a basin with water at 105°F. Assist the patient if needed. If the patient is incontinent, carefully clean and dry the area around the anus. Change bed linens as needed.

6. Take the container with the bowel movement to the bathroom. Use tongue blades to remove a specimen and place it in a specimen container (Figure 43-6). Do not contaminate the outside of the specimen container or the cover. If possible, take a sample (about 1 teaspoon) from each part of the specimen.

7. Empty the collection container into the toilet. Clean or dispose of the collection container according to facility policy. If the patient was incontinent, dispose of the soiled brief or padding as biohazardous waste. Place soiled linen in the proper hamper.

8. Remove and dispose of your gloves according to facility policy.

9. Wash your hands.

10. Cover the container and attach the completed label. Make sure the cover is on the container tightly. Place the container in a biohazard transport bag.

11. Take or send the specimen to the laboratory promptly. (Stool specimens are never refrigerated.)

12. Carry out procedure completion actions.

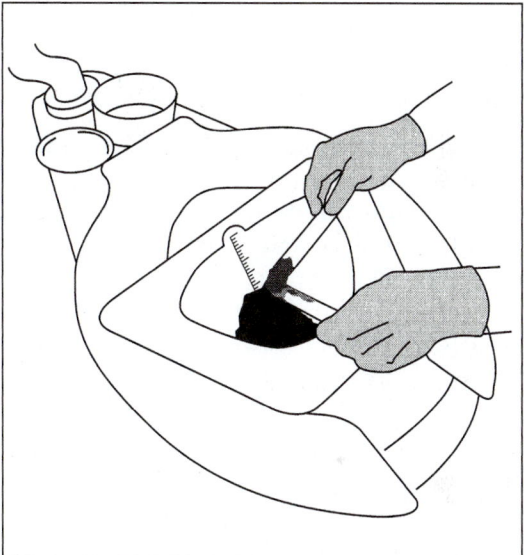

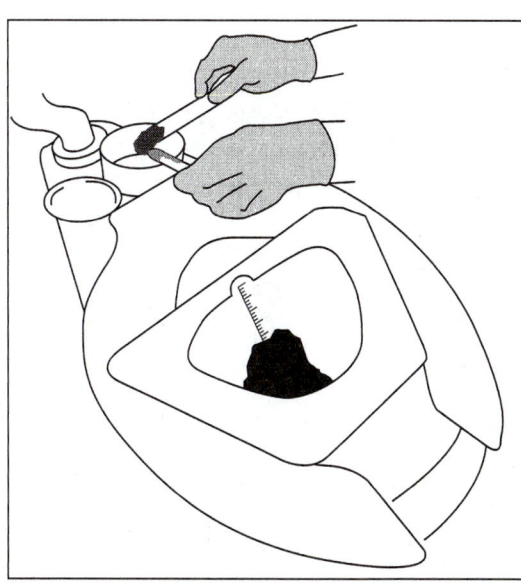

FIGURE 43-6 Use tongue blades to transfer the specimen from the collection device to the specimen cup.

SPECIAL DIAGNOSTIC TESTS

Some techniques used to diagnose problems of the gastrointestinal system include:

- Gastrointestinal (GI) series—a liquid called barium is either swallowed (upper GI series) or given as an enema (lower GI series). X-rays are then taken.
- Direct visualization procedures:
  - **Proctoscopy**—visualization of the rectum
  - **Sigmoidoscopy**—visualization of the sigmoid colon
  - **Gastroscopy**—visualization of the stomach

In preparation for the tests, the entire GI tract must be emptied before the x-rays.

- No food is permitted for 8 hours or longer.
- Enemas are given before the series until only the clear liquid returns.
- Laxatives are given the night before the test.

Cholecystogram (Gallbladder Series)

A gallbladder (GB) series is an x-ray examination similar to the GI series except that the dye tablets are swallowed. Orders for preparing patients for this test vary. Cleansing enemas are frequently ordered. A special diet may also be required beforehand.

Ultrasonography

Ultrasound is very high frequency sound that cannot be heard. When concentrated in a beam and directed at body organs and tissues, the ultrasound moves at different speeds through the tissues, because of the varying tissue density. This permits a picture to be made of the tissues being examined. Ultrasonography is the use of sound to produce an image of an organ or tissue.

ENEMAS

A cleansing **enema** is the technique of introducing fluid into the rectum to remove feces and flatus (gas) from the colon and rectum. (Refer to Procedures 111 and 112.) Enemas are given:

- to aid illumination during x-rays.
- before surgery.
- before testing.
- during bowel retraining programs.
- to relieve constipation and impaction.
- to instill drugs.

The fluids often used for enemas are:

- Soap solution (SSE)
- Salt solution (saline)
- Tap water (TWE)
- Phosphosoda

These solutions create a feeling of urgency in the patient's bowel. **Urgency** is the term used to describe the need to empty the bowel. Solutions are expelled a short time after they are given. When enemas are given in preparation for diagnostic x-rays or to instill drugs, the fluid is retained as long as possible.

General Considerations

Some general considerations to keep in mind are:

- Apply the principles of standard precautions. Avoid environmental contamination from your gloves.
- Administer an enema only upon the direction of a licensed nurse.
- If the patient is to get up following the enema and use the bathroom, make sure the bathroom is available and not in use before giving the enema.
- When possible, the enema should be given before the patient's bath or before breakfast.
- Do not give an enema within an hour following a meal.
- Consult the care plan or the nurse for the amount and type of solution to use, and any special instructions.

Tips: Avoid giving an enema within an hour after meals, because the increased peristalsis makes it difficult for the patient to retain the solution. Avoid administering an enema to a patient in a sitting position, such as on the toilet. The solution will not flow high into the colon when administered to a patient who is seated. It will cause the rectum to enlarge, causing rapid expulsion of the fluid.

Position

The best position for the patient to receive an enema is in the left Sims' position. Fluid flows into the bowel more easily when the patient is in this position. The left Sims' position and several alternative positions are shown in Figure 43-7.

At times, the enema may have to be administered with the patient on the bedpan in the supine position. The supine position can be used if the patient is unable to hold the fluid or to assume Sims' position.

- The patient's knees are flexed and separated.
- An orthopedic (fracture) bedpan is more comfortable than a regular bedpan. It may have to be padded when the patient is very thin.

Disposable Enema Units

Disposable enema units are available to give:

- Soap-solution enema
- Commercially prepared enema
- Phosphosoda enema
- Oil-retention enema

Administration of disposable enemas is simple. Time is saved in preparing and cleaning the equipment. The techniques for using reusable equipment for oil-retention or soap-solution enemas are the same. The procedures when using a prepackaged prepared solution follow.

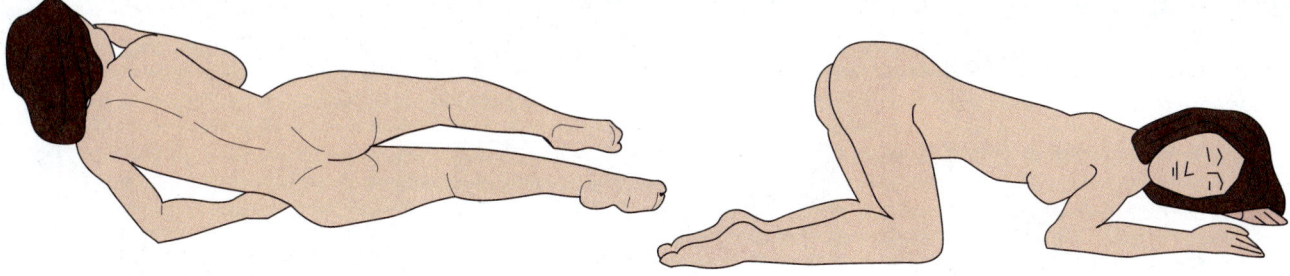

Sims' (left-lateral) Position

Knee-Chest Position

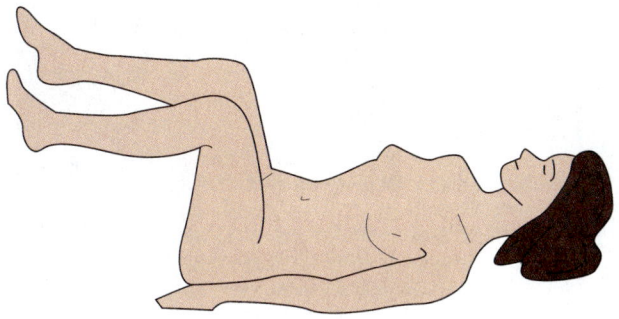

Position for Self-Administration

Child's Position

FIGURE 43-7 Alternative positions for enema administration.

PROCEDURE 111

GIVING A SOAP-SOLUTION ENEMA

 Note: *Be sure this is a nursing assistant procedure in your facility.*

1. Carry out beginning procedure actions.

2. Assemble equipment:
   - disposable gloves
   - disposable enema equipment, consisting of a plastic container, tubing with rectal tube, clamp, and lubricant (equipment is commercially available as a kit)
   - bedpan and cover
   - bed protector
   - toilet tissue
   - bath blanket
   - castile soap packet
   - towel, soap, basin

3. In the utility room:

a. Connect the tubing to the solution container (Figure 43-8A).

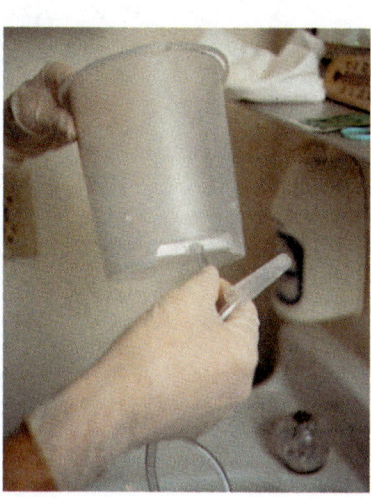

FIGURE 43-8A Attach the tubing to the container.

continues

PROCEDURE 111

continued

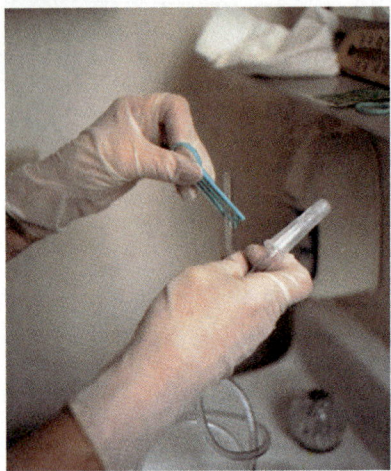

FIGURE 43-8B Slip the clamp over the tubing.

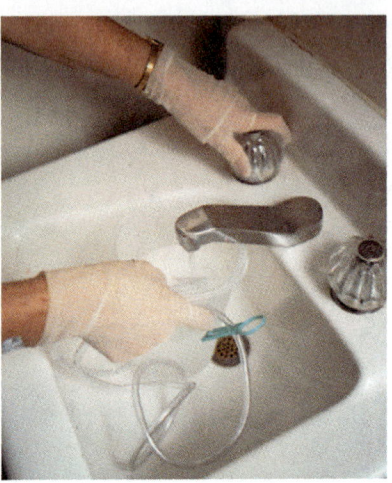

FIGURE 43-8C Fill the container with warm water.

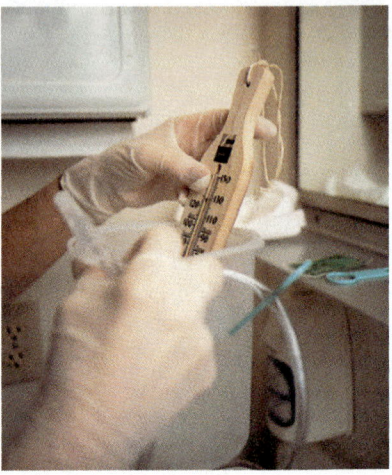

FIGURE 43-8D Use a bath thermometer to make sure the temperature is about 105°F.

b. Adjust the clamp on the tubing and snap it shut (Figure 43-8B).

c. Fill the container with warm water (105°F) to the 1,000-mL line (500 mL for children) (Figures 43-8C and D).

d. Open the packet of liquid soap and put the soap in the water (Figure 43-8E).

e. Using the tip of the tubing, mix the solution (mix gently so that no suds form) or rotate the bag to mix. Do not shake.

f. Run a small amount of solution through the tube to eliminate air and warm the tube (Figure 43-8F). Clamp the tubing (Figure 43-8G).

4. Place a chair at the foot of the bed and cover it with a bed protector. Place the bedpan on it.

5. Elevate the bed to a comfortable working height. Be sure the opposite side rail is up and secure for safety.

6. Cover the patient with a bath blanket and fanfold linen to the foot of the bed.

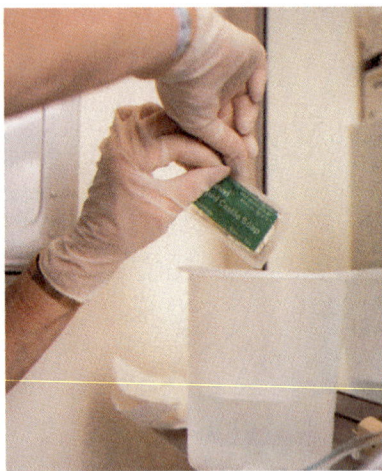

FIGURE 43-8E Add soap from the packet.

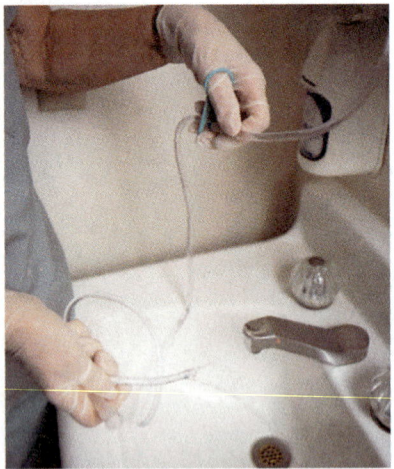

FIGURE 43-8F Run a small amount of water through the tubing to expel air.

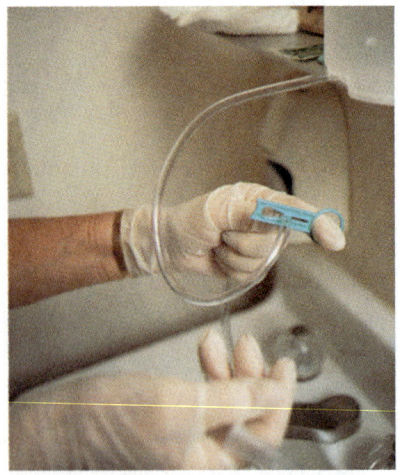

FIGURE 43-8G Clamp the tubing.

continues

PROCEDURE 111

continued

7. Wash your hands and put on gloves.

8. Place a bed protector under the patient's buttocks.

9. Help the patient turn to his left side and flex the knees.

10. Place the container of solution on the chair so the tubing will reach the patient.

11. Adjust the bath blanket to expose the anal area.

12. Expose the anus by raising the upper buttock.

13. Lubricate the tip of the tube. The patient should breathe deeply and bear down as the tube is inserted, to relax the anal sphincter. Insert the tube 2 to 4 inches into the anus.

14. Never force the tube. If the tube cannot be inserted easily, get help. There may be a tumor or a mass of feces blocking the bowel. The mass of feces is known as an *impaction*.

15. Open the clamp and raise the container 12 inches above the level of the anus so that the fluid flows in slowly (Figure 43-8H).

    • Ask the patient to take deep breaths to relax the abdomen.

    • If the patient complains of cramping, clamp the tube and wait until the cramping stops. Then open the tubing to continue the fluid flow.

16. Clamp the tubing before the container is completely empty.

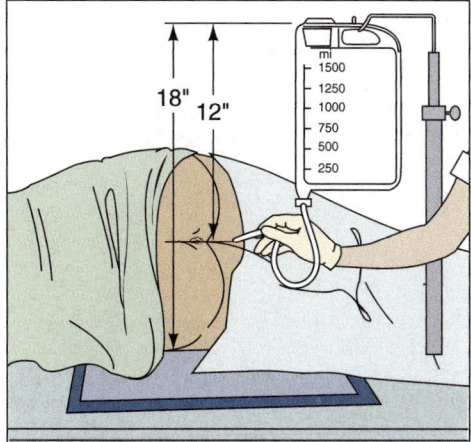

FIGURE 43-8H Raise the container above the anus so the flow of fluid is unobstructed.

17. Tell the patient to hold his breath while the upper buttock is raised and the tube is gently withdrawn.

18. Wrap the tubing in a paper towel. Put it in the disposable container.

19. Place the patient on a bedpan or assist him to the bathroom.

20. Using a paper towel, so your glove does not contaminate the control or crank, raise the head of the bed to a comfortable height if the patient is on the bedpan. Raise the side rail for safety if the bed is left in the higher horizontal position.

21. Place toilet tissue and the signal cord within reach of the patient. If the patient is in the bathroom, stay nearby. Caution the patient not to flush the toilet.

22. Discard disposable materials as biohazardous waste, according to facility policy.

23. Remove your gloves and discard according to facility policy. Wash your hands.

24. Return to the bedside. Put on fresh gloves.

25. Remove the bedpan. Place it on a bed protector on the chair and cover it.

26. Cleanse the anal area.

27. Remove the bed protector and discard according to facility policy.

28. Remove gloves and wash your hands.

29. Give the patient soap, water, and towel to wash and dry his hands.

30. Replace the top bedding and remove the bath blanket.

31. Put on gloves. Take the bedpan to the bathroom. Dispose of contents according to facility policy or, using a paper towel, flush the toilet.

32. Remove gloves and dispose of according to facility policy.

33. Wash your hands.

34. Air the room and leave the room in order.

35. Unscreen the unit.

36. Clean and replace all other equipment used according to facility policy.

37. Carry out procedure completion actions.

Giving an Enema with a Commercially Prepared Chemical Enema Solution

Commercially prepared enemas are convenient to administer and more comfortable for the patient. The enema may be either an oil-retention enema or a phosphosoda enema and is following by a cleansing (soap-solution) enema.

- The solution is already measured and ready to use.
- A small amount of fluid will remain in the container after administration.
- The solution in a phosphosoda enema draws fluid from the body to stimulate peristalsis.

- The oil-retention enema solution softens the feces, making them easier to expel.
- The amount of solution administered is about 4 ounces.
- The tip of the container is pre-lubricated.
- The enema solution is in an easy-to-handle plastic container.
- The solution is sometimes used at room temperature.
- You may be asked to warm the solution by placing the container in warm water before administration. Check with the nurse regarding your facility's policy.

PROCEDURE 112

GIVING A COMMERCIALLY PREPARED ENEMA

 Note: *Be sure this is a nursing assistant procedure in your facility.*

 Note: *This procedure may be followed when giving an oil-retention or a phosphosoda enema.*

1. Carry out beginning procedure actions.

2. Assemble equipment:
   - disposable gloves
   - disposable prepackaged enema
   - bedpan and cover
   - bed protector
   - pan of warm water (if enema solution is to be warmed)

3. Open the package and remove the plastic container of enema solution. Place the solution container in warm water (if it is to be warmed).

4. Lower the head of the bed to a horizontal position and elevate the bed to a comfortable working height. Raise the side rail on the opposite side of the bed for safety.

5. Put on gloves.

6. Place a bedpan and cover on the chair close at hand.

7. Assist the patient to turn to the left side and flex the right leg.

8. Place a bed protector under the patient.

9. Expose only the patient's buttocks by drawing the bedding upward in one hand.

10. Remove the cover from the enema tip (Figure 43-9). Gently squeeze to make sure the tip is undamaged (patent).

11. Separate the buttocks, exposing the anus, and ask the patient to breathe deeply and bear down slightly.

12. Insert the lubricated enema tip 2 inches into the rectum.

13. Gently squeeze and roll the container until the desired quantity of solution is administered (Figure 43-10). A small amount of solution will remain in the container. Avoid releasing pressure on the container, or the solution will return.

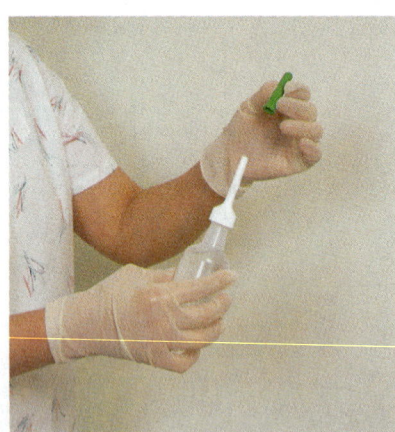

FIGURE 43-9 Remove the cover from the pre-lubricated tip of the container.

continues

PROCEDURE 112

continued

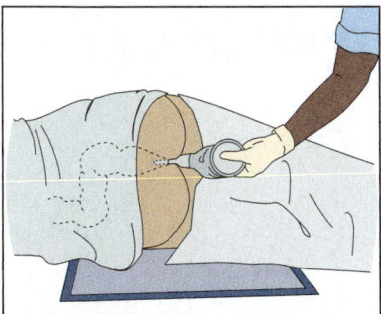

FIGURE 43-10 Squeeze the bottle from the bottom. A small amount of fluid will remain in the container.

14. Remove the tip from the patient and place the container in the box. Encourage the patient to hold the solution as long as possible.

15. Remove gloves and dispose of properly. Wash your hands.

16. Discard the used enema as biohazard waste.

17. Provide privacy. This enema should be retained for 20 minutes. Give the patient the call signal and leave.

18. When the patient feels the urge to defecate, lower the bed and assist the patient to the bathroom or commode, or position the patient on the bedpan.

19. Raise the head of the bed to a comfortable height if the patient is using a bedpan.

20. Place toilet tissue and the signal cord within reach of the patient. Raise the side rail for safety if the bed is left in high position. If the patient is in the bathroom, stay nearby. Caution the patient not to flush the toilet.

21. Return to the patient when signaled. Wash your hands. Lower the nearest side rail, if it is up. Put on gloves.

22. Remove the bedpan and place it on the bed protector covering the chair. Observe the contents of the bedpan. Cover the bedpan.

23. Clean the anal area of the patient, if required.

24. If the patient has used a commode or toilet:
    a. Clean the anal area, if required.
    b. Observe the contents of the commode or toilet.
    c. Flush the toilet using a paper towel, or cover the commode.
    d. Remove gloves and discard according to facility policy. Assist the patient into bed.

25. Put on gloves. Take the bedpan or commode container and equipment to the bathroom. Dispose of contents according to facility policy.

26. Remove and dispose of gloves properly. Wash your hands.

27. Give the patient soap, water, and a towel to wash her hands. Return equipment. Leave the side rails down unless needed for safety and leave the bed in low position.

28. Carry out procedure completion actions.

Rectal Suppositories

Rectal **suppositories** are used to stimulate bowel evacuation or to administer medication. Medicinal suppositories must be inserted by the nurse. You may be asked to insert the type of suppository that softens stool and promotes elimination. (See Procedure 113.) Check your facility policy to be sure this is a nursing assistant function. The suppository must be placed beyond the rectal sphincter (circular muscle that controls the anal opening) and against the bowel wall so it can melt and lubricate the rectum.

Rectal Tube and Flatus Bag

The rectal tube is used to reduce flatus (gas) in the bowel. Placing a rectal tube into the rectum provides a passageway for the gas to escape. Flatus distends the intestines, causing pain and stress on incisions.

You can assist the patient as follows:
- Encourage activity.
- Promote regularity.
- Accept the expulsion of gas as a natural body function. Do not contribute to the patient's embarrassment.
- Use flatus-reducing procedures when ordered.
- Insert a rectal tube with flatus bag if ordered. (Remember that your facility policies must state that nursing assistants can perform this procedure.) (See Procedure 114.)

The disposable tube is used once in a 24-hour period for no more than 20 minutes.
- Relief may occur as soon as the tube is inserted.
- Check the amount of abdominal distention (stretching).
- Question the patient about the amount of relief.

PROCEDURE 113

INSERTING A RECTAL SUPPOSITORY

 Note: *Be sure this is a nursing assistant procedure in your facility.*

1. Carry out beginning procedure actions.

2. Assemble equipment:
   - disposable gloves
   - suppository as ordered
   - toilet tissue
   - bedpan and cover, if needed
   - lubricant
   - bed protector

3. Wash your hands and put on gloves.

4. Help the patient turn on the left side and flex the right leg. Place a bed protector under the patient's hips.

5. Adjust bed linen to expose the buttocks only.

6. Unwrap the suppository.

7. With your left hand, separate the patient's buttocks, exposing the anus.

8. Apply a small amount of lubricant to the anus and to the suppository and insert the suppository. The suppository must be inserted deeply enough to enter the rectum beyond the sphincter (approximately 2 inches) (Figure 43-11).

9. Encourage the patient to take deep breaths and relax (until the need to defecate is felt in 5 to 20 minutes).

10. Remove gloves and dispose of properly. Wash your hands.

11. Adjust the bedding and help the patient to assume a comfortable position.

12. Place the signal cord near the patient's hand, but check every 5 minutes.

13. Wash your hands and put on gloves.

14. Assist the patient to the bathroom or commode, or position the patient on a bedpan.

15. Provide privacy. Once the patient is finished, assist with hygiene if necessary.

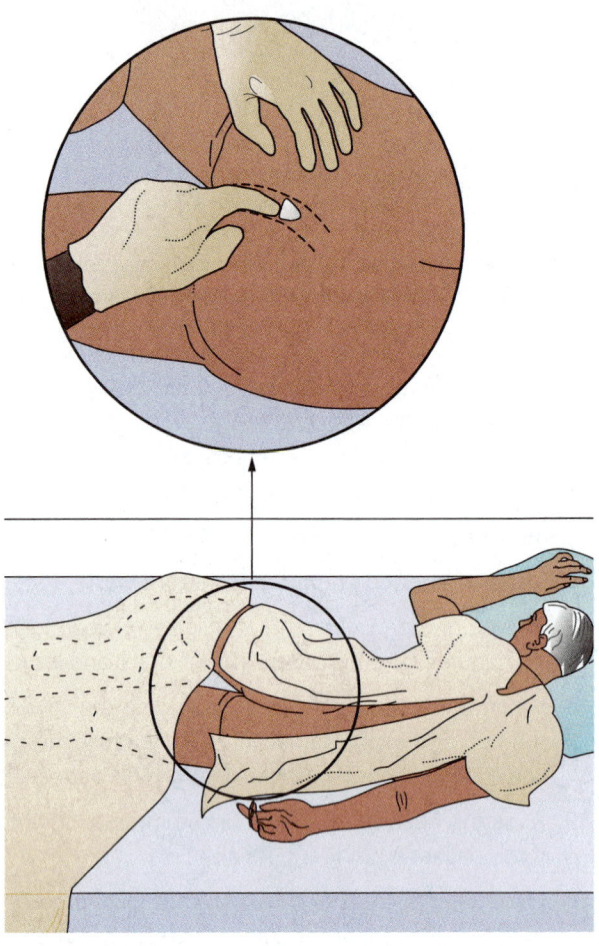

FIGURE 43-11 Lubricate the anus and insert the suppository beyond the sphincter muscle.

16. Observe results and note any unusual characteristics of the stool. If stool is unusual, save it and report to the nurse.

17. Dispose of stool and clean equipment according to facility policy. Store equipment as required.

18. Remove and dispose of gloves according to facility policy. Wash your hands.

19. Carry out procedure completion actions.

PROCEDURE 114

INSERTING A RECTAL TUBE AND FLATUS BAG

1. Carry out beginning procedure actions.

2. Assemble equipment:
   - disposable gloves
   - disposable rectal tube and flatus bag
   - bed protector
   - lubricant
   - tissue
   - tape
   - paper towel

3. Identify the patient and screen the unit. Explain what you plan to do.

4. Lower the head of the bed to horizontal position.

5. Wash your hands and put on gloves.

6. Assist the patient to turn to the left side and flex the right leg. Place a bed protector under the hips.

7. Adjust bed linen to expose only the patient's buttocks.

8. Lubricate the tip of the rectal tube.

9. Separate the buttocks, exposing the anus, and ask the patient to breathe deeply and bear down gently.

10. Insert the lubricated tip or rectal tube 2 to 4 inches.

11. Secure the rectal tube in place with a small piece of hypoallergenic adhesive (Figure 43-12).

12. Remove gloves and dispose of properly. Wash your hands.

13. Adjust the bedding and make the patient comfortable. Leave the unit neat and tidy. Place the signal cord within reach of the patient.

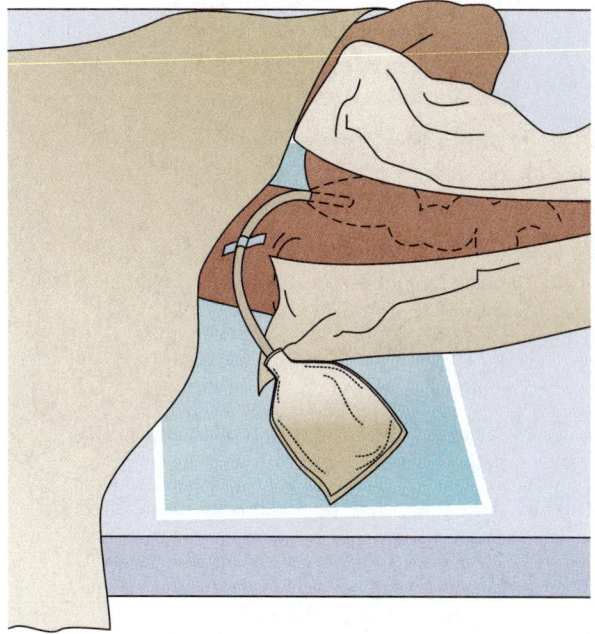

FIGURE 43-12 Secure the rectal tube, with flatus bag in place, using a small piece of hypoallergenic tape.

14. Return to the unit in 20 minutes. Wash your hands.

15. Put on gloves.

16. Gently remove the rectal tube and place it on a paper towel.

17. Clean the area around the anus as needed.

18. Dispose of the wrapped rectal tube and bag according to facility policy.

19. Remove and dispose of gloves according to facility policy. Wash your hands.

20. Carry out procedure completion actions.

REVIEW

A. True/False.

Mark the following true or false by circling T or F.

1. T F A herniorrhaphy is the surgery performed when there is bowel malignancy.

2. T F The drainage from a new cholecystectomy incision is normally yellowish-green.

3. T F The patient is placed on the left side, if possible, for the administration of an enema.

4. T F When administering an enema using a prepackaged chemical solution, approximately 4 ounces are given.

5. T F Be sure the bathroom is free before giving an enema.

6. T F A flatus tube is used to reduce abdominal distention from gas.

7. T F An enema may be given only upon direction from the nurse.

8. T F When giving a soap-solution enema, approximately 2,000 mL are used.

9. T F Gastric ulcers are located in the esophagus.

B. Matching.

Choose the correct word from Column II to match each word or phrase in Column I.

Column I	Column II
10. _____ gas	**a.** stool
11. _____ yellow discoloration of skin	**b.** flatus
	c. cholelithiasis
12. _____ large bowel	**d.** cyanosis
13. _____ feces	**e.** cholecystectomy
14. _____ gallstones	**f.** colon
	g. jaundice

C. Multiple Choice.

Select the one best answer for each of the following.

15. Signs of possible gastrointestinal malignancy might be
    a. good appetite.
    b. change in stool color.
    c. weight gain.
    d. pallor.

16. Your patient has just returned from surgery for gallstones. She will be most comfortable in the
    a. dorsal recumbent position.
    b. lithotomy position.
    c. semi-Fowler's position.
    d. left Sims' position.

17. Enemas are given
    a. after the patient showers.
    b. at bedtime.
    c. before diagnostic testing.
    d. after surgery.

18. The oil-retention enema is usually
    a. preceded by a soap-solution enema.
    b. retained one hour.
    c. followed by a soap-solution enema.
    d. given in the semi-Fowler's position.

19. Urgency is a term that means
    a. need to urinate.
    b. need to empty the bowel.
    c. pain from flatus.
    d. need to vomit.

D. Completion.

Complete the statements in the spaces provided.

20. The enema given to soften feces is known as _____ _____.

21. The purpose of a soap-solution enema is to _____ _____.

E. Nursing Assistant Challenge.

Mr. Rayburn has been admitted with a provisional diagnosis of gastric ulcers. He had been complaining of a burning sensation in his stomach halfway between meal times. He is scheduled for an upper GI series at 8 AM tomorrow morning. Answer the following questions regarding Mr. Rayburn and his care.

22. What acid is naturally found in Mr. Rayburn's stomach?

23. Before the GI series, will it be all right to serve Mr. Rayburn breakfast in the morning?

24. What procedure will you be asked to carry out before the test?

25. Will Mr. Rayburn swallow the barium, or will he be given a barium enema?

26. Will x-rays be taken?

EXPLORING THE WEB

Description	Location
American College of Gastroenterology	*http://www.acg.gi.org*
Combined Health Information Database	*http://chid.nih.gov/subfile/subfile.html*
Discovery Health	*http://health.discovery.com*
Dr. Greenson's Gastrointestinal and Liver Pathology	*http://www.pds.med.umich.edu*
Dr. Minocha's Page on Acid Reflux and Heartburn	*http://www.pds.med.umich.edu*
EnemaBag.com	*http://www.enemabag.com*
Johns Hopkins Gastroenterology and Hepatology Resource Center	*http://hopkins-gi.org*
Medline Plus Constipation	*http://www.nlm.nih.gov/medlineplus/constipation.html*
Medline Plus Fecal Impaction	*http://www.nlm.nih.gov/medlineplus/ency/article/000230.htm*
National Institute of Diabetes, Digestive, & Kidney Diseases	*http://www.niddk.nih.gov/index.htm*
Society of Gastroenterology Nurses and Associates	*http://www.sgna.org*
Wound, Ostomy, & Continence Nurses Society	*http://www.wocn.org*
Yahoo Health	*http://health.yahoo.com*

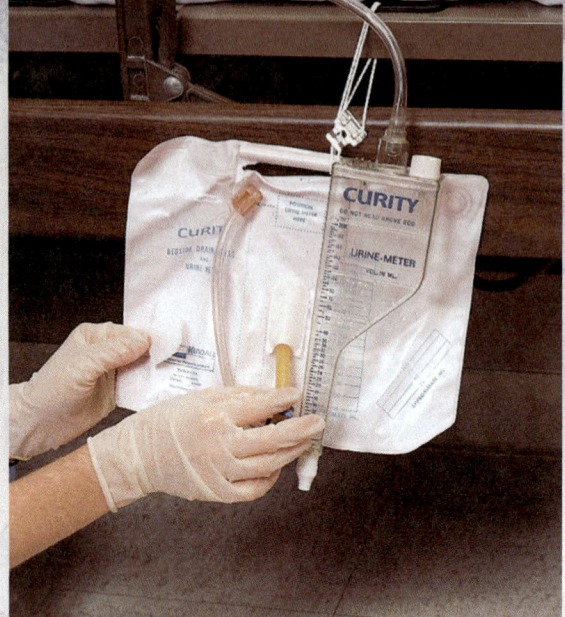

Urinary System

objectives

After completing this unit, you will be able to:

- Spell and define terms.
- Review the location and function of the urinary system.
- List five diagnostic tests associated with conditions of the urinary system.
- Describe some common diseases of the urinary system.
- Describe nursing assistant actions related to the care of patients with urinary system diseases and conditions.
- Demonstrate the following procedures:
  - Procedure 115 Collecting a Routine Urine Specimen
  - Procedure 116 Collecting a Clean-Catch Urine Specimen
  - Procedure 117 Collecting a 24-Hour Urine Specimen
  - Procedure 118 Testing Urine with the HemaCombistix®
  - Procedure 119 Routine Drainage Check
  - Procedure 120 Giving Indwelling Catheter Care
  - Procedure 121 Emptying a Urinary Drainage Unit
  - Procedure 122 Disconnecting the Catheter
  - Procedure 123 Applying a Condom for Urinary Drainage
  - Procedure 124 Connecting a Catheter to a Leg Bag
  - Procedure 125 Emptying a Leg Bag

vocabulary

Learn the meaning and the correct spelling of the following words and phrases:

Bowman's capsule	glomerulus	nephritis	suppression
catheter	hematuria	nephron	suprapubic catheter
condom catheter	hydronephrosis	pelvis	ureter
cortex	indwelling catheter	pyelogram	urethra
cystitis	intravenous	renal calculi	urinalysis
cystoscopy	pyelogram (IVP)	renal colic	urinary bladder
dialysis	kidney	retention	urinary incontinence
dysuria	lithotripsy	retrograde	urinary meatus
Foley catheter	medulla	pyelogram	void

INTRODUCTION

The urinary system consists of the kidneys, ureters, bladder, and urethra. The functions that this system performs are vital. It:

- excretes liquid wastes.
- manages blood chemistry.
- manages fluid balance.

Because the chemistry of the blood and urine reflect the chemistry of the cells, many tests are performed on urine specimens. It is important that urine samples be obtained and preserved properly.

STRUCTURE AND FUNCTION

The urinary system is shown in Figure 44-1. As the name implies, the organs of this system produce urine—liquid waste—that is excreted from the body. The urinary system also helps to control the vital water and salt balance of the body. Inability to secrete urine by the kidneys is known as **suppression**. Inability to excrete urine that has been produced by the kidneys is called **retention**. The organs of this system include:

- **Kidneys**: Organs that produce the urine.
- **Ureters**: Tubes that carry the urine from the kidneys to the urinary bladder. These tubes are 10 to 12 inches long and about ¼-inch wide.
- **Urinary bladder**: Holds the urine until expelled. The urge to urinate (micturate or void) occurs when 150 to 300 mL of urine are in the bladder, although the bladder can hold more urine than this.
- **Urethra**: The tube that carries the urine to the outside. The female urethra is about 1½ inches long. The male urethra is about 8 inches long. The opening to the outside is called the external **urinary meatus**. The meatus is guarded by a round sphincter muscle that relaxes to release the urine.

The Kidneys

The two bean-shaped kidneys are located behind the peritoneum. They are held in place by capsules of fat. Each kidney weighs about 5 ounces. The outer portion of the kidney is called the **cortex**. This area produces the urine. The middle area is known as the **medulla**. It is a series of tubes that drain the urine from the cortex. The **pelvis** of the kidney receives the urine and directs it to the ureter.

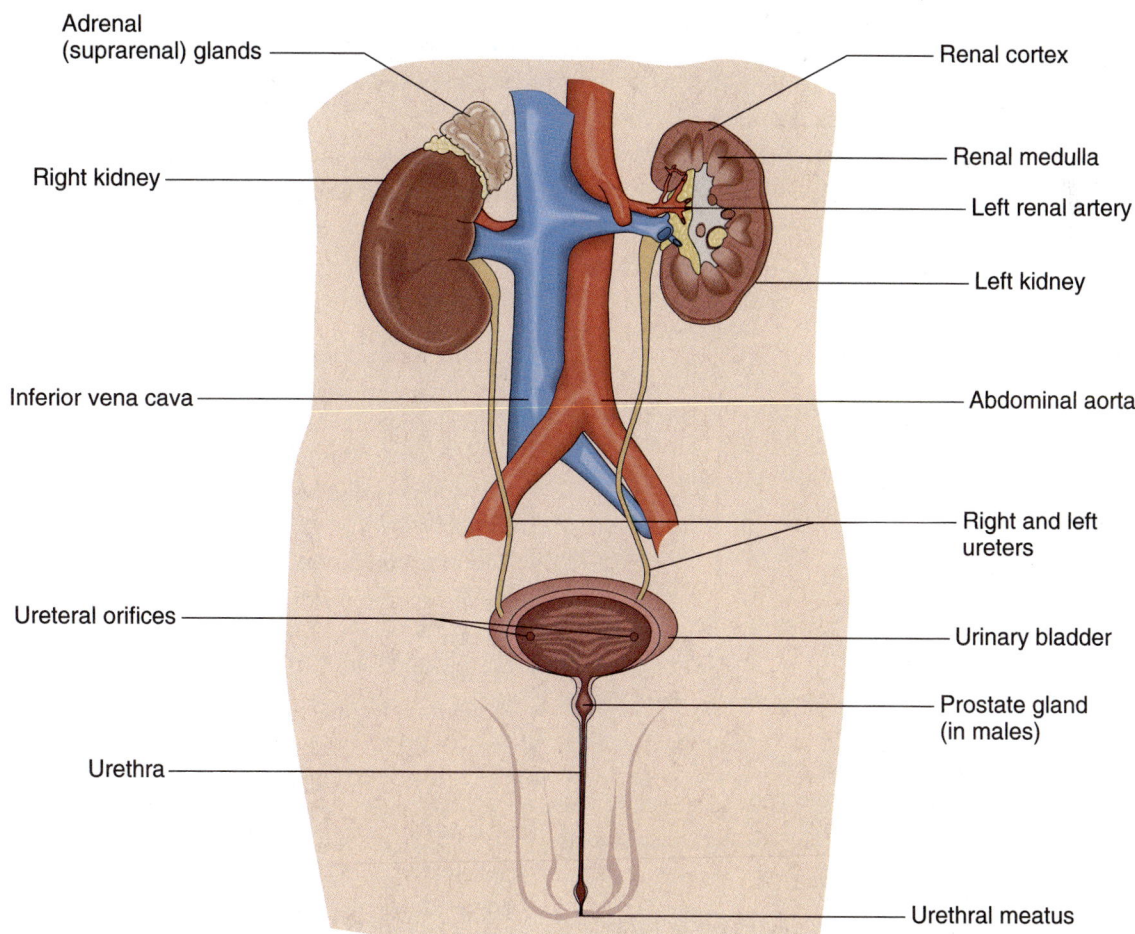

Adrenal (suprarenal) glands

Right kidney

Inferior vena cava

Ureteral orifices

Urethra

Renal cortex

Renal medulla

Left renal artery

Left kidney

Abdominal aorta

Right and left ureters

Urinary bladder

Prostate gland (in males)

Urethral meatus

FIGURE 44-1 Structures of the urinary system.

Urine Production. The renal arteries carry blood to each kidney. Their many branches pass through the medulla to the cortex. In the cortex, urine is produced in filtering units called **nephrons** (Figure 44-2). It is estimated that each kidney contains 1 million nephrons.

Blood arriving at the kidneys carries waste products such as acids and salts. These waste products must be eliminated from the body. Urine is a liquid waste solution containing water and dissolved substances. In the kidneys:

- Waste products, helpful products, and large quantities of water are passed (filtered) through the capillary walls of the **glomerulus** (capillary bed) into **Bowman's capsule**, forming a liquid called *filtrate*.
- The filtrate moves slowly along the convoluted tubules where some water and helpful substances like sugar are reabsorbed into the blood.
- The liquid remaining in the convoluted tubules is urine, which contains wastes.
- The urine passes into the collecting tubules of the medulla, then out of the kidney to the ureter and into the urinary bladder.
- Normal urine is acidic and pale to deep yellow in color.
- Dilute urine has more water and fewer dissolved substances, so it is colorless to pale yellow.
- Concentrated urine has less water and more dissolved substances, so it is darker in color and has a stronger odor.
- The amount of urine produced depends on the amount of intake and various physical conditions.

Inadequate water intake leading to dehydration results in a small amount of concentrated urine.

The substances in the urine provide good information about the chemistry of the body and how well it is functioning. Tests are frequently performed on the urine (**urinalysis**).

COMMON CONDITIONS

Common conditions affecting the urinary system include inflammations due to ascending or descending infections and obstructions to the normal flow of fluids through the tube structure.

Cystitis

Cystitis, or inflammation of the urinary bladder, is fairly common. It is particularly common in women because of the shortness of the female urethra. Signs and symptoms of cystitis include:

- Frequent urination
- **Hematuria** (blood in the urine)
- **Dysuria** (painful urination and/or burning upon urination)
- Bladder spasm

Treatment. Treatment is aimed at relieving the symptoms and eliminating the cause. Treatment includes:

- Sitz baths
- Rest
- Bacteriostatic agents
- Increased fluid intake
- Antibiotics

Nephritis

Nephritis means inflammation of the kidney. Nephritis:

- May follow an attack of infectious disease or may result from general arteriosclerosis. In either case, kidney cells are destroyed. This results in decreased urine production.
- May follow a disease course that is acute (rapid) or chronic (slow).
- Causes hypertension and edema.

Signs and symptoms of nephritis are:

- Edema
- Hematuria
- Proteinuria (protein in urine)
- Hypertension
- Oliguria (occasionally) (decreased urination)

Treatment. Treatment includes:

- Absolute bed rest
- Low-sodium diet
- Restricted fluid intake, at times
- Frequent checks on vital signs

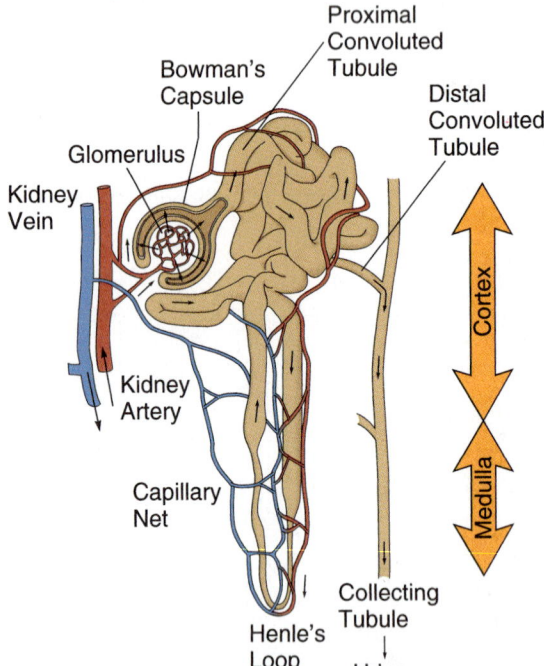

FIGURE 44-2 Nephron and related structures. Arrows indicate the flow of blood through the nephron. The urine produced by the nephron flows through the collecting tubule.

- Accurate intake and output (I/O) measurement
- Steroid medication in some cases

If both kidneys are involved, the patient will require regular dialysis until the diseased kidneys can be replaced with a healthy kidney (kidney transplant). Dialysis is the process of removing the waste products from the blood with a hemodialysis machine, commonly called an artificial kidney.

Many patients on dialysis receive treatment in a hospital dialysis unit or in special outpatient dialysis centers. Portable equipment is brought to the patient's bedside, if necessary. Other patients receive dialysis at home, using portable dialysis machines. The patient's overall physical condition is an important factor in determining if home dialysis is an option.

Renal Calculi

Renal calculi are kidney stones. They can cause obstructions when they become lodged in the urinary passageways. There may be no sign of the development of renal calculi until some obstruction develops. Then:

- The pain is sudden and intense. It is called renal colic.
- Calculi may be passed in the urine.
- As stones pass along the tract, tissue damage may occur, resulting in hematuria (blood in the urine).

Treatment. The goal of treatment is to relieve the blockage and eliminate the stones.

- Encouraging fluids increases urine output. This helps to move the stones along the tract.
- All urine must be strained through gauze or filter paper, which is inspected for stones before it is discarded (Figure 44-3). Stones that are found can be analyzed. With information from the stones, the diet can sometimes be changed to make the formation of stones less likely.
- When it is impossible for the patient to pass the stones, surgery may be necessary. This type of surgery can be done by passing a cystoscope through the urethra or through a surgical incision. With the cystoscope, the physician is able to see inside the bladder and locate the stones. The stones may then be crushed so they can be flushed out in the urine.
- At other times, the stones can be reached and removed only through a surgical incision. When a surgical incision is made, the patient usually returns from surgery with two drainage tubes in place. One tube is inserted in the urinary bladder. The other tube is inserted in the ureter or kidney.
  - The nurse will see that proper drainage is established.
  - In addition to routine postoperative care, you must check frequently to be sure the drainage is not blocked by kinks in the tubes or by the patient's body lying on the tubes.
  - The amount and type of drainage from each area should be carefully noted.

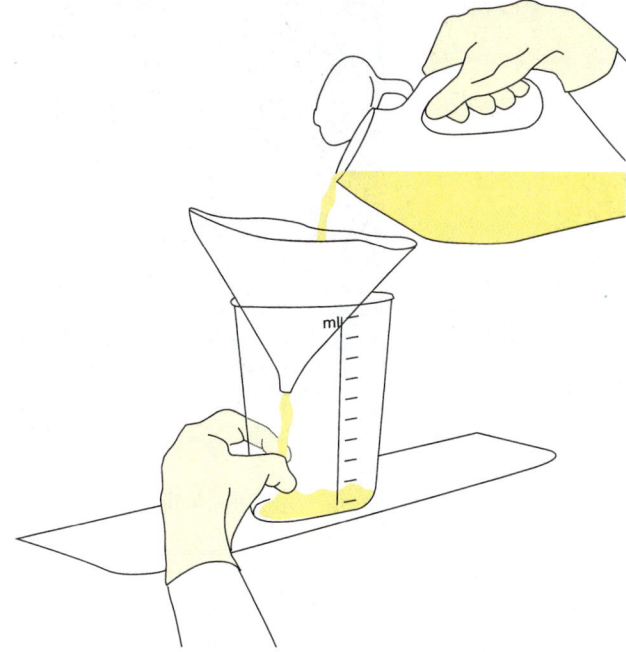

FIGURE 44-3 When the physician writes an order to strain urine, each voiding is poured through filter paper to retrieve kidney stones.

- Lithotripsy is a technique that uses carefully directed sound waves to crush the stones without the need for any surgical incision. The patient receiving this form of treatment is usually in the hospital less than 24 hours.

Hydronephrosis

Hydronephrosis results from accumulation of fluid within the kidney. The increasing amount of urine causes pressure on the kidney cells. As a result, kidney cells are destroyed. The fluid accumulates in the kidney because something is blocking its flow. The flow may be blocked by:

- Renal calculi
- Kinking or twisting of the ureters
- Tumors, especially benign prostatic hypertrophy
- Distended bladder

Symptoms may be acute and similar to those of renal calculi, or they may occur so gradually that they go unnoticed until much damage has been done.

Treatment. The condition is treated by draining the urine above the blockage to relieve pressure and then correcting the cause.

RESPONSIBILITIES OF THE NURSING ASSISTANT

Be sure you understand the orders for each individual patient before you assist in nursing care. Orders regarding positioning, drainage, and activity for urological (urinary) patients vary.

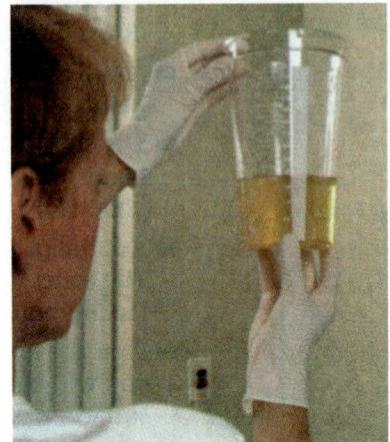

FIGURE 44-4
Accurately measure
and record intake
and output.

There are some important measures that will apply to most urinary patients in your care:

- Accurately measure intake and output (Figure 44-4).
- Promptly report signs and symptoms of:
  - Bleeding
  - Chilling
  - Elevated temperature
  - Reduced output
  - Increased edema
  - Pain
- Properly care for urinary drainage.
- Know the proper steps to take for encouraging fluid intake (forcing fluids) and for limiting fluids.
- When assisting with urination, collecting a urine sample, or recording I/O, note and report the following:
  - Amount of urine
  - Color of urine
  - Odor of urine
  - Presence and type of sediment

URINARY INCONTINENCE

Urinary incontinence (loss of control of urination) may be due to one or a combination of factors. It is not unusual to find more than one factor present at the same time.

- Any interruption of cerebral control can lead to incontinence, including stroke, brain damage that destroys the control centers or pathways, confusion and decreased awareness due to general cerebral degeneration, or aphasia leading to the patient's inability to communicate to others the need for help.
- Incontinence may occur simply because the patient is unable to reach the proper facilities in time. The condition may be related to fecal impaction. Fecal impaction acts as a mechanical obstruction, causing the urine to be retained. The incontinence in this case is actually overflow. Perhaps the most common reason for incontinence is infection. Inflammation irritates sensory nerve

guidelines *for*

Caring for the Patient with Incontinence

Nursing assistant responsibilities include:

- Assisting patients who need help to toilet regularly.
- Answering call lights promptly.
- Always being courteous and patient when assisting patients with toileting.
- Maintaining a positive attitude when changing soiled garments and bed linen and never being critical.
- Performing good perineal care and being sure skin is clean and dry.
- Checking the skin for signs of irritation whenever toileting or bathing a patient or performing perineal care.
- Giving special attention to patients who are confused or forgetful, because they may be unable to clearly state their need for assistance.
- Changing wet linen immediately. This limits discomfort and embarrassment of the patient. Prolonged exposure of the skin to urine is a major cause of skin breakdown. In addition, pathogens grow rapidly on the warmth and moisture and can quickly move upward through the urinary tract, causing life-threatening infection.
- Helping the patient become continent. Little reference should be made to the temporary incontinence. Nursing assistants can do much to give emotional support and reassurance to patients who are incontinent.

endings in the bladder. Mucosal and bladder contractions are increased, causing the incontinence.

- Incontinence may be temporary, lasting only a few days. For example, after a period of illness, continence may improve as the patient becomes more able to respond to the environment. Attention to the underlying causes and the temporary use of incontinence pads may be all that is needed. Every effort should be made to help the patient become continent as soon as possible, with little reference to the temporary incontinence. You can give a great deal of emotional support and reassurance to the patient.
- Incontinence of an established nature continues even though the patient is ambulatory. This is a more

difficult, but still not impossible, form of incontinence to treat. Drugs are sometimes used to achieve bladder control. Retraining may also be needed.

DIAGNOSTIC TESTS

Techniques used to diagnose problems of the urinary tract include:

- Magnetic resonance imaging (MRI)
- CAT scan
- Urinalysis—one common method of learning about the condition of the kidneys is to examine and test the urine.
- Cystoscopy—a test usually performed during surgery. It enables the physician to look inside the bladder. An instrument called a cystoscope is inserted through the urethra. Following this examination, frequency of urination is to be expected, but heavy bleeding or a complaint of sharp, intense pain should be reported at once.

- Pyelogram—an x-ray examination of the urinary tract, similar to the GB and GI series. The dye may be given intravenously (intravenous pyelogram or IVP) or inserted during cystoscopy (retrograde pyelogram) through the urethra. Preparation of the patient usually includes cleansing enemas. Satisfactory results of the x-ray examination depend largely on proper patient preparation.
- Blood chemistry tests
  - Blood urea nitrogen (BUN)
  - Creatinine

Urine Specimens

Routine Urine Specimen. Urinalysis is the most common laboratory test. The specimen is usually taken when the patient first voids (urinates) in the morning. (See Procedures 115 and 116.) The properties of fresh urine begin to change after 15 minutes. Therefore, it is important that you immediately take the sample to the laboratory or refrigerate it until delivery can be made.

PROCEDURE 115

COLLECTING A ROUTINE URINE SPECIMEN

1. Carry out beginning procedure actions.
2. Assemble equipment:
   - disposable gloves
   - bedpan/urinal with cover
   - bed protector
   - toilet tissue
   - small plastic bag
   - specimen container and cover
   - label, including:
     - patient's full name
     - room number
     - facility identification
     - date and time of collection
     - physician's name
     - examination to be done
     - other information requested or required
   - graduate pitcher
   - laboratory requisition slip, properly filled out
   - biohazard specimen transport bag

3. Completely fill out the label of the specimen container.
4. Wash your hands and put on disposable gloves.
5. If the patient cannot ambulate, offer the bedpan or urinal.
6. Instruct the patient not to discard toilet tissue in the pan with the urine. Provide a small plastic bag in which to place the soiled tissue.
7. After the patient has voided, cover the pan and place it on the bed protector on the chair. Offer wash water to the patient.
8. If the patient can ambulate to the bathroom, place a specimen collector in the toilet.
9. Assist the patient to the bathroom. Ask the patient to void into the specimen collector. Instruct the patient to discard soiled toilet tissue in the plastic bag provided. Tissue must not be placed in the collector.
10. Provide privacy.

continues

PROCEDURE 115

continued

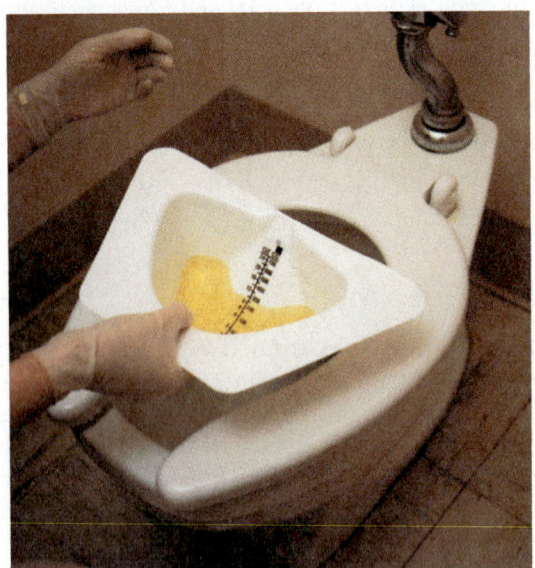

FIGURE 44-5 Remove the collection device. Note the total amount of urine if the patient is on I&O.

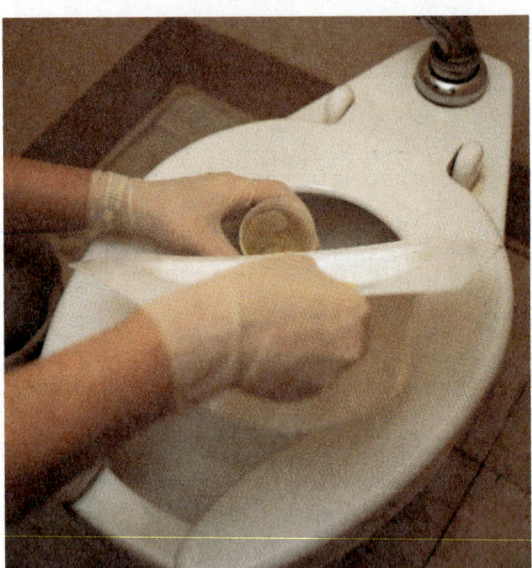

FIGURE 44-6 Carefully pour the specimen into the container.

11. Put on gloves. Remove the specimen collector from the toilet. If the patient is on I/O, note the amount of urine (Figure 44-5). If the patient used a bedpan, pour the urine into a graduate to measure it. Note the amount. Remove gloves and discard according to facility policy. Wash your hands.

12. Remove the cap from the specimen container, and place it (inside up) on a shelf or other flat surface in the bathroom or utility room. Do not touch the inside of the cap or container.

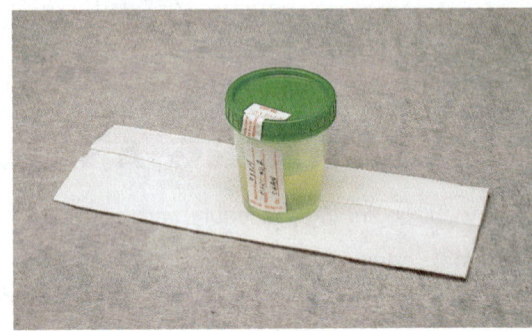

FIGURE 44-7 After placing the cap on the container, apply the label.

13. Put on gloves. Carefully pour about 120 mL of urine into the specimen container from the collector (Figure 44-6).

14. Remove and discard gloves according to facility policy.

15. Wash your hands.

16. Place the cap on the specimen container. Do not contaminate the outside of the container. Attach the completed label to the container (Figure 44-7). Place the specimen container in a biohazard specimen transport bag and attach a laboratory requisition slip (Figure 44-8).

17. Carry out procedure completion actions.

18. Follow facility policy for transporting the specimen to the laboratory.

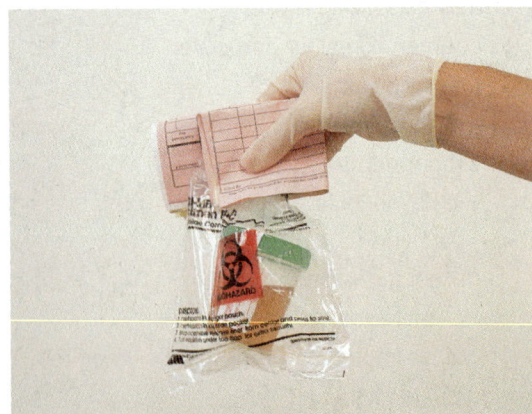

FIGURE 44-8 The properly labeled container is placed in a transport bag with the laboratory requisition attached.

PROCEDURE 116

COLLECTING A CLEAN-CATCH URINE SPECIMEN

1. Carry out beginning procedure actions.

2. Assemble equipment:
   - disposable gloves
   - small plastic bag
   - sterile specimen container and cover
   - label for container, with:
     - patient's full name
     - room number
     - facility identification
     - date and time of collection
     - physician's name
     - type of specimen test to be performed
     - any other information requested
   - gauze squares or cotton
   - antiseptic solution
   - laboratory requisition slip, properly filled out
   - biohazard specimen transport bag

3. Wash your hands and put on disposable gloves.

4. Wash the patient's genital area properly or instruct the patient to do so. If the area is soiled due to incontinence, perform perineal care.

   a. *For female patients:*

   i. Using the gauze or cotton and the antiseptic solution, cleanse the outer folds of the vulva (folds are also called *labia* or *lips*) from front to back. Use a separate cotton/gauze square for each side. Discard the gauze/cotton in the plastic bag.

   ii. Cleanse the inner folds of the vulva with two pieces of gauze and antiseptic solution, again from front to back. Discard used gauze/cotton in the plastic bag.

   iii. Cleanse the middle, innermost area (meatus or urinary opening) in the same manner. Discard the gauze/cotton in the plastic bag.

   iv. Keep the labia separated so that the folds do not fall back and cover the meatus.

   b. *For male patients:*

   i. Using the gauze/cotton and the antiseptic solution, cleanse the tip of the penis. Begin at the meatus, working outward and using a circular motion. Wash the remainder of the penis using downward strokes.

   ii. Discard the gauze/cotton in the plastic bag.

5. Open the container. Place the cap on the counter with the clean inside facing up. Do not touch the inside of the cup or lid with your hands.

6. Instruct the patient to void, allowing the first part of the urine to escape. Then:

   a. Catch the urine stream that follows in the sterile specimen container.

   b. Allow the last portion of the urine stream to escape.

   Note: If the patient is on I/O, or if the amount of urine passed must be measured, catch the first and last part of the urine in a bedpan, urinal, or specimen collection container.

7. Place the sterile cap on the urine container immediately to prevent contamination of the urine specimen.

8. Allow the patient to wash her hands.

9. With the cap securely tightened, wash the outside of the specimen container. Dry the container.

10. Remove and dispose of gloves according to facility policy.

11. Wash your hands.

12. Attach a completed label to the container and place the specimen in the transport bag.

13. Carry out procedure completion actions.

14. Follow facility policy for transporting the specimen to the laboratory.

Catheterized Urine Specimen. When a urine specimen is needed that is free of contamination from organisms found in areas near the urinary meatus (opening), the specimen may be collected by inserting a sterile tube (**catheter**). The nurse will perform this procedure.

Twenty-Four-Hour Specimen. If a 24-hour urine specimen is ordered, all urine excreted by the patient in a 24-hour period is collected and saved. (See Procedure 117.) A 24-hour urine specimen requires that the patient start the 24-hour time period with an empty bladder. For this reason, the first specimen is discarded.

- All urine is saved in a large, carefully labeled container that is supplied by the laboratory and may contain a preservative.
- The container is usually surrounded by ice. If the patient has an indwelling catheter, place the catheter bag in a container surrounded by ice. Empty the bag into the container supplied by the laboratory.

- The patient is asked to void. This first urine is discarded so that the bladder is empty at the time the test begins.
- All other urine is saved, including that voided as the test time finishes.
- No toilet tissue should be allowed to enter the container.
- If you or the patient forget to save a specimen during the test period, report it immediately to the nurse. The test must be discontinued and started again for another 24 hours.

Remember to put on disposable gloves and remove and dispose of them properly each time you collect a specimen.

Urine Testing

The HemaCombistix® is used to test for the presence of protein, blood, and glucose, and for pH (acidity) of urine. See Procedure 118.

PROCEDURE 117

COLLECTING A 24-HOUR URINE SPECIMEN

1. Carry out beginning procedure actions.

2. Assemble equipment:
- disposable gloves
- 24-hour specimen container (supplied by health care facility)
- label
- bedpan, urinal, or commode, or specimen collector for toilet
- plastic bag
- sign for patient's bed
- biohazard bag

3. Label the container with:
- patient's name
- room number
- test ordered
- type of specimen
- time started
- time ended

- date
- physician's name

4. Emphasize to the patient the necessity of saving all urine passed.

5. Place the specimen collection container in the bathroom in a pan of ice (Figures 44-9A and B). The ice will keep the specimen cool for 24 hours.

6. Put on disposable gloves.

7. Allow the patient to void.
- **a.** Assist with the bedpan or urinal as needed.
- **b.** Measure the amount of urine passed if the patient's I/O is being monitored.
- **c.** Discard the urine specimen.
- **d.** Note the date and time of voiding. This time will mark the start of the 24-hour collection.

8. Place a sign on the patient's bed to alert other health care team members that a 24-hour urine specimen is being collected. (The sign may read: *Save all urine—24-hour specimen.*)

continues

PROCEDURE 117

continued

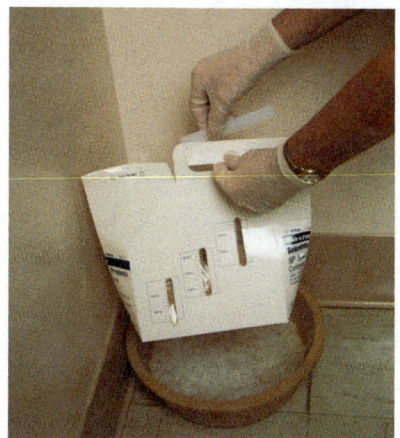

FIGURE 44-9A Close the container with the plastic fastener. Place the 24-hour specimen container in the patient's bathroom in a pan of ice.

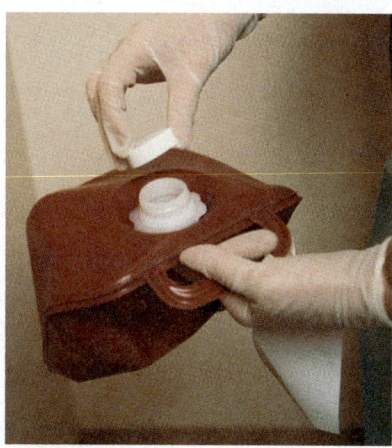

FIGURE 44-9B Some facilities use plastic containers for collecting a 24-hour specimen.

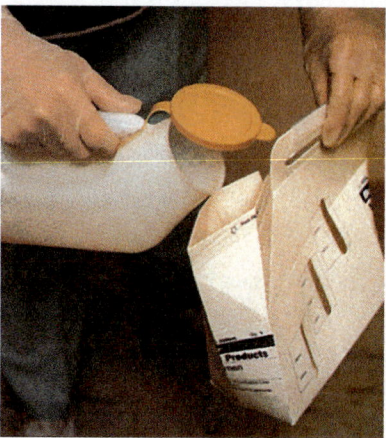

FIGURE 44-9C Open the mouth of the container wide to avoid spilling the specimen.

9. From this time on, for a period of 24 hours, all urine voided is added to the specimen container (Figure 44-9C). The container is kept on ice when not in use. Check facility policy regarding handling of the specimen container.

10. Instruct the patient not to discard toilet tissue into the specimen collection container. Provide small plastic bags for this purpose.

11. At the end of the 24-hour period:
    a. Put on disposable gloves.
    b. Ask the patient to void one last time.
    c. Add this urine to the specimen container.

12. Remove the sign from the patient's bed. Check the container label for accuracy and completeness. Attach the appropriate requisition slip.

13. Remove and dispose of gloves according to facility policy.

14. Place the specimen in a protective biohazard bag for transport.

15. Carry out procedure completion actions.

16. Clean and replace all equipment used, according to facility policy.

17. Follow facility policy for transporting the specimen to the laboratory.

OSHA *Alert*

Various types of test strips and reagent tablets are used for testing urine specimens. Some reagents are caustic and will cause chemical burns if handled with wet hands. Avoid contact with your hands, if possible. The products are also hazardous if ingested, or if they contact the mucous membranes of the eyes, mouth, or genital area. They should be stored in a cool, dry, locked area when not in use.

PROCEDURE 118

TESTING URINE WITH THE HEMACOMBISTIX®

1. Assemble equipment:
   - disposable gloves
   - bottle containing HemaCombistix® reagent strips
   - fresh sample of urine

2. Wash your hands and put on gloves.

3. Take reagent strips and the sample to the bathroom.

4. Remove the cap and place it on the counter with the top side down.

5. Shake the bottle gently until reagent strips protrude from the end.

6. Remove one reagent strip. Do not touch the test areas of the strip with your fingers. Be sure your gloves are dry.

7. Dip the reagent end of the strip in fresh, well-mixed urine—remove immediately.

8. Tap the edge of the strip against the urine container to remove excess urine.

9. Compare the reagent side of the test areas with the corresponding color charts on the bottle (Figure 44-10) at the time intervals specified (Table 44-1).

10. Remove and dispose of gloves according to facility policy. Wash your hands.

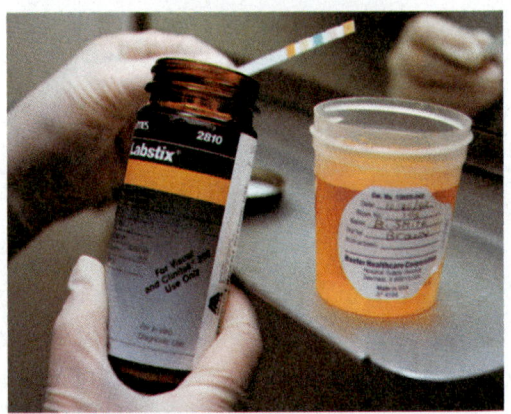

FIGURE 44-10 HemaCombistix® test results.

TABLE 44-1 HEMACOMBISTIX® RESULTS

Test	Reaction Time	Results
Blood	30 sec.	Light blue green to deep blue
Glucose	10–30 sec.	Light blue to dark brown
Protein	Immediately	Yellow to green
pH	Immediately	Orange to blue

RENAL DIALYSIS

As a result of disease or trauma, the kidneys may not be able to carry out their life-sustaining function of filtering impurities from the blood. In this case, mechanical dialysis is substituted to remove wastes from the blood.

Patients requiring this treatment usually have tubing permanently placed in the arm to make it easier to connect to the dialysis machine. The graft attaches to an artery and a vein to provide ready access to the blood circulatory system. When not in use, the tubing from the artery and the tubing from the vein are joined.

Note: The nursing assistant should never use the arm with a dialysis access site to measure blood pressure.

When dialysis is performed, the two sections of tubing are separated and attached to the dialysis machine. Blood passes from the artery to the machine, where impurities are filtered out. The blood is then returned to the patient's vein by way of the graft. The process takes six to eight hours. It is usually performed two to three times per week. Patients with chronic renal failure may be maintained in this manner for some time, often for more than one year.

Sometimes a compatible kidney can be obtained from a donor and transplanted into the person suffering from renal failure. If the kidney is not rejected, it will take on the life-sustaining role of the original kidneys.

URINARY DRAINAGE

Many patients with urinary problems will be on urinary drainage.

- Urine is drained from the bladder through a tube called a *catheter*.

- French catheters or straight catheters (Figure 44-11A) are hollow tubes. They are usually made of soft rubber or plastic. These catheters are used to drain the bladder. They do not remain in the bladder.
- Foley catheters (Figure 44-11B) have a balloon surrounding the neck. The balloon is inflated after the catheter is introduced into the bladder. This is known as an indwelling or retention catheter. Sometimes the patient will complain of feeling the urge to urinate after the catheter is inserted. This is due to the pressure of the balloon on the internal sphincter of the urethra. The pressure feels the same as the sensation of urine pressing on the sphincter. If the patient with a catheter complains of feeling the urge to void, notify the nurse.
- A suprapubic catheter (Figure 44-12) is inserted surgically through the abdominal wall directly into the bladder. A condom catheter is an external catheter used in males. It is applied over the penis and attached to drainage tubing.

The insertion of a catheter is a sterile procedure. It is performed by the nurse or advanced care provider. Closed urinary drainage systems protect the patient from infection. You have definite responsibilities when patients are using urinary drainage:

- Apply the principles of standard precautions.

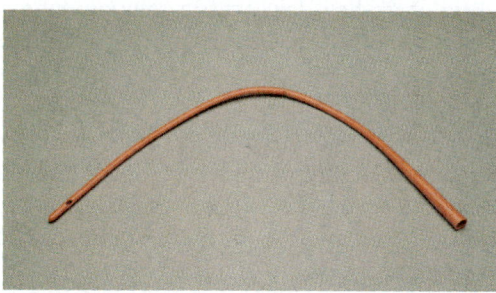

FIGURE 44-11A A straight catheter is inserted to collect a specimen, then removed.

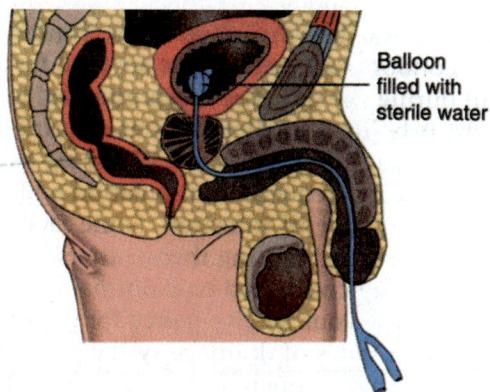

Balloon filled with sterile water

FIGURE 44-11B An indwelling (Foley) catheter is left in place to empty the bladder. The balloon is inflated with sterile water to hold the catheter in place.

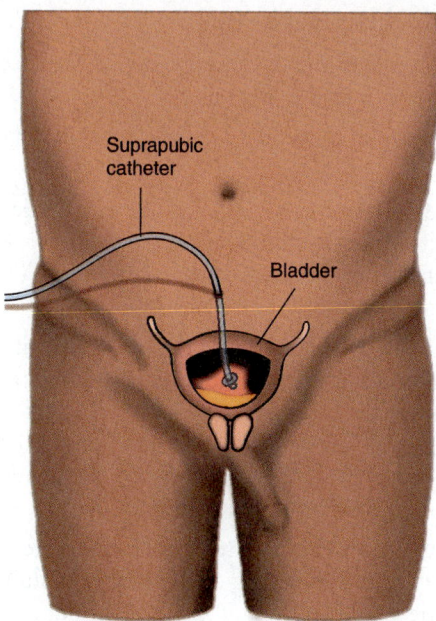

Suprapubic catheter

Bladder

FIGURE 44-12 The suprapubic catheter is surgically inserted through the abdominal wall. The urethra is not functional.

- Keep the urinary meatus clean.
- Wash the area around the meatus daily with a solution approved by your facility.
- Check regularly for signs of irritation or urinary discomfort and report them to the nurse.
- Secure the tubing so that there is no strain on the catheter or tubing. A catheter strap should be applied to the leg to secure the tubing.
- Maintain the drainage bag below the level of the bladder.
- When the patient is in bed, the closed drainage bag is attached to the frame of the bed, never the side rail.
- When the patient is in a chair or wheelchair, the closed drainage bag is attached to the frame of the chair.
- Many facilities use cloth catheter bags for privacy. The cloth bag is connected to the bed or chair frame, and the urinary drainage bag is placed in it.
- When the patient is ambulating, the tubing and drainage bag are carried below the level of the bladder.
- Secure the catheter with a strap or tape. Some facilities secure the catheter to the leg in women and the abdomen, using tape, in men. When securing the catheter to the leg, it is positioned on the top side. Avoid placing the catheter under the leg, which may pinch and obstruct the flow of urine. Know and follow your facility policy.
- Attach the tubing to the bed with a rubber band and plastic clip.
- Use care when lifting, moving, and transferring patients with catheters to avoid accidentally dislodging the catheter by pulling on the tubing.

- Do not open a closed system.
- Make sure the tubing is not kinked or obstructed. Never attach it to the side rail.
- Ensure that the collection bag does not touch the floor.
- Measure the amount of drainage in the collection bag at the end of each shift, note the character of the urine, and report and record the information. (See Procedure 121.)
- In certain medical conditions, the physician will order an hourly output measurement. In this situation, a catheter drainage bag with a *urimeter* (Figure 44-13) will be used. The urine drains into the small chamber. You will empty this chamber every hour and inform the nurse of the output measurement.
- Check the entire drainage setup each time care is given and at the beginning and end of your shift (see Procedure 119).
- Monitor the level of urine in the drainage bag. Most people excrete about 50 to 80 mL of urine each hour. If the level of urine in the bag does not change, if the catheter is leaking, if no urine is present in the bag, or if the urine has an abnormal color, odor, or appearance, inform the nurse.
- Notify the nurse if redness, irritation, drainage, crusting, or open areas are present at the catheter insertion site.

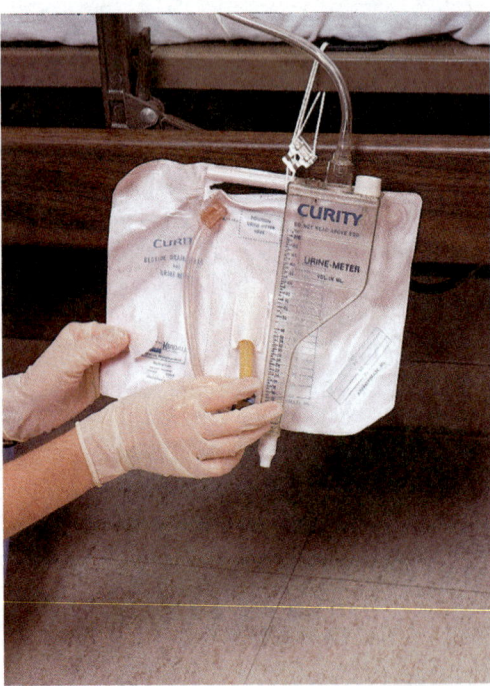

FIGURE 44-13 The drainage bag with a urimeter is used when the physician orders hourly output measurements.

DIFFICULT *Situations*

Unless the patient is on a fluid restriction, encourage the catheterized patient to drink fluids each time you are in the room. Make sure that ice in the water pitcher is refilled regularly. If the patient does not like to drink water, offer fluids of choice, as permitted. Increasing fluid consumption to 3,000 mL a day is best when the patient has an indwelling catheter. The increased fluid prevents sediment formation and flushes the catheter. Check the level of urine in the drainage bag each time you are in the room. Empty the bag if it is full.

- Notify the nurse if the patient complains of pain, burning, tenderness, or has other signs or symptoms of urinary tract infection.

Catheter Care

Once the Foley catheter is inserted, the urinary meatus must be kept clean and free of secretions. The area around the meatus is washed daily with a solution approved by your facility or with soap and water. In some facilities, this procedure may be performed on each shift. This care is called indwelling catheter care.

Indwelling catheter care may be performed during routine morning care, as part of perineal care, or as a separate procedure (see Procedure 120). Report signs of irritation or complaints of discomfort, and changes in the character or quantity of drainage.

Ambulating with a Catheter

When patients are ambulatory or using a geri-chair or wheelchair, you must be careful about the placement of the urinary drainage bag. Remember that the drainage bag must always be lower than the bladder so the urine cannot flow back into the bladder. The bag may be secured to the patient's leg or clothing when the patient ambulates.

When the patient is seated in a wheelchair, the tubing should run below and under the wheelchair so the drainage bag can be secured to the wheelchair back. The drainage bag or tubing must never touch the floor.

There are times when you will have to disconnect the catheter. Follow your facility policies for performing this procedure. In some facilities, a licensed nurse must give permission to disconnect a closed drainage system.

PROCEDURE 119

ROUTINE DRAINAGE CHECK

1. Carry out beginning procedure actions.

2. Wash your hands. Put on gloves.

3. Raise the bedding to observe the tubing.

4. Check the condition of the catheter and the meatus.

5. Keep the drainage tubing coiled on the bed so there is a direct drop to the collection bag (Figure 44-14).

6. The collection bag must be lower than the patient's hips.

7. Keep the end of the drainage tube above the urine level in the bag.

8. Be sure the drainage bag is attached to the bed frame (not the side rail).

9. Note the color, character, and flow of urine.

10. Measure urine using proper technique.

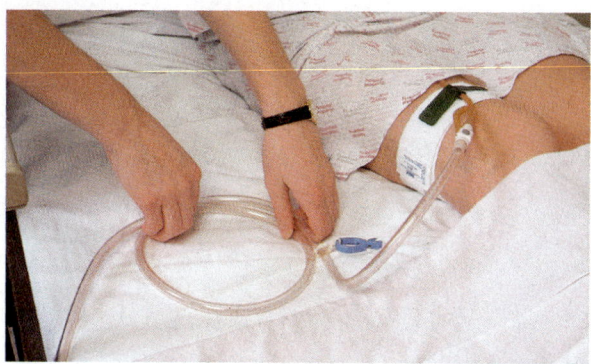

FIGURE 44-14 The Velcro® strap is used to fasten the catheter to the leg. Coil the tubing on the bed. These measures prevent the catheter from moving and accidentally being pulled out during movement or transfers.

11. Remove gloves and discard according to facility policy.

12. Carry out procedure completion actions.

PROCEDURE 120

GIVING INDWELLING CATHETER CARE

1. Carry out beginning procedure actions.

2. Assemble equipment:
   - disposable gloves
   - bed protector
   - bath blanket
   - plastic bag for disposables
   - daily catheter care kit (if available)
   - washcloth, towel, basin, and soap if kit is unavailable
   - antiseptic solution
   - sterile applicators
   - tape or Velcro strap

3. Raise the bed to a comfortable working height. Be

sure the opposite side rail is up and secure. Position the patient on his or her back, with legs separated and knees bent, if permitted.

4. Cover the patient with a bath blanket and fanfold bedding to the foot of the bed.

5. Ask the patient to raise the hips. Place a bed protector underneath the patient.

6. Position a bath blanket so that only the genitals will be exposed.

7. Arrange a catheter care kit on the overbed table. Open the kit. Position the open bag at the foot of the bed.

8. Wash your hands. Put on gloves and draw the drape or bath blanket back.

continues

PROCEDURE 120

continued

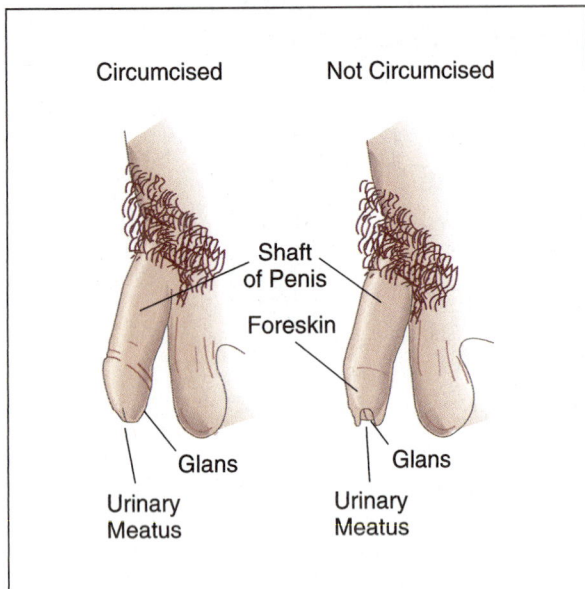

FIGURE 44-15 Comparison of circumcised and uncircumcised penis.

9. *For the male patient:*

- Gently grasp the penis and draw the foreskin back, if not circumcised (Figure 44-15).
- Using a new applicator dipped in antiseptic solution for each stroke, cleanse the glans from the meatus toward the shaft for approximately 4 inches.
- After each stroke, dispose of the used applicator in a plastic bag.
- **Alternate action:** Clean around the catheter first and then around the meatus and glans. Wash with soap and water, using a circular motion. Dry in the same manner. Make sure to return the foreskin (if not circumcised) to its proper position.

For the female patient:

- Separate the labia.
- Using a new applicator dipped in antiseptic for each stroke, cleanse from front to back. Begin at the center, then cleanse each side.

- After each stroke, dispose of the used applicator in a plastic bag.
- Clean the catheter down about 4 inches.
- Dry carefully.

10. Remove gloves and discard in plastic bag. Wash your hands.

11. Check the catheter to be sure it is secured properly to the leg (see Figure 44-14). Readjust the Velcro strap for slack, if needed. If a Velcro strap is not available, use tape (Figure 44-16).

12. Check to be sure the tubing is coiled on the bed and that it hangs straight down into the drainage container. Empty the bag and measure the contents, if necessary. Do not raise the bag above the level of the patient's hips.

13. Replace bedding and remove the bath blanket.

14. Fold the bath blanket and store, or put it in the linen hamper.

15. Lower the bed. Adjust side rails for safety.

16. Carry out procedure completion actions.

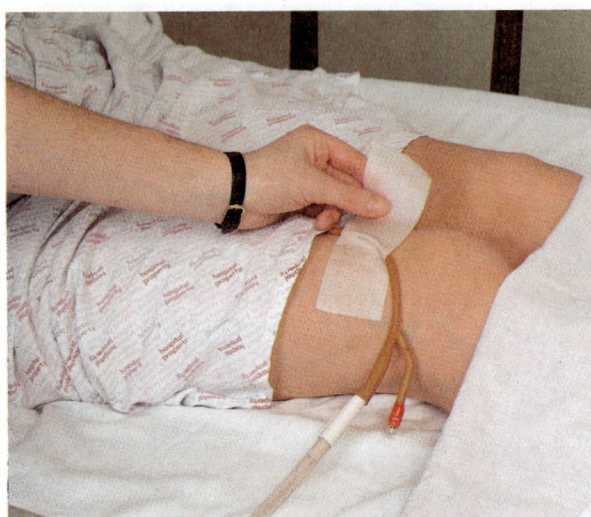

FIGURE 44-16 The catheter tubing may be taped to the thigh. The nurse may instruct you to tape the catheter to the abdomen in male patients.

PROCEDURE 121

EMPTYING A URINARY DRAINAGE UNIT

1. Carry out beginning procedure actions.

2. Assemble equipment:
   - disposable gloves
   - graduated container
   - sterile cap or sterile 4 × 4 pad (needed if container has no bottom drain tube)
   - antiseptic wipes

3. Wash your hands and put on gloves.

4. Place a paper towel on the floor under the drainage bag. Place a graduate on the paper towel under the drain of the collection bag.

5. Remove the drain from the holder (Figure 44-17) and open the drain. Allow the urine to drain into the graduate, using aseptic technique. Do not allow the tip of the tubing to touch the sides of the graduate (Figure 44-18).

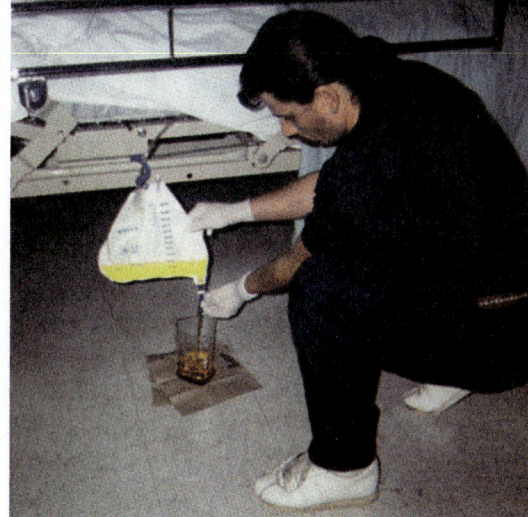

FIGURE 44-18 Center the graduate under the drainage spout. If the spout accidentally contacts your fingers or the edge of the graduate, wipe it with an alcohol sponge before returning it to the drainage bag.

6. Close the drain and replace it in the holder. If accidental contamination occurs, wipe the drain tip with an antiseptic wipe before returning it to the holder. Dispose of used antiseptic wipes in a plastic bag.

7. Check the position of the drainage tube.

8. Pick up the paper towel, touching the top surface only, and discard it.

9. Take the graduate to the bathroom and empty it.

10. Wash and dry the graduate and store it according to facility policy.

11. Record the amount of urine and note its character.

12. Remove gloves and discard according to facility policy.

13. Carry out procedure completion actions.

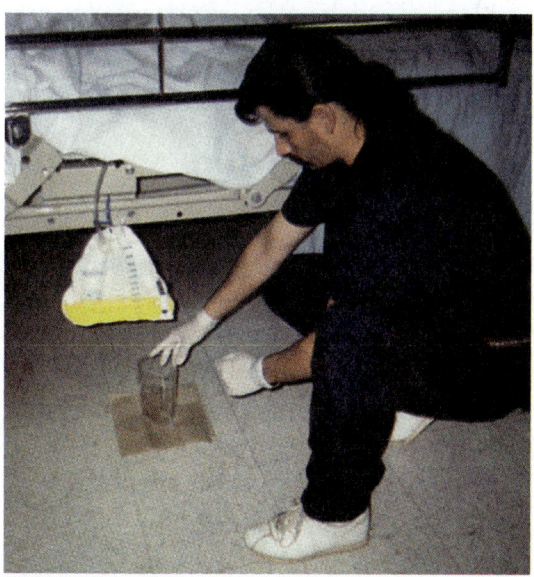

FIGURE 44-17 Place a paper towel on the floor under the drain.

Infection Risk

You must follow the procedure for disconnecting the catheter carefully. The patient who has an indwelling catheter is at risk for infection. There are several sites where infection can enter the drainage system (Figure 44-19):

- Urinary meatus, where the catheter is inserted
- Connection between the catheter and the drainage tube
- Connection between the drainage bag and the drainage tubing
- Opening used to empty the drainage bag

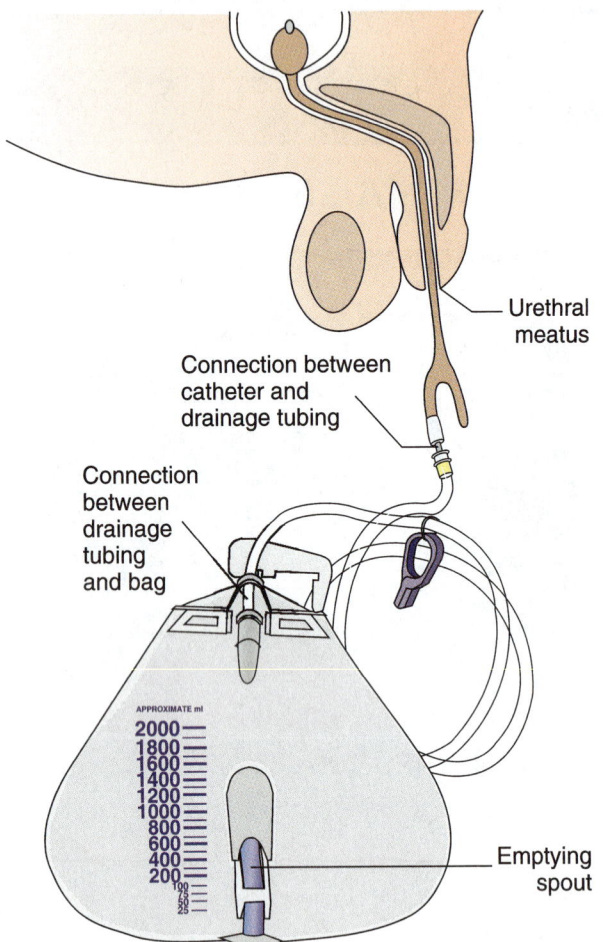

Urethral meatus

Connection between catheter and drainage tubing

Connection between drainage tubing and bag

APPROXIMATE ml

2000
1800
1600
1400
1200
1000
800
600
400
200

Emptying spout

FIGURE 44-19 Handle the closed drainage system carefully to avoid accidental contamination of these areas.

Disconnecting the Catheter

It is preferable never to disconnect the drainage setup, but at times it is necessary. If sterile caps and plugs are available, they should be used. If not, the disconnected ends must be protected with sterile gauze sponges. (See Procedure 122.)

External Drainage Systems (Male)

External urinary drainage systems are preferred for male patients who require long periods of urinary drainage. In external drainage, a catheter is not inserted in the urethra. Thus, there is less danger of infection. A condom (sheath) catheter is connected, or some other type of external drainage appliance is applied to the penis (see Procedure 123).

Other complications, ranging from minor irritation to circulatory impairment, can occur. The external catheter is applied over the penis. It is usually attached with an adhesive strip. The strip should always be wrapped in a spiral. If it completely encircles the penis, severe injury can result. Some external catheters have a self-adhesive film on the inside, making the adhesive strip on the outside unnecessary. About one inch of the catheter should extend beyond the tip of the penis and attach to the drainage tubing. Always apply the principles of standard precautions when caring for an external catheter.

The condom is attached to drainage tubing and a collection bag. The condom is removed every 24 hours and the penis is washed and dried. Different types of drainage systems are available. Urine may be collected in a bag that hangs from the bed or wheelchair or in a bag attached to the patient's leg.

PROCEDURE 122

DISCONNECTING THE CATHETER

1. Carry out beginning procedure actions.

2. Assemble equipment:
   - disposable gloves
   - antiseptic wipes
   - gauze sponges
   - sterile caps/plugs
   - clamps

3. Wash your hands and put on gloves.

4. Clamp the catheter.

5. Disconnect the catheter and drainage tubing. Do not put the ends down or allow them to

touch anything. If accidental contamination occurs, wipe the ends with antiseptic wipes before inserting the plug or placing the cap. Dispose of used antiseptic wipes in a plastic bag.

6. Insert a sterile plug in the end of the catheter. Place a sterile cap over the exposed end of the drainage tube (Figure 44-20).

7. Secure the drainage tube to the bed frame so that the tube will not touch the floor.

8. Remove and dispose of gloves according to facility policy. Wash your hands.

continues

PROCEDURE 122

continued

9. Carry out procedure completion actions.

📝 **Note:** *Reverse the procedure to reconnect the catheter. If you find an unprotected, disconnected tube in the bed or on the floor,* do not reconnect it. Report it at once.

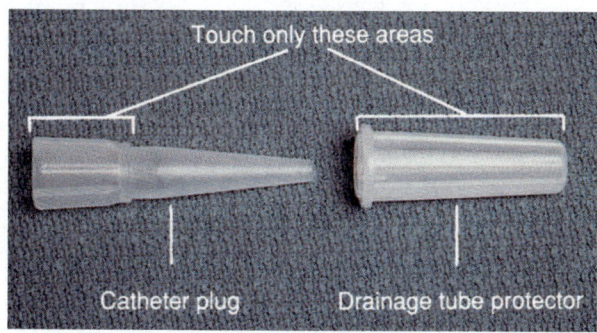

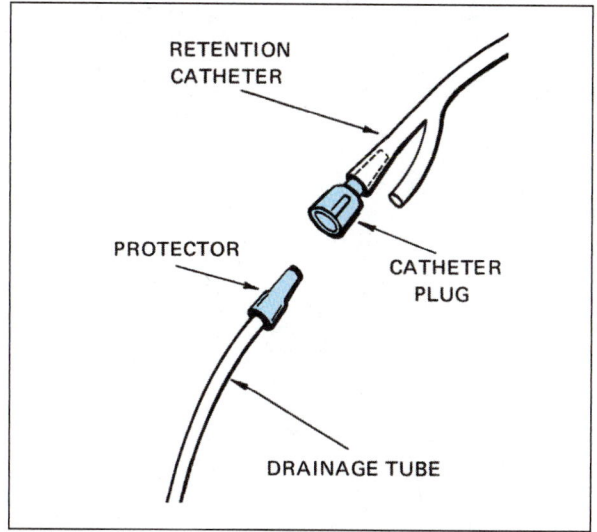

FIGURE 44-20 (Left) Sterile catheter plug and protective cap. (Right) Plug and protective cap in place.

PROCEDURE 123

APPLYING A CONDOM FOR URINARY DRAINAGE

1. Carry out beginning procedure actions.

2. Assemble equipment:
- disposable gloves
- basin of warm water
- washcloth
- towel
- condom with drainage tip
- bed protector
- bath blanket
- towel

3. Arrange equipment on the overbed table.

4. Raise the bed to a comfortable working height. Be sure the opposite side rail is up and secure for safety.

5. Lower the side rail on the side where you will be working.

6. Cover the patient with a bath blanket and fanfold bedding to the foot of the bed.

7. Wash your hands and put on gloves.

8. Place a bed protector under the patient's hips.

9. Adjust the bath blanket to expose the genitals only.

10. Carefully wash and dry the penis. Observe for signs of irritation. Check to see if the condom has a "ready stick" surface.

11. Apply the condom and drainage tip to the penis by placing the condom at the top of the penis and rolling toward the base of the penis. Leave space between the drainage tip and the glans of the penis to prevent irritation (Figure 44-21). If the patient is not circumcised, be sure that the foreskin is in normal position.

12. Spiral-wrap the tape provided with the condom to secure it to the penis (Figure 44-22).

13. The condom is now ready to be connected to drainage tubing leading to a collection bag.

continues

PROCEDURE 123

continued

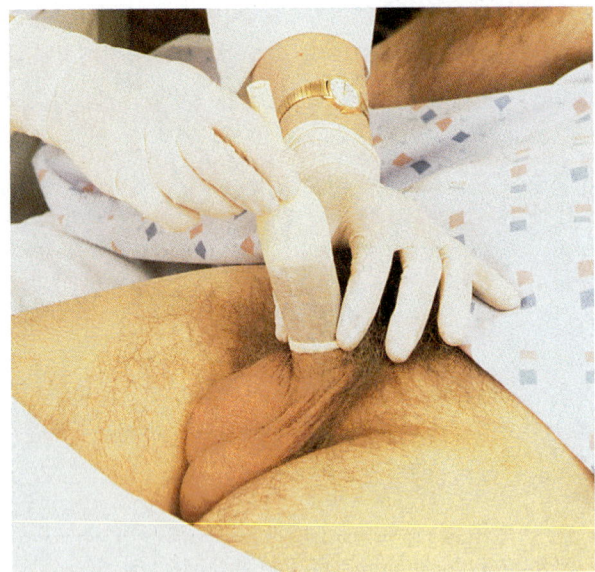

FIGURE 44-21 Leave room between the glans penis and the drainage tip on the condom to prevent irritation. Roll the condom down to the base of the penis.

14. Remove gloves and discard according to facility policy.

15. Wash your hands.

16. Adjust bedding and remove the bath blanket. Fold the bath blanket and store it in the room, or place it in the laundry hamper.

17. Lower the bed. Adjust the side rails for safety.

18. Carry out procedure completion actions.

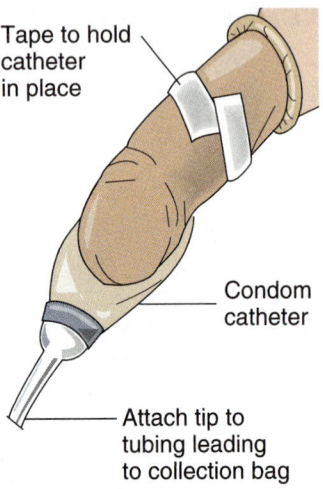

Tape to hold catheter in place

Condom catheter

Attach tip to tubing leading to collection bag

FIGURE 44-22 Correctly applied and secured condom catheter ready to be attached to the drainage tubing.

19. To change the catheter, remove the adhesive strip and roll the condom back over the tip of the penis. Discard it in a plastic bag, or according to facility policy.

   a. Observe the skin on the penis for redness, irritation, swelling, and open areas. If noted, report your observations to the nurse before applying a new condom catheter.

   b. After the catheter has been removed, it is not reapplied. A new catheter is used each time.

   c. Provide perineal care before applying another external catheter.

DIFFICULT *Situations*

Inspect the condom catheter periodically to make sure it is not twisted or obstructed. If the catheter becomes twisted, the urine will collect inside the catheter, causing irritation. As the urine accumulates, the catheter will expand until it eventually comes off.

Leg Bag Drainage

Some patients find it easier to ambulate when urine drainage is collected in a leg bag instead of the larger urinary drainage bag. (See Procedure 124.) The leg bag is held to the patient's leg by Velcro® straps, around either the thigh or the lower leg (Figure 44-23). Points to keep in mind when patients use a leg bag are:

- The leg bag is smaller and must be emptied more often (see Procedure 125).
- The bag must be placed so there is a straight drop down from the catheter.
- Tension on the catheter tubing must be minimal.
- Care must be taken not to introduce germs when connecting and disconnecting the bag and catheter.

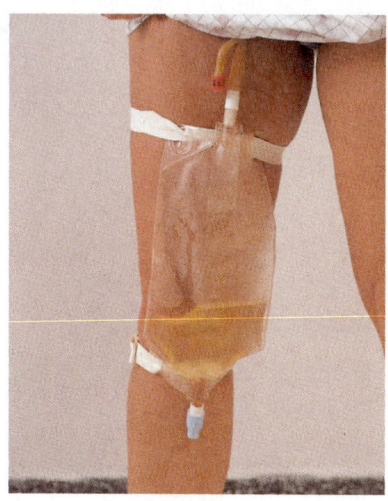

FIGURE 44-23 The leg bag is held in place by adjustable straps. The bag is smaller than a bed collection bag and must be emptied more often.

PROCEDURE 124

CONNECTING A CATHETER TO A LEG BAG

 Note: *Always check with the nurse before using a leg bag.*

1. Carry out beginning procedure actions.
2. Assemble equipment:
   - disposable gloves
   - antiseptic wipes
   - leg bag and tubing
   - emesis basin
   - bed protector
   - sterile cap/plug
   - clamp
3. Wash your hands and put on gloves.
4. Place a bed protector under the connection between the catheter and the drainage tube.
5. Clamp the catheter.
6. Disconnect the catheter and drainage tubing. Do not put them down or allow them to touch anything.
7. Insert a sterile plug in the end of the catheter. Place a sterile cap over the exposed end of the drainage tube.

 Note: *If accidental contamination occurs, wipe the area with antiseptic wipes before inserting a sterile plug or replacing a sterile cap over the exposed*

end of the drainage tubing. Dispose of used antiseptic wipes in a plastic bag.

8. Secure the drainage tube to the bed frame. The drainage tube must not touch the floor.
9. Remove the catheter plug.
10. Insert the end of the leg bag tubing into the catheter (Figure 44-24).

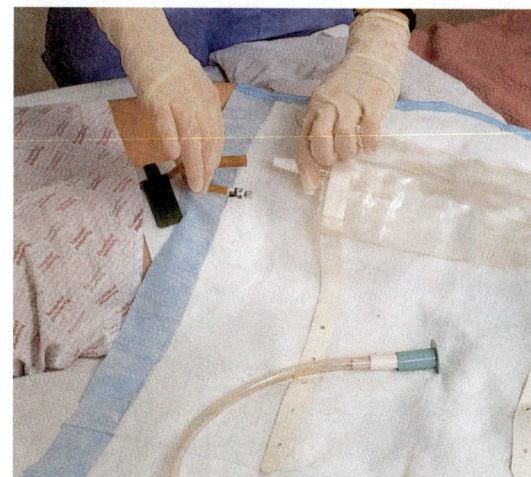

FIGURE 44-24 Carefully connect the catheter to the leg bag. Avoid touching anything against the end of the catheter. The drainage tubing on the bed bag is covered with a sterile cap that is left in place until it is reconnected to the catheter.

continues

PROCEDURE 124

continued

11. Release the catheter clamp.

12. Secure the leg bag with Velcro straps to the patient's leg so there is no tension on the tubing. Be sure there is a straight drop down from the catheter to the bag for urine flow. Check for leakage.

13. Remove the bed protector and discard it.

14. Remove gloves and discard according to facility policy. Wash your hands.

15. Assist the patient to get out of bed. The single-use leg bag should be discarded in a biohazardous waste container.

16. Carry out procedure completion actions.

 Note: To reconnect the regular drainage bag, reverse this procedure.

INFECTION CONTROL *Alert*

Avoid putting the patient to bed while he is wearing a leg bag. The urine may flow back into the bladder from the bag when the patient is in bed. Disconnect the leg bag and connect the catheter to the regular drainage bag when the patient is in bed.

PROCEDURE 125

EMPTYING A LEG BAG

1. Carry out beginning procedure actions.

2. Assemble equipment:
   - disposable gloves
   - antiseptic wipes
   - emesis basin
   - graduate pitcher
   - paper towels

3. Position the patient safely.

4. Wash your hands and put on gloves.

5. Release the Velcro straps holding the leg bag so the bag can be moved away from the patient's leg.

6. Place a paper towel on the floor under the drainage outlet of the leg bag.

7. Place a graduate on the paper towel under the drainage outlet.

8. Remove the cap, being careful not to touch the tip. Drain the collected urine into the graduate.

Do not put the cap down and do not touch the inside of the cap. If accidental contamination occurs, wipe the area with antiseptic wipes before replacing the cap. Dispose of used antiseptic wipes in a plastic bag.

9. Wipe the drainage outlet with an antiseptic wipe and replace the cap.

10. Refasten the straps to secure the drainage bag to the leg.

11. Make sure the patient is comfortable and safe.

12. Discard the paper towel.

13. Measure the urine and note the amount, if required.

14. Discard the urine. Clean the graduate and store it.

15. Remove gloves and discard according to facility policy.

16. Carry out procedure completion actions.

REVIEW

A. True/False.

Mark the following true or false by circling T or F.

1. T F Insertion of a sterile catheter into the urinary bladder is a routine nursing assistant task.

2. T F Gloves should be worn when emptying a urine collection bag.

3. T F It is preferable never to disconnect a urinary drainage setup.

4. T F The pain associated with kidney stones is referred to as renal colic.

5. T F If you find an unprotected, disconnected catheter or tubing on the floor, you should reconnect it immediately.

6. T F The hemodialysis machine takes the place of nonfunctioning kidneys.

7. T F Ample fluid intake encourages increased output, which is important in treating kidney stones.

8. T F A catheter with an inflatable balloon is called a French catheter.

9. T F French catheters are indwelling catheters.

10. T F Cystitis is a fairly common problem for women.

B. Matching.

Choose the correct term from Column II to match each phrase in Column I.

Column I

11. _____ indwelling catheter

12. _____ inability to expel formed urine

13. _____ urinate

14. _____ inflammation of the bladder

15. _____ blood in the urine

Column II

a. void

b. hematuria

c. cystitis

d. retention

e. dysuria

f. Foley catheter

g. suppression

C. Multiple Choice.

Select the one best answer for each of the following.

16. Your patient has a diagnosis of nephritis. Your care will include
 a. keeping the patient very active.
 b. serving a high-sodium diet.
 c. measuring I/O accurately.
 d. eliminating vital sign measurements so the patient can rest more.

17. Your patient has renal calculi. One of your care tasks will be
 a. saving all urine.
 b. straining urine.
 c. limiting fluids.
 d. inserting a catheter.

18. A common cause of hydronephrosis is
 a. renal calculi.
 b. pain in the bladder.
 c. bladder infection.
 d. drinking too much fluid.

19. Important signs and symptoms to note when there is a diagnosis involving the urinary system include
 a. hunger.
 b. thirst.
 c. temperature evaluation.
 d. voiding every 3 to 4 hours.

20. Indwelling catheter care is
 a. a licensed nurse responsibility.
 b. performed during AM care.
 c. safely omitted as long as the patient is in bed.
 d. performed twice a week.

D. Completion.

Complete the following statements.

21. The nursing assistant who finds a disconnected catheter in the bed should _____

22. A routine check of a patient who uses urinary drainage should include _____

E. Nursing Assistant Challenge.

Mr. Starkman is 68 years of age. An external urinary condom is to be applied. Answer the following regarding his care while the condom is being applied.

23. You should wear gloves to apply the condom.

 _____
 (yes) (no)

24. The condom should be applied by _____ of the penis.
 (pulling it up toward the tip) (rolling it down toward the base)

25. When applying the condom, you should _____ space between the drainage tip and the glans of the penis.
 (leave) (not leave)

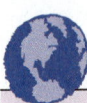 **EXPLORING THE WEB**

Description	Location
Digital Urology Journal	*http://www.duj.com*
Internet Pathology Laboratory—Urinalysis	*http://medlib.med.utah.edu*
Lab and Pathology Topics Index	*http://www.palpath.com*
LabTestsOnline	*http://www.labtestsonline.org*
Loyola University Department of Urology	*http://www.luhs.org*
Nephron Information Center	*http://www.nephron.com*
Society of Urologic Nurses and Associates	*http://suna.inurse.com*
Stanford Department of Urology	*http://www.med.stanford.edu*
UCLA Department of Urology	*http://www.urology.medsch.ucla.edu*
University of Michigan Department of Urology	*http://www.um-urology.com*
University of Virginia Urology	*http://www.healthsystem.virginia.edu*
Urology at Hopkins	*http://urology.jhu.edu*
Urology Nurses Online	*http://www.duj.com*
UrologyChannel	*http://www.urologychannel.com*

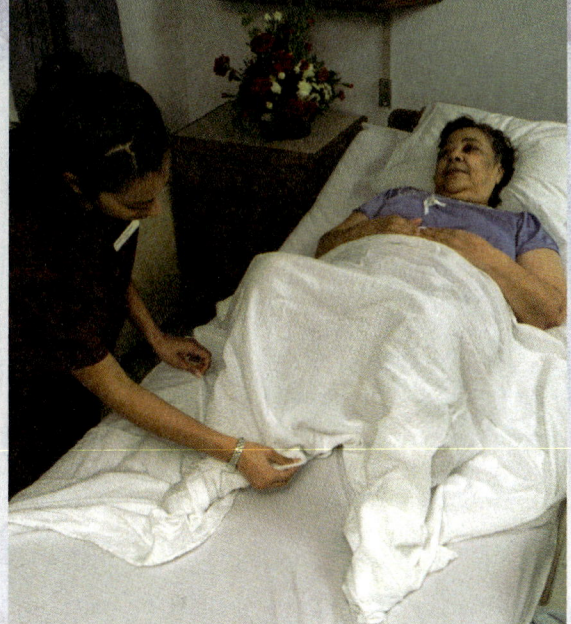

Reproductive System

objectives

After completing this unit, you will be able to:
- Spell and define terms.
- Review the location and functions of the organs of the male and female reproductive systems.
- Describe some common disorders and conditions of the male reproductive system.
- Describe some common disorders and conditions of the female reproductive system.
- List six diagnostic tests associated with conditions of the male and female reproductive systems.

- Describe nursing assistant actions related to the care of patients with conditions and diseases of the reproductive system.
- State the nursing precautions required for patients who have sexually transmitted diseases.
- Demonstrate the following procedures:
  - Procedure 126 Breast Self-Examination
  - Procedure 127 Giving a Nonsterile Vaginal Douche

vocabulary

Learn the meaning and the correct spelling of the following words and phrases:

amenorrhea	endometrium	metrorrhagia	salpingectomy
benign prostatic	epididymis	oophorectomy	seminal vesicles
hypertrophy	fallopian tubes	orchiectomy	sexually transmitted
biopsy	genitalia	ovary	disease (STD)
brachytherapy	gonorrhea	oviduct	simple mastectomy
chancre	hemorrhoid	ovulation	sperm
chlamydia	herpes simplex II	ovum	sterility
climacteric	hysterectomy	panhysterectomy	syphilis
clitoris	labia majora	Pap smear	testes
colporrhaphy	labia minora	pelvic inflammatory	trichomonas vaginitis
Cowper's glands	leukorrhea	disease (PID)	uterus
cystocele	lumpectomy	penis	vagina
dilatation and curettage	mammogram	prostatectomy	vas deferens
(D & C)	mastectomy	prostate gland	venereal warts
douche	menopause	puberty	vulva
dysmenorrhea	menorrhagia	radical mastectomy	vulvovaginitis
ejaculatory duct	menstruation	rectocele	

STRUCTURE AND FUNCTION

Both the male and female reproductive organs have dual functions. They:

1. Produce reproductive cells. The male produces **sperm**. The female produces the **ovum**.
2. Produce hormones that are responsible for sex characteristics.
   a. Males produce testosterone.
   b. Females produce estrogen and progesterone.

In the reproductive process, the:

- male and female engage in sexual intercourse.
- male ejaculates (propels) the sperm and the seminal fluid in which they swim into the female vagina.
- sperm and egg meet in the female fallopian tube. One sperm penetrates the egg and conception takes place.
- baby (fetus) develops in the uterus until birth.
- female breasts (mammary glands) produce milk to nourish the newborn.

The Male Reproductive Organs: Structure and Function

The male organs (Figure 45-1) include the:

- **Testes**: Two glandular organs located in the scrotum. The testes produce sperm and the hormone testosterone.

- **Epididymis**: A 20-foot-long coiled tube located on the top and back of each testis. The epididymis stores the sperm and allows them to mature.

- **Vas deferens**: A tube that leads from the epididymis. It carries the sperm upward into the pelvic cavity to the seminal vesicles during ejaculation. The vas deferens is accompanied by nerves and blood vessels. Together, they form the spermatic cord.

- **Seminal vesicles**: Located behind the bladder. They receive and store the sperm from the vas deferens. They contribute nutrients to the seminal fluid. The small ejaculatory duct leads from the seminal vesicles to the urethra just below the prostate gland.

- **Ejaculatory duct**: Carries the fluid produced in the seminal vesicles. Fluids are added as the sperm are propelled forward. The sperm and fluid form the seminal fluid or ejaculate. The fluid contains nutrients and other substances needed by the sperm.

- **Prostate gland**: Found just below the urinary bladder surrounding the urethra. It secretes a fluid that increases the ability of the sperm to move in the seminal fluid. Enlargement of the prostate gland may prevent urine from passing through the urethra. This is a fairly common occurrence in older men.

- **Cowper's glands**: Two small glands located beside the urethra. They produce mucus for lubrication.

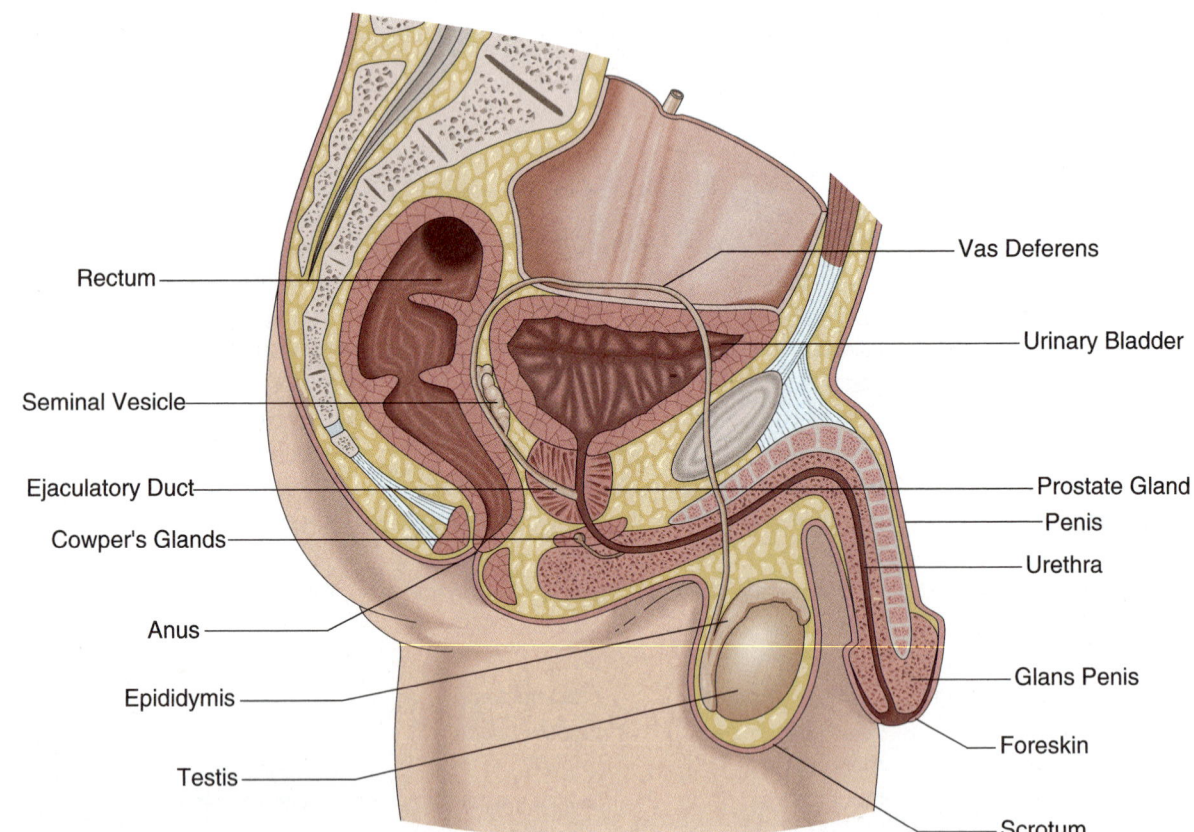

FIGURE 45-1 Cross-section of the male reproductive system.

- **Penis:** Composed of special tissue that can become filled with blood, making the organ enlarge and become stiffened so that it may enter the vagina to deposit seminal fluid. Loose-fitting skin (the prepuce or foreskin) covers the penis.

The male urethra passes through the penis and serves two purposes. It carries:

- Reproductive fluid during intercourse
- Urine during voiding

The two activities cannot occur at the same time because they are under the control of different parts of the nervous system.

The Female Reproductive Organs: Structure and Function

The external female structures (genitalia) (Figure 45-2) include the:

- **Vulva:** Made up of two liplike structures, the **labia majora** and **labia minora**. When the labia are separated, other external structures may be seen.
- **Clitoris:** A very sensitive structure found just behind the juncture of the labia minora. It functions during sexual stimulation to begin the rhythmic series of contractions associated with female climax (orgasm).
- Urinary meatus: The opening of the urethra to the outside.
- Vaginal meatus: The opening to the vagina or birth canal.

The Internal Female Structures

The internal female reproductive organs (Figures 45-3 and 45-4) include the following structures.

- **Ovaries:** Two small glands, found on either side of the uterus, at the ends of the oviducts (fallopian tubes) in the pelvis. They produce two hormones, estrogen and progesterone, and the egg (ovum). The eggs are contained in many little sacs called follicles. About once each month, a follicle matures and releases an ovum.

The ovum makes its way into one of the four-inch-long oviducts. This process is called ovulation. The cells of the follicles that are left produce progesterone. The progesterone causes changes within the uterus, readying it for the possibility of receiving a fertilized ovum.

- **Fallopian tubes** (**oviducts**): Two tubes, approximately four inches long, that serve as a pathway between the ovary and uterus. The sperm and egg meet in the tubes. Fertilization takes place here.
- **Uterus:** A hollow, pear-shaped organ. Its walls are made up of involuntary muscles. It is lined with special tissue called **endometrium**. The uterus has three main parts: the fundus, body, and cervix. The body and the fundus can stretch enough to hold a fetus, the amniotic sac, and the afterbirth (placenta). The cervix extends into the vagina. During labor, the cervix opens up to allow the baby to be delivered.
- **Vagina:** Found between the urinary bladder and the rectum. Its muscular walls are capable of much stretching. It is lined with mucous membrane. Two glands known as Bartholin's glands are found on either side of the external vaginal opening. They provide lubrication.

Menstruation and Ovulation

The menstrual cycle (female sexual cycle) begins at **puberty**. Puberty occurs in girls between the ages of 9 and 17. The cycle varies in length, usually between 25 and 30 days. The average is 28 days, which is why it is considered a monthly cycle.

During the menstrual cycle, a mature egg, or ovum (plural, ova):

- is released from one of the ovaries.
- travels from the ovary to one of the fallopian tubes.
- may be fertilized by a male sperm.

At the same time that the ovum is being matured and expelled from the ovary (ovulation), the lining of the uterus (endometrium) is being built up and made ready to receive

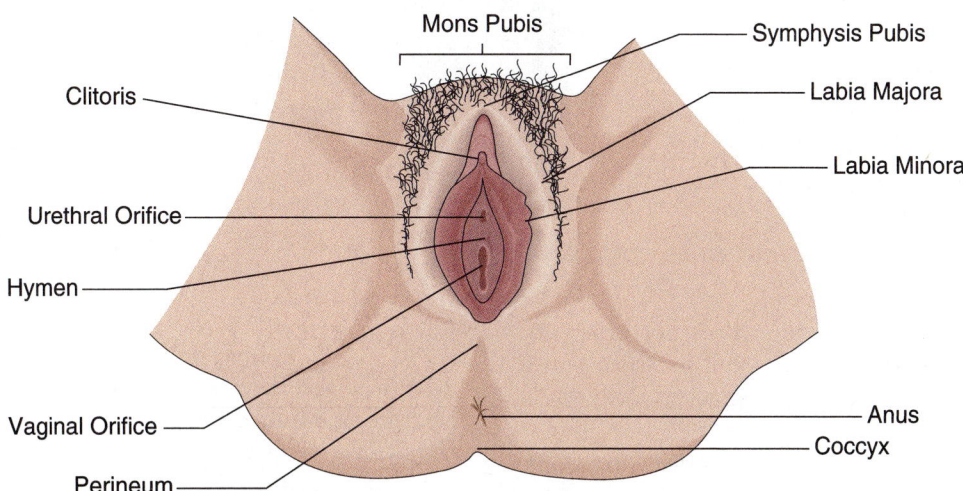

FIGURE 45-2 External female reproductive organs.

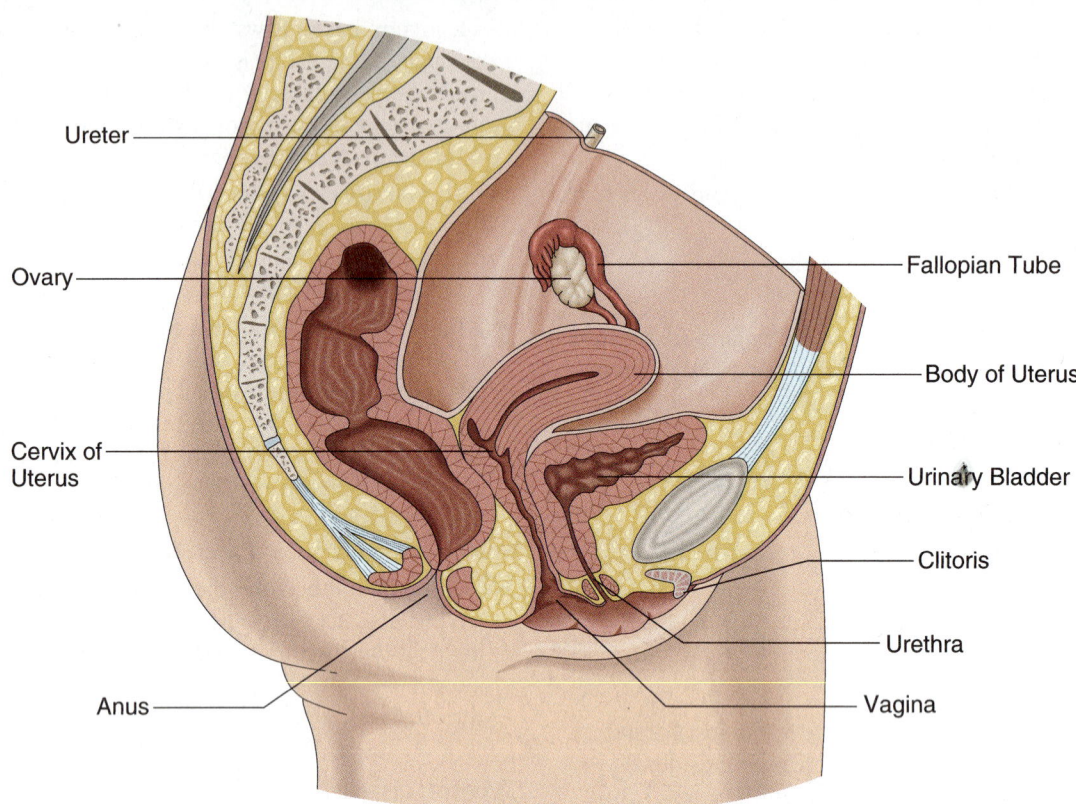

FIGURE 45-3 Cross-section of internal female reproductive system.

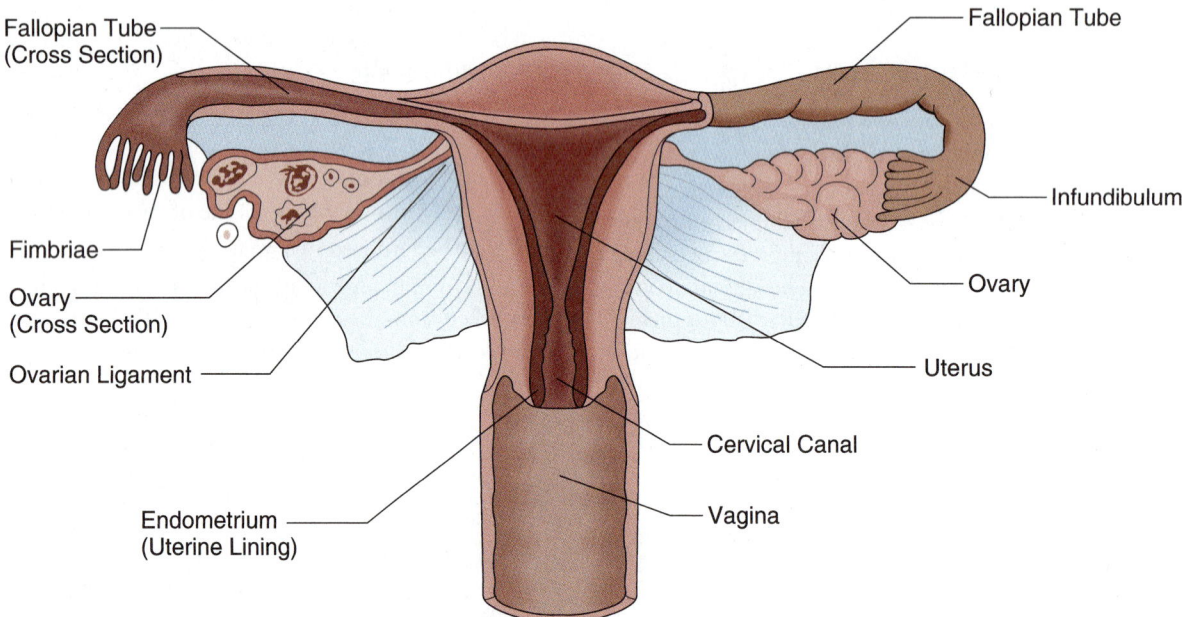

FIGURE 45-4 Anterior view of interior female reproductive organs.

the fertilized ovum. If fertilization does not occur, the endometrium is no longer needed, so it is carried out of the body as the menstrual flow. This process is known as **menstruation**.

Unlike the sperm cells, all the special cells that will become the ova exist when a woman is born. When the last ova are released, the menstrual cycle ceases and **menopause** begins.

Menopause

As women age, the menstrual cycle becomes irregular and gradually ceases altogether. This is called the menopause, or **climacteric**, or change of life.

Menopause usually occurs around the age of 55 and involves a natural series of changes that stops the menstrual cycle. These changes are not abrupt, but usually take place over a period of years. Because eggs are no longer being matured and released, pregnancy cannot occur.

Some women may undergo menopause earlier in life after surgical removal of the ovaries.

CONDITIONS OF THE MALE REPRODUCTIVE ORGANS

The male organs are subject to the same kinds of disease processes that affect other body parts. Examples of these conditions are tumors and infections. A very common problem experienced by many men involves the prostate gland.

Prostate Conditions

Benign prostatic (of the prostate gland) **hypertrophy** (Figure 45-5):

- is an enlargement of the prostate gland without tumor development.
- causes narrowing of the urethra, which passes through the center of the prostate gland.
- can cause sufficient enlargement to cause urinary retention.
- is noncancerous.

Signs and symptoms of prostate conditions include difficulty in starting the stream of urine or in emptying the bladder completely.

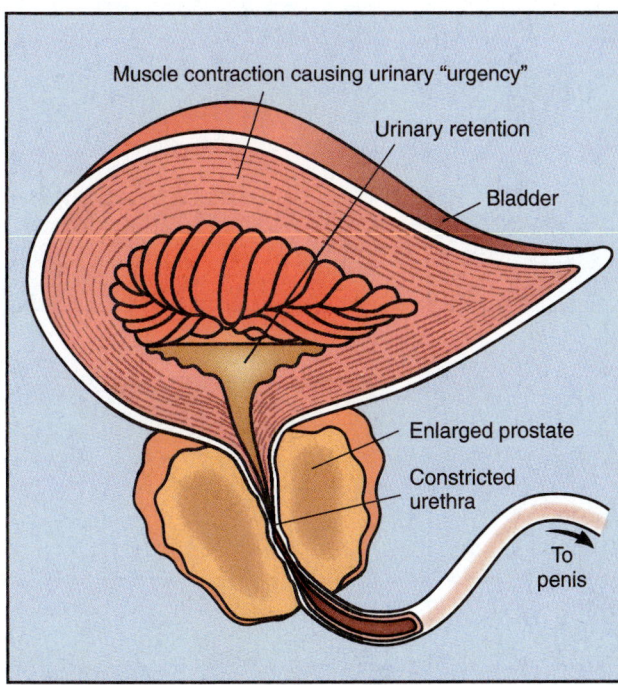

FIGURE 45-5 Cell growth causes the prostate to enlarge, constricting the urethra. The bladder may not empty completely, causing discomfort and increasing the risk of infection.

Prostate cancer is the second leading cause of cancer deaths in males. A blood test, the prostate specific antigen (PSA), is used to screen for abnormalities. Because of the widespread use of the blood test, many prostate cancers are caught early, and the outcome is usually favorable. Prostate cancer usually grows very slowly. In the early stages, there may be no symptoms. As the condition progresses, signs and symptoms develop. The most common are:

- difficulty with urination
- decreased force of the urine stream
- frequency of urination
- urgency (an intense need to urinate)
- urinary retention
- repeated urinary tract infections
- blood in the urine or semen

Treatment. Various surgical approaches are used to remove all or part of the prostate gland (**prostatectomy**) to relieve urinary retention.

- Transurethral prostatectomy (TURP)—only enough of the gland is removed, working from inside the urethra, to permit urine to pass.
- Perineal prostatectomy—the entire gland is removed through surgical incisions in the perineum.
- Suprapubic prostatectomy—an incision is made just above the pubis and part of the gland is removed.
- Radiation therapy consists of five to seven weeks of treatments in which radiation is directed to the prostate gland.
- **Brachytherapy** is another form of radiation therapy in which tiny radioactive seeds or pellets are implanted directly inside the prostate gland. This treatment is very successful and preferred over traditional radiation therapy because it has fewer side effects.
- Hormone therapy is used to treat some prostate cancers. This treatment suppresses the male sex hormone (testosterone) that stimulates the cancer to grow.

Patients are likely to be disturbed by the necessity of prostate surgery. Men often fear that they will not be able to have sexual intercourse after a prostatectomy. They feel that their manhood is threatened.

Urinary incontinence is also a common problem and a great concern. In most cases, the rate of leakage decreases over time. Nevertheless, incontinence has a substantial impact on quality of life.

Postsurgical Care. In addition to routine postoperative care, the prostatectomy patient:

- will have a Foley catheter in place following the surgery.
- may have a suprapubic drain through the suprapubic incision.
- may have a perineal drain in the perineal incision.

DIFFICULT *Situations*

After prostate surgery, the patient may have a three-way catheter with continuous irrigation. Inform the nurse if the bottle is low. Monitor the tubing for the presence of blood clots. Monitor the patient for signs of excess bleeding, cold or clammy skin, pallor, restlessness, falling blood pressure, or rapid pulse. If noted, report promptly.

The nursing assistant should:

- Wear personal protective equipment and apply the principles of standard precautions if contact with blood, body fluids, mucous membranes, or nonintact skin is likely.
- Be careful that the tubes do not become twisted, stressed, or dislodged when positioning the patient.
- Carefully note the amount and color of drainage from all areas.
- Report at once any sudden increase in bright redness or the appearance of clots that seem to block the tube.

- Report to the nurse if dressings become wet with urinary drainage.
- Be patient and understanding of the patient's emotional stress.
- Refer questions about possible sexual limitation and urinary incontinence to the nurse so that the patient can get information and support.

At times, it will be necessary to irrigate (wash out) the drainage tubes. This is a sterile procedure that will be carried out by the nurse or physician.

Cancer of the Testes

Cancer of the testes is fairly common. Treatment may require removal of the testicles (**orchiectomy**). This procedure is performed when there is testicular malignancy. When an early diagnosis is made, treatment can be started early. Orchiectomy can then be avoided.

Testicular self-examination (Figure 45-6) is an important way to locate lumps or changes in the testes. This procedure should be performed by all adult males:

- At least once each month
- During a warm shower so the scrotum will be relaxed
- With soapy fingers
- By palpating each testis between the fingers and thumb

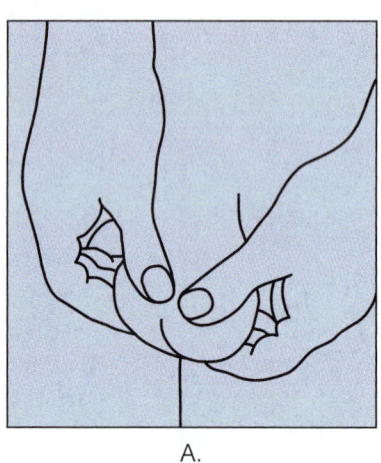

A.

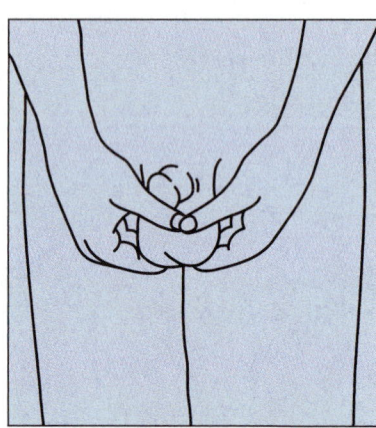

B.

FIGURE 45-6 TSE should be performed once a month after a warm bath or shower. The heat will relax the scrotum, making it easier to find abnormalities. A. Stand in front of the mirror. Look for swelling on the skin of the scrotum. B. Examine each testicle with both hands. Position your index and middle fingers under the testicle with the thumbs on top. Gently roll the testicle between your thumbs and fingers. (Having one testicle larger than the other is normal.) C. Find the epididymis (the soft, tubelike structure at the back of the testicle). Do not mistake the epididymis for an abnormal lump. D. If you find a lump, notify your doctor right away. Most lumps are found on the sides of the testicle, but some are located on the front. Testicular cancer is highly curable when detected early and treated promptly.

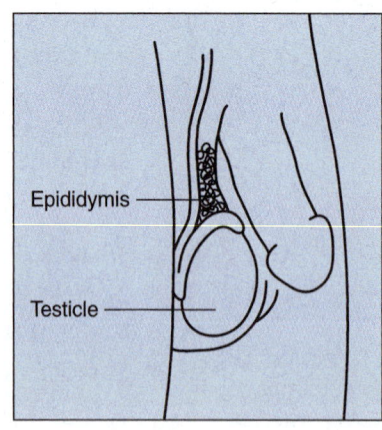

Epididymis

Testicle

C.

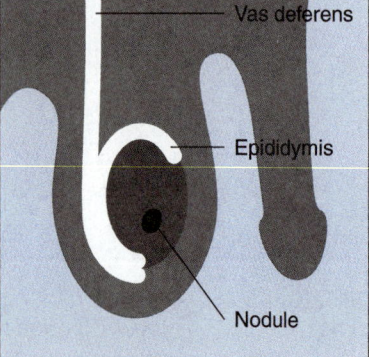

Vas deferens

Epididymis

Nodule

D.

CONDITIONS OF THE FEMALE REPRODUCTIVE ORGANS

Like the male organs, female reproductive organs are subject to disease processes, including tumors and infections.

Rectocele and Cystocele

Rectoceles and cystoceles are hernias. They usually occur at the same time.

- Rectoceles (Figure 45-7) are a weakening of the wall shared between the vagina and the rectum. These hernias frequently cause constipation and hemorrhoids (varicose veins of the rectum).
- Cystoceles (Figure 45-8) are a weakening of the muscles between the bladder and the vagina. Cystoceles cause urinary incontinence.

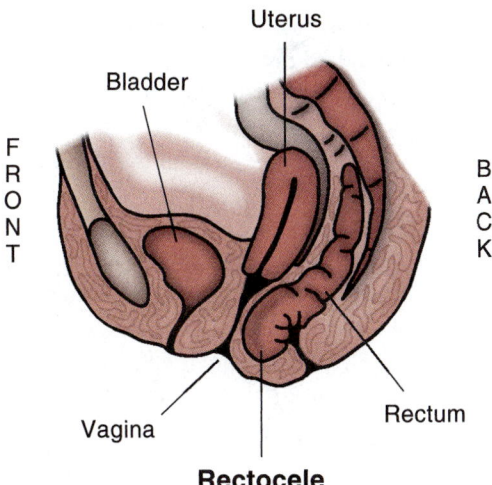

FIGURE 45-7 A rectocele causes the rectum to bulge into the vagina.

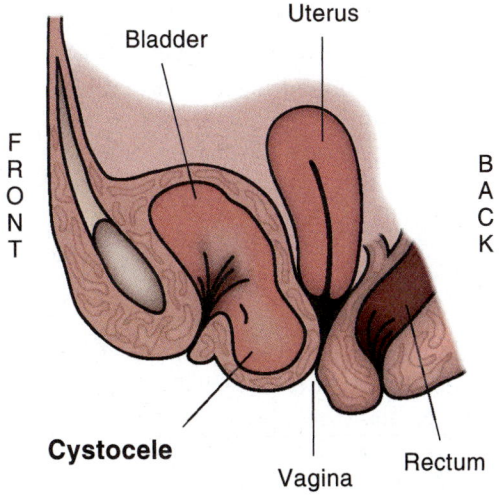

FIGURE 45-8 A cystocele causes the bladder to bulge into the vagina.

Treatment and Nursing Care. A surgical procedure called colporrhaphy tightens the vaginal walls.

In addition to routine postsurgical care, you may assist in:

- Applying ice packs
- Giving sitz baths
- Giving vaginal douches (irrigations) (see Procedure 127)
- Checking carefully for signs of excessive bleeding or foul discharge

Vulvovaginitis

Vulvovaginitis is most often caused by a fungal infection of *Candida albicans*.

- There is a thick, white, cheesy vaginal discharge.
- Inflammation and itching are intense.
- Douches are not given for this condition.
- Special drugs and creams are prescribed to fight the infection.

Tumors of Uterus and Ovaries

Benign and malignant tumors of the uterus and ovaries are frequent. Malignancies of the cervix are very common. The cure rate is very high if treated in time.

The most common indications of tumors of the uterus and ovaries are changes in the menstrual flow, such as:

- Menorrhagia (excessive flow)
- Amenorrhea (lack of menstrual flow)
- Dysmenorrhea (difficult or painful menstrual flow)
- Metrorrhagia (bleeding at completely irregular intervals)

Ovarian cancer is very dangerous because there are no symptoms until it is well advanced and has spread beyond the ovaries. Even then, the symptoms are often mild, such as bloating, and may be attributed to other problems. It usually cannot be detected by a pelvic examination. This cancer accounts for more deaths than any other cancer of the female reproductive system. The disease has a strong familial link, and is most common in women over age 50. Women who have never had children and those who have taken fertility drugs are also at high risk. Women who take birth control pills have a lower risk.

Signs and Symptoms of Ovarian Cancer. Signs and symptoms of ovarian cancer may include:

- abdominal discomfort and pain
- bloating
- nausea
- diarrhea
- frequent urination
- sudden weight gain or loss
- abnormal vaginal bleeding

Treatment. Several different types of procedures may be performed to treat tumors of the female reproductive tract, including chemotherapy, radiation, and surgery. Some surgical procedures are:

- Total hysterectomy—removal of the entire uterus, including the cervix.
- Oophorectomy—removal of an ovary. In younger women, at least a portion of the ovary is left to continue hormone production whenever possible.
- Salpingectomy—removal of a fallopian tube.
- Panhysterectomy—removal of the uterus and both ovaries and tubes. The surgical approach may be abdominal or vaginal. If a panhysterectomy is performed, the patient experiences surgically induced menopause. The more uncomfortable symptoms of menopause are usually relieved with hormone supplements.

Nonsurgical forms of treatment include:

- Radiation therapy, if cancer is present
- Chemotherapy, if cancer is present

Postoperative Care. In addition to the usual postoperative care, the care following a hysterectomy will include:

- caring for catheter drainage.
- possibly caring for a nasogastric tube, which may be in place to relieve abdominal distention and nausea.
- giving special attention to maintaining good circulation, because slowing of the blood supply to the pelvis may result in clot formation.
- introducing fluids and foods gradually after the initial nausea subsides.
- carefully observing the patient for low back pain.
- monitoring urine output and bleeding.
- checking both the abdominal incisional area and the vagina for presence and type of drainage.
- providing emotional support

Tumors of the Breast

Tumors, both benign and malignant, are commonly found in the breasts. Breast cancer is the second most common cancer in women. However, men can also develop breast cancer. Signs and symptoms of breast tumors include:

- Painless lump or mass
- Nipple discharge
- Retraction of nipple
- Scaly skin around nipple
- Dimpling of the skin
- Enlarged lymph nodes

Treatment. Mastectomy means removal of the breast. All or part of the breast tissue may be removed in a mastectomy.

- A simple mastectomy removes the breast tissue only.
- A radical mastectomy includes the breast tissue, underlying muscles, and the glands in the axillary area.

This procedure is not performed as often as it was previously.

- A lumpectomy removes the abnormal tissue and only a small amount of the breast tissue.

Nonsurgical forms of treatment include:

- radiation therapy
- chemotherapy
- hormonal chemotherapy, which blocks estrogen from entering the breast cancer cells

Any form of mastectomy requires a great deal of psychological adjustment for the patient. There is the fear of disfigurement and the fear of loss of femininity. Many excellent breast forms are now available to restore the outward physical appearance of the mastectomy patient. Breast implants are another way of restoring the physical form of the breast. There are also support groups to aid in the psychological adjustment.

Postoperative Care. In addition to routine postoperative care, you will:

- Wear personal protective equipment and apply the principles of standard precautions if contact with blood, body fluids, mucous membranes, or nonintact skin is likely.
- Avoid taking the blood pressure on the side where the surgery was done.
- Realize that because a large amount of blood can be lost during a mastectomy, transfusions are likely to be ordered. Monitor a blood transfusion as you would monitor an intravenous infusion.
- Check pressure dressings frequently for signs of excess bleeding.
- Check the bed linen, because blood may drain to the back of the dressing.
- Report immediately numbness or swelling in the arm of the operative side.
- Be ready to offer support; walking may be difficult for the patient, who may feel unbalanced.
- Offer your fullest emotional support.
- Assist the patient in rehabilitative exercises.
- Refer questions about disfigurement and loss of femininity to the nurse, who will see that the patient is provided with accurate information and support.

SEXUALLY TRANSMITTED DISEASE (STD)

Sexually transmitted diseases (STDs) affect both men and women. Although most sexually transmitted diseases can be treated and cured, patients do not develop immunity to repeated infections. It is possible to transmit the organisms causing STDs from:

- Mucous membrane to mucous membrane, such as from genitals to mouth or genitals

- Mucous membrane to skin, such as genitals to hands
- Skin to mucous membrane, such as hands to genitals

Using standard precautions correctly will protect the nursing assistant from contracting these diseases when caring for patients.

Any disease that is transmitted mainly in this way is an STD. There are many sexually transmitted diseases. Some are seen more commonly than others. It is important to realize that patients may:

- not always be aware that they have been infected.
- be too embarrassed to tell you about the problem.
- not realize the serious damage these infectious diseases can do to the body.

The most common sexually transmitted diseases are gonorrhea, herpes simplex II, and syphilis. Other sexually transmitted diseases are caused by chlamydia, human papilloma virus, HIV, and the trichomonas parasite.

Trichomonas Vaginitis

Trichomonas vaginitis is caused by a parasite, *Trichomonas vaginalis*. This condition:

- is sexually transmitted.
- may affect the male reproductive tract with no signs and symptoms.
- in females, causes a large amount of white, foul-smelling vaginal discharge called **leukorrhea**.
- can be controlled with medication.
- requires that both sex partners receive treatment.

Gonorrhea

Gonorrhea is a serious STD caused by the bacterium *Neisseria gonorrheae*. The disease causes an acute inflammation. In the male:

- Greenish-yellow discharge appears from the penis within two to five days after contact.
- There is burning on urination.
- The disease can spread throughout the reproductive tract, causing **sterility** (inability to reproduce).

In the female:

- 80% may have no signs or symptoms for quite a while. Thus, it is possible to spread the disease before the woman is aware of being infected.
- **Pelvic inflammatory disease** (**PID**) can lead to formation of abscesses and sterility.

It is important for all sex partners to be treated with antibiotics. When a pregnant woman has gonorrhea, her baby's eyes may be permanently damaged if they are contaminated by the disease during birth. As a preventive measure, all babies' eyes are routinely treated with silver nitrate drops or antibiotics shortly after birth.

Syphilis

Syphilis is caused by the microorganism *Treponema pallidum*. Both sexes show the same effects of the disease. If untreated, this disease passes through three stages.

1. First stage—a sore (**chancre**) develops within 90 days of exposure. The chancre heals without treatment. Because it is not painful, it may go entirely unnoticed.

2. Second stage—may be accompanied by a rash, sore throat, or other mild symptoms suggestive of a viral infection. Again, the signs and symptoms disappear without treatment. The disease is infectious during the first and second stages and may be transmitted to a sexual partner. By this time, the microorganisms have gained entrance into vital organs such as the heart, liver, brain, and spinal cord.

3. Third stage—permanent damage is done to vital organs, though the damage may not appear for many years.

An additional danger of syphilis during pregnancy is that the microorganism can attack the fetus, causing it to die or be seriously deformed.

Herpes

Herpes simplex II (genital herpes) is an infectious disease caused by the herpes simplex virus (Figure 45-9). It is transmitted primarily through direct sexual contact. The person who has herpes:

- may develop painful, red, blister-like sores on the reproductive organs.
- has sores that are associated with a burning sensation.
- usually has sores that heal in about two weeks.
- must remember that the fluid in the blisters is infectious.
- may transmit (shed) organisms even when an outbreak is not present.

People with the herpes infection may have only one episode or may have repeated attacks. In many cases, repeated attacks are milder. Individuals who have weakened immune systems often develop chronic cases of herpes (Figure 45-10). In addition to the local discomfort:

- There seems to be a greater incidence of cancer of the cervix and miscarriages among female sufferers than among women who do not have this condition.
- Newborn children can be infected when the mother gives birth.
- The baby of a mother with an active case of herpes simplex II is usually delivered by cesarean section.

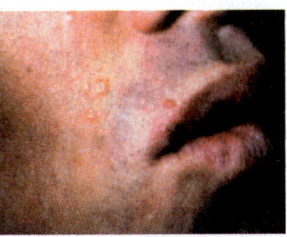

FIGURE 45-9 Oral herpes can be spread to the genital area, just as genital herpes can be spread to the mouth. *(Courtesy of Daniel J. Barbaro, MD, Fort Worth, Texas)*

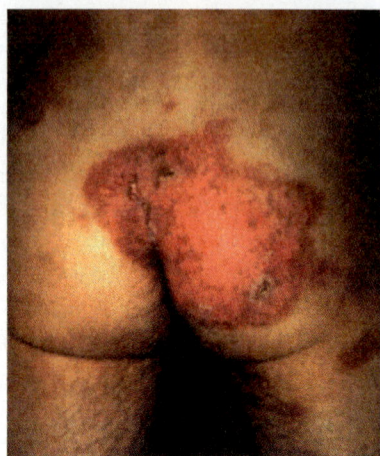

FIGURE 45-10
Chronic herpes in an AIDS patient. *(Courtesy of Daniel J. Barbaro, MD, Fort Worth, Texas)*

Because herpes is caused by a virus, there is no cure. Medications are available to stop the replication of the virus, which makes an outbreak subside more quickly. Topical creams are available to relieve discomfort and reduce the danger of spreading the infection.

Venereal Warts

Venereal warts are caused by a virus.

- Lesions develop on the genitals, on both skin and mucous membranes.
- The warts are cauliflower-shaped, raised, and darkened.
- They may be removed by ointments or surgery but often recur.
- They may cause discomfort during intercourse and may cause bleeding when dislodged.
- Warts predispose the patient to development of cancerous changes.
- Venereal warts are one of the most rapidly growing forms of STD.

Chlamydia Infection

Chlamydia are small infectious organisms that can invade mucous membranes of the body. These organisms can be:

- Introduced into the eyes, infecting the conjunctiva. This causes inflammation (conjunctivitis) and a more serious condition called trachoma. Trachoma can lead to blindness.
- Sexually transmitted; this commonly causes infections of the reproductive tract.
- The cause of serious pelvic inflammatory disease (PID), with scarring and even systemic infections. The scarring can result in sterility.
- Responsible for signs and symptoms similar to those of gonorrhea, except that the discharge is usually yellow to whitish in color.
- Treated with antibiotics.

Patients with pelvic infections are usually checked for gonorrhea. If they are found negative for gonorrhea, they are frequently diagnosed as having nongonorrheal urethritis (NGU) or nonspecified urethritis (NSU), because many different organisms may cause the infection. However, chlamydia organisms are the most common cause.

Human Immunodeficiency Virus (HIV) Disease

HIV is a viral disease. It is transmitted primarily through direct contact with the bodily secretions of an infected person. Therefore, it can be transmitted through direct sexual contact. HIV disease destroys the immune system. There is no cure for this condition, although drugs can slow the damage to the body. If the disease progresses, the immune system is severely weakened. This stage of HIV disease is called AIDS (acquired immune deficiency syndrome). A complete discussion of this disease is found in Unit 12.

DIAGNOSTIC TESTS

Techniques used to diagnose problems of the reproductive system include:

- Cultures for microorganisms.
- Urinalysis for hormone levels.
- **Pap smear**—test using cells from the cervix to detect possible cancer of the cervix. The test:
  - is painless.
  - can be performed in the physician's office during the routine pelvic examination.
  - should be done regularly.
- **Dilatation and curettage (D & C)**—a surgical procedure used to help diagnose conditions of the uterus, including tumors. In a D & C, the opening of the cervix is stretched open (dilated) and the uterus is scraped with a surgical instrument known as a curette.
- **Biopsy** (examining a sample of living tissue) is used to make a diagnosis. The biopsy sample is obtained through a needle. The procedure may be performed in the physician's office or in the hospital.
- Blood tests for cancer of the prostate.
- MRI and CT scans to help define the presence and extent of tumors.
- Ultrasound, a painless diagnostic tool that uses sound waves to diagnose ovarian cancer and other tumors.
- Cystoscopy—used to evaluate prostate conditions.
- Self-examination.

  Breast self-examination should be performed:
  - by all adult females (see Procedure 126).
  - each month on the last day of the menstrual flow.
  - on one selected day of the month, after menopause.
  - Faithfully in a routine manner.

  Testicular self-examination should be performed:
  - by all adult males.
  - at least once each month.

- during a warm shower so the scrotum will be relaxed.
- with soapy fingers.
- by palpating each testis between the fingers and thumb.
- Mammography—x-rays of the breasts. A mammogram:
  - can identify the presence of tumors up to two years before the tumor can be felt during self-examination.

- Should be performed when the woman is between the ages of 35 and 40 years, to provide a baseline evaluation.
- Thereafter, should be performed every one to two years until age 50.
- Should be performed yearly after age 50.

PROCEDURE 126

BREAST SELF-EXAMINATION

1. Disrobe above the waist and stand or sit in front of a mirror. Observe breasts for changes in shape or size (Figure 45-11A).

 Note: *Some women prefer to perform breast self-examination standing in the shower.*

2. Raise arms above your head and clasp your hands (Figure 45-11B). Press inward with your hands while observing your breasts. Note any "dimpling" of the breast tissue.

3. Fold a small towel.

4. Lie on the bed with the towel under your right shoulder.

5. Flex your right arm and bring it over your head.

6. With the fingers of the left hand, examine the right breast (Figure 45-11C).
   - Use your fingertips.
   - Use a rolling motion.
   - Start at the nipple and work around the entire breast so that all tissue is examined (Figure 45-11D).

7. Examine the right axilla in the same way.

8. Repeat the procedure with the opposite breast and axilla.

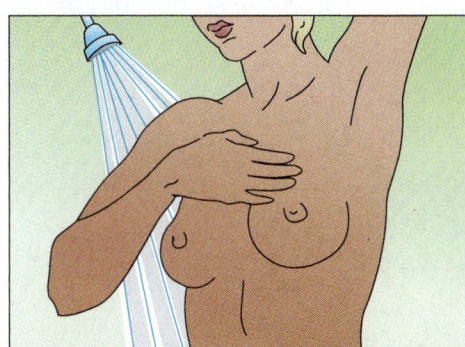
A

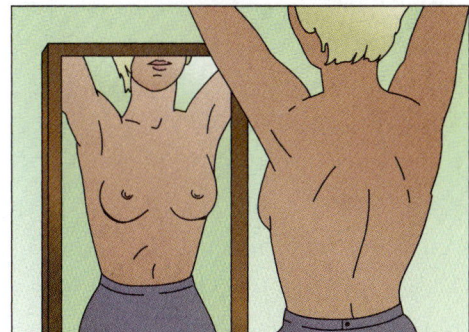
B

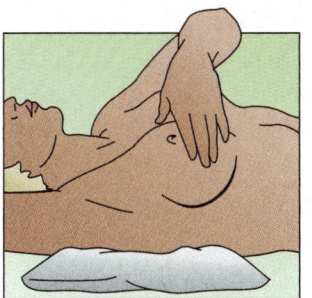 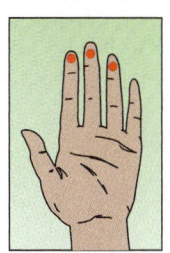
C

Finger pads

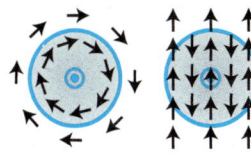 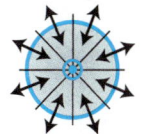
D

FIGURE 45-11 Breast self-examination. Each breast is examined systematically. A. With the fingers flat, check for a knot, lump, or thickening. B. Raise your arms and compare breast shape. C. Lie down with a small pillow under the shoulder and one arm behind the head. Check again for any knot, lump, or thickening. Move your fingers in a circular motion, inward toward the nipple. Use the pads of the fingers. D. Direction of motion of fingers over breast during examination. *(Courtesy of the American Cancer Society)*

VAGINAL DOUCHE

A vaginal **douche** is an irrigation of the vagina with fluid or medication. It is done by physician's order.

A vaginal douche requires standard precautions. When a douche is given to administer medications, it is given by the nurse. Other douches may be given by the nursing assistant if it is the policy of the facility. Be sure to check. Vaginal douches are given to:

- Remove odor or foul discharge
- Stop bleeding
- Relieve inflammation and pain
- Neutralize vaginal secretions
- Disinfect the vagina
- Cleanse the vagina before surgery or examination
- Administer antiseptic drugs

PROCEDURE 127

GIVING A NONSTERILE VAGINAL DOUCHE

1. Carry out beginning procedure actions.

2. Assemble equipment:
   - disposable gloves
   - disposable douche
   - bed protector
   - toilet tissue
   - bath blanket
   - cotton balls
   - disinfectant
   - cup
   - irrigating standard
   - bedpan and cover
   - plastic bag

3. Pour a small amount of the specified disinfecting solution over the cotton balls in the cup.

4. Measure water into the douche container. The temperature should be about 105°F. Add powder or solution as ordered.

5. Hang the douche bag on the standard. Close the clamp on the tubing. Leave the protector on the sterile tip.

6. Place a bed protector on the chair and assemble equipment where you can reach it. Screen the unit.

7. Elevate the bed to a comfortable working height and put up the side rails for safety.

8. Wash your hands and put on gloves. Lower the side rail on the working side.

9. Assist the patient into the dorsal recumbent position.

10. Place a bed protector beneath the patient's buttocks.

11. Remove the perineal pad (if used) from front to back and discard it in a plastic bag.

12. Drape the patient with a bath blanket (Figure 45-12). Fanfold top bedding to the foot of the bed.

13. Place a bedpan under the patient and ask her to void. Follow facility policies for emptying bedpan, if necessary.

14. Cleanse the patient's perineum.
    - Use one cotton ball with disinfectant for each stroke.
    - Cleanse from the vulva toward the anus.
    - Cleanse the labia majora first.

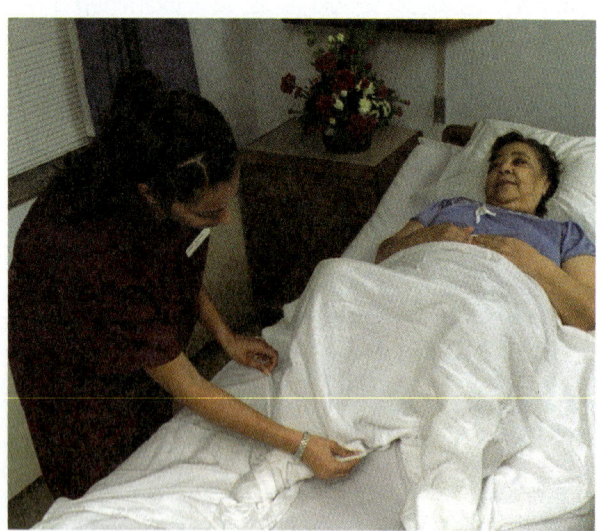

FIGURE 45-12 Drape the patient.

continues

PROCEDURE 127

continued

- Expose the labia minora with your thumb and forefinger and cleanse.
- Give special attention to folds.
- Discard used cotton balls in a plastic bag.

15. Replace the bedpan, if necessary. Position the patient in the dorsal recumbent position and readjust the bath blanket, if necessary. Elevate the head slightly for comfort, if desired.

16. Open the clamp to expel air. Remove the protector from the sterile tip of the disposable douche.

17. Allow a small amount of solution to flow over the inner thigh and then over the vulva. Do not touch the vulva with the nozzle.

18. Allow solution to continue to flow and insert the nozzle slowly and gently into the vagina, with an upward and backward movement, for about 3 inches.

19. Rotate the nozzle from side to side as solution flows.

20. When all solution has been given, remove the nozzle slowly and clamp the tubing.

21. Have the patient sit up on the bedpan to allow all the solution to return.

22. Remove the douche bag from the standard and place it on the bed protector.

23. Dry the perineum with tissue. Discard used tissue in the bedpan.

24. Cover the bedpan and place it on the bed protector on the chair.

25. Have the patient turn on her side. Dry her buttocks with tissue.

26. Place a clean pad over the vulva from front to back. Do not touch the inside of the pad.

27. Remove the bed protector and bath blanket. Replace with top bedding.

28. Observe the contents of the bedpan. Note the character and amount of discharge, if any. Discard the contents of the bedpan according to facility policy. Care for equipment according to facility policy. Remove gloves and dispose of them according to facility policy. Wash your hands.

29. Carry out procedure completion actions.

REVIEW

A. True/False.

Mark the following true or false by circling T or F.

1. T F D & C is a surgical procedure that can help establish a diagnosis related to the female reproductive system.

2. T F Following a panhysterectomy, you should check the patient for increased bleeding.

3. T F Salpingectomy means removal of the ovaries.

4. T F Foul-smelling leukorrhea is associated with the condition called trichomonas vaginitis.

5. T F The female with gonorrhea may not know she has been infected with the disease.

6. T F Untreated gonorrhea passes through three stages.

7. T F Syphilis is caused by a bacterium.

8. T F AIDS may be sexually transmitted.

9. T F The discharge in gonorrhea is white and very irritating.

B. Matching.

Choose the correct term from Column II to match each phrase in Column I.

Column I	Column II
10. _____ inability to reproduce	**a.** dysmenorrhea
11. _____ inflammation of the vagina	**b.** mastectomy
12. _____ painful menstruation	**c.** circumcision
13. _____ removal of a breast	**d.** leukorrhea
14. _____ whitish discharge	**e.** sterility
	f. vaginitis

C. Multiple Choice.

Select the one best answer for each of the following.

15. You are to give a nonsterile douche. You will remember to
  a. place the patient in a high Fowler's position.
  b. use a solution with a temperature of about 115°F.
  c. insert the nozzle about 3 inches into the vagina.
  d. allow the nozzle to touch the vulva.

16. Breast self-examination should be performed
  a. daily.
  b. weekly.
  c. monthly.
  d. yearly.

17. Your patient has just returned from a suprapubic prostatectomy. You know that
  a. there will be no incision.
  b. there will be a Foley catheter drain.
  c. the patient must be assisted to void every 2 hours.
  d. the patient will be NPO for 2 to 3 days.

18. Testicular self-examination should be
  a. done daily.
  b. performed while lifting the commode.
  c. performed with soapy fingers.
  d. performed only by males over age 50.

D. Completion.

Complete the following statements.

19. The type of precautions to be used when caring for patients with STD is _____.

20. Women over the age of 50 should have a mammogram _____.

21. Breast self-examination should be performed
_____.

E. Nursing Assistant Challenge.

Mrs. Forstein is 39 and has been admitted for a large pelvic mass. Her doctor suspects that she has a large tumor in her left ovary. She has experienced menorrhagia, dysmenorrhea, and pelvic pain. She is scheduled for an oophorectomy after tests are complete.

Briefly answer the following questions:

22. How else might you have described her menorrhagia and dysmenorrhea?

23. Does the doctor plan to remove the entire uterus, including the cervix?

24. What type of pain would be very significant following surgery?

25. What two areas would you check for drainage?

26. Why is it so important to maintain good circulation postoperatively?

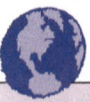 **EXPLORING THE WEB**

Description	Location
Andropause (Men's Health)	http://www.andropausecanada.com
Dr. Donnica's Woman's Health	http://www.drdonnica.com
Gynecologic Health Center	http://www.womens-health.com
Health Scout Men's and Women's Health Centers	http://www.healthscout.com
HIV Insite	http://hivinsite.ucsf.edu
HIV Positive	http://www.hivpositive.com
InterNational Council on Infertility Information Dissemination	http://www.inciid.org
The Hormone Foundation (Men's Health)	http://www.hormone.org
Johns Hopkins AIDS Service	http://www.inciid.org
Menopause Online	http://www.menopause-online.com

continues

EXPLORING THE WEB   *continued*

Description	Location
National Center for HIV, STD, and TB Prevention	*http://www.cdc.gov/nchstp/dstd/dstdp.html*
National Library of Medicine HIV Resources	*http://www.hivpositive.com*
National Women's Health Resource Center	*http://www.healthywomen.org*
New York Times Men's Health Center	*http://www.nytimes.com*
New York Times Women's Health Center	*http://www.nytimes.com*
Not for Men Only—The Male Health Center Education Site	*http://www.malehealthcenter.com*
Project Inform	*http://www.projinf.org*
University of Michigan Prostate Cancer Program	*http://www.cancer.med.umich.edu*

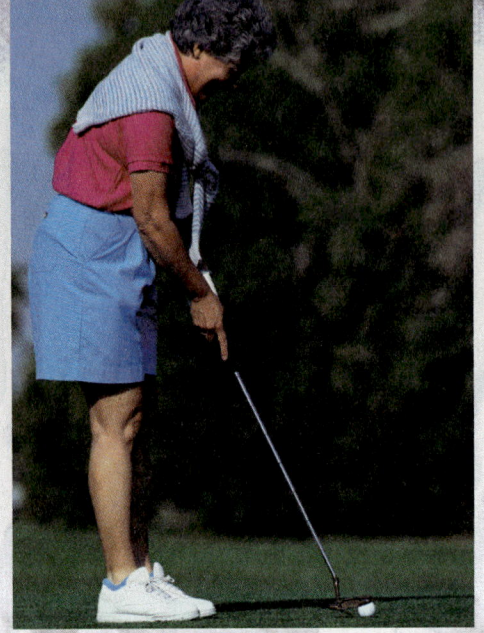

Caring for the Patient with Cancer

objectives

After completing this unit, you will be able to:

- Spell and define terms.
- List methods of reducing the risk of cancer.
- Explain the importance of good nutrition in cancer prevention and treatment.

- List seven signs and symptoms of cancer.
- Describe three types of cancer treatment.
- Describe nursing assistant responsibilities when caring for patients with cancer.

vocabulary

Learn the meaning and the correct spelling of the following words and phrases:

benign	carcinogen	malignant	radiation therapy
biopsy	chemotherapy	metastasis	
cancer	immunotherapy	palliative care	

INTRODUCTION

Cancer is a disease in which the normal mechanisms of cell growth are disturbed. Cells grow abnormally, invade surrounding tissues, and use oxygen and nutrition intended for normal cells. Cancers that stay in one location and do not spread are benign. Benign cancers usually grow slowly. Some types of cancer cells spread to other parts of the body through the blood and lymphatic systems. This is called metastasis. When metastasis occurs, a tumor will eventually grow in another area. Cancers that spread to other parts of the body are malignant. Many patients die from metastasis instead of the original tumor. Some malignant cancers spread very rapidly. A carcinogen is a substance that causes cancer. Tobacco is one common carcinogen. The incidence of cancer and death rates vary with geographic location, sex, race, and age.

Risk Factors

Many factors increase the risk of developing cancer. Some cancers tend to be genetic. This means they run in families. Breast cancer, ovarian cancer, and pancreatic cancer are examples of cancers that seem to have a hereditary component. Other common risk factors for cancer are:

- Age—this is the most common risk, with most cancers occurring in persons over the age of 55
- Lifestyle and habits:
  - smoking (Figure 46-1) and using smokeless or chewing tobacco
  - alcohol consumption
  - diet
- Family history, genetics
- Environmental pollution

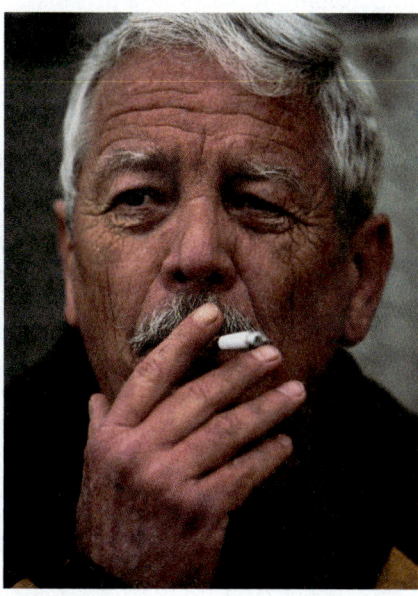

FIGURE 46-1 Lifestyle and habits such as cigarette smoking increase the risk of cancer.

- Harmful substances in the environment
  - asbestos
  - benzene
- Chemicals
- Radiation
- Prolonged sun exposure
- Infections and some viruses

Nutrition and Cancer

There is a direct relationship between intake of certain foods and the development of certain types of cancers. Table 46-1 lists various types of cancers and their relationship to certain food items. Obesity is associated with cancer of the gallbladder, uterus, colon, and breast. The American Cancer Society recommends following the food guide pyramid. These dietary guidelines will help prevent cancer:

- No more than 30% of total calories from fat
- Total cholesterol from diet should not exceed 300 mg a day
- At least 55% of total calories should come from complex carbohydrates, such as fruit, vegetables, cereals, and grains
- Salt from all food sources should not exceed 1 teaspoon a day

TABLE 46-1 CANCER AND FOOD	
Type of Cancer	**Relationship to Food**
Breast	High-fat diet
Prostate	High-fat diet
Colon	High-fat diet, low intake of fruits and vegetables, low fiber, low intake of complex carbohydrates
Esophagus	Low intake of fruits and vegetables, low fiber, low intake of complex carbohydrates, salt-cured foods; also drinking alcoholic beverages
Bladder	Low intake of fruits and vegetables, low fiber, low intake of complex carbohydrates
Stomach	Low intake of fruits and vegetables, low fiber, low intake of complex carbohydrates, high intake of salt-cured food
Larynx	Low intake of fruits and vegetables, low fiber, low intake of complex carbohydrates
Lung	Low intake of fruits and vegetables, low fiber, low intake of complex carbohydrates

CANCER PREVENTION AND DETECTION

The American Cancer Society recommends certain lifestyle changes and preventive measures. These include:

- not smoking
- limiting the intake of alcoholic beverages
- following the food guide pyramid and eating a healthy diet
- regular exercise (Figure 46-2)
- maintaining a healthy weight
- avoiding sun exposure, particularly between 10:00 AM and 3:00 PM.
- getting genetic testing and counseling if at risk for familial cancers

Some patients take various drugs to reduce the risk of cancer. Natural substances, such as vitamin E and selenium, are being researched for their cancer prevention properties.

Signs and Symptoms of Cancer

Each type of cancer has its own signs and symptoms. General signs and symptoms that may indicate cancer spell the word CAUTION:

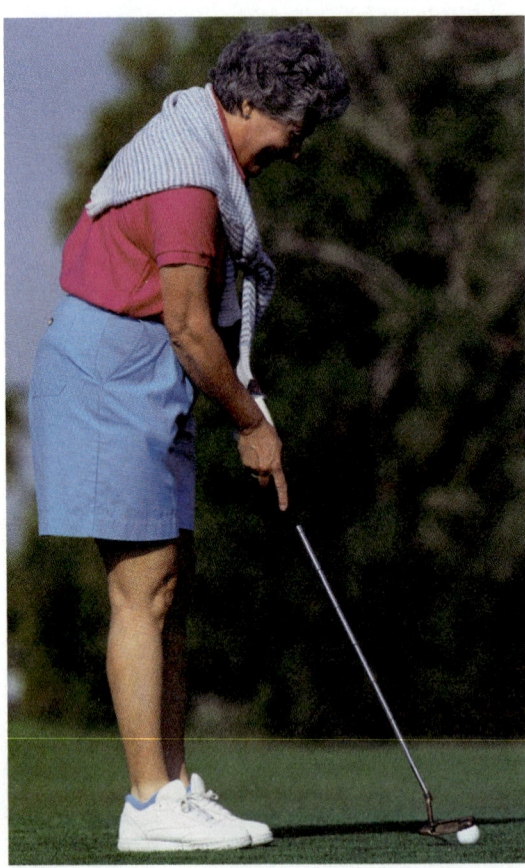

FIGURE 46-2 Regular exercise reduces the risk of cancer and many other diseases.

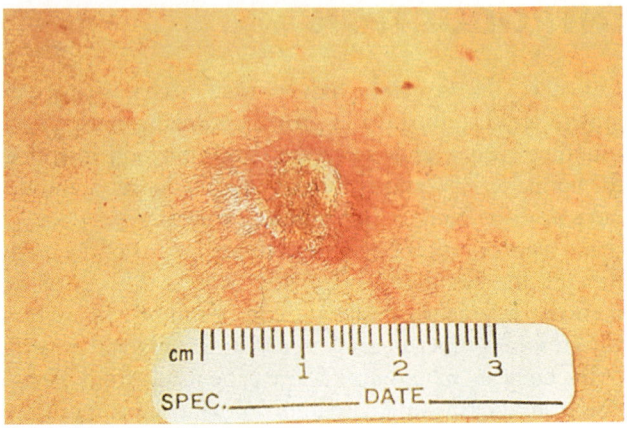

FIGURE 46-3 A sore that does not heal should be examined by the doctor.

C = Change in bowel or bladder habits

A = A sore that does not heal (Figure 46-3)

U = Unusual bleeding or discharge

T = Thickening or lump in the breast, testicles, or any part of the body

I = Indigestion or difficulty swallowing

O = Obvious change in a wart, mole, or skin condition (Figure 46-4)

N = Nagging cough or hoarseness

People with one or more of these warning signs should see a doctor right away.

Screening

Regular screening (Figure 46-5) for cancer is a key to survival, because the outcome is better if the disease is detected early. Many different professional organizations have guidelines for cancer screening. These vary slightly from one group to the next. Screening is based on a person's age, gender, risk factors, family history, ethnicity, and history of exposure to carcinogens in the environment. Some personal

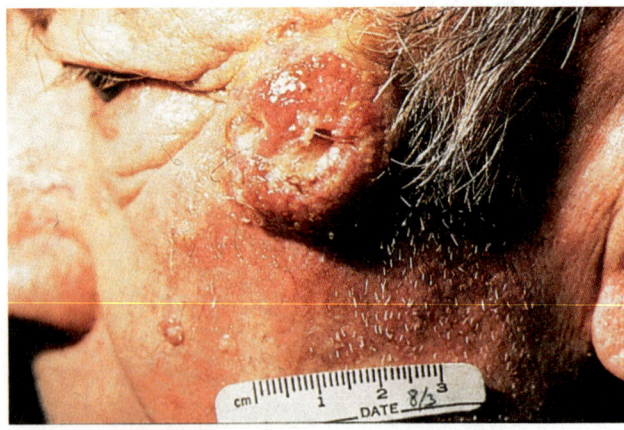

FIGURE 46-4 Change in a wart or mole warrants further investigation.

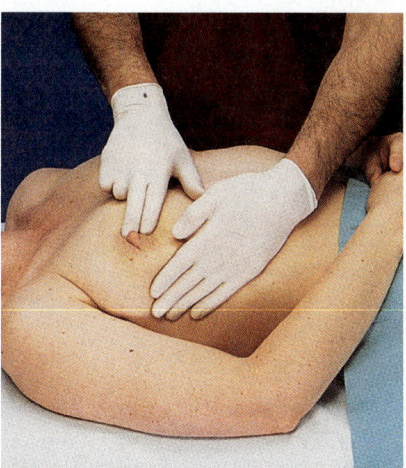

FIGURE 46-5 Regular health screening and early cancer detection are key to survival.

screening tests are recommended monthly, such as breast self-examination for women and testicular self-examination for men. Other routine screening tests are done by physicians. Examples of screening recommendations are listed in Table 46-2.

TREATMENT

Many different treatments are used for cancer. In addition, some people use alternative and complementary therapies. The type of treatment is determined by:

- the type of cancer
- location of the cancer
- whether the cancer is malignant
- the stage (how advanced the cancer is)
- general condition of the patient

Surgery

A **biopsy** is a minor surgery that is sometimes done to diagnose a cancer. A biopsy involves removing a small piece of tissue from a suspicious area. The tissue is sent for laboratory examination. If the biopsy is positive for cancerous cells, a surgical procedure is done with the goal of completely removing the cancer. This may involve removing all or part of an organ, such as a lung, breast, or the uterus. Lymph nodes in the area may also be removed. The surgeon removes as much cancerous tissue as possible.

TABLE 46-2 SCREENING RECOMMENDATIONS

Location	Screening Test	Age	Frequency of Test
Breast	Mammogram	35–39	Baseline examination
Breast	Mammogram	40 and over	Yearly
Prostate	Rectal exam PSA blood test	50 and over	Yearly
Testicular	Exam by doctor	15 and over	Yearly
Colon/rectal	Digital rectal exam Fecal occult blood test	40 and over	Yearly
Colon/rectal	Sigmoidoscopy	50 and over	Every 3 years
Colon/rectal	Colonoscopy	50 and over	Every 5 years
Cervix	Pap smear	18 and over or at onset of sexual activity	Yearly
Skin	Skin examination	20–39	Every 3 years
Skin	Skin examination	over 40	Yearly
Mouth	Oral examination	20–39	Every 3 years
Mouth	Oral examination	over 40	Yearly

If removing the entire cancerous area is not possible, a portion is left and is usually treated with other methods. Reconstructive surgery may be done for cosmetic repair of an area. Sometimes this is done early, or even with the initial surgery. Other times reconstruction is done long after the original surgery. An example of reconstructive surgery is breast reconstruction. Preventive surgery may involve a radical procedure that is done when there is a strong genetic link to cancer. For example, the breasts or ovaries may be removed because of a high risk of developing cancer. Preventive surgery is also done to remove areas, such as rectal polyps, that may develop into cancer later.

Chemotherapy

Chemotherapy uses medications or drugs to destroy the cancer. Unfortunately, healthy cells may also be destroyed. The goals of chemotherapy vary, depending on the type of cancer, stage, and situation. Goals might be to:

- completely eliminate the cancer.
- control and slow the growth of cancer to prolong the patient's life.
- reduce the size of the cancer to eliminate pain and improve quality of life.

Chemotherapy is given by many different routes. Some patients are able to take oral medications. Others must receive the drugs in the muscles, veins, or other organs and body cavities. If the drugs are given intravenously, a central intravenous catheter (Figure 46-6) is often inserted to avoid repeated needlesticks and reduce the risk of vein irritation and collapse. Chemotherapy drugs are very potent and can irritate the skin, eyes, and mucous membranes of caregivers. Because of this, special measures are used to handle the drugs. Never eat, drink, or chew gum in an area where chemotherapy is being prepared. If you accidentally contact a chemotherapy drug with your hands or mucous membranes, flush well with water and seek medical atten-

tion. These drugs and the containers they are dispensed in require special handling and disposal.

Side Effects of Chemotherapy. Chemotherapy targets rapidly regenerating cells, such as cancer cells. The drugs cannot differentiate cancer cells from normal cells, so other cells that regenerate rapidly may also be affected. Other cells in the body that are commonly affected are:

- blood cells, such as red blood cells, white blood cells, and platelets
- hair and nail cells
- gastrointestinal cells

Side effects of cancer drugs can range from mild to life-threatening. Patients receiving these drugs need special monitoring. Sometimes the dose and scheduling must be changed to reduce side effects. Common side effects are:

- Alopecia (hair loss). This commonly starts within two weeks after chemotherapy begins. It may take up to five or six months to regrow the hair.
- Nausea and vomiting, depending on the drugs used. Sometimes nausea occurs immediately, but it may be delayed until several days after the drug is given.
- Anorexia, or loss of appetite. This sometimes occurs because the drugs cause changes in the tastebuds. In other patients, loss of appetite is due to nausea.
- Anemia, a deficiency of the red blood cells. This is caused by changes in the body due to the chemotherapy drugs. Sometimes special medications are given to reverse the anemia.
- Fatigue. Patients often become very tired. Anemia and reduced number of red blood cells are the most likely cause.
- Low white blood cell count, which increases the risk of infection. This usually starts within a week of the beginning of therapy, and it may last a long time. Precautions are taken to prevent exposure to infection.
- A reduction in the number of platelets in the blood, which increases the risk of bleeding. Precautions must be taken to prevent injury.
- Destruction of the mucous membranes of the mouth. This causes burning, pain, redness, and breakdown inside the mouth.

Many other side effects are caused by chemotherapy drugs. The nurse will advise you what to watch for in each patient.

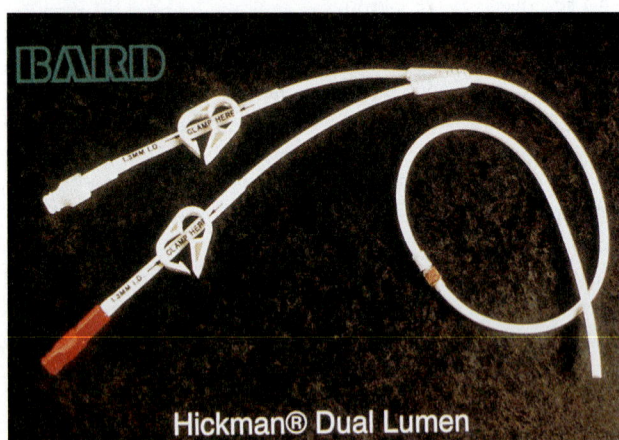

FIGURE 46-6 The central intravenous catheter is commonly inserted to deliver intravenous chemotherapy. *(Photo provided by Bard Access Systems. Hickman™ is a registered trademark of Bard Access Systems)*

DIFFICULT *Situations*

Monitor the chemotherapy patient for bruising and abnormal skin lesions. Inform the nurse promptly if fever is present. Encourage fluids of the patient's choice, as tolerated.

Disposal of Body Fluids and Wastes. Patients receiving chemotherapy may excrete the drugs in their waste and body fluids. Discard gloves and other protective apparel, if worn, in a leakproof container. Follow facility policies for discarding PPE in a biohazardous waste or other contaminated area. Because the drugs are excreted in body waste, linens that have contacted blood, body fluids, or excretions require special handling. Wear gloves when handling linen, and always apply the principles of standard precautions. Soiled items should be put in specially marked bags before you send them to the laundry.

Special Care of the Chemotherapy Patient. Observe chemotherapy patients for side effects of the drugs and report any possible problems to the nurse promptly. Provide nursing comfort measures, such as good mouth care and daily bathing. Routinely take precautions to prevent injuries and infection. For example, you may be instructed to remind the patient to cough and deep breathe to keep the lungs clear. You may be asked to take vital signs every 4 hours. Rectal temperatures should not be taken in some patients. Check with the nurse before taking a rectal temperature. Report a fever over 101°F or chilling to the nurse immediately. Other signs of infection to report are:

- swelling, redness, or irritation inside the mouth
- rectal pain or tenderness
- change in bowel or bladder habits
- pain or burning on urination
- redness, swelling, open area, or pain on the skin
- cough or shortness of breath
- decreased level of consciousness
- decreased urine output
- warm, flushed, dry skin
- hypotension (below 100/60, or as instructed)

Because of the risk of bleeding, patients may have to take special precautions, such as blowing the nose gently and using an electric razor. A very soft toothbrush will probably be necessary. Special mouthwash products may be ordered. The care plan and the nurse will provide special directions.

Promoting good nutrition and hydration is very important. You may be asked to serve the patient six small meals a day. High-protein drinks may also be ordered. Encourage fluids, and record intake and output, including emesis. Alternate periods of rest with periods of activity, to reduce fatigue. Plan your care to allow frequent rest periods. Inform the nurse if the patient:

- has nausea or vomiting
- is not eating or drinking
- complains of changes in the tastebuds, affecting the ability or desire to eat
- constipation or diarrhea
- has white patches or unusual areas inside the mouth (Figure 46-7)
- complains of signs of a vaginal infection
- develops bruising or bleeding (Figure 46-8)

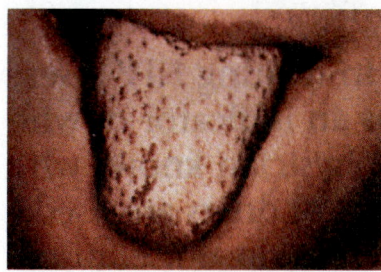

FIGURE 46-7
Monitor for and report white patches in the mouth to the nurse. *(Courtesy of Daniel J. Barbaro, MD, Fort Worth, Texas)*

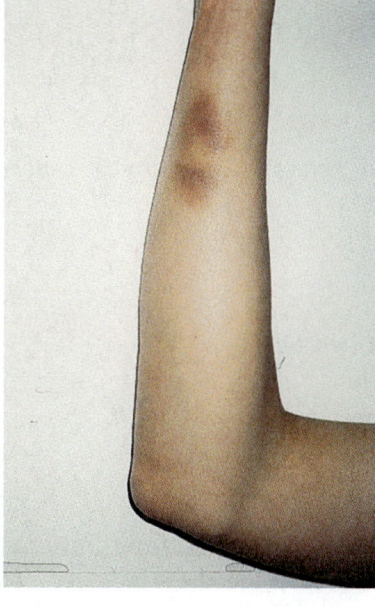

FIGURE 46-8
Report bruises to the nurse promptly.

Because the chemotherapy drugs are so toxic, you must observe the patient closely when he or she is receiving them. Inform the nurse promptly if:

- there are signs of intravenous (IV) infiltration, such as redness, swelling, or pain at the needle insertion site
- change in mental status
- change in vital signs

Assisting the Patient with Body Image. Cancer surgery and chemotherapy may change body appearance. This is often very upsetting to the patient. Hair loss may be especially traumatic, particularly in females. Be calm and reassuring. The hair will grow back, although the color or texture may be different. Assist the patient to wear a turban, scarf, or wig, if desired.

Radiation Therapy

Radiation therapy involves the use of high-energy, ionizing beams at the site of the cancer (Figure 46-9). The objective is to destroy the cancerous tissue without damaging healthy tissue. Several different types of radiation therapy may be used. Common side effects of radiation that should be reported to the nurse are:

- fatigue
- nausea, vomiting

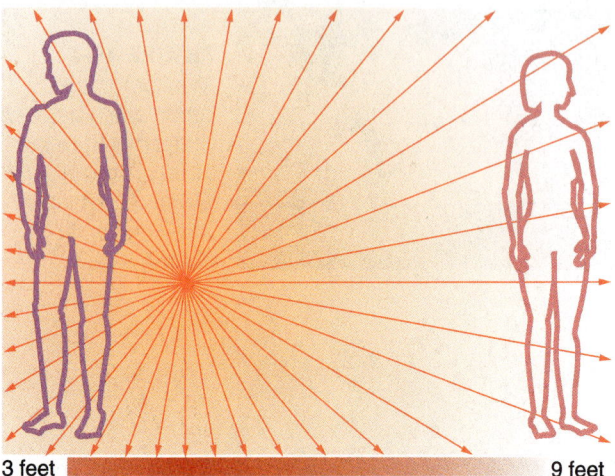

FIGURE 46-9 Radiation therapy is used to treat certain cancers.

- diarrhea
- skin redness, irritation, peeling
- change in ability to taste
- irritation of mucous membranes
- cough
- shortness of breath

Special Care of the Radiation Therapy Patient.
The patient may have markings on the skin at the site where radiation is delivered. Do not wash these off. The radiation may be very irritating to the patient's skin. Check the skin daily for problems and report them to the nurse, if found. Special skin care may be listed on the care plan. You may be instructed to:

- wash the patient with lukewarm water and mild soap; in some situations no soap is used.
- avoid rubbing or creating friction on the skin.
- avoid shaving areas near the treatment field.
- avoid tape on the patient's skin near the treatment field.
- avoid lotions and cosmetics near the treatment field.
- avoid tight fitting garments; dress the patient in loose, comfortable clothing.

Protecting Yourself from Radiation Exposure.
Sources of radiation are sometimes implanted inside the patient's body. If this is the case, you will be instructed in special precautions to follow to reduce your risk of radiation exposure. A list of precautions will be placed on the chart or elsewhere. Follow these instructions carefully. In general, you should:

- not remain in the patient's room any longer than necessary.
- stay at least 3 feet away from the patient unless direct care is being delivered.

- inform the nurse if an implant comes out of a body cavity (if so, do not touch it).
- find out if special precautions are necessary for handling soiled linens, tissues, or dressings.
- inform the nurse if you are pregnant, or suspect you may be pregnant.

Immunotherapy

Immunotherapy is another cancer treatment that is done to alter the patient's immune response and eliminate the cancer. Various biologic agents are given to change the normal immune response. The vital signs are regularly and closely monitored when these agents are given. Side effects of therapy usually cease within a week after treatment. Care of the patient receiving immunotherapy involves:

- monitoring vital signs every 4 hours, or more often if instructed.
- monitoring capillary refill as instructed.
- advising the patient to remain in bed if the systolic blood pressure is below 100, or according to the nurse's instructions.
- weighing the patient daily and informing the nurse of weight gain.

Notify the nurse promptly if the patient:
- has fever or chills
- has rapid pulse (over 100, or according to nurse's instructions), or rapid respirations (over 24, or according to nurse's instructions)
- becomes cyanotic
- is short of breath
- is restless or apprehensive
- has diarrhea, nausea, or vomiting
- complains of itching

PAIN

Pain is the most common symptom in patients with cancer. The pain may be caused by the cancer, or be a result of the treatment. The pain may cause difficulty sleeping, loss of appetite, depression, and anxiety. Pain over an extended period of time reduces the patient's quality of life. The World Health Organization (WHO) analgesic ladder (Figure 46-10) is used as a model for pain management.

Cancer patients should be evaluated for pain regularly. A pain scale (Units 8 and 10) is usually used. Narcotic pain-relieving medications may be necessary to control the pain. These are not withheld out of fear of addiction. The incidence of addiction in cancer patients is very low. Pain should be treated before it becomes severe and out of control. Notify the nurse promptly if a patient complains of pain.

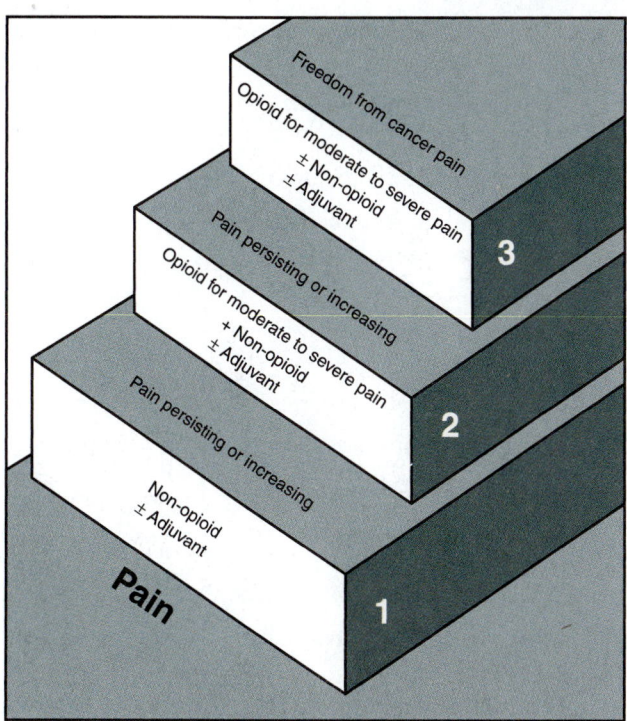

FIGURE 46-10 The WHO three-step analgesic ladder is used for a model in pain management. *(Courtesy of World Health Organization, Geneva, Switzerland. Used with permission)*

MENTAL AND EMOTIONAL NEEDS

Patients with cancer have a life-altering disease. They often fear dying. They may be anxious or depressed, and they often go through the grieving process (Unit 31). Nursing assistant measures to assist with mental and emotional needs include:

- spending as much time as possible with the patient if he wants to talk.
- allowing the patient to talk about feelings and fears.
- being proficient at providing physical care and assistance with ADLs.
- anticipating patients' needs before they ask.
- respecting the patient's beliefs and wishes.
- providing emotional support.
- respecting the patient's privacy if she wants to be alone.

COMMUNICATION *Highlight*

A cancer diagnosis evokes strong feelings and emotions in patients and their families. These may be difficult to understand and cope with. Patients or families may lash out in anger at you or their loved ones. They are not angry with you. They are angry with their circumstances. Avoid responding with anger. Keep your temper even, and do not take comments personally. Saying, "I see you are upset," or validating their feelings is the best way to respond. Providing compassionate care, listening, and giving sincere, solid, emotional support will help patients and family members cope with this difficult time.

- making the patient feel respected and valued as a person.

Avoid giving the patient false hope. If you think a patient is losing control, inform the nurse. Just being with the patient and allowing him to talk is very helpful.

PALLIATIVE CARE

Some patients with cancer elect to have **palliative care**. This care is designed to treat the symptoms of discomfort, but not the disease. The patient will have an advance directive and do not resuscitate (DNR) order. The patient is kept comfortable until death occurs. A hospice (Unit 31) may be involved in the patient's care. One goal of this care is to maintain the patient's quality of life for as long as possible.

Nursing Assistant Measures. Your care is designed to keep the patient clean and comfortable. Use nursing measures, such as positioning and backrubs, to enhance the patient's comfort. Spend time with the patient and allow her to talk, if she wants. Respect the patient's wishes. Provide emotional support. Inform the nurse if the patient is short of breath, anxious, or complains of pain.

REVIEW

A. True/False.

Mark the following true or false by circling T or F.

1. T F Benign tumors spread rapidly to other parts of the body.

2. T F A carcinogen is a cancer-producing substance.

3. T F Most cancers occur in persons over the age of 65.

4. T F In a healthy diet, no more than 30% of daily calories comes from fat.

5. T F Lifestyle modification may reduce the risk of cancer.

B. Matching.

Choose the correct word from Column II to match the word or phrase or statement in Column I.

Column I

6. ____ cancer that spreads

7. ____ tissue sample

8. ____ medications or drugs

9. ____ changes immune response

10. ____ comfort care

Column II

a. chemotherapy

b. malignant

c. palliative

d. biopsy

e. immunotherapy

C. Multiple Choice.

Select the one best answer for each of the following.

11. The most common risk factor for cancer is
   a. cigarette smoking.
   b. heredity.
   c. poor nutrition.
   d. age.

12. Complex carbohydrates should make up ____% of the daily caloric intake.
   a. 20%
   b. 30%
   c. 55%
   d. 85%

13. Lifestyle changes that will reduce the risk of cancer include
   a. drinking herbal tea daily.
   b. getting a complete physical exam every 5 years.
   c. a regular exercise program.
   d. consuming at least 800 mL of water daily.

14. Females should perform a breast self-examination
   a. weekly.
   b. monthly.
   c. every six months.
   d. yearly.

15. Males should perform testicular self-examination
   a. monthly.
   b. every three months.
   c. every six months.
   d. annually.

16. The use of medications to destroy cancer cells is
   a. brachytherapy.
   b. radiation therapy.
   c. chemotherapy.
   d. complementary therapy.

17. A deficiency of red blood cells that is a common side effect of cancer therapy is
   a. alopecia.
   b. anemia.
   c. anorexia.
   d. metastasis.

18. Radiation therapy is a cancer treatment that uses
   a. high-energy ionizing beams.
   b. chemicals.
   c. medication
   d. change in the immune response.

19. A patient returns from a radiation treatment with markings on the skin. You should
   a. wash the markings off with soap and water.
   b. scrub the area vigorously.
   c. apply lotion to the area.
   d. leave the markings alone.

20. The most common symptom of patients with cancer is
   a. nausea.
   b. vomiting.
   c. pain.
   d. alopecia.

D. Nursing Assistant Challenge.

Mr. Weiss is a 37-year-old patient who was recently diagnosed with breast cancer. He had a breast surgically removed and is undergoing chemotherapy. You take his vital signs early in the shift, but he refuses to speak to you. A few hours later, you bring his meal tray to the room and set it on the overbed table. Mr. Weiss sweeps the tray off the table with his arm and food and dishes fly everywhere. He yells at you, shouting "You know I am not hungry. Now get out of here and leave me alone."

21. Why do you think Mr. Weiss is acting this way?

22. Is he mad at you?

23. What action should you take immediately?

24. What will you report to the nurse?

25. Should you leave Mr. Weiss alone for the rest of the shift?

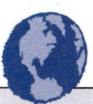 **EXPLORING THE WEB**

Description	Location
Cancer immunity	http://www.nlm.nih.gov/medlineplus/cancers.html
Cancer risk assessment	http://users.rcn.com
Oncology tools	http://www.fda.gov/cder/cancer
American Cancer Society	http://www.cancer.org
American Society of Clinical Oncology	http://www.asco.org
Breast Cancer Awareness Crusade	http://www.avoncompany.com
Canadian Breast Cancer Network	http://www.cbcn.ca
Cancer Clinical Services Quality Assurance Project	http://qap.sdsu.edu
Cancer News	http://www.cancernews.com
CancerEducation.com	http://www.cancereducation.com
CancerFacts.com	http://www.cancerfacts.com
CancerPage.com	http://www.cancerpage.com
CancerSource.com	http://www.cancersource.com
CancerTrack	http://www.cancertrack.com
CancerWeb	http://cancerweb.ncl.ac.uk
Combined Health Information Database	http://chid.nih.gov/subfile/subfile.html
Electronic Journal of Oncology	http://elecjoncol.org
International Cancer Alliance	http://www.icare.org
Jabboury Foundation for Cancer Research	http://www.jabboury.org
JNCI Cancer Spectrum	http://jncicancerspectrum.oupjournals.org
Medline Plus	http://www.nlm.nih.gov/medlineplus/cancers.html
National Cancer Institute	http://www.cancer.gov/cancerinfo/literature
National Foundation for Cancer Research	http://www.researchforacure.com
OncoLink	http://www.oncolink.com
Oncology Nursing Society	http://www.ons.org
RobertsReview	http://www.robertsreview.com

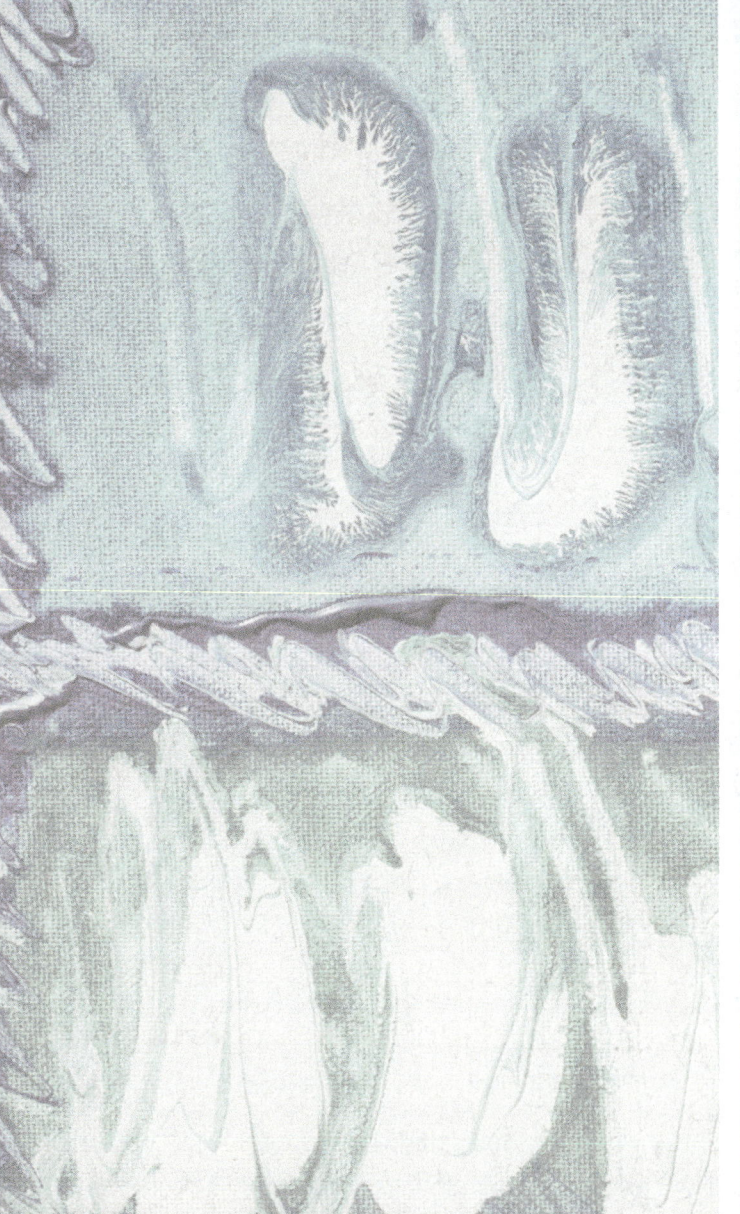

Expanded Role of the Nursing Assistant

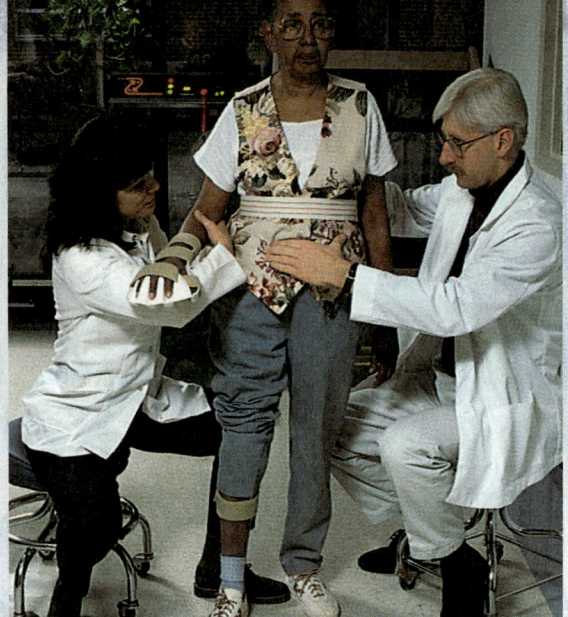

Rehabilitation and Restorative Services

objectives

After completing this unit, you will be able to:
- Spell and define terms.
- Describe the differences between rehabilitation and restorative care.
- List five members of the interdisciplinary team.
- Describe the role of the nursing assistant in rehabilitation.
- Describe the principles of rehabilitation.
- List the elements of successful rehabilitation/ restorative care.
- List six complications resulting from inactivity.
- Describe four perceptual deficits.
- Describe four approaches used for restorative programs.
- Describe the guidelines for implementing restorative programs.

vocabulary

Learn the meaning and the correct spelling of the following words and phrases:

activities of daily living (ADLs)	disability	mobility skills	rehabilitation
	geriatric	perceptual deficit	restorative
adaptive device	handicap	physiatrist	self-care deficit

INTRODUCTION TO REHABILITATION AND RESTORATIVE CARE

The term **rehabilitation** refers to a process in which the patient is assisted to reach an optimal level of ability. That means we are concerned with helping the patient be the best that he or she can be: physically, mentally, and emotionally. Rehabilitation and restorative care are similar processes, but there are some differences:

- Rehabilitation is usually more aggressive and intensive than restorative care (Figure 47-1). Therapies are planned for a period of several weeks. Restorative care is a slower process; it may be planned for weeks or months or go on indefinitely.

- Rehabilitation requires the skills of many disciplines, including nursing and various therapies. **Restorative** care is basically a nursing responsibility, carried out with consultation from therapists and other health professionals.

- Rehabilitation services may be provided in a general acute care hospital, in a rehabilitation center, in the skilled care facility, in a subacute care unit, or in the patient's home. Most restorative care is given in a skilled care facility or in the patient's home.

- OBRA regulations require that restorative services be provided to patients in skilled care facilities. Nursing assistants in these facilities must have the knowledge and skills to participate in this process.

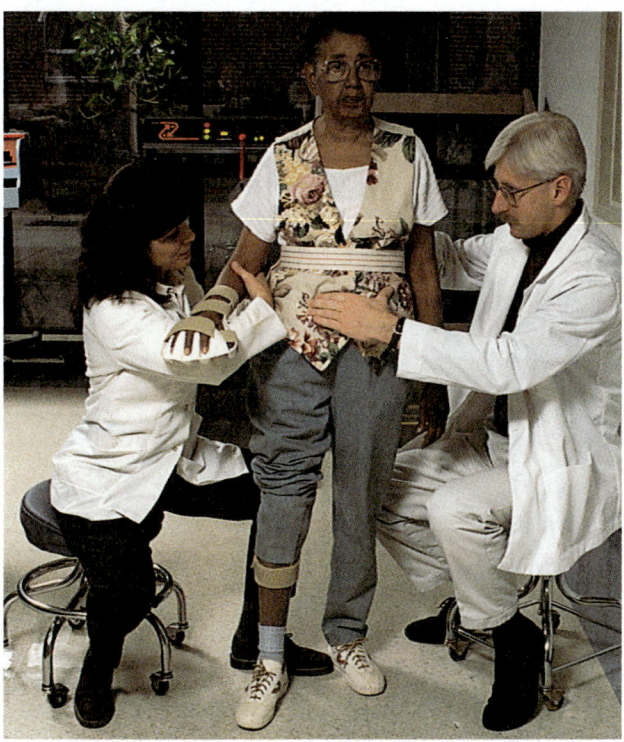

FIGURE 47-1 Rehabilitation is more aggressive and intensive than restorative care.

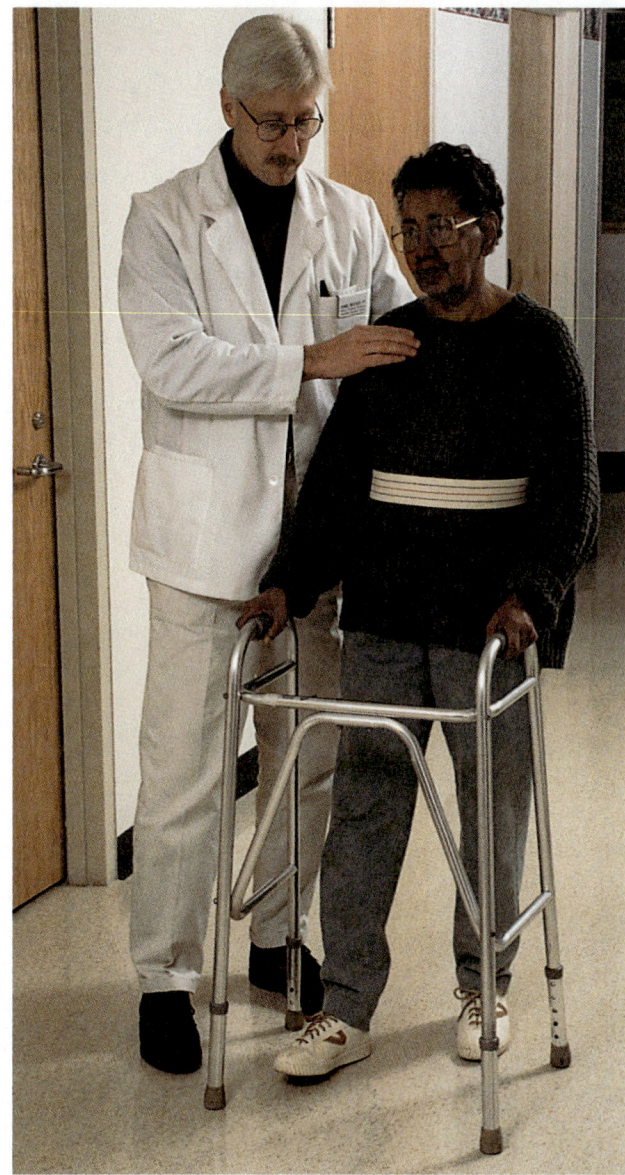

FIGURE 47-2 Rehabilitation and restorative nursing both work on increasing mobility and independence.

The goals of both rehabilitation and restorative care are to:

- Increase the patient's physical abilities. This may include **mobility skills** (Figure 47-2) and the ability to carry out **activities of daily living** (**ADLs**). Activities of daily living are the tasks that we learn as children and do throughout life. These tasks include: bathing, oral care, hair and nail care, dressing and undressing, eating, toileting, and mobility.

- Prevent complications such as pressure sores and contractures.

- Maintain the patient's current abilities.

- Help the patient adapt to limitations imposed by a disability.

- Increase the patient's quality of life.

The information in this unit applies to both rehabilitation and restorative care.

REASONS FOR REHABILITATION/ RESTORATIVE CARE

A person may need rehabilitation because of a **disability**. A disability exists when the person has an impairment that affects the ability to perform an activity that a person of that age would normally be able to do. Adults, for example, are able to dress and undress independently. If a person is unable to do this because of a disease or injury, a disability exists. A disability may be temporary or permanent.

A **handicap** exists if the disability limits or prevents the person from fulfilling a role that is normal for that person. This might include such functions as holding a job, managing a household, and raising a family.

If a disability is permanent, such as quadriplegia (paralysis from the neck down) from a spinal cord injury, it is unrealistic to expect that rehabilitation will enable the patient to walk again. In these situations, the interdisciplinary team will teach the patient to:

- adapt to the present circumstances.
- assume responsibility for personal well-being by directing others who give the care.
- use adaptive devices to increase independence.

Impairments or disabilities result from trauma or disease. Disorders of the musculoskeletal system, such as amputation (Figure 47-3) of an extremity or arthritis, may require rehabilitation. Stroke, spinal cord injury, and brain injuries are examples of nervous system disorders that will benefit from rehabilitation. A patient who has been in bed for a long time because of a serious illness, such as heart disease, may require rehabilitation for reconditioning or to restore the individual to a previous level of ability.

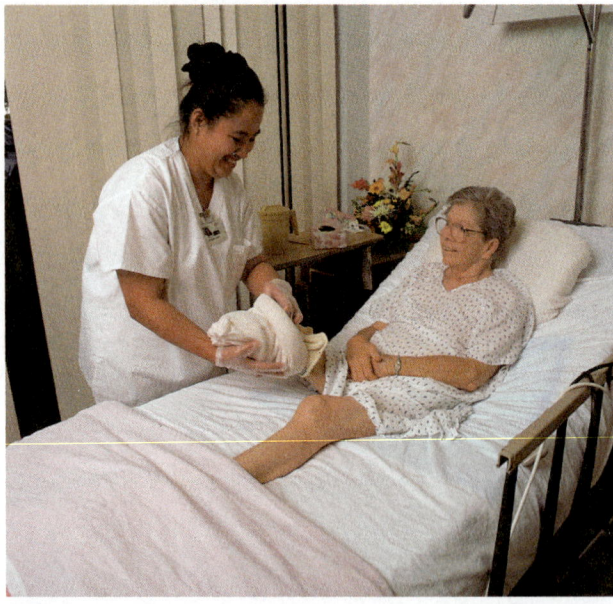

FIGURE 47-3 Patients who have had an amputation will often benefit from intensive rehabilitation.

THE INTERDISCIPLINARY HEALTH CARE TEAM

Physicians who specialize in rehabilitation are called **physiatrists**. Nurses and nursing assistants who work in rehabilitation receive additional training and education. Many other disciplines may be involved in the rehabilitation process. For instance, a person who has had a stroke may receive:

- physical therapy to learn how to walk again.
- occupational therapy to relearn the activities of daily living.
- speech therapy to learn new communication methods.
- nursing services for bowel and bladder training, prevention of pressure ulcers, and other complications.
- dietitian services to help the patient learn to manage new dietary restrictions for a low-sodium diet (to reduce blood pressure), and to plan and prepare meals.
- psychological support to adapt to the sudden changes brought about by the stroke.
- social services to plan for the impending discharge.

Each discipline has specific responsibilities, but all disciplines work together with the patient and family to resolve problems and to plan care.

There are many subspecialties in rehabilitation. Health care professionals may choose to work in **geriatric** (care of the elderly) or pediatric rehabilitation. Others may specialize in the care of patients with strokes, spinal cord injuries, brain injuries, amputations, or arthritis.

The Role of the Nursing Assistant in Rehabilitation

The nursing assistant who works in rehabilitation will assist the nurses with

- procedures to prevent complications: passive range-of-motion exercises and positioning.
- mobility skills: transfers and ambulation.
- bathing and personal care procedures.
- bowel and bladder training programs.
- maintaining the patient's nutritional status.
- programs to increase the patient's independence.

PRINCIPLES OF REHABILITATION

Four principles form the foundation of successful rehabilitation or restorative care.

- *Treatment begins as soon as possible.*

  This means that plans for maintaining or increasing abilities begin as soon as the patient's condition is stable. For example, if a patient has had a stroke, passive exercises and positioning techniques are initiated in the critical care unit to prevent contractures, pressure ulcers, and other complications that would prohibit or delay rehabilitation.

- *Stress the patient's ability, not disability.*

  Care providers must think in terms of what the patient can do, not what the patient cannot do. The patient's strengths are used to help in adapting to any limitations. A *strength* refers to anything the patient is able to do. Perhaps a patient whose dominant hand is paralyzed cannot use that hand to feed himself—but instead of having nursing staff feed him, he can be taught to use the other, stronger hand.

- *Activity strengthens and inactivity weakens.*

  Complications result from physical and mental inactivity. These can cause further disability or even be life-threatening. A rehabilitation or restorative plan of care always includes approaches and goals for both physical and mental activity.

- *Treat the whole person.*

  When we are giving care to patients, we are not concerned only with their physical well-being. We also must attend to their emotional and mental health needs (Figure 47-4). An angry or depressed patient will not be able to concentrate on the work involved in rehabilitation. We must also work with the patients' families. They directly influence the emotional and mental health of the patients.

The elements of successful rehabilitation/restorative care require that members of the team:

- have a positive attitude about the patients and their capabilities.
- have confidence in their own abilities as caregivers.
- be willing to learn from other care providers, patients, and their families.

- use problem-solving skills in place of unproductive coping methods.
- use all available tools and resources to give effective care.
- work with other staff as team members.
- realize that ideal working situations seldom exist, but strive to bring ideal and real closer together.
- continually learn and acquire new skills by participating in educational programs.
- accept the need for change to improve the quality of care for all patients.

Keys to success in rehabilitation and restorative nursing programs are:

- Use of the care plan. All staff are familiar with the patient's problems, goals, and approaches to use.
- Consistency of care. All staff use the same approaches (as listed on the care plan) when caring for the patient.
- Continuity of care. There is a smooth progression and flow between caregivers and between shifts.
- Good communication among all caregivers, the patient, and interested family members.

COMPLICATIONS FROM INACTIVITY

People with disabilities may be unable to move about at will. The inactivity or immobility can result in numerous complications affecting body systems:

1. Musculoskeletal system.
   - Muscles become weak and atrophy (decrease in size and strength).
   - Contractures can form, making any movement impossible. A contracture (Figure 47-5) occurs when a joint is in a permanent state of flexion.
   - Disuse osteoporosis develops. This means that calcium drains from the bones, causing them to become brittle. Fractures can occur even without trauma.

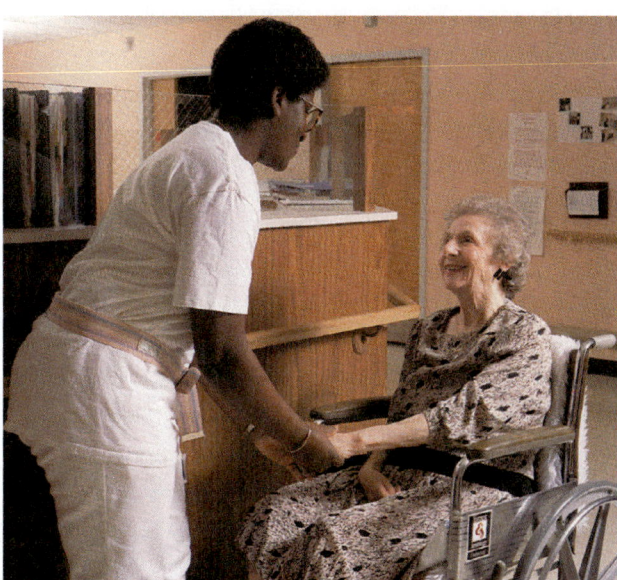

FIGURE 47-4 The patient's mental and emotional state are as important as her physical condition.

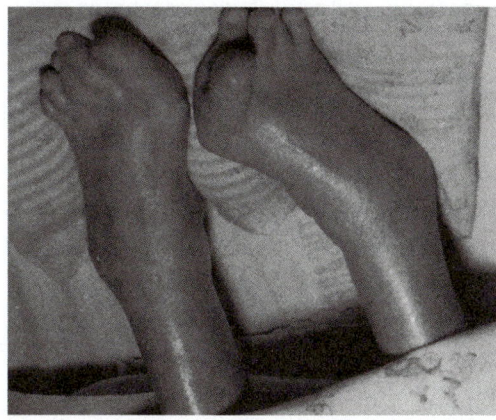

FIGURE 47-5 Contractures often result from immobility. This patient has foot drop, a serious contracture of the feet.

2. Integumentary system.
   - Pressure sores develop over bony prominences.
3. Cardiovascular system.
   - The heart takes longer to return to a normal pace after activity.
   - Blood does not circulate as efficiently. This can lead to thrombus (blood clot) and embolus (a blood clot that moves through the circulatory system).
   - Edema may be caused by lack of movement.
   - The heart must work harder to pump blood through the body.
   - Changes in the blood vessels may cause dizziness and fainting when the patient is placed in the upright position.
4. Respiratory system.
   - The lungs do not expand. Secretions collect in the lungs and cause pneumonia.
   - Respiratory tract infections are more common.
5. Gastrointestinal system.
   - Appetite decreases, causing weight loss.
   - The risk of pressure sores increases with weight loss and lack of nutrition.
   - Peristalsis slows down, causing indigestion and constipation.
   - Indigestion and heartburn may result if the patient is not positioned properly during and after meals.
   - The patient is at risk of choking unless positioned upright during and after meals.
6. Urinary system.
   - The bladder does not empty completely. This increases the risk of bladder infection.
   - Incontinence can result from inability to get to the bathroom.
   - Urinary stones may develop from calcium in the bloodstream resulting from osteoporosis.
7. Nervous system.
   - Weakness and limited mobility.
   - Insomnia may result from sleeping too much during the day, then being unable to sleep at night.
8. Psychosocial reaction.
   - Depression can occur from physical and mental inactivity and feelings of helplessness.
   - Inactivity and lack of sensory stimulation can cause disorientation.
   - Irritability, boredom, and lethargy may result from the patient's frustration.

Activities of Daily Living

One purpose of restorative care is to increase the patient's physical abilities. This includes mobility skills and the ability to carry out activities of daily living.

These tasks or skills are taught to us as children. Healthy adults do these tasks automatically. If the patient cannot complete any or all of the ADLs, a **self-care deficit** exists. Adults may have self-care deficits because of:

- Diseases such as multiple sclerosis, post polio syndrome, arthritis, Parkinson's disease, or Alzheimer's disease
- Injuries causing damage to the extremities, brain, or spinal cord
- Vision impairment
- Emotional illness

Deficits are caused by problems that limit the patient's ability to do self-care. Examples of these problems are:

- Decreased strength
- Lack of endurance
- Limited range of motion
- Depression

DIFFICULT *Situations*

Disabilities can take many forms. Some forms, such as speech, hearing, or language problems, interfere with communication. Other problems, such as physical impairments, may make you uncomfortable. You may be unsure of how to avoid offending the patient. Individuals who are newly disabled are more sensitive to their problems than people who have lived with a disability for a long time. People with disabilities are like you are. They have the same wants and needs. Their problems are no different from yours. However, having a disability makes living with these same problems much more difficult and creates additional problems. People with disabilities can do many of the same things you can. However, they may need to adapt the environment to do them. Changing things to meet a patient's needs is called providing *reasonable accommodation*. People with disabilities may perform a task differently than you do. However, the outcome of a task is the same. Their bodies just work differently! As a rule, persons who have disabilities do not want to be treated differently from anyone else. Many are self-sufficient. All are valuable and equal members of society. Emphasize the uniqueness, value, and worth of each patient. Avoid comparing the differences between people. Treat people with disabilities the way you like to be treated.

- Disorientation
- Perceptual deficits

There are many types of **perceptual deficits**. These usually occur because of damage to the brain from disease or injury. Here are some examples of perceptual deficits:

- An inability to organize a task. ADLs cannot be completed unless the individual is able to prepare for the task, get the necessary items together, and then do it.
- An inability to sequence a task. When putting on clothing, for example, a slip must go on before the dress and socks before shoes.
- Lack of judgment. This deficit may be noted if a patient puts on a wool coat in hot weather (when appropriate clothing is available).
- An inability to identify common objects, such as eating utensils and grooming items (*agnosia*). The patient may try to use a fork to comb her hair, for example.
- An inability to use common items (*apraxia*). The patient may be able to identify the item but be unable to use it (even though there is no physical reason such as paralysis).
- An inability to initiate a task.

Patients with self-care deficits are evaluated by therapists and nurses. The results of evaluation will determine whether a patient's functional (physical) abilities can be increased. In other words, can the interdisciplinary team help this person to relearn an activity of daily living? This is discussed with the patient and the family.

RESTORATIVE PROGRAMS

If the patient has the potential to relearn an ADL and is motivated to try, a restorative program is planned. These programs are sometimes called retraining programs or ADL programs.

When the patient is unable to do any of the ADLs independently, it is generally best to concentrate on just one at a time. The first step is to find out what the patient wants to work on first. The interdisciplinary team then works with the patient and family to plan the process. They will:

- Establish goals. Each ADL consists of several steps, as shown in Table 47-1. The patient will not be able to do all steps right away. Some patients may never be able to do all of the steps. Goals, therefore, are very small. For example, if the patient is in a restorative program for eating, the first goal may be to hold a glass and drink from it. All goals are functional. Instead of saying the patient will walk 30 feet, the goal will state: "Patient will walk to the dining room for breakfast."
- Plan approaches. The approaches include the techniques and procedures carried out by the interdisciplinary team. The approaches are planned to help the patient relearn the ADL.

TABLE 47-1 FUNCTIONAL STEPS OF ACTIVITIES OF DAILY LIVING

Bathing	• Gets to tub/sink/shower • Regulates water flow and temperature • Washes/rinses upper body • Washes/rinses lower body • Dries body
Dressing/Undressing	• Obtains/selects clothing • Puts on/takes off slipover top • Puts on/takes off cardigan-style top • Manages buttons, snaps, ties, zippers • Puts on/takes off skirt/pants • Buckles belt • Puts on socks/shoes
Eating	• Gets to table • Uses spoon, fork, knife appropriately • Opens/pours • Brings food to mouth • Chews, swallows • Uses napkin
Toileting	• Gets to commode/toilet • Manipulates clothing • Sits on toilet • Eliminates in toilet • Cleans self • Flushes toilet • Gets clothing back in place • Washes hands
Mobility	• Gets self to side of bed • Maintains upright position • Comes to standing position • Places self in position to sit in chair • Locks wheelchair brakes • Turns body to sit • Lowers self into chair • Propels wheelchair • Repositions self in chair • Raises self from chair • Places self in position to sit on edge of bed • Walks alone/with assistance • Uses assistive device

Approaches Used in Restorative Programs

The approach to use should be indicated on the care plan. It is important that the same approach be used consistently.

- *Setup.* Patients with self-care deficits are not able to set up or prepare for activities of daily living. You may need to provide the setup (Figure 47-6). Example for bathing: collect all needed items, prepare the bathtub or shower, help the patient into the tub or shower.
- *Verbal cues.* The care provider uses short, simple phrases to prompt the patient. Example: give the patient a prepared washcloth and then say, "Please wash your face" (Figure 47-7). If a complete task, such as washing the entire face, is overwhelming, break it down into a series of smaller tasks, such as washing the forehead, then the left cheek, and so forth.
- *Hand-over-hand techniques.* Example for eating program: Place a glass in the patient's hand. Place your hand over the patient's hand. Guide the glass to the patient's mouth (Figure 47-8).
- *Demonstration.* Act out what you want the patient to do. Example: Before giving the patient a toothbrush, make the motions of brushing your teeth with the toothbrush (Figure 47-9).

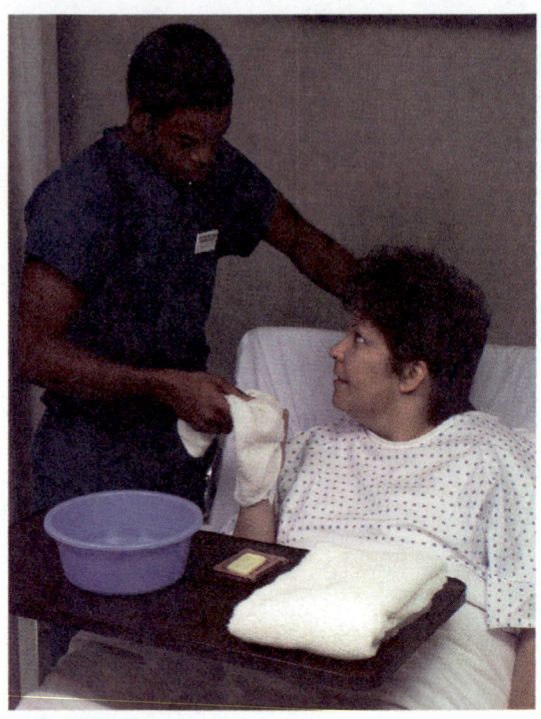

FIGURE 47-7 The nursing assistant uses verbal cues to assist the patient with ADLs.

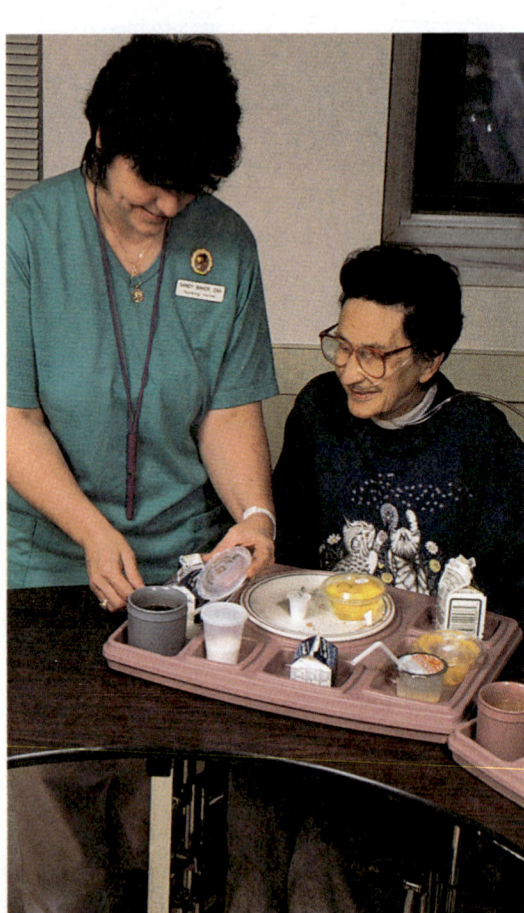

FIGURE 47-6 This patient is able to feed herself if the nursing assistant sets up the tray.

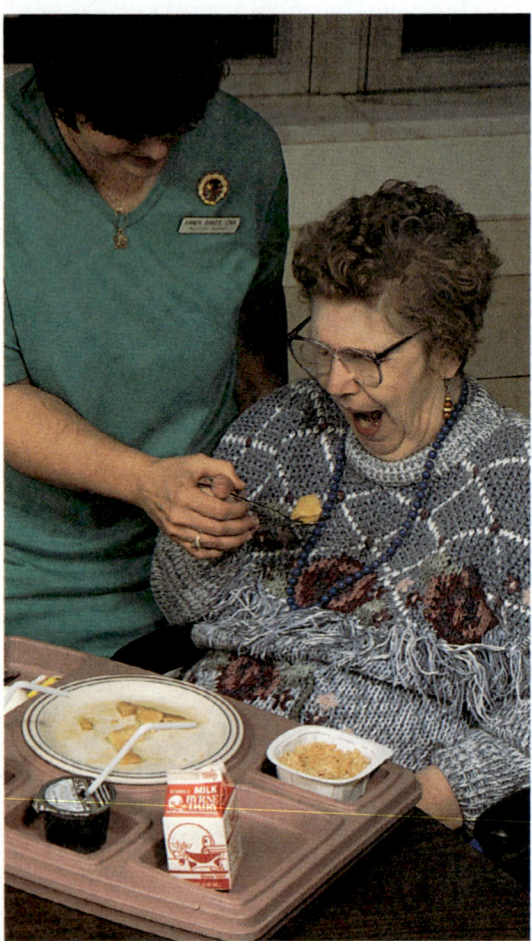

FIGURE 47-8 Hand-over-hand technique is another approach that helps patients relearn essential skills.

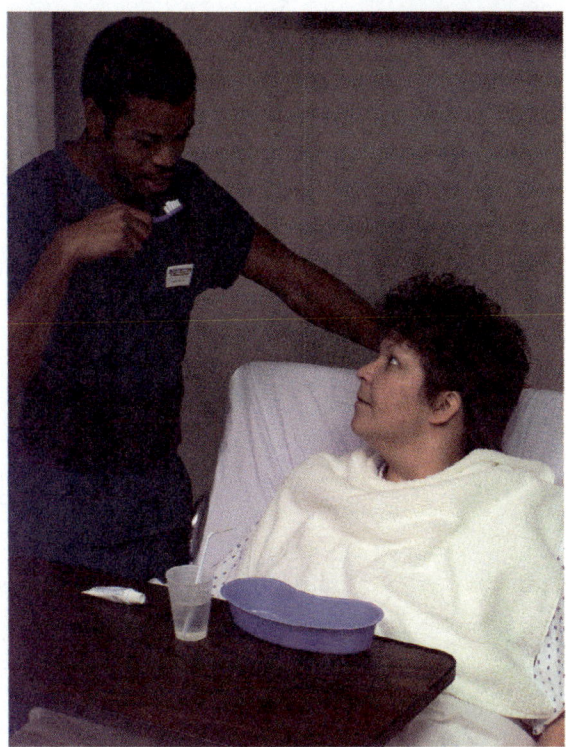

FIGURE 47-9 Demonstrating the activity is a good way to help the patient understand the directions.

Adaptive devices are sometimes used to simplify an ADL. **Adaptive devices** are ordinary items that have been modified for use by patients with various types of problems.

Not all patients are candidates for restorative programs. For those who are not, the goals are to prevent complications and maintain remaining abilities as long as possible. Some patients reach the point where even maintenance is difficult. We are then basically concerned with preventing complications.

The Restorative Environment

All patients benefit from living in an environment that attempts to improve the quality of life. The interdisciplinary team can help promote this environment:

- Give the patient a sense of control and opportunities to make decisions.
- Remember that mental and physical activity are essential to the patient's well-being.
- Encourage and assist patients to be well dressed and well groomed.
- Use touch freely in appropriate ways with patients.
- Provide cues for orientation throughout the building.
- Respect the patients' identity, individuality, and privacy at all times.
- Respect and understand the patient's sexuality and need for intimacy.
- Give patients opportunities to help others.
- Encourage and assist patients to remain a part of the community.
- Create an environment that is safe, serene, and colorful.

guidelines *for*

Implementing Restorative Programs

- Know why the patient has the self-care deficit.
- Keep your directions simple but not childish.
- Avoid distractions. Do the ADL in a private area.
- Be consistent. Read the care plan and follow the specific directions each time you work with the patient.
- Use adaptive devices consistently and correctly.
- Do not show impatience. Be encouraging and give praise.
- Treat the patient with dignity at all times.
- Realize that the patient's progress may be uneven and inconsistent.

REVIEW

A. True/False.

Mark the following true or false by circling T or F.

1. T F Rehabilitation services are provided only in special hospitals.

2. T F OBRA regulations require that restorative services be provided to patients in skilled care facilities.

3. T F Rehabilitation and restorative services both strive to prevent complications.

4. T F Persons with disabilities will never recover their lost skills.

5. T F All persons with disabilities are considered to be handicapped.

B. Multiple Choice.

Select the one best answer for each of the following.

6. A patient with a permanent disability is
   a. taught to adapt to the present circumstances.
   b. not a good candidate for rehabilitation.
   c. given much sympathy.
   d. encouraged to be helpless.

7. Disabilities may result from
   a. too much exercise.
   b. getting inadequate sleep.
   c. spinal cord injury.
   d. not drinking enough water.

8. A patient who is unable to communicate verbally will be treated by a
   a. physical therapist.
   b. occupational therapist.
   c. nursing assistant.
   d. speech and language therapist.

9. Physical inactivity can cause
   a. pressure ulcers.
   b. dehydration.
   c. pain.
   d. infection.

10. Agnosia is a perceptual deficit in which the patient cannot
   a. organize a task.
   b. identify common items.
   c. sequence a task.
   d. initiate a task.

11. Adaptive devices are
   a. inappropriate for patients receiving rehabilitation.
   b. used by nursing assistants to feed patients.
   c. ordinary items modified for use by patients with self-care deficits.
   d. used only by occupational therapists.

12. Placing your hand over the patient's hand to guide the patient's actions is an approach called
   a. giving verbal cues.
   b. demonstration.
   c. hand-over-hand technique.
   d. setting up.

C. Completion.

Complete the statements by choosing the correct word from the following list.

   activities of daily living
   atrophy
   contracture
   disability
   disuse osteoporosis
   embolus
   geriatric
   handicap
   mobility skills
   physiatrist
   rehabilitation
   self-care deficit
   verbal cues

13. The process used to help a patient reach an optimal level of ability is _____.

14. Ambulation and transfers are examples of _____.

15. Dressing and undressing are examples of _____.

16. An impairment that affects the ability to perform an activity that a person of that age would normally be able to do is called a/an _____.

17. When the impairment limits or prevents the person from fulfilling a role that is normal for that person, a/an _____ exists.

18. A person who chooses to work with rehabilitation of the elderly is specializing in _____ rehabilitation.

19. A physician who specializes in rehabilitation is called a/an _____.

20. A/An _____ occurs when a joint is in a permanent state of flexion.

21. _____ occurs when a muscle shrinks and loses strength.

22. Physical inactivity can cause calcium to drain from the bones, resulting in _____.

23. A/An _____ is a blood clot that moves through the circulatory system.

24. A/An _____ exists when an adult cannot complete one or more activities of daily living.

25. Using short, simple phrases to prompt the patient to complete an activity of daily living is called _____.

D. Nursing Assistant Challenge.

You are working as a nursing assistant in the rehabilitation unit of a subacute care section of a skilled nursing facility. Think about what you have learned in this unit and answer the following questions:

26. What types of patients will you see?

27. What kinds of disabilities will the patients have?

28. What may be the cause of the self-care deficits experienced by your patients?

29. What kinds of problems can limit a patient's ability to do self-care?

30. What are the differences between rehabilitation and restorative care?

31. What are the responsibilities of the nursing assistant when giving restorative care?

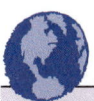 **EXPLORING THE WEB**

Description	Location
Gait belt procedure	*http://www.texashste.com*
Advance for Nursing	*http://www.advancefornurses.com*
Ambulation Program for Restorative Nursing	*http://www.mpcrf.org*
American Occupational Therapy Organization	*http://www.aota.org*
American Physical Therapy Association	*http://www.apta.org*
Association of Rehabilitation Nurses	*http://www.rehabnurse.org*
Physical Therapist Online	*http://physicaltherapist.com*
Physical Therapy Clinical Toolbox	*http://physicaltherapy.about.com*
Rehabilitation Nursing—What? Why? How?	*http://www.rcna.org.au*
Restorative Nursing PowerPoint Presentation	*http://www.michigan.gov/documents/ cis_bhs_fhs_restorative_nursing_36960_7.ppt*

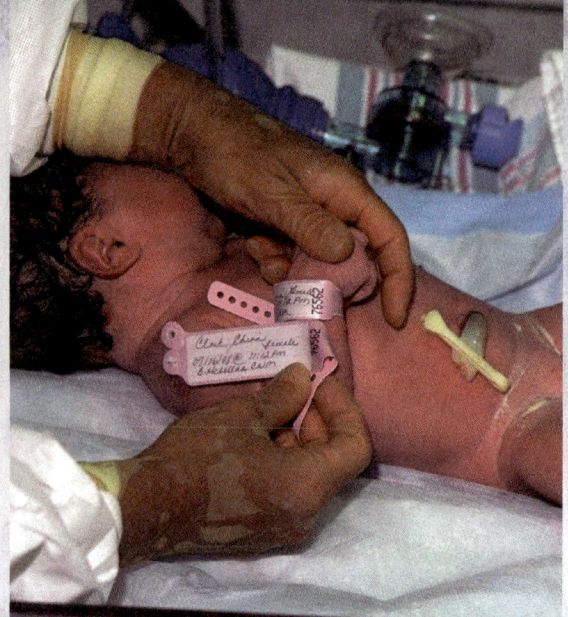

Obstetrical Patients and Neonates

LEGAL *Alert*   By state law, you may not be permitted to perform some of the advanced procedures discussed in this section. Consult with your instructor or supervisor to be sure you know your legal responsibilities. Do not perform or assist in any procedure you are not permitted by law to do.

objectives

After completing this unit, you will be able to:

- Spell and define terms.
- Assist in the prenatal care of the normal pregnant woman.
- List reportable observations of patients in the prenatal period.
- Assist in care of the normal postpartum patient.
- Properly change a perineal pad.
- Recognize reportable observations of patients in the postpartum period.
- Recognize reportable signs and symptoms of urine retention in the postpartum patient.
- Assist in care of the normal newborn.
- Demonstrate three methods of safely holding a baby.
- List measures to prevent inadvertent switching, misidentification, and abduction of infants.
- Assist in carrying out the discharge procedures for mother and infant.
- Demonstrate the following procedures:
  - Procedure 128 Changing a Diaper
  - Procedure 129 Bathing an Infant

vocabulary

Learn the meaning and the correct spelling of the following words and phrases:

amniocentesis	engagement	isolette	quickening
amniotic fluid	episiotomy	labor	rooming-in
amniotic sac	expulsion stage	lactation	status
Apgar score	fetal monitor	lochia	trimester
cesarean	fetoscopy	neonate	ultrasound
circumcision	fetus	obstetrical	umbilical cord
colostrum	foreskin	placenta	vaginal examination
dilation stage	fundus	placental stage	
efface	gestational age	postpartum	
endoscope	involution	prenatal	

INTRODUCTION

When a baby is ready to be born, it is normally upside down in the mother's uterus with its head toward the birth canal (Figure 48-1). Before the baby is born, it is known as a **fetus**. It is surrounded by a membranous bag called an **amniotic sac**. The fetus floats in a liquid called **amniotic fluid**.

The fetus gets nourishment from the mother through the **umbilical cord**. The umbilical cord is attached to the fetus and the **placenta** (afterbirth). The placenta is attached to the wall of the mother's uterus.

After the baby is born and separated from the umbilical cord, the placenta, amniotic sac, and remaining cord are expelled as the afterbirth. After a period of time, the mother's uterus, or womb, which was greatly stretched to accommodate the pregnancy, will return to its normal size and shape.

There are three phases of pregnancy:

- **Prenatal** (before birth)
- Labor and delivery
- **Postpartum** (after birth)

The nursing assistant, who is specially trained, helps provide care and support throughout each phase.

PRENATAL CARE

The care of the mother begins in the prenatal period, when she first learns she is pregnant. You may meet her as you work in a doctor's office or in an **obstetrical** (pregnancy) clinic.

A normal pregnancy lasts about 280 days and is divided into **trimesters** (3 months). Each trimester is noted by specific signs and symptoms:

First trimester (1 through 12 weeks)

- Absence of menstrual period
- Nausea and vomiting (usually in the morning)
- Swelling and tenderness of breasts
- Frequent urination
- Constipation
- Positive pregnancy test within 7 to 10 days after conception
- Softening of uterus and cervix, and bluish color of vagina noted by examiner
- Increased vaginal secretions

Second trimester (13 through 27 weeks)

- Weight gain
- Abdominal enlargement
- Stretch marks may be noted on abdominal skin
- Breast enlargement—colostrum may be noted at about 20 weeks
- Hemorrhoids may be noted
- Uterus and fetus enlargement noted by examiner— mother will feel **quickening** (movements of fetus) about the 20th week

Third trimester (28th through 40th week)

- Mother feels occasional painless uterine contractions (the contractions are strengthening the uterus for labor)
- Uterus and fetus increase in size; this may cause indigestion, insomnia, and shortness of breath
- Mother may have backaches related to posture changes due to weight of fetus
- Edema of ankles may be present
- Varicose veins may appear

The care of the mother throughout pregnancy is important to ensure the birth of a healthy baby. The first trimester is an especially critical time. During the first three months, the fetus is very susceptible to the negative effects of tobacco, alcohol, caffeine, and other drugs, as well as to viruses and bacteria. Exposure to any of these may cause physical and/or mental harm to the developing fetus.

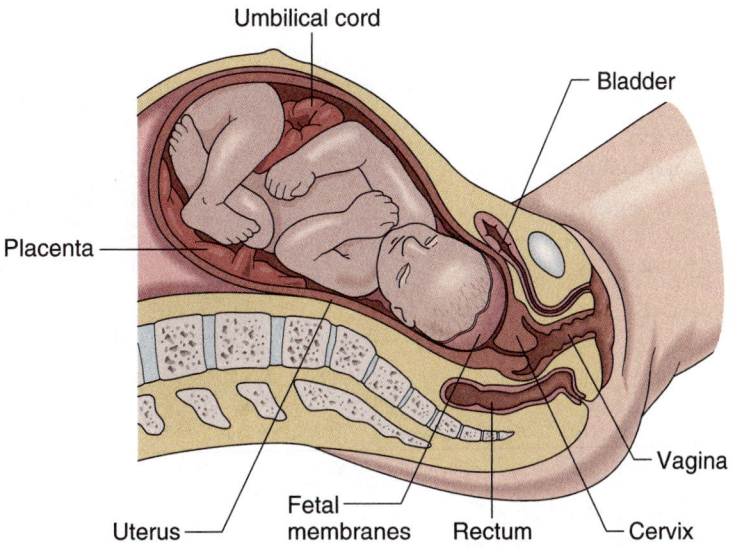

FIGURE 48-1 The usual position of the fetus at birth. This is known as the vertex position.

The pregnant woman is usually advised to visit the physician, nurse practitioner, or midwife at least once a month during the first trimester. During the first visit, the examiner will complete a very thorough history and physical examination, which will include:

- Routine information: age, occupation (to determine exposure to any hazards), education, race (some genetic diseases such as sickle cell anemia are found only in certain races), religion (this may affect mother's health care practices)
- History of menstruation, contraception, pregnancies
- Medical and family history
- Nutritional status
- Examination of fetus

Visits become more frequent as the pregnancy progresses. Routine procedures during the visits include:

- Weighing the mother
- Taking the blood pressure and pulse
- Urine testing
- Counseling and teaching the mother about diet, lifestyle, and signs and symptoms that she should report to the physician
- Palpating the abdomen to check fetal size
- Listening for fetal heart tones

You should call anything unusual to the attention of the nurse. Examples of items to report are:

- Complaints of persistent headache
- Elevated blood pressure
- Vaginal bleeding
- Complaints of dizziness
- Swelling of the hands and feet

PREPARATION FOR BIRTH

Both parents are encouraged to participate fully in the birth of their baby. Special training for the birth begins in the prenatal period. It prepares the parents to participate in the birthing process. Many parents choose to participate in natural childbirth. This technique of birthing:

- allows the mother to be awake and fully participate in the birth.
- encourages the father or an alternative support person to act as coach for the mother.
- necessitates little, if any, pain-controlling medication. One of the most popular of these methods is called the Lamaze method.

Training Classes

In birth training classes:

- The father or some other person learns to act as a coach for the mother.
- The mother learns ways of cooperating with her body during labor and delivery, using special breathing and relaxation techniques.

- The couple sees films of the birth process.
- Vaginal and cesarean deliveries are discussed.
- There are opportunities to ask questions of a trained professional.

PRENATAL TESTING

Congenital abnormalities (those present at birth) can sometimes be identified through prenatal testing. Testing methods include:

- **Ultrasound**—a technique of using sound waves to identify **gestational age** (time of development) and defects in the structure of fetal organs (Figure 48-2).
- **Amniocentesis**—a procedure in which a sterile needle is inserted into the fetal sac and cells are withdrawn for examination. Some genetic defects may be identified in this way.
- **Fetoscopy**—a direct visualization of the fetus in the uterus through a small visualization instrument (**endoscope**). Blood abnormalities may also be identified from samples of the fetal blood that is withdrawn.

LABOR AND DELIVERY

At the end of 40 weeks (within 2 weeks more or less), the signs of impending **labor** will be noted:

- **Engagement** or lightening (the fetus moves downward—sometimes referred to as "dropping")
- Mucous plug is expelled from cervix
- Dilation of cervix begins
- Amniotic membranes may rupture just before actual labor begins, or may rupture during labor
- Uterine contractions begin
  - Irregular at first
  - Stronger, more regular, and closer together as labor progresses

The mother is taught during her pregnancy when she should go to the hospital.

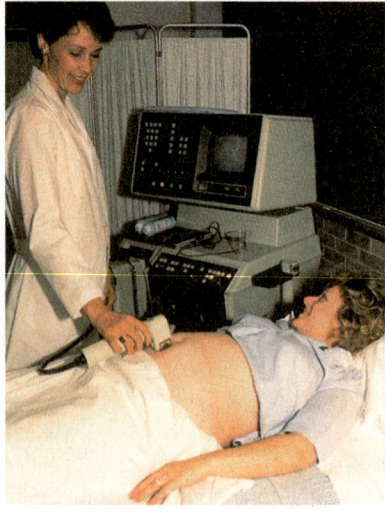

FIGURE 48-2 The ultrasound test is done to check fetal development and detect defects in development of fetal organs. *(Courtesy of Jackson Community College, Jackson, MI)*

Dilation

The **dilation** (opening) **stage** begins with the first regular uterine contractions. It ends when the cervix is fully dilated or opened. This may take 18 to 24 hours in a first pregnancy. As the labor progresses, the cervix also thins (**effaces**) so that the fetus may move downward into the birth canal and out of the mother's body. The degree of dilation at any given time is measured by the nurse or physician. The nurse or physician places a gloved finger in the patient's vagina and measures (approximately) the size of the cervical opening and amount of effacement. This procedure is called **vaginal examination**.

Relief of Discomfort

Drugs may be given to the mother in the labor and delivery phase to reduce pain. Three approaches are frequently employed for a vaginal delivery:

1. Epidural—this is the most common technique. The anesthetic drug is introduced into the epidural space around the spinal cord. Because the drug is not introduced into the cerebrospinal fluid, its effect is more localized in the reproductive organs. The patient's legs can move, but they are weak. Women who are pregnant for the first time may be given this relief when they have reached 5 to 6 cm cervical dilation. Women who have had more than one pregnancy may have it started at 3 to 4 cm dilation without slowing the progress of labor. Controlled introduction of drugs through the epidural route offers relief throughout the delivery. Patients receiving epidural pain relief must be carefully monitored for changes in pulse and blood pressure. Report a drop in blood pressure to the nurse at once.

2. Regional caudal block—this technique introduces the anesthetic drug into the cerebrospinal fluid. It affects a somewhat larger area, but the legs can still move. This form of relief is commonly known as a *saddle block*. This is usually given in the delivery room.

3. Pudendal block—this technique specifically blocks the function of the nerves in the perineum. This medication is usually administered in the delivery room.

When any of these procedures is used, the patient will not feel an episiotomy or its repair, but she will still be able to move her legs. The type of pain relief given to the mother during labor and delivery determines the postpartum care she will receive.

Fetal Monitors

In most hospitals, a **fetal monitor** (instrument to check the well-being of the baby during labor) (Figure 48-3) is attached either to the mother's abdomen or to the baby's head.

Expulsion

Expulsion stage is the period extending from the point of full cervical dilation until the baby is delivered. This may be 1 to 2 hours or more.

The baby moves down the birth canal. The mother is encouraged to help the process by "bearing down" with her abdominal muscles with each contraction. Figures 48-4 and 48-5 show the baby being assisted in delivery and rotated as the shoulders are presented.

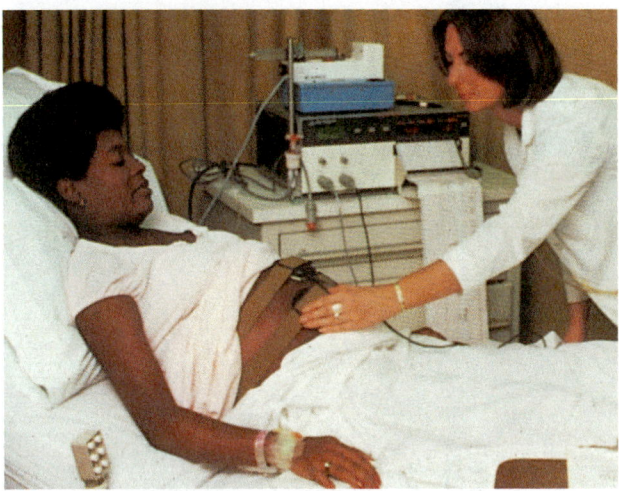

FIGURE 48-3 The fetal monitor enables the staff to evaluate the infant's condition during labor. *(Courtesy of Memorial Medical Center of Long Beach, CA)*

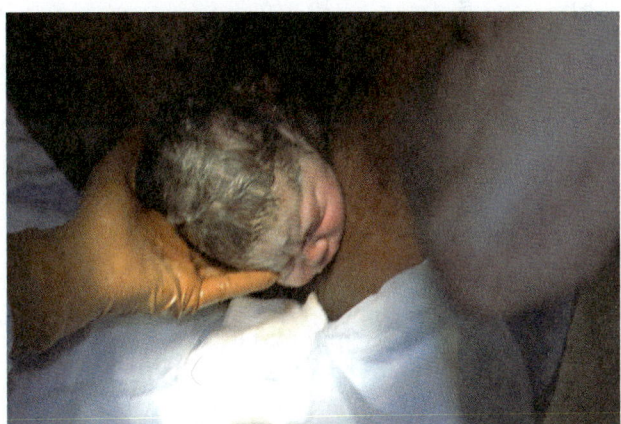

FIGURE 48-4 The baby's head emerges.

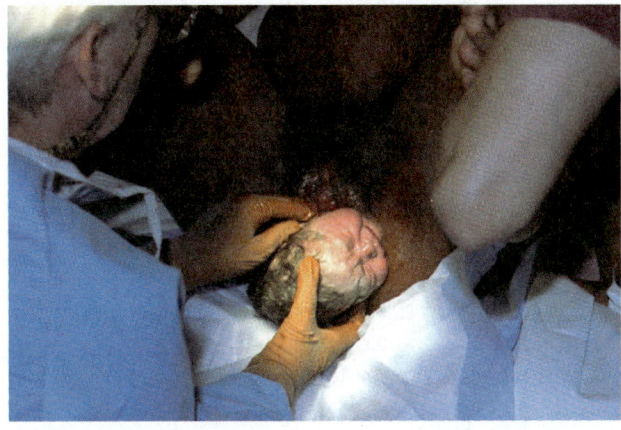

FIGURE 48-5 After the shoulders are delivered, the rest of the body is readily delivered.

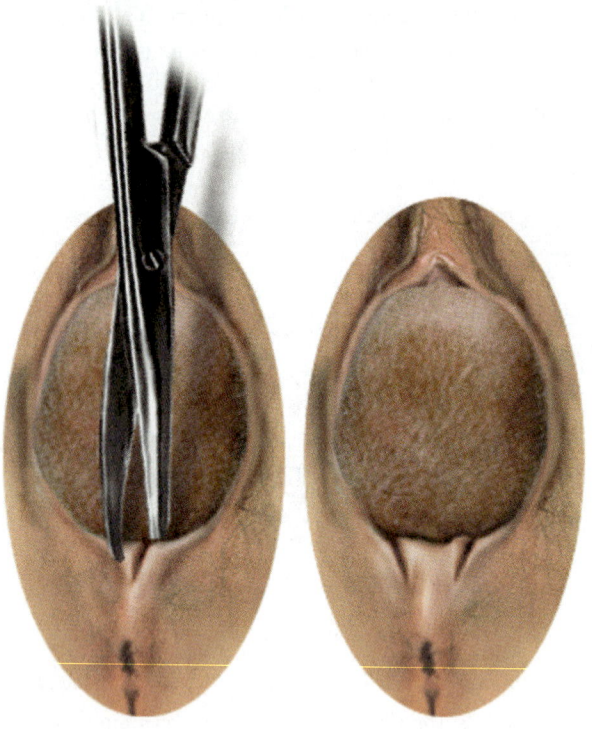

FIGURE 48-6 An episiotomy may be done to prevent tearing of the perineum.

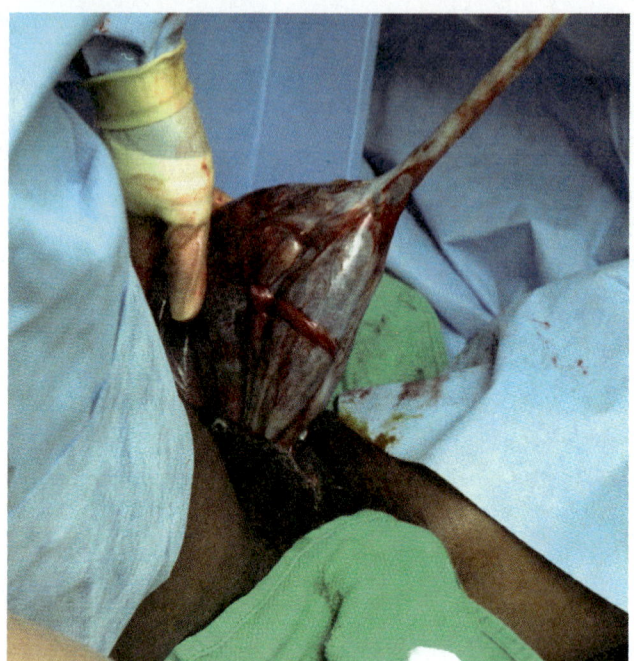

FIGURE 48-7 The placenta is delivered.

During delivery, it may be necessary to enlarge the vaginal opening. This is done by making a cut in the perineum. The cut is called an **episiotomy** (Figure 48-6) The episiotomy is sutured (sewn up) after delivery.

Forceps may be used at this stage to assist in delivery of the head. Once delivered, the baby is held head down to clear the respiratory tract. The baby is then usually placed on the mother's abdomen while the cord is clamped and cut. In addition:

- An **Apgar score** is determined. The Apgar score is used to evaluate a newborn on five qualities at 1 minute, 5 minutes. and 10 minutes after delivery. The higher the score, the better the baby's condition.

- The mother is encouraged to hold her newborn, now called a **neonate**, to establish emotional bonding. This is done even when the baby is delivered by cesarean section.

Placental Stage

The **placental stage** lasts from delivery of the baby through the delivery of the placenta (Figure 48-7). This is a short period. The placenta is usually delivered within an hour of the delivery of the baby.

In this stage, the placenta separates from the wall of the uterus. Uterine contractions push it downward and out through the birth canal. After delivery of the placenta:

- If an episiotomy was needed, it is repaired.

- The mother's uterus is checked for firmness. Drugs may be given to help it contract to control bleeding.

- Both mother and child are identified with name tags (Figure 48-8) before being separated.

- The baby is footprinted (Figure 48-9) along with the mother's thumbprint.

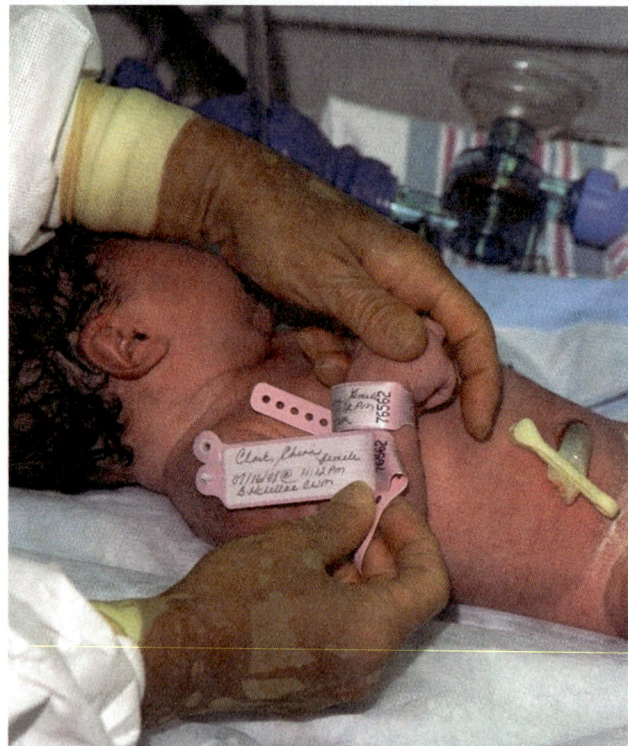

FIGURE 48-8 The mother and infant are given identifying bands. In some hospitals, fathers are also given an identification band. This is a security feature to reduce the risk of an infant abduction.

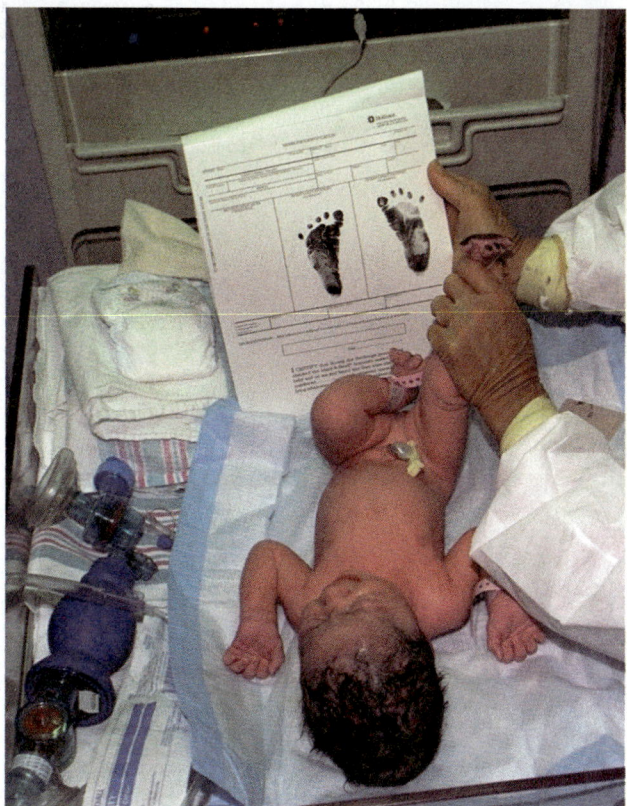

FIGURE 48-9 The infant's footprints are taken soon after delivery.

- The baby's eyes are treated to prevent infection (Figure 48-10).

In most hospitals today, the labor, delivery, and postpartum (period after delivery) care are all carried out in the same room. Keeping the newborn in the same room with the mother is called **rooming-in**. The baby can be taken to the nursery if the mother has complications or is unable to rest with the baby in the room. The usual length of stay for the new mother and baby is about two days unless there are complications. After the mother has recovered from anesthesia and any medications that were given during labor, she is encouraged to do as much self-care as possible. She is allowed to get out of bed soon after delivery if there are no complications.

The father or another supportive person who has attended the prenatal classes with the pregnant woman is encouraged to participate in the labor, delivery, and care of the newborn. The baby's siblings, grandparents, and other family members are allowed to visit during the postpartum period and to hold and love the baby (Figure 48-11). Many hospitals serve the new parents a special, private meal the evening before discharge.

In the last several years there has been a trend toward:

- making the delivery a family affair.
- having the delivery take place at home or in a homelike environment.
- continuing to provide for the safety of both mother and infant.

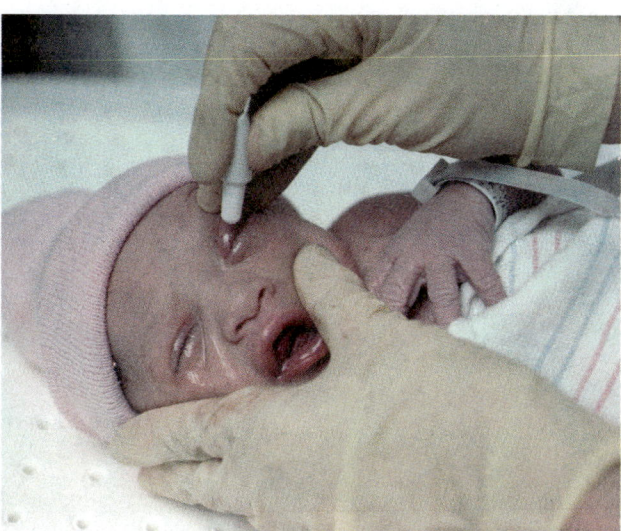

FIGURE 48-10 Silver nitrate is placed in the eyes to reduce the risk of infection that the infant may have contracted during the birthing process.

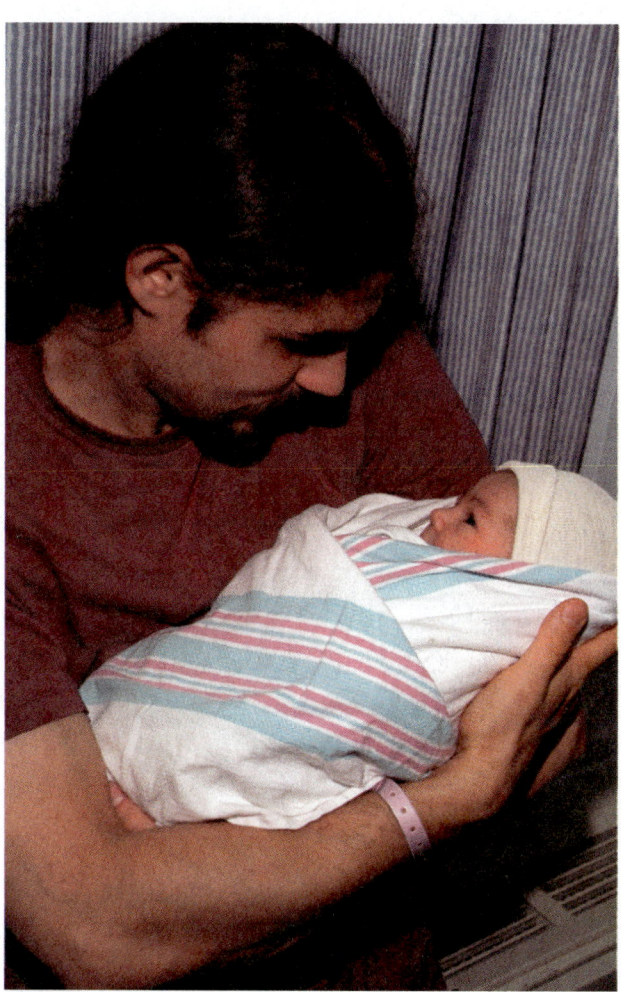

FIGURE 48-11 The father is getting to know the infant. Note the father's identification band.

CESAREAN BIRTH

Cesarean section is another way of delivering a baby. The baby is delivered through an incision in the abdomen rather than through the birth canal. Between 20 and 30% of all births in the United States occur in this way.

A spinal or epidural anesthetic is administered before the surgery. This type of procedure introduces the drugs into the cerebrospinal fluid and blocks sensation from the upper abdomen down to the toes. Until the anesthetic wears off, the patient will not be able either to feel or move her legs.

After the delivery, the mother sometimes is given a general anesthetic that allows her to sleep during the rest of the procedure.

Cesarean deliveries may be performed when there is:

- Fetal distress
- A preterm infant
- Breech (non-headfirst) presentation
- Prolonged rupture of the membranes
- Prolapsed cord
- Genital herpes
- Premature separation of the placenta
- Placenta previa
- Failure of labor to progress
- A mother who has already had a cesarian section

The incision in the abdominal wall may be:

- Vertical, along the midplane
- Transverse, across the lowest and narrowest part of the abdomen (bikini cut)

The mother's coach or partner is encouraged to be in the operative area to offer emotional support while the cesarean is being done. The same basic activities are carried out in the operating room as are followed after a vaginal delivery.

After the surgery is complete, the baby is usually admitted to the nursery (Figure 48-12). The mother is moved to the

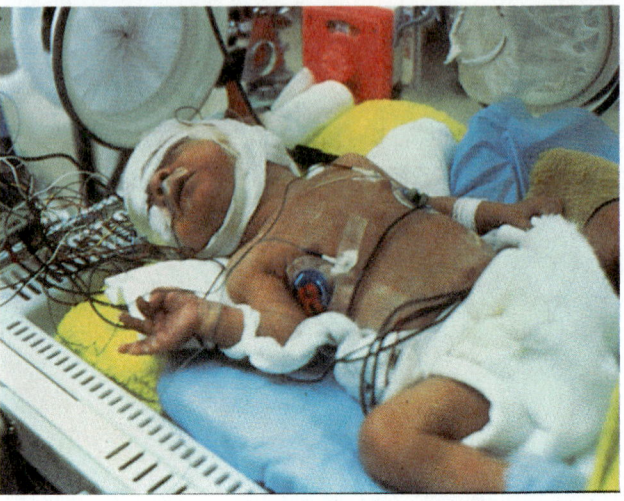

FIGURE 48-13 This infant has been moved to the neonatal intensive care unit. The eyes are covered to protect them. *(Courtesy of Memorial Medical Center of Long Beach, CA)*

recovery room for immediate post-anesthesia care. If the infant is in distress, she will be taken to the neonatal intensive care unit (Figure 48-13).

POSTPARTUM CARE

You may be assigned to assist in caring for the mother during the postpartum period.

With other team members, you will assist the mother from the stretcher into bed. A protective pad (Chux) may be placed under the patient's buttocks.

Always wear gloves and follow standard precautions when caring for the postpartum patient. There is a high probability of contact with blood, mucous membranes, urine, and breast milk. All of these body fluids are considered potentially infectious.

Anesthesia

If an anesthetic was used, follow the procedures for postoperative care of surgical patients, which were covered in Unit 29.

- Keep the patient flat on her back.
- Make sure the patient has a fresh gown and clean bed linen.
- Check blood pressure, pulse, and respirations as ordered until the patient is stable.
- Continue to monitor vital signs every 4 hours for 24 hours.
- If the patient complains of being cold, an extra blanket may provide comfort. If the patient does not become comfortable, inform the nurse.
- Record the first voiding. Inform the nurse if the patient has not voided by the end of your shift.

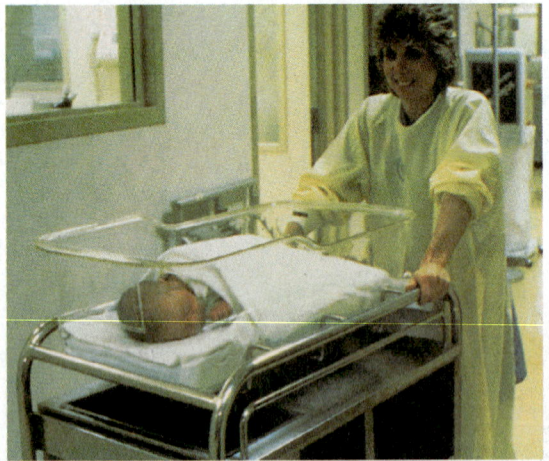

FIGURE 48-12 Babies are transported in their own bassinets from the delivery room to the nursery. *(Courtesy of Memorial Medical Center of Long Beach, CA)*

Drainage

Carefully check the condition of the perineum and the perineal pad for the amount and color of drainage.

- When removing the pad, always lift it away from the body from front to back.
- Red vaginal discharge, called **lochia**, is expected. *Lochia rubra* is the name given to the discharge that occurs during the first three days after delivery. The amount of discharge and any clotting should be reported.

Initially, the lochia is bright red and moderate in amount (Figure 48-14). Over the next week, the lochia will lessen and become pink to pink-brown in color. A discharge that is yellowish-white or brown may continue for 1 to 3 weeks after delivery and then stop. Note and report:

- Signs of tenderness
- Signs of inflammation
- Presence of an episiotomy
- Presence of large blood clots
- Foul-smelling lochia
- Saturation of a pad in 15 to 30 minutes (Figure 48-15)

The Uterus

The size and firmness of the uterus should be checked and reported. A soft and enlarging uterus indicates excessive bleeding.

Massaging. The top of the uterus, the **fundus**, is massaged in a circular fashion while the opposite hand is held against the pubic bone (Figure 48-16). Massaging the fundus stimulates the uterine muscles to contract, firming the uterus.

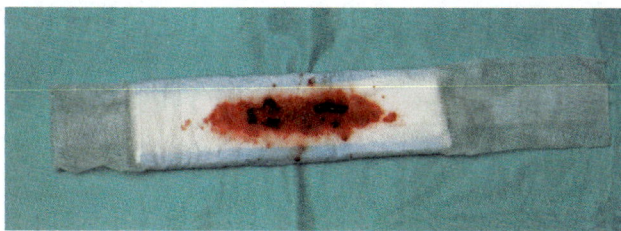

FIGURE 48-14 Moderate lochia is normal during the first few days.

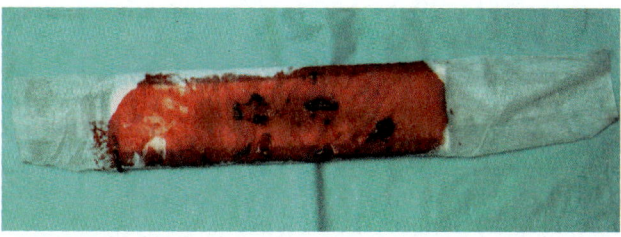

FIGURE 48-15 Heavy lochia must be promptly reported to the nurse.

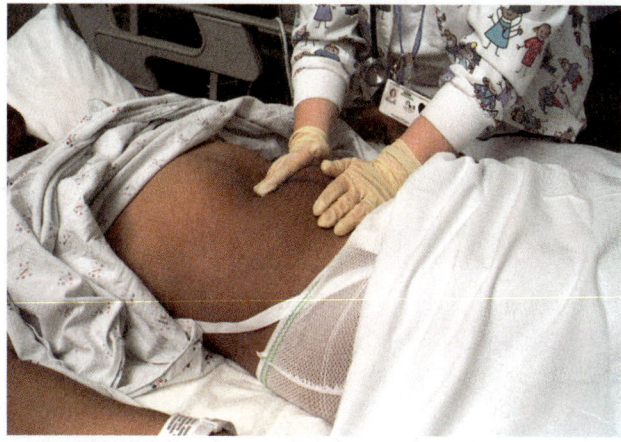

FIGURE 48-16 Both hands are used to massage the fundus.

Measuring Height of Uterus. The level of the fundus is measured by placing the fingers lengthwise across the abdomen between the fundus and the navel. On the first postpartal day, the level of the fundus is usually at the umbilicus or one to two fingers'-width below.

Cramping. As the uterus begins to return to its normal size (**involution**), the patient may experience strong uterine contractions or cramps. Cramping may also be associated with breast feeding. This is normal, but be sure to report any complaints of pain to your team leader, who can administer medication for relief.

Voiding

The new mother should be encouraged to void within the first 6 to 8 hours after the delivery. Check carefully for signs of urine retention. These include:

- A uterus that is unusually high or pushed to one side
- Swelling just above the pubis
- Complaints of urgency (the need to void), but with voidings of 200 mL or less

Be sure to report:

- Signs of possible urine retention immediately, so the patient's recovery will not be impeded
- Any inability to void within the first 8 hours postpartum
- Voidings of less than 100 mL

This is important because a full bladder can cause postpartum hemorrhage.

TOILETING AND PERINEAL CARE

The mother may be:

- Provided with a squeezable bottle filled with warm tap water.
- Instructed to rinse the genitals and perineum after voiding or defecating.

INFECTION CONTROL *Alert*

Infection occurs in about 6% of all postpartum patients. When assisting patients with toileting, have the patient stand up before flushing the toilet. This prevents spraying with contaminated water. Inform the nurse promptly if a patient has an elevated temperature, chills, foul-smelling lochia, or other signs and symptoms of infection.

- Instructed to gently pat, not wipe, the perineal area containing the stitches with tissue or special medicated pads—once only, from front to back. The tissue is discarded in the toilet.
- Taught to wash her hands before applying a fresh perineal pad.
- Taught not to touch the inside of the perineal pad.

If the perineum is very uncomfortable:

- Specially medicated pads may be used for cleansing. The procedure is always the same—front to back and discard.
- Anesthetic sprays may be ordered.
- Ice packs may be used to reduce edema and give comfort.

Patients should be cautioned to apply anesthetics and ointments after cleansing.

Sitting may be uncomfortable when an episiotomy has been performed. Instruct the mother to squeeze her buttocks together and hold them in this position until she is seated upright. This reduces tension on the suture line.

BREAST CARE

The mother's first milk is called colostrum. The colostrum:

- Is watery.
- Carries protective antibodies to the child.
- Usually begins to flow about 12 hours after delivery. Lactation, the flow of milk, does not begin until the second or third postpartum day.

Keeping the breasts clean is especially important when the mother is planning to breast-feed her baby.

- The mother's hands and nipples should be washed just prior to feeding the baby.
- During the shower, the mother should wash the breasts, using a circular motion from the nipples outward.
- Creams are sometimes used between feedings to help the nipples remain supple.

- Breast pads absorb milk leakage. They should be changed frequently.
- The breasts should be supported by a well-fitted brassiere.

Even if the mother chooses not to breast-feed, the breasts should be washed daily with soap and water. The breasts should also be supported continuously by a well-fitted brassiere. Medication to suppress milk production is sometimes ordered.

When delivery is uncomplicated, mothers and healthy newborns do not stay in the hospital very long. They are usually able to go home within two days.

NEONATAL CARE

After the newborn is admitted to the nursery, some procedures not carried out in the delivery room are completed. The physician or nurse will examine the baby and make an evaluation of the baby's condition, or status.

Apgar Scoring

The Apgar score is an evaluation of the neonate. It is made at 1 minute, 5 minutes, and 10 minutes after birth. The areas evaluated are:

- Heart rate
- Respiratory effort
- Muscle tone
- Reflex, irritability
- Color

A number value is applied to each assessment and recorded on a special form. For example, the neonate who has a heart rate of less than 100, has slow respirations, offers slight resistance to limb extension, has a weak cry, and is pale and cyanotic would be rated as follows:

Heart rate	1
Respiratory effort	1
Muscle tone	1
Reflex, irritability	1
Color	0
Total	4

Totals indicate the infant's condition. A score of 7 to 10 indicates that the infant is in good condition. A score of 4 to 6 indicates a fair condition. A score of 0 to 4 indicates a poor condition.

Care of the Newborn Infant

In the nursery the baby's vital signs are determined. Measurements of length and weight are also taken. The infant's axillary temperature is monitored and recorded every 30 to 60 minutes until stable, then every 4 hours or according to the nurse's instructions.

When the newborn's status becomes stable:

- If the eyes were not treated with silver nitrate drops or antibiotics in the delivery room, or the footprints were not taken, these procedures are done at this time.
- The baby is cleaned. Sometimes an admission bath using an antiseptic soap or oil is administered, but procedures for bathing newborns vary from hospital to hospital. In some hospitals, the bath is omitted and the cheesy material known as *vernix caseosa* is allowed to remain on the skin. The area around the umbilical cord is carefully cleaned with a solution prescribed by the facility (Figure 48-17).
- The baby must be kept warm because a newborn's temperature has not yet stabilized. The baby is dressed according to facility policy. A stockinette cap is placed on the head because much body heat can be lost through this surface.
- The baby is placed in a crib or **isolette** (Figure 48-18).

- Feeding is not usually started for 4 to 6 hours after birth. During these hours, the baby is monitored and observed carefully for successful, independent life. After 4 to 6 hours, the baby is either taken to breast-feed or started on feedings of glucose and water. Babies whose mothers are unable to feed will be fed in the nursery.
- Male babies may be circumcised before discharge. In **circumcision**, the excess tissue (**foreskin**) is cut from the tip of the penis (Figure 48-19). This procedure is usually performed based on the parents' personal choices, as well as cultural, ethnic, and religious traditions. For members of some faiths, circumcision is a religious ceremony performed at another location within the first few weeks of life.
- Babies who are jaundiced may have their eyes protected and be placed under a special light (bili light) to help clear the levels of bilirubin in the skin.

Handling the Infant

Take care when lifting, carrying, and positioning an infant. Remember to:

- Lift the baby by grasping the legs securely with one hand while slipping the other hand under the baby's back to support the head and neck (Figures 48-20A to D).

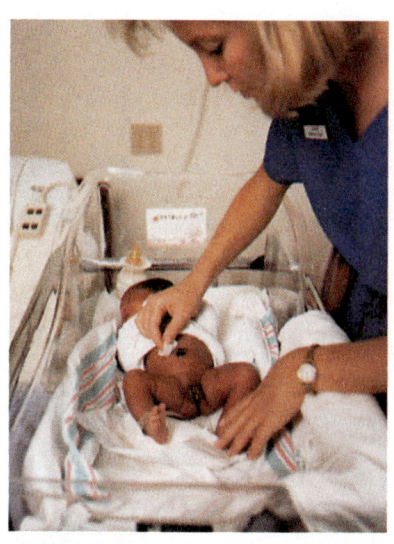

FIGURE 48-17
The cord is carefully cleaned to cause it to dry and to prevent infection.

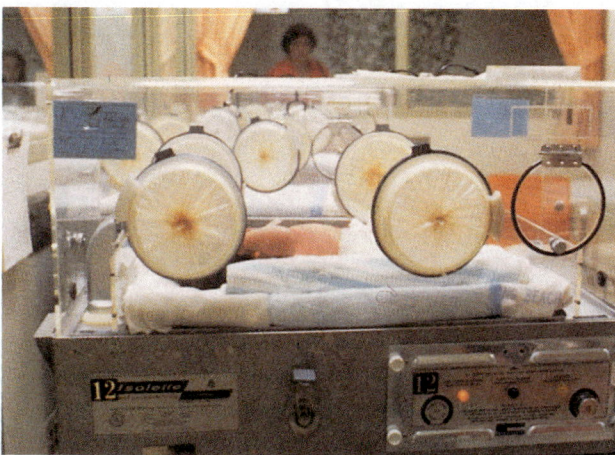

FIGURE 48-18 Some babies are cared for in the controlled environment of the isolette. *(Courtesy of Memorial Medical Center of Long Beach, CA)*

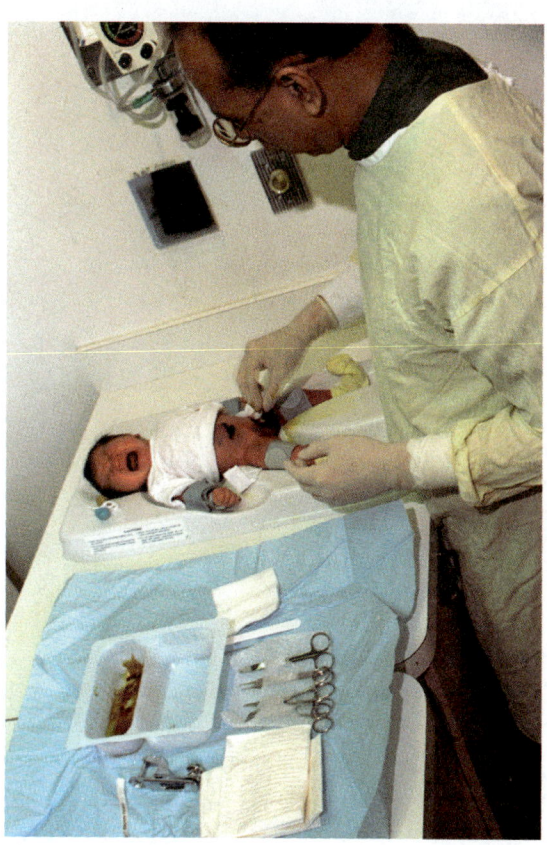

FIGURE 48-19 The infant is circumcised shortly after birth at the parents' request.

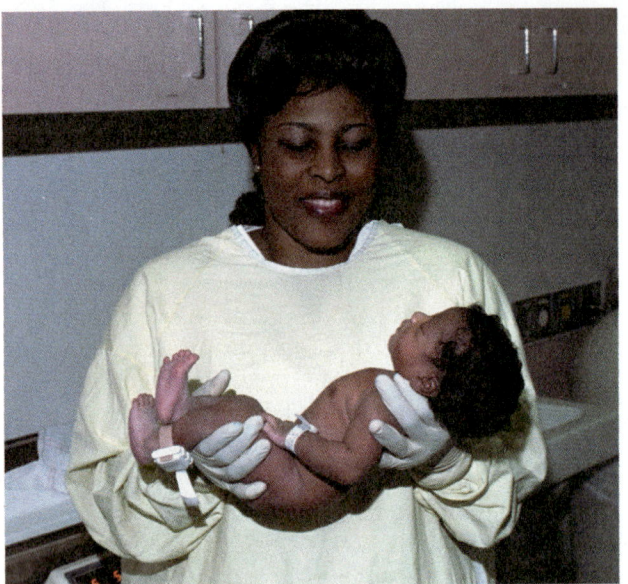

FIGURE 48-20A Always support the infant's bottom and neck.

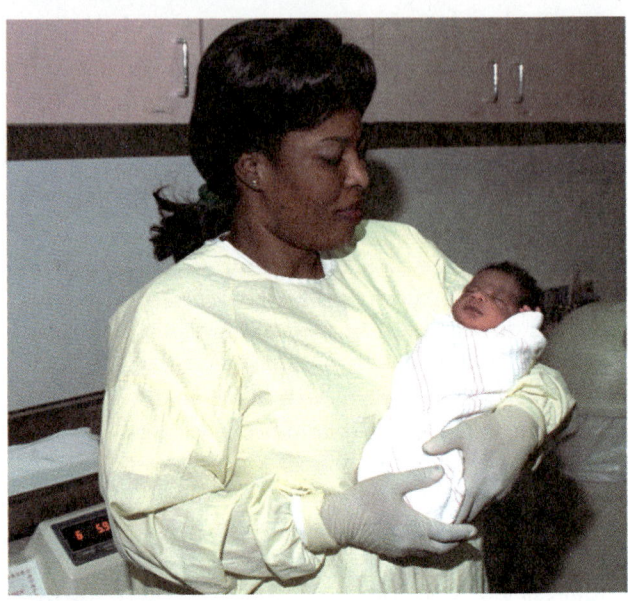

FIGURE 48-20B Cradle hold.

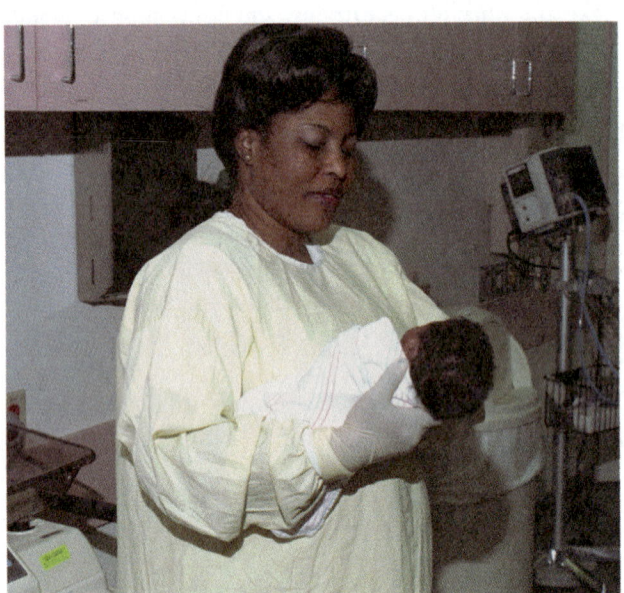

FIGURE 48-20C Football hold.

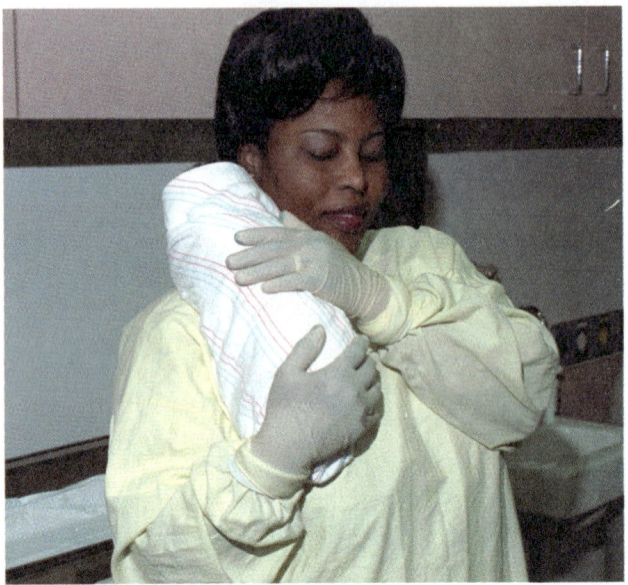

FIGURE 48-20D Shoulder hold.

- Hold the baby securely.
- Support the head, neck, and back at all times.
- Back through doorways when carrying a baby.
- Never turn your back on an infant when the infant is on an unprotected surface.

PKU Test

The baby's blood is tested to detect the presence of phenyl-ketonuria (PKU). PKU is a congenital, hereditary abnormality. It may lead to mental retardation if undetected and not treated early. In PKU, normal protein digestion is not possible. The disorder cannot be cured, but it can be controlled by a special diet.

Eye Care

This procedure is performed by the nurse. Silver nitrate ($AgNO_3$) in a 1% solution is commonly used, but other medications such as antibiotics may be ordered.

Elimination

The passage of urine and stool in a newborn infant are important observations. A normal newborn will urinate 6 to 10 times a day. Elimination activity is recorded and the color of stool documented. Stools should change from dark, meconium stools (Figure 48-21A) to brown-yellow, pasty transitional stools, then finally to yellow stools that are slightly loose (Figure 48-21B).

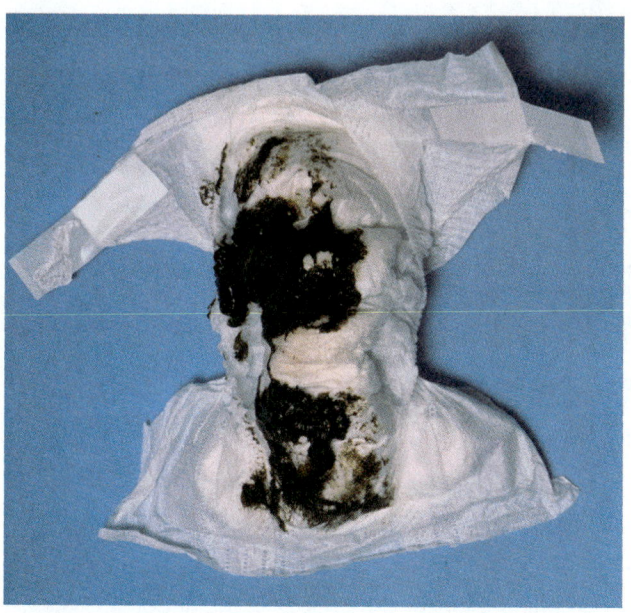

FIGURE 48-21A The first stools are meconium stools.

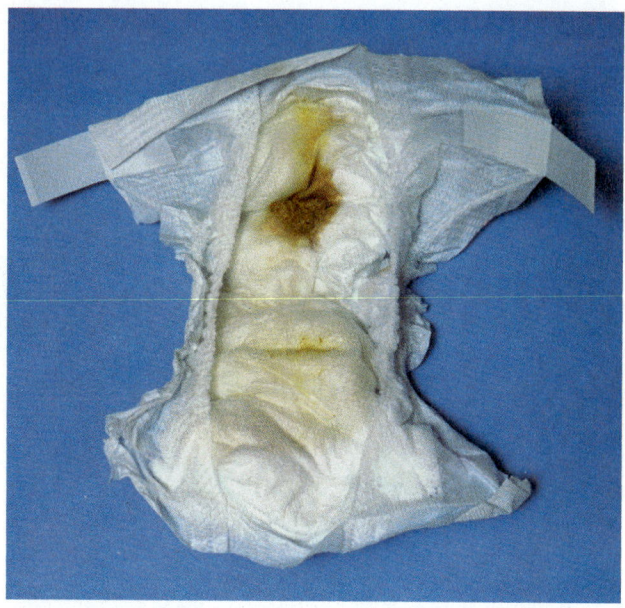

FIGURE 48-21B A yellow stool from a breast-fed infant.

PROCEDURE 128

CHANGING A DIAPER

1. Carry out beginning procedure actions.

2. Assemble equipment:
   - clean diaper
   - gloves
   - plastic bag or container for trash
   - damp washcloths, wipes, or cotton balls for cleansing
   - mild soap, if used
   - supplies for cord care and/or circumcision care, according to facility policy

3. Remove the soiled diaper and observe for color, consistency, and quantity of elimination.

4. Roll the soiled diaper so the clean outer side faces out. Put it in the trash or place it out of reach of the infant.

5. Cleanse the diaper area with wipes or a damp washcloth. Clean from the front toward the back

in a female infant, and from the tip of the penis toward the scrotum for a male infant. Cleanse all folds of the groin and anus. Discard the wipes or washcloth.

6. Lift the buttocks with one hand and slide the new, open diaper underneath.

7. Pull the diaper between the legs. Fold the top edge of the diaper down so it is positioned under the umbilical cord. Fasten the tape snugly on each side.

8. Perform cord care with alcohol or antiseptic according to facility policy.

9. Change other clothing, blanket, or crib linen if soiled or wet.

10. Discard the soiled diaper and your gloves, if not done previously.

11. Carry out procedure completion actions.

Post-Circumcision Care

The circumcision should be checked each time the diaper is changed and should be a routine part of that care. Observe the incision site for bleeding and report anything unusual. The crib identification should note the new circumcision. A note should also be included on the nursery record as to the condition of the circumcision and first voiding after circumcision.

Bathing the Infant

The infant may be bathed after the temperature has stabilized. Bathing is done daily, and as needed. The nurse will teach the parents how to bathe the infant as part of the discharge instructions.

PROCEDURE 129

BATHING AN INFANT

Note: *Before beginning the procedure, check with the nurse to make sure the infant's temperature is stable enough for bathing. Keep the infant warm throughout the procedure.*

1. Carry out beginning procedure actions.

2. Assemble equipment:
   - clean diaper
   - gloves (if this is the infant's first bath, wear gloves for the entire procedure; change them before contact with mucous membranes or nonintact skin, according to the principles of standard precautions)
   - washbasin with warm water (98°F to 100°F)
   - plastic bag or container for trash
   - washcloths (2–3)
   - towel
   - cotton balls
   - liquid infant cleanser/shampoo
   - supplies for cord care and/or circumcision care, according to facility policy
   - blankets
   - sheet

3. Place the infant in a bassinet with sides. Arrange the supplies within reach.

4. Check the infant's skin for dryness, peeling, or signs of infection. If present, notify the nurse and obtain instructions for care.

5. Check the site of the umbilical cord for redness, drainage, drying, and bleeding. If present, notify the nurse and obtain instructions for care.

6. Remove the infant's clothing. Cover the infant with a blanket for warmth.

7. Moisten a cotton ball with plain water. Cleanse the eye from inner to outer canthus, in one wipe. Repeat with a new cotton ball for the other eye.

8. Wash the external ears with plain water and a cotton ball or twisted end of the washcloth.

9. Make a mitt with the washcloth. Wash the face and neck with plain water, with attention to areas behind the ears and creases in the neck.

10. Pat the face and neck dry with a towel.

11. Pull the blanket down to expose the upper body.

12. Cleanse the upper body with soap and a washcloth. Rinse soap from the hands quickly, then rinse the remainder of the upper body. Pat dry with a towel.

13. Cleanse the area around the umbilicus. Rinse the area. Keep the cord dry. Pat dry. Follow the nurse's instructions for cord care.

14. Cover the upper body with the blanket. Pull blanket up to expose the lower body.

15. Wash the legs and outer buttocks with soap and water. Rinse well and pat dry.

16. Obtain a fresh washcloth.

17. Cleanse the genitalia with plain water.
    - *Female infant:*
      - Spread labia gently. Wash from front to back toward the anus. Turn the washcloth so a separate part is used for each wipe.
      - Wash the remaining portions of the labia and the folds in the groin.
      - Rinse and pat dry.
    - *Uncircumcised male infant:*
      - Avoid retracting the foreskin.
      - Wash from the urethra outward, then down toward the scrotum.
      - Wash the remaining portions of the scrotum and the folds in the groin.
      - Rinse and pat dry.

continues

PROCEDURE 129

continued

- *Circumcised male infant:*
  - Care for the circumcision according to the nurse's instructions.
  - Check for bleeding.
  - Gently cleanse the area with warm water and cotton balls.
  - Apply petroleum jelly gauze dressing, or according to facility policy.

18. Cleanse the anal area with soap. Rinse and pat dry.

19. Diaper the infant (see Procedure 128).

20. Wrap the infant in the blanket.

21. Pick up the infant, using the football hold. Hold the head over the basin.

22. Wet the scalp well with a washcloth and water.

23. Lather and gently wash the scalp with baby shampoo or gentle cleanser.

24. Rinse the scalp by pouring water from a small cup over the scalp and into the washbasin, or rinse well using a washcloth.

25. Pat dry.

26. Comb the infant's hair. Cover the head, according to facility policy.

27. Dress the infant.

28. Replace the damp blanket and sheets.

29. Carry out procedure completion actions.

SECURITY

All infants must be identified to prevent inadvertent switching, misidentification, and abduction. The nurse will apply identification bands to the infant's wrist and ankle while in the delivery room. The mother is given a matching wrist band. In some facilities, the father is also given a wrist band. The identification bands must be checked each time the infant is brought to the mother for feeding or rooming-in. Crib cards and other documents are also used for infant identification. Each facility has policies for checking identification. In some, the identification is also checked at the beginning and end of each shift.

Infant Abduction

Unfortunately, a number of infant abductions occur each year. Nursing personnel will be expected to wear an identification badge. Reinforce your identity and position to the mothers each time you provide care. The mother will be instructed not to hand the infant over to someone she does not know. Hospitals have various security measures in place to prevent abduction. Some apply magnetic-sensor ankle bands in the delivery room. An alarm will sound if the infant is removed from the unit, similar to an anti-shoplifting device. The mother's written permission may be required for other friends or relatives to hold or feed the infant. If the infant must be transported to another area of the hospital, nursing staff must remain with the child, then return him or her to the original location.

Each hospital has a policy and procedure to follow in the event of an infant abduction. You must become familiar with the procedures to follow in case this occurs. Taking a proactive position is best, however. Be aware of safety and security measures, and practice them daily.

DISCHARGE

To carry out the discharge procedure from a facility:

- Match the baby's identification with the mother's.
- Dress the child in his or her own clothing (Figure 48-22). This may be done in the nursery or in the mother's room.
- Wrap the baby in a blanket, using the technique of "papoosing," as shown in Figure 48-23A through D.

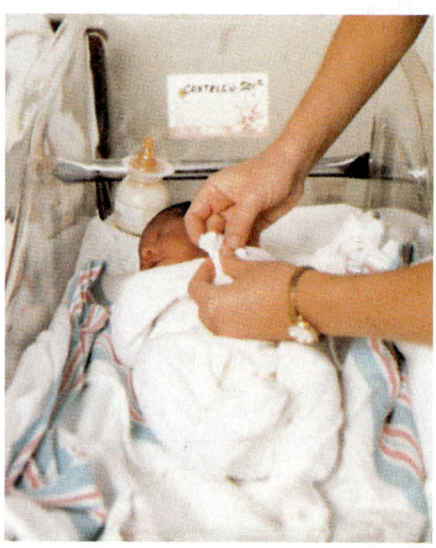

FIGURE 48-22 Dress the infant in his or her own clothing.

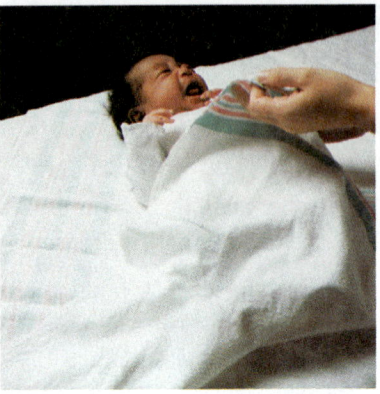

FIGURE 48-23A
Position the receiving blanket under the infant so the corners are at the head and feet. Bring the bottom corner up over the infant.

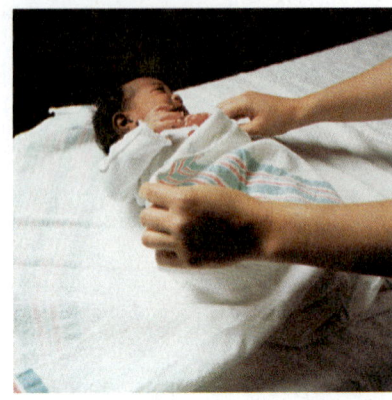

FIGURE 48-23B
Fold one side corner over the infant.

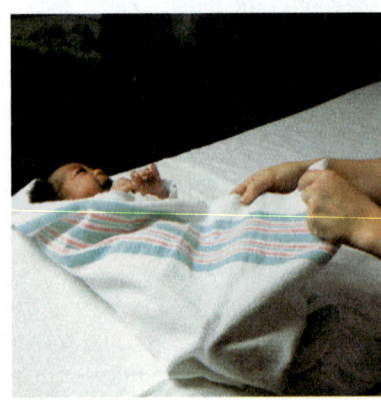

FIGURE 48-23C
Bring the corner from the other side over the infant.

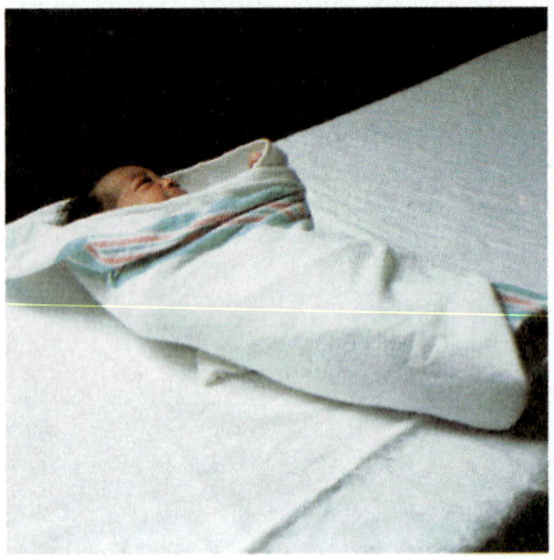

FIGURE 48-23D
Tuck the final corner under the infant, who is now ready for discharge.

- Check to be sure that the mother has received and understands any special discharge instructions. If not, inform the nurse.
- Check to be sure equipment or needed formula is ready when the parents and newborn are ready to go home (Figure 48-24).
- Transport the mother, carrying her baby, by wheelchair to the discharge area. Make sure the infant is strapped into a properly secured car seat. Stay with them until they leave.
- Record the discharge information on the charts of both mother and child. Include the condition of each and the time of release.

Home Care

The discharged mother faces many new challenges. It will take approximately six weeks for her reproductive organs to recover. Home care of the mother includes:

- Providing adequate nutrition
- Allowing for sufficient rest
- Attending to proper elimination

- Providing emotional support during any transitory depression
- Providing breast care, if she is nursing the baby

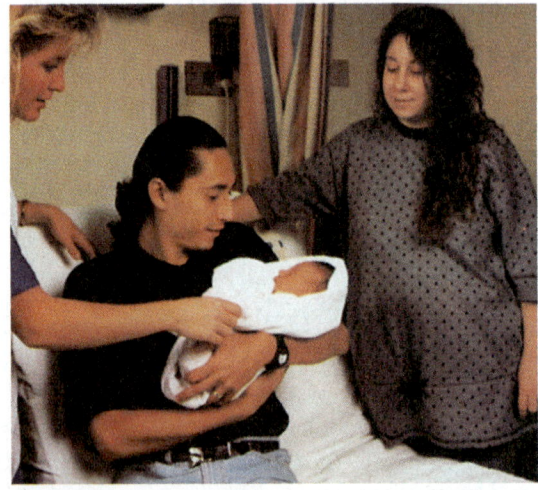

FIGURE 48-24 Parents prepare to leave the hospital with the newborn.

REVIEW

A. True/False.

Mark the following true or false by circling T or F.

1. T F You are responsible for noting and reporting the first postpartal voiding.

2. T F Care of the mother begins in the prenatal period.

3. T F The nurse or physician monitors the progress of labor by performing a vaginal examination.

4. T F Immediate postpartum lochia should be yellowish-white.

5. T F Massaging the cervix stimulates the uterine muscles to contract.

6. T F A congenital abnormality is one that is present at birth.

7. T F Ultrasound is a technique used to examine the baby before birth.

8. T F In the first pregnancy, the period of labor and delivery called expulsion lasts 18 to 24 hours.

9. T F As labor progresses, the uterine cervix becomes more and more tightened.

10. T F The shoulder hold is a safe way to hold and support an infant.

11. T F The first feeding for the newborn is usually given 12 hours after birth.

12. T F The mother's hands and nipples should be washed before she nurses the baby.

B. Matching.

Choose the correct term from Column II to match each phrase in Column I.

Column I

13. _____ surgery to remove the foreskin

14. _____ maintains an even temperature for the fetus

15. _____ mother's first postpartum breast secretions

16. _____ attachment between baby and placenta

17. _____ vaginal discharge following delivery

Column II

a. lochia

b. umbilical cord

c. fundus

d. lactation

e. colostrum

f. circumcision

g. vernix caseosa

h. isolette

i. placenta

C. Nursing Assistant Challenge.

You are working in a prenatal clinic for a nurse practitioner. One of the patients is Mrs. McDonnel, who is coming in today for her first appointment. She tells you she has missed two menstrual periods. Answer the following questions.

18. What signs and symptoms do you expect to see today and for the next month or so?

19. Because this is the patient's first visit, what equipment and supplies do you need to have ready for the nurse practitioner?

20. What signs and symptoms will you observe during the second trimester?

21. What signs and symptoms will you observe during the third trimester?

22. Which procedures would be completed at each visit?

23. What statements by the patient would you report immediately?

EXPLORING THE WEB

Description	Location
American College of Nurse Midwives	*http://www.acnm.org*
American College of Women's Health, Obstetric, and Neonatal Nurses	*http://www.awhonn.org*
Circumcision Information and Resource Page	*http://www.cirp.org*
Combined Health Information Database	*http://chid.nih.gov/subfile/subfile.html*
JHPIEGO (Johns Hopkins)	*http://www.jhpiego.org*
Mother Care	*http://www.jsi.com*
Neonatal Resuscitation Program	*http://www.aap.org*
Prime Intrah (maternal and public health issues)	*http://www.intrah.org*
U.S. Department of Health and Human Services	*http://www.hhs.gov*
Weyerhauser Family Foundation	*http://www.wfamilyfoundation.org*

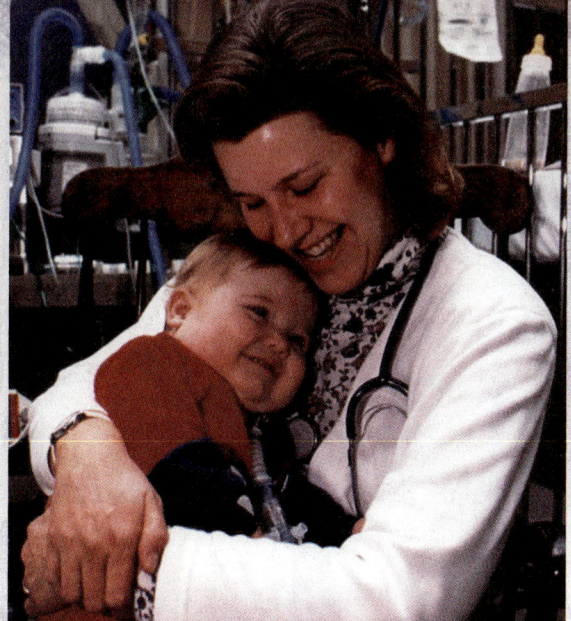

Pediatric Patients

objectives

After completing this unit, you will be able to:

- Spell and define terms.
- Describe the major developmental tasks for each pediatric age group.
- Describe how to foster growth and development of hospitalized pediatric patients.
- Describe how to maintain a safe environment for the pediatric patient.
- Discuss the role of parents and siblings of the hospitalized pediatric patient.
- Demonstrate the following procedures:
  - Procedure 130 Admitting a Pediatric Patient
  - Procedure 131 Weighing the Pediatric Patient
  - Procedure 132 Changing Crib Linens
  - Procedure 133 Changing Crib Linens (Infant in Crib)
  - Procedure 134 Measuring Temperature
  - Procedure 135 Determining Heart Rate (Pulse)
  - Procedure 136 Counting Respiratory Rate
  - Procedure 137 Measuring Blood Pressure
  - Procedure 138 Bottle-Feeding an Infant
  - Procedure 139 Burping (Method A)
  - Procedure 140 Burping (Method B)

vocabulary

Learn the meaning and the correct spelling of the following words and phrases:

adolescence	developmental	foster parent	regress
adoptive parent	milestones	initiative	stepparent
autonomy	developmental tasks	legal custody	
biological parent	family	legal guardian	

INTRODUCTION

Children, like adults, get sick and need hospitalization for diagnosis and treatment of their illnesses. But children are different. They are not just small adults. Children can differ in age, size, and developmental level. When you work with children, you will also be working with the people who are most important to them—their parents or those responsible for their upbringing. When a child is sick and hospitalized, the illness affects the entire family. The family is an important part of the child's life regardless of the child's age. When working with pediatric patients, you will need to include the parents in giving care to the child.

In today's society, the words *parents* and *family* can have different meanings. A child may live with one or both parents. The words *biological*, *adoptive*, *foster*, and *step* can refer to the various types of parents that may be part or all of a child's family. The terms are defined as follows:

- **Biological parent**—birth (genetic) parent
- **Adoptive parent**—person who has legally assumed responsibility for parenting
- **Foster parent**—person who carries out parenting duties under the authority of a legal agency
- **Stepparent**—person who assumes the parenting role by marrying a birth or adoptive parent

Families may also include combinations of parents. For example, a child may live with a biological father and an adoptive mother or stepmother. Or a child may live with a single parent, who could be either biological, adoptive, or foster. Other family arrangements may include the child living with a relative while the parent maintains legal custody of the child. **Legal custody** refers to the person who has the right to give consent for hospitalization and for the procedures that may be needed while the child is hospitalized. This person is known as the **legal guardian**. The child may live with someone other than the legal guardian.

The word **family** refers to the household unit in which the child lives. Members of the family may include the parents, siblings (biological, adoptive, or step), and/or other relatives or persons in the household.

As a member of the health care team, it is important for you to identify the child's caretakers as well as the person who has legal custody. Depending on the child's age, some hospitals require at least one family member to remain at the hospital during the child's stay. This person may be required to stay in the room at all times, and cannot leave the child alone.

This unit provides guidelines for care of the hospitalized child. The nursing assistant must recognize that hospitalization may interrupt the child's normal growth and development. This is a traumatic time for the child. Suggestions are given to show how the nursing assistant can assist and encourage the child's development during hospitalization.

Safety is an important part of providing care. This unit presents guidelines for creating a safe environment for each pediatric age group. Because families are important, suggestions are also made on creating a family-centered approach to pediatric health care.

PEDIATRIC UNITS

Pediatric units are typically set up in one of two ways:

1. According to specific age groups of children
2. According to the types of patients, such as surgical, orthopedic, cardiac, and so on

You may have the opportunity to work with children in a specific age group, or you may work with children in a variety of age groups (Figure 49-1). Regardless of the ages of the children, working in pediatrics will offer you many rewards and challenges.

When a child is admitted to the hospital, you may be involved in the admission procedure. A nurse will obtain a medical and social history from the parents. Information obtained will include the child's nickname, the ages and names of siblings, the child's likes and dislikes, and normal times and routines for meals, naps, and bedtimes. Any information that will make the child's hospital stay easier is marked in the history. Once the history is complete, you can continue with the admission procedure (see Procedure 130).

This unit gives guidelines for caring for children by age groups. The groups are:

- Infancy (0–1 year)
- Toddler (1–3 years)
- Preschooler (3–6 years)
- School-age (6–12 years)
- Adolescent (13–18 years)

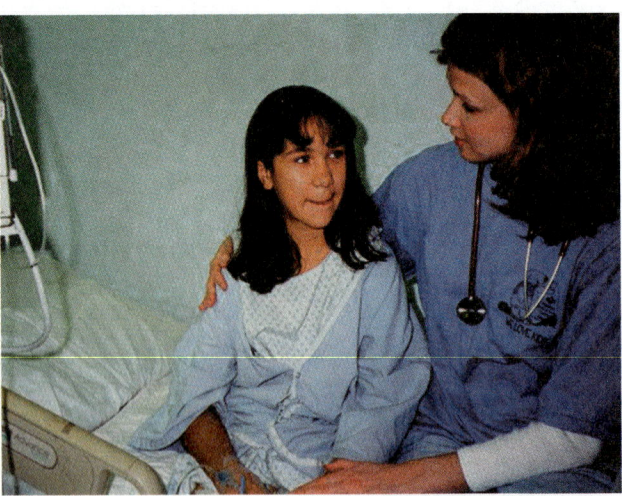

FIGURE 49-1 Make the child feel comfortable during the admission process.

PROCEDURE 130

ADMITTING A PEDIATRIC PATIENT

1. Introduce yourself to the child and his parents.

2. Show them all to the child's room and familiarize them with the unit.

3. Explain what you will do.

4. Wash your hands.

5. Place an identification band on the child.

6. Dress the child in his own pajamas or hospital clothing.

7. Obtain the child's height and weight. Record according to hospital policy. (Refer to Procedure 131.)

8. Measure the child's vital signs. (Refer to Procedures 134 through 137.)

9. Obtain a urine specimen. (Refer to Unit 44.)

10. Wash your hands.

11. Assist the physician or nurse with examination of the child as necessary.

12. Explain rooming-in and visiting policies to the parents.

13. If the parents leave, stay with the child to provide comfort.

DEVELOPMENTAL TASKS

For each age group, it is expected that the child will have reached a certain developmental level. Each level is characterized by physical and psychological tasks that the average child in the group can perform. If you understand the developmental tasks for each age group, it will be easier to find ways to help and encourage the child's development during hospitalization. The approaches suggested here should be personalized for each patient. Some children may appear younger than their stated age due to medical and/or emotional problems. It is also normal for children to regress (go backward) when hospitalized.

CARING FOR INFANTS (BIRTH–1 YEAR)

During the first year of life, the normal infant will:
- Double her birth length.
- Triple her birth weight.
- Show progress in gaining mastery over gross motor behavior, beginning with the head and moving down the trunk toward the feet.

The normal infant begins by gaining head control. The infant then progresses to rolling over, sitting up, crawling, and walking. These motor skills generally occur within specific weeks or months of the infant's life. Achievement of these skills is referred to as the infant's developmental milestones. These milestones are outlined from birth through two years of age in Table 49–1.

Learning to trust is the primary psychosocial developmental task for the infant. All infants depend on others for survival; others must meet all their basic needs. How the infant's needs are met lays the foundation for the infant's developing personality.

Normally, the mother is the caregiver and prime source for developing trust. However, when the infant is hospitalized, the hospital caregivers may assume the role of substitute mother. A caregiver can continue to develop the infant's trust by responding to her cry and her needs. Trust is fostered by feeding, holding, touching, and talking to the infant (Figure 49-2), in addition to keeping her warm and dry.

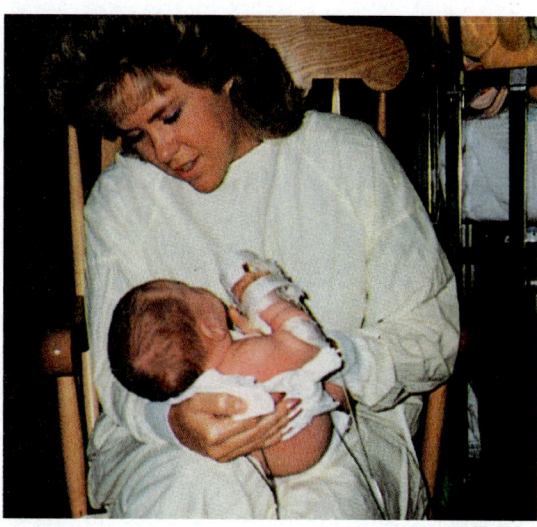

FIGURE 49-2 Holding the infant and making good eye contact promotes trust, security, and affection.

TABLE 49-1 NORMAL AGE FOR ATTAINMENT OF MAJOR DEVELOPMENTAL MILESTONES

Age	Motor Skill	Language	Adaptive Behavior
4–6 wks.	Head lifted from prone position and turned from side to side	Cries	Smiles
4 mo.	No head lag when pulled to sitting from supine position Tries to grasp large objects	Sounds of pleasure	Smiles, laughs aloud, and shows pleasure re familiar objects or persons
5 mo.	Voluntary grasp with both hands	Primitive sounds: "ah goo"	Smiles at self in mirror
6 mo.	Grasps with one hand Rolls prone to supine Sits with support	Range of sounds greater	Expresses displeasure and food preference
8 mo.	Sits without support Transfers objects from hand to hand Rolls supine to prone	Combines syllables: "baba, dada, mama"	Responds to "No"
10 mo.	Sits well Creeping Stands holding onto support Finger-thumb opposition in picking up small objects		Waves "bye-bye," plays "patty-cake" and "peek-a-boo"
12 mo.	Stands holding onto support Walks with support	Says two or three words with meaning	Understands names of objects Shows interest in pictures
15 mo.	Walks alone	Several intelligible words	Requests by pointing Imitates
18 mo.	Walks up and down stairs holding support Removes clothes	Many intelligible words	Carries out simple commands
2 yrs.	Walks up and down stairs by self Runs	Two- to three-word phrases	Organized play Points to some parts of body

Source: Mary Fran Hazinski, *Nursing Care of the Critically Ill Child* (St. Louis: C.V. Mosby Company, 1984, p. 387).

It is important for the infant to have consistent mothering. Therefore, it is ideal to have the mother room-in with her infant. If this is not possible, an alternative approach is to use the same caregivers for an infant. This means that every time a nurse or nursing assistant works, he will care for the same infants. Besides being consistent for the infant, it also allows the caregiver to become familiar with the infant as a unique person. Consistency is especially important when an infant is between six and seven months of age. At this age, the infant normally begins to display a fear of strangers.

Communicating with Infants

Working with infants can be challenging because the infant cannot tell the caregiver in words what he wants or needs. The infant communicates with his cry and body movements. The cry can vary depending on needs. Just as a mother learns to interpret the sound of her infant's cry, the caregiver will also learn to interpret the meanings of the cry by caring for the infant.

Infants respond to voices, faces, and touch. You should talk to the infant (Figure 49-3) whenever you are giving personal care such as bathing, feeding, or holding.

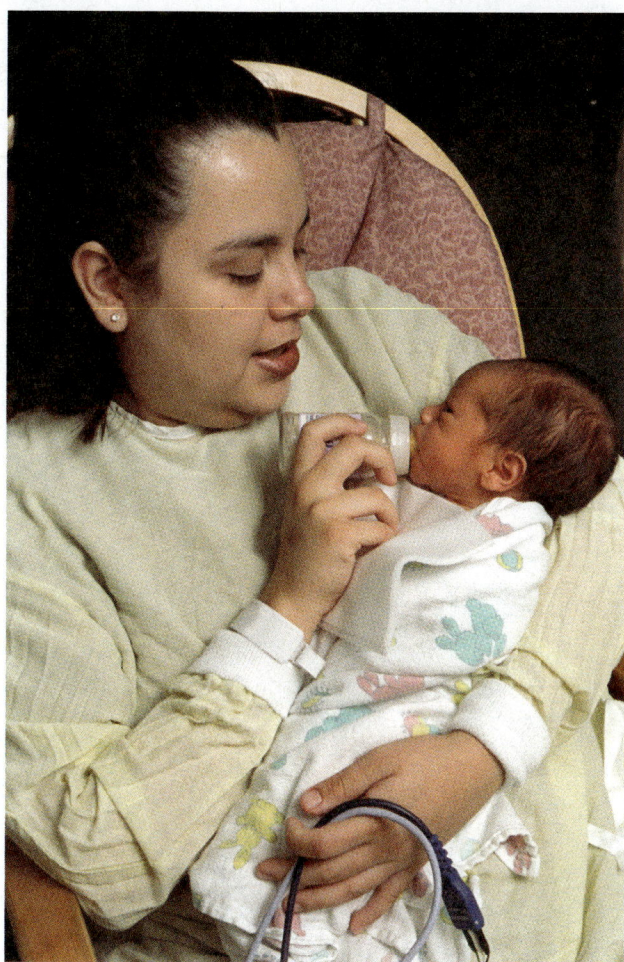

FIGURE 49-3 Talk to the infant each time you provide care.

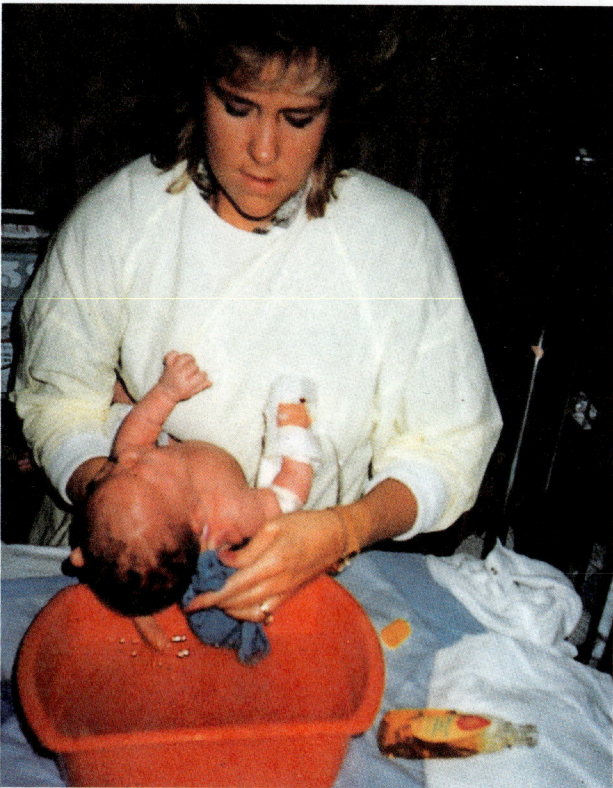

FIGURE 49-4 Hold the infant properly when giving care. The nursing assistant is supporting the head during the bath.

The Waking Hours

When the infant is awake, she needs to explore the environment. Age-appropriate toys are provided so that the infant can continue development while in the hospital. Appropriate toys include colorful mobiles, rattles, and mirrors.

Importance of Families

Siblings of the infant should be allowed to visit while the infant is hospitalized. Toddlers and preschoolers engage in "magical thinking." In other words, they believe that if they wish the infant to be sick, it happens, or if they wish the baby to be gone she won't be back. Therefore, it is important for both toddlers and preschoolers to see their infant sibling. If the mother is rooming-in with the infant, it is also important for toddlers and preschoolers to see and talk to their mother.

Routine Procedures

When carrying out routine care of the infant, be sure that you hold the infant properly (Figure 49-4). (Refer to Unit 48.)

Before feeding the infant, organize his care so that he can be allowed to digest his food and sleep after he has eaten. You should not move him unnecessarily, as it may cause him to vomit what he has just eaten. In organizing the care, you would weigh him, bathe him, diaper him, and dress him. Then change the crib linens, weigh him, and feed him.

The routine procedures covered here may apply to all pediatric patients. They include:

- Procedure 131—Weighing the pediatric patient (infant and older children)
- Procedure 132—Changing crib linens
- Procedure 133—Changing crib linens (infant in crib)
- Procedure 134—Measuring temperature (rectal, oral, and axillary)
- Procedure 135—Determining heart rate (pulse)
- Procedure 136—Counting respiratory rate
- Procedure 137—Measuring blood pressure

Weighing the Infant

Routine care includes weighing the infant. This procedure should also be done before feeding.

Tips: Put clean paper on the scale before using it, to prevent chilling. Balance the scale with the paper in place. Keep your hand on the infant to prevent accidents. Work quickly to prevent heat loss in the infant. Disinfect the scale each time it is used, to prevent cross-contamination.

PROCEDURE 131

WEIGHING THE PEDIATRIC PATIENT

Infant

1. Wash your hands.

2. Place a small sheet or receiving blanket on the scale and balance the scale with the blanket on it.

3. Check the infant's previous weight.

4. Check the infant's identification band.

5. Remove the infant's diaper and shirt.

6. Place the infant on the scale, keeping a hand over the infant to prevent falling (Figure 49-5).

7. Move the bar to the correct weight until the scale balances.

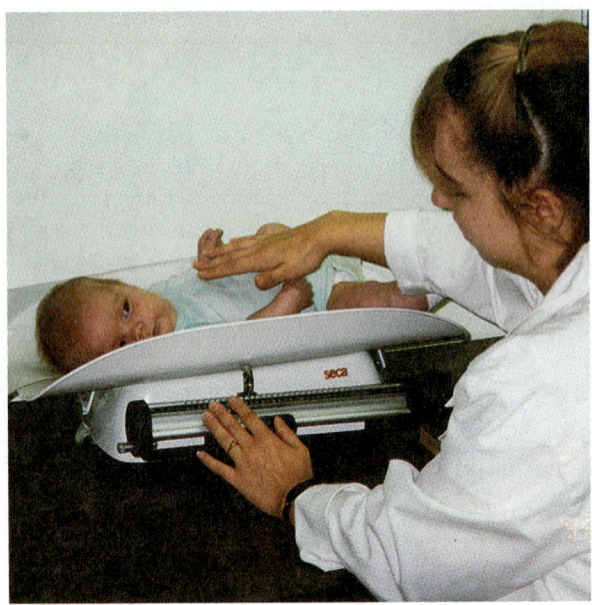

FIGURE 49-5 Maintain light hand contact with the infant while adjusting the weights with the other hand.

8. Return the infant to the crib. Diaper and dress the infant.

9. Record the infant's weight according to hospital policy.

10. Remove the linen from the scale and place it in a laundry receptacle.

11. Return the scale to its proper storage place.

12. Wash your hands.

Toddler to Adolescent

1. Use an upright scale if the child is able to stand. Bring the scale to the bedside, if possible, and balance it.

2. Wash your hands.

3. Check the child's identification band.

4. Check the child's previous weight.

5. Weigh the child in as few clothes as possible. Remove any diaper and shoes or slippers.

6. Have the child stand on the scale. Move the bar to the correct weight until the scale balances.

7. Record the weight according to hospital policy.

8. Return the child to bed.

9. Return the scale to its proper storage place.

10. Wash your hands.

Alternate Action: If the toddler is unable to stand on his own, pick him up and step on the scale. Obtain the combined weight. Put the toddler back in bed, weigh yourself, and subtract your weight from the combined weight. The toddler's weight is the difference in weights.

PROCEDURE 132

CHANGING CRIB LINENS

1. Wash your hands.

2. Gather supplies:
   - disposable gloves
   - sheet
   - blanket
   - shirt
   - diaper
   - pad

   Do steps 1 and 2 before bathing the infant.

3. When bathing the infant, apply the principles of standard precautions as you would with an adult.

4. After bathing the infant, diaper and dress her.

5. Place the infant in a stroller, playpen, or other safe place.

6. Strip the linen from the crib. Wear gloves if linen is soiled. Dispose of soiled or used linen according to facility policy.

7. Remove gloves and discard according to facility policy.

8. Wash your hands.

9. Place clean linen on the bed and open the sheet, hem side down.

10. Make one side of the crib, miter the corners top and bottom, and tuck in the side (Figure 49-6A).

11. Pull down the crib top (Figure 49-6B). Pull up the crib side (Figure 49-6C).

12. Repeat step 10 on the opposite side of the crib.

13. Place a diaper pad on top of the sheet, according to hospital policy.

14. Place a clean blanket at the bottom of the bed.

15. Arrange bumper pads around the sides of the crib.

16. Wash your hands.

17. Return the infant to the crib, cover her with the blanket (if appropriate), and pull up the crib side.

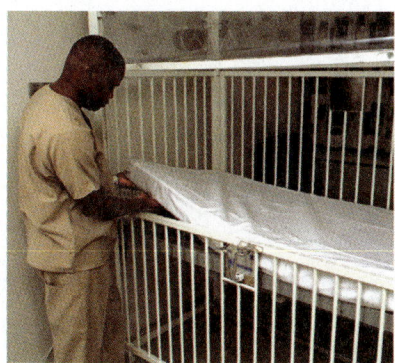

FIGURE 49-6A Make one side of the crib. Miter the corners at the top and bottom and tuck the sheet under the mattress.

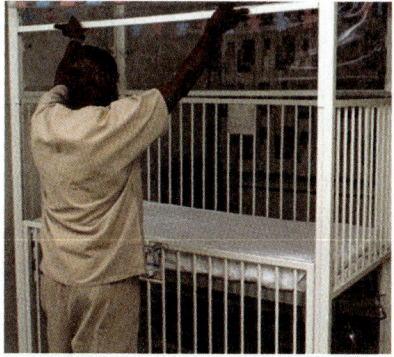

FIGURE 49-6B Pull the crib top down.

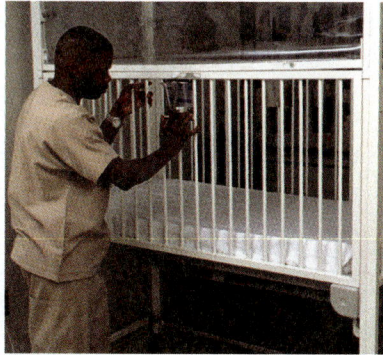

FIGURE 49-6C Pull the side up and check for security.

PROCEDURE 133

CHANGING CRIB LINENS (INFANT IN CRIB)

1. Wash your hands.
2. Gather linens
   - sheet
   - blanket
   - shirt
   - diaper
   - bathing equipment
   - disposable gloves

   Do steps 1 and 2 before bathing the infant.
3. After bathing the infant, diaper and dress him.
4. Pick up the infant and hold him in one arm.
5. With your free hand, strip the old linen off the crib. Wear gloves if linen is soiled.
6. Place the clean linen on the mattress and open the sheet, placing the hem side down. Place the infant on the sheet.
7. Place one hand on the infant and keep it on him at all times.
8. Make one side of the crib. Miter the corners, top and bottom, and tuck in the side.
9. Remove your hand from the infant and pull up the crib side.
10. Go around to the other side of the crib.
11. Take down the crib side, place one hand on the infant, and repeat step 8.
12. Place a diaper pad under the infant and cover him with the blanket, if appropriate.
13. Arrange bumper pads around the crib, if appropriate.
14. Pull up the crib side.
15. Wash your hands.

Determining Vital Signs

The infant's vital signs must be measured as outlined in the care plan. It is normal for an infant's heart to beat faster than an adult's. The normal ranges of heart rates and respiratory rates for each age group are listed in Table 49-2. An increase in the infant's heart and respiratory rates can be caused by stress (crying, fever, or infection). Therefore, the pulse and respiratory rates should be taken when the infant is quiet, either awake or sleeping.

TABLE 49-2 NORMAL VITAL SIGNS

| Age | Heart Rate | Respirations | Blood Pressure | |
			Systolic	Diastolic
Infants	120–160	30–60	74–100	50–70
Toddlers	90–140	24–40	80–112	50–80
Preschoolers	80–110	22–34	82–110	50–78
School–age	75–100	18–30	84–119	54–80
Adolescents	60–90	12–16	94–119	62–88

Note: Pulse and respiration are taken for a full minute. The apical pulse is used with infants and young children.

PROCEDURE ⬤134

MEASURING TEMPERATURE

Temperatures on children 5 years of age and under are usually taken rectally or by the tympanic method unless there is a medical reason not to. Axillary temperature can be taken in place of rectal temperatures.

Rectal Temperature

All other vital signs should be measured before the temperature if a rectal temperature is to be measured.

1. Wash your hands and put on gloves.

2. Check the patient's identification band.

3. Explain to the parents and child what you are going to do.

4. Inspect the thermometer for breaks.

5. Shake down the thermometer.

6. Cover the thermometer with a disposable sheath.

7. Lubricate the thermometer sheath, if it is not prelubricated.

8. Lay the child on his back on bed (Figure 49-7A) or on her stomach across your lap (Figure 49-7B).

9. Insert the thermometer ½ inch into the child's rectum and hold. Hold the child securely and gently so the child does not move about.

10. Leave the thermometer in place for the required amount of time (3 to 5 minutes). See your hospital policy.

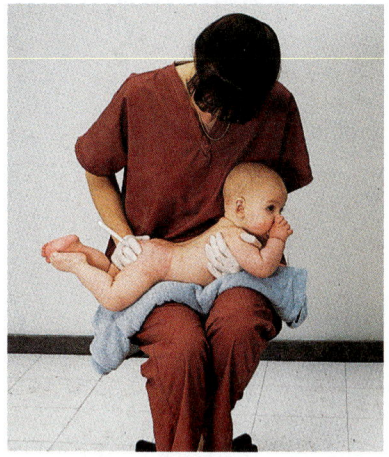

FIGURE 49-7B
Infant in prone position.

11. Remove the thermometer. Discard the sheath according to facility policy.

12. Remove gloves and wash your hands.

13. Record.

14. Report any deviations from normal according to hospital policy.

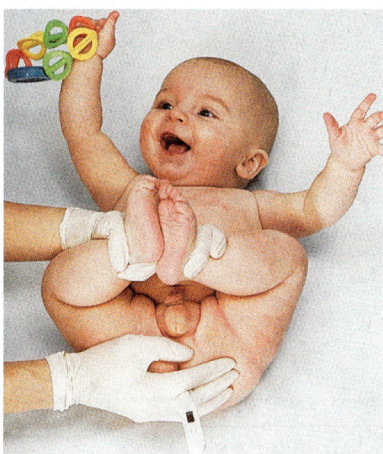

FIGURE 49-7A
Infant in supine position.

SAFETY *Alert*

Check with the nurse before taking a rectal temperature on a newborn infant. In some facilities, the first rectal temperature must be taken by the nurse, to ensure that the rectum is patent. After that, axillary or tympanic temperature may be the method of choice. Know and follow your facility policy. When taking a rectal temperature, grasp the child's ankles gently, but firmly, with one hand. Cover the penis of a male infant with a diaper. Insert the lubricated thermometer while holding the ankles. Continue to hold the ankles with one hand and the thermometer with the other throughout the procedure.

continues

PROCEDURE 134

continued

Oral Temperature

1. Explain to the parents and child what you will be doing.

2. Check the patient's identification band.

3. Wash your hands.

4. Inspect the thermometer for breaks.

5. Shake down the thermometer.

6. Cover the thermometer with a disposable sheath.

7. Apply gloves.

8. Instruct the child to hold the thermometer under his tongue. If the child cannot hold the thermometer in his mouth, then obtain either a rectal, tympanic, or axillary temperature.

9. Leave the thermometer under the child's tongue for the required amount of time (usually 5 to 8 minutes).

10. Remove the thermometer. Discard the sheath according to facility policy.

11. Read the thermometer.

12. Remove gloves and discard according to facility policy.

13. Wash your hands.

14. Record the temperature.

15. Report any deviations from normal according to hospital policy.

Axillary Temperature

1. Explain to the parents and child what you are going to do.

2. Check the patient's identification band.

3. Wash your hands.

4. Inspect the thermometer for breaks.

5. Shake down the thermometer.

6. Cover the thermometer with a disposable sheath.

7. Place the thermometer in the child's armpit.

8. Hold the child's arm close to her chest for the required amount of time (10 minutes).

9. Remove the thermometer. Discard the sheath according to facility policy.

10. Read the thermometer.

11. Wash your hands and record the temperature value.

12. Report any deviations from normal according to hospital policy.

 Note: *If an electronic thermometer is used, follow the manufacturer's directions supplied with the equipment.*

Tympanic Temperature

1. Explain to the parents and child what you are going to do.

2. Check the patient's identification band.

3. Wash your hands.

4. Check the lens on the thermometer to make sure it is clean and intact.

5. Set the appropriate mode on the thermometer.

6. Place a clean probe cover on the probe.

7. Position the patient so you will have access to the ear you will be using.

8. If the patient is under age 3, pull the ear straight back, then down. In children over age 3, pull the ear up and back. While gently tugging the ear, fit the probe snugly into the canal, aiming at the tympanic membrane. Point the probe tip at the midpoint between the eyebrow and sideburn on the opposite side of the face. The probe tip should penetrate at least one-third of the ear canal and form a complete seal.

9. Press the activation button. Leave the thermometer in place until the display blinks or signals that the temperature is final.

10. Remove the thermometer. Discard the probe cover.

11. Wash your hands and record the temperature.

12. Report any deviations from normal according to hospital policy.

DIFFICULT *Situations*

When taking vital signs on an infant or small child, take the rectal temperature *last*. Taking the rectal temperature first may cause the infant to cry, which will accelerate the pulse and respirations.

PROCEDURE 135

DETERMINING HEART RATE (PULSE)

With infants and children, the easiest way to find the heart rate is to place the stethoscope over the heart (Figure 49-8). This is called the apical pulse. It should be done when the child is quiet or at rest because stress and crying can result in a reading that is higher than normal.

1. Wash your hands.

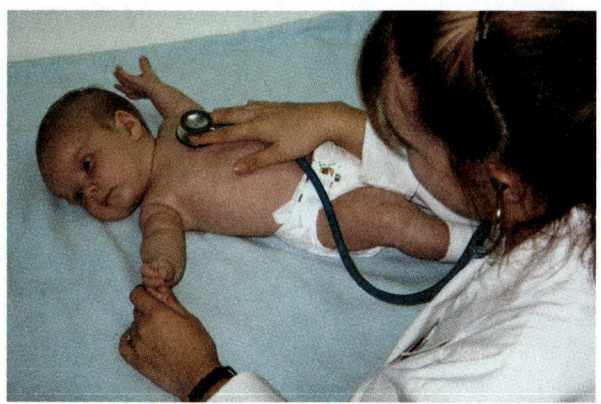

FIGURE 49-8 Measuring the apical pulse.

2. Check the patient's identification band.

3. Explain the procedure to the patient and/or his parents. Clean stethoscope earpieces and diaphragm with an antiseptic wipe and dry them. (Allow a child to play with the stethoscope first.)

4. Rub the diaphragm of the stethoscope to warm it so that it will not be cold when placed on the infant's chest.

5. Place the stethoscope over the infant's heart and count the number of beats you hear in a minute.

6. Clean the stethoscope earpieces and diaphragm with an antiseptic wipe and dry them.

7. Wash your hands and record the results.

8. Report rates higher or lower than the normal for the appropriate age group, according to hospital policy.

Note: The radial pulse can be used for children 6 years and over. The procedure used is the same as for adults. Refer to Procedure 42 in Unit 19.

PROCEDURE 136

COUNTING RESPIRATORY RATE

Infants and toddlers use their abdominal muscles for breathing. To count the respiratory rate for this age group, look at the abdomen and chest and count the respirations for a minute.

To obtain the respiratory rate for preschoolers and older children, follow Procedure 44 in Unit 19, as for adults, but count the respirations for a full minute.

PROCEDURE (137)

MEASURING BLOOD PRESSURE

A blood pressure measurement may not always be required for all pediatric patients. If blood pressure is to be recorded, you must have the correct size cuff for the child. The cuff should cover two-thirds of the upper arm.

1. Select the correct cuff size for the patient.

2. Assemble all equipment. Clean stethoscope earpieces and diaphragm with an antiseptic wipe and dry them.

3. Wash your hands.

4. Check the patient's identification band.

5. Explain the procedure to the child, using language such as, "This will feel like a tight hug on your arm."

6. Wrap the cuff securely around the upper arm.

7. Feel for the brachial pulse.

8. Place the stethoscope earpieces in your ears and place the diaphragm near the pulse point.

9. Pump up the cuff until you no longer hear the pulse. Release the valve and listen for systolic and diastolic sounds.

10. Wash your hands and record the results according to hospital policy.

Feeding

Feeding is important to the infant because it satisfies her hunger and sucking needs. Sucking provides the infant with a pleasant sensation, whether she receives food with her sucking or not. The amount of time an infant needs to suckle will vary with each infant. Always provide the infant with the opportunity to suck. This is even more important if the infant cannot eat.

When feeding an infant:

- Hold the infant unless there is a medical reason not to.
- If an infant cannot be held, you should still hold the bottle for her while she eats.
- An infant should never be left in a crib with a bottle propped in his mouth. This is dangerous because the infant could get too much formula at one time, vomit, and choke.

- Holding the infant during a feeding also allows close, physical contact with the person feeding her.
- During feeding and following feeding, the infant should be burped.

Note: If an infant cannot be fed, she should still be held and allowed to suck on a pacifier unless a medical reason prevents removal of the infant from the crib.

INFECTION CONTROL *Alert*

The formula and bottle should be sterile for bottle-feeding a newborn infant. Wash your hands well before feeding the infant. Avoid touching the nipple or the inside of the cap with your hands. Keep the nipple covered with the cap until you are ready to begin feeding. Check the expiration date on the bottle to make sure the formula has not expired.

SAFETY *Alert*

Shake the bottle slightly to ensure that the formula is mixed well. Invert the bottle and drop a few drops of formula on your wrist to check for temperature of formula and patency of the nipple. Formula should drip freely, but not come out in a stream. If the formula runs out in a stream, change the nipple before proceeding. Elevate the child's head and shoulders slightly during feeding to prevent aspiration of formula and allow air to rise to the top of the stomach, where it is expelled more readily. Keep the nipple filled with formula at all times, to prevent ingestion of air. A steady stream of bubbles should rise in the bottle during feeding. If the infant pushes the nipple out with her tongue, reinsert it. This is a normal reflex and does not mean the child is full or does not want to eat.

PROCEDURE 138

BOTTLE-FEEDING AN INFANT

1. Wash your hands.

2. Gather the infant's formula and diaper pad, washcloth, or bib.

3. Check the infant's identification band.

4. Pick up the infant and hold her to feed her, unless there is a medical reason not to.

5. Sit in a chair or rocker.

6. Hold the infant in the crook of your arm, with the infant's head slightly raised (Figure 49-9).

7. Place a diaper, washcloth, or bib under the infant's chin, covering the chest.

8. Tip the bottle so the nipple is filled with formula.

9. Stroke the side of the infant's cheek closest to you. The infant will automatically turn toward the side stroked and open her mouth. Place the nipple in the infant's mouth.

10. If the nipple is in the mouth but the infant is not sucking, gently lift up under the infant's chin to close her mouth on the nipple.

11. Hold the bottle so the nipple stays filled with formula while the infant feeds.

12. Feed the infant the ordered amount of formula and burp according to the infant's age and hospital policy. (See Procedures 139 and 140.)

 Note: *Bottle-fed infants swallow a lot of air while sucking. Burping is important to remove the air from their stomachs.*

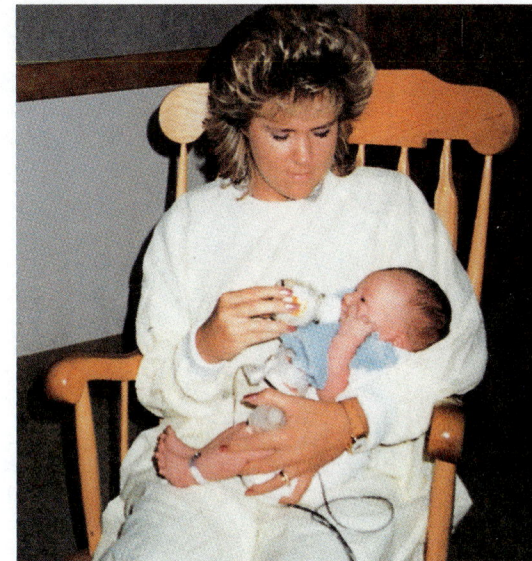

FIGURE 49-9 Hold the infant with the head elevated during bottle feeding. Keep the nipple filled with fluid while the infant sucks.

13. If the infant starts to vomit while feeding, remove the bottle and turn the infant to the side, with her head lowered, to prevent aspiration. Seek help as needed.

14. After feeding, return the child to the crib and place her on her back or side.

15. Pull up the crib side.

16. Wash your hands.

17. Record the amount of formula the infant took, according to hospital policy.

Burping

The frequency with which you burp the infant will depend on the infant's age and medical condition. Burping is important because bottle-fed infants swallow a lot of air while sucking. The infant can be burped as frequently as after every half-ounce of formula. Older infants can be burped after 1 to 2 ounces during feeding and at the conclusion of feeding. Refer to your hospital policy for the frequency of burping. There are two methods of burping an infant. (See Procedures 139 and 140.)

Breast-Feeding

If the rooming-in or visiting mother is breast-feeding, she should be directed to an area where she can be assured of privacy as well as comfort. As a nursing assistant, you may be responsible for weighing the infant before and after feeding, according to your hospital policy. Refer to the steps for weighing in Procedure 131.

When returning the infant to his crib after feeding, place him on his back or side. A rolled blanket can be used to keep him on his side.

PROCEDURE 139

BURPING (METHOD A)

1. Place a diaper or cloth over your shoulder.

2. Lift the infant up to your shoulder, holding the infant close to your chest (Figure 49-10).

3. Holding the infant in place with one hand, use the other hand to gently rub or pat the infant's back until the infant burps.

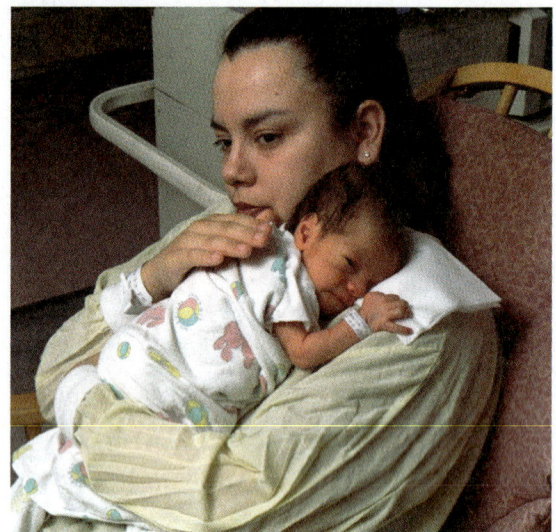

FIGURE 49-10 Burping the infant during and after feeding helps eliminate swallowed air. Gently rub or pat the infant's back.

PROCEDURE 140

BURPING (METHOD B)

1. Place a diaper, cloth, or bib under the infant's chin.

2. Place the child in a sitting or upright position. Put one hand on the infant's chest, supporting the infant's weight (Figure 49-11). With the other hand, gently rub or pat the infant's back until the infant burps.

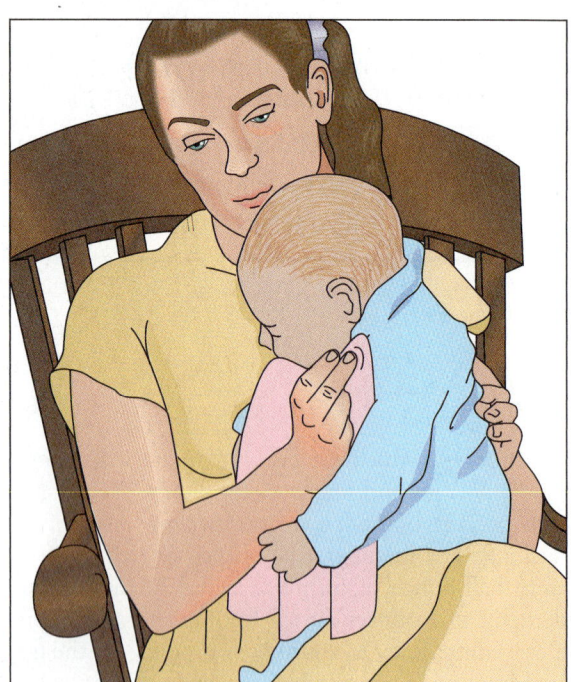

FIGURE 49-11 An alternative method of burping is to sit the infant on your lap with a cloth or bib under the chin.

Restraints

It is generally not necessary to obtain a physician's order to restrain an infant or a child. The infant or child is considered to be incompetent. Restraints can be used for the child's safety. Restraints are used to protect the child from injury to herself or to others, or to protect the child from injury by equipment used in care. Any child who is restrained in any way should be freed from the restraints every 2 hours and allowed to exercise the extremities under supervision. Restraints should never be tied to a crib side or bed rail, only to the bed or crib frame.

A *jacket restraint* is a sleeveless cloth garment. It is fitted to the child's chest and crosses in the back, out of the child's reach. It has long straps that can be tied under the mattress or through a chair. When tied this way, the child can move the extremities, sit up, lie down in bed, or turn side-to-side without falling.

An *extremity restraint* may be used on the child's arms, hands, legs, or feet. Commercial restraints are available in sheepskin, Velcro, or disposable materials. This restraint is placed on the child's extremity according to hospital policy and procedure and manufacturers' directions. The ties are tied to the frame of the crib. For very small infants, the ties may be pinned to the mattress.

Summary of Nursing Assistant Tasks and Responsibilities When Caring for Infants

- Maintain a safe environment.
- Provide information to the health team through monitoring of vital signs (temperature, pulse, respiration), weight, intake, and output.
- Provide routine care such as bathing, feeding, and changing.
- Collect and test specimens.
- Assist with treatments, examinations, and procedures.
- Provide warmth, security, and affection.

SAFETY *Alert*

Avoid use of restraints whenever possible. Consider alternatives, such as distraction, before applying restraints. If restraints are necessary, the nurse should make the decision regarding the type of restraint to use. Remove and reapply the restraint every 2 hours. Elevate the head of the bed every 30 minutes. Offer comfort measures, including food, fluids, and toileting as appropriate. Provide distraction and touch.

guidelines *for*

Ensuring a Safe Environment for Infants

- Always keep crib side rails up.
- Always keep one hand on the infant when the crib side rail is down.
- Use crib bumpers or rolled blankets to prevent injury.
- Never tie balloons or toys to cribs.
- Never use toys with small removable parts or pointed objects.
- Never prop bottles.
- Never tape pacifiers in an infant's mouth.

CARING FOR TODDLERS (1–3 YEARS)

The years between 1 and 3 can be a difficult time for a child to be hospitalized. This is the age when a child is trying to be independent and in control. Between 1½ and 3 years of age, the child:

- Increases motor coordination
- Becomes more verbal
- Becomes more curious about the world

At the same time, her parents are trying to toilet-train her. They also are beginning to set limits on her behavior. The developmental task for the toddler is **autonomy** (independent action).

When caring for the toddler, allow her as much independence and choice as possible (within hospital policy guidelines). Avoid situations that could create a struggle between the caregiver and the child. Expect delays when the toddler is feeding herself or bathing. Be sure to allow the toddler time to do these activities.

The Hospital Environment

When a toddler is hospitalized, it is important to provide an environment that allows as much independence and control as possible while ensuring safety. An example of this is the choice of bed (crib) for the toddler. If a crib is to be used, it should have a top and sides to prevent the child from climbing out and possibly falling (Figure 49-12). If the child has been sleeping in a bed at home, then it is more appropriate to provide a child-sized hospital bed with side rails, if available. Hospital policies vary, so check your hospital policy with reference to toddlers.

If the child is toilet-trained, it is important to know the words the child uses for urination and bowel movements.

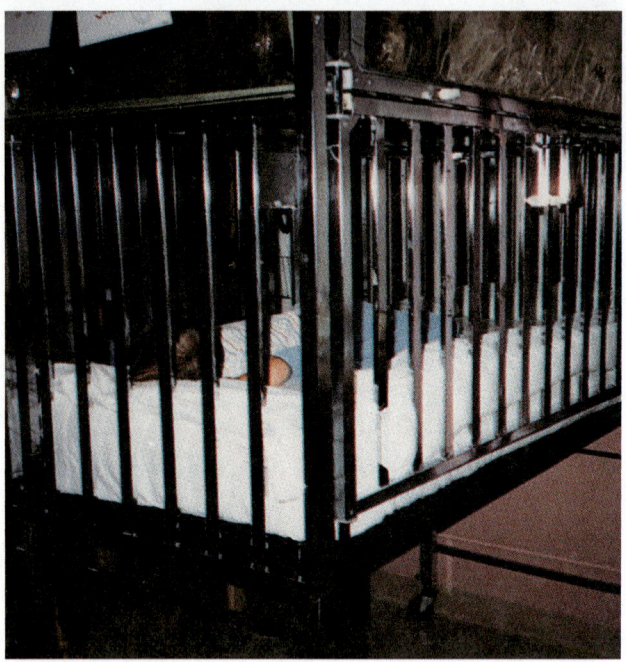

FIGURE 49-12 The crib must provide a safe environment, yet be large enough to allow freedom of movement.

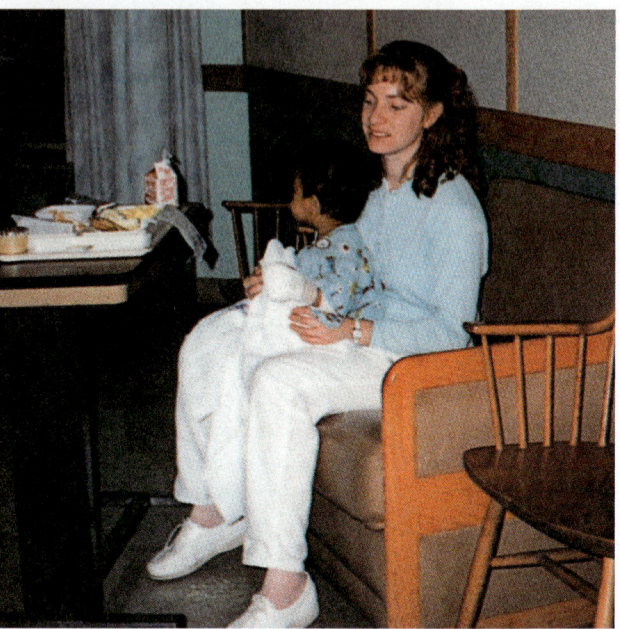

FIGURE 49-13 The nursing assistant must help the toddler when necessary, but allow the toddler as much independence as possible. Avoid rushing.

It is also important to know if the child uses a potty chair or the toilet at home. You should try to provide the same arrangement for toileting in the hospital. It is not uncommon for a hospitalized child to regress. You should not be surprised if a toddler who is toilet-trained starts to have "accidents" while in the hospital. Do not scold the child if this happens. The incident should be treated in a matter-of-fact manner. In addition, a hospitalized toddler may ask for a bottle or pacifier. Even though the toddler may have been weaned from them, treat the request as normal. Do not try to reason with the child.

The Toddler's Need for Autonomy

The toddler is learning to be independent. He may want to feed, dress, and wash himself while in the hospital. It will be your responsibility to help the toddler with these activities (Figure 49-13). You should allow him his independence. At the same time, you must keep him safe. For example, when bathing the toddler in the bathtub, you must never leave him alone, even for a minute. Before you put the toddler in the tub, check the temperature of the bath water.

Emotional Reaction to Illness

Another important area in the care of toddlers concerns their feelings of responsibility for their own illnesses. You must stress that the illness is not the toddler's or anyone else's fault.

To overcome anxiety about routine procedures, allow the toddler to handle equipment whenever possible. A few extra minutes spent to familiarize the toddler with the

equipment to be used may make the difference between a frightened child and an interested one (Figure 49-14).

The toddler will have a difficult time if separated from the mother. One way to prevent this is to permit the mother to

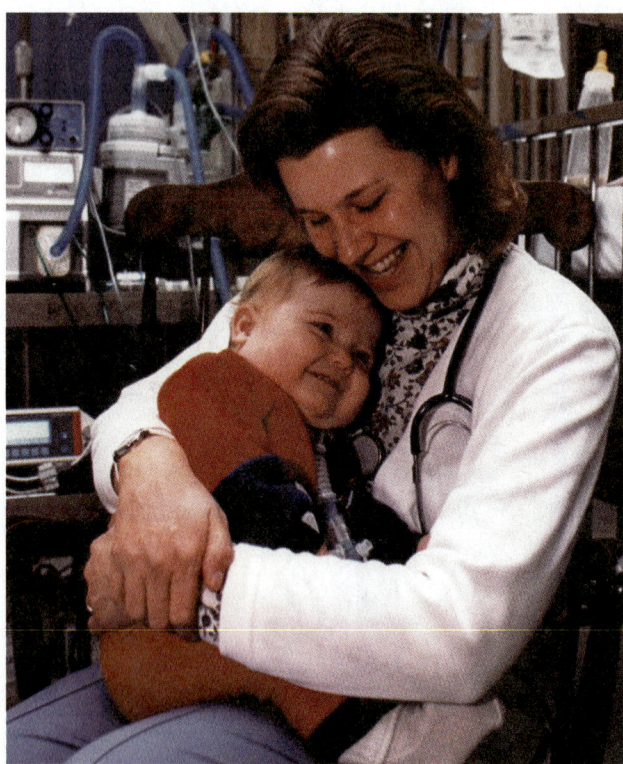

FIGURE 49-14 Showing affection and allowing the toddler to become familiar with your equipment will help relieve anxiety.

room-in. If this cannot happen, either because a parent cannot stay or because hospital policy does not permit it, then parents should be encouraged to visit frequently. If a parent is not going to stay:

- Reassure the child that she will not be alone.
- Tell her the names of the people who will care for her.
- Encourage each person caring for the toddler to introduce himself when entering the room.
- Whenever possible, place the toddler who does not have a parent staying with her in a room near the nurses' station.
- Encourage parents who cannot visit to call, or you can call the parents so the child can talk to them.

Routine Activities

Routines are important to toddlers. Ask the parents to describe the child's normal day. Try to follow the child's usual schedule as much as possible for eating, naps, toileting, and other activities. Ask the parents about the child's nickname, likes, dislikes, names of siblings and pets, and anything else the parents feel the nursing assistant should know about the child.

Toddlers love to play but, because they have short attention spans, they cannot play with one toy for a long time. Plan a variety of activities to keep the toddler amused. For example:

- Finger painting
- Moving toy cars or trucks
- Coloring
- Handling blocks
- Push-pull toys
- Reading of stories

Educational toys that teach how to dress, button, and zip can also be fun for the toddler. Stethoscopes, masks, and gloves make good hospital toys because they can allow the toddler to work out his fears. Do not leave the child alone with these items, because of the risk of accident or injury.

Toddlers will not play together, but they will play near or next to each other.

Temper tantrums are common with toddlers. If they occur, ignore the tantrum as long as the child cannot hurt herself or others. If a toddler is misbehaving, set limits in a firm, consistent manner.

When working with the toddler, remember that he is trying to be independent. Allow the toddler as much choice as possible. For example, at snack time ask if he wants an apple or a cracker. If no choice can be given, be firm and say what will occur. For example, "It's time to take your nap now." It is best to be truthful and to give simple explanations to toddlers. If the child is having a blood test, tell him just before it happens. It does not do any good to prepare toddlers in advance because they do not have any concept of time. Such advance warning only increases their anxiety.

guidelines *for*

Ensuring a Safe Environment for Toddlers

- All poisonous liquids should be kept in a locked container or cabinet.
- All open electrical sockets should have protective covers. Never leave toddlers unattended or unsupervised.
- Never leave toddlers alone in the bathtub or bathroom.
- Keep thermometers out of toddlers' reach.
- Keep crib sides and side rails up when the toddler is in bed.
- Never allow toddlers to play with balloons unless supervised.
- Avoid toys with sharp edges, long strings, or small removable parts.
- Keep doors to stair, kitchen, treatment, and storage areas closed and locked whenever possible.
- Keep doors to linen chutes locked.

The toddler has great natural curiosity and loves to explore. It is important to maintain a safe environment in the hospital.

Summary of Nursing Assistant Tasks and Responsibilities When Caring for Toddlers

- Maintain a safe environment.
- Apply standard precautions if contact with blood, body fluids, mucous membranes, or nonintact skin is likely.
- Provide information to the health team through monitoring of vital signs (temperature, pulse, and respiration), weight, intake, and output.
- Supervise and assist with routine care such as bathing, feeding, and dressing.
- Collect and test specimens.
- Assist with treatments, examinations, and procedures.
- Provide and assist with opportunities for play.
- Provide warmth, security, and affection.
- Promote independence by providing opportunities for choices.

CARING FOR PRESCHOOL CHILDREN (3–6 YEARS)

Developmental Tasks

Between the ages of 3 and 6 years, the child's language, fine motor skills, and gross motor skills continue to increase with activity. The preschooler continues to develop independence, but the primary developmental task for the age group is initiative (doing things themselves). Children in this age group need to be able to initiate physical and intellectual activities to feel more competent. The preschooler learns her sex role in life by imitating the behavior of the same-sex parent.

The preschooler needs his independence, but he still needs to feel safe and secure. The caregiver must provide the correct balance of independence and control for the preschooler. This is normally the job of the parents, but when the preschooler is hospitalized, you will be considered the caregiver.

Emotional Reactions to Illness

Preschoolers normally have many fears. One fear is that their body parts will be injured or changed. For example, a preschooler may fear that if an adhesive bandage is taken off, some of her will "leak out." Preschoolers cannot tell the difference between a "good hurt" and a "bad hurt"; that is, pain from a procedure versus pain from a spanking. Therefore, it is important to use simple, honest explanations when telling the preschooler what to expect.

Fear of the dark, of night time, and of being alone are other normal fears for a preschooler. You can help reduce this fear by leaving a nightlight on. Another child in the room can also ease his fears. Be sure to leave the call bell within reach. Sitting with him until he falls asleep will also help. Like the toddler, the preschooler can also benefit from having his mother room-in, because he still fears separation.

"Magical thinking" and fantasy are still present in this age group. Therefore, it is important to stress to the preschooler that it is not her fault that she is sick, and that she is not sick because she was bad. The preschooler needs to know that she will return home. She will not be forgotten and left in the hospital. Siblings should be allowed and encouraged to visit. In addition to easing separation from the family, this can also be a way of assuring the child that no one is taking her place at home.

Explaining Procedures

When telling a preschooler what to expect, simple, honest explanations work best. Choose your words carefully because the preschooler takes things literally (exactly as said).

- If surgery is being planned, show and tell the child what parts of his body will be involved in the procedure.
- Preschoolers have a limited concept of time, so when you explain when something will occur, use time references that are familiar to the child (such as meal time, nap time, or the time of a favorite TV show). For example, if the child is scheduled for an x-ray in the late morning, tell her that she will have it after breakfast or before lunch.
- Always explain to the preschooler what you are going to do. Do not assume that he will remember what you told him before. The preschooler needs to maintain some control. Therefore, allow him to make as many decisions as possible. Give him the opportunity to make a choice.
- Allow the preschooler to do as much of her own care as she can, to make her feel independent.

Activities

Imagination and fantasy are part of the preschooler's world. Imaginary playmates are normal for the preschooler. These playmates may find their way to the hospital with the child. The playmates can vary in age and sex. They often have different or unusual-sounding names. If the child talks about his imaginary friend, treat it matter-of-factly and listen. However, you need to be realistic. Do not say that you see or hear this playmate. Just say that you know this playmate exists only in the child's imagination.

Play is important for the hospitalized preschooler. Play may give you clues about what the preschooler is thinking. The preschooler is more coordinated and can enjoy activities such as puzzles, coloring, and drawing. The preschooler enjoys imitating roles and playing with other children. Playing house and doctor is especially fun for this age group. Hand puppets are also a good way to talk to preschoolers, because they relate easily to the character of the puppet.

You can help the preschooler deal with her hospital stay by maintaining consistency in her schedule and in the limits put on her behavior. Positive reinforcers such as hugs or stickers should be used as rewards for appropriate behavior.

guidelines *for*

Ensuring a Safe Environment for Preschoolers

- Keep toys from cluttering walkways to prevent falls.
- Keep side rails on the bed up at night.
- Keep beds in low position.
- Keep doors to kitchen and storage areas closed.
- Keep a nightlight on.
- Never leave the child unattended in the tub.
- Never allow children to run with popsicles or lollipops in their mouths.

Summary of Nursing Assistant Tasks and Responsibilities When Caring for Preschoolers

- Maintain a safe environment.
- Apply standard precautions if contact with blood, body fluids, mucous membranes, or nonintact skin is likely.
- Provide information to the health team through monitoring of vital signs (temperature, pulse, and respiration), weight, intake, and output.
- Supervise and assist with routine care such as bathing, feeding, and dressing.
- Collect and test specimens.
- Assist with treatments, examinations, and procedures.
- Provide and assist with opportunities for play.
- Provide warmth, security, and affection.

CARING FOR SCHOOL-AGE CHILDREN (6–12 YEARS)

In general, the school-age years are a time of exceptionally good health (Figure 49-15). School-age children are more active, stronger, and steadier than younger children. They have either had most of the childhood illnesses or have been immunized against them. The most common problems of these times involve the gastrointestinal system (for example, stomach aches) and the respiratory system (for example, colds and coughs).

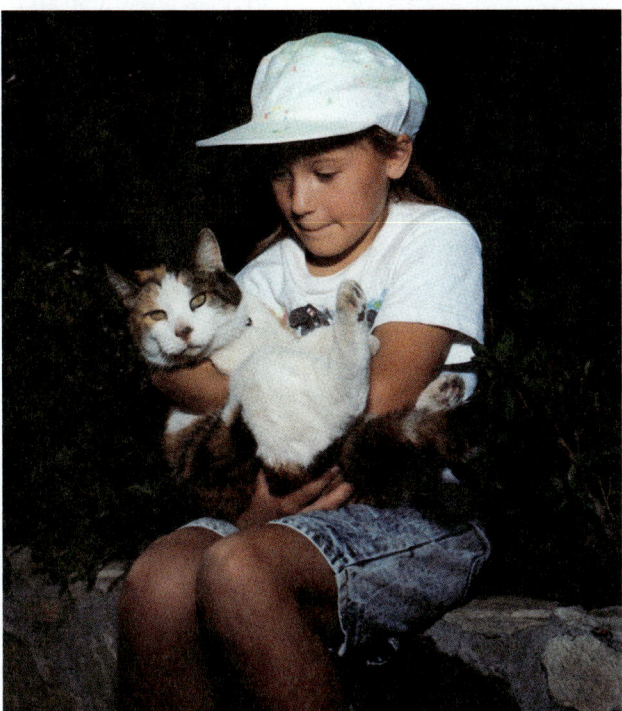

FIGURE 49-15 School-age children tend to be healthier than younger children, but complain primarily of colds and stomach aches.

Developmental Tasks

In this period, the child is striving to achieve a sense of accomplishment through an increasing number of tasks and completion of projects. He also continues to increase control over his environment and his independence. It is important to remember these tasks when caring for the school-age child.

The school-age child's reaction to hospitalization will be significantly different from that of the younger child. The school-age child is better able to handle the stress of illness and hospitalization. In fact, hospitalization presents the school-age child with an opportunity to:

- Explore a new environment
- Meet new friends
- Learn more about her body

Psychosocial Adjustment

Separation from parents will not be as difficult for the school-age child. However, those just entering this period may regress to a preschool level. These children will need their parents' presence.

The school-age child has left the security of home and entered the school system. In school, the child has begun to develop relationships with other children. In the hospital, she may respond more to the separation from her peers than from her parents. It is important to give these children opportunities to communicate with their schoolmates. For example, they can be helped to write letters and make phone calls. When possible, friends can visit.

The older school-age child may welcome the opportunity to be away from his parents. In this situation, the child can test newly developed skills and increase independence. Children of this age group also need privacy—but if the parents are there, they may not get it. Some parents may need to have their child's opposition to their staying explained in this context, because they may think the child is angry with them.

Roommate selection is especially important for this age group. A roommate of approximately the same age will act as a diversion. With a roommate of the same age, the child will be able to continue work on the developmental task of learning to get along with others. Because the school-age child is seeking more independence, she may be reluctant to ask for help even when she needs it. Her feelings may show themselves in different ways, such as:

- Irritability.
- Hostility toward her siblings.
- Other behavior problems. It is important that you, as a caregiver, observe and note these behaviors and bring them to the attention of your supervisor.

Resistance to bedtime may also become a problem during these years. In the hospital, it is important to be aware of the parents' rules and follow them. Learning rules is another developmental task of the school-age years.

Adjustment to Illness

Fears or stresses associated with an illness and subsequent hospitalization contribute to the school-age child's feelings of loss of control. By involving the child in her own care, you will help her to be a more cooperative patient (Figure 49-16). Procedures that we routinely do without explanation or without providing options, such as using the bedpan, are particularly upsetting to the school-age child. This child is trying hard to act grown up but is not being given the chance. It is also important for this child's self-esteem that you do not scold him when he does lose control. It is best to just overlook the episode.

The school-age child is able to reason. She also understands the impact of her illness and the potential for disability and death. These children take an active interest in health and enjoy acquiring knowledge. You can help them gain information and deal with their fears by explaining all procedures in simple terms. This is also an appropriate age for playing with hospital equipment such as a stethoscope.

Pain is passively accepted by the school-age child. He is able to tell you where his pain is located and what it feels like. This child will hold rigidly still, bite his lip, or clench his fists when in pain, in an effort to keep in control and to act brave. This child does well with distraction during painful procedures. During procedures, you should stay with him whenever possible to talk him through them. This child also tries to postpone all major procedures. For example, when it is time to go to a test, he will need to go to the bathroom. The caregiver needs to put limits on the number of postponements the child is allowed.

Activities

Increased physical and social activities are characteristic of this period. Hospitalization does not usually provide school-age children with adequate diversions. School-age children may also miss the activities of school, although they usually deny this.

You should allow these children time during the day for their own work. This includes school work and visits with

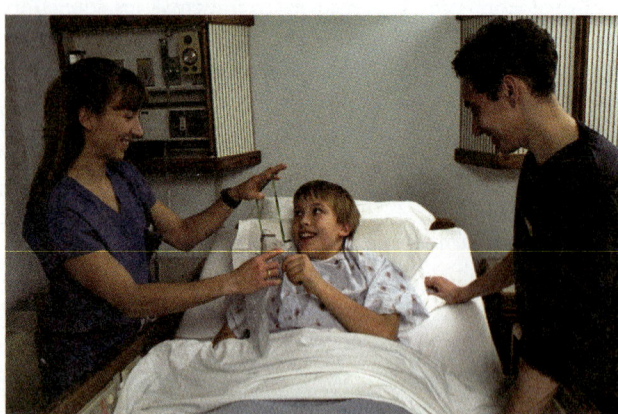

FIGURE 49-16 Explain procedures to the school-age child to give her a feeling of participating in her care.

friends and other patients. Competitiveness is also characteristic of this period. It adds to the school-age child's need to stay up-to-date with school work. Having the play therapist at the hospital provide appropriate activities will help to reduce the stress the child feels.

Caregivers should encourage the child to take part in her own care as part of her work. Helping to make her bed or clean her room will make her feel useful. She should be held responsible only for tasks that are within her capabilities.

Physically, this child has entered a period of slow, steady growth. Although growth has slowed, it is still important to maintain a balanced diet. School-age children tend to be less picky about what they eat and they are more willing to try new foods.

Summary of Nursing Assistant Tasks and Responsibilities When Caring for School-Age Children

- Maintain a safe environment.
- Apply standard precautions if contact with blood, body fluids, mucous membranes, or nonintact skin is likely.
- Provide information to the health care team through monitoring of vital signs (temperature, pulse, and respiration), weight, intake, and output.
- Supervise and assist with routine care.
- Collect and test specimens.
- Assist with treatments, examinations, and procedures.
- Provide explanations using proper names of body parts, drawings, and books.
- Encourage socialization with other children in the same age group.
- Provide time for school work and tutors.

CARING FOR THE ADOLESCENT (13–18 YEARS)

Adolescence is the transitional period from childhood into adulthood. Like school-age children, adolescents are relatively healthy. The major health problems of this period are usually related to the drastic physical changes that occur during this time, to accidents, to sports injuries, or to chronic and/or permanent disabilities.

Psychosocial Development

Dealing with adolescents is especially difficult for health care providers because:

- The adolescent is developing an identity and becoming increasingly independent.
- Being hospitalized forces the adolescent into a situation where she is now dependent on others to meet her needs. Because of this, it is important to allow the adolescent to make as many of her own decisions as possible. When this is not possible, keep the adolescent involved in the decision-making process.
- Adolescents have a difficult time with authority figures (Figure 49-17). As the caregiver, you will represent authority to this child. You should not get into struggles with the adolescent. Limit the restrictions on them whenever appropriate.
- Adolescents are usually uncooperative. The best approach is to let the adolescent know, in a nonthreatening way, what the rules of the unit are. It is best to do this at the time of his admission. Speak to adolescents as you would to adults. Be as flexible as possible. For example, instead of struggling through the morning trying to get the adolescent up and washed, give him a list of things that have to be accomplished by a certain time. Then allow him the freedom to do things his way and in his order. At the time you decided on, check back with the adolescent to see that the tasks have been completed.

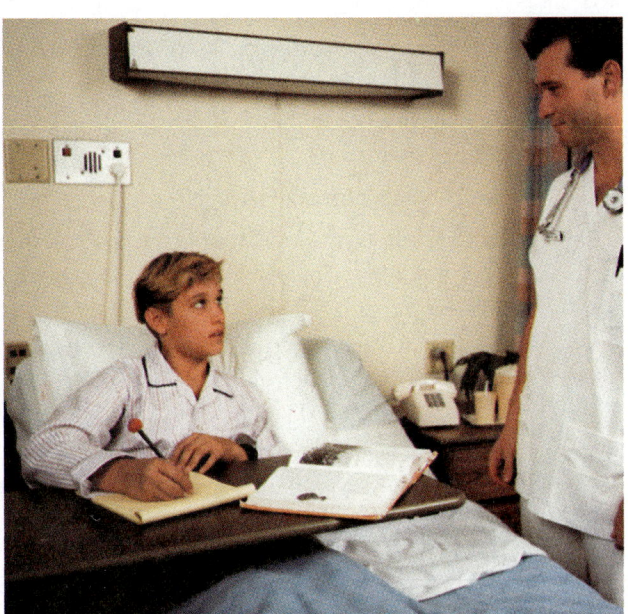

FIGURE 49-17 Adolescents may have difficulty with authority figures and tend to be uncooperative. Be firm, patient, and persistent.

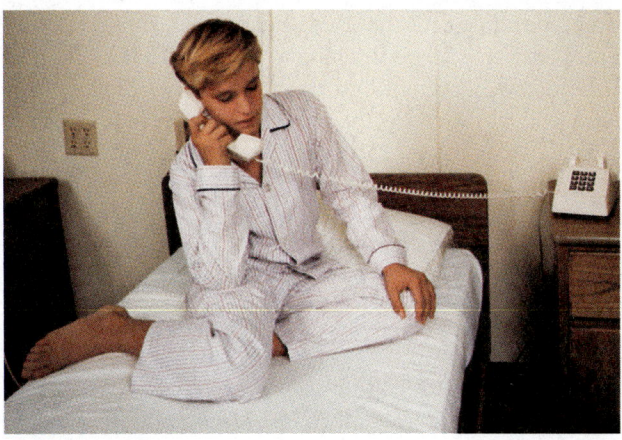

FIGURE 49-18 Allowing the adolescent to stay in touch with friends is important.

The most important people to adolescents are their friends. A hospital stay makes it more difficult for the adolescent to see friends. It is essential that you:

- allow the adolescent time for visits.
- permit phone calls (Figure 49-18).
- introduce them to other patients their age.

Recognize that adolescents may not want to visit with others if illness has changed their appearance in any way. Body image is important at this age. You can promote a positive image by encouraging the adolescent to continue a normal grooming routine in the hospital. Also encourage the adolescent to wear clothes or her own pajamas. This will make her look and feel better about herself. Use the opportunity to teach good hygiene practices if the hospitalized adolescent does not already practice them. Ask a nurse to help you if you note that this is a problem for your patient.

Keep in mind that the adolescent is very aware of the changes taking place in his body, whether they can be seen or not. It is important to provide the adolescent with privacy. Keep him covered as much as possible during procedures and examinations.

Nutrition and Activity

Adolescents go through a growth spurt. Girls are usually two years ahead of boys. Adequate nutrition and rest continue to be important. In the hospital, the importance of proper eating habits should be stressed to the adolescent. You should:

- Permit the adolescent to continue to make decisions about what and when she will eat, unless it is medically unsafe.
- Recognize that adolescent girls are often on diets. Emotional problems related to weight are common.
- Be aware that adolescents frequently skip breakfast.

The adolescent often stays up late and likes to sleep late in the morning. Sleep requirements are decreased, but a good night's sleep is essential. It is important to explain the routines of the unit and yet provide flexibility for the adolescent. For example, if the television must be turned off at a certain time, the adolescent should be encouraged to find another quiet activity (such as listening to music with headphones) if he does not want to go to sleep. Many hospitals have lounges exclusively for the use of this age group, for their own activities and for socializing. Check with your supervisor to find out if there is a specific area for adolescents.

Summary of Nursing Assistant Tasks and Responsibilities When Caring for Adolescents

- Maintain a safe environment.
- Apply standard precautions if contact with blood, body fluids, mucous membranes, or nonintact skin is likely.
- Orient the adolescent to unit and hospital rules.
- Provide information to the health team through monitoring of vital signs (temperature, pulse, and respiration), weight, intake, and output.
- Provide simple explanations to the adolescent.
- Assist with body hygiene to help maintain positive self-image.
- Collect and test specimens.
- Assist with treatment, examinations, and procedures.
- Promote independence. Allow adolescents as much control as possible over schedule of treatments, procedures, and so on.
- Encourage socialization with other adolescents.

guidelines *for*

Ensuring a Safe Environment for Adolescents

- Carefully check all electrical equipment that the adolescent brings to the hospital—radios, hair dryers, and so on—to ensure that it is appropriate and safe to use. Review hospital guidelines regarding use of electrical equipment with the patient.
- Review smoking policies with all adolescents.
- Reinforce to adolescents that alcohol and other drugs are illegal and are not permitted.
- Provide assistance with showers and bathing if the patient is incapacitated or weakened in any way. The adolescent may not ask for assistance.
- Reinforce the use of shoes or slippers to prevent injuries to the feet.
- Remind adolescents to keep staff informed of their whereabouts.
- Keep beds in low position to prevent falls.

REVIEW

A. True/False.

Mark the following true or false by circling T or F.

1. T F It is normal for a child to regress when hospitalized.

2. T F The nursing assistant can foster an infant's sense of trust by keeping him warm and dry.

3. T F The nursing assistant may assume the role of substitute mother.

4. T F Between the ages of 6 and 7 months, the infant loses her fear of strangers.

5. T F Following a feeding, the infant should be encouraged to play.

6. T F Routine weighing of the infant should be carried out right after the 10 AM feeding.

7. T F Pulse and respirations should be measured when the child is quiet or asleep.

8. T F The school-age child has an average heart rate of 90 to 140 beats per minute.

9. T F The respiratory rate of the toddler averages 30 to 60 respirations per minute.

10. T F The systolic blood pressure of the child increases with age.

11. T F Preschoolers normally have many fears.

12. T F The preschooler learns his or her sex role in life by imitating the behavior of the opposite-sex parent.

13. T F The most common physical complaints of a school-age child are stomach aches and colds.

14. T F The school-age child would be most comfortable sharing a room with a teenager.

15. T F It is best to overlook the loss of self-control exhibited by the school-age child.

16. T F The best way to measure a pulse rate in an infant or child is the apical method.

17. T F The temperature of a child under 5 years of age should be measured using the rectal method.

18. T F Sucking should be encouraged only when the infant is hungry.

19. T F It is proper to prop a bottle so the infant can eat in his crib if you are very busy.

20. T F After a feeding, the infant should be placed carefully on her back.

21. T F To entertain an infant, tie a bright red balloon to the crib.

22. T F The toddler should be placed in a crib with a top and sides as a safety measure.

23. T F It is permissible to allow a toddler to play unsupervised in a bathtub for a short time before bathing him, as long as the water is warm.

24. T F Adolescents have a difficult time dealing with authority figures.

25. T F Adolescents are particularly sensitive about changes in their body images.

B. Matching.

Choose the correct word from Column II to match each phrase in Column I.

Column I

26. _____ physical and psychological achievements

27. _____ achievement of skills characteristic of a specific age group

28. _____ a person married to a biological parent

29. _____ to move backward developmentally

30. _____ person who has the right to consent to procedures and hospitalization of a minor

31. _____ birth parent

32. _____ self-determination

Column II

a. autonomy

b. regress

c. legal guardian

d. developmental tasks

e. biological parent

f. developmental milestone

g. stepparent

C. Nursing Assistant Challenge

You are assigned to take vital signs. The nurse manager just asked the maintenance department to check a problem with the tympanic thermometer, so it is not available. An electronic thermometer is available on the unit, as are oral and rectal glass thermometers. Select the appropriate thermometer and route or method for taking temperatures on these patients:

33. Joey, a 3-week-old infant who was admitted for surgery.

34. Brittany, a 15-month-old child who was admitted with an upper respiratory infection.

35. David, a 4-year-old child who was admitted with diarrhea.

36. Maria, a 6-year-old with cystic fibrosis, who is having difficulty breathing.

37. Lisa, an 8-year-old admitted with leukemia.

38. Robert, a 13-year-old who had his appendix removed earlier today.

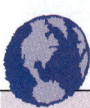

EXPLORING THE WEB

Description	Location
Bandaids and Blackboards	*http://www.faculty.fairfield.edu*
Child & Family Canada	*http://www.cfc-efc.ca*
Cincinnati Children's Patient Education Program	*http://www.cincinnatichildrens.org*
Combined Health Information Database	*http://chid.nih.gov/subfile/subfile.html*
Dr. Greene's House Calls	*http://www.drgreene.com*
KidsHealth.org	*http://kidshealth.org*
Kimmel Cancer Center at Jefferson	*http://www.kcc.tju.edu*
National Enuresis (Bedwetting) Society	*http://www.peds.umn.edu*
PEDBASE Pediatric Database	*http://www.icondata.com*
Pediatric Info—A Pediatric Information Library	*http://www.pedinfo.com*
Pediatric Surgery Update	*http://www.icondata.com*
Vanderbilt Pediatric Interactive Digital Library	*http://www.mc.vanderbilt.edu*
Virtual Children's Hospital	*http://www.vh.org*
The Virtual PNP	*http://home.earthlink.net*
Wong on the Web: WOW Papers	*http://www.us.elsevierhealth.com*

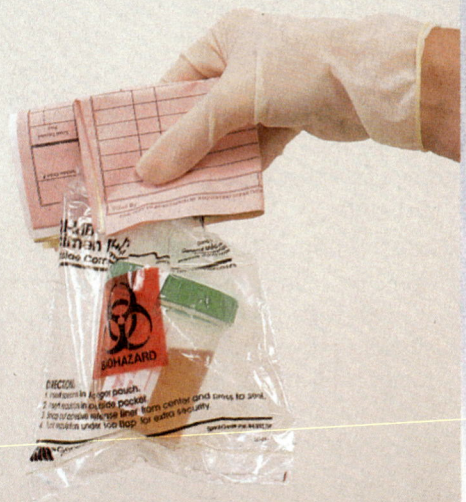

Special Advanced Procedures

> **LEGAL** *Alert* By state law, you may not be permitted to perform some of the advanced procedures discussed in this section. Consult with your instructor or supervisor to be sure you know your legal responsibilities. Do not perform or assist in any procedure you are not permitted by law to do.

objectives

After completing this unit—and with advanced training—you will be able to:

- Spell and define terms.
- State the reasons for removing an indwelling catheter as soon as possible.
- List the guidelines for caring for an ostomy.
- List at least six procedures in which sterile technique is used.
- Demonstrate the following procedures:
  - Procedure 141 Testing for Occult Blood Using Hemoccult® and Developer
  - Procedure 142 Collecting a Urine Specimen Through a Drainage Port
  - Procedure 143 Removing an Indwelling Catheter
  - Procedure 144 Giving Routine Stoma Care (Colostomy)
  - Procedure 145 Routine Care of an Ileostomy (with Patient in Bed)
  - Procedure 146 Setting Up a Sterile Field Using a Sterile Drape
  - Procedure 147 Adding an Item to a Sterile Field
  - Procedure 148 Adding Liquids to a Sterile Field
  - Procedure 149 Applying and Removing Sterile Gloves
  - Procedure 150 Using Transfer Forceps

vocabulary

Learn the meaning and the correct spelling of the following words and phrases:

appliance	ileostomy	port
colostomy	ostomy	stoma

INTRODUCTION

The responsibilities of nursing assistants vary throughout the nation. The scope and type of assignments that are given to nursing assistants are influenced by:

- Basic preparation
- Experience
- Specific advanced training in procedural skills
- Facility policy
- State laws that specify the range of practice of nursing assistants

Important principles to keep in mind are that:

- Some procedures that are considered routine for some workers would not be appropriate or permitted in other situations. Even basic procedures such as bed bathing might be restricted to nurses if the situation or patient conditions warrant such precautions.
- Under no circumstances can it be assumed that because the following procedures are included in this textbook, they should be assigned to all nursing assistants.
- Each facility has established policies and supervisory practices that are consistent with legal regulations and that ensure competency on the part of the caregiver and safety for the patient/resident.
- These procedures are to be carried out only after adequate practice, with supervision, and only in accord with specific facility policy. Additional information supporting these advanced procedures may be found in the units indicated.

OSHA *Alert*

Apply the principles of standard precautions when performing the advanced procedures in this unit involving contact with urine and feces. Although gloves are used routinely, you must think about potential contact with your uniform and other parts of your body, and select the appropriate protective equipment before beginning. For example, in caring for an ostomy, there may be potential for contact with your uniform. If this is the case, put on a gown before beginning. If there is potential for contact with the mucous membranes on your face, you should also wear a mask and eye protection.

URINE AND STOOL TESTS

Special tests performed on urine and stool samples may be part of your responsibility. Refer to Procedures 141 and 142. Additional information appears in Units 43 and 44.

PROCEDURE 141

TESTING FOR OCCULT BLOOD USING HEMOCCULT® AND DEVELOPER

1. Wash your hands and assemble equipment:
   - disposable gloves
   - bedpan with fresh specimen
   - Hemoccult® slide packet
   - Hemoccult® developer
   - tongue blade
   - paper towel

2. Place the paper towel on a flat surface and open the flap of the Hemoccult® packet, exposing the guaiac paper.

3. Put on gloves.

4. Using a tongue blade, take a small sample of feces and smear it on the paper area marked *A* (Figure 50-1A).

5. Repeat the procedure, taking the fecal sample from a different part of the specimen and making a smear in area *B*.

6. Close the tab and turn the packet over.

7. Open the back tab.

8. Apply two drops of Hemoccult® developer directly over each smear (Figure 50-1B). Time the reaction.

9. Read the results 30 to 60 seconds later.

continues

PROCEDURE 141

continued

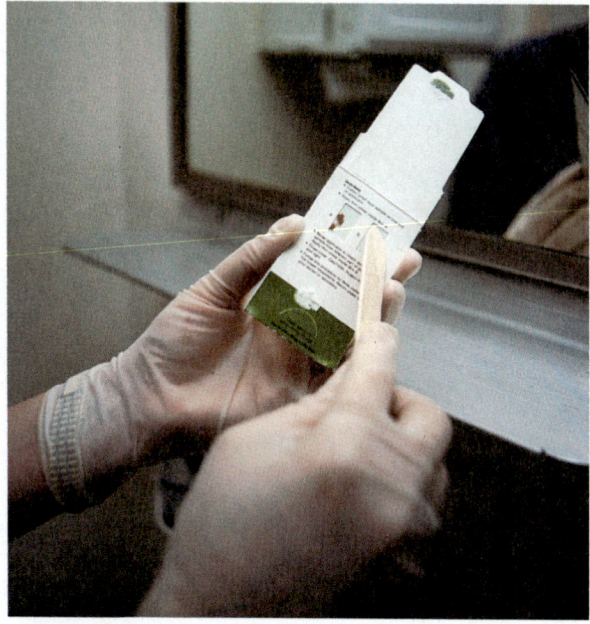

FIGURE 50-1A A small stool specimen is placed on a special area of the card for an occult blood test.

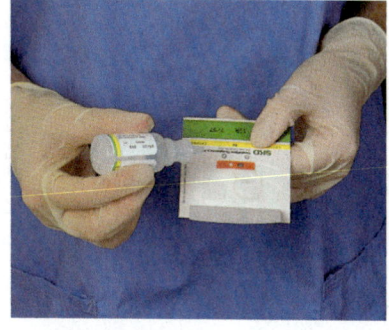

FIGURE 50-1B Apply drops of Hemoccult® developer on the exposed guaiac paper.

10. The presence of blood is indicated by a blue discoloration around the perimeter of the smear.

11. Dispose of the specimen.

12. Clean the bedpan according to facility policy and dispose of the paper towel, packet, and tongue blade.

13. Remove and dispose of gloves according to facility policy. Wash your hands.

Collecting a Specimen from a Closed Urinary Drainage System

At some time, it may be necessary to collect a fresh specimen of urine when the patient is on a closed urinary drainage system. Keep in mind that the:

- urine sample must be fresh.
- urine in the bag has accumulated over a period of time.

- the specimen may not be taken from the bag.
- the specimen must be taken from the catheter.

The procedure to be followed is determined by the type of Foley catheter that is in place. If the catheter has a **port** (opening) for fluid withdrawal, follow Procedure 142. The procedure must be carried out using proper techniques, to avoid introducing infectious organisms into the system.

PROCEDURE 142

COLLECTING A URINE SPECIMEN THROUGH A DRAINAGE PORT

1. Carry out beginning procedure actions.

2. Assemble equipment:
   - disposable gloves
   - tube clamp
   - laboratory requisition
   - completed label

   - emesis basin
   - 10-mL syringe
   - specimen cup and lid
   - 21-gauge or 22-gauge needle
   - sharps container
   - alcohol wipe

continues

PROCEDURE 142

continued

INFECTION CONTROL *Alert*

Unless you are instructed otherwise, select a sterile specimen collection cup for this procedure. Avoid touching the inside of the cup and the lid with your hands. When you open the cup, place the lid with the clean, inner side up on the table. Make sure the clamp is removed from the drainage tube before you leave the room after collecting the specimen, or urine will back up into the patient's bladder, causing discomfort and increasing the potential for infection and other complications.

- bed protector
- biohazard specimen transport bag

3. Go to the bedside half an hour before sample is to be collected.

4. Clamp the drainage tube.

5. Wash your hands. Return to the bedside after 30 minutes.

6. Put on gloves.

7. Place a bed protector on the bed and place an emesis basin on the bed protector under the catheter drainage port.

8. Wipe the drainage port with an alcohol wipe (Figure 50-2).

9. Carefully remove the cap on the syringe. Do not contaminate the tip.

10. Attach the needle carefully. Do not contaminate the needle tip.

11. Open the package with the specimen container. Remove the lid and lay it, inside up, on the bedside stand. Do not touch the inside of the cup or the lid with your hands.

12. Insert the needle into the port and withdraw the specimen (Figure 50-3).

13. Carefully withdraw the needle.

14. Wipe the port with the alcohol wipe.

15. Transfer the urine sample to the specimen container (Figure 50-4).

16. Handling the lid by the top only, cover the container.

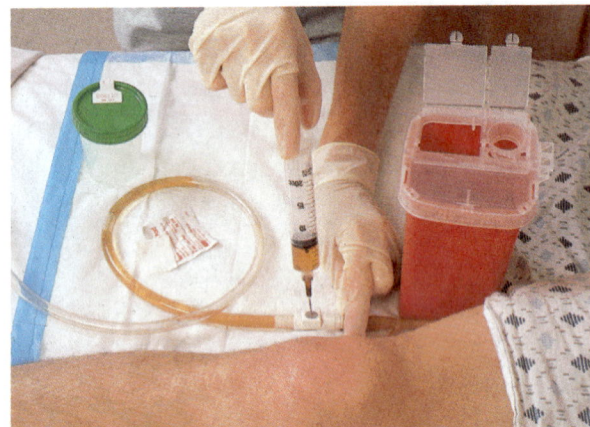

FIGURE 50-3 Draw the specimen into the needle.

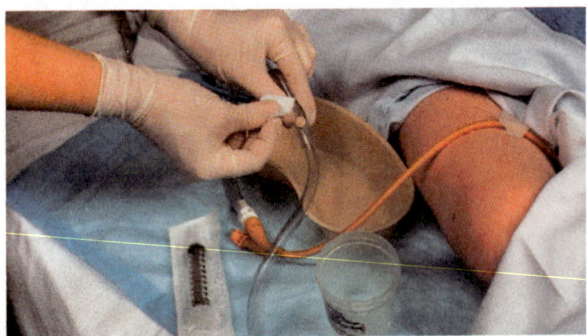

FIGURE 50-2 Wipe the port with an antiseptic wipe or alcohol sponge.

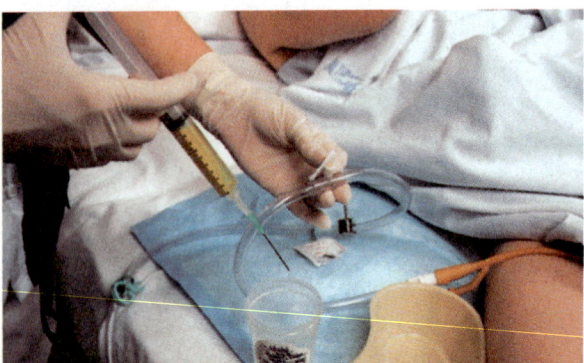

FIGURE 50-4 Transfer the specimen to the container.

continues

PROCEDURE 142

continued

17. Do not recap the needle. Do not detach the needle from the syringe. Discard the needle and syringe into the sharps container at the bedside.

18. Remove gloves and dispose of according to facility policy. Wash your hands.

19. Remove the catheter clamp.

20. Complete the information on the label and put the label on the container. Compare the label to the requisition to be sure that the information is complete and accurate.

21. Place the specimen container in a biohazard transport bag, seal the bag, and attach the completed laboratory requisition (Figure 50-5).

22. Carry out procedure completion actions.

23. Follow instructions for care and transport of the specimen.

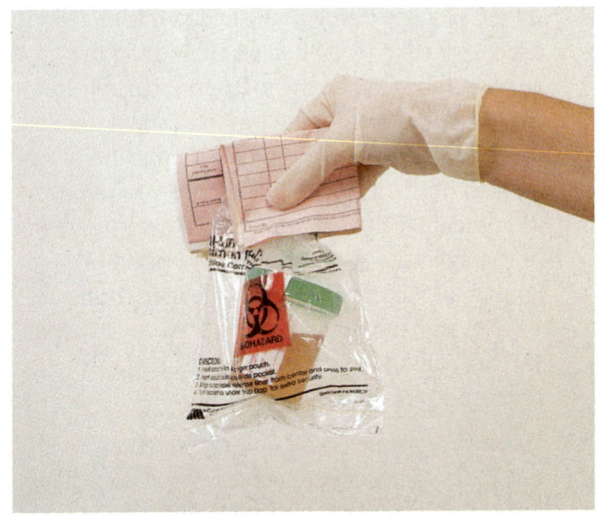

FIGURE 50-5 Place the specimen in the biohazard transport bag, seal the bag, and attach the laboratory requisition.

REMOVING AN INDWELLING CATHETER

An indwelling catheter is removed as soon as possible to reduce the risk of infection. A catheter must also be removed if it is obstructed, or for a routine change ordered by the physician. If a new catheter is not reinserted by the nurse, you must monitor the patient's voiding after catheter removal. Follow your facility policy for reporting to the nurse. If the patient has not voided within 6 to 8 hours, or if he or she complains of abdominal pain, notify the nurse.

PROCEDURE 143

REMOVING AN INDWELLING CATHETER

1. Carry out beginning procedure actions.

2. Assemble equipment:
   - disposable exam gloves, 2 pair
   - 10-mL syringe
   - underpad
   - plastic bag for used supplies
   - washcloth
   - towel
   - washbasin
   - soap

3. Position the underpad under the patient's buttocks.

4. Remove the tape or Velcro strap that secures the catheter to the leg.

5. Manipulate the tubing so that any urine in the tubing flows into the drainage bag.

6. Open the syringe. Attach the syringe to the inflation port.

7. Allow the inflation balloon to deflate into the syringe on its own. Follow facility policy for pulling

continues

PROCEDURE 143

continued

on the plunger to withdraw fluid. If this method is used, pull very gently to avoid collapsing the inflation tube. (When the inflation tubing is collapsed, deflation of the balloon cannot occur.) The amount of fluid in the balloon may be marked on the catheter. Make sure you remove this amount. Depending on the catheter used, the port may flatten when the fluid is withdrawn. Empty the fluid from the syringe, reinsert the needle, and attempt to remove fluid again. When you are satisfied that the balloon is empty, proceed to the next step.

8. Grasp the catheter close to the perineum. Gently pull the catheter. If you feel resistance, stop. The balloon may not be completely deflated. Repeat steps 6 and 7.

9. If no resistance is met, withdraw the catheter. Observe the tip for the presence of sediment, blood, or mucus. If present, inform the nurse. He or she may request a culture.

10. Disconnect the catheter from the drainage tubing. Discard the catheter in the plastic bag, or according to facility policy.

Note: Some facilities culture the tip of the catheter after it is removed. If this will be done, you will need a sterile specimen cup and sterile scissors. After removing the catheter, hold the end over the open specimen cup, and clip it 3 inches from the tip. Cover the cup and discard the remainder of the catheter.

11. Remove gloves and discard in the plastic bag.

12. Wash your hands.

13. Apply clean gloves.

14. Perform perineal care according to facility policy.

15. Empty the catheter bag and measure output. Discard the empty bag in the plastic bag, or according to facility policy.

16. After the catheter is removed, instruct the patient to drink fluids, if permitted. Offer to take the patient to the bathroom, or offer the bedpan or urinal in 2 to 4 hours. Inform the nurse if the patient cannot void, or has complaints of urgency, pain, or burning.

17. Carry out procedure completion actions.

OSTOMIES

The surgical removal of a section of diseased bowel requires the creation of an artificial opening (**ostomy**) in the abdominal wall for elimination of solid waste and flatus.

Care of the Patient with a Colostomy

When the colon is brought through the abdominal wall, the opening is called a **colostomy**. The mouth of the opening is called a **stoma** (Figure 50-6). The ostomy may be temporary or permanent. The location of the ostomy (Figure 50-7) determines if the feces are formed, soft and mushy, semiliquid, or liquid.

The patient with a colostomy does not have normal sphincter control. This means the patient cannot voluntarily control emptying of the bowel in the same manner as emptying through the anus. If the colostomy is located in the bowel where stool is formed, regularity of elimination may be established. As elimination is controlled, the stoma may be covered with a simple dressing between evacuations. Liquid to mushy fecal drainage from a stoma is collected in a disposable drainage pouch, called an **appliance**, that is attached over the stoma. (Refer to Procedure 144.)

Proper stoma care is required to maintain healthy tissue, because the area around the opening comes into contact with the liquid or semiliquid stool. At the stoma, there may be problems of:

• Leakage

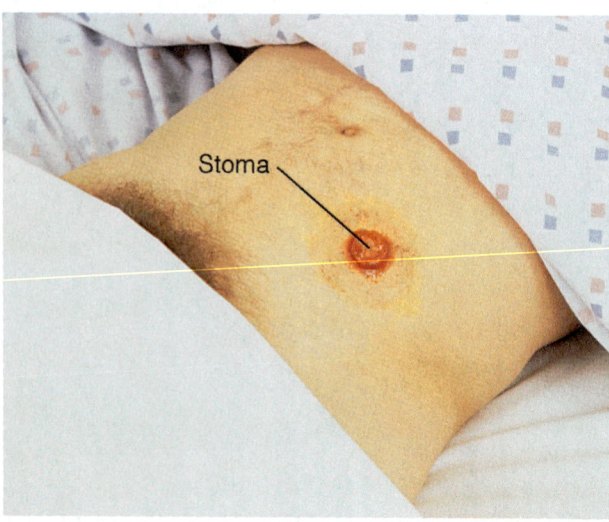

FIGURE 50-6 Typical colostomy stoma.

PROCEDURE 145

continued

to drain (note the clamp in Figure 50-12). Note the amount and character of drainage.

9. Wipe the end of the drainage sheath with toilet paper and move it out of drainage. Place used tissue in the bedpan. Cover the bedpan.

10. Disconnect the belt from the appliance and remove the belt from the patient. Place it on paper towels.

11. With a dropper, apply a small amount of solvent around the ring of the appliance. This will loosen it so it can be removed. Wait a few seconds. Do not force the appliance free.

12. Cover the stoma with gauze.
    - Carefully inspect the skin area around the stoma.
    - If the area is irritated or the skin is broken, cover the patient with a bath blanket, raise the side rail, and lower the bed.
    - Remove gloves and dispose of properly.
    - Wash your hands.
    - Report to the nurse for instructions.

- Put on fresh gloves before continuing any procedure.

13. Remove the gauze from the stoma and place it on paper towels.

14. If an appliance is used with a Karaya ring, moisten the ring, allow it to become sticky, and apply it to the stoma. If the appliance uses a paper-covered adhesive strip around the stoma opening, remove the paper and apply the strip around the stoma.

15. Clamp the appliance bag and apply it to the ring.

16. Remove gloves and dispose of properly. Wash your hands.

17. Adjust a clean belt in position around the patient and connect it to the appliance.

18. Remove the bath blanket and assist the patient to wash hands.

19. Wash your hands. Put on gloves.

20. Clean the patient's bathroom. Wash the belt and appliance, if reusable, and allow them to dry.

21. Carry out procedure completion actions.

STERILE TECHNIQUE

In many facilities, only licensed nursing personnel perform procedures using sterile technique. However, there are times when a nursing assistant may be asked to assist with a sterile procedure. Common nursing procedures in which sterile technique is used are:

- all invasive procedures
- procedures in which the skin is broken, such as injections and insertion of intravenous needles or catheters
- procedures in which body cavities are entered, such as catheterization and tracheal suctioning
- changing surgical dressings
- changing dressings on central intravenous catheters (see Unit 35)
- procedures involving patients with severe destruction of the skin, such as burns and trauma

Only sterile supplies contact the patient's body during sterile procedures. Sterile gloves are worn. Masks are worn during some sterile procedures. Follow the guidelines in Procedure 2 for applying a mask. In some procedures, the patient also wears a mask. In others, a mask is not necessary. Check with the nurse if you are not sure whether to wear a mask.

Environmental Conditions

Before using a sterile item, or creating a sterile field, check the environment. The surface on which you open the sterile package must be clean, dry, flat, and stable. The area must be free from airborne contamination. Patients can accidentally contaminate sterile supplies and trays. Explain the procedure to the patient before beginning. Instruct him or her to avoid touching sterile supplies, crossing over the sterile field, or talking, coughing, or sneezing over sterile articles. Remind the patient during the procedure, as necessary.

Setting Up a Sterile Field

A *sterile field* is a sterile surface that you create to use as a work area for sterile procedures. A 1-inch border around the outside edge of the field is considered not sterile. Avoid placing sterile items in this border area. Only the top surface of the work area is considered sterile. A sterile drape often hangs over the edges of the table. The area below the table top is not sterile. Sterile supplies can touch only the sterile field. Avoid touching the field or items on it with your hands.

guidelines *for*

Sterile Procedures

- Always wash your hands before beginning a sterile procedure.
- Check the expiration date on the package. Avoid using items that are beyond the expiration date.
- If the sterility of an item is in doubt, consider it unsterile and avoid using it.
- If a sterile package is cracked, cut, or torn, it is contaminated and should not be used.
- If a sterile item or package becomes wet, it is contaminated.
- If a sterile item contacts an unsterile item, the sterile item is contaminated.
- Follow your facility policy. You may be asked to sanitize and dry the table or other surface that sterile supplies will be placed on before establishing a sterile field.
- The outside of a sterile wrapper is not sterile. It may be handled with your hands. Avoid touching the inside of the wrapper or items inside the package with your hands.

- The inside of a sterile package can be used as a sterile field.
- Never turn your back on a sterile field.
- Avoid reaching across or touching a sterile field. If you must add an item to the sterile field, drop it onto the field from the sterile package.
- Avoid touching unsterile articles when wearing sterile gloves. Avoid touching the outside of sterile packages when wearing sterile gloves. Make sure you can see your hands at all times. Keep them above your waist. Avoid touching your clothing or body. If the gloves become torn or contaminated, change them immediately.
- If sterile gloves touch an unsterile item, such as the outside of a package, they are contaminated. Change them before proceeding.
- Keep sterile items above waist level.
- Avoid talking, coughing, or sneezing over a sterile field.

PROCEDURE 146

SETTING UP A STERILE FIELD USING A STERILE DRAPE

1. Wash your hands.

2. Open the sterile package containing the sterile drape.

3. With the thumb and index finger of your dominant hand, grasp the folded top edge of the drape.

4. Lift the drape out of the package. Extend your arm, holding the drape away from your body. Allow it to unfold. Make sure it does not touch any other surface, your body, or clothing as it unfolds.

5. Pick up the top corner on the other side of the drape after it is unfolded. Avoid touching the drape to your body, clothing, or other surfaces.

6. Beginning with the side opposite your body, slowly lay the drape across the table (Figure 50-13).

7. Open the other packages, and add necessary items to the sterile field.

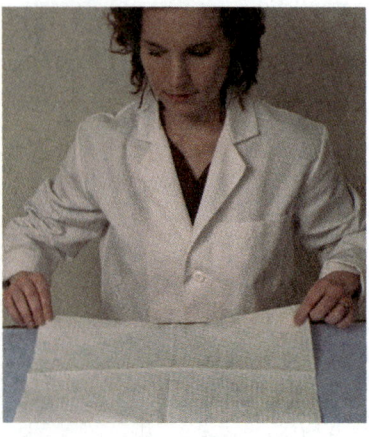

FIGURE 50-13
Beginning on the opposite side of the table, slowly position the drape.

PROCEDURE 147

ADDING AN ITEM TO A STERILE FIELD

1. Wash your hands.
2. Open the sterile package.
3. With one hand, grasp the package from the bottom. Using your free hand, pull the sides of the package away from the sterile field (Figure 50-14A). If you are using a peel-away package, peel the sides apart and drop the inner package onto the sterile field (Figure 50-14B).
4. Drop the sterile item onto the sterile field. Avoid touching the sterile field with the package wrapper.
5. Discard the wrapper.

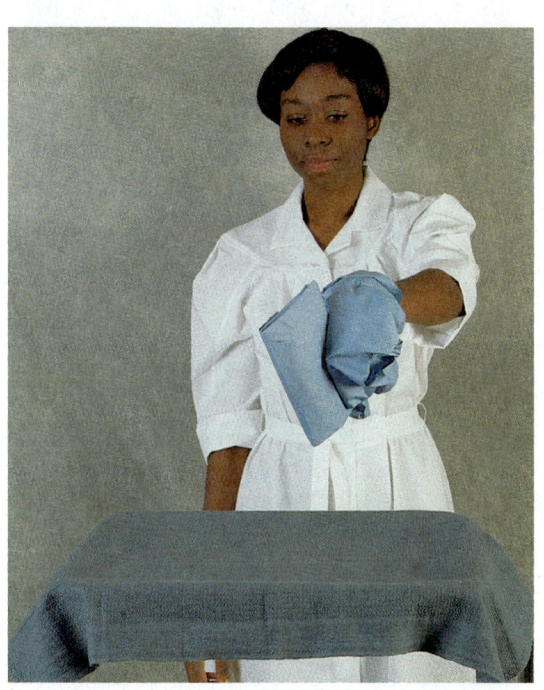

FIGURE 50-14A Pull the sides of the outer wrap back so they do not touch the sterile field. Drop the inner sterile package onto the sterile field.

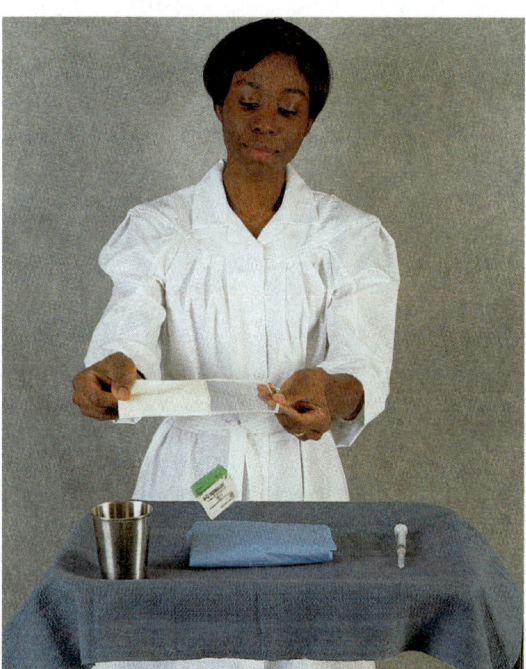

FIGURE 50-14B Peel the sides of the outer package back, then drop the sterile inner package onto the sterile field.

PROCEDURE 148

ADDING LIQUIDS TO A STERILE FIELD

1. Wash your hands.
2. Inspect the container. The seal should be intact, and the container should not be broken or cracked.
3. Open the container of liquid.
4. Place the cap upright on the table, with the outside of the cap resting on the table surface and the clean inner side facing up.

continues

PROCEDURE 148

continued

5. Pour a small amount of the solution into the sink or wastebasket to rinse the lip. When adding the solution to the sterile field, pour from the same side of the container. This is done to remove any microbes that might be on the lip.

6. Hold the bottle at an angle, 6 to 8 inches above the sterile bowl or other sterile container. Avoid reaching across the sterile field with your arm or hand.

7. From the clean side of the container, slowly pour the liquid to prevent splashing (Figure 50-15). If the liquid is spilled or splashed, the field is contaminated because moisture soaks through to the nonsterile surface beneath.

8. Replace the cap on the bottle.

9. Write the date and time the container was opened on the bottle. Write on the label, or use a separate piece of tape. Avoid writing directly on

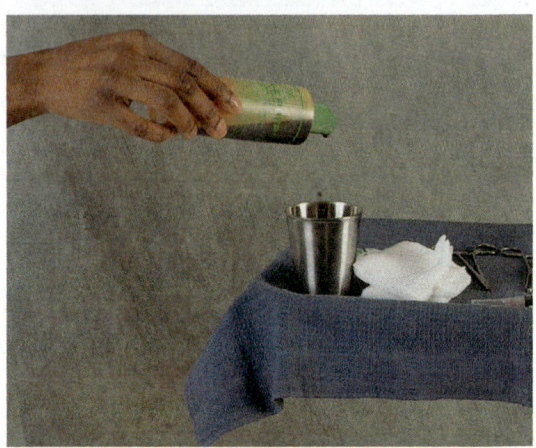

FIGURE 50-15 Pour the liquid slowly into the cup to prevent splashing.

the plastic bottle. The ink from a pen or marker may bleed through the plastic, contaminating the solution.

If a small surface is needed, the inside of a sterile package can be used as a sterile field. If a larger surface is needed, a sterile drape is used as the foundation for the sterile field.

Sterile Gloves. Using sterile gloves is essential when using aseptic (sterile) technique. Wearing sterile gloves permits you to touch sterile items without contaminating them.

PROCEDURE 149

APPLYING AND REMOVING STERILE GLOVES

1. Wash your hands.

2. Check the glove package for sterility.

3. Open the outer package by peeling the upper edges back with your thumbs.

4. Remove the inner package containing the gloves and place it on the inside of the outer package.

5. Open the inner package, handling it only by the corners on the outside (Figure 50-16).

6. Pick up the cuff of the right-hand glove using your left hand (Figure 50-17). Avoid touching the area below the cuff.

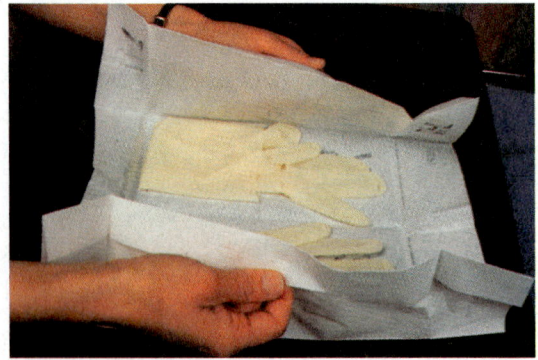

FIGURE 50-16 Carefully fold the edges of the package back without touching the inside of the package or the gloves.

continues

PROCEDURE 149

continued

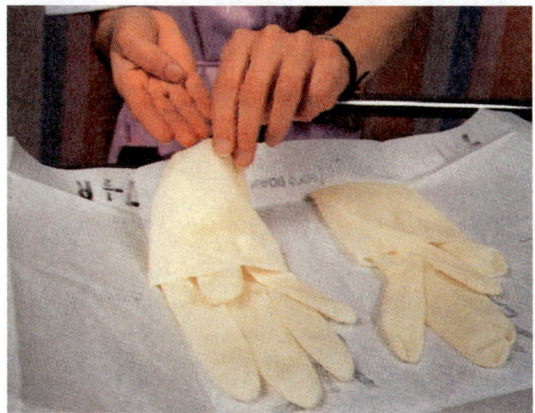

FIGURE 50-17 With your fingertips, carefully lift the edges of the cuff, then slide the opposite hand into the glove.

7. Insert your right hand into the glove. Spread your fingers slightly, sliding them into the glove fingers. If the glove is not on correctly, do not attempt to straighten it at this time.

8. Insert the gloved fingers of your right hand under the cuff of the left glove (Figure 50-18).

9. Slide your fingers into the left glove, adjusting the fingers of the gloves for comfort and fit. Because both gloves are sterile, they may touch each other. Avoid touching the cuffs of the gloves.

10. Insert your right hand under the cuff of the left glove and push the cuff up over your wrist (Figure 50-19). Avoid touching your wrist or the outside of the cuff with your glove.

11. Insert your left hand under the cuff of the right glove and push the cuff up over your wrist. Avoid touching your wrist or the outside of the cuff with your glove.

12. You may now touch sterile items with your sterile gloves. Avoid touching unsterile items.

To remove the gloves:

13. Grasp the outside of the glove on your nondominant hand at the cuff. Pull the glove off so that the inside of the glove faces outward. Avoid touching the skin of your wrist with the fingers of the glove.

14. Place this glove into the palm of the gloved hand.

15. Put the fingers of the ungloved hand *inside* the cuff of the gloved hand. Pull the glove off inside out. The first glove removed should be inside the second glove.

16. Discard the gloves into a covered container or trash, according to facility policy.

17. Wash your hands.

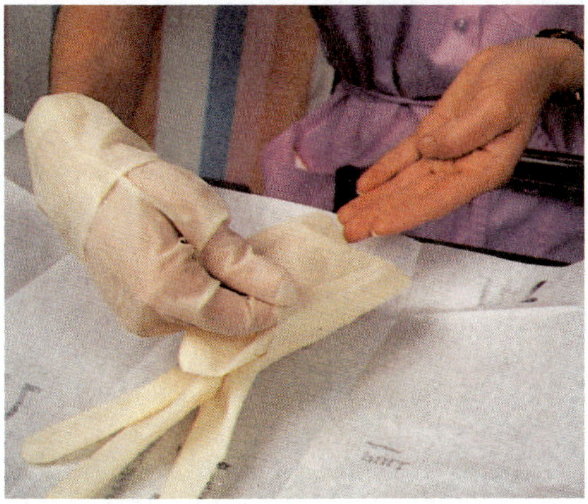

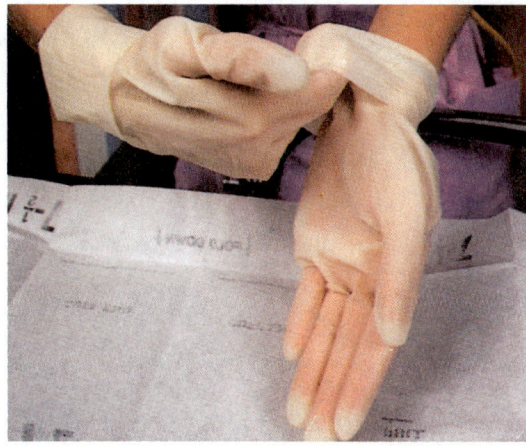

FIGURE 50-18 Protect the right-hand glove by sliding the fingers under the cuff of the left glove. Slide your left hand into the glove. Once both hands are gloved, adjust both gloves for comfort and fit.

FIGURE 50-19 Carefully adjust the cuffs. Avoid touching your wrists.

Transfer Forceps.   Some facilities use sterile transfer forceps to add supplies to the sterile field (Figure 50-20). When the sterile tray is packaged, the cup for liquids is turned on its side. The transfer forceps are also used to turn the cup without contaminating the sterile tray. The forceps are used for one procedure, then sterilized after use. Using transfer forceps eliminates the need to use sterile gloves to handle sterile supplies.

The handle of the sterile forceps is contaminated because you have touched it with your hands. Avoid touching the end of the forceps. The tips must be kept sterile to contact sterile items. After using the forceps, the tips must rest on a sterile surface to keep them sterile until the end of the procedure.

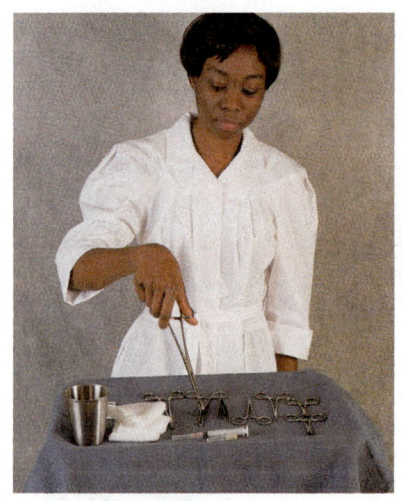

FIGURE 50-20 Use sterile transfer forceps to add sterile items to a sterile field. Do not allow the tips of the forceps to touch unsterile surfaces or objects.

PROCEDURE 150

USING TRANSFER FORCEPS

1. Wash your hands.
2. Open the package of sterile supplies in the normal manner.
3. Grasp the needed item with the tips of the forceps.
4. Pick the item up, moving it to the sterile field.
5. Lay the tips of the forceps within the sterile field. Keep the handles on the outside of the field. If the forceps are needed again during the procedure, you can pick them up by the handles to use them again.

REVIEW

A. True/False.

Mark the following true or false by circling T or F.

1. T F A stool with occult blood will appear bloody.

2. T F The Hemoccult® test is used to determine the presence of bile in the feces.

3. T F Gloves must be used when doing tests on feces or urine.

4. T F The proper amount of time to observe a Hemoccult® packet after placing a fecal smear and adding the developer is 5 minutes.

5. T F The drainage tube should be clamped for half an hour before you collect a sample from a drainage port.

6. T F Odor control can be a problem when a patient has an ostomy.

7. T F Drainage from a colostomy is always watery.

8. T F Nursing assistants should follow established policies of their own facilities in carrying out assigned tasks.

9. T F Nursing assistants should not carry out any procedure they have not been taught and for which they have not received supervision.

10. T F It is impossible to safely collect a sample of urine from a closed urinary drainage system.

11. T F The nursing assistant should reinsert the catheter if the patient does not void within 4 hours of catheter removal.

12. T F Apply the principles of standard precautions when caring for an ostomy.

13. T F The patient may be asked to wear a mask during some procedures.

14. T F The outside of a sterile package is always sterile.

15. T F Nonsterile items can be added to the edges of a sterile field.

16. T F You may handle sterile items if you are wearing sterile gloves.

17. T F You may reach across the sterile field to add supplies.

18. T F Waste products from an ostomy are discarded in the biohazardous trash.

B. Matching.

Choose the correct term from Column II to match each phrase in Column I.

Column I	Column II
19. _____ opening	**a.** occult
20. _____ artificial opening in large intestine	**b.** ileostomy
	c. stoma
21. _____ artificial opening in small intestine	**d.** appliance
	e. colostomy
22. _____ hidden	**f.** contamination
23. _____ drainage pouch	**g.** port

C. Multiple Choice.

Select the one best answer for each of the following.

24. An artificial opening in the colon is known as a/an
   a. tracheostomy.
   b. colostomy.
   c. ileostomy.
   d. proctostomy.

25. The reaction time for a Hemoccult® test is
   a. 2 to 4 seconds.
   b. 30 to 60 seconds.
   c. 2 to 3 minutes.
   d. 90 to 120 seconds.

26. The port of a closed urinary drainage system should be cleaned before withdrawal with
   a. soap and water.
   b. a paper towel.
   c. antiseptic.
   d. a sterile 4 × 4 gauze pad.

27. During routine care, the area around a colostomy should
   a. never be cleaned.
   b. be covered with petroleum jelly.
   c. be washed with soap and water.
   d. be cleaned with an antiseptic.

28. An ileostomy as compared to a colostomy
   a. has more formed stool.
   b. tends to be more irritating.
   c. has drainage containing blood clots.
   d. has a larger stoma.

29. You are giving routine stoma care to a patient with a colostomy and find the stoma red and irritated. You should
   a. complete the procedure.
   b. clean the area with alcohol.
   c. apply powder and attach the ostomy bag.
   d. cover the area and notify the nurse.

30. If the skin around an ileostomy stoma is broken, you should
   a. wipe it with alcohol.
   b. wash it with soap and water.
   c. cover it with a 4 × 4 gauze pad.
   d. inform the nurse.

31. Sterile technique is used for
   a. colostomy care.
   b. changing surgical dressings.
   c. routine pressure ulcer care.
   d. administering enemas and suppositories.

32. Which of the following statements are true?
   a. A sterile package may be used up to 30 days after the expiration date.
   b. Always wash your hands before applying sterile gloves.
   c. The sterile area of the sterile drape includes the top and area hanging over the edge.
   d. Regular exam gloves are worn when assisting with a sterile dressing change.

33. When pouring liquid into a cup on a sterile field, a small amount splashes onto the sterile drape. The drape is
   a. contaminated.
   b. clean.
   c. sterile.
   d. aseptic.

34. You are using pickup forceps to add supplies to a sterile field. You expect to add more supplies before the procedure is finished. Which of the following is true?
   a. The handle to the forceps is sterile.
   b. The forceps must be stored in liquid disinfectant solution so they remain sterile.
   c. The tip of the forceps must be placed on a sterile area until the procedure is finished.
   d. The forceps may be used for 24 hours after the package is opened.

35. When removing an indwelling catheter
   a. cut the inflation port close to the catheter to remove fluid from the balloon.
   b. tell the patient to take a deep breath, then quickly remove the catheter with the balloon inflated.
   c. withdraw fluid from the inflation port with a needle and syringe.
   d. remove half the fluid from the balloon before removing the catheter.

D. Nursing Assistant Challenge.

Mrs. Knight, who is 60 years old, was in an accident and received a broken right leg and two broken wrists. She has a long-standing colostomy, but because of her injuries cannot provide her own colostomy care. Answer the following questions about her care.

36. Will you need to wear gloves to give her colostomy care?

37. What will you use to remove feces from around the stoma?

38. What will happen if you apply too much lotion around the stoma?

39. How will the ostomy bag be held in place?

40. What are the three major problems associated with having a stoma?

EXPLORING THE WEB

Description	Location
Female urinary catheter care suggestions	*http://www.urologyclinicofhouston.com*
Home care of urinary catheters	*http://www.childrenshc.org*
Suprapubic urinary catheter suggestions	*http://www.urologyclinicofhouston.com*
Urinary catheter care instructions	*http://www.chclibrary.org*
Continent Ostomy Centers	*http://www.ostomy.com*
Family Practice Notebook—Urinary Catheter	*http://www.fpnotebook.com*
International Ostomy Association	*http://www.ostomyinternational.org*
Society of Urologic Nurses and Associates	*http://suna.inurse.com*
United Ostomy Association	*http://www.uoa.org*
Urinary Indwelling Catheter	*http://www.nmh.org*
World Ostomy Resource	*http://homepage.powerup.com.au*
Wound, Ostomy, & Continence Nurses Society	*http://www.wocn.org*

Response to Basic Emergencies

UNIT 51

Response to Basic Emergencies

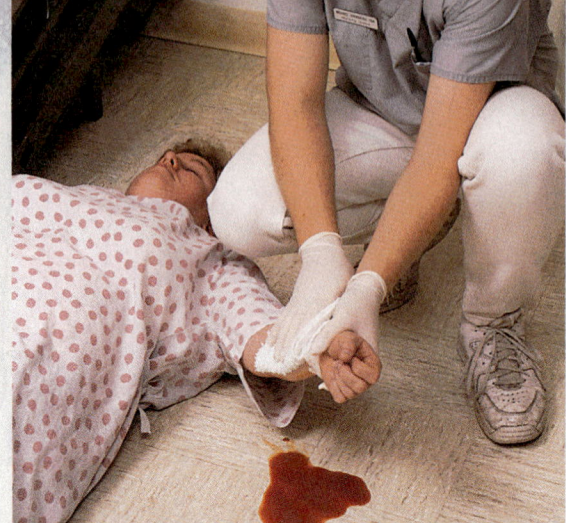

Response to Basic Emergencies

objectives

After completing this unit, you will be able to:
- Spell and define terms.
- Recognize emergency situations that require urgent care.
- Be able to evaluate situations and determine the sequence of appropriate actions to be taken.
- Describe how to maintain the patient's airway and breathing during respiratory failure and respiratory arrest.
- Recognize the need for CPR.
- List the benefits of early defibrillation.
- Identify the signs, symptoms, and treatment of common emergency situations such as:
  - Cardiac arrest
  - Choking
  - Bleeding
  - Shock
  - Fainting
  - Heart attack
  - Brain attack (stroke)
  - Seizure
  - Vomiting and aspiration
  - Thermal injuries
  - Poisoning
  - Known or suspected head injury
- Demonstrate the following procedures:
  - Procedure 151 Head-Tilt, Chin-Lift Maneuver
  - Procedure 152 Jaw-Thrust Maneuver
  - Procedure 153 Mask-to-Mouth Ventilation
  - Procedure 154 Adult CPR, One Rescuer
  - Procedure 155 Adult CPR, Two-Person
  - Procedure 156 Positioning the Patient in the Recovery Position
  - Procedure 157 Heimlich Maneuver— Abdominal Thrusts
  - Procedure 158 Assisting the Adult Who Has an Obstructed Airway and Becomes Unconscious
  - Procedure 159 CPR for Infants
  - Procedure 160 Obstructed Airway: Conscious Infant
  - Procedure 161 Obstructed Airway: Unconscious Infant
  - Procedure 162 CPR for Children, One Rescuer
  - Procedure 163 Child with Foreign Body Airway Obstruction

vocabulary

Learn the meaning and the correct spelling of the following words and phrases:

adjunctive devices	dislocation	head-tilt, chin-lift	respiratory arrest
automatic external	emergency	maneuver	respiratory failure
defibrillator (AED)	emergency care	Heimlich maneuver	shock
cardiac arrest	Emergency Medical	hemorrhage	sprain
cardiopulmonary	Services (EMS)	jaw-thrust maneuver	strain
resuscitation (CPR)	first aid	pocket mask	ventilation
defibrillation	fracture	recovery position	victim

DEALING WITH EMERGENCIES

All emergency situations develop rapidly and unpredictably. Emergency situations can occur at any time to anyone. Examples include:

- Automobile accidents
- Brain attacks (strokes)
- Suddenly feeling weak
- Fainting and falling

An **emergency** is any unexpected situation that requires immediate action and medical attention. In a true emergency, prompt action is needed to prevent further complications

guidelines *for*

Responding to an Emergency

- Always remember the priorities of any emergency as the ABCs:
  - **A**irway: obstructed or unobstructed?
  - **B**reathing: is the victim able to breathe?
  - **C**irculation: is the heart beating, is there bleeding?
- Stay calm. Nothing is accomplished and more problems will result if the people at the scene of the emergency become flustered and agitated. If you are calm, you will be a calming influence on the victim.
- Know what to do to summon immediate help; you need to get the nurse to the scene as soon as possible. Stay with the victim and call out for help. If you are out in the community, tell the closest person to call Emergency Medical Services (EMS).
- Do not move the victim unless the person will be endangered by staying where he is.
- Stay with the victim until the person in charge gives you permission to leave.
- Know your limitations. Be aware of what procedures you are qualified to perform in an emergency. Never attempt to render treatment unless you have received the appropriate training.
- Know the procedures to follow for emergencies. Health care facilities have code names for various emergencies. Know what these are and how to announce a code. If you are out in the community, know the appropriate first aid to apply in emergency situations.
- Know the procedures for activating the **Emergency Medical Services** (**EMS**) system (Figure 51-1). In most parts of the country, this is done by dialing 911 (Figure 51-2). You will need to:
  - give the address
  - describe what happened (e.g., the person was burned or has no heartbeat)
  - the person's name (if you know this information)
  - telephone number where the call is being made from

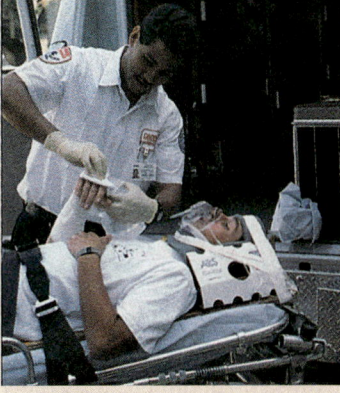

FIGURE 51-1 Know the procedure for activating the EMS system in your community.

  - number of persons needing help
- Keep the person warm. Cover with blankets.
- Do not give the person any fluids or food.
- If the person starts to vomit, turn her head to one side to avoid aspiration.
- If the person is conscious, assure him that help has been called and is on the way.
- Protect the person's privacy. Keep other people away from the scene unless they are qualified to assist.
- In all situations, apply standard precautions to prevent exposure to blood, body fluids, mucous membranes, and nonintact skin during the emergency.

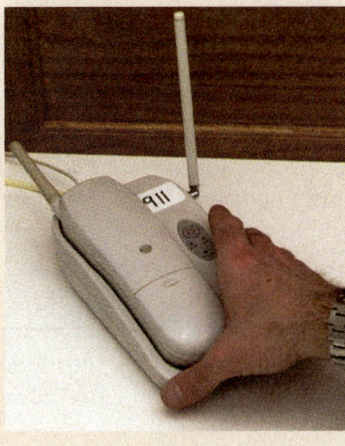

FIGURE 51-2 The EMS system is activated by dialing 911 in most communities in the United States.

and to save the life of the victim (person needing help). It is important that you know the signs and symptoms of an emergency and that you be able to take immediate action. The following guidelines are basic actions to remember for any emergency.

BEING PREPARED

While working in the hospital or long-term care facility, you are always close to professional medical help. When you witness an accident away from the medical facility, however, professional help is not always readily available. Whatever course of action you choose, the victim should not be further endangered.

FIRST AID

First aid includes:

- Immediate care for victims of injuries or sudden illness
- Care needed later if medical help is delayed or is not available

First aid will be needed for different conditions in a variety of situations. These conditions can range from the minor to the very severe. When you give first aid, you deal with the:

- Victim's emotional state
- Victim's physical injuries
- Management of the whole accident situation

Persons in life-threatening situations must be given immediate attention. Life-threatening situations include those in which a person:

- Has no airway
- Has stopped breathing
- Is in shock
- Has been poisoned
- Is choking
- Is bleeding profusely

Evaluating the Situation

At the scene of an accident, assess the situation and find out the extent of injuries. Quickly determine the number of victims, their potential injuries, and any dangerous factors at the scene.

For example, at the scene of an auto accident, there may be several victims. Some may be trapped in their vehicles, others may be lying on the highway. There may be cars burning and the danger of explosion. In this situation, you must first get yourself and the victims away from further danger.

In the medical facility, unless there is a fire, you usually will be dealing with a single victim. You will be able to focus on the needs of that individual. For example, you might enter a patient's room and find a patient lying on the floor, despite the fact that the bed side rails are up. Quickly evaluate the situation as you signal for help, giving the patient's name and location and describing the scene.

EMERGENCY CARE

Emergency care is care that must be given right away to prevent loss of life.

- Whether you are out in the community or in the health care facility, ask someone nearby to summon help.
- Do not leave people who need urgent care to get help yourself. (Exception—CPR; see CPR directions.)
- As help is on the way, check, in the following order, the victim for:
  - Degree of reponsiveness
  - Airway/breathing capability
  - Presence and rate of heartbeat
  - Signs of bleeding
  - Signs of shock
- Do not move the person if you do not have to.
- Do not allow the person to get up and walk around.
- Check for other injuries.

MAINTAINING THE PATIENT'S BREATHING

The normal respiratory rate is determined by age. Normal respiratory rates for various age groups are listed in Table 51-1.

TABLE 51-1 NORMAL RESPIRATORY RATES	
Age	**Normal Respiratory Rate per Minute**
Infant	30–60
Toddler	24–40
Preschool child	22–34
School-age child	18–30
Teenager	12–16
Adult	12–20

TABLE 51-2 MONITORING FOR BREATHING ADEQUACY

- The patient can talk, respirations are between 12 and 20, and there is no apparent distress.

- The rhythm is regular.

- The patient's color is normal, with no cyanosis or gray coloration.

- Look at the patient's chest. It should expand equally with each inspiration.

- Listen for breath sounds, by placing your ear next to the patient's nose and mouth, if necessary. The sounds should be quiet, without gurgling, wheezing, gasping, or other abnormal sounds.

- Feel for breath movement on your cheek and ear.

TABLE 51-3 SIGNS AND SYMPTOMS OF INADEQUATE BREATHING TO REPORT TO THE NURSE IMMEDIATELY

- Movement in the chest is absent, minimal, or irregular.

- Breathing movement appears to be in the abdomen, not the lungs.

- Air movement cannot be detected by listening and feeling for breath sounds on your cheek and ear.

- Respiratory rate is too slow or rapid.

- Respirations are irregular, gasping, very deep, or shallow.

- Respirations appear labored.

- The patient is short of breath.

- The patient's skin, lips, tongue, earlobes, mucous membranes, or nailbeds are blue or gray.

- The patient is unable to speak at all, or cannot speak in sentences because he is short of breath.

- Respirations are noisy.

- Nasal flaring is present during inspiration.

- The muscles below the ribs and/or above the clavicles retract inward during respiration.

Respiratory failure occurs when breathing is insufficient to sustain life. **Respiratory arrest** occurs when breathing stops. It is caused by many conditions, including heart attack, brain attack (stroke or CVA), overdose, drowning, electrocution, poisoning, and traumatic injuries. Follow the criteria in Table 51-2 to determine if the patient's breathing is adequate. Abnormal respirations are often a warning of an impending crisis. Stay with the patient and use the call signal or telephone to request assistance if the patient is in distress. Report problems to the nurse immediately. Signs and symptoms to report are listed in Table 51-3.

Opening the Airway

If you discover a patient who is in respiratory failure or respiratory arrest, remain in the room and signal or call for immediate help. You must open the patient's airway if she cannot do this independently. The most common cause of airway obstruction is the tongue falling back into the throat. Opening the airway lifts the tongue from the back of the throat, making breathing easier. This procedure, as well as some other emergency procedures in this unit, is most effective when the patient is lying in the supine position. Always remove the pillow. Position the patient on the back before beginning.

Because of the nature of the situation, you may not have time to wash your hands or perform other beginning procedure actions. Immediately after the patient is safe, wash your hands well. Avoid contact with the patient's secretions if you are not wearing gloves or other personal protective equipment.

The **head-tilt, chin-lift maneuver** (Procedure 151) is the most common method of opening the airway. If the patient

has a neck injury, do not perform this procedure. Instead, use the jaw-thrust maneuver.

The **jaw-thrust maneuver** (Procedure 152) is used to open the airway of patients with known or suspected neck injuries, and in those whose airways cannot be opened using the head-tilt, chin-lift method. In some facilities, this procedure is used for patients with head and facial injuries. This is because patients with injuries of the head and face often have neck injuries as well. The purpose of the procedure is to open the airway without moving the head or neck.

Mask-to-Mouth Resuscitation

When a patient stops breathing, his respirations must be sustained by artificial means to prevent brain damage and other complications. If you have taken a CPR class previously, you may have learned mouth-to-mouth **ventilation**. This is a technique of breathing for the patient. Most health care facilities discourage staff from using this method on patients because of the risk of disease transmission. Various **adjunctive devices** are used instead. An airway adjunct is a

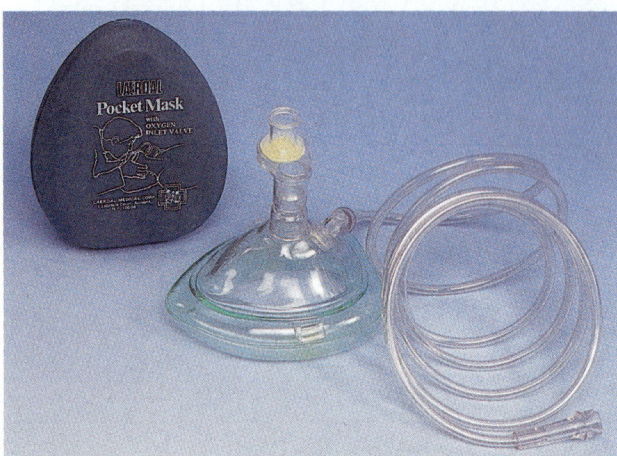

FIGURE 51-3 A pocket mask is a simple, efficient device that provides a one-way barrier in the event that mouth-to-mouth (mask) ventilation is necessary. Supplemental oxygen may be added by connecting tubing to the male adapter on the mask.

secondary device used to maintain respirations. This is done by a trained and qualified health care professional.

Mask-to-mouth ventilation is performed using a **pocket mask** (Figure 51-3). This is a temporary measure until more advanced airway support is available. The mask has a special valve that prevents the patient's exhaled air and secretions from entering the caregiver's mouth. This infection control feature protects the user. Room air contains approximately 21% oxygen. You do not use all the oxygen you take in when you breathe. You exhale extra oxygen, so there is more than enough for the patient to use. He or she must be positioned in the supine position with the airway open for effective ventilation. The mask covers both the nose and the mouth. It can be turned upside down for infant resuscitation. (Refer to Procedure 153.)

Most pocket masks are clear plastic. This enables you to see the position of the patient's mouth. Monitoring the color of the patient's lips will help you see how well the patient is being oxygenated. Sometimes the patient will vomit during artificial ventilation. You will see this in the mask. If vomiting occurs, quickly turn the patient on his or her side, then clear the mouth and continue ventilation. A licensed professional will suction the patient when suction is available.

CARDIAC ARREST

A person may stop breathing but still have a heartbeat. This is called **respiratory arrest**. If the situation is not reversed, the heart will stop beating. **Cardiac arrest** is the term used when the heart has stopped beating and respirations have ceased. When the heart and lungs are not functioning, blood and oxygen are not circulated to the brain and the rest of the body. The person is clinically dead. Permanent damage to the brain and other organs occurs within 4 to 6 minutes. Indications of cardiac arrest are:

- No response from the victim
- No breathing can be detected
- No pulse

Cardiopulmonary resuscitation (CPR) is a procedure used to maintain blood circulation throughout the body until the EMS can respond to the emergency. *You must never perform CPR unless you have completed an approved course, taught by an approved instructor.* The American Heart Association and the American Red Cross both offer such courses in communities across the country. **The information in this book is not intended to take the place of an approved course.** (Refer to Procedures 154 and 155.)

In the health care facility, you must know whether CPR is to be initiated. A patient who is very elderly or who has a terminal illness may not wish to be resuscitated if cardiac arrest occurs. In these cases the physician must write an order "do not resuscitate" (DNR) or "no code" (Figure 51-4). If there is no DNR order, full life support measures are given for cardiac arrest.

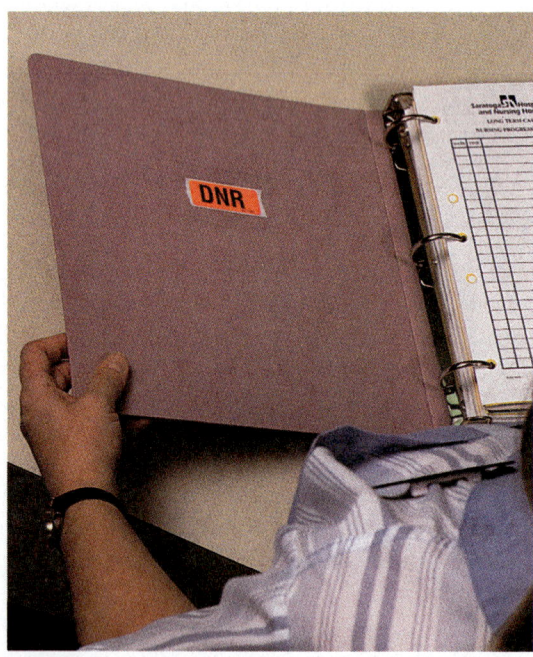

FIGURE 51-4 A DNR on the patient's chart means the patient does not wish to be resuscitated in the event of cardiac arrest.

PROCEDURE 151

HEAD-TILT, CHIN-LIFT MANEUVER

1. Place one hand on the forehead. Place the fingers of the opposite hand below the center of the jaw bone, directly under the chin.

2. Tilt the head back gently.

3. With your fingertips, lift the lower jaw forward (Figure 51-5). The lower teeth should almost touch the upper teeth. Avoid pressing on the neck, which may worsen the airway obstruction.

4. Keep the patient's mouth open. If necessary, pull the patient's lower lip forward. Avoid inserting your fingers into the mouth.

5. If the patient cannot maintain this position, maintain the airway manually, by holding your hands in place, if necessary.

6. As soon as the patient is safe, and the nurse or other professionals have assumed responsibility for care, wash your hands well.

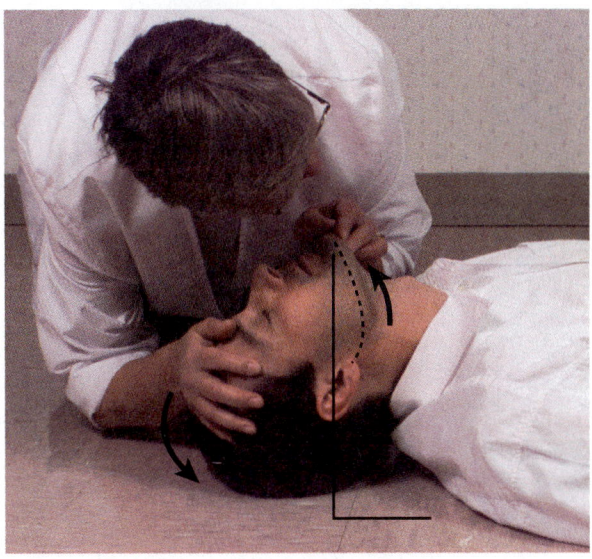

FIGURE 51-5 Use the head-tilt, chin-lift technique to open the airway unless head injury is suspected.

SAFETY *Alert*

The jaw-thrust maneuver is the only method that should be used for opening the airway when neck or spinal cord injuries are suspected.

PROCEDURE 152

JAW-THRUST MANEUVER

1. Move the patient into the supine position as a single unit. Avoid twisting the neck, back, or spine during movement.

2. Pull the head of the bed away from the wall.

3. Position yourself above the patient's head.

4. Position your elbows on the mattress.

5. Using your forearms, stabilize the sides of the head to prevent movement.

6. Place one hand on each side of the lower jaw, just below the ears (Figure 51-6).

continues

PROCEDURE 152

continued

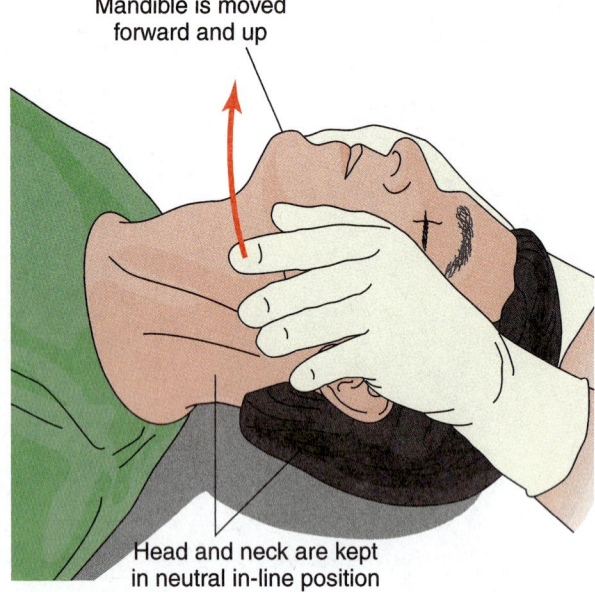

Mandible is moved forward and up

Head and neck are kept in neutral in-line position

FIGURE 51-6 Position your fingers at the angle of the jaw, pushing it upward and forward.

7. Use the tips of your index fingers to push the lower jaw forward.

8. Keep the patient's mouth open. If necessary, pull the patient's lower lip forward. Avoid inserting your fingers into the mouth.

9. If the patient cannot maintain this position, maintain the airway manually, by holding your hands in place, if necessary.

10. As soon as the patient is safe, and the nurse or other professionals have assumed responsibility for care, wash your hands well.

PROCEDURE 153

MASK-TO-MOUTH VENTILATION

Supplies needed:
- disposable exam gloves
- pocket mask with anti-reflux (one-way) valve

1. Pull the head of the bed away from the wall.

2. Apply gloves.

3. Open the patient's airway using the head-tilt, chin-lift method or the jaw-thrust maneuver.

4. Position yourself at the patient's head.

5. Position the mask on the patient's face, with the small end over the bridge of the nose and the wide end on the patient's chin. The ventilation port should be centered over the patient's mouth.

6. Seal the mask to the patient's face by positioning your thumbs on the top of the mask and fingers at the sides. Hold the airway in the open position.

7. Take a deep breath, then seal your mouth over the ventilation port, exhaling into the mask. The ventilation should take 1 to 1½ seconds in infants and children, and 2 seconds in adults. During the ventilation, look at the patient's chest. It should rise as you blow air in.

8. Remove your mouth from the mask and allow the patient to exhale passively. Continue to breathe into the mask once every 4 to 5 seconds.

PROCEDURE 154

ADULT CPR, ONE RESCUER

Standard precautions should be followed if at all possible. This means gloves should be worn and a barrier device used. If the victim is bleeding, a gown and mask may also be necessary. These items should be readily available in a health care facility.

Careful evaluation is required before CPR is administered.

1. Gently shake the person and ask him, "Are you okay?" Call the victim's name if you know it (Figure 51-7).

2. Call out for help. If someone responds to your call, send her to call the EMS system. If no one responds to your call, call the EMS system yourself and return to the victim as soon as possible.

3. Turn the victim on his back as a unit, supporting the head and back (Figure 51-8). For CPR to be effective, the victim must be lying on his back on a hard surface.

4. Open the airway, using a head-tilt, chin-lift technique (see Procedure 151).

5. Maintain the open airway with the head-tilt, chin-lift technique or jaw-thrust maneuver (see Procedure 152). Place your ear near the victim's mouth. At the same time, observe the victim's

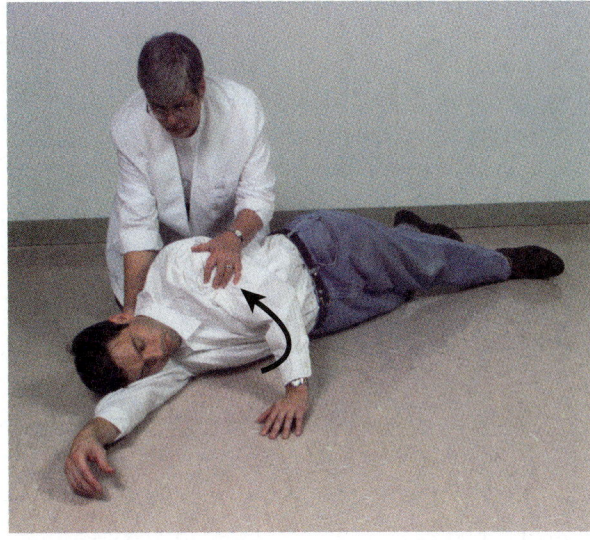

FIGURE 51-8 Support the head and back while turning the patient as a unit.

chest. You are looking, listening, and feeling for any signs that the victim may be breathing. You should look, listen, and feel for 3 to 5 seconds (Figure 51-9). If the victim is breathing, maintain an open airway, monitor his breathing, and call EMS if that was not done earlier.

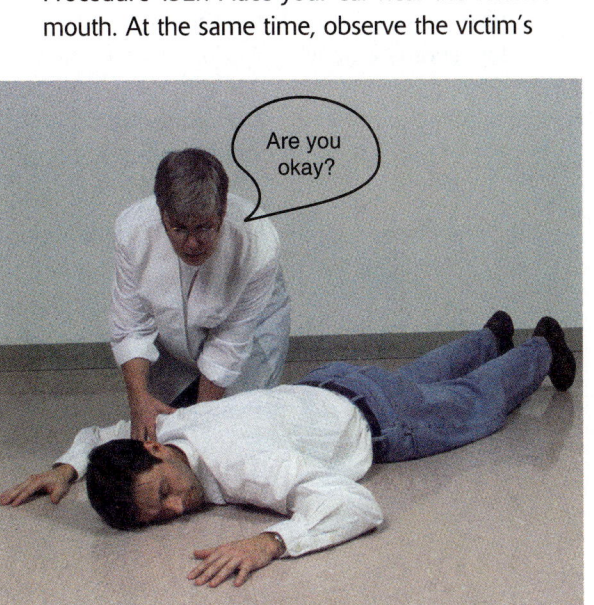

FIGURE 51-7 Gently shake the patient and ask, "Are you okay?"

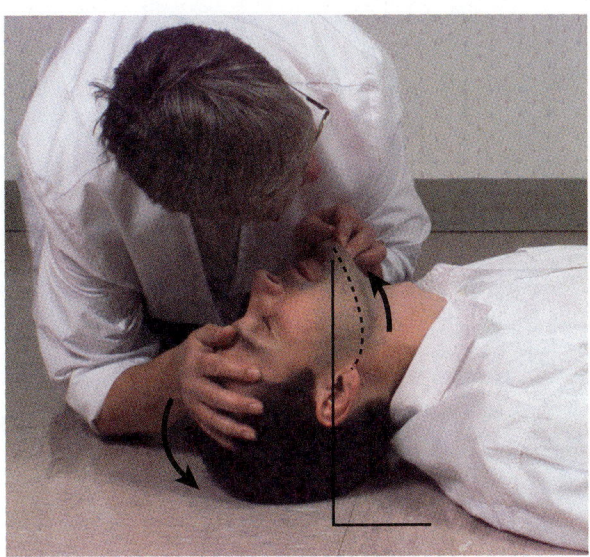

FIGURE 51-9 Take 3 to 5 seconds to look, listen, and feel for respirations on your cheek and ear.

continues

PROCEDURE 154

continued

6. If there are no signs of breathing, seal the victim's nose with your thumb and forefinger and seal the victim's mouth, using your mouth or a barrier device.

7. Ventilate 2 times, taking 2 seconds for each ventilation (Figure 51-10). Allow the chest to deflate between ventilations. Watch the chest rise to determine if enough air is getting through.

8. After the ventilations, check for the presence of a heartbeat. Maintain the open airway, using the head-tilt technique, with one hand. With the other hand, feel for the victim's carotid pulse on the near side of the victim (Figure 51-11). Take 5 to 10 seconds to determine whether there is a pulse. If there is a pulse, but no respirations, continue with ventilations at the rate of 1 every 4 to 5 seconds. Continue to check periodically for a pulse.

9. If there is no pulse, begin chest compressions at the ratio of 15 compressions to 2 ventilations. Kneel by the victim's shoulders and determine proper hand placement. Your shoulders should be over the victim's sternum. Using correct hand placement and technique, compress the victim's chest 1½ to 2 inches. While doing compressions, you must:

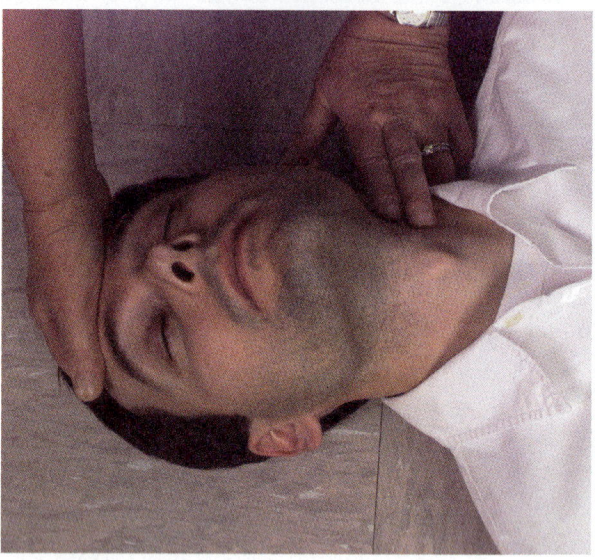

FIGURE 51-11 Check the carotid pulse in the notch on either side of the neck.

- locate the "landmark" hand position (Figure 51-12). Run your fingers up the lower margins of the ribs, and locate the xiphoid process. Hold your index and middle fingers over the xiphoid process to keep your place. Proper hand placement is very important to prevent injury.

- place the heel of your other hand on the chest next to your fingers (Figure 51-13). Next, place the landmark hand on top of the other hand,

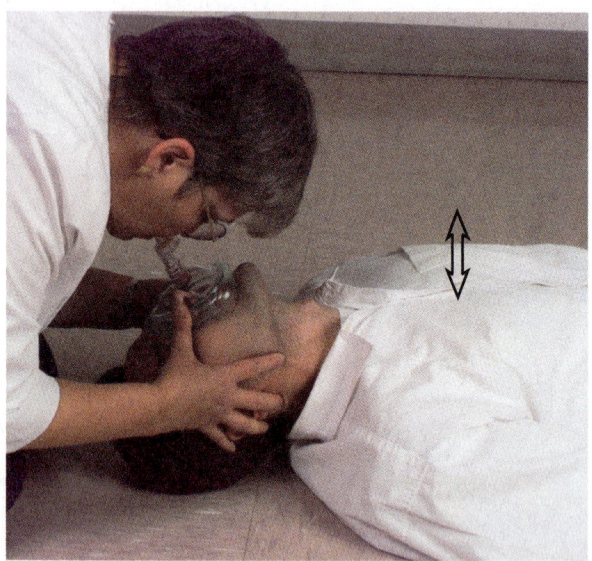

FIGURE 51-10 Give 2 full ventilations, allowing for exhalation between each. Make sure the chest rises and falls with each ventilation.

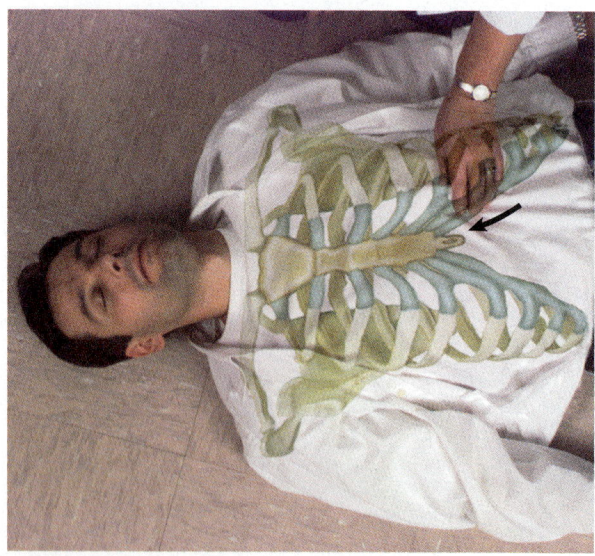

FIGURE 51-12 Proper hand placement is very important to prevent further injury.

continues

PROCEDURE 154

continued

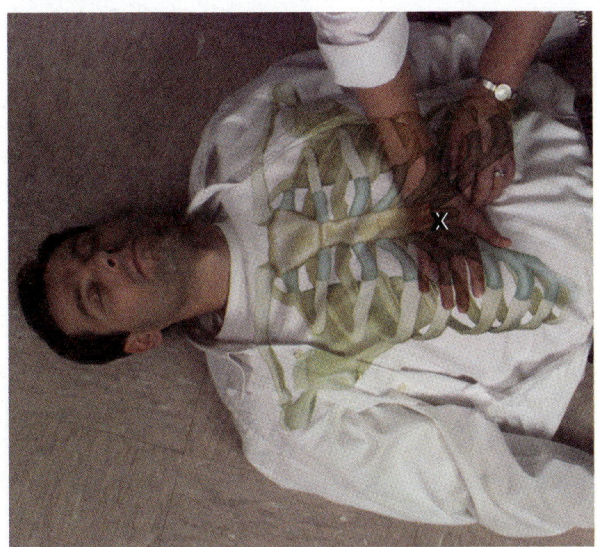

FIGURE 51-13 Place two fingers of your landmark hand in the sternal notch. Position the heel of the other hand on the chest next to the landmark.

interlacing the fingers (Figures 51-14 and 51-15A). Lock your elbows.

- keep your elbows straight, with your shoulders directly over the victim's sternum (Figure 51-15B).
- compress the sternum straight down 1½ to 2 inches at a rate of 100 compressions a minute. (This is *not* 100 actual compressions

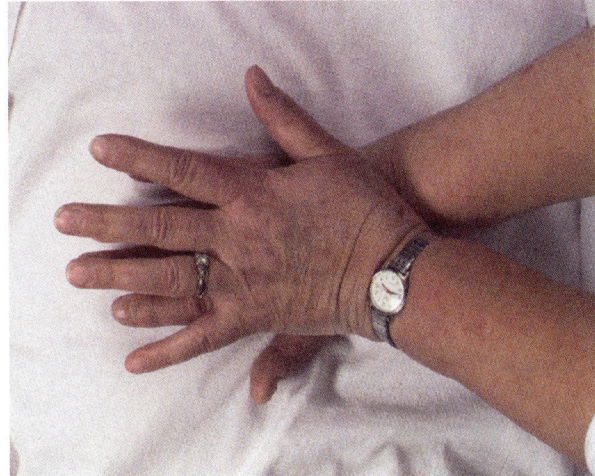

FIGURE 51-14 Now position the heel of the landmark hand on top of the other hand. Only the heel of the hands should touch the chest. Avoid applying pressure on the ribs with your fingers.

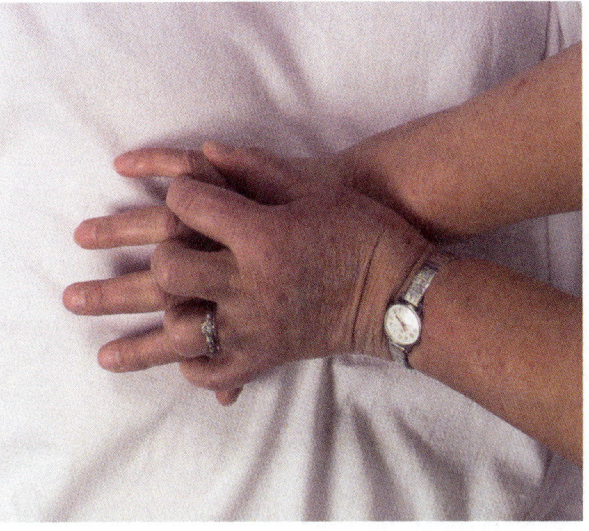

A

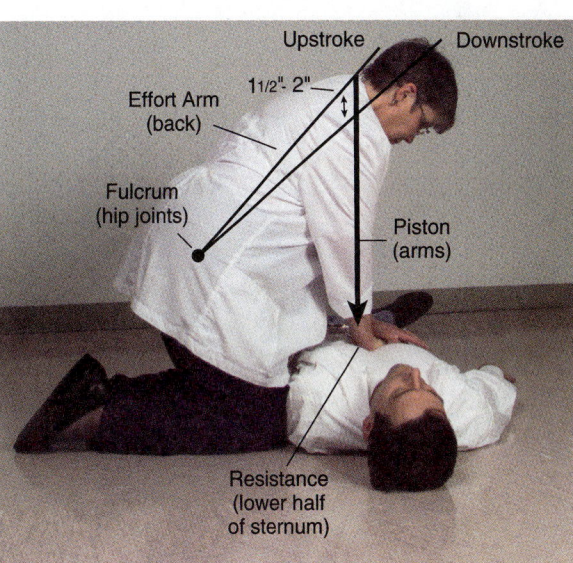

B

FIGURE 51-15 Lock your elbows. Position your shoulders directly over the sternum.

a minute, but rather a *rate* of 100 per minute, meaning more than one compression per second.)

- Downward pressure should be on the sternum only. Avoid pressing on the ribs with your fingers.
- Keep the fingers interlaced and slightly elevated from the chest.
- Compressions should be smooth and rhythmic.

continues

PROCEDURE 154

continued

- Completely release pressure, but maintain hand contact with the chest between each compression. The release in pressure allows the heart to refill with blood.
- Count out loud during compressions: one and, two and, three and, —

10. Do 15 compressions to 2 ventilations per cycle.

11. Do four cycles:
    - 15 compressions and 2 ventilations for each cycle
    - Take 2 seconds for each ventilation
    - Observe chest rise to check for effectiveness of ventilations
    - Use a compression rate of 100 compressions per minute

12. At the end of four cycles, feel for the carotid pulse for 5 seconds. If there is no pulse, ventilate 2 times.

13. Continue to repeat the cycle of 15 compressions to 2 ventilations. Feel for the carotid pulse every few minutes.

14. If the victim resumes breathing but is unconscious, and if there is no evidence of trauma, place the victim in recovery position on his side.

15. If the heart is beating but there is no breathing, continue ventilations at the rate of 1 every 5 seconds or 12 times per minute.

16. If there is no heartbeat and no breathing, continue with chest compressions and ventilations at the ratio of 15 compressions to 2 ventilations.

PROCEDURE 155

ADULT CPR, TWO-PERSON

The techniques for two-person CPR are exactly the same as for one person. The compression to ventilation rate is 15 compressions to every 2 ventilations. Chest compressions are done at the rate of 100 per minute. The two rescuers should be on opposite sides of the victim if possible.

1. If CPR is in progress:
   a. The second rescuer comes in after the first rescuer has completed a cycle of 15 compressions and 2 breaths.
   b. One rescuer moves to the victim's head, opens the airway, and says, "Stop CPR." She checks for spontaneous return of the pulse when no compressions are performed.
   c. The other rescuer finds the correct hand position.
   d. If the pulse is absent, say, "No pulse." The ventilator gives 2 breaths and the compressor begins chest compressions, counting "one and, two and, three and, four and, five." At the end of the 15th compression, the compressor

pauses to allow the other rescuer to give two ventilations (Figure 51-16).

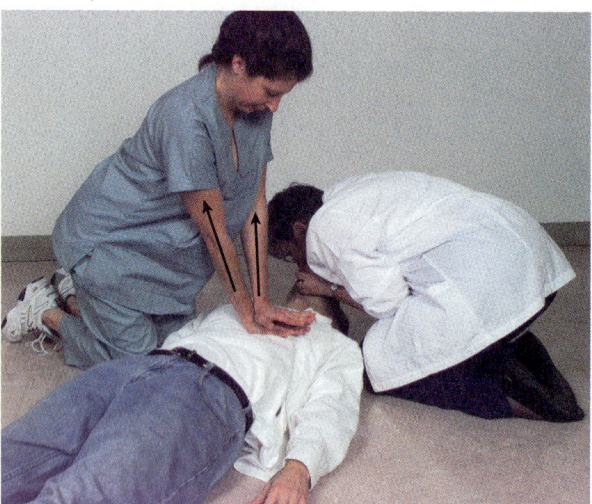

FIGURE 51-16 The rescuer doing compressions at the chest pauses briefly at the end of each 15 compressions so the other rescuer can give 2 breaths.

continues

PROCEDURE 155

continued

e. The cycles continue with periodic pulse checks. The ventilator is responsible for reevaluating the patient. Palpate the carotid pulse during the second rescuer's chest compressions. You will feel a pulse if the compressions are effective. Signal the compressor periodically to pause for 5 seconds for a reassessment of pulse and respirations.

2. If no CPR is in progress and both rescuers arrive on the scene at the same time:

a. Both rescuers must decide what needs to be done, and they must start immediately.

b. One rescuer calls the EMS system while the other person begins one-rescuer CPR.

c. One rescuer goes to the head of the victim and
   – determines unresponsiveness
   – positions the victim
   – opens the airway
   – checks for victim's breathing
   – if breathing is absent, says "no breathing" and gives 2 ventilations
   – checks for pulse; if no pulse, says "no pulse"

d. Second rescuer (at the same time as first rescuer does above procedure)
   – finds location for chest compressions
   – places hands in proper position
   – initiates external chest compressions after first rescuer says "no pulse"

e. During the cycle, the ventilator should monitor the pulse during compressions and breathing to determine the effectiveness of these procedures.

f. The compressor gives 15 compressions at the rate of 100 a minute, then pauses briefly, keeping the hands in place on the chest. The ventilator gives 2 ventilations. The cycle resumes with 15 compressions to 2 ventilations and repeats indefinitely until further help arrives, the victim regains consciousness, or the rescuers are exhausted and unable to continue.

g. Chest compressions should be stopped for 5 seconds at the end of the first minute and every few minutes thereafter to determine if the victim has resumed spontaneous breathing and circulation.

To Switch Sides

3. When the rescuers are on opposite sides of the victim:

a. The change of positions takes place without interrupting the 15:2 sequence (Figures 51-17A–D).

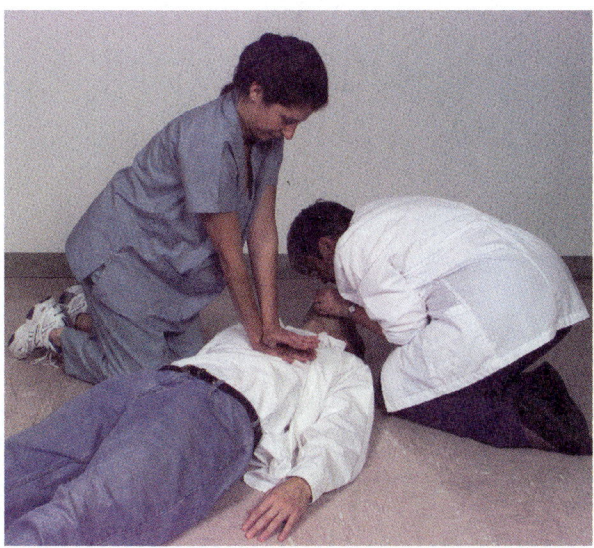

A. The person at the chest signals that it is time to change positions.

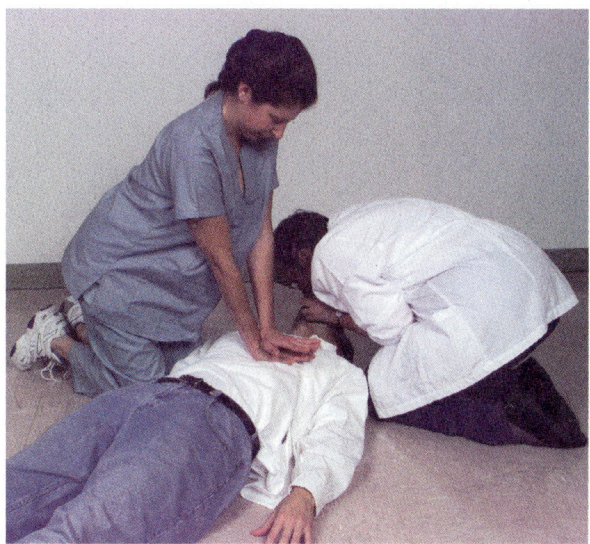

B. The rescuer at the head gives 2 full breaths after the 15th ventilation, then moves down to the chest.

FIGURE 51-17A and B Rescuers can change positions without interrupting the sequence.

continues

PROCEDURE 155

continued

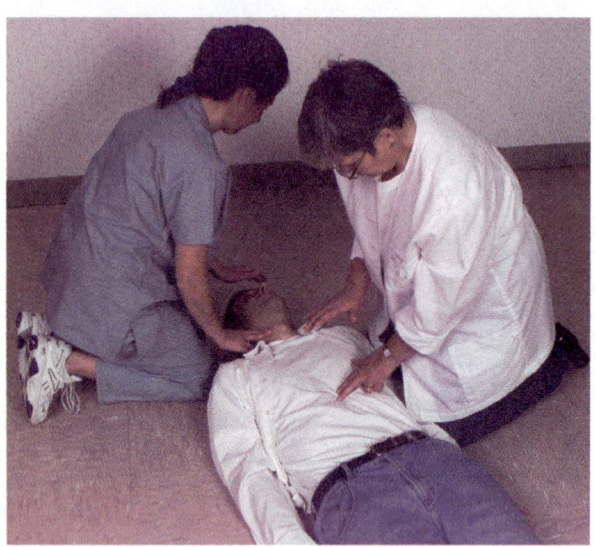

FIGURE 51-17C After moving to the chest, the rescuer finds the landmark and places hands in position. The person at the head checks for return of pulse and respiration.

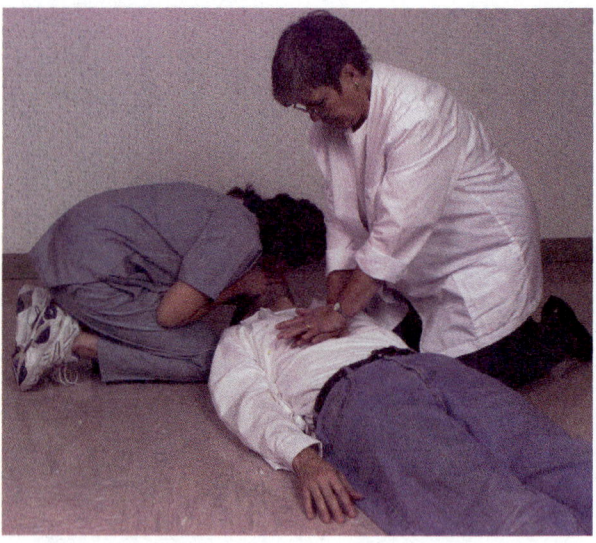

FIGURE 51-17D If the pulse is absent, the rescuer at the head gives 2 breaths, signaling the rescuer at the chest to begin compressions.

 b. The rescuer performing compressions directs when the switch takes place, at the end of a 15:2 sequence.

  – The ventilator gives 2 breaths, assumes the position for compressions, and locates the proper hand position.

  – The compressor, after the 15th compression, moves to the victim's head and checks the carotid pulse for 5 seconds.

  – If there is no pulse, the rescuer at the victim's head gives 2 breaths and tells the rescuer at the chest to continue with CPR.

  – If there is a pulse but no breathing, continue with ventilations and monitor the pulse.

4. When the rescuers are on the same side of the victim:

 a. The compressor initiates the switch by saying so while continuing chest compressions.

 b. The ventilator gives 2 ventilations after the 15th compression.

 c. After the ventilations, the ventilator moves quickly behind and around the compressor and assumes the compressor position.

 d. The compressor moves to the victim's head to check the pulse and to become the new ventilator.

 e. The new compressor gets in position beside the victim's chest, assumes the correct hand position, and waits to begin compressions.

 f. The new ventilator quickly moves to the victim's head, does a pulse and breathing check, and resumes with the correct procedure, if needed.

5. Remember, if the victim resumes breathing and the pulse returns, place the victim in the recovery position (Procedure 156).

THE RECOVERY POSITION

If the patient is unresponsive, but is breathing and has a pulse, he should be positioned in the **recovery position** to prevent complications. The recovery position is a modified lateral position (Figure 51-18). The patient's position must:

- be stable

- avoid pressure on the chest
- avoid pressure on the lower arm
- allow the airway to remain open.

Continue to monitor the patient according to facility policy to ensure that the pulse and respirations remain adequate. Take vital signs according to the nurse's instructions.

PROCEDURE 156

POSITIONING THE PATIENT IN THE RECOVERY POSITION

1. Kneel beside the patient and straighten his legs.
2. Place the arm nearest you above the patient's head with the palm up and the elbow bent slightly.
3. Position his opposite arm across his chest.
4. Place your lower hand on the patient's thigh on the far side of the body. Pull the thigh up slightly, closer to the center of the patient's body.
5. Place your upper hand on the patient's shoulder on the opposite side of the body.
6. With one hand on the thigh and the other on the shoulder, roll the patient onto his side, facing you.

7. Move the patient's upper hand close to the cheek, bending the elbow. This hand should be close to the face, but not under the body. Adjust the upper body so that the hip and knee are at right angles.
8. Tilt the patient's head back slightly to keep the airway open. Now place his upper hand, palm facing down, under the cheek to maintain the head position.
9. Continue to monitor the patient closely for adequate breathing.

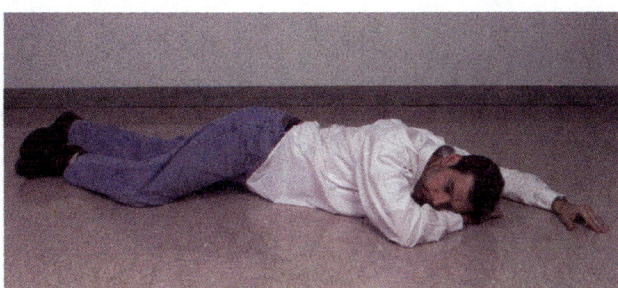

FIGURE 51-18 If the victim is breathing but not conscious, place him in the recovery position.

EARLY DEFIBRILLATION

Public access to defibrillation has proven to be highly successful. Defibrillation is a method of treatment that uses an electric shock to reverse disorganized activity in the heart during cardiac arrest. Early defibrillation has proven to be critical to survival in a victim with cardiac arrest. Defibrillators are placed in various locations in the community and are used by trained rescuers in the event of cardiac arrest. Some studies have shown that the chance of survival doubles when early access to defibrillation is available. The speed with which defibrillation is performed is the key to success. Early defibrillation (within 5 minutes) is a high-priority goal in the community. In health care facilities, the goal is to defibrillate within 3 minutes.

Automatic external defibrillators (AEDs) are computerized devices that are simple to learn and operate. The AED is used *only* when a patient is unresponsive, not breathing, and pulseless. When the device is attached to the victim's

chest, the unit determines if an electrical shock is necessary to reestablish or regulate the heartbeat. Several different models are available, and the operating instructions are slightly different for each. The four basic steps to using the AED are:

1. Turn the power to the unit on.
2. Apply the electrode pads to the patient's chest.
3. All rescuers stand back to allow the machine to analyze the heart rhythm.
4. All rescuers continue to stand back; the operator of the unit presses the shock button and/or follows the unit's instructions, which are usually audible through a voice-synthesized message.

Hospitals normally use manual, portable defibrillators for caring for patients who are in cardiac arrest. These defibrillators are operated by qualified, licensed personnel. The AED is not routinely used in the hospital. However, hospitals with large campuses and some large hospitals have purchased AED units for public areas, such as the lobby and cafeteria. If your facility purchases an AED, employees will be trained in its use. Although the AED is simple to operate, only those who are properly trained may use it. CPR and use of the AED are included in basic life support classes for health care professionals.

CHOKING

A person chokes when the throat is occluded (closed up or blocked) and air cannot get into the airway. In this situation, you must take quick, decisive action. (Refer to Procedures 157 and 158.)

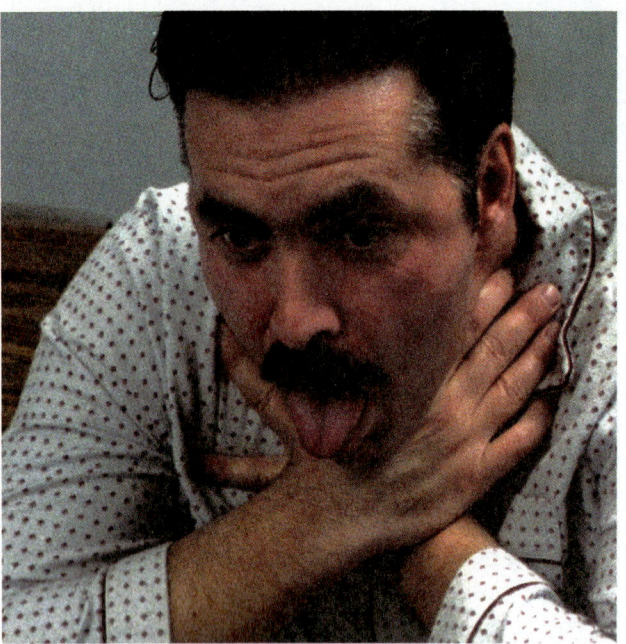

FIGURE 51-19 The universal distress signal for choking is one or both hands at and around the throat.

- The airway can be blocked by accumulation in the back of the throat of:
  - Any foreign body
  - Blood
  - Food
  - Vomitus
- Tilting the head back can sometimes clear the airway, because positioning in this way pulls the tongue forward.
- If the person can speak and is coughing vigorously, do not intervene. Coughing is the most effective way to dislodge materials from the airway. Stay close by and encourage coughing.
- A complete blockage is signaled by the person being unable to speak, high-pitched sounds on inhalation, and grasping the throat in the universal distress signal (Figure 51-19).
- Apply standard precautions, if possible, when assisting a patient who is choking. This involves using gloves and a special mask or face shield during rescue breathing. Know where this equipment is kept and follow your facility policies for use of this equipment in an emergency.

PROCEDURE 157

HEIMLICH MANEUVER—ABDOMINAL THRUSTS

1. Ask the person if she is choking.

2. If the person starts to cough, wait.

3. If the person cannot speak, cough, or breathe, but is conscious, apply subdiaphragmatic abdominal thrusts (**Heimlich maneuver**) until the foreign body is expelled.

   a. Stand behind the victim and wrap your arms around the victim's waist.

   b. Clench your fist, keeping the thumb straight (Figure 51-20A).

   c. Place your fist, thumb side in, against the victim's abdomen slightly above the navel and below the tip of the xiphoid process.

   d. Grasp your clenched fist with your opposite hand (Figure 51-20B).

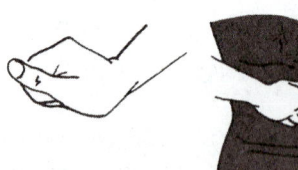

FIGURE 51-20A
Clench your fist, keeping the thumb straight.

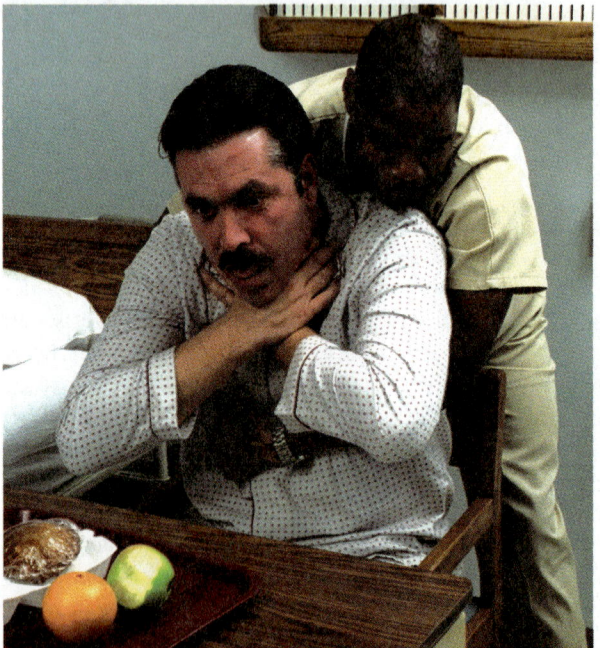

FIGURE 51-20B Grasp the clenched fist with your opposite hand. Avoid pressing against the ribs with your forearms.

continues

PROCEDURE 157

continued

e. Avoid pressing on the patient's ribs with your forearms. This could cause serious injury to the internal structures, including the liver.

f. Thrust forcefully with the thumb side of your fist against the midline of the victim's abdomen, slightly above his navel, inward and upward (Figure 51-20C). Keep your elbows bent and extended away from your

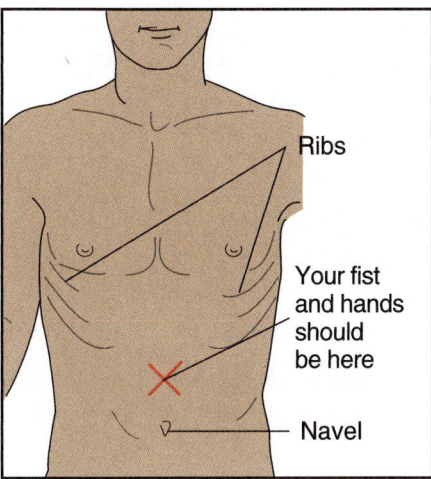

Ribs

Your fist and hands should be here

Navel

FIGURE 51-20C Thrust forcefully, inward and upward with the thumb side of your fist just above the navel.

body. You do not want to "hug" the victim because the thrust will not be as effective. Be sure you are below the tip of the sternum (xiphoid process).

4. Keep thrusting if the object is not dislodged. If the person begins to cough forcefully, wait.

5. Activate the EMS system.

6. Continue the Heimlich maneuver until the obstruction is expelled or the victim becomes unconscious. If the victim becomes unconscious, place the victim in supine position. Proceed with Procedure 158.

Alternative Action: Chest thrusts are used when pressure to the abdomen would be harmful or impossible. Chest thrusts are used if the choking person is in late pregnancy or if the victim is so large you are unable to get your arms around him. Follow steps 1 and 2, then stand behind the victim, place arms directly under the victim's armpits, and around the victim's chest. Place the thumb side of your fist in the middle of the breastbone (avoid ribs and xiphoid process). Grab your fist with your other hand and perform thrusts until the foreign body is expelled or the victim becomes unconscious.

PROCEDURE 158

ASSISTING THE ADULT WHO HAS AN OBSTRUCTED AIRWAY AND BECOMES UNCONSCIOUS

1. Activate the EMS system.

2. Apply gloves.

3. Turn the victim on his back.

4. To remove a foreign object from the airway, follow these steps:

   a. With the victim's face up, grasp the tongue and jaw between your thumb and fingers.

   b. Pull upward, opening the mouth and drawing the jaw forward.

   c. Insert the index finger of your other hand down along in inside of one cheek, toward the base of the tongue.

   d. Bend your finger and sweep in from the side with a hooking motion. Do not poke straight in, because that may push the object further down. Use the hooking action, across toward the other cheek, to loosen and remove the object.

   e. Try to bring the foreign object up into the mouth if you can see it.

continues

PROCEDURE 158

continued

    f. Be careful not to force the object deeper into the throat.

    g. If the object can be brought into the mouth, remove it.

5. If the victim is not breathing, give 1 slow breath through a pocket mask or barrier device. If the air does not go in, reposition the victim's head and try again. If the air still does not go in, begin with 5 abdominal thrusts.

6. Straddle the victim's thighs (Figure 51-21) and administer 5 abdominal thrusts, as follows:

    a. Place the heel of one hand on the victim's abdomen slightly above the navel. Your hand

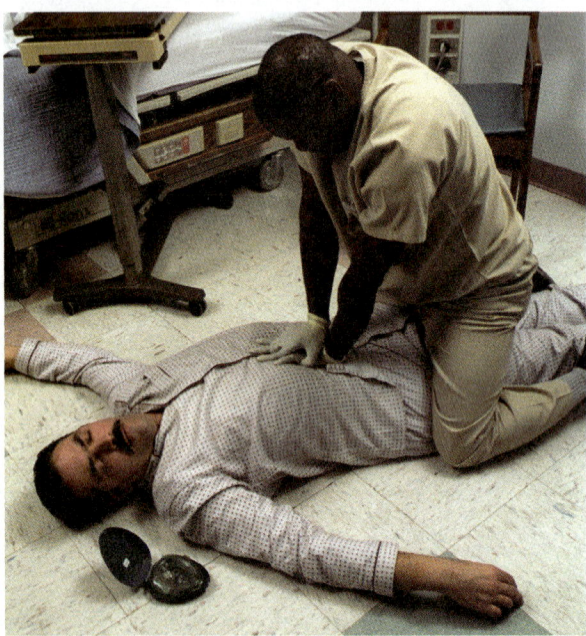

FIGURE 51-21 Straddle the thighs, position your hands, and deliver 5 inward, upward thrusts.

should be flat with the fingers pointing toward the victim's head.

    b. Place your other hand in a similar position over the first.

    c. Keep your elbows straight, with your shoulders directly over the victim's abdomen. Press inward and upward with 5 quick thrusts. Keep your hands centered on the victim's abdomen.

7. If the obstruction is not relieved, continue to repeat the procedure until the obstruction is relieved or more advanced health care professionals arrive:

    a. Tongue-jaw lift

    b. Finger sweep

    c. Attempt to ventilate

    d. If the last breath is ineffective, reposition the head and attempt to ventilate again.

    e. 5 abdominal thrusts

8. If the obstruction is removed, keep the airway open and check to make sure the patient is breathing.

    a. If breathing, position the victim in the recovery position.

    b. If not breathing, give 2 slow breaths.

    c. Check the pulse. If the pulse is absent, begin CPR.

    d. If the pulse is present, continue rescue breathing once every 4 to 5 seconds.

Note: *A victim who is given mouth-to-mouth breathing or abdominal thrusts may vomit. Roll a victim who vomits away from you onto one side and clean out the mouth with your fingers. Then roll the victim back and continue the procedure.*

CPR AND OBSTRUCTED AIRWAY PROCEDURES FOR INFANTS

The following procedures for infants (Procedures 159 to 161) and children (Procedures 162 and 163) are only guidelines for CPR and emergency treatment of an obstructed airway. An *infant* is a baby from birth to approximately 1 year of age. A *newly born* infant (newborn) is from the time of birth to approximately 1 month of age. You *must*

successfully complete an approved course before you perform these procedures.

CPR AND OBSTRUCTED AIRWAY PROCEDURES FOR CHILDREN

A child is considered to be between 1 and 8 years of age. If the child is more than 8 years old, adult CPR and obstructed airway procedures are used.

PROCEDURE 159

CPR FOR INFANTS

Note differences between CPR on infants and adults:

- The ratio is 1 rescue breath (ventilation) to 3 compressions in a newly born infant. It is 1 breath to every 5 compressions in an infant up to 1 year of age.

- The ratio of compressions to ventilations is 3:1 in a *newly born* or premature infant in the hospital. It is 5 compressions to 1 ventilation in other infants. The rate is 100 compressions a minute. Remember, this is the *speed* of the compressions, and not the *actual number* of compressions delivered.

- Breaths are given with the rescuer's mouth covering the infant's nose *and* mouth.

- Breaths must be *gentle*.

- Circulation is assessed by taking the brachial pulse rather than the carotid pulse.

- To find the landmark in an infant, draw an imaginary line through the nipples. The landmark is approximately one finger's width below this line, in the lower half of the chest. Do not press on the xiphoid process.

- If there are two rescuers, the preferred hand placement for chest compressions in an infant is to encircle the chest and back with the hands, then compress downward with the thumbs. If you are alone or size does not permit encircling the chest, use the tips of your second and third fingers to apply compressions.

- The depth of compressions is approximately one-third of the depth of the child's body. Compressions should be deep enough to produce a palpable pulse during compression.

- Compressions should be smooth and rhythmic.

- Reevaluate for the return of a pulse every 30 seconds. Continue compressions until the infant can sustain a heart rate of more than 60 beats per minute.

1. Determine unresponsiveness by tapping the shoulder (Figure 51-22A).

2. Call out for help. If a second rescuer is present, have him activate the EMS system.

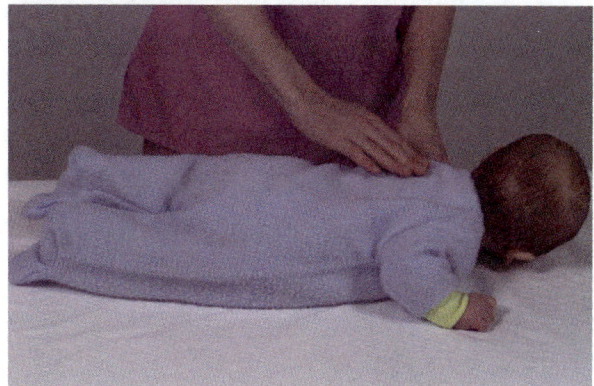

FIGURE 51-22A Determine unresponsiveness by tapping the shoulder.

3. Support the infant's head and shoulders and place the infant on his back on a firm surface.

4. Use the head-tilt, chin-lift technique to open the airway. Be careful not to tilt the head back too far (Figure 51-22B).

5. Maintain an open airway and place your head in position over the infant's chest to look, listen, and feel for breathing (Figure 51-22C). If the infant is breathing and there are no signs of trauma, place the infant in recovery position.

6. If the infant is not breathing, maintain an open airway and give 2 slow breaths with your mouth completely covering the infant's nose and mouth. The breaths must be gentle because of an infant's

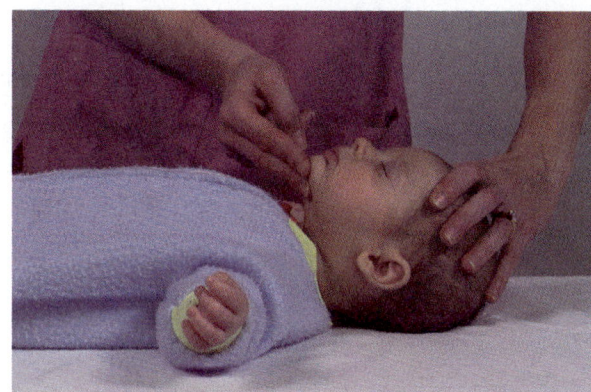

FIGURE 51-22B Open the airway with the head-tilt, chin-lift maneuver. Avoid tipping the head back too far.

continues

PROCEDURE 159

continued

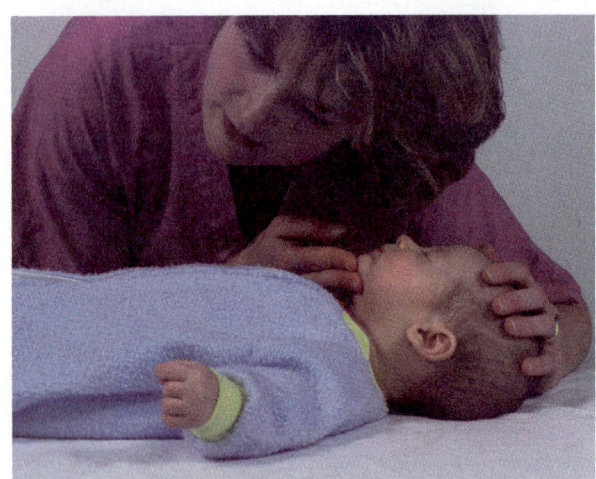

FIGURE 51-22C Look, listen, and feel for breathing.

small size. If the breaths do not cause the chest to rise, reposition the head and attempt to ventilate again.

7. Assess for signs of circulation, such as coughing, movement, and color. Determine lack of pulse by feeling for the brachial pulse with two fingers, while maintaining an open airway (Figure 51-22D).

8. If there is no pulse, begin chest compressions:
   - Draw an imaginary line between the nipples.
   - If there are two rescuers, encircle the chest with your hands. Use your fingertips to support the

back. Position your thumbs one finger-width below the imaginary line in the middle of the sternum. If this is not possible, or if you are alone, place your index finger below the imaginary line in the middle of the chest. Place your middle and ring fingers next to the index finger. Use these fingers to compress the sternum at that point (Figure 51-22E). *Do not compress over the xiphoid process.*
   - Compress the sternum about ½ to 1 inch at a rate of 100 times per minute.
   - Give 1 rescue breath for every 5 compressions.

9. Do 20 cycles of compressions and rescue breaths.

10. Check the brachial pulse.

11. If you are alone, activate the EMS system now.

12. If there is no pulse, continue rescue breaths and compressions.

13. Check for a pulse every 30 seconds. If the pulse returns, check for breathing. If there is no breathing, give 1 rescue breath every 3 seconds (20 breaths per minute). Monitor the pulse. If breathing is present, place the infant in the recovery position and maintain an open airway. Monitor breathing and pulse.

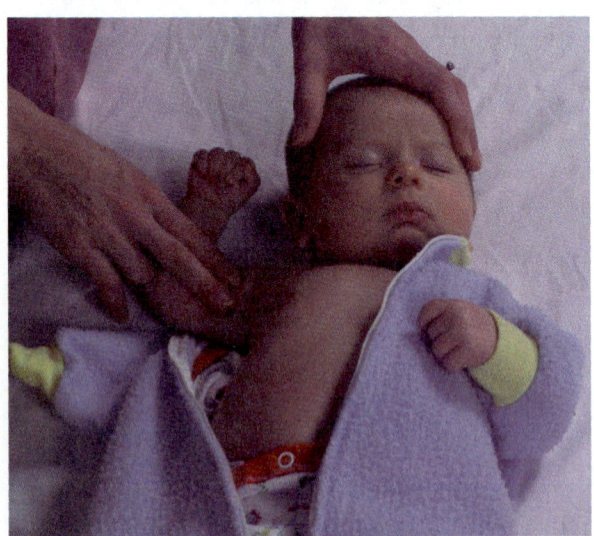

FIGURE 51-22D Check the brachial pulse.

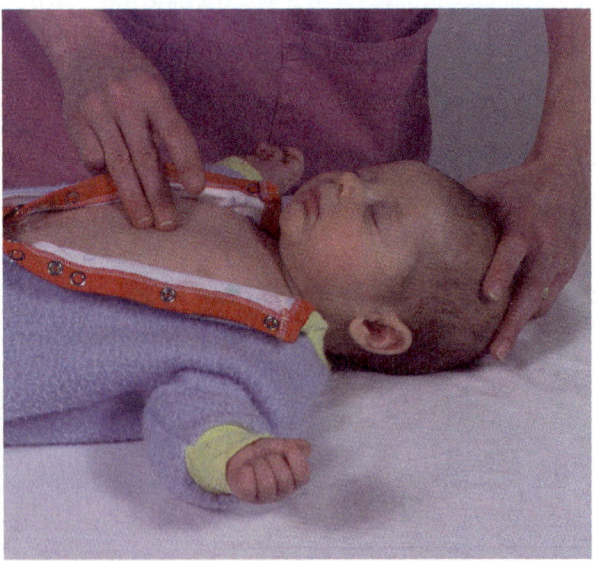

FIGURE 51-22E Compress the sternum with two or three fingers.

PROCEDURE 160

OBSTRUCTED AIRWAY: CONSCIOUS INFANT

Perform this procedure only if the airway of the conscious infant is completely obstructed and someone has witnessed or strongly suspects that there is a foreign body obstruction. If the infant cannot breathe because of an infection, the infant should be rushed to the nearest life support facility. Procedures to clear the airway *should not be performed*. Allow the infant with respiratory distress to find and maintain the most comfortable position.

1. Determine whether there is airway obstruction by observing breathing difficulties, weak or absent cry, or ineffective cough.

2. Supporting the infant's head and neck with one hand, position the infant face down with head lower than trunk, over one arm (support your arm on your thigh) and deliver up to 5 back blows (Figure 51-23A).

3. Supporting the infant on your arm, turn the infant face up and deliver up to 5 chest thrusts in the midsternal region (using landmarks for positioning as for chest compressions) (Figure 51-23B). Do chest thrusts more slowly than chest compressions at a rate of 1 per second.

4. Repeat steps 2 and 3 until the foreign body is expelled or the infant becomes unconscious.

If the Infant Becomes Unconscious

5. Call out for help. If someone responds, have that person call the EMS system. Place the infant on his back.

6. Perform a tongue-jaw lift. Do not perform a blind finger sweep, but remove the foreign body if you can see it.

7. Open the airway with the head-tilt, chin-lift method and try to give rescue breaths.

8. Reposition the infant's head and try again to give rescue breaths.

9. Deliver up to 5 back blows.

10. Deliver up to 5 chest thrusts.

11. Perform a tongue-jaw lift and remove the foreign body if you can see it.

12. Maintain an open airway with the head-tilt, chin-lift method and try again to give rescue breaths.

13. Repeat steps 8 through 12 until successful.

14. If you are alone and your efforts are unsuccessful, activate the EMS system after trying to clear the airway for about one minute.

15. When the obstruction is removed, check for breathing. If there is no breathing, give rescue breaths. If there is no pulse, give 2 breaths and start cycles of compressions and rescue breaths. If a pulse is present, open the airway with the head-tilt, chin-lift manuever and check for breathing. If there is breathing, place the infant in the recovery position. Monitor breathing and pulse while maintaining an open airway. If the infant is not breathing, give 1 rescue breath every 3 seconds (20 breaths per minute). Monitor pulse.

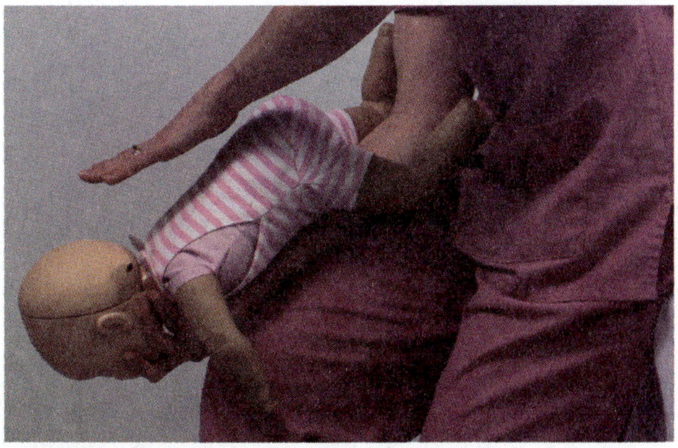

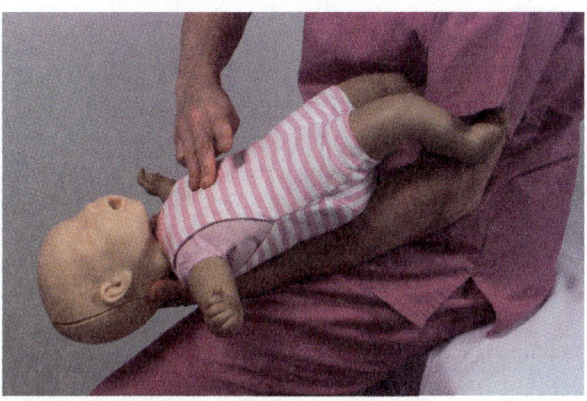

FIGURE 51-23A Position the infant face down, with face lower than trunk. Deliver up to 5 back blows.

FIGURE 51-23B Turn the infant face up and deliver up to 5 chest thrusts.

PROCEDURE 161

OBSTRUCTED AIRWAY: UNCONSCIOUS INFANT

1. Determine unresponsiveness as directed in Procedure 160.

2. Call out for help.

3. Support the head and neck and turn the infant on her back on a firm, hard surface.

4. Use the head-tilt, chin-lift method to open the airway. Do not tilt the head too far back.

5. Determine lack of breathing by maintaining an open airway and looking, listening, and feeling for breathing.

6. Try to give rescue breaths by placing your mouth over the infant's nose and mouth.

7. Reposition the head, check your mouth seal, and try again to give rescue breaths.

8. Activate the EMS system. If someone else is available, have that person make the call.

9. Deliver up to 5 back blows.

10. Deliver up to 5 chest thrusts.

11. Do a tongue-jaw lift and remove the foreign body if you can see it. If you do not see the object, do not perform blind finger sweeps.

12. Try to do rescue breaths again.

13. Repeat steps 9 through 12 until successful.

14. If you are alone and your efforts are unsuccessful, activate the EMS system after about one minute of effort.

15. Check for pulse and respirations when the obstruction is removed.

16. If the infant is breathing, place the infant in the recovery position. Maintain an open airway and monitor pulse and breathing. If there is no breathing, give 20 rescue breaths per minute and monitor the pulse.

17. If there is no pulse, give 2 rescue breaths and start cycles of compressions and breaths. If there is a pulse, open the airway and check for breathing.

PROCEDURE 162

CPR FOR CHILDREN, ONE RESCUER

1. Establish unresponsiveness by tapping the shoulder and calling the child's name.

2. If another person is available, have that person activate the EMS system. If another person is not present, give one minute of rescue support and then activate the EMS system.

3. Use the head-tilt, chin-lift method or jaw-thrust method to open the airway. Check for breathing by looking, listening, and feeling. If the child is breathing or begins breathing, place the child in the recovery position.

4. If there is no breathing, give 2 slow breaths, taking 1 to 1½ seconds per breath. Pause briefly

after the first breath to take a deep breath, then deliver the second breath. Observe the child's chest for rising. Allow the chest to deflate between breaths.

5. Assess for signs of circulation, such as coughing, movement, and color. Assess for heartbeat by taking the carotid pulse. If pulse is present but there is no breathing, do rescue breathing of 1 breath every 3 seconds (20 breaths per minute).

6. If there is no pulse, locate the landmark by using the imaginary line between the nipples. Put the heel of one hand on the chest one finger-width below this line. Give 5 chest compressions (at

continues

PROCEDURE 162

continued

a rate of 100 compressions per minute). The compression depth is approximately one-half the depth of the child's chest, or 1 to 1½ inches. Keep the heel of your hand in contact with the chest and avoid bounding. Make sure you are directly on the sternum, not on the ribs or xiphoid

process. Open the airway and provide 1 slow breath. Repeat the cycle.

7. After about one minute of rescue support, check pulse. If there is no pulse, continue the cycle of 5 compressions to 1 breath.

PROCEDURE 163

CHILD WITH FOREIGN BODY AIRWAY OBSTRUCTION

Conscious Child

1. Ask "Are you choking?"

2. Give abdominal thrusts, using the same hand placement as you would for an adult, slightly above the navel and well below the xiphoid process. Do not rest your forearms on the ribcage, as this can cause injury.

3. Repeat thrusts until the foreign body is removed or the victim becomes unconscious.

If the Child Becomes Unconscious

4. If another person is present, have that person activate the EMS system.

5. Perform a tongue-jaw lift. If you see the foreign body, perform a finger sweep to remove it. If you do not see the object, do not perform blind finger sweeps.

6. Open the airway and try to do rescue breathing. If still obstructed, reposition the child's head and try to do rescue breathing again.

7. Straddle the child's hips and give up to 5 inward, upward abdominal thrusts.

8. Repeat steps 5 through 7 until effective. If the child is breathing or begins breathing, place the child in the recovery position.

9. If the airway obstruction is not relieved after about one minute, activate the EMS system.

Unconscious Child

1. Establish unresponsiveness. If another person is present, have that person activate the EMS system.

2. Open the airway and try to ventilate. If unsuccessful, reposition the child's head and try ventilations again.

3. Give up to 5 abdominal thrusts.

4. Perform a tongue-jaw lift. Remove the foreign body only if you can see it.

5. Repeat steps 2 to 4 until effective. If the child is breathing or resumes breathing, place the child in the recovery position.

6. If the airway obstruction is not relieved after about one minute, activate the EMS system.

OTHER EMERGENCIES

For some of the emergencies described here, a patient at home or in a long-term care facility may need to be transported to a hospital emergency room. Be sure, if the patient is at home, that you know:

- Initial emergency actions to perform

- How and when to notify the EMS system
- How and when to notify your supervisor
- How, when, and which family members to notify in the event of emergency

If the patient is in a long-term care facility, know the initial emergency actions to perform and the procedure to follow for emergencies.

guidelines *for*

Non-Cardiac Facility Emergencies

- Anticipate and prevent emergencies whenever possible. Think safety and evaluate the patient and environment for potential safety hazards when you enter the room and again when you leave the room.

- If you discover a patient who is ill or injured, stay with the patient and call for help. Your facility will teach you the procedure for getting help. Some facilities instruct employees to call out. Others instruct you to pull the call signal or bathroom emergency signal. Some instruct you to use the telephone in the patient's room.

- Know facility procedures, phone numbers, and names for various code situations for reporting emergencies and completing incident reports.

- Do not move patients who have fallen to the floor unless they are in immediate danger. Movement may worsen an injury. The nurse will check the patient and give permission for the move.

- Stay calm and do not panic. Reassure the patient.

- Start emergency measures that you are trained to do while you are waiting for help to arrive.

- Do not give the patient anything to eat or drink.

- Know the location of emergency equipment and supplies on your unit. You may be instructed to get emergency supplies.

- Many emergencies involve bleeding. Remember that the potential for contact with blood, body fluid, secretions (except sweat), excretions, mucous membranes, and nonintact skin exists. Always remember and apply the principles of standard precautions. Carry extra gloves in your pockets if you are working in an area where they are not immediately available. Know where personal protective equipment is kept.

- Once the nurse arrives, do as he or she directs.

BLEEDING

Remember that if the person is conscious, the extent of injuries is likely to be far less severe than if the person is unconscious. With the unconscious person, the next imminent threat to life is the loss of blood. Apply gloves and follow standard precautions if you see or suspect that the patient is bleeding. Bleeding is usually easy to see. Sometimes, however, the bleeding is internal. Internal bleeding will only be shown by the signs of shock (described in the next section). Examine the person for evidence of bleeding. Take the following steps to prevent additional loss:

SAFETY *Alert*

Do not be distracted by copious bleeding in an unconscious patient. Always check the adequacy of the patient's airway first. If airway, breathing, and circulation are adequate, quickly apply gloves and take measures to stop the bleeding.

- Identify the area that is bleeding.
- Have the victim apply continuous pressure over the bleeding area, if able.
- If the victim is not able, apply continuous, direct pressure over the bleeding area with a pad and your gloved hand, if necessary (Figure 51-24).
- Call for help.
- If seepage occurs, increase the padding and pressure.
- If there are no broken bones and there is no pain, raise the wounded area above the level of the heart, but do not release pressure. This will help to reduce bleeding.
- Support the elevated area.
- Use binding of some kind to hold the padded pressure if there is bleeding from more than one area.
- If you have learned the location of the major blood vessels that control blood flow to an area, and direct pressure seems ineffective, apply pressure over the appropriate pulse point to control **hemorrhage** (heavy bleeding) (Figure 51-25).
- Keep the person comfortably warm and quiet until help arrives.

Note: Persons who are bleeding are often very frightened. Their anxiety contributes to the development of shock. Continuous reassurance is essential.

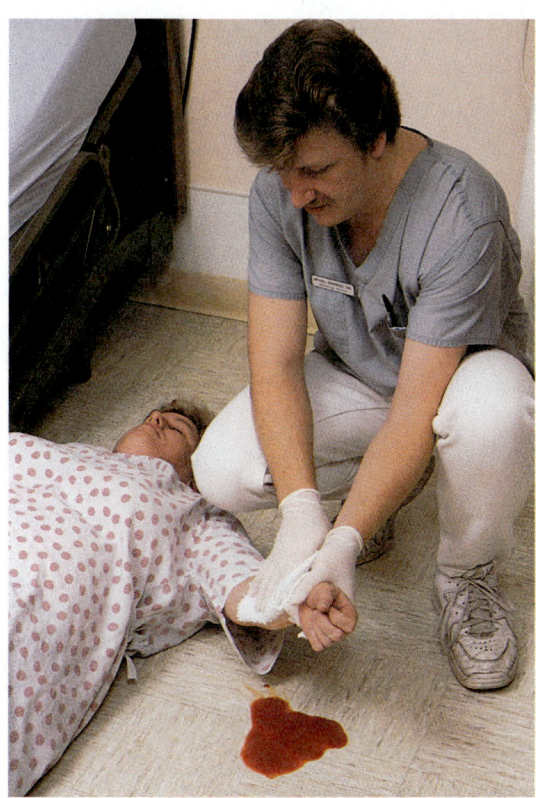

FIGURE 51-24 Apply firm hand pressure over the bleeding area with a pad and your gloved hand.

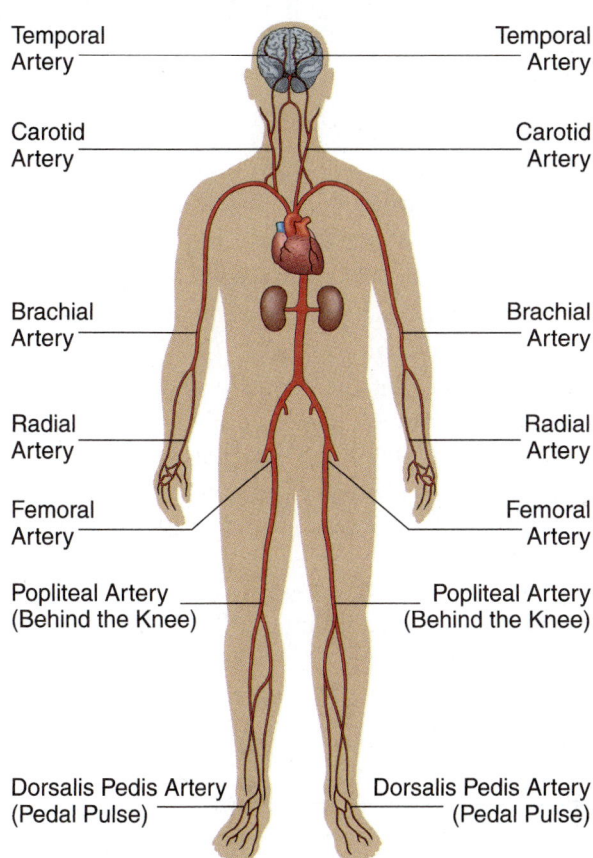

Temporal Artery

Carotid Artery

Brachial Artery

Radial Artery

Femoral Artery

Popliteal Artery (Behind the Knee)

Dorsalis Pedis Artery (Pedal Pulse)

Temporal Artery

Carotid Artery

Brachial Artery

Radial Artery

Femoral Artery

Popliteal Artery (Behind the Knee)

Dorsalis Pedis Artery (Pedal Pulse)

FIGURE 51-25 Pressure is applied at pulse points.

SHOCK

Shock is defined as a disturbance of the oxygen supply to the tissues and return of blood to the heart. It can follow:

- Any severe injury
- Cardiac arrest
- Acute hemorrhage
- Severe pain
- Excessive loss of body fluids (as in severe burns)
- Serious infection

Signs and Symptoms of Shock

Early signs and symptoms include:

- Pale, cold skin that is moist to the touch
- Complaints of weakness
- Weak, rapid pulse
- Rapid and irregular breathing
- Restlessness and anxiety
- Perspiration

Later signs of shock include:

- Mottled skin
- Lack of response
- Sunken eyes with pupils that are dilated, and vacant expression
- Loss of consciousness
- Drop in body temperature
- Low blood pressure

Preventive Measures

Anxiety aggravates the situation, but shock can be prevented if steps are taken early. Prevention of shock includes controlling situations that could trigger it.

- Call for help—activate the emergency medical system.
- Keep the person lying down and quiet.
- Maintain normal body temperature. Provide light warmth if needed.
- Position person with the feet and legs slightly higher than body and head (Trendelenburg position), unless contraindicated by specific injury. This ensures improved circulation to vital organs.
  - Burned areas should be elevated unless it causes the person pain.
  - If fractures are involved, make sure the part is splinted (braced) before positioning the person, to prevent shock.
- The patient may complain of thirst. Do not give her anything to eat or drink.
- Intravenous fluids to improve circulatory volume and low volumes of oxygen will be given.

- This equipment will be available in a care facility.
- In the community, the emergency personnel answering the call will bring the supplies necessary to manage fluid and oxygenation.
- Continue to monitor pulse and respirations.

Unless shock is controlled, death can occur. Until help arrives, your care can often make the difference between life and death.

FAINTING

When the blood supply to the brain is reduced for a short time, the person loses consciousness. This is called fainting. Fainting is usually a temporary condition. It is corrected as soon as blood flow to the brain is restored.

Unfortunately, when consciousness is lost, the person is likely to fall and injuries can occur. Patients who are ambulating for the first time should be assisted. If fainting occurs and the patient falls, do not try to hold the patient upright. Ease the patient to the floor to prevent injury. Assist patients who are *feeling* faint to a safe position.

The patient who is sitting and feels faint, light-headed, dizzy, and nauseated should be encouraged to lower her head between her knees. Pallor, cold skin, perspiration, or visual changes also signal fainting. To provide assistance to a fainting person, the nursing assistant should:

- Help the patient to assume a protected position, sitting or lying down
- Loosen tight clothing
- Position head lower than heart to encourage cerebral blood flow
- Allow person to rest for at least 10 minutes
- Maintain normal body temperature
- Call for additional help
- Monitor pulse and respirations
- Do not give the patient anything to eat or drink

HEART ATTACK

Heart attacks can occur in any age group, but the high-risk group includes those who:

- Are overweight
- Smoke
- Have atherosclerosis
- Remain immobile for long periods
- Are older
- Have diabetes
- Have a history of heart disease

Signs and Symptoms

Signs and symptoms of heart attack include:

- Crushing pain that can radiate up the jaw and down the arm, or heaviness in chest

- Perspiring, skin cold and clammy
- Nausea and vomiting
- Pale to grayish color of the face
- Difficulty breathing or absence of breathing
- Loss of consciousness
- Irregular pulse or loss of pulse (the loss of heart function is called cardiac arrest)

At other times, the pain of the attack may resemble indigestion and the person remains conscious. Do not be fooled into thinking that the degree of pain indicates the severity of the attack. Both victims need immediate attention.

Action

In the health care facility:

- Immediately signal for help.
- Stay with the patient if the patient is conscious.
- Have the patient stop any activity and assume a comfortable position.
- Help keep the patient calm.
- Elevate the head of the bed to assist breathing.
- Provide oxygen, if available.

If the patient is unconscious:

- Check for breathing and heartbeat.
- If necessary, institute CPR (if you have been trained) until a professional takes charge.

In the community, and if the person is conscious, proceed as follows.

1. Evaluate the situation.
2. Activate the EMS.
3. Allow the person to sit up or assume a comfortable position. Loosen clothing about the neck.
4. Keep onlookers away.
5. Provide fresh air but keep the person comfortably warm.
6. Monitor pulse and respirations.
7. Be prepared to initiate CPR.

In the community, if the person is unconscious, follow steps 1 and 2. Then:

3. Check for breathing and heartbeat.
4. If heartbeat is present but breathing has ceased, establish an open airway and institute mask-to-mouth resuscitation.
5. If breathing and heartbeat have ceased (cardiac and respiratory arrest), institute CPR until a professional takes charge.

BRAIN ATTACK

A brain attack (cerebral vascular accident or CVA), also called a *stroke*, occurs when there is interference with normal blood circulation to the brain. It usually is caused by a clot that has lodged in a cerebral vessel or by a blood vessel that has ruptured.

Signs and Symptoms

The person with a severe brain attack usually:

- Experiences seizure activity
- Loses consciousness
- Experiences difficulty breathing
- Develops paralysis on one side of the body and of the muscles on either side of the face
- Has unequal pupil reaction

The patient with a less severe brain attack may experience:

- Disorientation
- Dizziness
- Headache
- Slurred speech
- Memory loss
- Loss of consciousness

Action

First aid includes:

- Maintaining an airway
- Providing mask-to-mouth breathing as needed
- Administering CPR, if needed (by a trained, qualified individual)
- Positioning the victim on one side so fluids will drain from the mouth
- Maintaining normal body temperature
- Keeping the person quiet until help arrives or transportation to a medical facility can be arranged

SEIZURES

Seizures or convulsions are sometimes seen when there is:

- Drug overdose
- Head injury
- Degenerative brain disease
- Stroke
- Infectious disease and fevers
- Tumors
- Hypoglycemic reactions
- Seizure disorder. Seizure disorder now is largely controlled with medication, but unusual stress, missed medication doses, and other factors can cause a convulsion

Signs and Symptoms

Seizures do not always follow the same pattern. Their range may be:

- A momentary loss of contact with the environment (absence seizure, or *petit mal*), in which there are no random or uncontrolled movements but the person seems to stare blankly.

- A generalized tonic-clonic seizure, or *grand mal* form in which:
  - consciousness is lost.
  - the person falls.
  - the person becomes rigid.
  - uncontrolled voluntary movements occur.
  - frothing at the mouth occurs.
  - the person becomes cyanotic.
  - the person loses control of bladder and/or bowel function.

Gradually the seizure lessens and the person recovers. The person is usually:

- Confused
- Disoriented for a period of time
- Very tired

Action

If you witness a seizure, take the following steps:

- Wear gloves and apply standard precautions, because there is a high probability of contact with blood and body fluids when caring for a patient with a seizure.
- Do not restrain the person's movements.
- Protect the person from injury. For example, move any objects that might break or cause bruising.
- Loosen clothing around the neck.
- Maintain an airway by positioning. Do not try to put anything in the mouth.
- Cradle the person's head.
- Observe the seizure.

After seizure activity stops:

- Turn the person to the side so fluid or vomitus can drain freely after the movements subside.
- Give mask-to-mouth resuscitation if breathing is not resumed following the seizure.
- Allow the person to rest undisturbed.
- Stay with the person but summon medical assistance.
- Report and record seizure activity: time, length of seizure, body parts or activity involved.

VOMITING AND ASPIRATION

Food and air are both taken into the body through the mouth. The passageway in which food and air enter is shared. The ability to swallow is made less efficient by some diseases and by aging. Occasionally food, water, vomitus, or other objects accidentally go down the trachea and into the lungs. This is called *aspiration*, and can occur when a patient is vomiting, bleeding, eating, or drinking. Thick secretions from the mouth may also enter the lungs. Aspiration can cause serious complications.

Signs and Symptoms

Signs and symptoms of aspiration include:

- Coughing
- Choking on food or liquid
- Cyanosis
- Vomiting, especially when lying flat in the supine position
- Inability to swallow
- Inability to spit out vomitus, blood, or secretions from the mouth

Action

If a patient has aspirated anything:

- Stay with the patient and call for help.
- Use standard precautions and select personal protective equipment appropriate to the procedure.
- Do not give the patient any liquids.
- Keep the patient's head elevated if allowed.
- Turn the patient's body to the side if he or she is vomiting while lying down. If turning the patient's body is not possible, turn the head to the side.
- Provide an emesis basin if the patient is vomiting.
- If the patient begins choking and an airway obstruction occurs, follow the procedure for clearing the obstructed airway.
- After the episode, assist the patient with mouth care.

Make observations as possible and report to the nurse:

- Observe any vomitus for color, odor, presence of undigested food, blood, or coffee-ground appearance (coffee-ground appearance suggests blood in the stomach). Save the emesis for the nurse to inspect.
- Measure or estimate the amount of vomitus or blood, and record on the intake and output record.

ELECTRIC SHOCK

Electric shock can occur in the:

- community, when high-tension wires are knocked down in accidents or storms, or when electrical appliances are misused or malfunction.
- health facility, because of frayed wires and faulty outlets or fixtures.

Severe burns and cardiac and respiratory arrest can result from electric shock. You must protect yourself as you try to rescue the victim.

Action

- Turn off the electricity at the terminal source, such as at a fuse box, before touching the victim, if possible.

OSHA Alert

Evaluate the environment carefully. Make sure you are in a safe zone before approaching the patient, away from sources of electricity and water.

- If the source of electricity cannot be controlled, try to move the victim away with some nonconductive material. Dry wood (a broom handle, for example) is a good nonconductor.
- Once free of the electrical source, check the victim for breathing and pulse.
- Summon medical help.
- Administer CPR, if necessary.
- Once breathing and heart function are restored, check for burns and other injury. Keep the person lying down and comfortable.
- Give first aid for burns or other injuries.

BURNS

Burns result in loss of skin integrity. They may be caused by heat, chemicals, or radiation. There is a high risk of infection with any burn. Burns are classified as partial thickness or full thickness, depending on the degree of injury. Partial thickness burns are:

- First-degree burns—involve only the top layer (epidermis) of skin. There is redness, temporary swelling, and pain. There is usually no permanent scarring. This burn looks like a sunburn. The skin is not broken or blistered.
- Second-degree burns—involve both epidermis and dermis. The skin color may vary from pink or red to white or tan. Blistering, pain, and some scarring occur.

Full thickness burns are:

- Third-degree burns—involve epidermis, dermis, and subcutaneous tissue. The tissue is bright red to tan and brown. There may be no pain initially because nerve endings have been destroyed. Later, pain and scarring will result.

Emergency Treatment for Burns

1. Call the nurse immediately.
2. If the patient's clothing is on fire, use a coat or blanket to smother the flames.

3. Cool water may be applied to lower skin temperature and to stop further tissue damage. Remove wet clothing (follow nurse's instructions).

4. Third-degree burns usually require extensive treatment.

ORTHOPEDIC INJURIES

Orthopedic injuries include injuries to bones, joints, muscles, and ligaments.

- A **fracture** is a break in a bone.
- A **sprain** is an injury to a ligament caused by sudden overstretching. A sprained ankle may occur, for example, if a person falls and turns the ankle quickly while falling. Swelling may be noted shortly afterward.
- A **strain** is excessive stretching of a muscle that results in pain and swelling of the muscle. You may strain the muscles in your back if you use incorrect lifting and moving techniques.
- A **dislocation** occurs in a joint, when one bone is displaced from another bone. This can occur in a paralyzed arm that is allowed to hang without support. The weight of the arm pulls the upper arm bone out of position in the shoulder joint. A dislocation can also be caused by improperly lifting a patient under the arms.

Treatment for Orthopedic Injuries

If you suspect a patient has suffered a fracture:

- Stay with the patient.
- Do not attempt to move the patient.
- Call the nurse immediately.
- If the patient is on the floor and a fracture is suspected, the nurse will instruct you to put the patient to bed after the nursing assessment. Have plenty of help available. One staff member should be responsible for immobilizing and moving the fractured extremity while others move the rest of the body. Roll the patient onto a sheet, blanket, or backboard and then lift him into bed. This is less traumatic for the patient and reduces the risk of worsening the injury.
- Monitor the patient's vital signs as instructed. Report changes to the nurse.

If a fracture is suspected, x-rays will be taken of the injury. If a fracture is present, the physician will put a cast on the affected extremity, place the patient in traction, or do surgery.

If you suspect that a patient has suffered a sprain, strain, or dislocation, notify the nurse at once. You may be instructed to:

- elevate the injured extremity.
- apply ice packs to the area.
- after 24 hours, you may be instructed to apply warm packs to the area.

HEAD INJURY

A patient with a known or suspected head injury always requires close observation and monitoring. Bleeding inside the skull commonly occurs when the head strikes a broad, hard object, such as the floor, causing internal bleeding. Some serious complications of head injuries may not be apparent until 72 hours after a head injury. This is particularly true in the elderly. As people age, the brain shrinks slightly. This does not affect the patient mentally. The space between the brain and the skull allows extra room for swelling and bleeding. Signs and symptoms of an acute bleeding problem may not be apparent for several days until the problem progresses to a point where it increases pressure on the brain. It can take up to six weeks before the patient shows symptoms from a very tiny "bleed." This is usually long after the original injury has been forgotten.

Signs and Symptoms

Signs and symptoms of a possible head injury include:

- Change in the patient's level of alertness or consciousness
- Change in orientation (ability to recognize time, place, person)
- Memory loss
- Unequal pupils
- Visual disturbances
- Blood or clear fluid leaking from ears or nose
- Change in ability to speak or make self understood
- Change in ability to follow directions
- No response to verbal stimulation
- Weakness of arms or legs, difficulty maintaining balance
- Headache
- Nausea and/or vomiting

Remember that signs and symptoms of a problem may not occur for several days.

Action

If you think a patient has suffered a head injury:

- Stay with the patient and call for help.
- Monitor pulse and respirations while waiting for the nurse to arrive.
- Keep the environment quiet and calm.
- Do not give the patient anything to drink.
- Reassure and orient the patient.
- Elevate the head on a pillow.
- Do not move the patient if he is on the floor.
- Monitor vital signs regularly after the injury, as instructed.

ACCIDENTAL POISONING

Immediate attention is needed if a patient is the victim of accidental poisoning. All potentially harmful substances must be kept in locked cupboards. If you suspect that a poisoning has happened:

- Call the nurse immediately.

- Try to determine what the patient has taken and save the container.
- The nurse may administer a substance that will cause vomiting. (Not all substances can be safely removed from the patient's body by vomiting.)
- Know where to find the telephone number for the regional poison control center.

REVIEW

A. True/False.

Mark the following true or false by circling T or F.

1. T F You need no special training to give CPR.

2. T F CPR is needed if breathing and circulation fail.

3. T F The Heimlich maneuver is used to stop bleeding.

4. T F The person in shock should be kept quiet and lying down.

5. T F When controlling bleeding, the bleeding part should be elevated.

6. T F Vomiting should be induced for anyone who has swallowed a poisonous substance.

7. T F Immediate treatment for burns may include applying cold water to lower skin temperature.

8. T F A dislocation occurs when one bone is displaced from another bone.

9. T F For orthopedic injuries, immediate treatment includes the application of warm packs.

10. T F Third-degree burns only involve the epidermis.

B. Matching.

Choose the correct term from Column II to match each phrase in Column I.

Column I	Column II
11. ____ person needing first aid	**a.** arrest
	b. first aid
12. ____ excessive bleeding	**c.** victim
13. ____ care given when victim has no breathing or heartbeat	**d.** CPR
	e. contraindicated
14. ____ signaled by a drop in blood pressure	**f.** hemorrhage
	g. splintered
15. ____ emergency care	**h.** shock

C. Multiple Choice.

Select the one best answer for each of the following.

16. An organization that offers instruction in CPR is the
- **a.** American Diabetes Association.
- **b.** American Association of Nurses.
- **c.** Association for Resuscitation.
- **d.** American Heart Association.

17. First aid is care given
- **a.** for nausea and vomiting.
- **b.** only upon a physician's order.
- **c.** if medical help is delayed.
- **d.** for cough, cold, or sore throat.

18. Which of the following is a life-threatening situation requiring intervention? A person who
- **a.** broke a finger.
- **b.** fell and bruised a knee.
- **c.** is in shock.
- **d.** is coughing.

19. The first step you should take when arriving on the scene of an accident is to
- **a.** stop a passerby.
- **b.** evaluate the situation.
- **c.** move the victims to one side.
- **d.** help the victims get up and walk.

20. To assist a person who has fainted,
- **a.** help the person to stand up and walk to circulate the blood.
- **b.** cover the person with several blankets.
- **c.** loosen tight clothing.
- **d.** position the person's head higher than the heart.

21. To assist the person who is experiencing a seizure, you should
- **a.** keep the person as active as possible.
- **b.** restrain the person's movements.
- **c.** keep the head straight.
- **d.** maintain an airway and protect the person from injury.

22. You suspect that a patient is in shock because the
    a. blood pressure is elevated.
    b. face is flushed.
    c. skin is cold and clammy.
    d. pulse is full and bounding.

23. The overstretching of a ligament can result in a
    a. fracture.
    b. sprain.
    c. strain.
    d. dislocation.

24. For one-person CPR, the ratio of chest compressions to ventilations is
    a. 15 compressions to 2 ventilations.
    b. 5 compressions to 1 ventilation.
    c. 5 compressions to 2 ventilations.
    d. 15 compressions to 1 ventilation.

25. If a victim of cardiac arrest resumes breathing but is unconscious, you should place the victim
    a. in recovery position.
    b. on his back.
    c. on his abdomen.
    d. in a chair.

26. The first action to take when an adult is choking and is conscious is to tell the person what you are going to do and then
    a. slap the person on the back.
    b. give abdominal thrusts.
    c. begin artificial respirations.
    d. begin chest compressions.

27. The first priority in an emergency is
    a. airway.
    b. bleeding.
    c. circulation.
    d. level of consciousness.

28. When a person suffers cardiac arrest,
    a. the heart has stopped beating.
    b. the respirations are less than 12 per minute.
    c. biological death has occurred.
    d. unconsciousness occurs in about 4 minutes.

29. In the health care facility, you would initiate CPR for cardiac arrest unless
    a. the patient has a DNR order.
    b. you think the patient would not want to be revived.
    c. the patient is very old.
    d. the death is unexpected.

30. If you are working in a patient's home and CPR is initiated, you must
    a. call the EMS system yourself if you are alone.
    b. drive the patient to the closest hospital.
    c. do CPR for 20 minutes and if the patient does not respond, call the EMS system.
    d. go next door to have the neighbor call the EMS system.

31. CPR on an infant is always done with a ratio of
    a. 1 ventilation to 5 compressions.
    b. 5 ventilations to 1 compression.
    c. 15 ventilations to 1 compression.
    d. 15 compressions to 2 ventilations.

32. The procedure to clear an obstructed airway on a conscious infant is to position the infant and
    a. deliver 5 abdominal thrusts followed by 5 back blows.
    b. deliver 5 back blows followed by 5 chest thrusts.
    c. perform a blind finger sweep.
    d. perform 2 ventilations followed by 5 compressions.

33. When performing CPR on a child, the procedure is
    a. done as it is on an adult.
    b. done as it is on an infant.
    c. done with a ratio of 1 ventilation to 5 chest compressions.
    d. done with a ratio of 2 ventilations to 15 chest compressions.

34. During CPR on a child, the pulse is checked by taking the
    a. carotid pulse.
    b. brachial pulse.
    c. radial pulse.
    d. femoral pulse.

35. The preferred treatment for external bleeding is to
    a. apply continuous, direct pressure.
    b. apply a tourniquet.
    c. apply pressure to pulse points.
    d. apply a heat pack.

D. Nursing Assistant Challenge.

You and a friend are driving home from work. A car immediately ahead of you goes through a stop sign and is hit on the passenger side by a car going through the intersection. You and your friend park your car to see if your help is needed in this emergency. The people in the other car are conscious, alert, and deny having any injuries. The passenger in the car that ran the stop sign is unconscious and begins to vomit. You see blood coming from the person's right arm. The driver is conscious but dazed and seems to be disoriented. List, in sequence, the actions you would take.

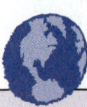 # EXPLORING THE WEB

Description	Location
ACLS.net	*http://www.acls.net*
American Association of Critical Care Nurses	*http://www.aacn.org*
American Heart Association	*http://www.americanheart.org*
Combined Health Information Database	*http://chid.nih.gov/subfile/subfile.html*
Emergency Nurses Organization	*http://www.ena.org*
Learn CPR	*http://depts.washington.edu*
MediSmart Online Emergency Tutorials	*http://medi-smart.com/tutorials.htm*
Neonatal Resuscitation Program	*http://www.aap.org*
New York Emergency Room RN	*http://www.nyerrn.com*

Moving Forward

UNIT 52

Employment Opportunities and
Career Growth

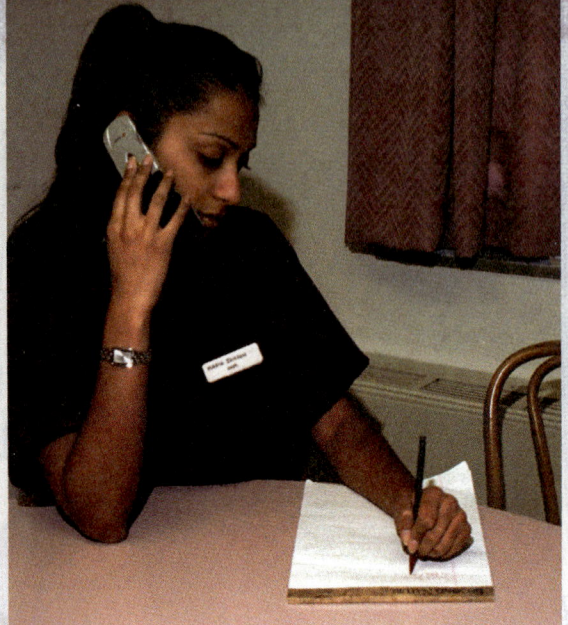

Employment Opportunities and Career Growth

objectives

After completing this unit, you will be able to:

- Spell and define terms.
- List nine objectives to be met in obtaining and maintaining employment.
- Follow a process for self-appraisal.
- Name sources of employment for nursing assistants.
- Prepare a résumé and a letter of resignation.
- List the steps for a successful interview.
- List the requirements that must be met when accepting employment.
- List steps for continuing development in your career.

vocabulary

Learn the meaning and the correct spelling of the following words and phrases:

job interview	networking	reference	résumé

INTRODUCTION

Having completed a nursing assistant program, you are now ready to look for employment. You will want to be as successful as an employee as you were as a student. If you meet the objectives presented in this unit, the task will be made much easier.

Searching for and obtaining a job requires several steps:

- Completing a self-appraisal
- Searching for employment opportunities
- Assembling a résumé
- Validating your references
- Making specific applications for work
- Participating in interviews
- Deciding whether to take the job

OBJECTIVE 1: SELF-APPRAISAL

The first objective is to determine your personal assets and limitations that could influence your choice of employment. To do this:

- Divide a piece of paper into three columns.
- Title one column *assets*, one *limitations*, and one *solutions*.
- Review all the positive contributions you can make in an employment situation and list them. For example:
  - Your preference in the care of certain patients
  - Your caring attitude
  - Special skill you have with particular patients
  - Your personal appearance
- Honestly review all the limitations that might make certain employment less obtainable. For example, consider:
  - Home responsibilities
  - Specific hours you can work
  - Transportation problems
  - Physical limitations
- Think of possible solutions so that you reduce the number of limitations. The fewer limitations you have at the beginning of your job search, the more you expand the possibilities for employment.

Make your lists, review them, and add to them over several days.

OBJECTIVE 2: SEARCH FOR ALL EMPLOYMENT OPPORTUNITIES

Having thought through your assets and limitations and found as many solutions to the limitations as possible, you are ready to search for employment. Possible sources for the search process are all the agencies or facilities that employ nursing assistants:

- Physicians' offices
- Blood banks
- Clinics
- Hospices
- Homes for aged or disabled, assisted living, or personal care facilities
- Long-term care facilities
- Hospitals
- Home health care agencies
- Rehabilitation centers
- Telephone directory—select facilities that meet your specific needs for available transportation or specific type of care
- Classified ads found in the newspaper
  - Look for facilities in your area.
  - Consider the type of work you are willing to do.
  - Consider the shifts that have openings.
  - Note the person to contact for an interview or additional information.
- Facility in which you received your clinical experience
  - Administrators sometimes offer jobs to new nursing assistants who trained in their facility.
  - Job openings may be posted on the employee bulletin board.
- Friends and colleagues
  - Friends may know of job openings.
  - Colleagues may put you in touch with others who have potential job connections (Figure 52-1).
  - A current term for these activities is **networking**.

Finding employment is a full-time job. You must wake up early and set a time to begin looking for work. It may be helpful to list the steps involved in looking for a job, and preparations you need to make, such as ironing a shirt, finding a babysitter, and preparing a résumé. Apply for jobs early in the day. This makes a good impression and gives you enough time to fill out applications, take tests, or have interviews. Applying at several facilities in the same area will help you organize your time and save time and travel.

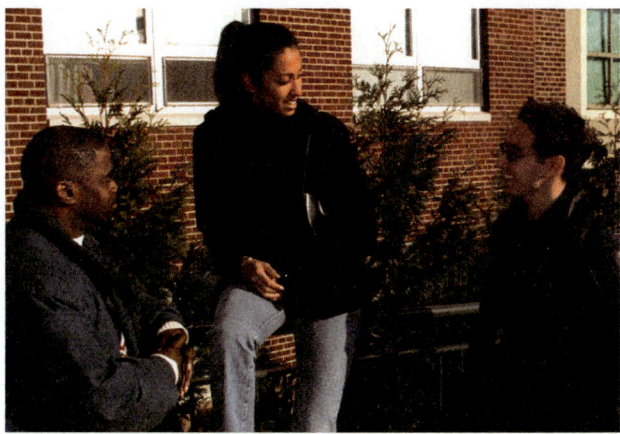

FIGURE 52-1 Friends and classmates are valuable sources of information about potential jobs.

Follow up on all job leads right away. If you hear of a job opening late in the day, call and schedule an appointment for the next day.

OBJECTIVE 3: ASSEMBLE A PROPER RÉSUMÉ

A résumé is a written summary of work and educational history. You should:

- Prepare several copies
- Always keep a copy for yourself
- Type the résumé for a neat appearance
- Carry a copy whenever you seek employment
- Use the résumé as a ready reference when you fill out forms
- Update the résumé regularly

The résumé should be carefully prepared to include:

- Your name, address, and telephone number
- Your educational background
  - List your most recent education first.
  - Give dates.
  - Include a brief summary of the content.
- Your work history over the last five years, especially if it gives evidence of successful experiences in the same or related areas as the job for which you are applying
- Proof of being on the State Nurse Aide Registry
- List of any continuing education classes you have attended
- Other experiences you have had; include jobs that show initiative, reliability, trustworthiness, and worthwhile ways you have spent your time
- References—a list of three people who know you and can verify your abilities
- Some personal information that indicates your interests and activities

It is not necessary to include the following in your résumé, although some of this information may be shared during the interview:

- Age
- Marital status
- Religion
- Sex
- Height
- Weight

OBJECTIVE 4: VALIDATE REFERENCES

References are people who know you and who would be willing to comment, either in writing or verbally over the telephone, about you and your abilities. Be sure to include accurate titles, names, addresses, and telephone numbers when listing references.

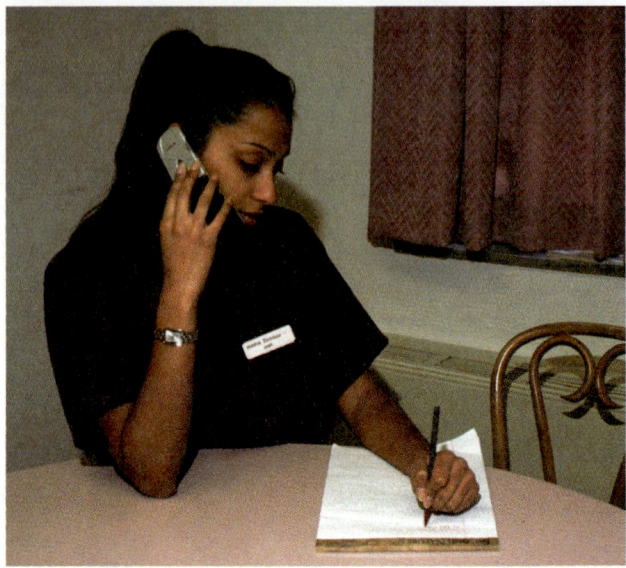

FIGURE 52-2   Get permission before using names for references.

Anyone you use as a reference:

- should give you permission to use their names (Figure 52-2).
- should know you well enough to make an honest evaluation.
- should not be related to you.
- may need to have their memories refreshed about dates of employment or experiences you have stated in your résumé.

OBJECTIVE 5: MAKE SPECIFIC APPLICATIONS FOR WORK

Handle this part of the job search process in a businesslike way:

- Select three facilities that interest you most.
- Call and ask for the director of nursing or personnel department.
- Tell the person who answers that you are interested in learning if there are any openings for a nursing assistant, and if so, what application procedure is to be followed.
- Be prepared to answer questions about your preparation and experience. Have your résumé in your hand.
- Make an appointment for an interview, if possible. A job interview is an opportunity for the person applying for a job and the employer's representative to learn about each other. Each person has the opportunity to ask questions to determine if the job seeker has qualifications that match the needs of the job available.
- Fill out an application form (Figure 52-3). Use your résumé to be sure you complete the form. Read the

EMPLOYMENT APPLICATION
(PLEASE TYPE OR PRINT IN INK)

CHARTER SUBURBAN HOSPITAL
16453 South Colorado Avenue
Paramount, California 90723

PERSONAL DATA

LAST NAME	FIRST		TELEPHONE ( )	DATE

ADDRESS	STREET	CITY	STATE	ZIP	HOW LONG?

PREVIOUS ADDRESS	STREET	CITY	STATE	ZIP	HOW LONG?

OTHER NAMES UNDER WHICH YOU HAVE WORKED	HOW WERE YOU REFERRED TO US FOR EMPLOYMENT?

POSITION DESIRED:

1ST CHOICE: 2ND CHOICE:

DATE YOU CAN START:

SHIFT YOU CAN WORK:

☐ DAYS ☐ P.M.s ☐ NIGHTS ☐ WEEKENDS

ARE YOU APPYING FOR: ☐ FULL-TIME ☐ PART-TIME

☐ ON CALL/FLOAT ☐ TEMPORARY

SOCIAL SECURITY NUMBER | DO YOU HAVE THE LEGAL RIGHT TO WORK IN THIS COUNTRY? ☐ YES ☐ NO

ARE YOU UNDER 18 YEARS OLD? ☐ YES ☐ NO

LIST FRIENDS & RELATIVES (STATE RELATIONSHIP) EMPLOYED BY THIS HOSPITAL

TRANSPORTATION AVAILABLE? ☐ YES ☐ NO

HAVE YOU EVER BEEN CONVICTED OF A FELONY? IF YES, DESCRIBE THE CIRCUMSTANCES:
(A FELONY CONVICTION WILL NOT AUTOMATICALLY DISQUALIFY YOU FOR EMPLOYMENT) _____

EDUCATION

	NAME AND LOCATION	CIRCLE LAST YEAR COMPLETED	DATE LAST ATTENDED	MAJOR FIELD OF STUDY	DIPLOMA OR DEGREE RECEIVED
HIGH SCHOOL		1 2 3 4			
COLLEGE OR UNIVERSITY		1 2 3 4			
PROFESSIONAL TRAINING		YEARS ATTENDED			
GRADUATE SCHOOL					
OTHER					

OFFICE SKILLS (CLERICAL APPLICANTS ONLY)

☐ TYPING_____ WPM
☐ SHORTHAND/SPEEDWRITING _____ WPM
☐ 10 KEY ADDING MACHINE

☐ DICTAPHONE
☐ KEYPUNCH
☐ PBX

☐ MEDICAL TERMINOLOGY
☐ OTHER_____

PROFESSIONAL LICENSURE

TYPE	LICENSE NUMBER	STATE	EXPIRATION DATE

AP1018

FIGURE 52-3 Complete the application form neatly, correctly, and completely. *(Courtesy of Charter Suburban Hospital)*

directions on the application carefully. Fill out all information. If something on the application does not apply, put N/A (not applicable) in the space rather than leaving it blank. List all your previous employers, even if they were health care providers. If you skip an employer, it looks as if you are hiding something.

EMPLOYMENT (LIST MOST RECENT FIRST)

MAY WE CONTACT PRESENT EMPLOYER? ☐ YES ☐ NO

FROM MO YR	TO MO YR	EMPLOYER'S NAME	POSITIONS & DUTIES	PRESENT OR LAST SALARY	REASON FOR LEAVING
		STREET ADDRESS CITY STATE			
		PHONE NO. ( )	SUPERVISOR'S NAME & TITLE		

FROM MO YR	TO MO YR	EMPLOYER'S NAME			
		STREET ADDRESS CITY STATE			
		PHONE NO. ( )	SUPERVISOR'S NAME & TITLE		

FROM MO YR	TO MO YR	EMPLOYER'S NAME			
		STREET ADDRESS CITY STATE			
		PHONE NO. ( )	SUPERVISOR'S NAME & TITLE		

FROM MO YR	TO MO YR	EMPLOYER'S NAME			
		STREET ADDRESS CITY STATE			
		PHONE NO. ( )	SUPERVISOR'S NAME & TITLE		

FROM MO YR	TO MO YR	EMPLOYER'S NAME			
		STREET ADDRESS CITY STATE			
		PHONE NO. ( )	SUPERVISOR'S NAME & TITLE		

DO YOU HAVE A MEDICAL/PHYSICAL CONDITION WHICH COULD LIMIT YOUR JOB PERFORMANCE?

☐ YES ☐ NO, IF "YES", PLEASE EXPLAIN: _____

_____

_____

I CERTIFY THAT ALL STATEMENTS MADE ON THIS APPLICATION ARE TRUE AND THAT ANY MISSTATEMENTS MAY BE CAUSE FOR TERMINATION OR DENIAL OF EMPLOYMENT WITH CHARTER SUBURBAN HOSPITAL. PERMISSION IS GRANTED TO INVESTIGATE AND VERIFY EMPLOYMENT AND EDUCATION. I UNDERSTAND THAT EMPLOYMENT WITH CHARTER SUBURBAN HOSPITAL IS CONTINGENT UPON PASSING AN ANNUAL HEALTH ASSESSMENT THEREAFTER.
CHARTER SUBURBAN HOSPITAL IS AN EQUAL OPPORTUNITY EMPLOYER.

_____   _____
SIGNATURE   DATE

FIGURE 52-3 *continued*

Complete the application in its entirety. Do not write "see résumé." Although you may attach your résumé to the application, there are legal reasons why you must complete the application. Make sure the information is accurate, spelled correctly, complete, and neat. Use a pen to complete the application. The application represents you on paper. A messy application sends a negative message.

- Learn the names of the persons to whom you speak.
- Thank the person speaking with you by name.

Repeat the steps until you land the job.

OBJECTIVE 6: PARTICIPATE IN A SUCCESSFUL INTERVIEW

After you have investigated job leads and completed applications, an employer may contact you to schedule an interview. You will be given a date and time to meet. The interview is very important. Most hiring decisions are made during the interview. How you present yourself in the interview is as important as your training, experience, and ability to do the job.

Approach the interview in three steps.

Preparation.
- Plan what you will wear.
- Do not overdress, but be neat and clean.
- Check your clothes for loose or lost buttons or stains.
- Be sure to take a bath and use deodorant.
- Brush your teeth.
- Make sure your fingernails are short and clean.
- Polish your shoes.
- Make sure your hair is neat.
- If you have a beard or a mustache, be sure it is trimmed.
- Do not chew gum.
- Prepare a list of questions you want to ask.
- Have your résumé in hand.

Actual Interview. Be prepared when going to an interview. Bring pens and pencils, papers, a map, reference information, and your résumé with you. You will also need a photo identification, such as a driver's license, and your Social Security card. If you have completed a CNA program, bring a copy of your certificate and state certification. Go to the interview alone. Arrange for babysitters and transportation ahead of time. It is a good idea to arrive a little early so you can complete paperwork, if requested.

- Offer a firm handshake.
- Stand until you are invited to sit.
- Remember that you are "selling" yourself.
- Be careful of body language.
- Make good eye contact with the interviewer. Your eyes should send a message such as, "I like you."
- Listen carefully to the interview questions and be sure you understand them before you answer. If you do not understand, ask for clarification. Your answers to questions should reflect your positive features.
- Share information willingly with the interviewer.

- Use your list to learn information important to you such as:
  - Responsibilities (ask for a job description)
  - Hours of work
  - Dress code
  - Opportunities for future assistance or financial aid to further your education
  - Starting salary
  - Fringe benefits such as health insurance
  - Schedule of raises

At the end of the interview, thank the interviewer, whether you are hired or not. Leave a copy of your résumé for future reference.

After the Interview. When you get home:
- Write a short thank-you note to the person who interviewed you, thanking her for her time and the opportunity to be considered for the job.
- Review the interview in your mind. Plan changes you would make to improve future interviews.

OBJECTIVE 7: ACCEPT A JOB

Before accepting a job, think carefully about your employer's expectations of your abilities and job performance. If you accept the job, you must be prepared to follow the policies and procedures of the facility. For example, if the interviewer told you that nursing assistants are scheduled to work every other weekend, do not take the job unless you are willing to do this. There are certain specific requirements you will have to complete as you begin your job, as we discuss in this section.

Orientation

Orientation is designed to help you safely perform the duties listed in your job description. It is mandatory and all new employees are required to attend. Keep in mind that

LEGAL *Alert*

To work in the United States, you must complete an I-9 form, which proves your legal eligibility to work. To do this, you must provide a copy of your Social Security card and a picture identification. The employer may make a copy of these documents. He or she will also have to sign the form to verify that the facility has verified your identity and work eligibility.

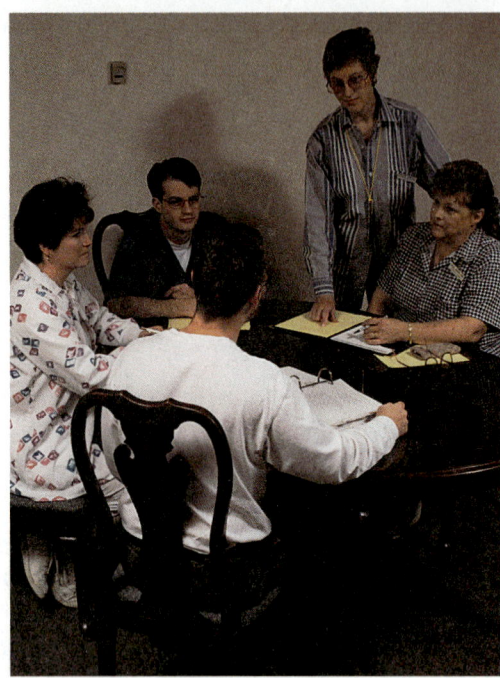

FIGURE 52-4 Orientation is an important part of your employment.

even if you were hired to work an evening or night shift, orientation classes may be held during the day. Orientation generally consists of two parts. You will spend at least a day in the classroom learning about the policies and procedures of the employer (Figure 52-4). You will be given employee handbooks that you can refer to in the future. Information presented during the class may include:

- Policies for scheduling and making assignments
- What to do during fire and other emergencies
- How and when performance evaluations are completed
- The organizational chart of the facility
- Safety policies and procedures

A clinical orientation is provided on the nursing unit. An instructor, another nurse, or an experienced competent nursing assistant will work with you the first few days so that you may learn

- The routine of the unit
- The location of equipment and supplies
- How to do specific procedures as required by the employer

Health and Safety Requirements

State and federal regulations require new employees to:

- Obtain a physical examination within a specified number of days (some employers will require this before you begin work).
- Receive a two-step Mantoux (tuberculosis) test within a specified number of days (this too may be required before you begin work).

- Indicate whether they wish to receive the hepatitis B vaccine. Health care employers are required by law to offer this vaccination without cost to direct-care employees. It is the employee's choice whether to take the vaccine. If the employee refuses it at the time of orientation, it can be given at another time if the employee changes her mind.

Some employers require employees to wear back supports while working. These are generally issued to you by the employer.

Health Care Worker Background Check

Some states require that a criminal background check be performed on all health care workers. If you work in one of these states, the procedure should be explained to you during the interview.

Drug Testing

Many employers require that drug testing be performed before you begin work. This procedure too should be explained during the interview.

LEGAL *Alert*

Drug testing is usually done by means of a urine sample. Some prescription drugs, foods, and vitamins may interfere with the urine test results. You will be asked to list prescription and nonprescription medications you are taking. Be honest, and list everything. Collection of the urine specimen is generally monitored to prevent tampering. Some agencies check the temperature of the urine immediately after the specimen is obtained, as a further safeguard. Some facilities will not allow you to take personal items into the bathroom when providing the specimen. Access to water may also be limited, because it is possible to dilute a sample. Some facilities seal the container with tamper-evident tape, which is signed by both the employee and the nurse who assists with specimen collection. Your employer may also have a policy requiring random drug testing if you are involved in a work-related injury, or any time use of illicit substances is suspected.

Uniform Requirements

Most health care employers have dress codes that indicate:

- Color and style of uniform to be worn on duty
- Acceptable jewelry that can be worn with the uniform
- Type of shoes and stockings that are safe to wear
- Acceptable hairstyles and makeup (including whether nail polish is permitted)

Remember that these policies are for purposes of safety and infection control. Some employers will issue the uniforms to you either at no charge or for a charge that is deducted from your paycheck over a period of time.

OBJECTIVE 8: KEEP THE JOB

You can make your new position secure if you:

- Arrive on time prepared to work. Good attendance is very important. Be at work when you are scheduled and avoid calling off unless you are ill. If you will be unable to work your next scheduled shift, notify your facility as far in advance as possible so they can find a replacement.
- Follow the policies and procedures outlined in your orientation.
- Follow the rules of ethical and legal conduct.
- Recognize your limitations and seek help.
- Have an open and positive attitude.

OBJECTIVE 9: CONTINUE TO GROW THROUGHOUT YOUR CAREER

You will continue to grow if you take advantage of each new experience and opportunity you find.

- Keep your certificate current.
- Seek out knowledgeable staff members and watch and learn by their example.
- Do not be afraid to ask questions at appropriate times.
- Use the nursing medical literature to learn more about the patients' conditions.
- Participate in care conferences with an open mind so that each conference can be a learning experience for you.
- Complete 12 hours of continuing education each year (Figure 52-5), or follow the requirements in your state.
- Investigate the possibilities of advancing your formal education by:
  - Enrolling in general education courses offered at the high school or college in your area.
  - Taking courses in communication, listening, English, and psychology.

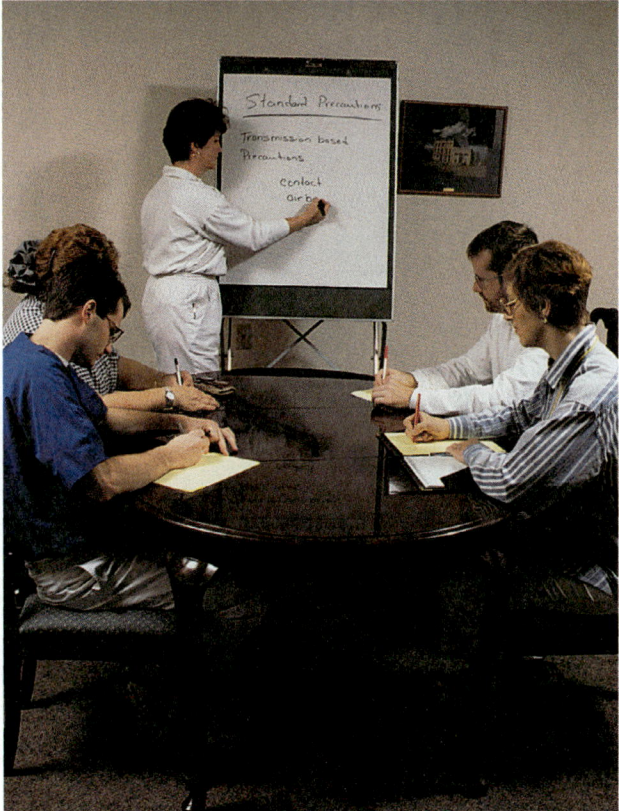

FIGURE 52-5 Take advantage of staff development programs to further your knowledge.

  - Participating in in-service education programs at your facility or at nearby hospitals.
  - Enrolling in minicourses offered by hospitals on subjects of general public interest, such as hypertension, weight control, and diabetes.
  - Selecting books at the library that pertain to health issues.
  - Researching programs that can prepare you for professional advancement into the ranks of LVN or RN.

Career Ladders

Many facilities have career ladders available for nursing assistants. The career ladder enables the assistant to progress to a higher position within the organization, such as a restorative assistant. One professional nursing organization has developed the End-of-Life Nursing Education Consortium (ELNEC) Project, which enables direct caregivers, including nursing assistants, to achieve advanced status in providing end-of-life care. Additional education is usually required to move up the career ladder. Completing specialized certificate programs is an excellent way to advance in your career. Explore the possibilities within your facility. Community and junior colleges in your area may also have classes available.

OBJECTIVE 10: RESIGN PROPERLY FROM EMPLOYMENT

When you are ready to leave your present situation, you should do so pleasantly and properly.

- Give as much notice as possible—usually equal to the time of the pay period.
- Submit a letter of resignation and include:

– Date

– Salutation (greeting) to the director of nursing

– Brief explanation of your reasons for leaving

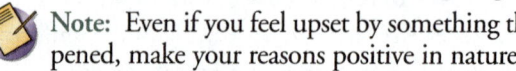 **Note:** Even if you feel upset by something that happened, make your reasons positive in nature.

– Date your resignation is to be effective

– Thank for the opportunity to have worked and grown with the experience of working in that facility

– Your signature

REVIEW

A. True/False.

Mark the following true or false by circling T or F.

1. T F The employer may ask your religion during an interview.

2. T F In making a self-appraisal, you only need to list the things you could offer an employer.

3. T F What you wear to an interview is not important.

4. T F The availability of transportation should be considered when you are choosing a job.

5. T F The interview should provide you with information about the exact responsibilities you will have.

6. T F Checking for job possibilities with the administrator of the facility in which you had your clinical experience is proper.

7. T F If you fail to get the job after the interview, there is nothing left for you to do about the situation.

8. T F At the end of every interview, you should thank the interviewer, even if you did not get the job.

9. T F Participation in care conferences can be a way to continue to grow.

10. T F When resigning, give ample notice.

B. Multiple Choice.

Select the one best answer for each of the following.

11. The first step in finding a job is
  a. making phone calls.
  b. doing a self-assessment.
  c. looking in the paper.
  d. writing letters to friends.

12. A self-appraisal includes
  a. reading classified ads.
  b. networking with friends.
  c. caring for patients.
  d. listing assets, limitations, and solutions.

13. A compilation of your work history is called a/an
  a. résumé.
  b. interview.
  c. summary.
  d. application.

14. Which of the following would you include in your résumé?
  a. Marital status
  b. Religion
  c. Weight
  d. Address

15. Before putting a reference name down,
  a. ask permission.
  b. call the prospective employer.
  c. tell the person you are going to use his name.
  d. get the phone number and birth date.

C. Nursing Assistant Challenge.

You have made it! You have completed your course and are eagerly looking forward to employment. Answer these questions.

16. What information will you need to have when completing an application for employment?

17. What items do you need to have with you when you go for your interview?

18. How will you dress for the interview?

19. The interview comes to a close and the interviewer has not given you any information concerning wages and benefits. How would you handle this?

EXPLORING THE WEB

Description	Location
Career Nurse Assistant Program	*http://www.cna-network.org*
CNA Inservices (Frontline)	*http://www.frontlinepub.com*
Direct Care Alliance	*http://www.directcarealliance.org*
End-of Life Nursing Education Consortium (ELNEC) Project	*http://www.aacn.nche.edu*
Health Care Hiring	*http://www.healthcarehiring.com*
Institute for Caregiver Education	*http://www.innernet.net*
Job Ready Sample Assessment	*http://www.nocti.org*
Job Task Analysis	*http://www.co.stanislaus.ca.us*
Mature Professionals in the Workplace	*http://www.advancefornurses.com*
Med Careers	*http://www.medcareers.com*
Net Guide to Health Care and Medical Employment	*http://members.aol.com*
Nurse Aide State Registries	*http://www.cahf.org*
Paraprofessional Healthcare Institute	*http://www.paraprofessional.org*
Promissor	*http://www.promissor.com*
VisaScreen Credentials Assessment	*http://www.cgfns.org*

Guidelines for Hand Hygiene

INTRODUCTION

In 2002, the CDC published the results of extensive handwashing studies, as well as new recommendations for cleansing hands. Each recommendation is categorized on the basis of existing scientific data, theoretical rationale, applicability, and economic impact. The CDC system for categorizing recommendations is:

Category IA. Strongly recommended for implementation and strongly supported by well-designed experimental, clinical, or epidemiologic studies.

Category IB. Strongly recommended for implementation and supported by certain experimental, clinical, or epidemiologic studies and a strong theoretical rationale.

Category IC. Required for implementation, as mandated by federal or state regulation or standard.

Category II. Suggested for implementation and supported by suggestive clinical or epidemiologic studies or a theoretical rationale.

No recommendation. Unresolved issue; practices for which insufficient evidence or no consensus regarding efficacy exist.

RECOMMENDATIONS

1. Indications for handwashing and hand antisepsis
   - When hands are visibly dirty or contaminated with proteinaceous material, or are visibly soiled with blood or other body fluids, wash hands with either a non-antimicrobial soap and water or an antimicrobial soap and water (IA).
   - If hands are not visibly soiled, use an alcohol-based hand rub for routinely decontaminating hands in all other clinical situations described in items (IA).
   - Alternatively, wash hands with an antimicrobial soap and water in all clinical situations (IB).
   - Decontaminate hands before having direct contact with patients (IB).
   - Decontaminate hands before donning sterile gloves when inserting a central intravascular catheter (IB).
   - Decontaminate hands before inserting indwelling urinary catheters, peripheral vascular catheters, or other invasive devices that do not require a surgical procedure (IB).
   - Decontaminate hands after contact with a patient's intact skin (e.g., when taking a pulse or blood pressure, and lifting a patient) (IB).
   - Decontaminate hands after contact with body fluids or excretions, mucous membranes, nonintact skin, and wound dressings if hands are not visibly soiled (IA).
   - Decontaminate hands if moving from a contaminated-body site to a clean-body site during patient care (II).
   - Decontaminate hands after contact with inanimate objects (including medical equipment) in the immediate vicinity of the patient (II).
   - Decontaminate hands after removing gloves (IB).
   - Before eating and after using a restroom, wash hands with a non-antimicrobial soap and water or with an antimicrobial soap and water (IB).
   - Antimicrobial-impregnated wipes (i.e., towelettes) may be considered as an alternative to washing hands with non-antimicrobial soap and water. Because they are not as effective as alcohol-based hand rubs or washing hands with an antimicrobial soap and water for reducing bacterial counts on the hands of health care workers, they are not a substitute for using an alcohol-based hand rub or antimicrobial soap (IB).
   - Wash hands with non-antimicrobial soap and water or with antimicrobial soap and water if exposure to Bacillus anthracis is suspected or proven. The physical action of washing and rinsing hands under such circumstances is recommended because alcohols, chlorhexidine, iodophors, and other antiseptic agents have poor activity against spores (II).
   - No recommendation can be made regarding the routine use of nonalcohol-based hand rubs for hand hygiene in health-care settings. Unresolved issue.

2. Hand-hygiene technique
   - When decontaminating hands with an alcohol-based hand rub, apply product to palm of one hand and rub hands together, covering all surfaces of hands and fingers, until hands are dry (IB).
   - Follow the manufacturer's recommendations regarding the volume of product to use.
   - When washing hands with soap and water, wet hands first with water, apply an amount of product recommended by the manufacturer to hands, and rub hands together vigorously for at least 15 seconds, covering all surfaces of the hands and fingers. Rinse hands with water and dry thoroughly with a disposable towel. Use towel to turn off the faucet (IB).
   - Avoid using hot water, because repeated exposure to hot water may increase the risk of dermatitis (IB).
   - Liquid, bar, leaflet, or powdered forms of plain soap are acceptable when washing hands with a non-antimicrobial soap and water. When bar soap is used, soap racks that facilitate drainage and small bars of soap should be used (II).
   - Multiple-use cloth towels of the hanging or roll type are not recommended for use in health-care settings (II).

3. Surgical hand antisepsis
   - Remove rings, watches, and bracelets before beginning the surgical hand scrub (II).
   - Remove debris from underneath fingernails using a nail cleaner under running water (II).
   - Surgical hand antisepsis, using either an antimicrobial soap or an alcohol-based hand rub with persistent activity, is recommended before donning sterile gloves when performing surgical procedures (IB).
   - When performing surgical hand antisepsis using an antimicrobial soap, scrub hands and forearms for the length of time recommended by the manufacturer, usually 2–6 minutes. Long scrub times (e.g., 10 minutes) are not necessary (IB).
   - When using an alcohol-based surgical hand-scrub product with persistent activity, follow the manufacturer's instructions. Before applying the alcohol solution, prewash hands and forearms with a non-antimicrobial soap and dry hands and forearms completely. After application of the alcohol-based product as recommended, allow hands and forearms to dry thoroughly before donning sterile gloves (IB).
4. Other recommendations
   - Do not add soap to a partially empty soap dispenser. This practice of "topping off" dispensers can lead to bacterial contamination of soap (IA).

- Provide workers with hand lotions or creams to minimize the occurrence of irritant contact dermatitis associated with hand antisepsis or handwashing (IA).
- Do not wear artificial fingernails or extenders when having direct contact with patients at high risk (e.g., those in intensive care units or operating rooms) (IA).
- Keep natural nails tips less than ¼-inch long (II).
- Wear gloves when contact with blood or other potentially infectious materials, mucous membranes, and nonintact skin could occur (IC).
- Remove gloves after caring for a patient. Do not wear the same pair of gloves for the care of more than one patient, and do not wash gloves between uses with different patients (IB).
- Change gloves during patient care if moving from a contaminated body site to a clean body site (II).
- No recommendation can be made regarding wearing rings in health-care settings. Unresolved issue.
- Monitor workers' adherence to recommended hand-hygiene practices and provide personnel with information regarding their performance (IA).
- Encourage patients and their families to remind workers to decontaminate their hands (II).
- Store supplies of alcohol-based hand rubs in cabinets or areas approved for flammable materials (IC).

Guidelines for Infection Control in Health Care Personnel

INTRODUCTION

Two agencies are responsible for establishing infection control guidelines and legislating the practices of workers in all health care facilities. The Occupational Safety and Health Agency (OSHA) is a section of the Department of Labor of the federal government. OSHA legislates the practices of employers to protect the well-being of the workers. OSHA oversees the safety and health of all employees, not just those in health care. The Centers for Disease Control and Prevention (CDC) is also a federal government agency. CDC has no power to legislate but establishes guidelines for the prevention of disease in health care facilities. These guidelines set the standards for practice.

The information presented in Units 12 and 13 is based on the laws and guidelines of these two agencies. This appendix includes additional information on infection control that has been distributed by CDC. These guidelines apply to all settings: hospitals, long-term care facilities, the patient's home, clinics, and physicians' offices.

Responsibilities of the Health Care Employee

Your role as a health care worker requires that you:

- participate in educational programs about the principles of infection control
- report any infectious exposure or infectious disease that you may have to the proper person in your facility.
- follow the recommendations of your physician or health care provider and facility policies regarding your treatment for exposure or presence of disease.
- follow the guidelines and procedures established by the employer for the prevention of the spread of disease.

PREVENTION OF INFECTIOUS DISEASE: IMMUNIZATIONS

Table 12-2 of this text lists several immunizations recommended by the U.S. Public Health Service's Advisory Committee on Immunization Practices. Individual states have regulations on the vaccination of health care workers. Screening tests are available to determine susceptibility to certain diseases (hepatitis B, measles, mumps, rubella, and varicella [chicken pox]). Your employer may require that you be tested. Additional diseases are listed below for which vaccines are available for health care workers in special circumstances.

Name: BCG vaccine (for tuberculosis)
Primary/ booster dose schedule: One dose, no booster dose recommended.
Indications: Health care workers in communities where drug-resistant TB is prevalent, a strong likelihood of infection exists, and full implementation of TB infection control precautions has been inadequate in controlling the spread of infection.
Major precautions: Immunocompromised state and pregnancy.
Special considerations: TB control efforts are directed toward early identification and treatment of cases of active TB and toward preventive therapy for converters.

Name: Hepatitis A vaccine
Primary/booster dose schedule: Two doses of vaccine either 6–12 months apart or 6 months apart (depending on type of vaccine).
Indications: Recommended only for employees who work with the virus in a laboratory setting.
Major precautions: Contraindicated if history of allergic reaction to preservatives in vaccine, pregnancy.
Special considerations: Health care workers who travel internationally to certain areas should be evaluated for vaccination.

Name: Meningococcal polysaccharide vaccine
Primary/booster dose schedule: One dose, need for boosters is unknown.
Indications: Not routinely indicated for health care workers in the United States.
Major precautions: Vaccine safety in pregnant women has not been evaluated.
Special considerations: May be useful in certain outbreak situations.

Name: Polio vaccine
Primary/booster dose schedule: Two doses given 4–8 weeks apart followed by third dose 6–12 months after second dose.
Indications: Health care workers in close contact with persons who may be excreting virus and laboratory personnel who may be exposed to the virus.
Major precautions: Allergic reaction after receiving streptomycin or neomycin, pregnancy.
Special considerations: Use only inactivated polio vaccine for immunocompromised persons or workers who care for these patients.

Name: Rabies vaccine

Primary/booster dose schedule: Two different vaccines are given one each on days 0, 7, 21, or 28. Booster doses based on frequency of exposure.

Indications: Workers in contact with rabies virus or with infected animals in diagnostic or research activities.

Major precautions: None.

Special considerations: None.

Name: Tetanus and diphtheria (Td)

Primary/booster dose schedule: Two doses 4 weeks apart, third dose 6–12 months after second dose, booster every 10 years.

Indications: All adults, tetanus prophylaxis in wound management.

Major precautions: First trimester of pregnancy, history of neurological reaction or allergic reaction or severe local reaction.

Special considerations: None.

Name: Typhoid vaccine

Primary booster/dose schedule: One dose, booster doses depend on route of administration and rate of exposure.

Indications: Workers in laboratories who frequently work with Salmonella typhi.

Major precautions: History of severe local or systemic reaction, certain types of the vaccine should not be given to immunocompromised persons.

Special considerations: Vaccine should not be considered as an alternative to proper procedures.

Name: Vaccinia vaccine (smallpox)

Primary/booster dose schedule: One dose, boosters every 10 years.

Indications: Laboratory workers who work with animals or cultures with these viruses.

Major precautions: Pregnancy, presence or history of eczema, immunocompromised persons.

Special considerations: Vaccine may be considered for health care workers who have direct contact with contaminated dressings or other infectious material from volunteers in clinical studies involving the virus.

Postexposure Prophylaxis

Postexposure prophylaxis refers to actions that are taken after an employee is exposed to an infectious disease while working in the health care setting. The purpose of these measures is to prevent further transmission of infection. Postexposure prophylaxis through antibiotics or vaccines may be required for these diseases: diphtheria, hepatitis A, hepatitis B, HIV, meningococcal disease, pertussis (whooping cough), rabies, and varicella-zoster virus. Work restrictions may be imposed on an employee after exposure or infection with infectious disease. Decisions on work restrictions are based on how the disease is transmitted and the epidemiology of the disease. Work restrictions may include any or all of these restrictions:

- patient contact.
- contact with patient's environment.
- food-handling.
- care of high-risk patients.
- care of infants, newborns.
- immunocompromised patients and their environments.
- performance of invasive procedures.
- exclude from duty (exclusion from the health care facility and from any health care activities outside the facility, no contact with susceptible persons in facility or in the community).
- Exposure or infection with any of these diseases may require work restrictions:
  - conjunctivitis (eye infection)
  - hepatitis A
  - hepatitis B
  - hepatitis C
  - herpes simplex
  - human immunodeficiency virus (HIV)
  - measles
  - rubella
  - streptococcal infection group A
  - varicella zoster
  - cytomegalovirus infections
  - diarrhea
  - diphtheria
  - enteroviral infections
  - meningococcal infections
  - mumps
  - pediculosis (lice)
  - pertussis
  - scabies
  - tuberculosis
  - viral respiratory infections

Health Counseling

Health care workers should receive counseling regarding:

- the risk and prevention of infections acquired while working.
- the risk of illness or other problems after exposure to infectious disease.
- actions to take after exposure to infectious disease, including postexposure prophylaxis procedures.
- possible consequences of exposure or diseases for family members, patients, and other workers both inside and outside the health care facility.

Records

Employers must maintain records for all employees regarding medical evaluations, immunizations, exposures, postexposure prophylaxis, screening tests, and exposure to bloodborne pathogens. Employees have the right to review these records and to expect that all information in the file will be kept confidential. Information cannot be disclosed or reported without the written consent of the employee to any person within or outside the work place except as required by law.

INFECTIONS/INFECTIOUS DISEASES

Several infectious diseases are described in this section in addition to those included in the text on pages 156–163: Remember that standard precautions are followed with *all patients*. Isolation precautions may also be required Follow your employer's procedures and policies. Anyone exposed to any of these diseases should report this fact to the proper facility authority before going to work. Work restrictions may be imposed, depending on the disease.

Conjunctivitis

Conjunctivitis (pink eye) is an infection of the clear membrane that covers the front of the eye and the inside of the eyelid. It may be caused by either bacteria or a virus. The eye is inflamed and there may be a purulent discharge. Contaminated hands are a major source of transmission. Handwashing, glove use, and disinfection of instruments can prevent transmission.

Cytomegalovirus

Cytomegalovirus (CMV) may be found in health care institutions, in infants and young children infected with the virus, and in immunocompromised patients such as persons with AIDS. The disease is transmitted through close, intimate contact, through contact with secretions or excretions like saliva or urine, or through the hands.

Diphtheria

Diphtheria is currently a rare disease in the United States, because immunizations are given during infancy. It is caused by bacteria, affects the lining of the throat, and is highly contagious. The disease is transmitted by contact with respiratory droplets or contact with skin lesions of infected patients.

Acute Gastrointestinal Infections

Infections of the gastrointestinal tract may be caused by bacteria, virus, or protozoa. Symptoms include vomiting, diarrhea, or both, with or without fever, nausea, and abdominal pain. The microorganisms are transmitted through contact with infected individuals, from consuming contaminated food, water, or other beverages. The most common gastrointestinal infection is that caused by Salmonella.

Herpes Simplex

The herpes simplex virus causes infections of the fingers and around the mouth (cold sores). The virus also causes genital herpes. There have been no reports that workers with genital herpes have transmitted the disease to patients. Transmission occurs through contact with lesions or secretions such as saliva, vaginal secretions, or amniotic fluid. Exposed areas of the skin are the most likely sites of infection, especially when cuts, abrasions or other skin lesions are present.

Measles

Measles is caused by a virus and is characterized by a rash on the body and fever. It is highly contagious. Measles is transmitted by large droplets during close contact with infected persons and by the airborne route. Workers born after 1957 should be considered immune to measles if they have had physician-diagnosed measles or appropriate vaccine on or after their first birthday, or have been proven immune through testing. Persons born and immunized between 1957 and 1984 were given only one dose of vaccine during infancy and may require a second dose. Persons born before 1957 are generally considered to be immune.

Meningococcal Disease

Transmission of meningococcal disease occurs through droplets during contact with respiratory secretions or through handling laboratory specimens. Transmission in health care settings is uncommon.

Mumps

Mumps (infection of parotid glands) is caused by a virus and is transmitted by droplets through contact with respiratory secretions, including saliva. Vaccination prevents mumps transmission. Workers are considered immune if they have had physician-diagnosed mumps, appropriate vaccination after their first birthday, or have been proven immune through testing. Persons born before 1957 may be considered immune.

Parvovirus

Parvovirus is the cause of erythema infectiosum (Fifth disease), a common rash illness that is usually acquired during childhood. The virus is transmitted through contact with infected persons, fomites, or large droplets. Transmission to workers from infected patients appears to be rare.

Pertussis

Pertussis (whooping cough) is caused by a bacteria and is highly contagious. Symptoms include cough, mild fever, and loss of appetite. Transmission occurs by contact with respiratory secretions or large droplets from the respiratory tracts of infected persons.

Poliomyelitis

The last cases of acquired poliomyelitis were reported in 1979. Poliomyelitis is caused by a virus and is transmitted through contact with feces or urine of infected persons but can be spread by contact with respiratory secretions and in rare cases, through feces.

Rabies

Human rabies occurs primarily from exposure to rabid animals. Theoretically, rabies may be transmitted to health care workers from exposures to saliva from infected patients, but no cases have been documented to prove this.

Rubella

Rubella (three-day measles) is characterized by a rash and is transmitted by contact with droplets from the nose and throat of infected persons. Rubella is usually a mild disease but can cause congenital defects in the fetus of a pregnant woman. Persons are considered susceptible to rubella if they have not had appropriate immunization or if laboratory tests do not give evidence of immunity.

Scabies and Pediculosis

Scabies is caused by a mite that burrows into the skin, leaving "tracks." This results in intense itching. Scabies is easily transmitted through skin-to-skin contact. The disease is treated with applications of topical creams or lotions (scabicides).

Pediculosis (lice) may infest the human body, the human head, or the pubic area. Head lice are transmitted by head-to-head contact with infested fomites such as combs or brushes. Body lice are usually associated with poor personal hygiene and unclean environments and are transmitted by contact with the skin or clothing of an infested person. Pubic lice can also be found in the axilla, eyelashes, or eyebrows. Transmission is primarily through intimate or sexual contact.

Staphylococcus aureus

Staphylococcus aureus (staph) is a common bacteria that can cause infections in the skin, the lungs, the blood, and the urinary bladder. Food poisoning is frequently caused by staph. The major sources of staph are infected and colonized patients. A colonized patient is one who harbors the microorganism but has no symptoms. The most common sites are the nose, hands, axilla, perineum, and throat. Transmission of the bacteria usually occurs through the hands of workers, which can become contaminated by contact with colonized or infected body sites of patients. Staph infections are treated with antibiotics. In the last few years staph microorganisms have become resistant to many antibiotics. Methicillin-resistant staphylococcus aureus (MRSA) is an example. Infection with a resistant microorganism can be a dangerous situation for patients who are already at risk for infections.

Streptococcus, group A

Group A Streptococcus (GAS) can cause infections in the throat (strep throat), the skin, the blood, and other body organs. GAS can be transmitted from patients to health care workers after contact with infected secretions.

Vaccinia

The World Health Organization (WHO) declared the world free of small pox in 1980. The smallpox vaccine is still available in the United States. Laboratory workers who are in contact with certain viruses need to be vaccinated every 10 years. Susceptible persons may acquire vaccinia from a recently vaccinated person through contact with the vaccination site for 2–21 days after vaccination. This can be prevented by covering the site and with thorough handwashing after contact with the site.

Varicella

Varicella (chicken pox) is caused by a virus and is characterized by blister like skin lesions. Herpes zoster (shingles) is caused by the same microorganism. Herpes zoster occurs in persons who have had chicken pox. The virus lies dormant in the body and later erupts in the form of shingles. The virus is transmitted by contact with infected lesions and in health care facilities, airborne transmission has occurred from patients with chicken pox or shingles to susceptible persons who had no direct contact with the infected patient. Tests are available for determining a person's immunity to varicella. A vaccine was licensed for use in 1995.

Viral Respiratory Infections

Included in this group of infections are influenza and respiratory syncytial virus (RSV). There are several different viruses that can cause respiratory infections. Transmission is by person to person contact with an infected individual and by droplet. This may be from patients to workers, from workers to patients and between workers. Visitors may also be a source of infection. Persons at risk for complications include the elderly, residents of long-term care facilities, persons with chronic lung or heart problems, and persons with diabetes. Influenza vaccine given to health care workers before the beginning of the flu season can help reduce the risk of infection.

PREGNANT HEALTH CARE WORKERS

Pregnant health care workers are generally no more or no less at risk for acquiring work-related infections than are other workers. However, infections are of special concern to female health care workers of childbearing age for several reasons. Some infections may be more severe during pregnancy and some infections may affect the fetus. Women of childbearing age are strongly encouraged to receive immunizations for vaccine-preventable diseases before they are pregnant.

LATEX HYPERSENSITIVITY

Health care workers are at risk for developing latex allergy because they frequently use latex gloves. Many of the products used in patient care contain latex, as do many household and personal items. Persons who have hay fever, hand dermatitis, and food allergies (to foods such as bananas, avocados, kiwi fruits, and chestnuts) are at increased risk of latex allergy. The amount and type of exposure needed to cause latex sensitivity is not known, although it is believed that wearing latex gloves when a rash is present on the hands increases the risk. A skin rash is often the first sign that a worker is becoming sensitive to latex. Some of the most common items that may contain latex are listed in Table B-1. Table B-2 is a more complete listing of items found in a health care facility that may contain latex.

Three types of reactions can occur in persons who use latex products:

- Irritant contact dermatitis or contact dermatitis—the development of dry, itchy, irritated areas on the skin, usually the hands. However, this problem may have many other causes as well, so one should not assume that a latex sensitivity is present without further diagnostic testing. *Irritant contact dermatitis is not a true allergy.*
- Allergic contact dermatitis (delayed hypersensitivity)—this is a sensitivity to the chemicals used during the manufacturing process. The reaction is similar to the symptoms of poison ivy.
- Latex allergy is a serious reaction to latex. This type of allergy is diagnosed with a blood or skin test. Even low exposure to latex can cause sensitive individuals to react. Reactions usually begin shortly after exposure to latex, but they can occur

TABLE B-1 COMMON ITEMS THAT MAY CONTAIN LATEX

This list is for example only and is not all-inclusive (For additional information see http://www.niosh.gov)

Emergency Equipment

Blood pressure cuffs
Stethoscopes
Disposable gloves
Oral and nasal airways
Endotracheal tubes
Tourniquets
Intravenous tubing
Syringes
Electrode pads

Personal Protective Equipment

Gloves
Surgical masks
Goggles
Respirators
Rubber aprons

Office Supplies

Rubber bands
Erasers

Hospital Supplies

Anesthesia masks
Catheters
Wound drains
Injection ports
Rubber tops of multidose vials
Dental dams

Household Objects

Automobile tires
Motorcycle and bicycle handgrips
Carpeting
Swimming goggles
Racquet handles
Shoe soles
Expandable fabric (waistbands)
Dishwashing gloves
Hot water bottles
Condoms
Diaphragms
Balloons
Pacifiers
Baby bottle nipples
Underwear (elastic in legs and waist)

hours later. Mild reactions cause hives, itching, and skin redness. More severe reactions include respiratory symptoms, including runny nose, sneezing, itchy eyes, difficulty breathing, and wheezing. Shock is the most severe reaction. This type of shock is similar to that experienced by persons who are allergic to bee stings.

Preventing Latex Allergy

Many health care facilities have latex-free carts. Some facilities are becoming completely latex-free. Health care workers should take the following steps to protect themselves from latex exposure and allergy in the workplace:

1. Use nonlatex gloves for activities that are not likely to involve contact with infectious materials (food preparation, routine housekeeping, maintenance, etc.). If latex gloves are used, avoid powdered gloves, which increase sensitivity through inhalation of latex proteins when gloves are removed.

2. Barrier protection is necessary when handling known or potentially infectious materials. If you use latex gloves, use powder-free gloves. Hypoallergenic latex gloves do not reduce the risk of latex allergy. However, they may reduce reactions to chemical additives in the latex (allergic contact dermatitis). Cloth stethoscope covers provide an excellent barrier against latex exposure, but can be a potential source of contamination to patients. Make sure your stethoscope cover is laundered regularly to reduce the potential risk of transmission.

3. Avoid oil-based hand creams or lotions (which can cause glove deterioration) unless they have been shown to reduce latex-related problems and maintain glove barrier protection.

4. After removing latex gloves, wash your hands with a mild soap and dry them thoroughly.

5. Attend educational classes about latex exposure provided by your employer.

6. Become familiar with procedures for preventing latex allergy.

7. Learn to recognize the symptoms of latex allergy: skin rashes; hives; flushing; itching; nasal, eye, or sinus symptoms; asthma; and shock.

8. If you develop symptoms of latex allergy, avoid direct contact with latex gloves and other latex-containing products until you can see a physician experienced in treating latex allergy.

9. If you have latex allergy, consult your physician regarding precautions to use, such as:
   - avoiding contact with latex gloves and other latex-containing products.
   - avoiding areas where you might inhale the powder from latex gloves worn by other workers.
   - informing your employer and your health care providers (physicians, nurses, dentists, etc.) that you have latex allergy.
   - wearing a medical alert bracelet.

10. Carefully follow your physician's instructions for dealing with allergic reactions to latex.

AMERICANS WITH DISABILITIES ACT

The Americans with Disabilities Act affects infection control policies for health care workers as well as other disabilities. An employer can evaluate applicants for their qualifications to perform the tasks required of the job for which they are being considered. The applicant may be asked about the ability to perform specific job functions but may not be asked about the existence, nature, or severity of a disability. Applicants with certain communicable diseases who are otherwise qualified for the job may justifiably be denied employment until they are no longer infectious.

INFECTION CONTROL PRACTICES

Unit 13 in the text describes the measures that are used to prevent the spread of infection. Remember that *standard precautions are used for **all patients***. Special precautions are implemented when a patient has a known infectious disease. These precautions are based on the means by which the disease is transmitted. In

TABLE B-2 COMMON ITEMS IN THE HEALTH CARE FACILITY THAT CONTAIN LATEX

Note: This list is not all-inclusive.

Adhesives, skin

Anesthesia circuits, bags, oxygen masks

Bandaids

Blood pressure cuff, tubing

Bulb syringe

Catheters:

    cardiac

    condom

    coude

    feeding

    indwelling

    pulmonary

    straight

    systems

    vascular

CPR manikins and medical training aids

Crutch tips, axillary pads, hand grips

Dental braces with rubber bands

Diapers, rubber pants

Dressings:

    Action Wrap

    Airstrips (some)

    BDF Elastoplast

    Bioclusive

    Centurion brief

    Coban (3M)

    Comfeel (Coloplast)

    Duoderm (Squibb)

    Dyna-flex, butterfly closures (J&J)

    Lyofoam (Acme)

Metalline

Montgomery strap (J&J)

Opraflex (Lohmann)

Opsite

PinCare (Hollister)

Reston foam (3M)

Selopor

Spandage (Medi-tech)

Venigard

Webril (Kendall)

Xerofoam (Sherwood)

Note: latex in package only: Active Strips (3M), CURAD, Nu-Derm (J&J), Steri-strip wound closure system, Tegaderm, Tegasorb

Elastic on underwear, socks, clothing

Elastic wrap: ACE, Dyna-flex, Elastikon (J&J)

Electrode bulbs, pads, grounding

Enemas, ready-to-use (Fleet Pediatric and Mineral Oil have latex valve, but will soon change)

Foods handled with latex gloves

G-tubes, buttons

Gloves: clean, orthodontic, sterile, surgical

ID bracelets

Incentive deep breathing exerciser

IV access: injection ports, Y-sites, bags, pumps, buretrol ports, PRN adapters, needleless systems

IV ports or syringes

Mattresses, therapeutic

Medication vial stoppers

Penrose drains

Pulse oximeters

Reflex hammers

Respirators

Resusitators, manual

Shoe covers

Spacer (for metered dose inhalers)

Sphygmomanometer (blood pressure cuff)

Stethoscope tubing

Storage bags, zippered plastic

Suction tubing

Syringes, disposable

Tapes:

    adhesive felt (Acme)

    cloth

    moleskin

    pink

    Waterproof (3M, J&J)

    Zonas

Tourniquets

Theraband (also strip, tube), other OT supplies

Thermometer probes

Vascular stockings (Jobst)

Wheelchair cushions, tires

---

addition to contact transmission, droplet transmission, and airborne transmission, there is common vehicle transmision (microorganisms transmitted by contaminated items such as food, water, medications, devices, and equipment) and vectorborne transmission (occurs when vectors such as mosquitoes, flies, rats, and other vermin transmit microorganisms).

The fundamentals of infectious disease prevention include: handwashing, gloving, patient placement, transport of infected patients, use of personal protective equipment, correct handling of equipment, supplies, and linens. These procedures are explained in Unit 13.

abbreviation   shortened form of a word or phrase.

abdominal distention   a condition in which the abdomen is bloated and enlarged.

abduction   movement away from midline or center.

abduction pillow   pillow used to maintain separation between the legs of a patient who has had hip surgery.

abrasion   injury that results from scraping the skin.

absence seizure   another name for a petit mal seizure.

abuse   improper treatment or misuse.

accelerated   increased or faster motion, as in pulse or respiration.

acceptance   coming to terms with a situation and awaiting the outcome calmly; final stage of dying which some people, but not all, reach.

acetone   colorless liquid produced during the metabolism of fats because glucose cannot be oxidized in the blood; has a sweet, fruity odor; appears in blood and urine of persons with diabetes.

acquired immune deficiency syndrome (AIDS)   a progressive disease of the immune system caused by the human immunodeficiency virus; initially an extremely high mortality rate was the norm for the disease; now combination drug therapy can slow the disease process and lengthen life expectancy of those infected with HIV.

activities of daily living (ADLs)   the activities necessary to fulfill basic human needs.

acupuncture   insertion of tiny, thin needles in various parts of the body to correct imbalances in energy and treat disease.

acute disease   disease that comes on suddenly, requires urgent treatment, and is usually resolved.

acute exacerbation   an increase in the severity of signs and symptoms of a chronic disease.

acute illness   illness that comes on suddenly; requires intensive, immediate treatment.

adaptations   adjustments.

adaptive device   item altered to make it easier to use by those with functional deficits to perform any activity of daily living.

Addison's disease   disease caused by underfunctioning of the adrenal glands.

adduction   movement toward midline or center.

adjunctive devices   secondary devices used to maintain the airway and respirations.

ADLs   *See* **activities of daily living**

admission   procedure carried out when a patient first arrives at a facility.

adolescence   teenage years.

adoptive parent   person who is a parent through a legal adoption procedure.

adrenal glands   endocrine glands; one is located on the top of each kidney; secrete hormones including epinephrine.

advance directive   document signed before the diagnosis of a terminal illness, when the individual is still in good health, indicating the person's wishes regarding care during dying.

AEM   *See* **Anthroposophically Extended Medicine**

afterbirth   *See* **placenta**

agitation   mental state characterized by irregular and erratic behavior.

aiding and abetting   not reporting dishonest acts that are observed.

AIDS   *See* **acquired immune deficiency syndrome**

airborne precautions   procedures used to prevent the spread of airborne pathogens.

airborne transmission   method of spreading disease by breathing tiny pathogens that remain suspended in the air for long periods of time.

akinesia   difficulty and slowness in carrying out voluntary muscular activities.

alcoholism   a dependency on alcohol.

alignment   *See* **body alignment**

allergen   substance that causes sensitivity or allergic reactions.

allergy   abnormal and individual hypersensitivity.

alopecia   absence of hair where hair normally grows.

alternative   choice; option.

alternative medical systems   therapeutic or preventive health care practices that are used instead of conventional health care; often involves the use of natural products rather than those derived from chemicals. These systems do not follow generally accepted methods and may not have a scientific explanation for their effectiveness.

alveoli   tiny air sacs that make up most of the lungs.

Alzheimer's disease   neurological condition in which there is a gradual loss of cerebral functioning.

AM care   care given in the early morning when the patient first awakens.

ambulate   to walk.

ambulation   the process of walking.

amenorrhea   without menstruation.

amino acids   basic components of proteins.

amniocentesis   transabdominal perforation of the amniotic sac to obtain a sample of the amniotic fluid.

amniotic fluid   fluid in which the fetus floats in the mother's womb.

amniotic sac   sac enclosing the fetus and amniotic fluid.

amputation   removal of a limb or other body appendage.

amulet   charm used to ward off evil.

amyotrophic lateral sclerosis (ALS)   a progressive neuromuscular disease that causes muscle weakness and paralysis.

analgesic   pain-relieving medication.

anaphylactic shock   extreme, sometimes fatal, sensitivity or allergic reaction to a specific antigen.

anatomic position   standing erect, facing observer, feet flat on floor and slightly separated, arms at sides, palms forward.

anatomy   study of the structure of the human body.

anemia   deficiency of quality or quantity of red blood cells in the blood.

aneroid gauge   device for measuring and registering blood pressure.

anesthesia   loss of feeling or sensation.

anger feeling of hostility, rage.

angina pectoris acute pain in the chest caused by interference with the supply of oxygen to the heart.

animal-assisted therapy pet therapy; pets visiting in a health care facility for a therapeutic purpose.

anorexia lack or loss of appetite for food.

anterior in anatomy, in front of the coronal or ventral plane.

Anthroposophically Extended Medicine (AEM) a holistic system of natural medicine that treats the whole person and not just the disease or symptoms; treatment is designed to harmonize the relationship of body, mind, and spirit.

antibiotic medication used to treat bacterial infection.

antibodies proteins produced in the body in response to invasion by a foreign agent (antigen); react specifically with the foreign agent.

anticoagulant medication that thins the blood and increases the risk of bleeding.

anti-embolism hose elasticized stockings used to support the leg blood vessels.

antigen marker on cells that identifies a cell as self or nonself; antigens on foreign substances that enter the body, such as pathogens, stimulate the production of antibodies by the body.

Apgar score method for determining an infant's condition at birth by scoring heart rate, respiratory effect, muscle tone, reflex irritability, and color.

aphasia language impairment; loss of ability to comprehend normally.

apical pulse pulse rate taken by placing a stethoscope over the tip of the heart.

apnea period of no respiration.

appliance device used with colostomy or ileostomy to collect drainage from a stoma.

approaches actions used by the health care team to help resolve a patient's problems; steps taken to reach a goal.

Aquamatic K-Pad® brand name of a unit for applying heat or cold.

aromatherapy use of natural scents and smells to promote health and well-being.

art therapy using art and the various senses to express oneself.

artery vessel through which oxygenated blood passes away from the heart to various parts of the body.

arthritis joint inflammation.

ascites fluid accumulation in the abdomen.

asepsis without infection.

aspirate to withdraw.

aspiration drawing of foreign materials into the respiratory tract.

assault attempt or threat to do violence to another.

assessment act of evaluating.

assignment specific list of duties; tells you which patients you will care for during your shift and the specific procedures to be performed.

assimilate to absorb.

assisted living situation in which a person primarily cares for himself or herself but has some help in meeting health care needs; may reside in a facility that provides health care supervision.

assistive devices equipment used to help people be more effective in their physical activity.

asthma chronic respiratory disease characterized by bronchospasms and excessive mucus production.

atelectasis collapse of lung tissue.

atheroma degeneration or thickening of artery walls due to formation of fatty plaque and scar tissue.

atherosclerosis degenerative process involving the lining of arteries, in which the lumen eventually narrows and closes; a form of arteriosclerosis.

atrium one of the two upper chambers of the heart.

atrophy shrinking or wasting away of tissues.

attitude an external expression of inner feelings about oneself or others.

aura peculiar sensation preceding the appearance of more definite symptoms in a convulsion or seizure.

auscultatory gap sound fadeout for 1–15 mm Hg (mercury) pressure, after which sound begins again; sometimes mistaken for the diastolic pressure.

autoclave machine that sterilizes articles.

autoimmune presence of antibodies against component(s) of body.

automatic external defibrillator (AED) computerized device that uses an electric shock to reverse disorganized activity in the heart during cardiac arrest.

autonomic dysreflexia potentially life-threatening complication of spinal cord injury; indicates uncontrolled sympathetic nervous system activity.

autonomy self-determination.

autopsy examination of body after death to determine cause of death.

avulsion fracture fracture caused by a bone fragment pulling off at the point of ligament or tendon attachment.

axilla armpit.

axon extension of neuron that conducts nerve impulses away from the cell body.

Ayurveda a natural system of medicine based on the belief that disease is due to an imbalance in the consciousness. Uses lifestyle interventions, natural therapies, and rebalancing among the body, mind, and environment.

bacillus (plural bacilli) rod-shaped bacterium.

bacteremia bacterial infection in the bloodstream; also known as *septicemia*.

bacterium (plural bacteria) a form of simple microbes.

balance bar section of an upright scale that holds the weights used to determine a patient's weight.

bandages fabric, gauze, net, or elasticized material used to cover dressings and keep them securely in place.

bargaining stage of the grieving process in which the individual seeks to make a deal or form a pact that will delay death.

baseline measurement of patient's vital signs or other body functions upon admission; future measurements are compared to baseline measurements to track the patient's progress.

baseline assessment initial observations of the patient and his or her condition.

battery an unlawful attack upon or touching of another person.

belief idea based on commonly held opinions, knowledge, and attitudes.

benign nonmalignant (tumor).

benign prostatic hypertrophy noncancerous enlargement of prostate gland.

bile   substance produced by the liver that prepares fats for digestion.

binders   fabric or elastic wraps that encircle the abdomen; may be used to hold dressings in place or support a surgical site.

biofeedback   a method of retraining the mind to control various physical problems and stresses that one would not normally be aware of.

biohazard   laboratory specimens or materials, and their containers contaminated by body fluids; these have the potential to transmit disease.

biological parent   natural parent who contributed sperm or an ovum to the development of the fetus.

biological therapy   biologically based practices using natural substances and products to promote or regain health.

biopsy   removal and examination of a piece of tissue from a living body.

bioterrorism   the use of biological agents, such as pathogenic organisms or agricultural pests, for terrorist purposes.

bisexuality   having sexual interest in both genders.

blood pressure   pressure of blood exerted against vascular walls.

body alignment   position of a human body in which the body can properly function.

body-based therapy   practices based on direct body contact, such as manipulation or movement.

body core   center of the body (internal).

body language   use of facial expression, body positions, and vocal inflections to convey a message.

body shell   outer surface of the body.

bolus   soft mass of food that is ready to be swallowed.

Bowman's capsule   tubule surrounding the glomerulus of the nephron.

box (square) corner   one type of corner used in the making of a hospital bed.

brachial artery   main artery of the arm.

brachytherapy   a form of radiation therapy in which tiny radioactive seeds or pellets are implanted directly inside the prostate gland.

bradycardia   unusually slow heartbeat.

braille   method of communication used by persons with visual impairments, who use fingertips to feel a series of raised dots representing letters and numbers.

brain attack   interference with the supply of blood to the brain; also known as *stroke* or *cerebral vascular accident*.

brain stem   base of the brain; enlarged extension of the spinal cord, located in the cranium; includes medulla oblongata, diencephalon, pons, and midbrain.

bridging   supporting the body on either side of an affected area to relieve pressure on the area.

bronchi   tubal structures connecting the trachea to the lungs.

bronchioles   smaller subdivisions or branches at end of the bronchi, located in the lungs.

bronchitis   inflammation of the bronchi.

bruxism   grinding of the teeth.

burnout   loss of enthusiasm for and interest in an activity.

bursae   small sacs of fluid found around joints.

bursitis   condition in which the bursae become inflamed and the joint becomes very painful.

cachexia   state of malnutrition, emaciation, and debility, usually resulting from a prolonged illness.

CAM   *See* **complementary/alternative medicine**

cancer   a disease in which the normal mechanisms of cell growth are disturbed. Cells grow abnormally, invade surrounding tissues, and use nutrition targeted for normal cells.

cannula   an indwelling tube inserted through a stoma to maintain patency.

CAPD   *See* **continuous ambulatory peritoneal dialysis**

capillary   hairlike blood vessel; link between arterioles and venules.

capillary refill   quick and painless method of checking a patient's peripheral circulation and oxygenation status; done by pressing on a fingernail and noting the time needed for skin color to return to normal when pressure is released.

carbohydrates   energy foods; used by the body to produce heat and energy for work.

carbon dioxide   gas that is a waste product in cellular metabolism.

carcinogen   a cancer-causing substance.

carcinoma   malignant tumor made up of connective tissue enclosing epithelial cells.

cardiac arrest   sudden and often unexpected stoppage of effective heart action.

cardiac cycle   all (mechanical and electrical) events that occur between one heart contraction and the next.

cardiac decompensation   another name for congestive heart failure.

cardiac muscle   muscle that forms the heart wall.

cardiopulmonary resuscitation (CPR)   emergency medical procedure undertaken to restart and sustain heart and respiratory functions.

care plan   nursing plan for care of a resident in a long-term care facility.

care plan conference   meeting of members of an interdisciplinary health care team to develop approaches and a plan of care.

caries   tooth decay or cavities.

carrier   person who hosts infectious organisms without having symptoms of disease.

cartilage   type of body tissue.

cataract   opacity of the lens of the eye, resulting in loss of vision.

catastrophic reaction   severe and unpredictable violent behavior of a person with dementia.

catheter   tube for evacuating or injecting fluids.

causative agent   etiology of a specific disease process.

cavity   enclosed area; space within the body that contains organs.

celibate   has no sexual intercourse.

cell   basic unit in the organization of living substances.

cellulose   basic substance of all plant foods, which can supply the body with roughage.

Celsius scale   scale for measuring temperature.

centimeter   one-hundredth of a meter.

central venous (CV) catheter   tube inserted into a large vein in the area of the clavicle.

cerebellum   portion of the brain lying beneath the occipital lobe; coordinates muscular activities and balance.

cerebrospinal fluid (CSF)   water cushion protecting the brain and spinal cord from shock.

cerebrovascular accident (CVA)   more commonly called *brain attack* or *stroke*; disorder of the blood vessels of the brain resulting in impaired cerebral circulation and often causing motor and cognitive deficits.

cerebrum   largest part of the brain, consisting of two hemispheres separated by a deep longitudinal fissure; controls all mental activities.

certification   an inspection process for facilities that accept state or federal funds as payment for health care.

cervical traction   use of weights to apply traction in the area of the cervical vertebrae.

cesarean   method of delivering fetus through a surgical incision in the abdominal wall and uterus.

chain of infection   process of events involved in the transmission and development of an infectious disease.

chancre   shallow, craterlike lesion; primary lesion of syphilis.

charting   entering information (documentation) in a patient's medical record (chart).

chelation therapy   intravenous injection of an amino acid by a licensed professional; commonly used to treat serious circulatory problems, heavy metal poisoning, and reduced blood flow in the legs.

chemical restraint   use of medications to control behavior.

chemotherapy   use of medications to treat disease.

chest tubes   sterile, clear plastic tubes that are inserted through the skin of the chest, between the ribs, and into the space between the lung and chest wall; used after surgery to drain bloody fluid from the chest and allow air to escape if there is a small leak of air at the suture line after lung surgery.

Cheyne-Stokes respiration   periods of apnea alternating with periods of dyspnea.

CHF   *See* **congestive heart failure**

chiropractic care   manual adjustments to keep the vertebrae in good alignment, relieving pressure on nerves, muscles, and joints.

chlamydia   type of sexually transmitted disease.

cholecystectomy   surgical removal of a diseased gallbladder and stones.

cholecystitis   inflammation of the gallbladder.

cholelithiasis   formation of stones in the gallbladder.

chronic disease or **illness**   incurable illness or disease, but treatable; requires ongoing care.

chronic obstructive pulmonary disease (COPD)   any condition, such as emphysema or bronchitis, that interferes with normal respiration over a long period of time.

chronologic   in sequential order by date or age.

chyme   semiliquid form of food as it leaves the stomach.

CircOlectric® bed   special kind of bed used when a patient cannot be turned within the bed.

circumcision   removal of the end of the prepuce by a circular incision.

citation   written notice that informs a facility of violations of OSHA rules.

clear liquid diet   diet of water and high-carbohydrate fluids given every 2 to 4 hours.

client   person receiving care; depending upon the health care setting, also known as *patient* or *resident*.

client care record   documentation of care provided in the home situation.

Client's Rights   document spelling out rights of persons receiving home health care.

climacteric   menopause; the combined phenomena accompanying cessation of the reproductive function in the female or reduction of testicular activity in the male.

clinical thermometer   instrument used to measure body temperature.

clitoris   small, cylindrical mass of erotic tissue; part of the external female reproductive organs analogous to the penis in the male.

closed bed   bed with sheets and spread positioned to the head of the bed; unoccupied.

closed (simple) fracture   fracture in which bones remain in proper alignment.

coccus (plural cocci)   round bacteria.

cochlea   spiral-shaped organ in the inner ear that receives and interprets sounds.

coercion   forcing a patient to do something against his or her wishes.

cognitive impairment   deficit in intellect, memory, or attention.

coitus   sexual intercourse; copulation.

cold pack   a type of thermal application used to lower the temperature of a portion of the body; often a commercially prepared, disposable item.

colon   large intestine.

colony   group of organisms derived from a single organism.

color therapy   alternative health care practices that use color to affect mood, emotions, relationships, and sense of well-being.

colostomy   artificial opening in the abdomen for the purpose of evacuation of feces.

colostrum   secretion from the lactiferous glands of the mother before the onset of true lactation two or three days after delivery of a baby.

colporrhaphy   suturing of the vagina; surgical procedure used to tighten vaginal walls.

combining form   word part that can be used with other word parts to form a variety of new words.

comfort   a state of well-being in which the patient is calm and relaxed, and is not in pain or upset.

comminuted fracture   fracture in which the bone is broken or crushed into small pieces.

communicable disease   disease caused by pathogenic organism; can be transmitted from person to person, either directly or indirectly.

communication   exchange of messages.

community   people who live in a common area and share common health needs.

compartment syndrome   a painful condition that occurs when pressure within the muscles builds up, preventing blood and oxygen from reaching muscles and nerves; a very serious complication that may develop following an injury or surgical procedure.

compensate   to seek a substitute for something unattainable or unacceptable.

complementary/alternative medicine (CAM)   a group of diverse systems, practices, and products that are not presently considered part of conventional medicine.

complementary medicine   a treatment regimen in which alternative practices are combined with conventional health care.

complete fracture   a break across the entire cross-section of the bone.

complication   situation that makes original condition more serious.

compound (open) fracture   fracture in which part of the broken bone protrudes through the skin.

compression fracture   break in a bone with crushing of the bone fragments.

concurrent cleaning   daily, routine cleaning of patient unit.

condom catether   latex sheath that fits over the penis; used for urinary drainage when connected to a urinary collection bag.

confidential   keeping what is said or written to oneself; private; not shared.

congenital   condition present at birth.

congestive heart failure (CHF)   condition resulting from cardiac output inadequate for physiological needs, with shortness of breath, edema, and abnormal retention of sodium and water in body tissues.

conjunctiva   mucous membrane that lines the eyelids and covers the eye.

connective tissue   tissue that holds other tissues together and provides support for organs and other body structures.

connective tissue cells   cells that form connective tissue.

constipation   difficulty in defecating.

contact precautions   practices used to prevent spread of disease by direct or indirect contact.

contact transmission   spread of disease by direct or indirect contact with infected person or contaminated objects.

contagious   communicable or easily spread.

contagious disease   disease that is communicable; disease that is caused by a pathogenic organism.

contaminated   unclean; impure; soiled with microbes.

continuous ambulatory peritoneal dialysis (CAPD)   a form of dialysis that removes waste products from the patient's blood; performed in subacute care centers.

continuous passive motion (CPM)   a therapy that prevents stiffness and improves circulation by delivering a form of passive range-of-motion exercise so that the joint is moved without the patient's muscles being used.

continuous positive airway pressure (CPAP)   oxygen therapy in which a mask is placed on the patient's face, then connected to a device that creates low levels of pressure.

continuum   continuous related series of events or actions.

contracture   permanent shortening or contraction of a muscle due to spasm or paralysis.

contraindicated   not recommended; disallowed; situation in which a remedy or treatment is not called for because of the patient's condition.

contraindication   situation in which a treatment or action is inappropriate.

contusion   mechanical injury (usually caused by a blow) resulting in hemorrhage beneath the unbroken skin.

convulsion   involuntary muscle spasm.

COPD   *See* **chronic obstructive pulmonary disease**

coping   handling or dealing with stress.

cornea   transparent portion of the eye through which light passes.

coronary embolism   blood clot lodged in a coronary artery.

coronary occlusion   closing off of a coronary artery.

coronary thrombosis   blood clot within a coronary vessel.

corporal punishment   use of painful treatment to change or correct behavior.

cortex   outer portion of a kidney.

countertraction   providing opposing balance to traction; used in reduction of fractures.

Cowper's glands   pair of small glands that open into the urethra at the base of the penis; part of the male reproductive system.

CPAP   *See* **continuous positive airway pressure**

CPM   *See* **continuous passive motion**

CPR   *See* **cardiopulmonary resuscitation**

critical list   list that patients are placed on when they are dangerously or terminally ill.

critical (clinical) pathways   written documents that detail the expected course of treatment and expected outcomes for a DRG.

cross-trained   educated in many different skills across (health care) disciplines.

crust   scab made of dried exudate.

CSF   *See* **cerebrospinal fluid**

culture   views and traditions of a particular group.

culture and sensitivity   test to determine type of microorganisms causing a disease and the specific antibiotics that can be used to treat the disease.

cupping   use of warmed glass jars to create suction on certain points of the body.

Cushing's syndrome   condition that results from an excess level of adrenal cortex hormones.

cutaneous membrane   skin.

cuticle   base of the fingernail.

CV catheter   *See* **central venous catheter**

CVA   *See* **cerebrovascular accident**

cyanosis   dusky, bluish discoloration of skin, lips, and nails caused by inadequate oxygen.

cyanotic   relating to the condition of cyanosis.

cystitis   inflammation of the urinary bladder.

cystocele   bladder hernia.

cystoscopy   procedure that uses an instrument (cytoscope) for visualization of the urinary bladder, ureter, and kidney.

D & C   *See* **dilatation and curettage**

dance therapy   use of dance to express oneself.

dangling   sitting up with legs hanging over the edge of the bed.

debilitating   weakening.

debride   to remove foreign material and necrotic tissue.

decubitus ulcer   older term for a pressure ulcer; open area that develops on the skin over a bony prominence as the result of pressure.

deep vein thrombosis (DVT)   blood clot that commonly occurs in the femoral vein, the large blood vessel in the groin.

defamation   something harmful to the good name or reputation of another person; slander.

defecation   bowel movement that expels feces.

defense mechanism psychological reaction or technique for protection against a stressful environmental situation or anxiety.

defibrillation using an electric shock to reverse disorganized activity in the heart during cardiac arrest.

degenerative joint disease (DJD) deterioration of the tissues of the joints.

dehydration excessive water loss.

delirium acute, reversible mental confusion due to illness and medical problems.

delusion false belief.

dementia progressive mental deterioration due to organic brain disease.

dendrite branch of a neuron that conducts impulses toward the cell body.

denial unconscious defense mechanism in which an occurrence or observation is refused recognition as reality in order to avoid anxiety or pain.

dentures artificial teeth.

depilatory substance used to remove body hair.

depressant drug that slows down body functions.

depressed fracture fracture in which the bone is depressed and fragments are driven inward; seen only in fractures of the skull and face.

depression morbid sadness or melancholy.

dermal ulcer pressure sore; pressure ulcer.

dermis layer of tissue that lies under the epidermis.

development gradual growth.

developmental milestones achievement of specific skills at a particular age level.

developmental tasks in psychology, normal steps in personality development.

diabetes mellitus disorder of carbohydrate metabolism.

diagnosis related groups (DRGs) method used by Medicare to determine the number of hospital days required for specific illnesses.

dialect local terminology and usage of a group's common language.

dialysis movement of dissolved materials through a semipermeable membrane, passing from an area of higher concentration to an area of lower concentration; means of cleansing waste or toxic materials from the body.

diaphoresis profuse sweating.

diarrhea a condition in which the patient has multiple, watery stools.

diastole period during which the heart muscle relaxes and the chamber fills with blood.

diastolic pressure blood pressure during period of cardiac ventricular relaxation.

diathermy treatment with heat.

digestion process of converting food into a form that can be used by the body.

digital thermometer hand-held, battery-operated device that registers temperature and displays reading as numbers.

dilatation and curettage (D & C) procedure in which the cervical canal is expanded and tissue is scraped from the lining of the uterus.

dilation stage stage of labor in which the opening to the cervix enlarges.

diplo- arranged in pairs, such as diplococci (bacteria that are arranged in groups of two).

dirty anything that has been exposed to pathogens.

disability persistent physical or mental deficit or handicap.

discharge procedure carried out as a patient leaves the facility.

disease definite, marked process of illness having characteristic symptoms.

disinfection process of eliminating pathogens from equipment and instruments.

dislocation displacement of the ends of a joint.

disorientation loss of recognition of time, place, or people.

disposable not reusable after one use.

disruption interference with the normal progress of events.

distal farthest away from a central point, such as point of attachment of muscles.

distended condition in which a body part, particularly the abdomen, becomes very large and tender.

distention the state of being stretched out (distended).

diuresis increase in output of fluids by the kidneys.

diverticula small blind pouches that form in the lining and wall of the colon.

diverticulitis inflammation of diverticula.

diverticulosis presence of many diverticula.

DJD *See* **degenerative joint disease**

DNR do not resuscitate when cardiac and respiratory arrest occur.

Doctor of Osteopathy (D.O.) a physician who receives a complete medical education similar to that of a medical doctor (MD). Additionally, the D.O. learns how to manipulate the spine for a therapeutic response in the body.

document legal record; recording observations and data about a patient's condition.

dorsal posterior or back.

dorsal lithotomy position position in which the patient is on the back with knees flexed and well separated; feet are usually placed in stirrups.

dorsal recumbent position position in which the patient is flat on the back with knees flexed and slightly separated, with feet flat on the bed.

dorsiflexion toes pointed up.

douche irrigation of the vaginal canal with medicated or normal saline solution.

drainage systematic withdrawal of fluids and discharges from wounds, sores, or body cavities.

draw sheet sheet folded under the patient, extending from above the shoulder to below the hips.

dressings gauze, film, or other synthetic substances that cover a wound, ulcer, or injury.

DRGs *See* **diagnosis related groups**

droplet precautions procedures used to prevent spread of disease by droplets in air.

droplet transmission a method of spreading infection by inhaling the droplets of a patient's respiratory secretions. The droplets do not travel more than three feet from the source patient.

duodenal resection surgical removal of a portion of small intestine (duodenum).

duodenal ulcer ulcer on the mucosa of the duodenum due to the action of gastric juice.

durable power of attorney for health care document stating that a person appointed by the patient can make health care decisions when the patient is unable to do so for himself or herself.

DVT *See* **deep vein thrombosis**

dyscrasia abnormality or disorder of the body.

dysentery infection in lower bowel.

dysmenorrhea painful menstruation.

dysphagia difficulty swallowing food and liquids.

dyspnea difficult or labored breathing.

dysuria painful voiding.

E. coli 0157:H7 a strain of *Escherichia coli* (not found in humans); a pathogen that multiplies rapidly and produces large amounts of toxins that cause serious illness and death.

ecchymosis bruising.

edema excessive accumulation of fluid in the tissues.

efface thinning of the cervix during labor.

ejaculatory duct part of the male reproductive system extending down from the seminal vesicles to the urethra.

elasticity ability to stretch.

electric bed bed operated by electricity.

electromagnetic therapy use of various forms of electrical energy to correct imbalances in the electric and magnetic fields, which are believed to cause illness and disease.

electronic thermometer battery-operated clinical thermometer that uses a probe and records the temperature on a viewing screen in a few seconds.

eloping wandering away from the health care facility.

embolus mass of undissolved material carried in the bloodstream; frequently causes obstruction of a vessel.

emergency situation requiring immediate attention or medical treatment.

emergency care medical treatment and nursing care provided to emergency patients.

Emergency Medical Services (EMS) treatment and care provided by specially trained health care personnel during emergencies.

emesis vomiting.

emotional lability unstable emotional status with frequent changes in emotions and mood.

empathy understanding how someone else feels.

emphysema chronic obstructive pulmonary disease in which the alveolar walls are destroyed.

EMS *See* **Emergency Medical Services**

enabler a device that empowers patients and assists them to function at their highest possible level.

enabling reacting to a patient in a manner that shields the patient from experiencing the full impact or consequences of his or her actions or behavior.

endocardium lining of the heart.

endocrine gland gland that secretes hormonal substances directly into the bloodstream; ductless gland.

endometrium mucous membrane lining the inner surface of the uterus.

endoscope instrument for examining the interior of the body.

enema injection of water and/or medications into the rectum and colon; used to help the bowels eliminate feces.

energy therapy alternative and complementary practices that involve working with the energy field that reportedly surrounds and penetrates the body.

engagement time when the fetus moves downward in the uterus in preparation for delivery (dropping).

enteral feeding giving nutrition through a tube inserted into the digestive tract.

enuresis bedwetting.

environmental safety adaptation of the environment to prevent incidents and injuries.

epidermis top layer of skin.

epididymis elongated, cordlike structure along the posterior border of the testes, in the ducts of which sperm is stored.

epidural catheter tube inserted into spinal area for delivery of medication.

epilepsy noninfectious disorder of the brain manifested by episodes of motor and sensory dysfunction, which may or may not be accompanied by convulsions and unconsciousness.

episiotomy incision of the perineum at the end of the second stage of labor to avoid tearing of the perineum.

epithelial cells structures that form protective coverings (epithelial tissue) and sometimes produce body fluids.

epithelial tissue structure formed from epithelial cells; protects, absorbs and produces fluids, excretes wastes.

ergonomics process of adapting the environment and using techniques and equipment to prevent worker injuries.

erythrocyte red blood cell.

eschar slough of tissue produced by burning or by a corrosive application.

essential nutrients foods required for normal growth and development and to maintain health.

estrogen hormone produced by the ovaries.

ethical standards guides to moral behavior.

ethnic relating to customs, languages, and traditions of specific groups of people.

ethnicity special groupings within a race.

etiology cause of a disease.

eustachian tube auditory tube; leads from the middle ear to the pharynx.

evaluation judgment.

eversion turning outward.

exacerbation worsening of a chronic medical condition.

exchange list list of measured foods that allows equivalent exchanges between foods within a designated food group.

excoriation superficial loss of substance, such as that produced by scratching the skin.

excrete to eliminate wastes from body.

expectorate to spit (to bring up sputum).

expiration exhalation.

exposure incident an occurrence during which there is possible personal contact with infectious material.

expressive aphasia inability to use verbal speech.

expulsion stage stage of labor and delivery during which the fetus is expelled.

extension movement by which the two ends of any jointed part are drawn away from each other.

face shield   type of personal protective equipment; protects mucous membranes of eyes, nose, and mouth from pathogens.

facility (health care)   an agency that provides health care.

Fahrenheit scale   system used in the United States and England to express temperature.

fallopian tube   *See* **oviduct**

false imprisonment   unlawfully restraining another.

family   group of persons (usually related by blood or marriage) with common values and traditions.

fasting   not eating.

fat   nutrient used to store energy.

fecal impaction   the most serious form of constipation, in which stool is retained in the rectum, where water is absorbed. Over time, the stool becomes hard and dry, and the patient is unable to pass it.

fecal material   another term for feces, stool, or solid body waste (bowel movement or BM). Normally brown, but color can be affected by certain foods, medications, and diseases. A BM is normally soft and formed.

feces   stool; semisolid waste eliminated from the body.

fetal monitor   device used to register activity and health status of the unborn fetus during labor.

fetoscopy   examination of the fetus while in the uterus.

fetus   child in the uterus from the third month to birth.

fibromyalgia   a common pain syndrome for which there is no known cause.

fingerstick blood sugar (FSBS)   a method of checking blood sugar by collecting a sample of capillary blood with a lancet.

first aid   emergency care and treatment of an injured person before complete medical and surgical care can be secured.

fistula   abnormal communication between two hollow organs or between a hollow organ and the exterior.

flaccid paralysis   loss of muscle tone and absence of tendon reflexes.

flagged   marked in a special way to call attention to it.

flatulence   excessive gas in the stomach and intestines.

flatus   gas or air in the stomach or intestines; air or gas expelled by way of any body opening.

flexion   decreasing the angle between two bones.

flora   normal population of organisms found in a given area.

flow sheet   clinical record of ongoing patient care and progress.

fluid balance   balance between fluid intake and fluid output.

Foley catheter   indwelling catheter placed in the urinary bladder to remove urine continuously.

fomite   any object contaminated with germs and thus able to transmit disease.

foot drop   tightening of leg muscles that causes the foot to point downward.

footboard   appliance placed at the foot of the bed so the feet rest firmly against it and are kept at right angles to the legs.

force fluids   notation meaning that the patient must be encouraged to take as much fluid as possible.

foreskin   prepuce; loose tissue covering the penis and clitoris.

foster parent   parent figure assigned by an agency.

Fowler's position   position in which the patient lies on the back with backrest elevated 45 to 60 degrees.

fracture   break in the continuity of bone.

friction   rubbing of the skin against another surface, such as bed linen.

FSBS   *See* **fingerstick blood sugar**

full liquid diet   diet consisting of all types of fluids.

full weight-bearing   able to stand on both legs.

fundus   portion of the uterus above the point of entrance of the oviducts.

fungus (plural fungi)   class of organisms to which molds and yeasts belong.

fusion   combination into a single unit.

gait   manner of walking.

gait belt   belt placed around the patient's waist to assist in ambulation.

gait training   teaching the patient to walk.

gastrectomy   surgical removal of part or all of the stomach.

gastric resection   surgical removal of part of the stomach.

gastric ulcer   erosion of the lining of the stomach.

gastroscopy   procedure to examine the inside of the stomach, using a scope for visualization.

gastrostomy feeding   nutrition given through a tube inserted into the stomach through the abdominal wall.

gatch bed   bed fitted with a jointed backrest and knee rest; patient can be raised to a sitting position and kept in that position by adjusting the bed.

general anesthetic   medication that induces a state of unconsciousness and reduces or eliminates ability to feel pain.

generalized tonic-clonic seizures   another name for grand mal seizures.

genetic   pertaining to or carried by a gene or genes.

genitalia   reproductive organs.

geriatric   relating to age or the elderly.

geriatrics   care of the elderly.

gestational age   age of development of a new individual within the uterus from conception to birth.

Glasgow Coma Scale   a system used to monitor neurologic problems after trauma, stroke, and other illnesses and injuries; uses a point score to rank the patient's responses to stimuli.

glaucoma   a condition in which the pressure is increased within the eye. Untreated, it will lead to blindness.

global aphasia   loss of all language ability.

glomerulus   blood vessels that branch to form a ball of capillaries in the cortex of the kidney.

glucagon   hormone produced by pancreas that increases blood sugar level.

glucose   simple sugar; also called *dextrose*.

glycogen   polysaccharide that is the chief carbohydrate storage material.

glycosuria   sugar in the urine.

goal   an outcome resulting from implementation of a care plan.

goggles   type of personal protective equipment used with standard precautions to protect the eyes.

gonads   reproductive organs; ovaries and testes.

gonorrhea   sexually transmitted disease that causes an acute inflammation.

gout   a metabolic disease that results in increased uric acid deposits in the joints, which causes pain.

graduate   container marked for milliliters, used to measure liquids.

graft   body tissue used for transplantation.

grand mal seizure   major epileptic seizure attended by loss of consciousness and convulsive movements.

greenstick fracture   breaking of a bone on one side only; most often seen in children.

grievance   situation in which a consumer feels there are grounds for complaint.

growth   physical changes that take place in body during development.

guided imagery   a practice in which the patient focuses on and visualizes positive changes, so as to cause the changes to occur.

halitosis   bad breath.

handicap   inability of person to fulfill a normal role due to disability.

hand-over-hand technique   method in which an instructor or caregiver places his or her hand over the hand of a learner or patient to guide an activity.

hantavirus   a virus spread by contact with rodents (rats and mice) or their excretions; causes serious illness or death.

harvest   to remove donor organs.

head-tilt, chin-lift maneuver   a procedure used to open a patient's airway if no neck injury is suspected; pressure is placed on the forehead while the jaw is lifted up.

health   state of physical, mental, and social well-being.

health care consumer   person requiring health care services.

health maintenance organization (HMO)   one type of prepaid health insurance provider.

heart block   condition in which conduction of electrical impulses from atrium to ventricles is impaired and pumping action of heart is slowed down (change in rhythm of heart).

Heimlich maneuver   procedure that uses abdominal thrusts to relieve obstruction in the trachea.

hematoma   a localized mass of blood that is confined to one area.

hematuria   blood in the urine.

hemianopsia   visual impairment due to stroke; affects one-half of visual field in one or both eyes.

hemiplegia   paralysis on one side of the body.

hemodialysis   method for circulating blood through semipermeable membranes to remove liquid body wastes.

hemoptysis   expectoration of blood.

hemorrhage   escape of blood from blood vessels.

hemorrhoids   varicose veins in the rectum.

HEPA   *See* **high efficiency particulate air respirator**

hepatitis   inflammation of the liver.

herbal therapy   use of herbs to treat pain and illness.

herbs   medicines made from plants.

hernia   protrusion or projection of a stomach organ through the wall or cavity that normally contains it.

herniorrhaphy   surgical operation for hernia.

herpes simplex II   an acute infectious viral disease.

heterosexuality   sexual attraction between persons of opposite genders.

high efficiency particulate air (HEPA) respirator   a mask used by health care workers that prevents the spread of airborne infection.

high Fowler's position   position in which backrest of bed is elevated to 90 degrees, with patient on back.

HIV   *See* **human immunodeficiency virus**

HMO   *See* **health maintenance organization**

holistic care   practices that consider the whole person, including mind, body, and spirit.

home health assistant   nursing assistant who practices under supervision in a client's home.

homemaker aide   person hired to perform light housekeeping tasks in a client's home.

homemaker assistant   person who provides home management help to a client in the client's home.

homeopathy   alternative medicine system that uses a wide range of natural (plant and mineral) substances to stimulate the body's immune system to fight disease.

homosexuality   sexual attraction between persons of the same gender.

hormone   secretion of endocrine gland; substance produced by an endocrine gland.

hospice   special facility or arrangement to provide care of terminally ill persons.

hospice care   health care for persons who are dying.

hospital   facility for care of the sick or injured.

host   animal or plant that harbors another organism.

human immunodeficiency virus (HIV)   virus that causes acquired immune deficiency disease (AIDS).

humidifier   a water bottle that moistens oxygen for comfort and prevents drying of the mucous membranes in the nose, mouth, and lungs; used when oxygen is administered at flow rates of 5 liters a minute and over.

hydrochloric acid   acid produced by the stomach.

hydronephrosis   increased pressure of urine on the kidney cells that results in their destruction.

hyperalimentation   technique in which high-density nutrients are introduced into a large vein.

hypercalcemia   excess calcium in the bloodstream.

hyperglycemia   excessive level of blood sugar.

hypersecretion   excessive secretion.

hypersensitivity   state of altered reactivity in which the body reacts to a foreign agent more strongly than normal or in an abnormal way.

hypersomnia   disorder characterized by sleeping very late in the morning and napping during the day; causes can be physical or psychological.

hypertension   high blood pressure.

hyperthyroidism   excessive functioning of the thyroid gland.

hypertrophy   increase in the size of an organ or structure that does not involve tumor formation.

hypnotherapy   practice used to create an altered state of consciousness in which the patient is more open to suggestion.

hypoallergenic tape   tape that reduces the incidence of skin reactions in patients who are allergic to adhesive backing.

hypochondriasis   abnormal concern about one's health.

hypoglycemia   abnormally low level of sugar in the blood.

hyposecretion   less than normal production of secretions.

hypotension low blood pressure.

hypothermia greatly reduced temperature.

hypothermia-hyperthermia blanket a fluid-filled blanket, the temperature of which can be raised or lowered.

hypothyroidism condition due to deficiency of thyroid secretion, resulting in a lower basal metabolism.

hypoxemia a condition in which there is insufficient oxygen in the blood.

hypoxia lack of adequate oxygen supply.

hysterectomy surgical removal of the uterus.

ice bag type of cold treatment.

IDDM *See* **insulin-dependent diabetes mellitus**

ileostomy incision in the ileum.

immune response response of the body to elements recognized as nonself, with the production of antibodies and rejection of the foreign material.

immunity ability to fight off infectious disease; state of being protected from a disease.

immunization process of making a person more resistant to an infectious agent.

immunosuppression condition in which the immune system is unable to respond to the challenge of infectious disease.

immunotherapy a cancer treatment that alters the patient's immune response to eliminate the cancer.

impacted fracture a fracture that occurs when the fragment from one bone is wedged into another bone.

impaction *See* **fecal impaction**

implementation putting into effect.

incarcerated (strangulated) hernia abnormal constriction of part of the intestinal tract that has herniated.

incentive spirometer apparatus used to encourage better ventilation.

incident an occurrence or event that interrupts normal procedures or causes a crisis.

incident report summary of information about an incident.

incomplete fracture a partial break in a bone.

increment amount of increase in measurements.

incubation development of bacteria in body between time of exposure and onset of signs and symptoms.

indwelling catheter Foley catheter that remains in the patient's bladder to drain urine.

infarction death of tissue.

infection invasion and multiplication of any organism and the damage this causes in the body.

infectious capable of transmitting disease.

inferior below another part.

infiltration passage of fluid into the tissues surrounding a vein that occurs when an IV needle or catheter comes out of the vein.

inflammation a localized protective reaction of tissue to irritation, injury, or infection; characterized by pain, redness, swelling, and sometimes loss of function.

informed consent permission given after full disclosure of the facts.

initiative action of taking the first step or initial action.

insertion distal point of attachment of skeletal muscle.

insomnia a chronic deprivation of quality or quantity of sleep because sleep is ended or interrupted prematurely.

inspiration drawing of air into the lungs; inhalation.

insulin active antidiabetic hormone secreted by the islets of Langerhans in the pancreas.

insulin-dependent diabetes mellitus (IDDM) form of diabetes mellitus that requires insulin administration as part of the therapy.

intake and output (I&O) recording of the amount of fluid ingested and the amount of fluid expelled by a patient.

integrative (integrated) health care using both mainstream medical treatments and CAM therapies to treat a patient.

integument the skin.

intention tremor involuntary movement of muscles (particularly hands) that increases when the patient attempts to use the muscles.

interdisciplinary health care team group of professionals from different health care disciplines who each contribute their expertise to the care of a single patient.

intermediate care health care provided to persons with medically stable conditions.

intermittent care care given periodically, at intervals.

interpersonal relationships how people interact with each other.

intervention actions that influence the eventual outcome of a situation.

intimacy feelings of closeness and familiarity.

intracranial pressure pressure exerted within the cranium.

intravenous (IV) infusion nourishment given through a sterile tube into a vein.

intravenous pyelogram (IVP) x-ray of urinary tract following injection of dye into vein.

invasion of privacy taking liberties with the person or personal rights of another.

invasive characterized by invading (penetrating into) or spreading.

inversion turning inward.

involuntary muscle muscle not under conscious control, mainly smooth muscle.

involuntary seclusion separation of patient from other patients and people, against the patient's will.

involution reduction in the size of the uterus following delivery.

I&O *See* **intake and output**

iodine element needed for proper function of the thyroid gland.

iris colored portion of the eye.

ischemia deficient blood supply to body tissues.

ischemic having inadequate blood flow to an area.

islets of Langerhans cells in the pancreas that produce insulin.

isolation place where a patient with easily transmitted disease is separated from others.

isolation technique special procedures carried out to prevent the spread of infectious organisms from an infected person.

isolation unit used for patients with communicable illness, for protection of other patients, staff, and visitors.

isolette environmentally controlled unit used to house a newborn infant.

IVP *See* **intravenous pyelogram**

jaw-thrust maneuver a method of opening the airway of patients with known or suspected neck injuries; involves pushing the jaw forward and upward.

JCAHO   *See* **Joint Commission for Accreditation of Healthcare Organizations**

job interview   discussion between employer and potential employee.

Joint Commission for Accreditation of Health Care Organizations (JCAHO)   an organization that inspects and accredits health care agencies that meet high quality standards.

Kaposi's sarcoma   a cancer that usually occurs in persons with HIV disease and men over 60 years of age.

Kardex   type of file in which nursing care plans are kept.

Kelly   a special clamp used to close tubes quickly.

kidney   glandular, bean-shaped organ, purplish-brown in color, situated in back of the abdominal cavity, one on each side of the spinal column; excretes waste matter in the form of urine.

kilogram   metric unit of weight measurement, equal to 1,000 grams or 2.2 pounds.

knee-chest position   position in which the patient is on the abdomen with knees drawn up toward the abdomen and legs separated; arms are brought up and flexed on either side of the head, which is turned to one side.

labia majora   two large, hair-covered, liplike structures that are part of the vulva.

labia minora   two hairless, liplike structures found beneath the labia majora.

labor   physiologic process by which the fetus is expelled from the uterus at term.

laceration   accidental break in skin, an injury.

lacrimal gland   produces tears.

lactation   secretion of milk.

laminectomy   surgical excision of the rear part of one or more vertebrae, usually to remove a herniated disk or lesion.

lancet   a tiny needle.

larynx   organ located at upper end of trachea; part of airway and organ of voice (voice box).

lateral   away from the midline.

legal custody   condition of having the responsibility for another person (including the right to consent to hospitalization and to give permission for procedures).

legal guardian   person who has the legal right to make decisions for another person.

legal standards   guides to lawful behavior.

lesions   abnormal changes in tissue formation.

leukemia   malignant disease of the blood-forming organs, characterized by abnormal proliferation and distortion of the leukocytes in the blood and bone marrow.

leukocyte   white blood cell.

leukorrhea   white vaginal discharge.

Lhermitte's sign   sharp, electrical-type sensation felt down spine when head is flexed; found in patients with multiple sclerosis.

liable   legally responsible.

libel   any written defamatory statement.

license   a state permit allowing a facility to operate.

licensed practical nurse (LPN); licensed vocational nurse (LVN)   graduate of a one-year certificate program, who must pass a state exam before being permitted to practice nursing.

life-sustaining treatment   treatment given to a critically ill or injured patient to maintain life and prevent death.

ligament   band of fibrous tissue that holds joints together.

light therapy   treatment in which patients are exposed to special lights covered with a plastic screen to block ultraviolet rays; used to treat mood and sleep disorders, jet lag, and depression.

lithotripsy   the crushing of calculi such as kidney stones.

living will   document describing the wishes of a terminally ill person, relating to health care.

local anesthetic   substance that blocks pain receptors or sensation in a specific area.

lochia   discharge from the uterus of blood, mucus, and tissue during the puerperal period.

long-term care   health care given to a person in a facility or the person's home for an extended period of time.

LPN   *See* **licensed practical nurse**

lumpectomy   excision of abnormal tissue, such as a "lump" in the breast.

LVN   *See* **licensed vocational nurse**

lymph   fluid found in lymphatic vessels.

lymphatic vessel   vessel that conveys electrolytes, water, and proteins.

macular degeneration   vision impairment due to damage to the macula located at the back of the eye, generally related to aging.

macule   flat, discolored spot on the skin.

maladaptive behavior   inappropriate reaction due to mental breakdown.

malignant   cancerous.

malodorous   having a bad or foul odor.

malpractice   improper, negligent, or unethical conduct that results in harm, injury, or loss to a patient.

mammogram   x-ray examination of the breasts.

managed care   methods used by insurance companies to reduce health care costs.

massage therapy   rubbing various areas of the body to stimulate circulation, promote relaxation, and provide pain relief. Massage increases feelings of well-being and reduces stress and fatigue.

mastectomy   excision of the breast.

masturbation   sexually stimulating self.

Material Safety Data Sheet (MSDS)   information provided by manufacturers about hazardous products; includes health hazards, safe use guidelines, and emergency procedures for chemical exposure.

mechanical lift   apparatus used to assist in lifting and transferring a patient.

mechanically altered diet   diet in which the consistency and texture of food are modified, making it easier to chew and swallow.

mechanical soft diet   a diet that includes ground meats; served to patients with no teeth, or those with serious dental problems.

medial   close to the midline of the body or structure.

Medicaid   federal- and state-funded program that pays medical expenses for those whose income is below a certain level.

medical asepsis   procedures followed to keep germs from being spread from one person to another.

medical chart   patient record containing all information about that patient.

medical diagnosis   name of disease; determination made by a physician.

Medicare   federal program that assists persons over 65 years of age with hospital and medical costs.

meditation   calming and quieting the mind by focusing attention.

medulla   forms part of the brain stem; also, the middle area of the kidney.

membranes   tissue sheets that line the body cavities.

memo   brief, written communication to relay information.

meninges   three-layered serous membranes covering the brain and spinal cord.

meningitis   inflammation of the meninges.

menopause   period when ovaries stop functioning and menstruation ceases; female climacteric.

menorrhagia   excessive bleeding during menstruation.

menstruation   loss of an unneeded part of the endometrium following the release of an ovum and lack of conception.

mental illness   behavioral maladaptations.

metabolism   sum total of the physical and chemical processes and reactions taking place in the body.

metastasis   spreading of cancer to other body parts or locations.

metastasize   to spread (cancer) to other body parts.

methicillin-resistant *Staphylococcus aureus* **(MRSA)**   bacteria resistant to most antibiotics.

metrorrhagia   abnormal discharge from the uterus.

MI   *See* **myocardial infarction**

microbe   tiny organism that can be seen only with a microscope.

microorganism   tiny organism that can be seen only with a microscope, particularly bacteria.

mind-body therapy   practices that use various techniques to enhance the mind's ability to affect bodily function and symptoms.

mineral   inorganic chemical compound found in nature; many minerals are important in building body tissues and regulating body fluids.

mitered corner   one type of corner used in making a facility bed.

mites   microscopic organisms that cannot be seen with the naked eye.

mobility   ability to move or to be moved easily from place to place.

mobility skills   ability to move about in bed, out of bed, and walking.

modalities   forms of treatment or uses of therapeutic agents or regimens.

mold   organism in fungus family.

Montgomery straps   long strips of adhesive attached to the skin on either side of a wound, then tied to hold a dressing in place.

mores   customs of ethnic groups.

moribund   dying.

movement therapy   treatment that combines nonaerobic exercise and breath control to give patients an awareness of how the body moves; alters posture and motion to reduce pain and stress.

moxibustion   burning of herbal substances on or near the body.

MRSA   *See* **methicillin-resistant** *Staphylococcus aureus*

MS   *See* **multiple sclerosis**

MSDS   *See* **Material Safety Data Sheet**

mucous membrane   epithelial tissue that produces fluid called mucus; lines body cavities that open to the outside of the body.

mucus   secretion of mucous membranes; thick, sticky fluid.

multiple sclerosis (MS)   disease characterized by hardened patches scattered throughout the brain and spinal cord that interfere with the nerves in those areas.

multisensory stimulation   intense stimulation of sight, sound, touch, smell, pressure, pain, and touch to help the patient to awaken and use previously unused portions of the brain.

muscle cells   form muscle tissue; have ability to shorten or lengthen and to change their shape and the position of parts to which they are attached.

muscle tissue   tissue that has the ability to shorten and lengthen.

music therapy   therapeutic use of music to address physical, psychological, or cognitive needs and/or social functioning.

myocardial infarction (MI)   formation of an infarct in the heart muscle due to interruption of the blood supply to the area.

myocardium   heart muscle.

N95 respirator   mask with small, tightly woven pores that protects the wearer from airborne infection.

NACEP   *See* **Nurse Aide Competency Evaluation Program**

narcolepsy   condition in which the patient has sudden, uncontrollable, unpredictable urges to fall asleep during daytime hours.

narcotic   drug that relieves pain and produces sleep.

nasal cannula   tubing inserted into nostrils to administer oxygen.

nasogastric feeding (NG feeding)   nourishment given through a tube inserted through the nose into the stomach.

nasogastric (NG) tube   soft rubber or plastic tube that is inserted through a nostril into the stomach.

National Institute of Occupational Safety and Health (NIOSH)   federal agency responsible for conducting research and making recommendations for the prevention of work-related disease and injury.

naturopathic medicine   a medical system that focuses on whole-person wellness, emphasizing prevention and self-care. The doctor looks for the cause of illness, rather than strictly treating symptoms.

nebulizer   device used to apply a liquid in the form of a fine spray or mist; may be used to administer medication.

necrosis   tissue death.

neglect   failing to provide services to patients to prevent physical harm or mental anguish.

negligence   failure to exercise the degree of care considered reasonable under the circumstances, resulting in an unintended injury to a patient. Negligence is carelessness that may be caused by hurrying or not focusing on the task at hand.

neonate   newborn baby.

neoplasm   new growth; tumor.

nephritis   inflammation of the kidney.

nephron   microscopic kidney unit that produces urine.

nerve   bundle of nerve processes (axons and dendrites) that are held together by connective tissue.

nerve cells   carry electrical messages to and from different parts of body.

nervous tissue highly specialized tissue capable of conducting nerve impulses.

networking communication between individuals with a common interest or goal.

neuron cell of the nervous system.

neurotransmitter chemical compound that transmits a nervous impulse across cells at a synapse.

NG *See* **nasogastric feeding; nasogastric tube**

NIDDM *See* **non–insulin-dependent diabetes mellitus**

NIOSH *See* **National Institute of Occupational Safety and Health**

no-code order an order not to resuscitate a patient.

nodule a small, knotlike protrusion; a small mass of tissue.

non–insulin-dependent diabetes mellitus (NIDDM) diabetes controlled by diet and sometimes oral medication, for which insulin is not needed.

noninvasive remaining localized and not spreading; not penetrating.

nonpathogen microorganism that does not produce disease.

nonrapid eye movement (NREM) sleep the phase that accounts for 75% of the sleep cycle, in which sleep progresses from light to deep.

nonverbal communication communication transmitted without spoken words, such as by facial expression and body language.

nonweight-bearing unable to stand or walk on one or both legs.

nosocomial pertaining to or originating in a facility.

nosocomial infection infection acquired in a facility.

NPO nothing by mouth.

nucleoplasty a minimally invasive surgical procedure to remove tissue from herniated discs.

Nurse Aide Competency Evaluation Program (NACEP) test taken by the nursing assistant which, when passed successfully, entitles the nursing assistant to certification.

nurse's notes section of medical record in which nursing staff records procedures, medications, and observations.

nursing assistant person who helps, under supervision, with the care of the sick and infirm.

nursing diagnosis statement of a patient's problems leading to nursing interventions.

nursing process framework for nursing action.

nursing team members of the nursing staff who provide patient care.

nutrient nourishing substance or food.

nutrition process by which the body uses food for growth and repair and to maintain health.

nutrition therapy evaluation and modification on the patient's diet and nutrient intake to promote optimal nutrition for health, wellness, and healing.

nystagmus constant involuntary movement of the eyeball.

obese overweight.

objective observation observation made through the senses of the observer.

oblique fracture *See* **closed fracture**

OBRA *See* **Omnibus Budget Reconciliation Act**

observation noticing something.

obstetric, obstetrical pertaining to pregnancy, labor, and delivery.

obstruction blockage in a passageway.

occult blood small quantity of blood that can be detected only by microscope or chemical means.

occupational exposure coming into contact with infectious materials during the performance of a person's job.

Occupational Safety and Health Administration (OSHA) federal agency that makes and enforces regulations to protect workers.

occupational therapy therapeutic use of work and activities to help patients regain self-care skills.

OJD *See* **osteoarthritic joint disease**

Omnibus Budget Reconciliation Act (OBRA) law that regulates the education and certification of nursing assistants in acute care and long-term care facilities.

OMT *See* **osteopathic manipulative treatment**

oncology study of cancer.

oophorectomy surgical excision of an ovary.

open bed bed with top bedding fanfolded to bottom, ready for occupancy.

open (compound) fracture fracture in which part of the broken bone protrudes through the skin.

open reduction/internal fixation (ORIF) surgical procedure to reduce a fractured bone. The skin is opened and the fracture realigned and held in place by screws, plates, and pins.

operative pertaining to an operation.

ophthalmoscope instrument for examining the eyes.

oral hygiene care of the mouth and teeth.

oral report verbal report.

orchiectomy excision of one or both of the testes.

organ any part of the body that carries out a specific function or functions, such as the heart.

organism any living thing, plant or animal.

organizational chart guide for communication; spells out lines of authority.

ORIF *See* **open reduction/internal fixation**

orifice body opening such as the nose or mouth.

origin proximal point of attachment to skeletal muscle.

orthopedic concerning the prevention or correction of deformities (orthopedics).

orthopnea need to sit upright in order to breathe without difficulty.

orthopneic position a position in which the patient must sit up to breathe comfortably. The patient sits as upright as possible and leans slightly forward, supporting herself with the forearms.

orthotic device (orthosis) a device that restores or improves function and prevents deformity.

OSHA *See* **Occupational Safety and Health Administration**

ossicles any small bones, such as one of the three bones in the ear.

osteoarthritic joint disease (OJD) degenerative disease of joints.

osteopathic manipulative treatment (OMT) a passive, thrusting motion used to restore normal body movement and enhance blood and oxygen flow; used in combination with regular medical treatment.

osteoporosis a metabolic disorder of the bones in which bone mass is lost, causing them to appear porous and spongy; affected bones are at very high risk for fracture.

ostomy   suffix meaning "to create a new opening"; for example, colostomy.

otitis media   inflamed condition of the middle part of the ear.

otosclerosis   formation of bone in the inner ear that causes the ossicles to become fixed.

otoscope   instrument used to examine the ear.

ovaries (singular **ovary**)   endocrine glands located in the female pelvis; female gonads.

oviduct   tube in the body between the ovary and the uterus through which an ovum travels; part of the female reproductive system.

ovulation   lunar monthly ripening and discharge of an ovum from the cortex of the ovary.

ovum (plural **ova**)   female egg.

oxygen   gas that is essential to cellular metabolism and life.

oxygen concentrator   device that removes impurities from room air and concentrates oxygen to be delivered to a patient.

oxygen mask   device to administer oxygen through nose and mouth; placed over patient's face.

oxygenation   movement of oxygen from the lungs into the blood, which carries the oxygen to body cells.

pacemaker   artificial device placed in the body to regulate the heartbeat.

PACU   *See* **postanesthesia care unit**

pain   a state of discomfort; a warning signal that something is wrong.

palliative care   comfort care; care that treats the symptoms of discomfort, but not the underlying disease.

pallor   less color than normal for the skin.

panhysterectomy   removal of the entire uterus.

Pap smear   simple test used to detect cancer of the cervix.

papule   solid, elevated lesion of the skin.

PAR   *See* **post-anesthesia recovery**

paralysis   loss or impairment of the ability to move parts of the body.

paranoia   state in which one has delusions of persecution and/or grandeur.

paraplegia   paralysis of the lower portion of the body and of both legs.

parasite   organism that lives within, upon, or at the expense of another organism known as the *host*.

parathormone   hormone produced by parathyroid glands that regulates calcium and phosphorus levels in the blood.

parathyroid glands   two pairs of endocrine glands situated on posterior of thyroid gland; produce the hormone parathormone.

paresis   weakness of an extremity.

Parkinson's disease   neurological disorder due to deficiency of dopamine, a neurotransmitter; progressive disease characterized by stiffness of muscles and tremors.

partial weight-bearing   unable to bear full weight on one or both legs.

partners in practice   a method of providing care in which a registered nurse works with a nursing assistant as a team.

PASS   acronym for fire extinguisher use meaning: *P*ull the pin; *A*im the nozzle; *S*queeze the handle; *S*weep back and forth.

pathogen   microorganism or other agent capable of producing a disease.

pathologic fracture   fracture in a diseased bone that occurs as a result of osteoporosis, a tumor, or cancer.

pathology   disease.

patient   person who needs care; *see also* **resident** and **client**.

patient-controlled analgesia (PCA)   administration of pain-relieving medication controlled by the patient, using a special device; amount of medication to be delivered is preset by the nurse.

patient focused care   attention given to mental, physical, and emotional aspects of a person's being.

Patient's Bill of Rights   document developed by the American Hospital Association that describes the basic rights to which a patient is entitled.

PCA   *See* **patient-controlled analgesia**

pediatric   patient from birth to 18 years of age.

pediculosis   body lice; parasites that feed on humans and animals.

pelvic belt traction   form of traction in which a belt that is secured around a patient's hips is attached to weights.

pelvic inflammatory disease (PID)   inflammation of the pelvic organs.

pelvis   lower portion of the trunk of the body; basin-shaped area bounded by the hip bones, the sacrum, and the coccyx.

penis   male organ of copulation and urinary elimination.

pepsin   enzyme produced in the stomach that begins protein digestion.

perceptual deficit   inability to reason, think systematically, make judgments, or use common items.

percussion hammer   instrument used to test reflexes.

pericardium   membrane that surrounds the heart.

perineal care   cleansing of genital and rectal areas.

perineum   in the male, the area between the anus and the scrotum; in the female, the area between the anus and the vagina.

perioperative   occurring in association with an operative procedure.

peripheral   pertaining to the outside or outer part.

peripheral intravenous central catheter (PICC)   intravenous line inserted into a vein in the arm and threaded through to a larger vein.

peristalsis   progressive, wavelike movement that occurs involuntarily in hollow tubes of the body, especially the alimentary canal.

peritoneal dialysis   removal of liquid waste by washing chemicals through the abdominal cavity.

peritoneum   serous membrane that lines the walls of the abdominal and pelvic cavities.

personal protective equipment (PPE)   equipment such as waterproof gowns, masks, gloves, goggles, and other equipment needed to protect a person from infectious material.

personal space   physical closeness that a person is comfortable with during interactions with others.

personality   sum of the behavior, attitudes, and character traits of an individual.

petechiae   small purplish spots on the body surface, caused by minute hemorrhages.

petit mal seizure   type of epileptic attack that is generally short in nature; "absence" attack.

PFR95 respirator   mask with very tiny pores that prevents the wearer from breathing in infectious airborne microorganisms.

phagocyte   white blood cell that destroys substances such as bacteria, protozoa, and cells.

phantom pain   pain experienced in a body part that has been removed from the body, as if the part were still attached.

pharynx   muscular, membranous tube between mouth and esophagus; throat.

phlebitis   inflammation of a vein.

physiatrist   medical doctor specializing in rehabilitation.

physical abuse   mistreatment by hitting or other physical contact.

physical restraint   device used to prevent a patient from moving about or having access to his or her own body.

physical therapy   structured exercise that assists patients to regain mobility skills.

physiology   the science that deals with the functioning of living organisms.

PICC   *See* **peripheral intravenous central catheter**

PID   *See* **pelvic inflammatory disease**

piggyback   procedure used to administer medication through a vein.

pigmentation   coloration of an area by pigment.

pineal body   pea-sized endocrine gland located in the brain.

pituitary gland   "master" endocrine gland located in brain at base of skull (attached to hypothalamus); produces hormones that regulate growth and reproduction.

pivot   to twist or turn in a swiveling motion.

placenta   structure within the womb through which the unborn child is nourished; the afterbirth.

placental stage   period of the delivery process during which the afterbirth is expelled from the uterus.

planning   establishing possible solutions for a patient's problems (as determined by nursing diagnoses).

plantar flexion   extending the foot in a downward movement.

plasma   liquid portion of blood.

pleura   membranes that surround the lungs.

pleural effusion   fluid that collects around the lungs in patients who have cancer.

PM care   care given to prepare a patient for sleep.

pneumonia   inflammation and infection of the lungs.

pocket mask   a barrier device used for providing "mouth"-to-mouth resuscitation that prevents the patient's exhaled air and secretions from entering the caregiver's mouth.

polydipsia   excessive thirst.

polyphagia   excessive ingestion of food.

polyuria   excessive excretion of urine.

port   opening.

portal of entry   area of body through which microbes enter and cause disease.

portal of exit   area of body through which disease-producing organisms leave the body.

position sense   ability to know one's position in space, including how extremities are positioned.

postanesthesia care unit (PACU)   room where patients receive immediate care following surgery.

post-anesthesia recovery (PAR)   area where patients are taken after surgery to recover from anesthesia.

posterior   back or dorsal.

postmortem   after death.

postmortem care   care given to the body after death.

postoperative   after surgery.

postpartum   after parturition; after birth.

post polio syndrome (PPS)   a neurologic disorder marked by increased weakness and/or abnormal muscle fatigue in persons who had paralytic polio many years earlier.

postural support   device used as an enabler that maintains body position and alignment.

potentially infectious material   material or equipment that could be a source of disease-producing organisms.

pound   unit of measurement of weight, equivalent to 16 ounces or 453.6 grams.

PPE   *See* **personal protective equipment**

PPS   *See* **post polio syndrome**

prayer   a connection with a person's higher power.

preadolescence   years between the ages of 12 and 14.

predisposing factor   condition that contributes to the development of disease.

prefix   word part that is placed before a word root that changes or modifies the meaning of the word root.

prenatal   before birth.

preoperative   period before surgery.

pressure ulcer   ulceration due to ischemia; pressure sore.

private room   room in a health care facility that contains only one patient at a time.

probe   as used in this text, a long, slender part of an instrument; that portion of the electronic or tympanic thermometer placed into the patient.

procedure   series of steps outlining how and in what order and manner to do something.

proctoscopy   inspection of the rectum using a proctoscope.

professional boundaries   limits on how a health care worker interacts with patients.

progesterone   hormone produced by female ovaries.

prognosis   probable outcome of a disease or injury.

projection   unconscious defense mechanism by which an individual denies his or her own emotionally unacceptable traits and sees them as belonging to another.

pronation   placing or lying in a face-downward position; as applied to the hand, indicates the palms facing backward.

prone   position in which the patient is on the abdomen, spine straight, legs extended, and arms flexed on either side of the head.

prostatectomy   removal of all or part of the prostate gland.

prostate gland   gland of male reproductive system that surrounds the neck of the urinary bladder and the beginning of the urethra.

prosthesis   artificial substitute for a missing body part, such as dentures, hand, leg.

protein   basic material of every body cell; an essential nutrient.

protocol   standards of procedure and care developed for preparation of a patient for diagnostic tests.

protozoan (plural **protozoa**)   microscopic unicellular organism.

proximal   closest to the point of attachment.

pseudomembranous colitis   disease caused by overgrowth of *Clostridium difficile*, often after antibiotic therapy has depleted normal bowel flora; results in severe diarrhea and may cause dehydration.

psychiatric   relating to mental illness.

psychological abuse   mistreatment by threatening, belittling, or otherwise causing mental or emotional harm or upset.

puberty   condition or period of becoming capable of sexual reproduction.

pubic   concerning the pubes.

pulmonary embolism   blood clot in the lungs.

pulse   wave of blood pressure exerted against the walls of the arteries in response to ventricular contraction.

pulse deficit   difference between contractions of the heart and pulse expansions of the radial artery.

pulse oximetry   procedure for measuring level of oxygen in arterial blood.

pulse pressure   difference between the systolic and diastolic pressures.

pupil   circular opening in the center of the iris; regulates light entering the eye.

pureed diet   diet in which foods are blended with gravy or liquid until they are the consistency of pudding.

push fluids   to encourage a patient to drink additional fluids.

pustule   circumscribed, pus-containing lesion of the skin.

pyelogram   *See* **intravenous pyelogram (IVP)**

pyloric sphincter   muscle at the exit point of the pylorus.

QA   *See* **quality assurance**

qigong   physical and mental activities to teach the patient to channel the *chi* (life force or energy), thereby improving health.

quadrant   one of the four imaginary sections of the surface of the abdomen.

quadriplegia   paralysis of all four limbs.

quality assurance (QA)   an internal review done by facility staff to identify problems and find solutions for improvement.

quickening   first movement of the fetus in the uterus that is felt by the mother.

race   classification of people according to shared physical characteristics.

RACE   acronym relating to fire emergency procedure, meaning: *R*emove patient from danger; *A*ctivate alarm; *C*ontain fire; *E*xtinguish fire.

radial deviation   wrists are turned toward the thumb side.

radial pulse   pulse that can be measured by palpating the radial artery.

radiation therapy   treatment of cancer with radiation.

radical mastectomy   removal of entire breast and adjacent lymph nodes.

rales   abnormal respiratory sound heard in auscultation of the chest.

range-of-motion (ROM) exercises   series of exercises specifically designed to move each joint through its full range.

rapid eye movement (REM) sleep   the part of the sleep cycle in which dreams occur.

rate   valuation based on comparison with a standard.

RCP   *See* **respiratory care practitioner**

reaction formation   repressing the reality of an anxiety-producing situation; the individual exhibits behaviors that are exactly opposite to the real feelings.

reality orientation   techniques used to help a person remain oriented to environment, time, and self.

receptive aphasia   inability to understand written or spoken language.

recovery position   a modified lateral position used when the patient is recovering from certain emergencies, such as unconsciousness.

recovery room   location where surgical patients are taken after surgery; they return to their rooms when their conditions stabilize.

rectocele   protrusion of part of the rectum into the vagina.

references   in a résumé, statements about abilities and characteristics; persons who give such statements.

reflex   activity performed without conscious thought.

reflexology   stimulating reflex areas in the hands and feet to reduce stress, stabilize body functions, and correct health problems.

registered nurse (RN)   specially educated person who is licensed to plan and direct the nursing care of patients.

regress   to move in a backward fashion.

rehabilitation   process of assisting ill or injured person to attain optimal level of well-being and function.

Reiki   using touch on various areas of the body to promote health and well-being, restore energy, and enhance the body's natural healing ability.

relaxation   techniques and methods of reducing stress.

reminiscing   thinking and talking about the past.

remission   times in which a chronic disease appears stable.

renal calculi   kidney stones.

renal colic   spasm in an area near the kidney, accompanied by pain.

repression   involuntary exclusion from awareness of a painful experience or conflict-creating memory, feeling, or impulse.

reservoir   storage area; biologically, an animal or source that maintains infectious organisms that periodically can be spread to others.

resident   person being cared for in a long-term care facility; *see also* **client** and **patient**.

Resident's Rights   document that spells out rights of residents receiving care in long-term care facilities.

respiration   process of taking oxygen into the body and expelling carbon dioxide.

respiratory arrest   cessation of breathing.

respiratory care practitioner (RCP)   a licensed professional who specializes in care of patients with disorders of the cardiopulmonary system, respirations, and sleep disorders that affect the patient's breathing.

respiratory failure   a condition that occurs when breathing is insufficient to sustain life.

respiratory therapy   the department that provides care for patients with disorders of the cardiopulmonary system, respirations, and sleep disorders.

rest   state of comfort, calmness, and relaxation.

restorative   returning to preexisting level or status.

résumé   short account of a job applicant's career and qualifications.

retention   inability to excrete urine that has been produced.

retinal degeneration   breakdown and functional loss of the nervous layer of the eye.

retrograde pyelogram   backward-moving x-ray picture of ureter and renal pelvis.

rheumatoid arthritis   autoimmune response that results in inflammation of the joints.

rhythm   the repeat interval of measured time or movement.

rigor mortis   rigidity of skeletal muscles, developing 6 to 10 hours after death.

risk factor   specific behavior or condition that promotes certain diseases.

ritual   ceremonial acts that reinforce faith.

RN   *See* **registered nurse**

ROM   *See* **range-of-motion exercises**

rooming-in   practice of having mother and baby share a single room after delivery.

rotation   act of turning about the axis of the center of a body, as in rotation of a joint.

rubra   unusual redness or flushing of the skin.

Sacrament of the Sick   last rites given by clergy to a person who is terminally ill (dying).

salpingectomy   surgical removal of the fallopian tubes.

sarcoma   connective tissue tumor, often highly malignant.

scope of practice   extent or range of permissible activities.

scrotum   saclike pouch that holds the male gonads.

sebaceous gland   gland that produces a lubricating substance for hairs.

seizure   a convulsion; a condition characterized by severe, involuntary shaking and jerking of the body.

self-care deficit   inability to perform an activity of daily living.

self-esteem   feeling of confidence about oneself.

self-identity   personal knowledge of who one is; personal view of self.

semicircular canal   three tubes in the inner ear containing fluid; the function is concerned with balance and detecting motion.

semi-Fowler's position   position in which the patient is on the back with knees slightly flexed, and the head of the bed is elevated 30 to 50 degrees.

seminal vesicles   pair of accessory male sex glands that open into the vas deferens before it joins the urethra; they secrete fluid into seminal fluid.

semiprivate room   room in a health care facility that is shared by two patients.

semiprone   patient is positioned between the side and the abdomen.

semisupine   patient is positioned between the side and the back.

senile purpura   dark purple bruises on the forearms and back of hands, common in elderly individuals.

sensitivity   ability to be aware of and appreciate personal characteristics of others; state of acute or abnormal response to stimuli or allergens.

sepsis   presence of pus-forming and other pathogens or their toxins in the blood.

sequential compression therapy   postoperative procedure in which pneumatic boots are applied to massage the legs using a milking, wavelike motion. Prevents blood clots.

seropositive   state in which antibodies to HIV exist in the bloodstream.

serous membrane   tissue that produces serous fluid, covers organs, and lines closed body cavities.

sexual abuse   use of physical means or verbal threats to force a person to perform sexual acts.

sexuality   maleness or femaleness of an individual.

sexually transmitted disease (STD)   disease that is passed from one individual to another through sexual contact.

sharps   needles, knife blades, etc.; items that can cut or puncture skin.

shearing   force on skin over bone when the skin remains at the point of contact while the bone moves; causes damage to skin.

shift report   information about patients passed from outgoing shift to oncoming shift.

shock   condition in which there is a disruption of circulation that results in dangerously low blood pressure and an upset of all bodily functions.

side rails   sliding metal bars that may be pulled up on each side of the bed to prevent the patient from falling out of bed.

sigmoidoscopy   direct examination of the interior of the sigmoid colon.

sign   any objective evidence of an abnormal nature in the body or its organs.

sign language   communication for persons with hearing impairment; uses gestures and signs made with the fingers and hands.

simple fracture   fracture that does not produce an open wound in the skin. *See also* **closed fracture**

simple goiter   thyroid gland hyperplasia unaccompanied by other signs or symptoms.

simple mastectomy   removal of the breast tissue without removal of the underlying muscles.

Sims' position   position in which the patient is on the left side with left leg extended and right leg flexed; left arm is extended and brought behind the back; right arm is flexed and brought forward.

singultus   hiccup.

sitting transfer   moving patient from one surface to another with patient sitting.

skeletal muscle   muscle that is attached to bone and provides voluntary movement.

skilled care   health care provided to persons who require professional services over a period of time.

skilled care facility   long-term care facility.

skin tear   shallow injuries in which the epidermis is ripped or torn.

slander   false oral statement that injures the reputation of another person.

sleep   a period of continuous or intermittent unconsciousness in which physical movements are decreased.

sleep apnea   a potentially serious condition in which airflow stops for 10 seconds or more.

sleep deprivation   prolonged sleep loss (inadequate quality or quantity of REM or NREM sleep).

smooth muscle   muscle located in internal organs, responsible for involuntary movement.

soft diet   intake consisting of low-residue, mildly flavored, easily digested foods.

somnambulism   sleepwalking.

source   person who has an infection that can be spread to others.

spastic paralysis   paralysis in which there is no voluntary movement. The extremities move in an involuntary pattern, similar to muscle spasms. The patient is aware of the movements, but cannot stop or control them.

spasticity sudden, frequent, involuntary muscle contractions that impair function.

spatial-perceptual deficit inability to distinguish between left and right and up and down.

speculum instrument used to dilate a body opening.

speech therapy treatment to assist a patient to regain communication skills.

sperm male reproductive cell.

sphygmomanometer instrument for determining arterial pressures; blood pressure gauge.

spica cast body cast.

spinal anesthesia technique of providing anesthesia by introducing drugs into the spinal canal.

spiral fracture a fracture that twists around the bone.

spirillum (plural **spirilla**) spiral-shaped bacteria.

spirituality feeling of wholeness resulting from filling the human need to feel connected to the world and to a power greater than oneself.

splint type of orthosis used to maintain position and prevent contractures of the arm and hand.

sprain injury to ligament, resulting in pain and swelling.

sputum matter brought up from the lungs; phlegm.

square corner *See* **box corner**

stable health condition is steady, predictable, without complications.

staff development process used to educate staff in health care facilities.

standard guide for performance by which performance is measured.

standard precautions practices used in health care facilities to prevent the spread of infection via blood, body fluids, secretions, excretions, mucous membranes, and nonintact skin.

standing transfer patient is moved from one surface to another while standing.

staphylo- prefix meaning "in clusters."

status condition or state of health.

status epilepticus a seizure that lasts for a long time, or repeats without recovery; a very serious medical emergency.

STD *See* **sexually transmitted disease**

stent device that keeps the arteries open.

stepparent person who is married to a child's natural parent.

stereotype rigid beliefs based on generalizations.

sterile absence of all microorganisms; incapable of reproducing sexually.

sterile field area considered free of all microbes.

sterility inability to produce offspring.

sterilization process that renders an individual incapable of reproduction; process of cleaning equipment to remove all microbes and make equipment sterile.

stertorous snoring-type respirations.

stethoscope instrument used in auscultation to make audible the sounds produced in the body.

stimulant agent that produces stimulation or elicits a response.

stimulus anything that provokes a response in a cell, tissue, or other structure.

stoma artificial, mouthlike opening.

stool another name for feces.

strain injury to a muscle, resulting in pain.

strepto- prefix meaning "in chains."

stressors situations, feelings, or conditions that cause a person to be anxious about his or her well-being.

stroke cerebrovascular accident or brain attack; damage to the blood vessels of the brain.

Stryker frame special kind of bed used when a patient cannot be turned within the bed.

subacute care comprehensive, goal-oriented care for individuals with acute illness, injury, or worsening of a chronic medical problem.

subcutaneous tissue connective tissue located under the dermis; attaches skin to muscle.

subjective observation observation based on ideas perceived only by the individual involved.

sudoriferous gland gland that secretes perspiration.

suffix word part added to the end of a word root that changes or modifies the meaning of the word root.

suicide self-destruction; killing oneself.

sundowning behavior in which a person becomes more agitated and disoriented during the evening hours.

superimpose put on top of something else.

superior toward the head; upward.

supination act of turning the palm upward.

supine position lying with the face upward.

supplement to add.

supplements nutritional substances used to make up a deficiency or strengthen the whole.

supportive care care given to a dying patient that avoids prolonging life but provides comfort measures only.

supportive device used to help maintain a patient's body in a specific position.

suppository medication used to help the bowels eliminate feces.

suppression consciously refusing to acknowledge unacceptable feelings and thoughts.

suprapubic catheter a urinary catheter that is inserted surgically through the abdominal wall directly into the bladder.

surgical bed bed prepared for a patient returning from surgery.

surgical mask mask worn by health care workers during surgery, sterile procedures, and work in a droplet precautions room.

survey a review and evaluation to ensure that the facility maintains acceptable standards of practice and quality of care.

surveyor a representative of a private or governmental agency who reviews facility policies, procedures, and practices for quality of care.

symbols signs, pictures, or other characters used to communicate.

symmetry matching or correspondence in size, form, and arrangement.

sympathectomy excision or interruption of a sympathetic nerve.

symptom any perceptible change in the body or its function that indicates disease or the phases of disease.

synapse space between the axon of one cell and the dendrites of others.

synovial membranes tissues that produce synovial fluid and line joint cavities.

syphilis   infectious, chronic, venereal disease characterized by lesions that may involve any organ or tissue; usually exhibits cutaneous manifestations; relapses are frequent; may exist asymptomatically for years.

system   group of organs organized to perform a specific body function or functions; for example, the respiratory system.

systole   contraction or period of contraction of cardiac muscle.

systolic pressure   blood pressure exerted by the ventricles during the heart's contraction phase.

tachycardia   unusually rapid heartbeat.

tachypnea   pattern of rapid, shallow respirations.

talisman   object used to ward off evil.

tasks   accomplishments throughout life that lead to healthy participation in society; work to be done.

tasks of personality development   growing stages through which personality is formed, as described by Erickson.

TCM   *See* **traditional Chinese medicine**

TED hose   support hose.

tendon   fibrous band of connective tissue that attaches skeletal muscle to bone.

TENS   *See* **transcutaneous electrical nerve stimulation**

tepid   lukewarm.

terminal   final; life-ending stage.

testes   male gonads; reproductive glands located in the scrotal sac.

testosterone   hormone produced by the testes.

tetany   nervous condition characterized by intermittent toxic spasms that are usually paroxysmal and involve the extremities.

THA   *See* **total hip arthroplasty**

theft   taking anything that does not belong to you; stealing.

therapeutic diet   treatment through specifically planned nutrition.

therapeutic touch (TT)   use of the hands to exchange energy and stimulate healing by restoring the energy field in the body. The practitioner's hands do not touch the patient.

therapy   treatment designated to eliminate disease or other bodily disorder.

thermal blanket   large, fluid-filled blanket used to raise or lower a patient's temperature.

thrombocyte   blood platelet that is formed in the bone marrow and is important in blood clotting.

thrombophlebitis   development of venous thrombi in the presence of inflammatory changes in the vessel wall.

thrombus (plural thrombi)   blood clot.

thyrocalcitonin   hormone produced in thyroid gland.

thyroid gland   endocrine gland situated in base of neck; has two lobes, one on either side of trachea; produces hormones thyrocalcitonin and thyroxine.

thyroxine   hormone of the thyroid gland that contains iodine.

TIA   *See* **transient ischemic attack**

time/travel records   records kept of the time spent with clients and the distance traveled between client locations.

tissue   collection of specialized cells that perform a particular function; piece of paper used for cleansing (for example, toilet tissue, facial tissue).

toddler   stage of childhood from 1 to 3 years of age.

total hip arthroplasty (THA)   surgical replacement of hip joint with a prosthesis.

total parenteral nutrition (TPN)   meeting an individual's entire nutritional needs by providing high-density nutrients directly into the bloodstream.

toxin   microbe that produces poisons that travel to the central nervous system and cause damage.

trachea   windpipe.

tracheostomy   opening made into anterior trachea.

traditional Chinese medicine (TCM)   a complete health care system that treats disease by restoring the balance between the internal body organs and the external elements of earth, fire, water, wood, and metal.

traditions   customs and practices followed by a culture and passed from generation to generation.

transcutaneous electrical nerve stimulation (TENS)   use of electrical stimulation to relieve pain.

transfer   procedure followed when changing a patient's location.

transfer belt   gait belt used to assist and support patients during ambulation.

transient ischemic attack (TIA)   temporary reduction of flow of blood to the brain.

transitional care   subacute care given after acute care.

transmission   transfer from one place or person to another.

transmission-based precautions   isolation practices that prevent the spread of infection by interrupting the way in which the disease is spread.

transverse fracture   a fracture that breaks completely across the bone.

trapeze   horizontal bar suspended overhead down the length of the bed.

trauma   wound or injury.

tremor   involuntary trembling.

Trendelenburg position   position in which the patient has the head lower than the feet.

trichomonas vaginitis   inflammation of vaginal tissues with vaginal discharge caused by a protozoan.

trimester   period of three months.

tripod position   a sitting position that makes the thorax larger on inspiration, enabling the patient to inhale more air.

trochanter roll   rolled sheet or bath blanket placed under the patient extending from waist to mid-thigh; positioned against the hip to prevent lateral hip rotation.

TT   *See* **therapeutic touch**

tubercle   small, rounded nodule formed by infection with *Mycobacterium tuberculosis*.

tuberculosis disease   condition occurring when tuberculosis bacteria enter body and damage tissue.

tuberculosis infection   condition in which tuberculosis bacteria enter body but are walled off and contained and do not cause disease.

tumor   neoplasm.

turning (moving) sheet   *See* **draw sheet**

tympanic membrane   membrane serving as the lateral wall of the tympanic cavity and separating it from the external acoustic meatus (outer ear).

tympanic thermometer   device used to measure temperature at the tympanic membrane in the ear.

ulcer   open sore caused by inadequate blood supply and broken skin.

ulcerative colitis   inflammation of the colon resulting in the formation of ulcers.

ulnar deviation   with hand in supination, lateral movement of the wrist.

ultrasound   high-frequency sound waves (mechanical radiant energy of a frequency greater than 20,000 cycles per second) used for noninvasive imaging and other procedures.

umbilical cord   attachment connecting the fetus with the placenta. It is severed artificially at the birth of the child.

umbilicus   depressed scar marking the site of entry of the umbilical cord in the fetus.

unilateral neglect   patient ignores one side of body, such as the affected side after a stroke.

upper respiratory infection (URI)   infection involving the organs of the upper respiratory tract.

ureter   narrow tube that conducts urine from the kidney to the urinary bladder.

urethra   mucus-lined tube conveying urine from the urinary bladder to the exterior of the body; in the male, the urethra also conveys the semen.

urgency   need to urinate.

URI   *See* **upper respiratory infection**

urinalysis   laboratory analysis of urine.

urinary bladder   receptacle for urine before it is voided.

urinary incontinence   inability to control urination.

urinary meatus   external opening to urethra.

uterus   organ of gestation; womb.

vaccine   artificial or weakened antigens that help the body develop antibodies to prevent infectious disease.

vagina   tube that extends from the vulva to the uterine cervix; female organ of copulation that receives the penis during sexual intercourse.

vaginal examination   examination of vaginal and pelvic organs.

validation therapy   techniques used to help individuals feel good about themselves.

vancomycin-resistant enterococci (VRE)   type of bacteria resistant to most antibiotics.

varicose vein   enlarged vein in the leg due to an impaired valve in the vein.

vas deferens   tube that carries sperm from the epididymis to the junction of the seminal vesicle; ductus deferens.

vascular   an area of the body that contains many blood vessels and bleeds readily.

vasoconstriction   decrease in the inner diameter of the blood vessels.

vasodilation   dilation of the blood vessels.

vector   carrier, such as an arthropod, that transmits disease.

vein   vessel through which blood passes on its way back to the heart.

venereal wart   viral condition that can be sexually transmitted.

ventilation   process of breathing in oxygen and breathing out carbon dioxide; also, a means of breathing for another person.

ventral   front; anterior.

ventricle   small cavity or chamber, as in the brain or heart.

verbal abuse   use of speech to humiliate, threaten, or cause fear or anxiety in another person.

verbal communication   transmitting messages using words.

vertebrae   bones surrounding the spinal cord; the backbone or spine.

vertigo   sensation of rotation or movement of or about the person.

vesicle   blister-like skin lesion.

victim   someone who is injured unexpectedly, as in an accident.

virus   tiny living organisms by which some infectious diseases are transmitted.

visceral muscles   muscles that operate without conscious control.

visualization   a form of guided imagery that uses the imagination to form mental pictures to reduce the stress, pain, and symptoms associated with many medical conditions.

vital signs   measurements of temperature, pulse, respiration, and blood pressure.

vitality   exuberant physical and mental strength; capacity for endurance.

vitamin   general term for various, unrelated organic substances, found in many foods in small amounts, that are necessary for normal metabolic function of the body.

vocal cords   tissue that stretches across the larynx and produces vocal sounds.

void   to release urine from the bladder.

volume   capacity or size of an object or of an area; measure of the quantity of a substance.

voluntary muscle   *See* **skeletal muscle**

vulva   external female genitalia.

vulvovaginitis   inflammation of the external female reproductive structures (vulva and vagina).

ward   patient unit for three or more people.

warm soak   method of applying moist heat.

weight-bearing   able to stand on one or both legs.

wet compress   method for applying moist heat or cold.

wheal   localized area of edema on the body surface, often associated with severe itching.

word root   word form with a basic meaning; used in forming new words by combining it with prefixes or suffixes.

work practice controls   procedures used to prevent the spread of disease.

workplace violence   any physical assault, threatening behavior, or verbal abuse occurring in the workplace.

yeast   one type of fungus.

yoga   system to promote union between mind and body; involves a combination of breath control, postures, relaxation, and meditation.

index